Mechanism of Action Illust

DRUGS WITH ILLUSTRATED MECHANISMS OF ACTION	DRUGS WITH MECHANISMS OF A...
etanercept	none
famotidine	cimetidine, nizatidine, ranitidine hydrochloride
hydrochlorothiazide	chlorothiazide, chlorothiazide sodium, chlorthalidone, indapamide, metolazone
ipratropium bromide	none
isosorbide dinitrate, isosorbide mononitrate	nitroglycerin
levodopa	none
linezolid	none
milrinone lactate	inamrinone (formerly amrinone lactate)
nateglinide	repaglinide
olmesartan medoxomil	irbesartan, losartan potassium, valsartan
omeprazole	esomeprazole magnesium, lansoprazole, pantoprazole sodium, rabeprazole sodium
orlistat	none
phenelzine sulfate	isocarboxazid, tranylcypromine sulfate
remifentanil hydrochloride	codeine phosphate, codeine sulfate, fentanyl citrate, fentanyl transdermal, fentanyl transmucosal, hydrocodone bitartrate and acetaminophen, hydrocodone and ibuprofen, hydromorphone hydrochloride, levomethadyl acetate hydrochloride, levorphanol tartrate, meperidine hydrochloride, methadone hydrochloride, morphine sulfate, oxycodone and acetaminophen, oxycodone hydrochloride, oxymorphone hydrochloride, propoxyphene hydrochloride
reserpine	guanadrel sulfate, guanethidine monosulfate
spironolactone	none
tacrine	donepezil hydrochloride, galantamine hydrobromide, rivastigmine tartrate
ticlopidine hydrochloride	clopidogrel bisulfate
tubocurarine chloride	atracurium besylate
vasopressin	desmopressin acetate, lypressin

Nurse's
Drug
Handbook
2004

Blanchard & Loeb Publishers

Nurse's Choice for Better Care™

Nurse's Drug Handbook 2004

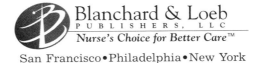

Blanchard & Loeb
PUBLISHERS, LLC
Nurse's Choice for Better Care™

San Francisco•Philadelphia•New York

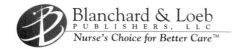
Blanchard & Loeb
PUBLISHERS, LLC
Nurse's Choice for Better Care™

Publishers: Ross Blanchard, Stanley E. Loeb
Clinical Director: Cindy Tryniszewski, RN, MSN
Clinical Project Manager: Marlene Ciranowicz, RN, MSN, CDE
Clinical Editors: Patricia Fischer, RN, BSN; Nancy F. Martin, RN, MSN;
Colleen Seeber-Combs, RN, MSN
Project Editor: Kevin D. Dodds
Book Editor: Doris Weinstock
Editors: Jennifer Bryant, Jane Cray, Catherine E. Harold, Deborah Lyons, Nancy Priff,
Michael Shaw
Copy Editors: Karen Comerford, Dolores Matthews
Indexer: Barbara Hodgson
Cover: Ray Keim
Interior Illustrations: Rolin Graphics, Inc.
Composition: Matrix Publishing Services

© 2004 Blanchard & Loeb Publishers, LLC

Printed in the United States of America

Blanchard & Loeb Publishers, LLC
333 Meadowlands Parkway
Secaucus, NJ 07096

Contents

Reviewers and Clinical Consultants

Reviewers

Peter J. Ambrose, PharmD
Associate Clinical Professor, Step III
Director
Los Angeles-Orange County Area Clerkships
University of California, San Francisco
San Francisco, CA

Donna Barto, RN, MA, CCRN
Nurse Educator
Helene Fuld School of Nursing
Blackwood, NJ
Staff Nurse
Virtua Memorial Hospital
Mount Holly, NJ

Edward M. Bednarczyk, PharmD
Clinical Assistant Professor
Pharmacy Practice and Nuclear Medicine
State University of New York at Buffalo
Buffalo, NY

Cristina E. Bello, PharmD
Assistant Professor of Pharmacy Practice
College of Pharmacy
Nova Southeastern University
Fort Lauderdale, FL

Scott M. Bonnema, PharmD
Consultant Pharmacist
Emissary Pharmacy and Infusion
Casper, WY

Felesia R. Bowen, RN, MS, PNP,C
Clinical Nurse Specialist
Children's Hospital at Robert Wood Johnson
University Hospital
New Brunswick, NJ

Cynthia Burman, PharmD
Clinical Assistant Professor
School of Pharmacy
Temple University
Philadelphia, PA

Kimberly A. Couch, PharmD
Clinical Pharmacy Specialist, Infectious
Diseases
Department of Pharmacy
Christiana Care Health System
Newark, DE

Brenda S. Frymoyer, RN, MSN
Clinical Nurse Specialist
Berks Cardiologists, Inc.
Reading, PA

Kimberly A. Galt, PharmD, FASHP
Associate Professor of Pharmacy Practice
Director
Drug Information Services
Co-Director
Center for Practice Improvement and Outcomes
Research
Creighton University
Omaha, NE

Deborah L. Green, RN, MSN
Director
Medical Telemetry-CHF Program
Moses H. Cone Health System
Greensboro, NC

Ronald L. Greenberg, PharmD, BCPS
Clinical Pharmacy Coordinator
Fairview Ridges Hospital
Burnsville, MN

Jan K. Hastings, PharmD
Assistant Professor
College of Pharmacy
University of Arkansas for Medical Science
Little Rock, AR

Michael D. Hogue, PharmD
Assistant Professor of Pharmacy Practice
McWhorter School of Pharmacy
Samford University
Clinical Coordinator
Walgreen Drug Store
Birmingham, AL

Kimberly A. Hunter, PharmD
Assistant Professor of Pharmacy Practice
Albany College of Pharmacy
Albany, NY

William A. Kehoe, Jr., PharmD, BCPS, FCCP
Professor of Clinical Pharmacy and Psychology
School of Pharmacy and Health Sciences
University of the Pacific
Stockton, CA

Julienne K. Kirk, PharmD, BCPS, CDE
Assistant Professor
Department of Family Medicine
School of Medicine
Wake Forest University
Winston-Salem, NC

Peter G. Koval, PharmD, BCPS
Clinical Pharmacist
Moses H. Cone Family Practice
Greensboro, NC

Lisa M. Krupa, RN,C, CEN, FNP
Nurse Practitioner
Medical Specialists
Munster, IN

Amista A. Lone, PharmD
Clinical Assistant Professor
College of Pharmacy
University of Arizona
Tucson, AZ

Jennifer L. Lutz, PharmD
Pharmacy Resident
Samuel S. Stratton Veterans Affairs Medical
Center
Albany, NY

T. Donald Marsh, PharmD, FASCP, FASHP
Director
Department of Pharmacotherapy
Mountain Area Health Education Center
Asheville, NC

Patrick McDonnell, PharmD
Assistant Professor of Clinical Pharmacy
School of Pharmacy
Temple University
Philadelphia, PA

Catherine M. Oliphant, PharmD
Assistant Professor of Pharmacy Practice
School of Pharmacy
University of Wyoming
Laramie, WY

Michael A. Oszko, PharmD, BCPS
Associate Professor
Dept. of Pharmacy
University of Kansas
Kansas City, KS

Vinita B. Pai, PharmD
Assistant Professor of Pharmacy Practice
College of Pharmacy
Idaho State University
Pocatello, ID

David J. Quan, PharmD
Clinical Pharmacist
University of California, San Francisco
San Francisco, CA

Susan M. Rao, RN, MSN
Staff Nurse
Intensive Care Unit
Saint Luke East
Fort Thomas, KY

Susan L. Ravnan, PharmD
Assistant Professor of Pharmacy Practice
School of Pharmacy and Health Sciences
University of the Pacific
Stockton, CA

Brenda M. Reap-Thompson, RN, MSN
Nurse Educator
Community College of Philadelphia
Philadelphia, PA
Nurse Consultant
Chauncey International, ETS
Princeton, NJ

Nancy Jex Sabin, RN, MSN, CFNP
Instructor
Hahn School of Nursing and Health Science
Family Nurse Practitioner
Student Health Center
University of San Diego
San Diego, CA

Melissa L. Sanders, PharmD
Assistant Professor of Clinical Pharmacy
School of Pharmacy
Temple University
Philadelphia, PA

Regina E. Silk, PharmD, RPh, BCPS
Assistant Clinical Professor
University of Connecticut Health Center
Farmington, CT

Elizabeth Sloand, RN, MSN, CPNP
Assistant Professor
School of Nursing
Johns Hopkins University
Baltimore, MD

Thomas F. Turco, PharmD
Clinical Pharmacist
Assistant Director of Pharmacy
Our Lady of Lourdes Medical Center
Camden, NJ

Lili Wang, PhD
Assistant Professor
School of Pharmacy
Memorial University of Newfoundland
St. Johns, NF, Canada

Craig Williams, PharmD
Clinical Specialist
Wishard Memorial Hospital
Assistant Professor of Clinical Pharmacy
School of Pharmacy
Purdue University
Indianapolis, IN

Clinical Consultants

Madeline Albanese, RN, MSN
Nurse Educator
Hospital of the University of Pennsylvania
Philadelphia, PA

Marlene Ciranowicz, RN, MSN, CDE
Independent Consultant
Huntingdon Valley, PA

Sheree M. Fitzgerald, RN,C, MSN, CNA
Program Coordinator
Ancora Psychiatric Hospital
Hammonton, NJ

Maryann Foley, RN, BSN
Independent Consultant
Flourtown, PA

Grace Hukushi, RN, BSN, LNC
Critical Care Nurse
Nursing Enterprises, Inc.
Brick, NJ

Sammie Justesen, RN, BSN
Independent Nurse Consultant
Providence, UT

Catherine T. Kelly, RN, PhD, CCRN, CEN, ANP
Faculty
School of Nursing
Mount Saint Mary College
Newburgh, NY

Sharon Kumm, RN, MN, CCRN
Assistant Professor
School of Nursing
University of Kansas
Kansas City, KS

Leanne McQuade, RN, BSN, CEN
Staff Nurse
Emergency Dept.
Doylestown Hospital
Case Manager
CAB Medical Consultant
Doylestown, PA

Pamela S. Ronning, RN, MPA
Program Coordinator
Kirkhof School of Nursing
Grand Valley State University
Allendale, MI

Maureen Ryan, RN,CS, MSN, FNP
Assistant Professor
Grand Valley State University
Allendale, MI
Nurse Practitioner
Emergency Dept.
St. Mary's Hospital
Grand Rapids, MI

Julie M. Smith, RN, BA
Staff Nurse
Radiology-Heart Station
Rancocas Hospital
Willingboro, NJ

Aaron J. Strehlow, RN,CS, FNP-C, NPNP
Administrator and Director of Clinical Services
UCLA School of Nursing
Health Center at the Rescue Mission
Los Angeles, CA

Maria Wilson, RN, MSN, CCRN
Staff Nurse
Emergency Dept.
Chestnut Hill Hospital
Philadelphia, PA

Blanchard & Loeb Publishers Nurse's Drug Handbook 2004, the Nurse's Choice for Better Care™, gives you what today's nurses and nursing students need: accurate, concise, and reliable drug facts. This book emphasizes the vital information you need to know before, during, and after drug administration. And the information is presented in easy-to-understand language and organized alphabetically, so you can find what you need quickly.

What's Special

In addition to the drug information you expect to find in each entry (see "Drug Entries" for details), *Nurse's Drug Handbook 2004* boasts these special features:

•**Practical trim size** allows the book to open flat so you can find the information you need without wrestling with a book that wants to close. You can hold the book in one hand, see complete pages at a glance, and use your other hand to document or perform other activities.

•**Introductory material** reviews essential general information you need to know to administer drugs safely and effectively, including an overview of pharmacology and the principles of drug administration. In addition, the five steps of the nursing process are explained and related specifically to drug therapy.

•**Colorful illustrations** throughout the text help you visualize selected mechanisms of action by showing how drugs work at the cellular, tissue, and organ levels. In addition, the inside front cover features a chart listing all the drugs whose mechanisms of action are illustrated as well as other drugs with the same mechanisms of action.

•**No-nonsense writing style** that speaks everyday language and uses the terms and abbreviations you typically encounter in your practice and your studies—although a few abbreviations may not be used in certain facilities. (See *Abbreviations,* pages

996 to 997.) And to avoid sexist language, we alternate between male and female pronouns throughout the book.

•**Up-to-date drug information,** including the latest FDA-approved drugs, new and changed indications, new warnings, and newly discovered adverse reactions.

•**Dosage adjustment,** highlighted in the text, alerts you to expected dosage changes for a patient with a specific condition or disorder, such as advanced age or renal impairment.

•**Warning,** highlighted in the text, calls attention to important facts that you need to know before, during, and after drug administration. For example, in the alatrofloxacin entry, this feature informs you that the drug usually is reserved for hospitalized patients and is given for no more than 2 weeks because of the high risk of severe liver damage.

•**Easy-to-use charts** for route, onset, peak, and duration and other charts in the appendices provide a timesaving way to track and check information. (See page xiii for details on route, onset, peak, and duration charts.) The appendices give an overview of the most important drug facts and nursing considerations for important drug groups, including insulin preparations and antihypertensive combination drugs. You'll also find handy information you can use every day in your practice and studies, such as instructions for calculating drug dosages and I.V. flow rates.

Drug Entries

Nurse's Drug Handbook 2004 clearly and concisely presents all the vital facts on the drugs that you'll typically administer. To help you find the information you need quickly, drug entries are organized alphabetically by generic drug name—from abciximab to zonisamide. For ease of use, every drug entry follows a consistent format. However, if specific details are unknown or don't apply, the heading isn't

FDA pregnancy risk categories

Each drug may be placed in a pregnancy risk category based on the FDA's estimate of risk to the fetus. If the FDA hasn't provided a category, the *Drug Handbook* notes that the drug is "Not rated." The categories range from A to X, signifying least to greatest fetal risk.

A Controlled studies show no risk

Adequate, well-controlled studies with pregnant women have failed to demonstrate a risk to the fetus in any trimester of pregnancy.

B No evidence of risk in humans

Adequate, well-controlled studies with pregnant women haven't shown increased risk of fetal abnormalities despite adverse findings in animals, or, in the absence of adequate human studies, animal studies show no fetal risk. The chance of fetal harm is remote, but remains possible.

C Risk can't be ruled out

Adequate, well-controlled human studies are lacking, and animal studies have demonstrated a risk to the fetus or are lacking as well. A chance of fetal harm exists if the drug is administered during pregnancy, but the potential benefits may outweigh the potential risk.

D Positive evidence of risk

Studies in humans, or investigational or post-marketing data, have demonstrated fetal risk. Nevertheless, potential benefits from the drug's use may outweigh potential risks. For example, the drug may be acceptable if needed in a life-threatening situation or serious disease for which safer drugs can't be used or are ineffective.

X Contraindicated in pregnancy

Studies in animals or humans, or investigational or post-marketing reports, have demonstrated positive evidence of fetal abnormalities or risks that clearly outweigh any possible benefit to the patient.

included so you can go right to the next section.

GENERIC AND TRADE NAMES

First, each entry identifies the drug's main generic name as well as alternate generic names. (For drugs prescribed by trade name, you can quickly check the comprehensive index, which refers you to the appropriate generic name and page.)

Next, the entry lists the most common U.S. trade names for each drug. It also includes common trade names available *only* in Canada, marked (CAN).

CLASS, CATEGORY, AND SCHEDULE

Each entry lists the drug's chemical and therapeutic classes. With this information, you can compare drugs in the same chemical class but in different therapeutic classes and vice versa.

The entry also lists the FDA's pregnancy risk category, which categorizes drugs based on their potential to cause birth defects. (For details, see *FDA pregnancy risk categories.*)

Where appropriate, the entry also includes the drug's controlled substance schedule. (For details, see *Controlled substance schedules,* page xiv.)

INDICATIONS AND DOSAGES

This section lists FDA-approved therapeutic indications. For each indication, you'll find the applicable drug form or route, age-group (adults, adolescents, or children), and dosage (which includes amount per dose, timing, and duration, when known and appropriate).

ROUTE, ONSET, PEAK, AND DURATION

Quick-reference charts show the drug's onset, peak, and duration (when known) for each administration route. The *onset of action* is the time a drug takes to be absorbed, reach a therapeutic blood level, and elicit an initial therapeutic response. The *peak therapeutic effect* occurs when a drug reaches its highest blood concen-

Controlled substance schedules

The Controlled Substances Act of 1970 mandated that certain prescription drugs be categorized in schedules based on their potential for abuse. The greater their abuse potential, the greater the restrictions on their prescription. The controlled substance schedules range from I to V, signifying highest to lowest abuse potential.

I High potential for abuse

No accepted medical use exists for Schedule I drugs, which include heroin and lysergic acid diethylamide (LSD).

II High potential for abuse

Use may lead to severe physical or psychological dependence. Prescriptions must be written in ink or typewritten and must be signed by the prescriber. Oral prescriptions must be confirmed in writing within 72 hours and may be given only in a genuine emergency. No renewals are permitted.

III Some potential for abuse

Use may lead to low-to-moderate physical dependence or high psychological dependence. Prescriptions may be oral or written. Up to five renewals are permitted within 6 months.

IV Low potential for abuse

Use may lead to limited physical or psychological dependence. Prescriptions may be oral or written. Up to five renewals are permitted within 6 months.

V Subject to state and local regulation

Abuse potential is low; a prescription may not be required.

MECHANISM OF ACTION

Set off by a box, this section concisely describes how a drug achieves its therapeutic effects at the cellular, tissue, and organ levels, as appropriate. Illustrations of selected mechanisms of action lend exceptional detail and clarity to sometimes complex processes.

INCOMPATIBILITIES

You'll be alerted to drugs or solutions that are incompatible with the topic drug when mixed in a syringe or solution or infused through the same I.V. line.

CONTRAINDICATIONS

An alphabetical list details the conditions and disorders that preclude administration of the topic drug.

INTERACTIONS

This section presents the drugs, foods, and activities (such as alcohol use and smoking) that can cause important, problematic, or life-threatening interactions with the topic drug. For each interacting drug, food, or activity, you'll learn the effects of the interaction.

ADVERSE REACTIONS

Organized by body system, this section highlights common, serious, and life-threatening adverse reactions in alphabetical order.

NURSING CONSIDERATIONS

Warnings, general precautions, and key information that you must know before, during, and after drug administration are detailed in this section. Examples include whether or not a pill can be crushed and how to properly reconstitute, dilute, store, handle, or dispose of a drug.

Patient teaching information is also included here. You'll find important guidelines for patients, such as how and when to take each prescribed drug, how to spot and manage adverse reactions, which cautions to observe, when to call the prescriber, and more. To save you time, how-

tration and the greatest amount of drug reaches the site of action to produce the maximum therapeutic response. The *duration of action* is the amount of time that a drug remains at a blood concentration that produces a therapeutic response.

Teaching your patient about drug therapy

Your teaching about drug therapy will vary with your patient's needs and your practice setting. To help guide your teaching, each drug entry provides key information that you must teach your patient about that drug. For all patients, however, you also should:

☑ Teach the generic and trade name for each prescribed drug that he'll take after discharge—even if he took the drug before admission.

☑ Clearly explain why each drug was prescribed, how it works, and what it's supposed to do. To help your patient understand the drug's therapeutic effects, relate its action to her disorder or condition.

☑ Review the drug form, dosage, and route with the patient. Tell him whether the drug is a tablet, suppository, spray, aerosol, or other form, and explain how to administer it correctly. Also, tell him how often to take the drug and for what length of time. Emphasize that he should take the drug exactly as prescribed.

☑ Describe the drug's appearance and explain that scored tablets can be broken in half for safe, accurate dosing. Warn the patient not to break unscored tablets because doing so may alter the drug dosage. If your patient has difficulty swallowing capsules, explain that she can open ones that contain sprinkles and take them with food or a drink but that she shouldn't do this with capsules that contain powder. Also, warn her not to crush or chew enteric-coated, extended-release, sustained-release, or similar drug forms.

☑ Teach the patient about common adverse reactions that may occur. Advise him to notify the prescriber at once if a dangerous adverse reaction, such as syncope, occurs.

☑ Warn her not to suddenly stop taking a drug if she's bothered by unpleasant adverse reactions, such as a rash and mild itching. Instead, encourage her to discuss the reactions with her prescriber, who may adjust the dosage or substitute a drug that causes fewer adverse reactions.

☑ Because many drugs cause some adverse reactions, such as dizziness and drowsiness, that can impair the patient's ability to perform activities that require alertness, help him develop a dosing schedule that prevents adverse reactions from interfering with such activities.

☑ Inform the patient which adverse reactions resolve with time.

☑ Teach the patient how to store the drug properly. Let him know if the drug is sensitive to light or temperature and how to protect it from these elements.

☑ Instruct the patient to store the drug in its original container, if possible, with the drug's name and dosage clearly printed on the label.

☑ Inform the patient which devices to use—and which ones to avoid—for drug storage or administration. For example, warn him not to take liquid cyclosporine with a plastic cup or utensils.

☑ Teach the patient what to do if she misses a dose. Generally, she should take a once-daily drug as soon as she remembers—provided that she remembers within the first 24 hours. If 24 hours have elapsed, she should take the next scheduled dose, but not double the dose. If she has questions or concerns about missed doses, tell her to contact the prescriber.

☑ Provide information that's specific to the prescribed drug. For example, if a patient takes a diuretic to manage heart failure, instruct him to weigh himself daily at the same time of day, using the same scale and wearing the same amount of clothing. Or if the patient takes digoxin or an antihypertensive drug, teach him how to measure his pulse and blood pressure and how to record the measurements. Then instruct him to bring the diary to his regular appointments so that the prescriber can monitor his response to the drug.

☑ Advise the patient to refill prescriptions promptly, unless she no longer needs the drug. Also instruct her to discard expired drugs because they may become ineffective or even dangerous over time.

☑ Warn the patient to keep all drugs out of the reach of children at all times.

ever, this section doesn't repeat basic patient-teaching points. (For a summary of
those, see *Teaching your patient about
drug therapy,* page xv.)

In short, *Blanchard & Loeb Publishers
Nurse's Drug Handbook 2004* is designed
expressly to give you more of what you
need. It puts vital drug information at your
fingertips and helps you remain ALWAYS
CURRENT in this critical part of your practice or studies.

Safe, effective drug therapy is one of your most important responsibilities. Not infrequently, a patient's life will depend on your ability to administer drugs accurately, safely, and effectively. In addition, you must keep up with the latest drug information, including newly approved drugs and recently reported life-threatening adverse reactions. Despite all the drug information that is available, medication errors remain one of the greatest threats to patients' well-being and a leading cause of lawsuits against nurses, physicians, and hospitals.

Your Responsibilities in Drug Therapy

Your basic responsibilities in drug therapy include:
• administering the right drug in the right dose by the right route at the right time to the right patient
• knowing the therapeutic use, dosage, interactions, adverse reactions, and warnings of each administered drug
• being aware of newly approved drugs that may be prescribed
• knowing about changes to existing drugs, such as new indications and dosages and recently discovered adverse reactions and interactions
• concentrating fully when preparing and administering drugs
• responding promptly and appropriately to serious or life-threatening adverse reactions, interactions, and other complications
• instructing each patient about the drug, how it's administered, which effects it causes or may cause, and which reactions to watch for and report to you or to the prescriber.

Several factors may reduce your ability to meet these basic responsibilities—and contribute to medication errors. First, hospitals and other health care facilities have budget restraints that may result in the elimination of professional nursing positions or the hiring of less qualified technicians to fill them. This forces the remaining nurses to care for more patients. Second, hospital patients are older and more acutely ill and typically receive more complex drug therapy than ever. Together, these factors place greater demands on you—increasing your stress level, reducing the time you have to concentrate on drug administration, and increasing your risk of making medication errors or overlooking serious adverse reactions or interactions.

The same factors reduce your time and energy for learning the latest drug facts—which you need to have at your command. You must have this information at your fingertips because your next patient may need a recently approved drug or a complex and unfamiliar drug regimen. How can you balance your limited time, on the one hand, with your need to know the latest developments, on the other?

Meeting Your Needs

Nurses and students need a reliable, accurate, easy-to-use, quick-reference drug book. They need a book clearly written by and for nurses that has been reviewed by experts in nursing and pharmacology. They need *Blanchard & Loeb Publishers Nurse's Drug Handbook 2004,* the Nurse's Choice for Better Care™, with its ALWAYS CURRENT features.

The content of *Nurse's Drug Handbook 2004* was developed, written, and edited by experienced practicing nurses. Expert consultants, reviewers, and advisors—both nurses and pharmacists—help ensure the accuracy and reliability of the information covered in each entry and help target that information to your needs. What's more, every drug fact is checked against the most prominent drug references today, including the *American Hospital Formulary Service Drug Information, Drug Facts and Comparisons, The Physicians' Desk Reference,* and the USP DI's *Drug Information for the Health Care Professional.*

In addition, to help you quickly access much-needed information, the book is organized alphabetically by generic drug name, follows a consistent format, and is concise.

To ensure that you're always current, *Blanchard & Loeb Publishers Nurse's Drug Handbook* is updated every year. This newest edition contains:
•more than 20 new drugs
•new drug facts on hundreds of existing entries, including updated information on new indications and dosages, new incompatibilities and interactions, new adverse reactions, and new nursing considerations
•scores of additional patient-teaching guidelines and suggestions
•completely new appendices on oral combination anti-diabetic agents and on vitamins
•updated facts in the existing appendices
•new illustrations for important mechanisms of action
•a comprehensive new index.

Even though the book is longer than last year's, you'll find the same highly readable type size that reduces eyestrain as you speed to the information you need.

Getting More from Your Drug Reference

Whether you work in or are preparing to work in acute care, home care, long-term care, or another health care setting, you'll want your own copy of *Nurse's Drug Handbook 2004*. That's because this book can help you:
•reduce your risk of medication errors because you'll have easy access to accurate, reliable drug information that's relevant to your practice
•stay current on the most up-to-date drug developments of the year
•improve your drug administration skills

and patient care before, during, and after drug therapy
•quickly detect and manage serious or life-threatening adverse reactions and complications or prevent them from occurring
•save time because you won't have to sift through volumes of information to find what you need, search for a book that's up-to-date, or look through several drug handbooks to get enough information
•increase your confidence about drug administration and enhance your professional interactions with other health care team members
•ensure the delivery of safe, effective care
•improve the depth and quality of your patient teaching.

Reaping the Rewards

Your patients deserve the best and safest care possible—and you deserve to have the tools to deliver that care. Whether you're a student or an experienced clinician, *Blanchard & Loeb Publishers Nurse's Drug Handbook 2004* will help you provide safe, effective drug therapy because of its practical, easy-to-understand, accurate, and reliable information on virtually all the drugs you're likely to administer. Take it with you to the clinical setting, share it with your peers, and use it to enhance your present and future position in the nursing profession.

Kathleen Dracup, RN, FNP, DNSc, FAAN
Dean and Professor
School of Nursing
University of California, San Francisco
San Francisco, CA

Understanding the basics of pharmacology is an essential nursing responsibility. Pharmacology is the science that deals with the physical and chemical properties, and biochemical and physiologic effects, of drugs. It includes the areas of pharmacokinetics, pharmacodynamics, pharmacotherapeutics, pharmacognosy, and toxicodynamics.

Nurse's Drug Handbook 2004 deals primarily with pharmacokinetics, pharmacodynamics, and pharmacotherapeutics— the information you need to administer safe and effective drug therapy (discussed below). *Pharmacognosy* is the branch of pharmacology that deals with the biological, biochemical, and economic features of naturally occurring drugs. *Toxicodynamics* is the study of the harmful effects that excessive amounts of a drug produce in the body; in a drug overdose or drug poisoning, large drug doses may saturate or overwhelm normal mechanisms that control absorption, distribution, metabolism, and excretion.

Drug Nomenclature

Most drugs are known by several names— chemical, generic, trade, and official— each of which serves a specific function. (See *How drugs are named.*) However, multiple drug names can also contribute to medication errors. You may find a familiar drug packaged with an unfamiliar name if your institution changes suppliers or if a familiar drug is newly approved in a different dose or for a new indication.

Drug Classification

Drugs can be classified in various ways. Most pharmacology textbooks group drugs by their functional classification, such as psychotherapeutics, which is based on common characteristics. Drugs can also be classified according to their therapeutic use, such as antipanic or antiobsessional drugs. Drugs within a certain therapeutic class may be further divided into subgroups based on their mechanisms of action. For example, the therapeutic class antineoplastics can be further classified as alkylating agents, antibiotic antineoplastics, antimetabolites, antimitotics, biological response modifiers, antineoplastic enzymes, and hormonal antineoplastics.

How drugs are named

A drug's chemical, generic, trade, and official names are developed at different phases of the drug development process and serve different functions. For example, the various names of the commonly prescribed anticonvulsant divalproex sodium are:
- Chemical name: Pentanoic acid, 2-propyl-, sodium salt (2:1) or ($C_{16}H_{31}O_4Na$)
- Generic name: divalproex sodium
- Trade name: Depakote
- Official name: Divalproex Sodium Delayed-Release Tablets, USP

A drug's *chemical name* describes its atomic and molecular structure. The chemical name of divalproex sodium—pentanoic acid, 2-propyl-, sodium salt (2:1), or $C_{16}H_{31}O_4Na$ (pronounced valproate semisodium)—indicates that the drug is a combination of two valproic acid compounds with a sodium molecule attached to only one side.

Once a drug successfully completes several clinical trials, it receives a *generic name,* also known as the nonproprietary name. The generic name is usually derived from but shorter than the chemical name. The United States Adopted Names Council is responsible for selecting generic names, which are intended for unrestricted public use.

Before submitting the drug for FDA approval, the manufacturer creates and registers a *trade name* (or brand name) when the drug appears ready to be marketed. Trade names are copyrighted and followed by the symbol ® to indicate that they're registered and that their use is restricted to the drug manufacturer. Once the original patent on a drug has expired, any manufacturer may produce the drug and market it with its own trade name.

A drug's *official name* is the name under which it's listed in the United States Pharmacopoeia (USP) and the National Formulary (NF).

Pharmacokinetics

Pharmacokinetics is the study of a drug's actions—or fate—as it passes through the body during absorption, distribution, metabolism, and excretion.

ABSORPTION

Before a drug can begin working, it must be transformed from its pharmaceutical dosage form to a biologically available (bioavailable) substance that can pass through various biological cell membranes to reach its site of action. This process is known as absorption. A drug's absorption rate depends on its route of administration, its circulation through the tissue into which it's administered, and its solubility—that is, whether it's more water-soluble (*hydrophilic*) or fat-soluble (*lipophilic*).

Although drugs may penetrate cellular membranes either actively or passively, most drugs do so by *passive diffusion,* moving inertly from an area of higher concentration to an area of lower concentration. Passive diffusion may occur through water or fat. Passive diffusion through water—*aqueous diffusion*—occurs within large water-filled compartments, such as interstitial spaces, and across epithelial membrane tight junctions and pores in the epithelial lining of blood vessels. Aqueous diffusion is driven by concentration gradients. Drug molecules that are bound to large plasma proteins, such as albumin, are too large to pass through aqueous pores in this way. Passive diffusion through fat—*lipid diffusion*—plays an important role in drug metabolism because of the large number of lipid barriers that separate the aqueous compartments of the body. The ability of a drug to move through lipid layers between aqueous compartments often depends on the pH of the medium—that is, the ability of the water-soluble or fat-soluble drug to form weak acid or weak base.

Drugs whose molecules are too large to readily diffuse may rely on *active diffusion,* in which special carriers on molecules, including peptides, amino acids, and glucose, transport the drug through the membranes. However, some molecules with selective membrane carriers can expel foreign drug molecules; this is why many drugs can't cross the blood-brain barrier.

Drug absorption begins at the administration route. The three main administration route categories are enteral, parenteral, and transcutaneous. Depending on its nature or chemical makeup, a drug may be better absorbed from one site than from another.

Enteral Administration

Enteral administration consists of the oral, nasogastric, and rectal routes.

Oral: Drugs administered orally are absorbed in the GI tract and then proceed by the hepatic portal vein to the liver and into the systemic circulation. Although generally considered the preferred route, oral drug administration has a number of disadvantages:

• The oral route doesn't always yield sufficiently high blood concentrations to be effective.

• Bioavailability may be less than optimal because of incomplete absorption and first-pass elimination (the part of metabolism that occurs during transit through the liver before the drug reaches the general circulation).

• Drug absorption may be incomplete if the drug is degraded by digestive enzymes or the acidic pH in the stomach or if it's excreted from the liver into the bile.

• Food in the GI tract, gastric emptying time, and intestinal motility may also impede drug absorption.

Nasogastric: Drugs administered through a nasogastric tube enter the stomach directly and are absorbed in the GI tract.

Rectal: Rectal drugs and suppositories also enter the GI tract directly after being inserted in the rectum and absorbed through the rectal mucosa. After being absorbed into the lower GI tract, rectal drugs enter the circulation through the inferior vena cava, bypassing the liver and thus avoiding first-pass metabolism. Suppositories, however, tend to travel upward into the rectum, where veins, such as the superior hemorrhoidal vein, lead to the liver. As a result, drug absorption by this route is often unreliable and difficult to predict.

Parenteral Administration

Parenteral routes may be used whenever enteral routes are contraindicated or inadequate. These routes include intramuscular (I.M.), intravenous (I.V.), subcutaneous (S.C.) and intradermal (I.D.) administration. Drug absorption is much faster and more predictable after parenteral administration than after enteral administration.

I.M.: Drugs administered by the I.M. route are injected deep into the muscle, where they're absorbed relatively quickly. The rate of drug absorption depends on the vascularity of the injection site, the physiochemical properties of the drug, and the solution in which the drug is contained.

I.V.: I.V. drug administration involves injecting or infusing the drug directly into the blood circulation, allowing for rapid distribution throughout the body. This route usually provides the greatest bioavailability.

S.C.: Drugs administered by the S.C. route are injected into the alveolar connective tissue just below the skin and are absorbed by simple diffusion from the injection site. The factors that affect I.M. absorption also affect S.C. absorption. Absorption by the S.C. route may be slower than by the I.M. route.

I.D.: Drugs administered intradermally, such as purified protein derivative (PPD), are injected into the dermis, from which they diffuse slowly into the local microcapillary system.

Transcutaneous Administration

Transcutaneous drug administration allows drug absorption through the skin or soft-tissue surface. Drugs may be inhaled, inserted sublingually, applied topically, or administered by the eyes, ears, nose, or vagina.

Inhalation: Inhaled drugs may be given as a powder and aerosolized or mixed in solution and nebulized directly into the respiratory tract, where they're absorbed through the alveoli. Inhaled drugs are usually absorbed quickly because of the abundant blood flow in the lungs.

Sublingual: Sublingual drug administration involves placing a tablet, troche, or lozenge under the tongue. The drug is absorbed across the epithelial lining of the mouth, usually quickly. This route avoids first-pass metabolism.

Topical: Topical drugs—creams, ointments, lotions, and patches—are placed on the skin and then cross the epidermis into the capillary circulation. They may also be absorbed through sweat glands, hair follicles, and other skin structures. Absorption by the skin is enhanced if the drug is in a solution.

Ophthalmic: Ophthalmic drugs include solutions and ointments that are instilled or applied directly to the cornea or conjunctiva as well as small, elliptical disks that are placed directly on the eyeball behind the lower eyelid. The movements of the eyeball promote distribution of these drugs over the surface of the eye. Although ophthalmic drugs produce a local effect on the conjunctiva or anterior chamber, some preparations may be absorbed systemically and therefore produce systemic effects.

Otic: Drops administered into the external auditory canal, otic drugs are used to treat infection or inflammation and to soften and remove ear wax. Otic solutions exert a local effect but may result in minimal systemic absorption with no adverse effects.

Nasal: Nasal solutions and suspensions are applied directly to the nasal mucosa by instillation or inhalation to produce local effects, such as vasoconstriction to reduce nasal congestion. Some nasal solutions, such as vasopressin, are administered by this route specifically to produce systemic effects.

Vaginal: Vaginal drugs include creams, suppositories, and troches that are inserted into the vagina, sometimes using a special applicator. These drugs are absorbed locally to treat such conditions as bacterial and fungal infections.

DISTRIBUTION
Distribution is the process by which a drug is transported by the circulating fluids to various sites, including its sites of action. To ensure maximum therapeutic effectiveness, the drug must permeate all membranes that separate it from its intended site of action. Drug distribution is influenced by blood flow, tissue availability, and protein binding.

METABOLISM
Drug metabolism is the enzymatic conversion of a drug's structure into substrate molecules or polar compounds that are either less active or inactive and are readily excreted. Drugs can also be synthesized to larger molecules. Metabolism may also convert a drug to a more toxic compound. Because the primary site of drug metabolism is the liver, children, the elderly, and patients with impaired hepatic function are at risk for altered therapeutic effects.

Biotransformation is the process of changing a drug into its active metabolite.

Compounds that require metabolic biotransformation for activation are known as *prodrugs.* During phase I of biotransformation, the parent drug is converted into an inactive or partially active metabolite. Much of the original drug may be eliminated during this phase. During phase II, the inactive or partially active metabolite binds with available substrates, such as acetic acid, glucuronic acid, sulfuric acid, or water, to form its active metabolite. When biotransformation leads to synthesis, larger molecules are produced to create a pharmacologic effect.

EXCRETION
The body eliminates drugs by both metabolism and excretion. Drug metabolites—and, in some cases, the active drug itself—are eventually excreted from the body, usually through bile, feces, and urine. The primary organ for drug elimination is the kidney. Impaired renal function may cause excessive elimination of a drug, thereby reducing the drug's therapeutic effect. Other excretion routes include evaporation through the skin, exhalation from the lungs, and secretion into saliva and breast milk.

A drug's elimination *half-life* is the amount of time required for half of the drug to be eliminated from the body. The half-life roughly correlates with the drug's duration of action and is based on normal renal and hepatic function. Typically, the longer the half-life, the less often the drug has to be given and the longer it remains in the body after it's discontinued.

Pharmacodynamics
Pharmacodynamics is the study of the biochemical and physiologic effects of drugs and their mechanisms of action. A drug's actions may be structurally specific or nonspecific. Structurally specific drugs combine with cell receptors, such as proteins or glycoproteins, to enhance or in-

hibit cellular enzyme actions. Drug receptors are the cellular components affected at the site of action. Many drugs form chemical bonds with drug receptors, but a drug can bond with a receptor only if it has a similar shape—much the same way that a key fits into a lock. When a drug combines with a receptor, channels are either opened or closed and cellular biochemical messengers, such as cyclic adenosine monophosphate or calcium ions, are activated. Once activated, cellular functions can be turned either on or off by these messengers. Structurally nonspecific drugs, such as biological response modifiers, don't combine with cell receptors; rather, they produce changes within the cell membrane or interior.

The mechanisms by which drugs interact with the body are not always known. Drugs may work by physical action (such as the protective effects of a topical ointment) or chemical reaction (such as an antacid's effect on the gastric mucosa), or by modifying the metabolic activity of invading pathogens (such as an antibiotic) or replacing a missing biochemical substance (such as insulin).

AGONISTS
Agonists are drugs that interact with a receptor to stimulate a response. They alter cell physiology by binding to plasma membranes or intracellular structures. *Partial agonists* can't achieve maximal effects even though they may occupy all available receptor sites on a cell. *Strong agonists* can cause maximal effects while occupying only a small number of receptor sites on a cell. *Weak agonists* must occupy many more receptor sites than strong agonists to produce the same effect.

ANTAGONISTS
Antagonists are drugs that attach to a receptor but don't stimulate a response; instead, they inhibit or block responses that would normally be caused by agonists. *Competitive antagonists* bind to receptor sites that are also compatible with an agonist, thus preventing the agonist from binding to the site. *Noncompetitive antagonists* bind to receptor sites that aren't occupied by an agonist; this changes the receptor site so that it's no longer recognized by the agonist. *Irreversible antagonists* work in much the same way that noncompetitive ones do, except that they permanently bind with the receptor.

Antagonism plays an important role in drug interactions. When two agonists that cause opposite therapeutic effects, such as a vasodilator and a vasoconstrictor, are combined, the effects cancel each other out. When two antagonists, such as morphine and naloxone, are combined, both drugs may become inactive.

Pharmacotherapeutics
Pharmacotherapeutics is the study of how drugs are used to prevent or treat disease. Understanding why a drug is prescribed for a certain disease can assist you in prioritizing drug administration with other patient care activities. Knowing a drug's desired and unwanted effects may help you uncover problems not readily apparent from the admitting diagnosis. This information may also help you prevent such problems as adverse reactions and drug interactions.

A drug's *desired effect* is the intended or expected clinical response to the drug. This is the response you start to evaluate as soon as a drug is given. Dosage adjustments and the continuation of therapy often depend on your accurate evaluation and documentation of the patient's response.

An *adverse reaction* is any noxious and unintended response to a drug that occurs at therapeutic doses used for prophylaxis, diagnosis, or therapy. Adverse reactions associated with excessive amounts of a drug are considered drug overdoses. Be prepared to follow your institution's policy for reporting adverse drug reactions.

An *idiosyncratic response* is a genetically determined abnormal or excessive response to a drug that occurs in a particular patient. The unusual response may indicate that the drug has saturated or overwhelmed mechanisms that normally control absorption, distribution, metabolism, or excretion, thus altering the expected response. You may be unsure whether a reaction is adverse or idiosyncratic. Once you report the reaction, the pharmacist usually determines the appropriate course of action.

An *allergic reaction* is an adverse response that results from previous exposure to the same drug or to one that's chemically similar to it. The patient's immune system reacts to the drug as if it were a foreign invader and may produce a mild hypersensitivity reaction, characterized by localized dermatitis, urticaria, angioedema, or photosensitivity. Allergic reactions should be reported to the prescriber immediately and the drug should be discontinued. Follow-up care may include giving drugs, including antihistamines and corticosteroids, to counteract the allergic response.

An *anaphylactic reaction* involves an immediate hypersensitivity response characterized by urticaria, pruritus, and angioedema. Left untreated, an anaphylactic reaction can lead to systemic involvement, resulting in shock. It's often associated with life-threatening hypotension and respiratory distress. Be prepared to assist with emergency life support measures, especially if the reaction occurs in response to I.V. drugs, which have the fastest rate of absorption.

A *drug interaction* occurs when one drug alters the pharmacokinetics of another drug—for example, when two or more drugs are given concurrently. Such concurrent administration can increase or decrease the therapeutic or adverse effects of either drug. Some drug interactions are beneficial. For example, when taken with penicillin, probenecid decreases the excretion rate of penicillin, resulting in higher blood levels of penicillin. Drug interactions may also occur when a drug's metabolism is altered, often owing to the induction of or competition for metabolizing enzymes. For example, H_2-receptor agonists, which reduce secretion of the enzyme gastrin, may alter the breakdown of enteric coatings on other drugs. Drug interactions due to carrier protein competition typically occur when a drug inhibits the kidneys' ability to reduce excretion of other drugs. For example, probenecid is completely reabsorbed by the renal tubules and is metabolized very slowly. It competes with the same carrier protein as sulfonamides for active tubular secretion and so decreases the renal excretion of sulfonamides. This particular competition can lead to an increased risk of sulfonamide toxicity.

Special Considerations
Although every drug has a usual dosage range, certain factors—such as a patient's age, weight, culture and ethnicity, gender, pregnancy status, and renal and hepatic function—may contribute to the need for dosage adjustments. When you encounter special considerations such as these, be prepared to reassess the prescribed dosage to make sure that it's safe and effective for your patient.

CULTURE AND ETHNICITY
Certain drugs are more effective or more likely to produce adverse effects in particular ethnic groups or races. For example, blacks with hypertension respond better to thiazide diuretics than do patients of other races; on the other hand, blacks also have an increased risk of developing angio-

edema associated with angiotensin-converting enzyme (ACE) inhibitors. A patient's religious or cultural background may also call for special consideration. For example, a drug made from porcine products may be unacceptable to a Jewish or Muslim patient.

ELDERLY PATIENTS
Because aging produces certain changes in body composition and organ function, elderly patients present unique therapeutic and dosing problems that require special attention. For example, the weight of the liver, the number of functioning hepatic cells, and hepatic blood flow all decrease as a person ages, resulting in slower drug metabolism. Renal function may also decrease with aging. These processes can lead to the accumulation of active drugs and metabolites as well as increased sensitivity to the effects of some drugs in elderly patients. Because they're also more likely to have multiple chronic illnesses, many elderly patients take multiple prescription drugs each day, thus increasing the risk of drug interactions.

CHILDREN
Because their bodily functions are not fully developed, children—particularly those under age 12—may metabolize drugs differently than adults. In infants, immature renal and hepatic function delay metabolism and excretion of drugs. As a result, pediatric drug dosages are very different from adult dosages.

The FDA has provided drug manufacturers with guidelines that define pediatric age categories. Use these categories as a guide when administering drugs, unless the manufacturer provides a specific age range:
•neonates—birth up to age 1 month
•infants—ages 1 month to 2 years
•children—ages 2 to 12
•adolescents—ages 12 to 16.

PREGNANCY
The many physiologic changes that take place in the body during pregnancy may affect a drug's pharmacokinetics and alter its effectiveness. Additionally, exposure to drugs may pose risks for the developing fetus. Before administering a drug to a pregnant patient, be sure to check its assigned FDA pregnancy risk category and intervene appropriately.

Principles of Drug Administration

Because there are thousands of drugs and hundreds of facts about each one, taking responsibility for drug administration can seem overwhelming. One way that you can enhance your understanding of the principles of drug administration is to *associate, ask,* and *predict* during the critical thinking process. For example, *associate* each drug with general information you may already know about the drug or drug class. *Ask* yourself why a drug is administered by a certain route and why it's given multiple times throughout the day rather than only once. Learn to *predict* a drug's actions, uses, adverse effects, and possible drug interactions based on your knowledge of the drug's mechanism of action. As you apply these principles to drug administration, you'll begin to intuitively know which facts you need to make rational clinical decisions.

Prescriptions for patients in hospitals and other institutions are typically written by the physician on forms called the *physician's order sheet* or are directly input into a computerized system with an electronic signature. Drugs are prescribed based not only on their specific mechanisms of action but also on the patient's profile, which commonly includes age, ethnicity, gender, pregnancy status, smoking and drinking habits, and use of other drugs.

"Rights" of Drug Administration

Always keep in mind the following "rights" of drug administration: the right drug, right time, right dose, right patient, right route, and right preparation and administration.

RIGHT DRUG

Many drugs have similar spellings, different concentrations, and several generic forms. Before administering any drug, compare the exact spelling and concentration of the prescribed drug that appears on the label with the information contained in the medication administration record or drug profile. Regardless of which drug distribution system your facility uses, you should read the drug label and compare it to the medication administration record at least three times:
• before removing the drug from the dispensing unit or unit dose cart
• before preparing or measuring the prescribed dose
• before opening a unit dose package (just prior to administering the drug to the patient).

RIGHT TIME

Various factors can affect the time that a drug is administered, such as the timing of meals and other drugs, scheduled diagnostic tests, standardized times used by the institution, and factors that may alter the consistency of blood levels and drug absorption. Before administering any p.r.n. drug, check the patient's chart to ensure that no one else has already administered it and that the specified time interval has passed. Also, document administration of a p.r.n. drug immediately.

RIGHT DOSE

Whenever you're dispensing an unfamiliar drug or in doubt about a dosage, check the prescribed dose against the range specified in a reliable reference. Be sure to consider any reasons for a dosage adjustment that may apply to your particular patient. Also, make sure you're familiar with the standard abbreviations your institution uses for writing prescriptions.

RIGHT PATIENT

Always compare the name of the patient on the medication record with the name on the patient's identification bracelet. When using a unit dose system, compare the name on the drug profile with that on the identification bracelet.

RIGHT ROUTE

Each prescribed drug should specify the administration route. If the administration route is missing, consult the prescribing physician. Never substitute one route for another unless you obtain a prescription for the change.

RIGHT PREPARATION AND ADMINISTRATION

For drugs that need to be mixed, poured, or measured, be sure to maintain aseptic technique. Follow any specific directions included by the manufacturer regarding diluent type and amount and the use of filters, if needed. Clearly label any drug that you've reconstituted with the patient's name, the strength or dose, the date and time that you prepared the drug, the amount and type of diluent that you used, the expiration date, and your initials.

Administration Routes

Drugs may be administered by a variety of routes and dosage forms. A particular route may be chosen for convenience or to maximize drug concentration at the site of action, to minimize drug absorption elsewhere, to prolong drug absorption, or to avoid first-pass metabolism. Different dosage forms of the same drug may have different drug absorption rates, times of onset, and durations of action. For example, nitroglycerin is a coronary vasodilator that may be administered by the I.V., sublingual, oral, or buccal route, or as a topical ointment or disk. The I.V., sublingual, and buccal forms of nitroglycerin provide a rapid onset of action, whereas the oral, ointment, and disk forms have a slower onset and a prolonged duration of action.

Drug administration routes include the enteral, parenteral, and transcutaneous routes.

ENTERAL

The enteral route consists of oral, nasogastric, and rectal administration. Drugs administered enterally enter the blood circulation by way of the GI tract. This route is considered the most natural and convenient route as well as the safest. As a result, most drugs are taken enterally, usually to provide systemic effects.

Oral

• *Tablets:* Tablets, the most commonly used dosage form, come in a variety of colors, sizes, and shapes. Some tablets are specially coated for various purposes. Enteric coatings permit safe passage of a tablet through the stomach, where some drugs may be degraded or may produce unwanted effects, to the environment of the intestine. Some coatings protect the drug from the destructive influences of moisture, light, or air during storage; some coatings actually contain the drug, such as procainamide; still others conceal a bad taste. Coatings are also used to ensure appropriate drug release and absorption. Some tablets shouldn't be crushed or broken because doing so may alter drug release.

• *Capsules:* Capsules are solid dosage forms in which the drug and other ingredients are enclosed in a hard or soft shell of varying size and shape. Drugs are generally released faster from capsules than from tablets.

• *Solutions:* Drugs administered in solution are absorbed more rapidly than those administered in solid form; however, they don't always produce predictable drug levels in the blood. Some drugs in solution should be administered with meals or snacks to minimize their irritating effect on the gastric mucosa.

• *Suspensions:* Suspensions are preparations consisting of finely divided drugs in a suitable vehicle, usually water. Suspensions should be shaken before administration to ensure the uniformity of the preparation and administration of the proper dosage.

Nasogastric

Drugs administered through a nasogastric or gastrostomy tube enter the stomach directly, bypassing the mouth and esophagus. They're usually administered in liquid form because an intact tablet or capsule could cause an obstruction in a gastric tube. Sometimes a tablet may be crushed or a capsule opened for nasograstic administration; however, doing so will affect the drug's release. You may need to consult a pharmacist to determine which tablets can be crushed or capsules opened.

Rectal

Some enteral drugs are administered rectally—as suppositories, solutions, or ointments—to provide either local or systemic effects. When inserted into the rectum, suppositories soften, melt, or dissolve, releasing the drug contained inside them. The rectal route may be preferred for drugs that are destroyed or inactivated by the gastric or intestinal environment or that irritate the stomach. It may also be indicated when the oral route is contraindicated because of vomiting or difficulty swallowing. The drawbacks of rectal administration include inconvenience, noncompliance, and incomplete or irregular drug absorption.

PARENTERAL

In parenteral drug administration, a drug enters the circulatory system through an injection rather than through GI absorption. This administration route is chosen when rapid drug action is desired; when the patient is uncooperative, unconscious, or unable to accept medication by the oral route; or when a drug is ineffective by other routes. Drugs may be injected into the joints, spinal column, arteries, veins, and muscles. However, the most common parenteral routes are the intramuscular (I.M.), intravenous (I.V.), subcutaneous (S.C.), and intradermal (I.D.) routes. Drugs administered parenterally may be mixed in either a solution or a suspension; those mixed in a solution typically act more rapidly than those mixed in a suspension. Parenteral administration has several disadvantages: The drug can't be removed or the dosage reduced once it has been injected, and injections are generally more expensive to administer than other dosage forms because they require strict sterility.

Intramuscular

I.M. injections are administered deep into the anterolateral aspect of the thigh (vastis lateralis), the dorsogluteal muscle (gluteus maximus), the upper arm (deltoid), or the ventrogluteal muscle (gluteus medius). I.M. injections typically provide sustained drug action. This route is commonly chosen for drugs known to be irritating to subcutaneous tissue. The drug should be injected as far as possible from major nerves and blood vessels.

Intravenous

In I.V. drug administration, an aqueous solution is injected directly into the vein—typically of the forearm. Drugs may be administered as a single, small-volume injection or as a slow, large-volume infusion. Because drugs injected I.V. don't encounter absorption barriers, this route produces the most rapid drug action, making it vital in emergency situations. Except for I.V. fat emulsions used as nutritional supplements, oleaginous preparations aren't usually administered by this route because of the risk of fat embolism.

Subcutaneous

The S.C. route may be used to inject small volumes of medication, usually 1 ml or less. S.C. injections are generally given below the skin in the abdominal area, lateral area of the anterior thigh, posterior surface of the upper arm, or lateral lumbar area. Injection sites should be rotated to minimize tissue irritation if the patient receives frequent S.C. injections—for example, a patient who takes insulin.

Intradermal
Common sites for I.D. injection are the arm and the back. Because only about 0.1 ml may be administered intradermally, this route is rarely used, except in diagnostic and test procedures, such as screening for allergic reactions.

TRANSCUTANEOUS
In transcutaneous administration, a drug crosses the skin layers, from either the outside (dermal) or the inside (mucocutaneous). This route includes sublingual (S.L.), inhalation, ophthalmic, otic, nasal, topical, and vaginal administration.

Sublingual
In S.L. administration, tablets are placed under the tongue and allowed to dissolve. Nitroglycerin is commonly administered by this route, which allows rapid drug absorption and drug action. The S.L. route also avoids first-pass metabolism.

Inhalation
Some drugs may be inhaled orally or nasally to produce a local effect on the respiratory tract or a systemic effect. Although drugs given by inhalation avoid first-pass hepatic metabolism, the lungs can also serve as an area of first-pass metabolism by providing respiratory conversion to more water-soluble compounds.

Ophthalmic
Ophthalmic solutions and ointments are applied directly to the cornea or conjunctiva for enhanced local penetration and decreased systemic absorption. These drugs are usually used in eye examinations and to treat glaucoma. Ophthalmic solutions pose a greater risk of drug loss through the nasolacrimal duct into the nasopharynx than ophthalmic ointments do.

Otic
Otic solutions are instilled directly into the external auditory canal for local penetration and decreased systemic absorption. These drugs, which include anesthetics, antibiotics, and anti-inflammatory drugs, usually require occlusion of the ear canal with cotton after instillation.

Nasal
Nasal solutions and suspensions are applied directly to the nasal mucosa for enhanced local penetration and decreased systemic absorption. These drugs are usually used to reduce the inflammation typically associated with seasonal or perennial rhinitis.

Topical
Topical drugs—including creams, ointments, lotions, and pastes—are applied directly to the skin. Transdermal delivery systems, usually in the form of an adhesive patch or a disk, are among the latest developments in topical drug administration. Because they provide slow drug release, these systems are typically used to avoid first-pass metabolism and ensure prolonged duration of action.

Vaginal
Vaginal troches, suppositories, and creams are inserted into the vagina for slow, localized absorption. Body pH that differs from blood pH causes drug trapping or reabsorption, which delays drug excretion through the renal tubules. Vaginal secretions are alkaline, with a pH of 3.4 to 4.2, whereas blood has a pH of 7.35 to 7.45.

A systematic approach to nursing care, the nursing process helps guide you as you develop, implement, and evaluate your care and ensures that you'll deliver safe, consistent, and effective drug therapy to your patients. The nursing process consists of five steps, including assessment, nursing diagnosis, planning, implementation, and evaluation. Even though documentation is not a step in the nursing process, you're legally and professionally responsible for documenting all aspects of your care before, during, and after drug administration.

Assessment

The first step in the nursing process, assessment involves gathering information that's essential to guide your patient's drug therapy. This information includes the patient's drug history, present drug use, allergies, medical history, and physical examination findings. Assessment is an ongoing process that serves as a baseline against which to compare any changes in your patient's condition; it's also the basis for developing and individualizing your patient's plan of care.

DRUG HISTORY

The patient's drug history is critical in your planning of drug-related care. Ask about his previous use of over-the-counter and prescription drugs as well as herbal remedies. For each drug, determine:
• the reason the patient took it
• the prescribed dosage
• the administration route
• the frequency of administration
• the duration of the drug therapy
• any adverse reactions the patient may have experienced and how he handled them.

Also determine if the patient has a history of drug abuse or addiction. Depending on his physical and emotional state,

you may need to obtain the drug history from other sources, such as family members, friends, other caregivers, and the medical record.

PRESENT DRUG USE

Ask about the patient's current use of over-the-counter and prescription drugs as well as herbal remedies. As you did in the drug history, find out the specific details for each drug (dosage, route, frequency, and reason for taking). Also ask the patient if he thinks the drug has been effective and when he took the last dose.

If the patient uses herbal remedies, similarly explore the use of these products because herbs may interact with certain drugs. Also ask about the patient's use of recreational drugs, such as alcohol and tobacco, as well as illegal drugs, such as marijuana and heroin. If the patient acknowledges use of these drugs, be alert for possible drug interactions. This information may also provide you with insight about the patient's response—or lack of response—to his current drug treatment plan.

Try to find out if the patient has any other problems that might affect his compliance with the drug treatment plan, and intervene appropriately. For instance, a patient who is unemployed and has no health insurance may fail to fill a needed prescription. In such a case, contact an appropriate individual in your facility who may be able to help the patient obtain financial assistance.

Be sure to ask the patient if his drug treatment plan requires special monitoring or follow-up laboratory tests. For example, patients who take antihypertensives need to have their blood pressure checked routinely, and those who take warfarin must have their prothrombin time tested regularly. Other patients must undergo periodic blood tests to assess their hepatic and renal function. Determine whether the patient has complied with this part of his treatment plan, and ask him if he knows the results of the latest monitoring or laboratory tests.

ALLERGIES

Find out if the patient is allergic to any drugs or foods. If he has an allergy, explore it further by determining the type of drug or food that triggers a reaction, the first time he experienced a reaction, the characteristics of the reaction, and other related information. Keep in mind that some patients consider annoying symptoms, such as indigestion, an allergic reaction. However, be sure to document a true allergy according to your facility's policy to ensure that the patient doesn't receive that drug or any related drug that may cause a similar reaction. Also, document allergies to foods because they may lead to drug interactions or adverse drug reactions. For example, sulfite is a food additive as well as a drug additive, so a patient with a known allergy to sulfite-containing foods is likely to react to sulfite-containing drugs.

MEDICAL HISTORY

While reviewing your patient's medical history, determine if he has any acute or chronic conditions that may interfere with his drug therapy. Certain disorders involving major body systems, such as the cardiovascular, GI, hepatic, and renal systems, may affect a drug's absorption, transport, metabolism, or excretion and interfere with its action; they may also increase the incidence of adverse reactions and lead to toxicity. For each disorder identified, try to determine when the condition was diagnosed, what drugs were prescribed, and who prescribed them. This information can help you determine whether the patient is receiving incompatible drugs and whether more than one prescriber is managing his drug therapy.

Ask a female patient if she is or may be pregnant or if she's breast-feeding. Many drugs are safe to use during pregnancy, but others may harm the fetus. Also, some drugs are distributed into breast milk. If your patient is or might be pregnant, check the FDA's pregnancy risk category for the prescribed drug and notify the prescriber if the drug may pose a risk to the fetus. If the patient is breast-feeding, find out if the drug is distributed in breast milk and intervene appropriately.

PHYSICAL EXAMINATION FINDINGS

As part of the physical examination, note the patient's age and weight. Be aware that age determines the dosage of certain drugs, such as sedatives and hypnotics, whereas weight determines the dosage of others, including some I.V. antibiotics and anticoagulants. As you perform the physical examination, note any abnormal findings that may point to body organ or system dysfunction. For example, if you detect liver enlargement and ascites, the patient may have impaired hepatic function, which can affect the metabolism of a drug he's taking and lead to harmful adverse or toxic effects. Also note whether a body organ or system appears to be responding to drug treatment. For example, if a patient has been taking an antibiotic to treat chronic bronchitis, thoroughly evaluate his respiratory status to measure his progress. And be sure to assess the patient for possible adverse reactions to the drugs he's taking.

Assess the patient's neurologic function to ensure that he can understand his drug regimen and carry out required tasks, such as performing a finger stick to obtain blood for glucose measurement. If a patient can't understand essential drug information, you'll need to identify a family member or another person who is willing to become involved in the teaching process.

Nursing Diagnosis

Based on information derived from the assessment and physical examination findings, the nursing diagnoses are statements of actual or potential problems that a nurse is licensed to treat or manage alone or in collaboration with other members of the health care team. They're worded according to guidelines established by the North American Nursing Diagnosis Association (NANDA).

One of the most common nursing diagnoses related to drug therapy is *knowledge deficit,* which indicates that the patient doesn't have sufficient understanding of his drug regimen. However, adverse reactions are the basis for most nursing diagnoses related to drug administration. For example, a patient receiving a narcotic analgesic might have a nursing diagnosis of *constipation* related to decreased intestinal motility or *ineffective breathing pattern* related to respiratory depression. A patient receiving long-term, high-dose corticosteroids may be at *risk for impaired skin integrity* related to cortisone acetate or *self-concept disturbance* related to physical changes from prednisone therapy. Many antiarrhythmics cause orthostatic hypotension and thus may place an elderly patient at *high risk for injury* related to possible syncope. Broad-spectrum antibiotics, especially penicillin, may lead to the overgrowth of *Clostridium difficile,* a bacterium that is normally present in the intestines. This overgrowth in turn may lead to pseudomembranous enterocolitis, characterized by abdominal pain and severe diarrhea. The nursing diagnoses in such a case might include *potential for infection* related to bacterial overgrowth, *alteration in comfort* related to abdominal pain, and *fluid balance deficit* related to diarrhea.

Planning

During the planning phase, you'll establish expected outcomes—or goals—for the patient and then develop specific nursing interventions to achieve them. Expected outcomes are observable or measurable goals that should occur as a result of nursing interventions and sometimes in conjunction with medical interventions. Developed in collaboration with the patient, the outcomes should be realistic and objective and should clearly communicate the direction of the plan of care to other nurses. They should be written as behaviors or responses for the patient, not the nurse, to achieve and should include a time frame for measuring the patient's progress. An example of a typical expected outcome is *The patient will accurately demonstrate self-administration of insulin before discharge.* Based on each outcome statement that you establish, you'd then develop appropriate nursing interventions, which might include drug administration techniques, patient teaching, monitoring of vital signs, calculation of drug dosages based on weight, and recording of intake and output.

Implementation

As you implement the nursing interventions, be sure to stringently follow the classic rule of drug administration: administer the right dose of the right drug by the right route to the right patient at the right time. Also, keep in mind that you have a legal and professional responsibility to follow institutional policy regarding standing orders, prescription renewal, and the use of nursing judgment. During the implementation phase, you'll also begin to evaluate the patient's expected outcomes and nursing interventions and make necessary changes to the plan of care.

Evaluation

Evaluation is an ongoing process rather than a single step in the nursing process. During this phase, you evaluate each expected outcome to determine whether or not it has been achieved and whether the original plan of care is working or needs to be modified. In evaluating a patient's drug treatment plan, you should determine whether or not the drug is controlling the signs and symptoms for which it was prescribed. You should also evaluate the patient for psychological or physiologic responses to the drug, especially adverse reactions. This constant monitoring allows you to make appropriate and timely suggestions for changes to the plan of care, such as dosage adjustments or changes in delivery routes, until each expected outcome has been achieved.

Documentation

You're responsible for documenting all your actions related to the patient's drug therapy, from the assessment phase to evaluation. Each time you administer a drug, document the drug name, dose, time given, and your evaluation of its effect. When you administer drugs that require additional nursing judgment, such as those prescribed on an as-needed basis, document the rationale for administering the drug and follow-up assessment or interventions for each dose administered.

If you decide to withhold a prescribed drug based on your nursing judgment, document your action and the rationale for it, and notify the prescriber of your action in a timely manner. Whenever you notify a prescriber about a significant finding related to drug therapy, such as an adverse reaction, document the date and time, the person you contacted, what you discussed, and how you intervened.

abciximab

ReoPro

Class and Category
Chemical: Fab fragment of chimeric 7E3 antibody
Therapeutic: Platelet aggregation inhibitor
Pregnancy category: C

Indications and Dosages
➤ *To prevent acute myocardial ischemic complications after percutaneous transluminal coronary angioplasty (PTCA) in patients at high risk for abrupt closure of treated coronary artery*

I.V. INFUSION OR INJECTION
Adults. 250-mcg/kg bolus 10 to 60 min before PTCA. *Maintenance:* 0.125 mcg/kg/min by continuous infusion for 12 hr. *Maximum:* 10 mcg/min.

➤ *To treat unstable angina in patients who haven't responded to conventional therapy and are scheduled for PTCA within 24 hr*

I.V. INFUSION OR INJECTION
Adults. 250-mcg/kg bolus, then 10 mcg/min by continuous infusion over 18 to 24 hr, concluding 1 hr after PTCA.

Route	Onset	Peak	Duration
I.V.	Unknown	Unknown	48 hr

Mechanism of Action
Binds to glycoprotein IIb/IIIa receptor sites on surface of activated platelets. Circulating fibrinogen can bind to these receptor sites and link platelets together, forming a clot that eventually blocks a coronary artery. By binding to receptor sites, abciximab prevents normal binding of fibrinogen and other factors and inhibits platelet aggregation.

Incompatibilities
Don't mix abciximab with other drugs. Administer it through separate I.V. line, whenever possible.

Contraindications
Active internal bleeding, arteriovenous malformation or aneurysm, bleeding disorders, CVA in past 2 years or that caused significant neurologic deficit at any time, GI or GU bleeding in past 6 weeks, hypersensitivity to abciximab, intracranial neoplasm, I.V. dextran therapy before or during PTCA, oral anticoagulant therapy in past 7 days unless PT is less than 1.2 times the control, severe uncontrolled hypertension, surgery in past 6 weeks, thrombocytopenia, vasculitis

Interactions
DRUGS
dipyridamole, heparin, NSAIDs, oral anticoagulants, thrombolytic drugs, ticlopidine: Increased risk of bleeding

Adverse Reactions
CNS: Confusion, dizziness, hyperesthesia
CV: Atrial fibrillation or flutter, bradycardia, embolism, hypotension, peripheral edema, pseudoaneurysm, supraventricular tachycardia, third-degree AV block, thrombophlebitis, weak pulse
GI: Dysphagia, hematemesis, nausea, vomiting
GU: Dysuria, hematuria, renal dysfunction, urinary frequency, urinary incontinence, urine retention
HEME: Anemia, bleeding, leukocytosis, thrombocytopenia
RESP: Bronchitis, bronchospasm, crackles, dyspnea, pleural effusion, pneumonia, pulmonary edema, pulmonary embolism, wheezing
SKIN: Pruritus, rash, urticaria
Other: Development of human antichimeric antibodies

Nursing Considerations
•Know that abciximab may be used with heparin and aspirin therapy.
•Inspect abciximab for particles; don't use if opaque particles are present.
•For continuous I.V. infusion, withdraw 4.5 ml from 2-mg/ml solution and inject prescribed amount into 250-ml bag of NS or D₅W, using an in-line sterile, nonpyrogenic, low–protein-binding 0.2- to 0.22-micron filter. Discard unused portion.
•Administer I.V. bolus using sterile, nonpyrogenic, low–protein-binding 0.2- to 0.22-micron filter.
•Avoid I.M. injections, venipunctures, and use of indwelling urinary catheters, NG tubes,

and automatic blood pressure cuffs during abciximab therapy to prevent bleeding. If appropriate, insert an intermittent I.V. access device to obtain blood samples.
•Monitor for GI, GU, and retroperitoneal bleeding and for bleeding at all puncture sites.
•**WARNING** If hemorrhage occurs, prepare to discontinue infusion immediately. Expect to treat severe thrombocytopenia with platelet transfusions if needed.
•Monitor for hypersensitivity reactions, such as rash, pruritus, wheezing, and dysphagia from laryngeal edema. If such reactions occur, discontinue infusion and notify prescriber immediately. If anaphylaxis occurs, administer epinephrine, antihistamines, and corticosteroids, as prescribed.
•Obtain platelet count 2 to 4 hours after initial bolus and every 24 hours thereafter during abciximab therapy as ordered. Expect platelet function to return to normal within 48 hours of conclusion of therapy.
•Monitor vital signs and continuous ECG tracings during treatment.
PATIENT TEACHING
•Teach patient about adverse reactions, including bleeding and hypersensitivity reactions, such as rash, urticaria, and dyspnea.
•Tell patient to prevent injury from falls by maintaining bed rest and from bleeding by keeping limb immobile while catheter sheath is in place.

acarbose

Precose

Class and Category
Chemical: Alpha-glucosidase inhibitor, oligosaccharide
Therapeutic: Antidiabetic
Pregnancy category: B

Indications and Dosages
➤ *To control blood glucose level in patients with type 2 (non–insulin-dependent) diabetes mellitus when the level can't be controlled by diet alone*
TABLETS
Adults. *Initial:* 25 mg t.i.d. with first bite of each meal. *Maintenance:* Increased to maximum at 4- to 8-wk intervals p.r.n. *Maximum:* 50 mg t.i.d. for patients who weigh 65 kg

(143 lb) or less; 100 mg t.i.d. for patients who weigh more than 65 kg.

Mechanism of Action
Inhibits action of alpha-amylase and alpha-glucoside enzymes. Normally, alpha-amylase hydrolyzes complex starches to oligosaccharides in small intestine, and alpha-glucoside hydrolyzes oligosaccharides, trisaccharides, and disaccharides to glucose and other monosaccharides in brush border of small intestine. In diabetic patients, acarbose inhibits these actions and delays glucose absorption, which reduces the blood glucose level after meals.

Contraindications
Chronic intestinal disease, cirrhosis, colonic ulceration, conditions that may deteriorate because of increased gas formation in intestines, diabetic ketoacidosis, digestive or absorption disorders, history of bowel obstruction, hypersensitivity to acarbose, inflammatory bowel disease

Interactions
DRUGS
calcium channel blockers, digestive enzymes (such as pancreatin), diuretics, estrogen, intestinal adsorbents (such as activated charcoal), isoniazid, nicotinic acid, oral contraceptives, phenothiazines, phenytoin, sympathomimetics, thyroid hormones: Possibly decreased therapeutic effects of acarbose
digoxin: Decreased serum level and therapeutic effects of digoxin
insulin, sulfonylureas: Decreased action of insulin, possibly increased risk of hypoglycemia

Adverse Reactions
GI: Abdominal distention and pain, diarrhea, flatulence

Nursing Considerations
•**WARNING** Be aware that acarbose isn't recommended for patients with significant renal dysfunction and a serum creatinine level above 2 mg/dl.
•If patient is receiving acarbose and a sulfonylurea or insulin to enhance glucose control, monitor his blood glucose level frequently, as appropriate.

A

•Store drug in sealed container in cool environment.
•Expect to decrease dosage to control GI upset.
•Monitor glycosylated hemoglobin level as ordered every 3 months for first year to evaluate glucose control and patient compliance.
•Monitor hematocrit and serum AST level every 3 months during first year of therapy and periodically thereafter, as ordered, because acarbose may decrease hematocrit and increase serum AST level.

PATIENT TEACHING
•Explain importance of self-monitoring glucose levels during acarbose therapy.
•Teach patient to recognize signs and symptoms of hypoglycemia and hyperglycemia.
•Warn patient that noncompliance with prescribed regimen can increase risk of diabetic complications, including neuropathy, retinopathy, and renal insufficiency.
•Explain that temporary insulin therapy may be needed if fever, trauma, infection, illness, surgery, or other stress alters blood glucose control.
•Warn patient not to take other drugs within 2 hours of taking acarbose unless specifically instructed by prescriber.
•Tell him to consult prescriber before taking OTC drugs during acarbose therapy.
•Advise patient who also takes another antidiabetic drug to carry glucose with him at all times in case hypoglycemia occurs.

acebutolol hydrochloride

Monitan (CAN), Sectral

Class and Category
Chemical: Beta$_1$-selective (cardioselective) adrenergic receptor blocker
Therapeutic: Antihypertensive, class II antiarrhythmic
Pregnancy category: B

Indications and Dosages
➤ *To treat hypertension*
TABLETS
Adults. *Initial:* 400 mg q.d. or 200 mg b.i.d. *Usual:* 200 to 800 mg q.d. Dosage increased to 1,200 mg/day in divided doses b.i.d. for severe hypertension or hypertension that isn't well controlled with usual dosage.
➤ *To treat premature ventricular arrhythmias*

TABLETS
Adults. *Initial:* 200 mg b.i.d. *Usual:* 600 to 1,200 mg/day.
DOSAGE ADJUSTMENT Maximum dosage of 800 mg q.d. for elderly patients. Dosage reduced by 50% for patients with creatinine clearance of less than 50 ml/min/1.73 m^2. Dosage reduced by 75% for patients with creatinine clearance of less than 25 ml/min/1.73 m^2.

Route	Onset	Peak	Duration
P.O.	1 to 1.5 hr	2 to 8 hr	24 hr or longer

Mechanism of Action
Inhibits stimulation of beta$_1$ receptors in heart, decreasing cardiac excitability, heart rate, cardiac output, and myocardial oxygen demand. Acebutolol also decreases kidneys' release of renin, which helps reduce blood pressure. Drug suppresses SA node automaticity and AV node conductivity, which suppresses atrial and ventricular ectopy. By decreasing myocardial oxygen demand, acebutolol decreases myocardial ischemia. At high doses, it inhibits stimulation of beta$_2$ receptors in lungs, which may cause bronchoconstriction.

Contraindications
Cardiogenic shock, heart failure unless caused by tachyarrhythmia, hypersensitivity to acebutolol, overt heart failure, second- and third-degree heart block, severe bradycardia

Interactions
DRUGS
alpha agonists, nasal decongestants: Increased risk of hypertension
aluminum salts, barbiturates, calcium salts, cholestyramine, colestipol, indomethacin, NSAIDs, penicillins, rifampin, salicylates, sulfinpyrazone: Decreased antihypertensive effects
anticholinergics, hydralazine, methyldopa, prazosin, reserpine: Increased risk of bradycardia and hypotension
beta$_2$ agonists, theophylline: Decreased bronchodilation
epinephrine: Increased risk of blocked sympathomimetic effects
ergot alkaloids: Increased risk of peripheral ischemia and gangrene

flecainide: Possibly increased effects of both drugs
lidocaine: Possibly increased serum lidocaine level, causing toxicity
oral contraceptives, quinidine: Possibly increased serum acebutolol level
sulfonylureas: Possibly decreased hypoglycemic effects
verapamil: Increased cardiac effects, leading to bradycardia and hypotension

Adverse Reactions
CNS: Abnormal dreams, anxiety, confusion, depression, dizziness, fatigue, fever, headache, insomnia
CV: Bradycardia, chest pain, edema, heart block, heart failure, hypotension
EENT: Abnormal vision, conjunctivitis, dry eyes, eye pain, pharyngitis, rhinitis
GI: Constipation, diarrhea, flatulence, hepatotoxicity, indigestion, nausea
GU: Dysuria, impotence, polyuria
MS: Arthralgia, myalgia
RESP: Bronchospasm, cough, dyspnea, wheezing
SKIN: Rash

Nursing Considerations
•Before therapy begins, obtain baseline renal function tests, as ordered.
•Check apical and radial pulses before giving acebutolol. Also, frequently monitor blood pressure and pulse rate, rhythm, and quality during treatment.
•Give acebutolol with food to prevent GI upset.
•Keep in mind that acebutolol may elevate uric acid, potassium, triglyceride, lipoprotein, and ANA levels; it also may interfere with accuracy of glucose tolerance tests.
•Monitor diabetic patient's blood glucose level to spot alterations.
•Notify prescriber if you detect a heart rate below 50 beats/min or signs of heart failure, such as dyspnea, crackles, unexplained weight gain, and jugular vein distention.
•Monitor patient for peripheral edema and evaluate fluid intake and output.
PATIENT TEACHING
•Tell patient that tablets may be crushed or swallowed whole.
•Warn him against discontinuing acebutolol abruptly, which could cause angina or dangerously high blood pressure.

•Instruct patient to take a missed dose as soon as possible up to 6 hours before next scheduled dose but not to double the next dose.
•Advise patient to consult prescriber before taking OTC drugs that contain alpha agonists, such as nasal decongestants and cold preparations.
•Instruct patient to report dizziness, confusion, and fever immediately.
•Encourage patient to maintain diet and lifestyle changes to help control blood pressure.

acetaminophen

Abenol (CAN), Acephen, Aceta Elixir, Acetaminophen Uniserts, Aceta Tablets, Apacet Capsules, Apacet Elixir, Apacet Extra Strength Tablets, Apacet Regular Strength Tablets, Aspirin Free Pain Relief, Exdol (CAN), Feverall, Feverall Sprinkle Caps, Genapap Infants' Drops, Genebs Extra Strength, Halenol Children's Junior Strength, Liquiprin Elixir, Liquiprin Infants' Drops, Meda Cap, Neopap, Oraphen-PD, Panadol, Panadol Infants' Drops, Redutemp, Robigesic (CAN), St. Joseph Aspirin-Free Infant Drops, Tapanol Extra Strength, Tempra, Tempra Drops, Tylenol, Tylenol Caplets, Tylenol Children's Chewable Tablets, Tylenol Extra Strength, Tylenol Gelcaps, Tylenol Infants' Drops

Class and Category
Chemical: Nonsalicylate, para-aminophenol derivative
Therapeutic: Antipyretic, nonnarcotic analgesic
Pregnancy category: B

Indications and Dosages
➤ *To relieve mild to moderate pain associated with headache, muscle ache, backache, minor arthritis, common cold, toothache, and menstrual cramps; to reduce fever*
CAPLETS, CAPSULES, CHEWABLE TABLETS, ELIXIR, E.R. CAPLETS, GELCAPS, LIQUID, SOLUTION, SPRINKLES, SUSPENSION, TABLETS
Adults. 325 to 650 mg q 4 to 6 hr, or 1,000 mg t.i.d. or q.i.d., or 2 E.R. caplets q 8 hr. *Maximum:* 4,000 mg/day.
Children over age 14. 650 mg q 4 hr. *Maximum:* 5 doses in 24 hr.
Children ages 12 to 14. 640 mg q 4 hr. *Maximum:* 5 doses in 24 hr.

Children age 11. 480 mg q 4 hr. *Maximum:* 5 doses in 24 hr.
Children ages 9 to 10. 400 mg q 4 hr. *Maximum:* 5 doses in 24 hr.
Children ages 6 to 8. 320 mg q 4 hr. *Maximum:* 5 doses in 24 hr.
Children ages 4 to 5. 240 mg q 4 hr. *Maximum:* 5 doses in 24 hr.
Children ages 2 to 3. 160 mg q 4 hr. *Maximum:* 5 doses in 24 hr.
Children age 1. 120 mg q 4 hr. *Maximum:* 5 doses in 24 hr.
Children ages 4 to 11 months. 80 mg q 4 hr. *Maximum:* 5 doses in 24 hr.
Children ages 0 to 3 months. 40 mg q 4 hr. *Maximum:* 5 doses in 24 hr.

SUPPOSITORIES
Adults and adolescents. 650 mg q 4 to 6 hr. *Maximum:* 4,000 mg/day.
Children ages 6 to 12. 325 mg q 4 to 6 hr. *Maximum:* 2,600 mg/day
Children ages 3 to 6. 120 to 125 mg q 4 to 6 hr. *Maximum:* 720 mg/day.
Children ages 1 to 3. 80 mg q 4 hr.
Children ages 3 to 11 months. 80 mg q 6 hr.

Route	Onset	Peak	Duration
P.O., P.R.	Varies	1 to 3 hr	3 to 4 hr

Mechanism of Action

Inhibits the enzyme cyclooxygenase, thereby blocking prostaglandin production and interfering with pain impulse generation in the peripheral nervous system. Acetaminophen also acts directly on the temperature-regulating center in the hypothalamus by inhibiting synthesis of prostaglandin E_2.

Contraindications

Hypersensitivity to acetaminophen or its components

Interactions

DRUGS
anticholinergics: Decreased onset of action of acetaminophen
barbiturates, carbamazepine, hydantoins, isoniazid, rifampin, sulfinpyrazone: Decreased therapeutic effects and increased hepatotoxic effects of acetaminophen

lamotrigine, loop diuretics: Possibly decreased therapeutic effects of these drugs
oral contraceptives: Decreased effectiveness of acetaminophen
probenecid: Possibly increased therapeutic effects of acetaminophen
propranolol: Possibly increased action of acetaminophen
zidovudine: Possibly decreased effects of zidovudine

ACTIVITIES
alcohol use: Increased risk of hepatotoxicity

Adverse Reactions

GI: Abdominal pain, hepatotoxicity, nausea, vomiting
HEME: Hemolytic anemia (with long-term use), leukopenia, neutropenia, pancytopenia, thrombocytopenia
SKIN: Jaundice, rash, urticaria
Other: Angioedema, hypoglycemic coma

Nursing Considerations

•Before and during long-term therapy, monitor liver function test results, including AST, ALT, bilirubin, and creatinine levels, as ordered.
•Monitor renal function in patient on long-term therapy. Keep in mind that blood or albumin in urine may indicate nephritis; decreased urine output, renal failure; and dark brown urine, presence of the metabolite phenacetin.
•Expect to reduce dosage for patients with renal dysfunction.
•Store suppositories under 80° F (26.6° C).

PATIENT TEACHING
•Tell patient that tablets may be crushed or swallowed whole.
•Instruct patient to read manufacturer's label and follow dosage guidelines precisely. Explain that infants' and children's acetaminophen liquid aren't equal in drug concentration and aren't interchangeable.
•Advise patient to use manufacturer's dropper or dosage cup only for liquid acetaminophen.
•Advise him to contact prescriber before taking other prescription or OTC drugs; they may contain acetaminophen and lead to toxicity.
•Teach patient to recognize signs of hepatotoxicity, such as bleeding, easy bruising, and malaise, which commonly occurs with chronic overdose.

acetazolamide

Acetazolam (CAN), Ak-Zol, Apo-Acetazolamide (CAN), Dazamide, Diamox, Diamox Sequels, Storzolamide

Class and Category

Chemical: Sulfonamide derivative
Therapeutic: Anticonvulsant, antiglaucoma, diuretic
Pregnancy category: C

Indications and Dosages

➤ *To treat chronic simple (open-angle) glaucoma*
S.R. CAPSULES, TABLETS, I.V. OR I.M. INJECTION
Adults. 250 to 1,000 mg/day (in divided doses for dosages above 250 mg).
➤ *As short-term therapy to treat secondary glaucoma and preoperatively to treat acute congestive (closed-angle) glaucoma*
S.R. CAPSULES, TABLETS, I.V. OR I.M. INJECTION
Adults. 250 mg b.i.d. or q 4 hr; or one S.R. capsule (500 mg) b.i.d.; or 500 mg initially, followed by 125 to 250 mg q 4 to 6 hr for severe acute glaucoma. To initially lower intraocular pressure rapidly, 500 mg I.V.; may repeat in 2 to 4 hr in acute cases, depending on patient response. Oral therapy usually initiated after initial I.V. dose.
S.R. CAPSULES, TABLETS
Children. 10 to 15 mg/kg/day in divided doses q 6 to 8 hr.
I.V. OR I.M. INJECTION
Children. 5 to 10 mg/kg/dose q 6 hr.
➤ *To induce diuresis in heart failure*
TABLETS, I.V. OR I.M. INJECTION
Adults. *Initial:* 250 to 375 mg or 5 mg/kg q.d. in morning. *Maintenance:* 250 to 375 mg or 5 mg/kg on alternate days or for 2 days followed by a drug-free day.
➤ *To treat drug-induced edema*
TABLETS, I.V. OR I.M. INJECTION
Adults. 250 to 375 mg q.d. for 1 to 2 days.
TABLETS, I.V. INJECTION
Children. 5 mg/kg/dose q.d. in morning.
➤ *To treat seizures, including generalized tonic-clonic, absence, and mixed seizures, and myoclonic jerk patterns*
TABLETS, I.V. OR I.M. INJECTION
Adults and children. 8 to 30 mg/kg/day in divided doses. *Optimal:* 375 to 1,000 mg/

day. When used with other anticonvulsants, 250 mg q.d.
➤ *To prevent or relieve symptoms of acute mountain sickness*
S.R. CAPSULES, TABLETS
Adults. 500 to 1,000 mg/day in divided doses, given 24 to 48 hr before ascent and continued for 48 hr or longer while at high altitude p.r.n. to control symptoms.

Route	Onset	Peak	Duration
P.O.	60 to 90 min	2 to 4 hr	8 to 12 hr
P.O. (S.R.)	2 hr	8 to 12 hr	18 to 24 hr
I.V.	2 min	15 min	4 to 5 hr

Mechanism of Action

Inhibits the enyzme carbonic anhydrase, which normally appears in the eyes' ciliary processes, brain's choroid plexes, and kidneys' proximal tubule cells. In the eyes, enzyme inhibition decreases aqueous humor secretion, which lowers intraocular pressure. In the brain, inhibition may delay abnormal, intermittent, and excessive discharge from neurons that cause seizures. In the kidneys, it increases bicarbonate excretion, which carries out water, potassium, and sodium, thus inducing diuresis and metabolic acidosis. This acidosis counteracts respiratory alkalosis and reduces symptoms of mountain sickness, including headache, dizziness, nausea, and dyspnea.

Contraindications

Chronic noncongestive closed-angle glaucoma; cirrhosis; hyperchloremic acidosis; hypersensitivity to acetazolamide; hypokalemia; hyponatremia; severe pulmonary obstruction; severe renal, hepatic, or adrenocortical impairment

Interactions
DRUGS
amphetamines, methenamine, phenobarbital, procainamide, quinidine: Decreased excretion and possibly toxicity of these drugs
corticosteroids: Increased risk of hypokalemia
cyclosporine: Increased cyclosporine level, possibly nephrotoxicity or neurotoxicity

diflunisal: Possibly significantly decreased intraocular pressure
lithium: Increased excretion and decreased effectiveness of lithium
primidone: Decreased serum and urine primidone levels
salicylates: Increased risk of salicylate toxicity

Adverse Reactions

CNS: Ataxia, confusion, depression, disorientation, dizziness, drowsiness, fatigue, fever, flaccid paralysis, headache, lassitude, malaise, nervousness, paresthesia, seizures, tremor, weakness
EENT: Altered taste, tinnitus, transient myopia
GI: Anorexia, constipation, diarrhea, hepatic dysfunction, melena, nausea, vomiting
GU: Crystalluria, decreased libido, glycosuria, hematuria, impotence, nephrotoxicity, phosphaturia, polyuria, renal calculi, renal colic, urinary frequency
HEME: Agranulocytosis, hemolytic anemia, leukopenia, pancytopenia, thrombocytopenia, thrombocytopenic purpura
SKIN: Photosensitivity, pruritus, rash, Stevens-Johnson syndrome, urticaria
Other: Acidosis, hyperuricemia, hypokalemia, weight loss

Nursing Considerations

• Use acetazolamide cautiously in patients with calcium-based renal calculi, diabetes mellitus, gout, or respiratory impairment.
• Know that acetazolamide may increase risk of hepatic encephalopathy in patients with hepatic cirrhosis.
• To avoid painful I.M. injections (caused by alkaline solution), administer acetazolamide by mouth or I.V. injection if possible.
• Reconstitute each 500-mg vial with at least 5 ml of sterile water for injection. Use within 24 hours because drug has no preservative.
• Monitor blood test results during acetazolamide therapy to detect electrolyte imbalances.
• Monitor fluid intake and output every 8 hours and body weight daily to detect excessive fluid and weight loss.

PATIENT TEACHING

• Inform patient that acetazolamide tablets may be crushed and suspended in chocolate or another sweet syrup. Alternatively, one tablet may be dissolved in 10 ml of hot water and added to 10 ml of honey or syrup.
• Advise patient to avoid potentially hazardous activities if dizziness or drowsiness occurs.
• Instruct patient who takes high doses of salicylates to notify prescriber immediately if signs of salicylate toxicity, such as anorexia, tachypnea, and lethargy, occur.
• Advise patient who plans to mountain climb to descend mountain gradually to avoid mountain sickness and to seek immediate medical care if symptoms of mountain sickness occur.

acetohexamide

Dimelor (CAN), Dymelor

Class and Category

Chemical: Sulfonylurea
Therapeutic: Antidiabetic
Pregnancy category: C

Indications and Dosages

➤ *To treat stable type 2 (non-insulin-dependent) diabetes mellitus*

TABLETS

Adults. *Initial:* 250 to 1,500 mg/day. Dosages of 1,000 mg or more daily may be divided and given b.i.d. before morning and evening meals.

DOSAGE ADJUSTMENT For patient being switched from another antidiabetic drug, acetohexamide dosage reduced to half the usual tolbutamide dosage or twice the usual chlorpropamide dosage. For patient being switched from insulin to acetohexamide monotherapy, dosages adjusted as follows: if insulin dosage is less than 20 U/day, acetohexamide begins at 250 mg/day and insulin is discontinued; if insulin dosage exceeds 20 U/day, acetohexamide begins at 250 mg/day and insulin is tapered by 25% to 30% before being reduced further according to patient response.

Route	Onset	Peak	Duration
P.O.	1 hr	Unknown	12 to 24 hr

Mechanism of Action
Stimulates insulin release from active beta cells in the pancreas, resulting in decreased blood glucose level. Improves insulin binding to insulin receptors. Increases the number of insulin receptors (with long-term administration). May reduce basal hepatic glucose secretion.

Contraindications
Diabetes mellitus complicated by ketoacidosis or pregnancy, hypersensitivity to acetohexamide, renal failure, sole therapy for type 1 (insulin-dependent) diabetes mellitus

Interactions
DRUGS
activated charcoal: Possibly reduced absorption and effectiveness of acetohexamide
androgens, anticoagulants, azole antifungals, chloramphenicol, clofibrate, fluconazole, gemfibrozil, H₂-receptor antagonists, magnesium salts, MAO inhibitors, methyldopa, probenecid, salicylates, sulfinpyrazone, sulfonamides, tricyclic antidepressants, urinary acidifiers: Enhanced hypoglycemic effect of acetohexamide
beta blockers, calcium channel blockers, cholestyramine, corticosteroids, diazoxide, estrogens, hydantoins, isoniazid, nicotinic acid, oral contraceptives, phenothiazines, rifampin, sympathomimetics, thiazide diuretics, thyroid drugs, urinary alkalizers: Decreased hypoglycemic effect of acetohexamide
digitalis glycosides: Possibly increased serum digitalis level

Adverse Reactions
CNS: Anxiety, chills, confusion, depression, dizziness, drowsiness, fatigue, headache, hyperesthesia, insomnia, malaise, nervousness, paresthesia, somnolence, syncope, tremor, vertigo, weakness
CV: Arrhythmias, edema, hypertension, vasculitis
EENT: Blurred vision, conjunctivitis, eye pain, pharyngitis, retinal hemorrhage, rhinitis, tinnitus
ENDO: Hypoglycemia
GI: Abdominal pain, anorexia, constipation, diarrhea, epigastric fullness, flatulence, heartburn, hepatitis, hepatotoxicity, indigestion, nausea, proctocolitis, vomiting
GU: Decreased libido, dysuria, polyuria
HEME: Agranulocytosis, aplastic anemia, eosinophilia, hemolytic anemia, leukopenia, pancytopenia, thrombocytopenia
MS: Abnormal gait, arthralgia, hypertonia, leg cramps
RESP: Dyspnea
SKIN: Diaphoresis, eczema, erythema multiforme, exfoliative dermatitis, flushing, jaundice, lichenoid reaction (skin thickening and accentuated lesions), maculopapular rash, photosensitivity, pruritus, rash, urticaria
Other: Disulfiram-like reaction (flushing, head throbbing, hypotension, nausea, tachycardia, vomiting), hyponatremia

Nursing Considerations
• Use acetohexamide cautiously in elderly patients and in those with cardiac, hepatic, or renal disease or thyroid dysfunction. The drug's duration of action is prolonged in patients with renal disease.
• Give acetohexamide 30 minutes before meals, crushing tablets if desired. If GI upset occurs, give in divided doses, as prescribed.
• Monitor for signs of hypoglycemia and hyperglycemia, especially after meals.
• Monitor blood glucose level frequently, as ordered. Provide additional insulin if needed during stressful periods, as prescribed.
• Monitor liver enzyme levels during therapy; acetohexamide may increase AST, ALT, and alkaline phosphatase levels.
• Store acetohexamide in tightly sealed container in a cool environment.
PATIENT TEACHING
• Stress importance of adhering to prescribed drug regimen, diet, and exercise program.
• Advise patient to take acetohexamide with food to avoid GI upset.
• Teach patient how to self-monitor blood glucose level and check urine for glucose and ketones, as appropriate.
• Teach patient to recognize and report signs of hypoglycemia and hyperglycemia.

acetohydroxamic acid

Lithostat

Class and Category

Chemical: Synthetic hydroxylamine and ethylacetate derivative
Therapeutic: Urease inhibitor
Pregnancy category: X

Indications and Dosages

➤ *As an adjunct to antimicrobial therapy to treat chronic UTIs caused by urea-splitting bacteria*

TABLETS

Adults. *Initial:* 12 mg/kg/day in divided doses q 6 to 8 hr. *Usual:* 250 mg t.i.d. or q.i.d. for a total daily dose of 10 to 15 mg/kg. *Maximum:* 1,500 mg/day.
Children. 10 mg/kg/day.
DOSAGE ADJUSTMENT Maximum dosage reduced to 1,000 mg/day or 500 mg q 12 hr for patients with serum creatinine level that exceeds 1.8 mg/dl.

Mechanism of Action

Inhibits urease, the enzyme that catalyzes urea's hydrolysis to carbon dioxide and ammonia in urine infected with urea-splitting bacteria. This action reduces the urine ammonia level and pH, enhancing antimicrobial drug effectiveness.

Contraindications

Contributing disorder that's treatable by surgery or appropriate antimicrobial therapy, hypersensitivity to acetohydroxamic acid, inadequate renal function (serum creatinine level above 2.5 mg/dl or creatinine clearance below 20 ml/min/1.73 m^2), risk of pregnancy, UTI caused by non–urease-producing organisms, UTI that can be controlled by appropriate antimicrobial therapy

Interactions

DRUGS

iron: Decreased intestinal absorption of iron, decreased effects of iron and acetohydroxamic acid

ACTIVITIES

alcohol use: Increased risk of severe rash 30 to 45 minutes after drinking alcohol

Adverse Reactions

CNS: Anxiety, depression, fever, lack of coordination, malaise, headache, nervousness, slurred speech, tiredness, tremor
CV: Calf pain (deep vein blood clot), palpitations, sudden chest pain
EENT: Pharyngitis, sudden change in vision
GI: Anorexia, nausea, vomiting
HEME: Reticulocytosis, unusual bleeding
RESP: Dyspnea
SKIN: Ecchymosis, hair loss, nonpruritic macular rash

Nursing Considerations

• Use acetohydroxamic acid cautiously in patients with severe chronic renal disease or anemia and those who've had phlebitis or thrombophlebitis.
• Be aware that risk of adverse psychomotor effects increases if patient drinks alcohol or takes drugs that affect alertness and reflexes, such as antihistamines, tranquilizers, sedatives, analgesics, and narcotics.
• Administer tablets with food or liquid, crushing them if needed.
• WARNING Acetohydroxamic acid chelates with dietary iron. If patient has iron deficiency anemia, expect to administer I.M. iron as needed during acetohydroxamic acid therapy.
• Monitor follow-up laboratory tests to check renal and hepatic function and urine pH, as ordered.

PATIENT TEACHING

• Instruct patient to take drug at same time each day, as prescribed.
• Tell patient to take a missed dose up to 2 hours after scheduled time. If more than 2 hours has passed, he should wait for next scheduled dose and shouldn't double that dose.
• Warn patient not to take drug with alcohol or iron and to consult prescriber before taking it with any other drug.
• Instruct patient to avoid hazardous activities during therapy.

acetylcysteine

Mucomyst, Mucosil

Class and Category

Chemical: N-acetyl derivative of cysteine

Therapeutic: Antidote (for acetaminophen overdose), mucolytic
Pregnancy category: B

Indications and Dosages

➤ *To liquefy abnormal, viscid, or thick-ened mucus secretions in chronic pul-monary disorders (including emphy-sema, bronchitis, tuberculosis, bronchi-ectasis, and cystic fibrosis) and in pneu-monia, pulmonary complications of thoracic or cardiovascular surgery, and tracheostomy care*

SOLUTION (DIRECT INSTILLATION INTO TRACHEOSTOMY)
Adults and children. 1 to 2 ml of 10% or 20% solution instilled q 1 to 4 hr, p.r.n.

SOLUTION (INHALATION)
Adults and children. 1 to 10 ml of 20% solution or 2 to 20 ml of 10% solution nebulized through face mask, mouthpiece, or tracheostomy q 2 to 6 hr. *Usual:* 3 to 5 ml of 20% solution or 6 to 10 ml of 10% solution t.i.d. or q.i.d.

➤ *To treat acetaminophen overdose*

SOLUTION (P.O.)
Adults and children. *Loading dose:* 140 mg/kg. *Maintenance:* 70 mg/kg 4 hr after loading dose and then q 4 hr to a total of 17 doses.

Mechanism of Action

Decreases viscosity of pulmonary secretions by breaking disulfide links that bind glycoproteins in mucus. Reduces liver damage from acetaminophen overdose. Usually, acetaminophen's toxic metabolites bind with glutathione in the liver, which detoxifies them. When acetaminophen overdose depletes glutathione stores, toxic metabolites bind with protein in liver cells, causing cellular necrosis. Acetylcysteine maintains or restores levels of glutathione or acts as its substitute, which reduces liver damage caused by acetaminophen overdose.

Incompatibilities

Don't administer acetylcysteine with nebulization equipment if drug can contact iron, copper, or rubber. Don't administer drug with amphotericin B, ampicillin sodium, chlortetracycline, chymotrypsin, erythromycin, hydrogen peroxide, iodized oil, oxytetracycline, tetracycline, or trypsin.

Contraindications

Hypersensitivity to acetylcysteine, no contraindications when used as antidote

Interactions
DRUGS
activated charcoal: Possibly adsorption and decreased effectiveness of acetylcysteine
nitroglycerin: Increased effects of nitroglycerin and possibly significant hypotension and headache

Adverse Reactions
CNS: Chills, dizziness, drowsiness, fever, headache
CV: Hypertension, hypotension, tachycardia
EENT: Rhinorrhea, stomatitis, tooth damage
GI: Anorexia, constipation, hepatotoxicity, nausea, vomiting
RESP: Bronchospasm, chest tightness, hemoptysis
SKIN: Clammy skin, pruritus, rash, urticaria
Other: Angioedema

Nursing Considerations
•If needed, dilute 20% instillation or inhalation solution with NS or sterile water if needed. The 10% solution may be used undiluted.
•To treat acetaminophen overdose, dilute 20% oral solution with cola or other soft drink to a concentration of 5% and use within 1 hour. Acetylcysteine is most effective if administered within 24 hours of acetaminophen ingestion.
•If patient vomits loading dose or any maintenance dose within 1 hour of administration, repeat dose as prescribed.
•Keep in mind that suicidal patient may not provide reliable information about vomiting. Watch such a patient to ensure that he ingests all of prescribed dosage.
•During treatment for acetaminophen overdose, monitor for signs of hepatotoxicity, such as prolonged bleeding time, altered coagulation, and easy bruising.
•Be aware that acetylcysteine may have a disagreeable odor, which disappears as treatment progresses.
•Because nebulization causes sticky residue on face and in mouth, have patient wash his face and rinse his mouth after each treatment.

- Be aware that an open vial of solution may turn light purple but that this doesn't alter its effectiveness.
- Refrigerate opened vials and discard after 96 hours.
- Assess type, frequency, and characteristics of patient's cough. Particularly note sputum. If cough doesn't clear secretions, prepare to perform mechanical suctioning.
- Monitor for tachycardia.

PATIENT TEACHING
- Instruct patient to notify prescriber immediately if he experiences nausea, rash, or vomiting.
- Warn patient about acetylcysteine's unpleasant smell; reassure him that it subsides as treatment progresses.
- To decrease mucus viscosity, encourage patient to consume 2 to 3 L of fluid daily unless contraindicated by another condition.

adenosine

Adenocard

Class and Category

Chemical: Monophosphorylated adenine riboside
Therapeutic: Antiarrhythmic
Pregnancy category: C

Indications and Dosages

➤ *To convert paroxysmal supraventricular tachycardia (PSVT) to normal sinus rhythm*

I.V. INJECTION

Adults and children who weigh 50 kg (110 lb) or more. *Initial:* 6 mg by rapid peripheral I.V. bolus over 1 to 2 sec. If PSVT continues after 1 to 2 min, 12 mg given as rapid bolus and repeated in 1 to 2 min if needed.
WARNING Don't give single doses of more than 12 mg.
Children who weigh less than 50 kg. *Initial:* 0.05 to 0.1 mg/kg as rapid central or peripheral I.V. bolus followed by saline flush. If PSVT continues after 1 to 2 min, additional bolus injections are given, incrementally increasing dose by 0.05 to 0.1 mg/kg. Follow each bolus with saline flush. Injections continue until PSVT converts to normal sinus rhythm or until patient reaches maximum single dose of 0.3 mg/kg.

Route	Onset	Peak	Duration
I.V.	Immediate	Immediate	Unknown

Mechanism of Action
Slows conduction time through the AV node and can interrupt reentry pathways through the AV node to restore normal sinus rhythm.

Incompatibilities
Don't mix adenosine with other drugs.

Contraindications
Atrial fibrillation or flutter; hypersensitivity to adenosine; second- or third-degree heart block or sick sinus syndrome, except in patients with a functioning artificial pacemaker; ventricular tachycardia

Interactions
DRUGS
carbamazepine: Increased degree of heart block
digoxin, verapamil: Possibly increased depressant effect on SA or AV node
dipyridamole: Increased effects of adenosine
methylxanthines, such as theophylline: Antagonized effects of adenosine
FOODS
caffeine: Antagonized effects of adenosine

Adverse Reactions
CNS: Apprehension, dizziness, headache, heaviness in arms, light-headedness, paresthesia
CV: Chest pain or pressure, hypotension, palpitations, prolonged asystole, transient hypertension, ventricular fibrillation, ventricular tachycardia
EENT: Blurred vision, metallic taste, throat tightness
GI: Nausea
MS: Neck and back pain
RESP: Dyspnea, hyperventilation
SKIN: Diaphoresis, facial flushing

Nursing Considerations
- Before administration, inspect adenosine for crystals. If solution isn't clear, don't administer it.
- Administer by rapid I.V. bolus over 1 to 2 seconds only. Slower administration can cause systemic vasodilation and reflex tachycardia.

• Expect prescriber to inject adenosine directly into a vein, if appropriate, to ensure that it reaches systemic circulation. If administered into an I.V. line, give as close to insertion site as possible and follow with rapid saline flush.
• Monitor heart rate and rhythm, blood pressure, and respiratory status frequently during adenosine therapy.
• Be aware that at the time of conversion to normal sinus rhythm, arrhythmias (such as PVCs, premature atrial contractions, sinus bradycardia, sinus tachycardia, and AV block) may occur for a few seconds but don't require intervention.
• **WARNING** Discontinue use and notify prescriber immediately if severe respiratory difficulties develop.
• Store adenosine at room temperature. Discard unused portion.

PATIENT TEACHING
• Instruct patient to report chest pain, palpitations, difficulty breathing, or severe headache during adenosine therapy.
• Warn patient that he may temporarily experience mild reactions, such as flushing, nausea, and dizziness.

alatrofloxacin mesylate
Trovan I.V.

trovafloxacin mesylate
Trovan

Class and Category
Chemical: Fluoroquinolone
Therapeutic: Antibacterial
Pregnancy category: C

Indications and Dosages
➤ *To treat life-threatening nosocomial pneumonia*
TABLETS, I.V. INFUSION
Adults. 300 mg I.V. q 24 hr followed by 200 mg P.O. q 24 hr when patient is stabilized for total of 10 to 14 days.
➤ *To treat life-threatening community-acquired pneumonia*
TABLETS, I.V. INFUSION
Adults. 200 mg I.V. q 24 hr followed by 200 mg P.O. q 24 hr when patient is stabilized for total of 7 to 14 days; or 200 mg P.O. q 24 hr for total of 7 to 14 days.

➤ *To treat complicated, life-threatening intra-abdominal infections, including postsurgical, gynecologic, and pelvic infections*
TABLETS, I.V. INFUSION
Adults. 300 mg I.V. q 24 hr followed by 200 mg P.O. q 24 hr when patient is stabilized for total of 7 to 14 days.
➤ *To treat complicated, life- or limb-threatening skin and soft-tissue infections, including diabetic foot infections*
TABLETS, I.V. INFUSION
Adults. 200 mg P.O. q 24 hr—or 200 mg I.V. q 24 hr followed by 200 mg P.O. q 24 hr when patient is stabilized—for total of 10 to 14 days.
DOSAGE ADJUSTMENT For patients with mild to moderate cirrhosis, 300-mg I.V. dosage reduced to 200 mg and 200-mg I.V. and P.O. dosage reduced to 100 mg.

Mechanism of Action
Interferes with DNA gyrase, the enzyme necessary for DNA replication in aerobic and anaerobic bacteria. May be active against pathogens that are resistant to such antibiotics as penicillins, cephalosporins, aminoglycosides, macrolides, and tetracyclines.

Incompatibilities
Don't mix alatrofloxacin with, or infuse it simultaneously through, same I.V. line as other drugs. Don't dilute it with NS or LR.

Contraindications
Hypersensitivity to alatrofloxacin, quinolone antimicrobial drugs, trovafloxacin, or their components

Interactions
DRUGS
antacids that contain aluminum, citric acid, magnesium, or sodium citrate; iron; morphine sulfate; sucralfate: Reduced absorption of trovafloxacin

Adverse Reactions
CNS: Dizziness, headache, light-headedness, seizures
CV: Hypotension
EENT: Hoarseness, throat tightness
GI: Abdominal pain, acute hepatic failure (evidenced by anorexia, dark urine, dysphagia, fatigue, jaundice, pale stool, and vomiting)
GU: Vaginitis
RESP: Dyspnea

SKIN: Photosensitivity, rash, urticaria or other skin reactions
Other: Angioedema

Nursing Considerations
•Infuse alatrofloxacin over 60 minutes; rapid or bolus I.V. injection may cause hypotension.
•Periodically assess liver function test results. Results may be elevated for up to 21 days after alatrofloxacin administration.
•WARNING Be aware that alatrofloxacin may cause severe liver damage, requiring liver transplantation or leading to death. Expect therapy to last no longer than 2 weeks because more prolonged therapy increases the risk of liver damage. Alatrofloxacin is reserved for hospitalized patients with life- or limb-threatening infections.

PATIENT TEACHING
•Instruct patient to report rash; urticaria; difficulty swallowing; swelling of the lips, face, or tongue; hoarseness; or throat tightness.

albuterol

(salbutamol)

Proventil, Ventolin

albuterol sulfate
(salbutamol sulphate)

AccuNeb, Airet, Gen-Salbutamol (CAN), Novo-Salmol (CAN), Proventil, Proventil Repetabs, Proventil Syrup, Ventolin, Ventolin HFA, Ventolin Syrup, Volmax

Class and Category
Chemical: Selective beta$_2$-adrenergic agonist, sympathomimetic
Therapeutic: Bronchodilator
Pregnancy category: C

Indications and Dosages
➤ *To prevent exercise-induced asthma*
INHALATION AEROSOL
Adults and children over age 4. 2 inhalations 15 to 30 min before exercise.

➤ *To treat bronchospasm in patients with reversible obstructive airway disease or acute bronchospastic attack*
E.R. TABLETS
Adults and children over age 12. *Initial:* 4 or 8 mg q 12 hr. *Maximum:* 32 mg/day in divided doses q 12 hr.
Children ages 6 to 12. *Initial:* 4 mg q 12 hr. *Maximum:* 24 mg/day in divided doses q 12 hr.

REPETABS
Adults and children over age 12. *Initial:* 4 to 8 mg q 12 hr. *Maximum:* 32 mg/day in divided doses q 12 hr.
Children ages 6 to 11. *Initial:* 4 mg q 12 hr. *Maximum:* 24 mg/day in divided doses q 12 hr.
SYRUP
Adults and children over age 14. *Initial:* 2 to 4 mg (1 to 2 tsp) t.i.d. or q.i.d. *Maximum:* 32 mg/day in divided doses.
Children ages 6 to 14. *Initial:* 2 mg (1 tsp) t.i.d. or q.i.d. *Maximum:* 24 mg/day in divided doses.
Children ages 2 to 6. *Initial:* 0.1 mg/kg t.i.d. (not to exceed 2 mg t.i.d.), increased to 0.2 mg/kg t.i.d. (not to exceed 4 mg t.i.d.).
TABLETS
Adults and children over age 12. *Initial:* 2 or 4 mg t.i.d. or q.i.d. *Maximum:* 32 mg/day in divided doses.
Children ages 6 to 12. *Initial:* 2 mg t.i.d. or q.i.d. *Maximum:* 24 mg/day in divided doses.
DOSAGE ADJUSTMENT For elderly patients, initial dosage reduced to 2 mg (1 tsp) of syrup t.i.d. or q.i.d. or 2 mg of tablets t.i.d. or q.i.d. (up to 32 mg/day).
INHALATION AEROSOL
Adults and children age 4 and older. 1 inhalation q 4 hr to 2 inhalations q 4 to 6 hr.
INHALATION CAPSULES (ROTOCAPS)
Adults and children age 4 and older. 200 mcg inhaled q 4 to 6 hr using inhalation device. *Maximum:* 400 mcg q 4 to 6 hr.
INHALATION SOLUTION
Adults and children age 12 and older. 2.5 mg t.i.d. or q.i.d. by nebulization over 5 to 15 min.
Children ages 2 to 12. *Initial:* 0.1 to 0.15 mg/kg t.i.d. or q.i.d. *Maximum:* 2.5 mg t.i.d. or q.i.d.

Route	Onset	Peak	Duration
P.O. (E.R. tab)	30 min	2 to 3 hr	12 hr
P.O. (syrup)	Rapid	2 hr	Unknown
P.O. (tab)	30 min	2 to 3 hr	4 to 8 hr
Inhalation (aerosol)	5 to 15 min	50 to 55 min	3 to 6 hr
Inhalation (rotocap)	5 to 15 min	0.5 to 3 hr	2 to 6 hr
Inhalation (solution)	5 to 15 min	1 to 2 hr	3 to 6 hr

Mechanism of Action

Albuterol attaches to beta$_2$ receptors on bronchial cell membranes, which stimulates the intracellular enzyme adenylate cyclase to convert adenosine triphosphate (ATP) to cAMP. This reaction decreases intracellular calcium levels. It also increases intracellular levels of cAMP, as shown. Together, these effects relax bronchial smooth-muscle cells and inhibit histamine release.

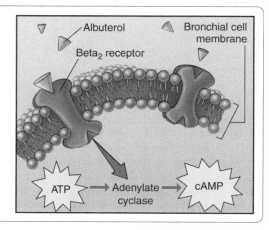

Contraindications

Hypersensitivity to albuterol or its components

Interactions

DRUGS

beta blockers: Inhibited effects of albuterol
bronchodilators (sympathomimetics), such as theophylline: Possibly adverse cardiovascular effects
digoxin: Decreased serum digoxin level
MAO inhibitors, tricyclic antidepressants: Increased vascular effects of albuterol
methyldopa: Increased vasopressor effect of methyldopa
potassium-lowering drugs: Possibly hypokalemia
potassium-wasting diuretics: Possibly increased hypokalemia

Adverse Reactions

CNS: Anxiety, dizziness, drowsiness, headache, hyperkinesia, insomnia, irritability, nervousness, tremor, vertigo, weakness
CV: Angina; arrhythmias, including tachycardia; hypertension; palpitations
EENT: Altered taste, dry mouth and throat, taste perversion
GI: Anorexia, diarrhea, dysphagia, heartburn, nausea, vomiting
RESP: Bronchospasm, cough, dyspnea, paradoxical airway resistance (with excessive inhalation), pulmonary edema
SKIN: Diaphoresis, flushing, pallor, pruritus, rash, urticaria
Other: Hypokalemia

Nursing Considerations

•Administer pressurized inhalations of albuterol during second half of inspiration, when airways are open wider and aerosol distribution is more effective.
•WARNING Use cautiously in patients with cardiac disorders, diabetes mellitus, digitalis intoxication, hypertension, hyperthyroidism, or history of seizures. Albuterol can worsen these conditions.
•Monitor serum potassium level because albuterol may cause transient hypokalemia.
•Be aware that drug tolerance can develop with prolonged use.

PATIENT TEACHING

•Teach patient how to use inhaler properly. Tell him to shake canister well before using and to check that a new canister is working properly by spraying it once into the air while looking for a fine mist.
•Instruct patient to wash mouthpiece with water once a week and allow it to air-dry.
•Advise patient to wait at least 1 minute between inhalations.
•Tell patient to check with his prescriber before using other inhaled drugs.
•Warn patient not to exceed prescribed dose or frequency. If doses become less effective, tell him to contact his prescriber.
•Tell patient to immediately report signs and symptoms of allergic reaction, such as difficulty swallowing, itching, and rash.

alendronate sodium

Fosamax

Class and Category

Chemical: Aminobisphosphonate

Therapeutic: Bone resorption inhibitor
Pregnancy category: C

Indications and Dosages

➤ *To prevent postmenopausal osteoporosis*

TABLETS

Adults. 5 mg q.d. or 35 mg once weekly in the morning with a full glass of water at least 30 min before first food, drink, or drug.

➤ *To treat postmenopausal osteoporosis*

TABLETS

Adults. 10 mg q.d. or 70 mg once weekly in the morning with a full glass of water at least 30 min before first food, drink, or drug.

➤ *To treat Paget's disease of the bone in patients whose alkaline phosphatase level is twice the upper limit of normal or higher and who are symptomatic and at risk for further complications*

TABLETS

Adults. 40 mg q.d. with a full glass of water for 6 mo.

DOSAGE ADJUSTMENT Dosage increased to 10 mg q.d. for postmenopausal women not receiving estrogen.

➤ *To increase bone mass in men with osteoporosis*

TABLETS

Adults. 10 mg q.d. or 70 mg once weekly in the morning with a full glass of water at least 30 min before first food, drink, or drug.

➤ *To treat glucocorticoid-induced osteoporosis in men and women who receive a daily glucocorticoid dosage equal to or greater than 7.5 mg of prednisone and who have low bone mineral density*

TABLETS

Adults. 5 mg q.d. in the morning with a full glass of water at least 30 min before first food, drink, or drug.

Route	Onset	Peak	Duration
P.O.	Unknown	Unknown	6 wk*

Contraindications

Esophageal abnormalities that delay esophageal emptying, such as stricture or achalasia; hypersensitivity to alendronate; hypocalcemia; inability to stand or sit upright for at least 30 minutes

---

* After single 5-mg dose for osteoporosis; 6 mo after single 5-mg dose for Paget's disease.

Mechanism of Action

Reduces the activity of cells that cause bone loss, slows the rate of bone loss after menopause, and increases the amount of bone mass. May act by inhibiting osteoclast activity on newly formed bone resorption surfaces, which reduces the number of sites where bone is remodeled. Bone formation then exceeds bone resorption at these remodeling sites, which gradually increases bone mass. May also inhibit bone dissolution by binding to hydroxyapatite crystals, which are composed of calcium, phosphate, and hydroxide and give bone its rigid structure.

Interactions

DRUGS

antacids, calcium, iron, multivalent cations: Decreased absorption of alendronate
aspirin: Increased risk of GI distress

FOODS

any food: Delayed absorption and decreased serum level of alendronate

Adverse Reactions

CNS: Headache
GI: Abdominal distention and pain, constipation, diarrhea, dysphagia, esophageal ulceration, esophagitis, flatulence, gastritis, heartburn, indigestion, melena, nausea, vomiting
MS: Arthralgia, bone pain, focal osteomalacia, muscle spasms, myalgia
SKIN: Rash
Other: Hypocalcemia

Nursing Considerations

• Monitor serum calcium level before, during, and after treatment. If hypocalcemia occurs, expect prescriber to order a calcium supplement before therapy begins.
• Ensure adequate dietary intake of calcium and vitamin D before, during, and after treatment.
• WARNING Alendronate may irritate upper GI mucosa, causing such adverse reactions as esophageal ulceration. To help minimize these reactions, have patient take it with a full glass of water and remain upright for at least 30 minutes.

PATIENT TEACHING

• Advise patient to take alendronate in the morning with a full glass of water. Explain that such beverages as orange juice, coffee, and mineral water reduce alendronate's effects.

• To help reduce esophageal irritation, tell patient not to chew or suck on tablet.
• Instruct patient to wait at least 30 minutes after taking alendronate to eat, drink, or take other drugs. Teach patient to remain upright for 30 minutes after taking alendronate *and* until consuming the first food of the day.

alglucerase

Ceredase

Class and Category
Chemical: Glucocerebrosidase beta-glucosidase
Therapeutic: Enzyme replacement
Pregnancy category: C

Indications and Dosages
➤ *To treat chronic nonneuropathic Gaucher's disease in patients with moderate to severe anemia, thrombocytopenia with bleeding tendencies, bone disease, or significant hepatomegaly or splenomegaly*

I.V. INFUSION
Adults and children. Up to 60 U/kg infused over 1 to 2 hr, usually q 2 wk.
DOSAGE ADJUSTMENT Highly individualized dosage based on body size and disease severity. Some patients may need infusion once every other day; others may need it once q 4 wk. Maintenance dosage progressively reduced every 3 to 6 mo to as low as 1 U/kg.

Route	Onset	Peak	Duration
I.V.	Up to 60 min	Unknown	Variable

Mechanism of Action
Catalyzes the normal hydrolysis of glucocerebroside to glucose and ceramide in membrane lipids. Gaucher's disease results from deficiency of the enzyme beta-glucocerebrosidase and causes the lipid glucocerebroside to accumulate in tissue macrophages.

Contraindications
Hypersensitivity to alglucerase

Adverse Reactions
CNS: Chills, dizziness, fatigue, fever, headache
CV: Transient peripheral edema, vasomotor irritability

EENT: Oral ulcerations
GI: Abdominal discomfort, diarrhea, nausea, vomiting
MS: Backache
Other: I.V. site burning, itching, or swelling

Nursing Considerations
• Before intitiating alglucerase therapy, expect to give antihistamines to patient who is hypersensitive to drug.
• On day that drug is administered, use aseptic technique to dilute alglucerase with NS to final volume of no more than 100 ml.
• Don't shake drug; shaking could inactivate it.
• Don't use alglucerase if it's discolored or contains precipitate.
• Be aware that drug doesn't contain preservatives. Discard unused portion.
• Infuse alglucerase with in-line I.V. particle filter.

PATIENT TEACHING
• Tell patient that he may experience flulike symptoms with each alglucerase dose.
• Instruct patient to report headache, hot flashes, nausea, and other adverse reactions.
• Inform patient that alglucerase is derived from pooled human placental tissue and poses a slight risk of viral contamination.
• Advise patient to keep appointments for scheduled doses of alglucerase.

allopurinol

Apo-Allopurinol (CAN), Lopurin, Purinol (CAN), Zyloprim

allopurinol sodium

Aloprim

Class and Category
Chemical: Hypoxanthine derivative, xanthine oxidase inhibitor
Therapeutic: Antigout
Pregnancy category: C

Indications and Dosages
➤ *To treat gout and hyperuricemia*
TABLETS
Adults. 200 to 600 mg/day in divided doses, depending on disease severity. *Usual:* 200 to 300 mg/day. *Maximum:* 800 mg/day.
➤ *To treat secondary hyperuricemia caused by neoplastic disease*
TABLETS
Children ages 6 to 10. 300 mg/day, adjusted

after 48 hr, depending on response to treatment.

Children under age 6. 150 mg/day, adjusted after 48 hr, depending on response to treatment.

➤ *To prevent gout attack*

TABLETS

Adults. 100 mg/day increased by 100 mg/wk until serum uric acid level is 6 mg/dl or less.

➤ *To prevent uric acid nephropathy during vigorous treatment of neoplastic disease*

TABLETS

Adults. 600 to 800 mg/day for 2 to 3 days, then adjusted to keep serum uric acid level within normal limits.

➤ *To treat recurrent calcium oxalate calculi*

TABLETS

Adults. 200 to 300 mg/day as a single dose or in divided doses, adjusted based on 24-hr urine urate level.

DOSAGE ADJUSTMENT For patient with impaired renal function, dosage adjusted to 200 mg/day if creatinine clearance is 10 to 20 ml/min/1.73 m^2, 100 mg/day if creatinine clearance is 3 to 10 ml/min/1.73 m^2, or 100 mg q.o.d. if creatinine clearance falls below 3 ml/min/1.73 m^2.

➤ *To treat increased serum and urine uric acid levels in patients with leukemia, lymphoma, and solid tumors whose cancer chemotherapy has increased those levels and who can't tolerate oral therapy*

I.V. INFUSION

Adults. 200 to 400 mg/m^2/day as a single infusion or in equally divided infusions q 6, 8, or 12 hr. *Maximum:* 600 mg/day.

Children. 200 mg/m^2/day as a single infusion or in equally divided infusions q 6, 8, or 12 hr.

Route	Onset	Peak	Duration
P.O.	2 to 3 days	1 to 3 wk*	1 to 2 wk

Incompatibilities

Don't combine I.V. allopurinol in solution with amikacin, amphotericin B, carmustine, cefotaxime sodium, chlorpromazine hydrochloride, cimetidine hydrochloride, clinda-

---

* For hyperuricemia; several months for gout attack prevention.

mycin phosphate, cytarabine, dacarbazine, daunorubicin hydrochloride, diphenhydramine hydrochloride, doxorubicin hydrochloride, doxycycline hyclate, droperidol, floxuridine, gentamicin sulfate, haloperidol lactate, hydroxyzine hydrochloride, idarubicin hydrochloride, imipenem-cilastatin sodium, mechlorethamine hydrochloride, meperidine hydrochloride, metoclopramide hydrochloride, methylprednisolone sodium succinate, minocycline hydrochloride, nalbuphine hydrochloride, netilmicin sulfate, ondansetron hydrochloride, prochlorperazine edisylate, promethazine hydrochloride, sodium bicarbonate, streptozocin, tobramycin sulfate, vinorelbine tartrate.

Mechanism of Action

Inhibits uric acid production by inhibiting xanthine oxidase, the enzyme responsible for converting hypoxanthine and xanthine to uric acid. Allopurinol is metabolized to oxipurinol, which also inhibits xanthine oxidase.

Contraindications

Hypersensitivity to allopurinol

Interactions

DRUGS

ACE inhibitors: Increased risk of hypersensitivity reactions

amoxicillin, ampicillin: Increased risk of rash

azathioprine, mercaptopurine: Inactivation of these drugs

chlorpropamide: Increased risk of hypoglycemia in patients with renal insufficiency

cyclophosphamide, other cytotoxic drugs: Enhanced bone marrow suppression

dicumarol: Increased half-life and anticoagulant action of dicumarol

thiazide diuretics: Possibly increased risk of allopurinol toxicity

uricosuric agents: Increased urinary excretion of uric acid

vitamin C (large doses): Possibly urine acidification and increased risk of renal calculus formation

Adverse Reactions

CNS: Chills, drowsiness, fever, headache, neuritis, paresthesia, peripheral neuropathy, somnolence

CV: Vasculitis

EENT: Epistaxis, loss of taste

GI: Abdominal pain, diarrhea, dysphagia, elevated liver function test results, gastritis, granulomatous hepatitis, hepatic necrosis, hepatomegaly, nausea, vomiting
GU: Exacerbation of renal calculi, renal failure
HEME: Agranulocytosis, aplastic anemia, bone marrow depression, eosinophilia, leukocytosis, leukopenia, thrombocytopenia
MS: Arthralgia, exacerbation of gout, myopathy
SKIN: Alopecia; ecchymosis; jaundice; maculopapular, scaly, or exfoliative rash (sometimes fatal); pruritus; urticaria

Nursing Considerations
• As ordered, obtain baseline CBC and uric acid level and review results of renal and liver function tests before and during allopurinol therapy.
• Reconstitute and dilute I.V. preparation to a concentration of 6 mg/ml or less.
• **WARNING** Discontinue allopurinol and notify prescriber immediately at first sign of hypersensitivity reaction, such as rash, which may precede more severe reactions.
• To decrease risk of calculus formation, maintain fluid intake of up to 3 L/day and monitor patient for output of 2 L/day. Also, don't give vitamin C.
PATIENT TEACHING
• Advise patient to take allopurinol after meals and to drink at least 10 large glasses of water daily.
• Instruct patient to report unusual bleeding or bruising, fever, chills, gout attack, numbness, and tingling.
• Inform patient that acute gout attacks may occur more frequently early in allopurinol treatment and that results may not be noticeable for 2 weeks or longer.
• Instruct patient not to drive or perform potentially hazardous tasks if drug causes drowsiness.

almotriptan malate

Axert

Class and Category
Chemical: Selective 5-hydroxytryptamine$_1$ (5-HT$_1$) receptor agonist
Therapeutic: Antimigraine drug
Pregnancy category: C

Indications and Dosages
➤ *To treat acute migraine*
TABLETS
Adults. *Initial:* 6.25 to 12.5 mg as a single dose, repeated in 2 hr p.r.n. *Maximum:* 2 doses/24 hr or 4 migraine treatments/mo.

DOSAGE ADJUSTMENT For patient with impaired renal or hepatic function, initial dose reduced to 6.25 mg with maximum daily dose of 12.5 mg.

> ### Mechanism of Action
> May stimulate 5-HT$_1$ receptors on intracranial blood vessels and sensory nerves in the trigeminal vascular system. By activating these receptors, almotriptan selectively constricts inflamed and dilated cranial blood vessels and inhibits the production of proinflammatory neuropeptides. The drug also interrupts the transmission of pain signals to the brain.

Contraindications
Basilar or hemiplegic migraine; cerebrovascular, peripheral vascular, or ischemic or vasospastic coronary artery disease (CAD); hypersensitivity to almotriptan or its components; hypertension (uncontrolled); use within 24 hours of other serotonin-receptor agonists or ergotamine-containing or ergot-type drugs

Interactions
DRUGS
ergotamine-containing drugs: Prolonged vasospastic reactions
erythromycin, itraconazole, ketoconazole, ritonavir: Possibly increased blood almotriptan level
MAO inhibitors, verapamil: Increased blood almotriptan level
selective serotonin reuptake inhibitors: Increased risk of hyperreflexia, lack of coordination, and weakness

Adverse Reactions
CNS: Dizziness, headache, paresthesia, somnolence, syncope
CV: Coronary artery vasospasm, hypertension, ischemia, MI, palpitations, vasodilation, ventricular fibrillation, ventricular tachycardia
EENT: Dry mouth
GI: Nausea

Nursing Considerations

•**WARNING** Because almotriptan therapy can cause coronary artery vasospasm, monitor patient with CAD for signs and symptoms of angina. Because drug also may cause peripheral vasospastic reactions, such as ischemic bowel disease, monitor patient for abdominal pain and bloody diarrhea.
•Expect to administer a lower dosage to patients with hepatic or renal dysfunction because of impaired drug metabolism or excretion.
•Monitor blood pressure regularly during therapy in patients with hypertension because almotriptan may produce a transient increase in blood pressure.

PATIENT TEACHING

•Inform patient that almotriptan is used to treat acute migraine attacks and that he shouldn't take it to treat nonmigraine headaches.
•Advise patient to consult prescriber before taking any OTC or prescription drugs.
•Advise patient not to take more than maximum prescribed dosage during any 24-hour period.
•Caution patient that drug may cause adverse CNS reactions, and advise him to avoid potentially hazardous activities until he knows how the drug affects him.
•Instruct patient to seek emergency care immediately if he experiences cardiac symptoms—such as heaviness, pain, pressure, or tightness in the chest, jaw, neck, or throat—after taking drug.

alosetron hydrochloride

Lotronex

Class and Category

Chemical: Selective serotonin 5-HT$_3$ receptor antagonist
Therapeutic: Antidiarrheal
Pregnancy category: B

Indications and Dosages

➤ *To treat women with severe diarrhea-predominant irritable bowel syndrome (IBS) who have failed to respond to conventional therapy*

TABLETS

Adult women. *Initial:* 1 mg q.d. for 4 wk, increased to 1 mg b.i.d., if needed, or discontinued if no response seen in first 4 wk of

therapy or if drug doesn't adequately control symptoms after 4 wk of b.i.d. regimen.

Mechanism of Action

Inhibits activation of 5-HT$_3$ non-selective cation channels found in enteric neurons in the GI tract, which increases visceral sensations, colonic transit, and secretions in the GI tract, resulting in reduced abdominal pain and hyperactivity of the GI tract, symptoms prominent in IBS.

Contraindications

Active diverticulitis; history of chronic or severe constipation or sequelae from constipation, Crohn's disease, diverticulitis, GI perforation or adhesions, hypercoagulable state, impaired intestinal circulation, intestinal obstruction or stricture, ischemic colitis, thrombophlebitis, toxic megacolon, or ulcerative colitis; known hypersensitivity to alosetron or its components

Interactions

None

Adverse Reactions

CNS: Anxiety, fatigue, headache, hypnagogic effects, malaise, temperature regulation disturbances
CV: Tachyarrhythmias
GI: Abdominal or GI discomfort and pain, abdominal distention, constipation, dyspepsia, hemorrhoids, GI spasms or lesions, hyposalivation, ileus, impaction, ischemic colitis, nausea, obstruction, perforation, regurgitation and reflux, small bowel mesenteric ischemia, ulceration
GU: Urinary frequency
RESP: Breathing disorders
SKIN: Rash, sweating, urticaria
Other: Nonspecific cramps or pain

Nursing Considerations

•Be aware that only physicians enrolled in Glaxo-SmithKline's prescribing program for alosetron should prescribe the drug and only patients who have read and signed the patient-physician agreement can receive the drug. Confirm that the agreement has been signed before initiating therapy.
•**WARNING** Monitor patient for constipation, especially those who are elderly or debilitated or who also take drugs that decrease gastrointestinal motility. Also monitor patient for

signs and symptoms of ischemic colitis, such as rectal bleeding, bloody diarrhea, or new or worsening abdominal pain. If these occur, discontinue drug immediately. Be aware that once alosetron is discontinued for ischemic colitis, drug should not be resumed later; however, a patient who no longer has constipation can resume the drug, if needed.

•Ensure that program stickers required by drug company are affixed to all prescriptions, including refills, before giving to patient.

PATIENT TEACHING
•Instruct patient to read the medication guide for alosetron, which outlines the risks and benefits of the drug.
•Advise patient to stop taking drug immediately and notify her prescriber if signs and symptoms of ischemic colitis or constipation occur. If constipation does not resolve after drug is stopped, instruct patient to notify her prescriber.
•Inform patient that drug will be discontinued after 4 weeks of 1 mg b.i.d. regimen if the drug isn't effective in controlling symptoms of IBS.

alpha₁-proteinase inhibitor (human)

(alpha₁-antitrypsin)

Prolastin

Class and Category
Chemical: Plasma protein
Therapeutic: Enzyme replacement
Pregnancy category: C

Indications and Dosages
➤ *To treat congenital alpha₁-antitrypsin deficiency in patients with signs of panacinar emphysema*

I.V. INFUSION
Adults. 60 mg/kg infused over 30 min (at rate of at least 0.08 ml/kg/min) once weekly.

Route	Onset	Peak	Duration
I.V.	In a few weeks	Unknown	Unknown

Contraindications
Hypersensitivity to alpha₁-proteinase inhibitor, selective immunoglobulin A (IgA) deficiency in patients with anti-IgA antibodies

Mechanism of Action
Replaces the enzyme alpha₁-antitrypsin, which normally inhibits the proteolytic enzyme elastase in patients with alpha₁-antitrypsin deficiency. Without alpha₁-proteinase inhibitor, elastase attacks and destroys alveolar membranes and causes panacinar emphysema.

Interactions
ACTIVITIES
smoking: Inactivation of alpha₁-proteinase inhibitor

Adverse Reactions
CNS: Dizziness, fever (up to 12 hours after treatment)
HEME: Mild, transient leukocytosis
Other: Flulike symptoms

Nursing Considerations
•Use alpha₁-proteinase inhibitor cautiously in patients at risk for circulatory overload because drug is a colloid solution that increases plasma volume.
•Give drug up to 3 hours after reconstitution. Don't refrigerate. Discard unused reconstituted drug.
•Administer by I.V. route only without other agents or drugs.
•**WARNING** Alpha₁-proteinase inhibitor is made from human plasma and may contain infectious agents, such as viruses. Ensure that patient is immunized against hepatitis B before giving drug. If time doesn't allow for antibody formation, give a single dose of hepatitis B immune globulin with hepatitis B vaccine, as prescribed.
•Monitor patient for delayed fever, which may occur up to 12 hours after therapy. Fever usually resolves within 24 hours.

PATIENT TEACHING
•Inform patient of potential risks of therapy, including infection, even though drug is treated to reduce the risk of infectious agent transmission.
•Stress the importance of receiving weekly doses to maintain an adequate antielastase barrier in the lungs. Explain that treatment must continue throughout the patient's lifetime.
•Warn patient not to smoke.

alprazolam

Apo-Alpraz (CAN), Novo-Alprazol (CAN), Nu-Alpraz, Xanax

Class, Category, and Schedule
Chemical: Benzodiazepine
Therapeutic: Antianxiety
Pregnancy category: D
Controlled substance: Schedule IV

Indications and Dosages
➤ *To control anxiety disorders, relieve anxiety (short-term therapy), or treat anxiety associated with depression*
TABLETS
Adults. *Initial:* 0.25 to 0.5 mg t.i.d., adjusted to patient's needs. *Maximum:* 4 mg/day in divided doses.
DOSAGE ADJUSTMENT In elderly or debilitated patients or patients with advanced hepatic disease, initial dosage adjusted to 0.25 mg b.i.d. or t.i.d. and increased gradually, as needed and tolerated.
➤ *To treat panic attack*
TABLETS
Adults. *Initial:* 0.5 mg t.i.d., increased q 3 to 4 days by no more than 1 mg/day, based on patient response. *Maximum:* 10 mg/day in divided doses.

Mechanism of Action
May increase the effects of gamma-aminobutyric acid (GABA) and other inhibitory neurotransmitters by binding to specific benzodiazepine receptors in the limbic and cortical areas of the CNS. GABA inhibits excitatory stimulation, which helps control emotional behavior. The limbic system contains many benzodiazepine receptors, which may help explain the drug's antianxiety effects.

Contraindications
Acute narrow-angle glaucoma, hypersensitivity to alprazolam, itraconazole or ketoconazole therapy

Interactions
DRUGS
antacids: Possibly altered rate of alprazolam absorption
cimetidine, disulfiram, fluoxetine, isoniazid, metoprolol, oral contraceptives, propoxyphene, propranolol, valproic acid: Possibly decreased elimination and increased effects of alprazolam
CNS depressants: Possibly increased CNS effects of both drugs

digoxin: Possibly increased serum digoxin level, causing digitalis toxicity
itraconazole, ketoconazole: Possibly profoundly inhibited metabolism of alprazolam
levodopa: Possibly decreased effects of levodopa
neuromuscular blockers: Possibly potentiated or antagonized effects of these drugs
phenytoin: Possibly increased serum phenytoin level, causing phenytoin toxicity
probenecid: Possibly faster onset or prolonged effects of alprazolam
ranitidine: Possibly reduced absorption of alprazolam
ACTIVITIES
alcohol use: Enhanced adverse CNS effects of alprazolam

Adverse Reactions
CNS: Agitation, confusion, depression, dizziness, drowsiness, fatigue, hallucinations, headache, insomnia, irritability, lack of coordination, light-headedness, memory loss, paresthesia, speech problems, syncope, tremor
CV: Chest pain, hypotension, nonspecific ECG changes, palpitations, tachycardia
EENT: Blurred vision, decreased or increased salivation, nasal congestion, tinnitus
GI: Abdominal discomfort, anorexia, constipation, diarrhea, elevated liver function test results, nausea, vomiting
GU: Decreased or increased libido, urinary hesitancy
MS: Dysarthria, muscle rigidity and spasms
RESP: Hyperventilation
SKIN: Dermatitis, diaphoresis, pruritus, rash
Other: Weight gain or loss

Nursing Considerations
•Expect to administer a higher dosage to patient with history of panic attacks that occur unexpectedly or during such situations as driving.
•Because alprazolam use can lead to dependency, expect to reduce dosage gradually when tapering off the drug. To prevent withdrawal symptoms, don't discontinue abruptly.
PATIENT TEACHING
•If alprazolam is prescribed to treat panic attacks, tell patient that drug isn't intended to relieve everyday stress.
•Warn patient not to stop taking drug abruptly because withdrawal symptoms may occur.

•Instruct patient never to increase the prescribed dosage because of the increased risk of dependency.
•Urge patient to avoid drinking alcohol during alprazolam therapy.
•Advise patient to avoid driving and activities that require alertness until alprazolam's effects are known.

alprostadil

Caverject, Edex, Muse

Class and Category

Chemical: Prostaglandin E_1
Therapeutic: Anti-impotence drug
Pregnancy category: C

Indications and Dosages

➤ *To treat erectile dysfunction due to vascular or psychogenic causes or both*
INTRACAVERNOUS INJECTION (CAVERJECT, EDEX)
Adults. *Initial:* 2.5 mcg. Dosage increased to 5 mcg if partial response is apparent or 7.5 mcg if no response is apparent, followed by incremental increases of 5 to 10 mcg until erection suitable for intercourse (not exceeding 1-hr duration) is achieved. No more than 2 doses, separated by 1 hr, should be given on a single day during initial titration phase. *Maximum:* 3 doses/week; each dose separated by 24 hr.
URETHRAL SUPPOSITORY (MUSE)
Adults. *Initial:* 125 to 250 mcg. If no response, dosage increased in stepwise increments to 500 or 1,000 mcg until erection suitable for intercourse (not exceeding 1-hr duration) is achieved. *Maximum:* 2 doses/24 hr.
➤ *To treat erectile dysfunction due to spinal cord injury*
INTRACAVERNOUS INJECTION (CAVERJECT, EDEX)
Adults. *Initial:* 1.25 mcg. Dosage increased to 2.5 mcg if partial response is apparent, then to 5 mcg, and increased in 5-mcg increments until erection suitable for intercourse (not exceeding 1-hr duration) is achieved. No more than 2 doses, separated by 1 hr, should be given on a single day during initial titration phase. *Maximum:* 3 doses/week; each dose separated by 24 hr.

Route	Onset	Peak	Duration
Intracavernous	5 to 20 min	Unknown	60 min
Intraurethral	5 to 10 min	Unknown	30 to 60 min

Contraindications

Anuria, balanitis (inflammation of head of penis), cavernosal fibrosis, hypersensitivity to alprostadil or its components, hyperviscosity syndrome, indwelling urethral catheter, leukemia, men for whom sexual activity is contraindicated, multiple myeloma, penile angulation, penile implants, Peyronie's disease, polycythemia, severe hypospadius (urethral opening on underside of penis), sickle cell anemia or trait, tendency to develop venous thrombosis, thrombocythemia, urethral obstruction or stricture, urethritis

Interactions

DRUGS
anticoagulants: Possibly increased risk of bleeding
cyclosporine: Possibly decreased blood cyclosporine level

Adverse Reactions

CNS: Dizziness, headache, syncope
CV: Hypertension, hypotension, tachycardia, vasodilation
EENT: Nasal congestion, sinusitis
GU: Pelvic pain; penile disorders, including edema, fibrosis, pain, and rash; priapism; prolonged erection; prostatic pain or enlargement; urethral abrasions; urethral bleeding
MS: Back pain
RESP: Cough, upper respiratory tract infection
Other: Flulike symptoms, injection site bruising or hematoma

Nursing Considerations

•Reconstitute solution with 1 ml of diluent, for a concentration of 5, 10, 20, or 40 mcg/ml, depending on vial strength. Gently swirl contents of reconstituted vial. Use reconstituted solution within 24 hours when stored at room temperature. Don't use any vials that contain precipitate or discolored solution. Discard unused portion of reconstituted solution.
•Using a ½-inch 27G to 30G needle, inject drug at a 90-degree angle into the proximal third of the spongy tissue that runs the length of the dorsolateral aspect of the penis, avoiding any visible veins. Rotate injection sites by alternating sides of the penis used for injection.
•Carefully examine the penis for signs and symptoms of penile fibrosis. Expect to discontinue treatment if patient develops cavernosal fibrosis, penile angulation, or Peyronie's disease (hardening of the corpora cavernosa,

Mechanism of Action

Alprostadil causes penile erection by increasing blood flow to the penis through relaxation of trabecular smooth muscles and dilation of cavernosal arteries. A naturally occurring prostaglandin, alprostadil interacts with specific membrane-bound receptors in the corpora cavernosa cells of the penis. This action activates intracellular adenyl cyclase, which in turn converts adenosine triphosphate (ATP) into cyclic adenosine monophosphate (cAMP). Increased intracellular levels of cAMP activate protein kinase, an enzyme that activates other enzymes to initiate a cascade of chemical reactions. These chemical reactions cause the trabecular smooth muscles to relax and the cavernosal arteries to dilate. Blood flow to the penis is then increased, which distends the penile lacunar spaces and compresses the veins, trapping blood in the penis and causing it to become enlarged and rigid.

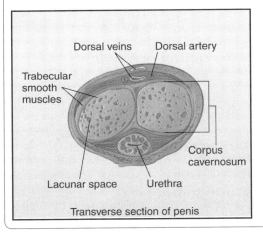

Transverse section of penis

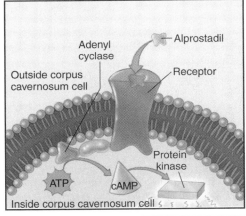

Inside corpus cavernosum cell

which causes the penis to become distorted when erect) during therapy.

•WARNING Assess patient for prolonged erection after drug administration. Notify prescriber and be prepared to treat patient for priapism if erection lasts longer than 4 hours.

•If patient is receiving an anticoagulant, such as warfarin or heparin, monitor him for bleeding at injection site because alprostadil may inhibit platelet aggregation.

PATIENT TEACHING

•Inform patient that initial therapy must be performed in the office setting. Teach him how to correctly administer intracavernous injections or urethral suppositories. Inform him that the goal of treatment is to produce an erection that lasts no longer than 1 hour.

•Advise patient to use alprostadil for injection no more than three times/week and to separate doses by 24 hours. Inform patient using urethral suppositories not to use more than two doses in a 24-hour period.

•Instruct patient to inform prescriber immediately of the development of nodules or hard tissue in the penis; an erection that persists for more than 4 hours; new or worsened penile pain; or persistent curvature, redness, swelling, or tenderness of the erect penis.

•Inform patient that common adverse reactions are mild to moderate pain immediately after injection, and burning after suppository insertion.

•Instruct patient using suppository form of drug to urinate just before inserting suppository and to insert suppository with the applicator supplied with drug. Tell patient to hold the penis upright after insertion and to roll it firmly between his hands to distribute drug.

•Tell patient to sit, stand, or walk for 10 minutes after inserting suppository to increase blood flow, which enhances erection.

•Inform patient that he can expect erection to occur 5 to 20 minutes after injecting drug or about 10 minutes after inserting suppository.

•Advise patient not to change drug dosage

without consulting prescriber and to keep regularly scheduled follow-up appointments to monitor progress.
• Warn patient that alprostadil offers no protection from sexually transmitted diseases. Urge him to use a condom to decrease risk of blood-borne disease exposure, because injection can cause a small amount of bleeding at the injection site.
• Instruct patient not to reuse or share needles or syringes. Inform him of proper procedure for sharps disposal.
• Warn patient taking suppository form not to engage in sexual intercourse with a pregnant woman unless a condom is used because the drug's effect on pregnancy is unknown.
• Advise patient who plans to travel not to check drug with airline baggage or store it in a closed car.

alteplase

(tissue plasminogen activator, recombinant)

Activase, Activase rt-PA (CAN)

Class and Category
Chemical: Purified glycoprotein
Therapeutic: Thrombolytic
Pregnancy category: C

Indications and Dosages
➤ *To treat acute MI*
ACCELERATED I.V. INFUSION
Adults who weigh more than 67 kg (148 lb). 15-mg bolus followed by 50 mg infused over next 30 min and then by 35 mg infused over next 60 min.
Adults who weigh 67 kg or less. 15-mg bolus followed by 0.75 mg/kg (up to 50 mg) infused over next 30 min and then 0.5 mg/kg (up to 35 mg) infused over next 60 min.
I.V. INFUSION
Adults who weigh more than 65 kg (143 lb). 100 mg infused over 3 hr as follows: 6 to 10 mg by bolus over first 1 to 2 min, 50 to 54 mg over remainder of first hr, 20 mg over second hr, and 20 mg over third hr.
Adults who weigh 65 kg or less. 1.25 mg/kg infused over 3 hr on similar administration schedule for those weighing more than 65 kg.
➤ *To treat acute ischemic CVA*
I.V. INFUSION
Adults. 0.9 mg/kg infused over 60 min, with

10% of total dose given as bolus over first min. *Maximum:* 90 mg.
WARNING To avoid acute bleeding complications, treatment for acute ischemic CVA must begin within 3 hr after onset of CVA symptoms and only after computed tomography or other diagnostic imaging method excludes intracranial hemorrhage.
➤ *To treat pulmonary embolism*
I.V. INFUSION
Adults. 100 mg infused over 2 hr.

Route	Onset	Peak	Duration
I.V.	Immediate	20 to 120 min	4 hr

Mechanism of Action
Binds to fibrin in a thrombus and converts trapped plasminogen to plasmin. Plasmin breaks down fibrin, fibrinogen, and other clotting factors, which dissolves the thrombus.

Incompatibilities
Don't add other drugs to solution that contains alteplase.

Contraindications
For all indications: Active internal bleeding, arteriovenous malformation or aneurysm, bleeding diathesis, intracranial neoplasm, severe uncontrolled hypertension
For acute MI and pulmonary embolism only: History of CVA, intracranial or intraspinal surgery or trauma in past 2 months
For acute ischemic CVA only: Recent head trauma, recent intracranial surgery, recent previous CVA, seizure activity at onset of CVA, subarachnoid hemorrhage, suspicion or history of intracranial hemorrhage

Interactions
DRUGS
drugs that alter platelet function, such as abciximab, acetylsalicylic acid, and dipyridamole; heparin; vitamin K antagonists: Increased risk of bleeding

Adverse Reactions
CNS: Cerebral edema, cerebral herniation, CVA, fever, seizure
CV: Arrhythmias (including bradycardia and electromechanical dissociation), cardiac ar-

rest, cardiac tamponade, cardiogenic shock, cholesterol embolism, coronary thrombolysis, heart failure, hypotension, mitral insufficiency, myocardial reinfarction or rupture, pericardial effusion, pericarditis, venous thrombosis and embolism
EENT: Epistaxis, gingival bleeding, laryngeal edema
GI: GI bleeding, nausea, retroperitoneal bleeding, vomiting
GU: GU bleeding
RESP: Pleural effusion, pulmonary edema, pulmonary reembolization
SKIN: Bleeding at puncture sites, ecchymosis, rash, urticaria
Other: Anaphylaxis

Nursing Considerations
•Immediately before use, reconstitute alteplase with sterile water for injection only. Swirl gently to dissolve powder; don't shake.
•Monitor for bleeding, especially at arterial puncture sites.
•Monitor blood pressure and heart rate and rhythm frequently during and after therapy.
•WARNING Alteplase therapy may cause arrhythmias from sudden reperfusion of the myocardium. Monitor continuous ECG for arrhythmias during drug therapy.
•Minimize bleeding from noncompressible sites by avoiding internal jugular and subclavian venous puncture sites.
•Discontinue alteplase immediately if serious bleeding occurs.
•After administering alteplase, apply pressure for at least 30 minutes, followed by a pressure dressing.
•Store reconstituted solution at room temperature (about 86° F [30° C]) or refrigerated (36° to 46° F [2.2° to 7.7° C]).
PATIENT TEACHING
•Tell patient to immediately report bleeding, including from the nose or gums.
•Advise patient to limit physical activity during alteplase administration to reduce risk of injury and bleeding.

aluminum carbonate
Basaljel

aluminum hydroxide
AlternaGEL, Alu-Cap, Alugel (CAN), Alu-Tab, Amphojel, Dialume

Class and Category
Chemical: Aluminum salt
Therapeutic: Antacid, phosphate binder
Pregnancy category: Not rated

Indications and Dosages
➤ *To treat hyperacidity associated with gastric hyperacidity, gastritis, hiatal hernia, peptic esophagitis, and peptic ulcers; to prevent phosphate renal calculus formation; to reduce hyperphosphatemia in chronic renal failure*
ALUMINUM CARBONATE CAPSULES, SUSPENSION, OR TABLETS
Adults. 2 capsules or tablets or 10 ml of suspension q 2 hr up to 12 times daily p.r.n.
ALUMINUM HYDROXIDE CAPSULES, SUSPENSION, OR TABLETS
Adults. 500 to 1,500 mg as capsules or tablets in divided doses 3 to 6 times daily, taken between meals and h.s.; 5 to 30 ml as suspension p.r.n., taken between meals and h.s.

Route	Onset	Peak	Duration
P.O.	Varies	Unknown	20 to 40 min*

Mechanism of Action
Neutralizes or reduces gastric acidity, resulting in increased stomach and duodenal alkalinity. Protects stomach and duodenum lining by inhibiting pepsin's proteolytic activity. Binds with phosphate ions in the intestine to form insoluble aluminum-phosphate compounds, which lower the blood phosphate level.

Contraindications
Hypersensitivity to aluminum

Interactions
DRUGS
allopurinol, chloroquine, corticosteroids, diflunisal, digoxin, ethambutol, H$_2$-receptor blockers, iron, isoniazid, penicillamine, phenothiazines, ranitidine, tetracyclines, thyroid hormones, ticlopidine: Decreased effects of these drugs
benzodiazepines: Increased effects of benzodiazepines

Adverse Reactions
CNS: Encephalopathy

---

* If fasting; at least 3 hr if given 1 hr after meals.

GI: Constipation, intestinal obstruction, white-speckled stool
MS: Osteomalacia, osteoporosis
Other: Aluminum accumulation in serum, bone, and CNS; aluminum intoxication; electrolyte imbalances

Nursing Considerations
• Don't administer aluminum hydroxide within 1 to 2 hours of other oral drugs.
• Be aware that two 0.6-g aluminum hydroxide tablets can neutralize 16 mEq of acid.
• Monitor serum levels of sodium, phosphate, and other electrolytes, as appropriate.

PATIENT TEACHING
• Instruct patient to chew tablets well before swallowing and then drink a full glass of water.
• Warn patient not to take maximum dosage for more than 2 weeks unless prescribed because this may cause stomach to secrete excess hydrochloric acid.
• Teach patient to prevent constipation with a high-fiber diet and increased fluid intake (2 to 3 L daily), if appropriate.
• If patient takes other prescription drugs, advise him to notify prescriber before taking aluminum because of risk of drug interactions.
• Advise patient to notify prescriber if symptoms worsen or don't subside.

amantadine hydrochloride

(adamantanamine hydrochloride)
Endantadine (CAN), Gen-Amantadine (CAN), Symmetrel

Class and Category
Chemical: Adamantane derivative
Therapeutic: Antidyskinetic, antiviral
Pregnancy category: C

Indications and Dosages
➤ *To manage symptoms of primary Parkinson's disease, postencephalitic parkinsonism, arteriosclerotic parkinsonism, and parkinsonism caused by CNS injury from carbon monoxide intoxication*

CAPSULES, SYRUP, TABLETS
Adults. *Initial:* 100 mg b.i.d. *Maximum:* 400 mg q.d. in divided doses.
➤ *To treat drug-induced extrapyramidal reactions*
CAPSULES, SYRUP, TABLETS
Adults. *Initial:* 100 mg b.i.d. *Maximum:* 300 mg q.d. in divided doses.
DOSAGE ADJUSTMENT For elderly patients, patients taking high doses of other antidyskinetics, and patients who have a serious medical condition (such as heart failure, epilepsy, or psychosis), initial dosage reduced to 100 mg q.d., with gradual titration to 100 mg b.i.d. after 1 to several wk. For patients with impaired renal function, dosage adjusted to 200 mg on day 1; and then to 100 mg q.d. if creatinine clearance is 30 to 50 ml/min/1.73 m^2; to 200 mg on day 1 and then to 100 mg q.o.d. if creatinine clearance is 15 to 29 ml/min/1.73 m^2; and to 200 mg q wk if creatinine clearance is less than 15 ml/min/1.73 m^2 or if patient is receiving hemodialysis.
➤ *To prevent and treat respiratory tract infection caused by influenza A*
CAPSULES, SYRUP, TABLETS
Adults and children age 12 and older. *Initial:* 200 mg q.d. or 100 mg b.i.d. *Maximum:* 200 mg/day.
DOSAGE ADJUSTMENT For patients with impaired renal function, dosage adjusted to 200 mg on day 1 and then to 100 mg q.d. if creatinine clearance is 30 to 50 ml/min/1.73 m^2; to 200 mg on day 1 and then to 100 mg q.o.d. if creatinine clearance is 15 to 29 ml/min/1.73 m^2; and to 200 mg q wk if creatinine clearance is less than 15 ml/min/1.73 m^2 or if patient is receiving hemodialysis.
Children ages 9 to 12. 100 mg q 12 hr. *Maximum:* 200 mg/day.
Children ages 1 to 9. 1.5 to 3 mg/kg q 8 hr or 2.2 to 4.4 mg/kg q 12 hr. *Maximum:* 150 mg/day.

Route	Onset	Peak	Duration
P.O.	In 48 hr*	Unknown	Unknown

Contraindications
Angle-closure glaucoma, hypersensitivity to amantadine or its components

---

* Antidyskinetic action; antiviral action unknown.

Mechanism of Action

Affects dopamine, a neurotransmitter that is synthesized and released by neurons leading from substantia nigra to basal ganglia and is essential for normal motor function. In Parkinson's disease, progressive degeneration of these neurons substantially reduces the supply of intrasynaptic dopamine. Amantadine may cause dopamine to accumulate in the basal ganglia by increasing dopamine release or by blocking dopamine reuptake into the presynaptic neurons of the CNS. Amantadine also may stimulate dopamine receptors or cause postsynaptic receptors to be more sensitive to dopamine. These actions help control alterations in involuntary muscle movements, such as tremors and rigidity, that are associated with Parkinson's disease.

Amantadine may inhibit influenza A viral replication by blocking the uncoating of the virus and the release of viral nucleic acid into respiratory epithelial cells. Amantadine also may interfere with early replication of viruses that have already penetrated cells.

Interactions

DRUGS

anticholinergics or other drugs with anticholinergic activity, other antidyskinetics, antihistamines, phenothiazines, tricyclic antidepressants: Possibly increased anticholinergic effects and risk of paralytic ileus
carbidopa-levodopa, levodopa: Increased effectiveness of these drugs
CNS stimulants: Excessive CNS stimulation, possibly causing arrhythmias, insomnia, irritability, nervousness, or seizures
hydrochlorothiazide, triamterene: Possibly decreased amantadine clearance and increased risk of toxicity
quinidine, quinine, trimethoprim-sulfamethoxazole: Increased blood amantadine level

ACTIVITIES

alcohol use: Possibly increased risk of CNS effects—including confusion, dizziness, and light-headedness—and orthostatic hypotension

Adverse Reactions

CNS: Agitation, anxiety, confusion, dizziness, drowsiness, fatigue, hallucinations, insomnia, irritability, light-headedness, mental impair-ment, nervousness, nightmares, suicidal ideation, syncope
CV: Orthostatic hypotension, peripheral edema
EENT: Blurred vision; dry mouth, nose, or throat
GI: Constipation, diarrhea, nausea
GU: Dysuria
HEME: Leukopenia, neutropenia
SKIN: Livedo reticularis (purplish, netlike rash)

Nursing Considerations

•Be aware that prophylactic therapy with amantadine should begin as soon as possible after exposure to persons infected with the influenza A virus and should continue for 10 days. During an influenza epidemic, expect drug to be given daily throughout the epidemic, which typically lasts 6 to 8 weeks. If patient has previously received the inactivated influenza A vaccine, prescriber may discontinue it when sure that patient has developed active immunity against the virus. If patient receives the inactivated influenza A vaccine at the same time amantadine therapy starts, expect amantadine to be given for 2 to 3 weeks.
•Expect amantadine therapy to start 24 to 48 hours after the onset of influenza A symptoms and to continue for 48 hours after their disappearance.
•Monitor patients who have a history of psychiatric illness or substance abuse because amantadine may worsen these conditions. Be aware that some patients taking amantadine have attempted suicide or had suicidal ideations.
•If patient has a history of heart failure or peripheral edema, monitor for weight gain and edema because drug may cause redistribution of body fluid.
•Be aware that amantadine may increase seizure activity in patients with a history of seizures.
•**WARNING** Monitor patient for signs and symptoms of neuroleptic malignant syndrome during dosage reduction or discontinuation of therapy. These include fever, hypertension or hypotension, involuntary motor activity, mental changes, muscle rigidity, tachycardia, and tachypnea. Be prepared to provide supportive treatment and additional drug therapy, as prescribed.
•Be aware that patients receiving more than 200 mg/day are more likely to experience adverse or toxic reactions.

•Monitor patient for decreased drug effectiveness over time. If therapeutic response declines, expect to increase dosage or discontinue drug temporarily, as ordered.

PATIENT TEACHING

•Instruct patient to take amantadine exactly as prescribed and not to stop taking it abruptly. Advise patient to notify prescriber if drug becomes less effective.

•Advise patient to notify prescriber if influenza symptoms don't improve after 2 to 3 days.

•**WARNING** Advise patient or family member to notify prescriber immediately if patient reveals thoughts of suicide.

•Encourage patient to avoid alcohol during amantadine therapy because alcohol may increase the risk of confusion, dizziness, lightheadedness, or orthostatic hypotension.

•Advise patient to avoid driving and other activities that require a high level of alertness until he knows how the drug affects him because it may cause blurred vision and mental impairment.

•Advise patient to change positions slowly to minimize effects of orthostatic hypotension.

•Tell patient to use ice chips or sugarless candy or gum to relieve dry mouth.

•Caution patient to resume physical activities gradually as signs and symptoms improve.

ambenonium chloride

Mytelase

Class and Category

Chemical: Synthetic quaternary ammonium compound
Therapeutic: Antimyasthenic, cholinergic
Pregnancy category: C

Indications and Dosages

➤ *To improve muscle strength in patients with myasthenia gravis in whom pyridostigmine or neostigmine are contraindicated*

TABLETS

Adults and adolescents. *Initial:* 5 mg t.i.d. or q.i.d., increased at 1- to 2-day intervals to optimum dosage based on patient response. *Usual:* Highly individualized but usually 5 to 50 mg t.i.d. or q.i.d.

Children. *Initial:* 0.3 mg/kg or 10 mg/m²/day in divided doses t.i.d. or q.i.d. *Maintenance:*

Up to 1.5 mg/kg or 50 mg/m²/day in divided doses t.i.d. or q.i.d.

Route	Onset	Peak	Duration
P.O.	20 to 30 min	Unknown	3 to 8 hr

Mechanism of Action

Attaches to acetylcholinesterase and blocks acetylcholine's breakdown. This action prolongs and exaggerates acetylcholine's effects, producing cholinergic responses, such as miosis, increased intestinal and skeletal muscle tone, bronchoconstriction, bradycardia, and increased salivary and sweat gland secretions.

Contraindications

Hypersensitivity to ambenonium, its components, or anticholinesterases; mechanical intestinal or urinary tract obstruction

Interactions

DRUGS

anesthetics, antiarrhythmics, corticosteroids, magnesium, methocarbamol: Decreased effects of ambenonium
aminoglycosides, anticholinesterase muscle stimulants, depolarizing muscle relaxants, ganglionic blockers, mecamylamine: Increased effects of ambenonium

Adverse Reactions

CNS: Dizziness, drowsiness, headache, loss of consciousness, seizures, syncope
CV: AV block, bradycardia, decreased cardiac output, hypotension
EENT: Dysphonia, increased salivation, laryngospasm
GI: Abdominal cramps, dysphagia, flatulence, increased gastric and intestinal secretions, increased peristalsis, mild diarrhea, nausea, vomiting
GU: Incontinence, urinary frequency or urgency
MS: Arthralgia, dysarthria, fasciculations, muscle spasms, muscle weakness
RESP: Bronchoconstriction, bronchospasm, dyspnea, increased tracheobronchial secretions, lung congestion, respiratory arrest or depression, respiratory muscle paralysis
SKIN: Diaphoresis, flushing, rash, urticaria

Nursing Considerations

•Increase dosage gradually as prescribed to avoid ambenonium accumulation and overdose.

•When increasing dosage to optimum level, note when no further increase in muscle strength is observed. Then expect to reduce dosage to previous effective level and to use this as maintenance dosage.

•Expect prescriber to order ephedrine (25 mg per ambenonium dose) or potassium chloride (1 to 2 g per ambenonium dose) to further improve muscle strength.

•WARNING Drug has a narrow margin between effectiveness and overdose. If patient receives more than 200 mg/day, monitor closely for signs of overdose (cholinergic crisis), such as abdominal cramps, diarrhea, nausea, vomiting, increased salivation, diaphoresis, difficulty swallowing, blurred vision, miosis, hypertension, fasciculations, and voluntary muscle paralysis.

•Assess neuromuscular status to detect progressive or recurrent muscle weakness in patient on long-term ambenonium therapy.

•If patient develops drug resistance during long-term therapy, expect to restore drug responsiveness by decreasing dosage or briefly discontinuing ambenonium under close medical supervision.

PATIENT TEACHING

•Instruct patient to swallow tablet with liquid or food to minimize GI irritation.

•Advise patient to consult prescriber before discontinuing drug—even if symptoms diminish or disappear.

amikacin sulfate

Amikin

Class and Category

Chemical: Aminoglycoside
Therapeutic: Antibiotic
Pregnancy category: D

Indications and Dosages

➤ *To treat serious gram-negative bacterial infections (including septicemia; neonatal sepsis; respiratory tract, bone, joint, CNS, skin, soft-tissue, intra-abdominal, burn, and postoperative infections; and serious, complicated, and recurrent UTIs) caused by* Acinetobacter, Enterobacter, Escherichia coli, Klebsiella, Proteus, Providencia, Pseudomonas, *and* Serratia; *and staphylococcal infections when penicillin is contraindicated*

I.V. INFUSION, I.M. INJECTION

Adults and children. 15 mg/kg/day in equal doses at equally spaced intervals (7.5 mg/kg q 12 hr or 5 mg/kg q 8 hr) for 7 to 10 days. *Maximum:* 1,500 mg/day.

DOSAGE ADJUSTMENT For patients with impaired renal function, loading dose of 7.5 mg/kg/day followed by maintenance dosage based on creatinine clearance and serum creatinine level and given q 12 hr. For morbidly obese patients, dosage not to exceed 1.5 g/day.

Neonates. *Loading dose:* 10 mg/kg. *Maintenance:* 7.5 mg/kg q 12 hr for 7 to 10 days.

➤ *To treat uncomplicated UTIs*

I.V. INFUSION, I.M. INJECTION

Adults. 250 mg b.i.d. for 7 to 10 days.

Route	Onset	Peak	Duration
I.V.	Immediate	Unknown	Unknown
I.M.	Rapid	Unknown	Unknown

Mechanism of Action

Binds to negatively charged sites on bacteria's outer cell membrane, disrupting cell integrity. Also binds to bacterial ribosomal subunits and inhibits protein synthesis. Both actions lead to cell death.

Incompatibilties

Don't mix or infuse amikacin with other drugs.

Contraindications

Hypersensitivity to amikacin or other aminoglycosides

Interactions

DRUGS

cephalosporins, enflurane, methoxyflurane, vancomycin: Increased nephrotoxic effects
general anesthetics: Increased risk of neuromuscular blockade
loop diuretics: Increased risk of ototoxicity
neuromuscular blockers: Possibly increased neuromuscular blockade and prolonged respiratory depression
penicillins: Possibly inactivation of or synergistic effects with amikacin

Adverse Reactions

CNS: Drowsiness, headache, loss of balance, neuromuscular blockade, tremor, vertigo
EENT: Hearing loss, ototoxicity, tinnitus
GI: Nausea, vomiting
GU: Azotemia, dysuria, nephrotoxicity, oliguria or polyuria, proteinuria

MS: Acute muscle paralysis; arthralgia; muscle fatigue, spasms, and weakness
RESP: Apnea
Other: Hyperkalemia

Nursing Considerations
•Expect to obtain results of culture and sensitivity testing before therapy begins.
•Prepare amikacin I.V. solution by adding contents of 500-mg vial to 100 to 200 ml of sterile diluent. Then infuse drug over 30 to 60 minutes.
•Administer I.M. injection in large muscle mass.
•Monitor for signs of ototoxicity, such as tinnitus and vertigo, especially during high-dosage or prolonged amikacin therapy.
•WARNING Because amikacin may produce nephrotoxic effects, assess renal function before and daily during therapy, as ordered. To minimize renal tubule irritation, maintain hydration during therapy.
•Be aware that amikacin may exacerbate muscle weakness in such conditions as myasthenia gravis and Parkinson's disease.
•Measure serum amikacin concentrations as ordered, usually 30 to 90 minutes after injection (for peak concentration) and just before administering next dose (for trough concentration).

PATIENT TEACHING
•Tell patient that daily laboratory tests are necessary during amikacin treatment.
•Instruct patient to report ringing in ears, hearing changes, headache, nausea, vomiting, and changes in urination.

amiloride hydrochloride
Midamor

Class and Category
Chemical: Pyrazine-carbonyl-guanidine
Therapeutic: Potassium-sparing diuretic
Pregnancy category: B

Indications and Dosages
➤ As adjunct to thiazide or loop diuretic in patient with heart failure or hypertension to correct diuretic-induced hypokalemia or to prevent diuretic-induced hypokalemia that increases the risk of arrhythmias or other complications

TABLETS
Adults. 5 to 10 mg/day as single dose; if hypokalemia persists, increased to 15 mg/day and then 20 mg/day.

Route	Onset	Peak	Duration
P.O.	2 hr	6 to 10 hr	24 hr

Mechanism of Action
Inhibits sodium reabsorption in distal convoluted tubules and cortical collecting ducts, causing sodium and water loss and enhancing potassium retention.

Contraindications
Hypersensitivity to amiloride; impaired renal function; serum potassium level above 5.5 mEq/L; therapy with another potassium-sparing diuretic, such as spironolactone or triamterene, or a potassium supplement

Interactions
DRUGS
captopril, enalapril, lisinopril, potassium products, spironolactone: Increased risk of hyperkalemia
digoxin: Decreased effectiveness of digoxin
lithium: Reduced renal clearance of lithium and increased risk of lithium toxicity
NSAIDs: Reduced diuretic effect of amiloride
sympathomimetics: Possibly reduced antihypertensive effects of amiloride
FOODS
high-potassium food: Increased risk of hyperkalemia

Adverse Reactions
CNS: Confusion, depression, dizziness, drowsiness, encephalopathy, fatigue, headache, insomnia, nervousness, paresthesia, somnolence, tremor, vertigo
CV: Angina, arrhythmias, orthostatic hypotension, palpitations
EENT: Dry mouth, increased intraocular pressure, nasal congestion, tinnitus, vision disturbances
GI: Abdominal pain or fullness, anorexia, appetite changes, constipation, diarrhea, GI bleeding, heartburn, indigestion, nausea, thirst, vomiting
GU: Bladder spasms, dysuria, impotence, loss of libido, polyuria
HEME: Aplastic anemia, neutropenia
MS: Arthralgia, muscle spasms or weakness
RESP: Cough, dyspnea
SKIN: Alopecia, jaundice, pruritus, rash
Other: Dehydration, hyperchloremia, hyperkalemia, hypernatremia, metabolic acidosis

Nursing Considerations
•Administer amiloride with food to reduce GI upset and early in the day to minimize sleep interference from polyuria.
•Monitor renal function test results, fluid intake and output, and weight. Also monitor serum potassium level to detect hyperkalemia.
•WARNING Don't administer amiloride with other potassium-sparing diuretics.

PATIENT TEACHING
•Warn patient to avoid high-potassium food and salt substitutes that contain potassium.
•Advise patient to consult prescriber before taking other drugs, including OTC remedies, especially sympathomimetics.
•Tell patient to report dizziness, trembling, numbness, and muscle weakness or spasms.
•Advise patient to increase fluid and fiber intake to prevent constipation.
•Warn patient to expect reversible hair loss and impotence.

aminocaproic acid

Amicar

Class and Category
Chemical: Aminohexanoic acid
Therapeutic: Antifibrinolytic, antihemorrhagic
Pregnancy category: C

Indications and Dosages
➤ *To treat excessive bleeding caused by fibrinolysis*
SYRUP, TABLETS
Adults. *Initial:* 5 g during first hour followed by 1.0 to 1.25 g/hr to sustain drug plasma level of 0.13 mg/ml. *Maximum:* 30 g/day.
I.V. INJECTION
Adults. 4 to 5 g in 250 ml of diluent over 1 hr followed by continuous infusion of 1 g/hr in 50 ml of diluent. Continue for 8 hr or until bleeding stops.

Route	Onset	Peak	Duration
P.O.	Rapid	Unknown	Unknown
I.V.	Immediate	Unknown	Under 3 hr

Mechanism of Action
Inhibits the breakdown of blood clots by interfering with plasminogen activator substances and producing antiplasmin activity.

Contraindications
Hypersensitivity to aminocaproic acid; signs of active intravascular clotting, as in disseminated intravascular coagulation; upper urinary tract bleeding

Interactions
activated prothrombin, prothrombin complex concentrates: Increased risk of thrombosis
estrogens, oral contraceptives: Increased risk of hypercoagulation

Adverse Reactions
CNS: CVA, delirium, dizziness, hallucinations, headache, malaise, weakness
CV: Bradycardia, cardiomyopathy, elevated serum CK level, hypotension, ischemia, thrombophlebitis
EENT: Nasal congestion, tinnitus
GI: Abdominal cramps and pain, diarrhea, elevated AST level, nausea, vomiting
GU: Elevated BUN level, intrarenal obstruction, renal failure
HEME: Agranulocytosis, leukopenia, thrombocytopenia
MS: Myopathy
RESP: Dyspnea, pulmonary embolism
SKIN: Pruritus, rash
Other: Elevated serum aldolase and potassium levels

Nursing Considerations
•Be aware that patients on oral therapy may need up to 10 tablets during the first hour of treatment and tablets around the clock during continued treatment.
•Mix aminocaproic acid solution with sterile water for injection, NS, D$_5$W, or Ringer's solution.
•WARNING Avoid rapid I.V. administration because of increased risk of hypotension and bradycardia.
•Monitor neurologic status for drug-induced changes. Note that increased clotting may lead to CVA.

PATIENT TEACHING
•Tell patient that he'll be closely monitored during I.V. therapy and will have blood drawn for laboratory tests before, during, and after treatment.
•Advise patient who takes aminocaproic acid at home to report adverse reactions, take drug exactly as prescribed, and keep follow-up appointments with prescriber.

aminoglutethimide

Cytadren

Class and Category

Chemical: Hormone
Therapeutic: Adrenal steroid inhibitor
Pregnancy category: D

Indications and Dosages

➤ *To suppress adrenal function in patients with Cushing's syndrome who are waiting for surgery or for whom other treatment can't be used*

TABLETS
Adults. *Initial:* 250 mg q 6 hr. Increased as needed by 250 mg/day q 1 to 2 wk. *Maximum:* 2,000 mg/day.

Route	Onset	Peak	Duration
P.O.	3 to 5 days	Unknown	72 hr

Mechanism of Action

Inhibits the conversion of cholesterol to delta-5-pregnenolone, which is needed to produce certain hormones, including adrenal glucocorticoids, mineralocorticoids, estrogens, and androgens.

Contraindications

Hypersensitivity to aminoglutethimide or glutethimide

Interactions

DRUGS
antidiabetic drugs, dexamethasone, digoxin, medroxyprogesterone, synthetic glucocorticoids, theophylline, warfarin and other oral anticoagulants: Decreased effects of these drugs

Adverse Reactions

CNS: Dizziness, drowsiness, fever, headache
CV: Hypotension, orthostatic hypotension, tachycardia
ENDO: Adrenal insufficiency, hypothyroidism, masculinization
GI: Anorexia, nausea
SKIN: Hair growth, morbiliform rash, pruritus, urticaria

Nursing Considerations

•Expect to reduce aminoglutethimide dosage or discontinue treatment if extreme drowsiness, severe rash, or excessively low cortisol level occurs.

•**WARNING** Monitor for signs of hypothyroidism, including lethargy, dry skin, and slow pulse. If prescribed, administer thyroid hormone supplement.
•Monitor blood pressure for orthostatic or persistent hypotension.
PATIENT TEACHING
•Teach patient to recognize signs and symptoms of orthostatic hypotension, including dizziness and weakness when moving from sitting to standing position, and how to avoid this condition, such as by rising slowly from a supine to an upright position. dizziness and weakness when moving from sitting to standing position, and how to avoid this condition, such as by rising slowly from a supine to an upright position.
•Tell patient to report dizziness, appetite loss, nausea, headache, or severe drowsiness. Warn him to avoid driving if drowsiness occurs.
•Instruct patient to take a missed dose as soon as remembered and to evenly space out the day's remaining doses.
•Advise patient that rash, sometimes accompanied by fever, may appear on day 10 of treatment and should subside by day 15 or 16. Tell him to report severe rash or one that doesn't disappear.

aminophylline

(theophylline ethylenediamine)

Phyllocontin, Truphylline

Class and Category

Chemical: Xanthine
Therapeutic: Bronchodilator
Pregnancy category: C

Indications and Dosages

➤ *To relieve acute bronchospasm*
I.V. INFUSION
Adults (nonsmokers) not currently receiving theophylline products. *Initial:* 6 mg/kg (equal to 4.7 mg/kg anhydrous theophylline), not to exceed 25 mg/min. *Maintenance:* 0.7 mg/kg/hr for first 12 hr, then 0.5 mg/kg/hr.
Children ages 9 to 16 not currently receiving theophylline products. *Initial:* 6 mg/kg (equal to 4.7 mg/kg anhydrous theophylline), not to exceed 25 mg/min. *Maintenance:* 1 mg/kg/hr for first 12 hr, then 0.8 mg/kg/hr.

Children ages 6 months to 9 years and young adult smokers not currently receiving theophylline products. *Initial:* 6 mg/kg (equal to 4.7 mg/kg anhydrous theophylline), not to exceed 25 mg/min. *Maintenance:* 1.2 mg/kg/hr for first 12 hr, then 1 mg/kg/hr.

Adults and children currently receiving theophylline products. *Initial:* If possible, determine the time, amount, administration route, and form of last dose. The loading dose is based on the principle that each 0.63 mg/kg (0.5 mg/kg anhydrous theophylline) administered as a loading dose raises the serum theophylline level by 1 mcg/ml. Defer loading dose if serum theophylline level can be readily obtained. If this isn't possible and patient isn't exhibiting obvious signs of theophylline toxicity, prescriber may order 3.1 mg/kg (2.5 mg/kg anhydrous theophylline), which may increase the serum theophylline level by about 5 mcg/ml. *Maintenance:* For adults (nonsmokers), 0.7 mg/kg/hr for first 12 hr, then 0.5 mg/kg/hr. For children ages 9 to 16, 1 mg/kg/hr for first 12 hr, then 0.8 mg/kg/hr. For children ages 6 months to 9 years and young adult smokers, 1.2 mg/kg/hr for first 12 hr, then 1 mg/kg/hr.

DOSAGE ADJUSTMENT For elderly patients and those with cor pulmonale, dosage reduced to 0.6 mg/kg for 12 hr, then 0.3 mg/kg. For patients with heart failure and hepatic disease, dosage reduced to 0.5 mg/kg for 12 hr, then 0.1 to 0.2 mg/kg.

➤ *To prevent or treat reversible bronchospasm from asthma, chronic bronchitis, and emphysema and to maintain patent airways*

E.R. TABLETS, ORAL LIQUID, TABLETS, SUPPOSITORIES
Adults and children. *Initial (rapidly absorbed forms):* 16 mg/kg/day or 400 mg/day (whichever is less) in divided doses q 6 to 8 hr. *Maintenance:* Daily dosage increased in increments of 25% q 3 days, as tolerated, until clinical response is achieved or maximum dose is reached. When maximum dose is reached, dosage adjusted according to peak serum theophylline level. *Initial (E.R. forms):* 12 mg/kg/day or 400 mg/day (whichever is less) in divided doses q 8 to 12 hr. *Maintenance:* Daily dosage increased in increments of 2 to 3 mg/kg q 3 days. When maximum dose is reached, dosage adjusted according to peak serum theophylline level.

Route	Onset	Peak	Duration
P.O. (E.R.)	Unknown	Unknown	8 to 12 hr
P.O. (tab)	Unknown	Unknown	6 to 8 hr
I.V.	Immediate	Unknown	4 to 8 hr

Mechanism of Action
Inhibits phosphodiesterase enzymes, causing bronchodilation. Normally, these enzymes inactivate cAMP and cGMP, which are responsible for bronchial smooth-muscle relaxation. Other mechanisms of action may include translocation of calcium, prostaglandin antagonism, stimulation of catecholamines, inhibition of cGMP metabolism, and adenosine receptor antagonism.

Incompatibilities
Don't add other drugs to prepared bag or bottle of aminophylline. Don't mix aminophylline in same syringe with doxapram. Also avoid administering amiodarone, ciprofloxacin, diltiazem, dobutamine, hydralazine, or ondansetron into the Y-port of a continuous infusion of aminophylline.

Contraindications
Active peptic ulcer disease, hypersensitivity to aminophylline, rectal or lower intestine irritation or infection (suppository form), underlying seizure disorder

Interactions
DRUGS
activated charcoal, aminoglutethimide, barbiturates, ketoconazole, rifampin, sulfinpyrazone, sympathomimetics: Decreased serum theophylline level
allopurinol, calcium channel blockers, cimetidine, corticosteroids, disulfiram, ephedrine, influenza virus vaccine, interferon, macrolides, mexiletine, nonselective beta blockers, oral contraceptives, quinolones, thiabendazole: Increased serum theophylline level
benzodiazepines: Antagonized sedative effects of benzodiazepines
beta agonists: Increased effects of aminophylline and beta agonist
carbamazepine, isoniazid, loop diuretics: Increased or decreased serum theophylline level
halothane: Increased risk of cardiotoxicity
hydantoins: Decreased serum hydantoin level
ketamine: Increased risk of seizures

lithium: Decreased serum lithium level
nondepolarizing muscle relaxants: Reversed neuromuscular blockade
propofol: Antagonized sedative effects of propofol
tetracyclines: Enhanced adverse effects of theophylline

FOODS

all foods: Altered bioavailability and absorption of E.R. aminophylline, leading to toxicity
high-carbohydrate, low-protein diet: Decreased theophylline elimination and prolonged aminophylline half-life
low-carbohydrate, high-protein diet; charcoal-broiled beef: Increased theophylline elimination and shortened aminophylline half-life

ACTIVITIES

alcohol abuse: Increased effects of aminophylline
smoking (1 or more packs/day): Decreased effects of aminophylline

Adverse Reactions

CNS: Dizziness, fever, headache, insomnia, irritability, restlessness, seizures
CV: Arrhythmias (including sinus tachycardia and life-threatening ventricular arrhythmias), hypotension, palpitations
EENT: Bitter aftertaste
ENDO: Hyperglycemia, syndrome of inappropriate ADH secretion
GI: Anorexia, diarrhea, epigastric pain, heavy feeling in stomach, hematemesis, indigestion, nausea, rectal bleeding or irritation (suppositories), vomiting
GU: Diuresis, proteinuria, urine retention in men with prostate enlargement
MS: Muscle twitching
RESP: Respiratory arrest, tachypnea
SKIN: Alopecia, exfoliative dermatitis, flushing, rash, urticaria

Nursing Considerations

•**WARNING** Because aminophylline has a narrow therapeutic window (10 to 20 mcg/ml), closely monitor serum theophylline level and observe for signs of toxicity, such as tachycardia, tachypnea, nausea, vomiting, restlessness, and seizures. Keep in mind that acetaminophen, furosemide, phenylbutazone, probenecid, theobromine, coffee, tea, soft drinks, and chocolate can produce inaccurate serum theophylline level.
•To determine peak serum theophylline level, draw blood sample 15 to 30 minutes after administering I.V. loading dose.

•Give immediate-release and liquid forms with food to reduce GI upset. Give E.R. form 1 hour before or 2 hours after meals because food can alter drug absorption.

PATIENT TEACHING

•Advise patient to avoid excessive intake of caffeine (in coffee, tea, soft drinks, and chocolate), which can falsely elevate the theophylline level.
•Inform patient that blood tests may be needed to monitor aminophylline's effect.

aminosalicylate sodium
(para-aminosalicylate, PAS)

Nemasol Sodium (CAN), PAS

Class and Category

Chemical: Para-aminobenzoic acid analogue
Therapeutic: Antitubercular
Pregnancy category: C

Indications and Dosages

➤ *To treat tuberculosis as adjunct to isoniazid, streptomycin, or both and in patients with multidrug-resistant tuberculosis or when therapy with rifampin and isoniazid isn't possible because of resistance or intolerance*

TABLETS

Adults. 14 to 16 g/day in two or three divided doses.
Children. 275 to 420 mg/kg/day in three or four divided doses.

Mechanism of Action

Inhibits the incorporation of para-aminobenzoic acid into folic acid and prevents the synthesis of folic acid, a compound necessary for bacterial growth. Aminosalicylate sodium is bacteriostatic against *Mycobacterium tuberculosis*, and it delays bacterial resistance to streptomycin and isoniazid.

Contraindications

Hypersensitivity to aminosalicylate sodium, severe renal disease

Interactions

DRUGS

digoxin: Decreased serum digoxin level
probenecid: Increased serum aminosalicylate level
rifampin: Decreased serum rifampin level

Adverse Reactions

CNS: Encephalopathy, fever
CV: Vasculitis
ENDO: Goiter with or without myxedema
GI: Abdominal pain, diarrhea, hepatitis, nausea, vomiting
HEME: Agranulocytosis, hemolytic anemia, leukopenia, thrombocytopenia
SKIN: Jaundice, various types of eruptions
Other: Infectious mononucleosis-like syndrome, Loeffler's syndrome (anorexia, breathlessness, fever, and weight loss)

Nursing Considerations

• Administer aminosalicylate with food to reduce GI upset.
• **WARNING** Protect drug from water, heat, and sunlight to prevent rapid deterioration. Don't administer tablets with brown or purple discoloration—a sign of deterioration.

PATIENT TEACHING
• Teach patient to discard aminosalicylate that appears brown or purple.
• Instruct patient to take drug with food.

amiodarone hydrochloride

Cordarone, Pacerone

Class and Category

Chemical: Iodinated benzofuran derivative
Therapeutic: Class III antiarrhythmic
Pregnancy category: D

Indications and Dosages

➤ *To treat life-threatening, recurrent ventricular fibrillation and hemodynamically unstable ventricular tachycardia when these arrhythmias don't respond to other drugs or when patient can't tolerate other drugs*

TABLETS
Adults. *Loading:* 800 to 1,600 mg/day in divided doses for 1 to 3 wk. *Maintenance:* 600 to 800 mg/day in divided doses for 1 mo; then if cardiac rhythm is stable, 400 mg/day in one or two doses. Use of lowest possible dose is recommended.

I.V. INFUSION
Adults. *Loading:* 150 mg over 10 min (15 mg/ min) followed by 360 mg infused over 6 hr (1 mg/min). *Maintenance:* 540 mg infused over 18 hr (0.5 mg/min); then after the first 24 hr, 720 mg infused over 24 hr (0.5 mg/min) with dosage continued up to 96 hr or until

rhythm is stable. Therapy should change to oral form as soon as possible.

Route	Onset	Peak	Duration
P.O.	2 days to 3 wk	1 to 5 mo	Weeks to months
I.V.	Hours to 3 days	1 to 3 wk	Weeks to months

Mechanism of Action

Acts directly on cardiac cell membranes, prolonging repolarization and the refractory period and increasing ventricular fibrillation threshold. Amiodarone relaxes vascular smooth muscles, mainly in the coronary circulation, and improves myocardial blood flow. It also relaxes peripheral vascular smooth muscles, which decreases peripheral vascular resistance and myocardial oxygen consumption.

Incompatibilities

Amiodarone is incompatible with heparin. To prevent precipitate formation, avoid combining amiodarone admixed with D_5W to a concentration of 4 mg/ml with aminophylline, cefamandole nafate, cefazolin sodium, or mezlocillin sodium, and avoid mixing amiodarone concentrations of 3 mg/ml with sodium bicarbonate.

Contraindications

Bradycardia that causes syncope (unless pacemaker is present), cardiogenic shock, hypersensitivity to amiodarone or its components, hypokalemia, hypomagnesemia, SA node dysfunction, second- and third-degree AV block (unless pacemaker is present)

Interactions

DRUGS
anticoagulants: Increased anticoagulant response, which can result in serious bleeding
beta blockers: Increased serum levels of beta blockers with increased risk of hypotension and bradycardia
calcium channel blockers: Increased serum levels of calcium channel blockers with increased risk of AV block or hypotension
cholestyramine: Decreased serum amiodarone level
cimetidine: Increased serum amiodarone level
cyclosporine: Increased serum cyclosporine level

digoxin: Increased serum digoxin level and risk of digitalis toxicity
disopyramide: Increased serum disopyramide level with QT prolongation and increased risk of arrhythmias
fentanyl: Increased serum fentanyl level with increased risk of bradycardia, decreased cardiac output, and hypotension
flecainide: Increased serum flecainide level
hydantoins: Increased serum hydantoin level with long-term use and reduced serum amiodarone level
lidocaine: Increased serum lidocaine level with increased risk of seizures
methotrexate: Increased serum methotrexate level with long-term use and increased risk of methotrexate toxicity
procainamide: Increased serum procainamide or N-acetylprocainamide level
quinidine: Increased serum quinidine level with risk of life-threatening arrhythmias
ritonavir: Increased serum amiodarone level with increased risk of cardiotoxicity
theophylline: Increased serum theophylline level with increased risk of theophylline toxicity

Adverse Reactions
CNS: Abnormal gait, ataxia, dizziness, fatigue, headache, insomnia, involuntary motor activity, lack of coordination, malaise, paresthesia, peripheral neuropathy, sleep disturbances, tremor
CV: Arrhythmias (including bradycardia, electromechanical dissociation, and ventricular tachycardia), cardiac arrest, cardiogenic shock, edema, heart failure, hypotension, vasculitis
EENT: Abnormal salivation, abnormal taste and smell, blurred vision, corneal microdeposits, dry eyes, halo vision, lens opacities, macular degeneration, optic neuritis, optic neuropathy, papilledema, permanent blindness, photophobia, scotoma
ENDO: Hyperthyroidism, hypothyroidism
GI: Abdominal pain, anorexia, constipation, diarrhea, elevated liver function test results, hepatitis, nausea, vomiting
GU: Decreased libido, epididymitis
HEME: Coagulation abnormalities, spontaneous bruising, thrombocytopenia
RESP: Acute respiratory distress syndrome; infiltrates that lead to dyspnea, cough, pulmonary fibrosis, pulmonary intersitital pneumonitis, crackles, and wheezing; pneumonia

SKIN: Alopecia, bluish gray pigmentation, flushing, photosensitivity, rash
Other: Angioedema

Nursing Considerations
•**WARNING** Be aware that amiodarone is sometimes used to treat ventricular arrhythmias in children. However, this is not an FDA-approved use and may lead to serious or life-threatening adverse reactions. Infusing amiodarone, especially at high concentrations and low flow rates, may allow plasticizers, such as di-(2-ethylhexyl) phthalate (DEHP), to leach out of the the I.V. tubing and adversely affect reproductive tract development in male infants and toddlers. Also, because amiodarone I.V. contains benzyl alcohol, it may cause a fatal gasping syndrome; monitor neonates for gasping respirations, hypotension, bradycardia, and shock.
•Monitor vital signs frequently during amiodarone treatment. Keep emergency equipment and drugs nearby.
•Monitor continuous ECG tracings and check for increased PR and QRS intervals, increased arrhythmias, and heart rate below 60 beats/min.
•Monitor serum amiodarone level, which normally ranges from 1.0 to 2.5 mcg/ml.
•Monitor liver enzyme and thyroid hormone levels. Be aware that amiodarone inhibits conversion of T_4 to T_3.
PATIENT TEACHING
•Inform patient that frequent monitoring and laboratory tests will be needed during treatment.
•Advise patient to report swollen hands and feet and signs of respiratory problems, such as wheezing, dyspnea, and cough.
•Instruct patient to report abnormal bleeding or bruising.

amitriptyline hydrochloride
Apo-amitriptyline (CAN), Elavil, Endep, Levate (CAN), Novotriptyn (CAN)

Class and Category
Chemical: Tertiary amine
Therapeutic: Tricyclic antidepressant
Pregnancy category: D

Indications and Dosages
➤ *To relieve depression, especially when accompanied by anxiety and insomnia*

TABLETS

Adults and children over age 12. *Outpatient:* 75 mg/day in divided doses, increased to 150 mg/day, if needed. *Inpatient:* 100 mg/day, gradually increased to 300 mg/day, if needed. *Maintenance:* 40 to 100 mg/day h.s.

DOSAGE ADJUSTMENT Maintenance dosage reduced to 10 mg t.i.d. plus 20 mg h.s. for adolescent and elderly patients.

I.M INJECTION

Adults and children over age 12. *Initial:* 20 to 30 mg q.i.d. Therapy should change to oral form as soon as possible.

Route	Onset	Peak	Duration
P.O.	14 to 21 days	Unknown	Unknown

Contraindications

During acute recovery phase after MI, hypersensitivity to amitriptyline, MAO inhibitor therapy within 14 days

Interactions

DRUGS

anticholinergics, epinephrine, norepinephrine: Increased effects of these drugs
barbiturates: Decreased serum amitriptyline level
carbamazepine: Decreased serum amitriptyline level and increased serum carbamazepine level, which increases therapeutic and toxic effects of carbamazepine
cimetidine, disulfiram, fluoxetine, fluvoxamine, haloperidol, H_2-receptor antagonists, methylphenidate, oral contraceptives, paroxetine, phenothiazines, sertraline: Increased serum amitriptyline level
cisapride: Possibly prolonged QT interval and increased risk for arrhythmias
clonidine, guanethidine, and other antihypertensives: Decreased antihypertensive effects
dicumarol: Increased anticoagulant effect of dicumarol
levodopa: Decreased levodopa absorption; sympathetic hyperactivity, sinus tachycardia, hypertension, agitation
MAO inhibitors: Possibly seizures and death
thyroid replacement drugs: Arrhythmias and increased antidepressant effects

ACTIVITIES

alcohol use: Enhanced CNS depression
smoking: Decreased amitriptyline effects

Mechanism of Action

Normally, when an impulse reaches adrenergic nerves, the nerves release serotonin and norepinephrine from their storage sites. Some serotonin and norepinephrine reaches receptor sites on target tissues. Most is taken back into the nerves and stored by the reuptake mechanism, as shown below.

Amitriptyline blocks serotonin and norepinephrine reuptake by adrenergic nerves. By doing so, it raises serotonin and norepinephrine levels at nerve synapses, as shown below. This action may elevate mood and reduce depression.

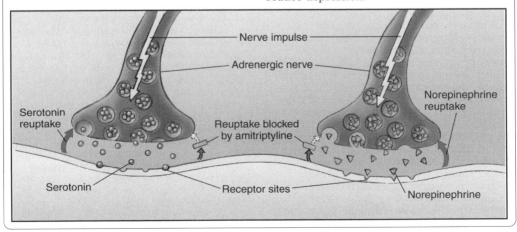

Adverse Reactions
CNS: Anxiety, ataxia, coma, chills, delusions, disorientation, drowsiness, extrapyramidal reactions, fatigue, fever, headache, insomnia, nightmares, peripheral neuropathy, tremor
CV: Arrhythmias (including prolonged AV conduction, heart block, and tachycardia), hypertension, MI, nonspecific ECG changes, orthostatic hypotension, palpitations
EENT: Abnormal taste, black tongue, blurred vision, dry mouth, increased salivation, nasal congestion, tinnitus
ENDO: Gynecomastia, increased or decreased blood glucose level, increased prolactin level, syndrome of inappropriate ADH secretion
GI: Abdominal cramps, constipation, diarrhea, flatulence, ileus, increased appetite, nausea, vomiting
GU: Impotence, libido changes, menstrual irregularities, testicular swelling, urinary hesitancy, urine retention
HEME: Agranulocytosis, bone marrow depression, eosinophilia, leukopenia, thrombocytopenia
SKIN: Alopecia, flushing, purpura
Other: Weight gain

Nursing Considerations
•Because of amitriptyline's atropine-like effects, use it cautiously in patients with a history of seizures, urine retention, or angle-closure glaucoma.
•**WARNING** Don't give an MAO inhibitor within 14 days of amitriptyline therapy because of the risk of seizures and death.
•Closely monitor patient with cardiovascular disorder because amitriptyline may cause arrhythmias, such as sinus tachycardia.
•Monitor blood pressure and assess patient for hypotension or hypertension.
•Stay alert for behavior changes, such as decreased interest in personal appearance and obvious hallucinations. Be aware that schizophrenic patients may develop psychosis, and paranoid patients may develop increased symptoms.
•Avoid abrupt withdrawal of amitriptyline after prolonged therapy; otherwise, nausea, headache, vertigo, and nightmares may occur.
PATIENT TEACHING
•Instruct patient to take amitriptyline at bedtime to avoid daytime drowsiness.
•Instruct patient to avoid using alcohol or OTC drugs that contain alcohol during ami-

triptyline therapy because alcohol enhances CNS depressant effects.

amlodipine besylate
Norvasc

Class and Category
Chemical: Dihydropyridine
Therapeutic: Antianginal, antihypertensive
Pregnancy category: C

Indications and Dosages
➤ *To control hypertension*
TABLETS
Adults. *Initial:* 5 mg/day, increased gradually over 10 to 14 days p.r.n. *Maximum:* 10 mg/day.
DOSAGE ADJUSTMENT Initial dosage of 2.5 mg/day for elderly patients or patients with impaired hepatic function. Dosage increased gradually over 7 to 14 days based on response.

➤ *To treat chronic stable angina and Prinzmetal's (variant) angina*
TABLETS
Adults. 5 to 10 mg/day.
DOSAGE ADJUSTMENT 5 mg/day only for elderly patients and patients with impaired hepatic function.

Route	Onset	Peak	Duration
P.O.	Unknown	Unknown	24 hr

Mechanism of Action
Binds to dihydropyridine and nondihydropyridine cell membrane receptor sites on myocardial and vascular smooth-muscle cells and inhibits the influx of extracellular calcium ions across the slow calcium channels of these cells. This decreases the intracellular calcium level, which inhibits smooth-muscle cell contractions and causes relaxation of coronary and vascular smooth muscles, decreased peripheral vascular resistance, and reduced systolic and diastolic blood pressure. Decreased peripheral vascular resistance also decreases the workload of the myocardium and myocardial oxygen demand, which may relieve angina. Also, by inhibiting coronary artery muscle cell contractions and restoring blood flow, amlodipine may relieve Prinzmetal's angina.

Contraindications
Hypersensitivity to amlodipine or its components

Interactions
DRUGS
beta blockers: Possibly excessive hypotension
fentanyl: Increased risk of severe hypotension and increased fluid volume requirements during surgery

Adverse Reactions
CNS: Anxiety, dizziness, fatigue, headache, lethargy, light-headedness, paresthesia, somnolence, syncope, tremor
CV: Arrhythmias, hot flashes, hypotension, palpitations, peripheral edema
EENT: Dry mouth, pharyngitis
GI: Abdominal cramps, abdominal pain, constipation, diarrhea, esophagitis, indigestion, nausea
GU: Decreased libido, impotence, urinary frequency
MS: Myalgia
RESP: Dyspnea
SKIN: Dermatitis, flushing, rash
Other: Weight loss

Nursing Considerations
• Use amlodipine cautiously in patients with heart block, heart failure, impaired renal function, or hepatic disorder.
• Monitor blood pressure while titrating amlodipine, especially in patients with heart failure.
PATIENT TEACHING
• Instruct patient to take missed dose as soon as it's remembered and take next dose in 24 hours.
• Tell patient to immediately notify prescriber of dizziness, arm or leg swelling, difficulty breathing, hives, or rash.
• Suggest taking amlodipine with food to reduce GI upset.
• Advise patient to routinely have his blood pressure checked to monitor for hypotension.

ammonium chloride

Class and Category
Chemical: Ammonium ion
Therapeutic: Acidifier
Pregnancy category: C

Indications and Dosages
➤ *To treat hypochloremia and metabolic alkalosis*

I.V. INFUSION
Adults. Individualized, based on serum bicarbonate level. *Usual:* 100 to 200 mEq added to 500 or 1,000 ml of NS, infused at 5 ml/min or less (about 3 hr for an infusion of 1,000 ml).

Route	Onset	Peak	Duration
I.V.	1 to 3 min	3 to 6 hr	Unknown

Mechanism of Action
Is converted to urea and hydrochloric acid in the liver. During the conversion, the drug is dissociated into ammonium and chloride ions, and hydrogen ions are released. These ions enter the blood and extracellular fluid, where hydrogen reacts with bicarbonate ions to form water and carbon dioxide. This process decreases bicarbonate ions and increases chloride ions in the blood and extracellular fluid, which decreases blood and urine pH and corrects alkalosis.

Incompatibilities
Don't mix I.V. ammonium chloride with codeine, levorphanol, or methadone.

Contraindications
Hypersensitivity to ammonium chloride or its components, markedly impaired renal or hepatic function, metabolic alkalosis caused by vomiting of hydrochloric acid and accompanied by sodium loss caused by sodium bicarbonate excretion in urine

Interactions
DRUGS
amphetamines, salicylates, sulfonylureas, tricyclic antidepressants: Decreased therapeutic blood level of ammonium
chlorpropamide: Increased effects of ammonium

Adverse Reactions
CNS: Fever, headache
CV: Phlebitis or thrombosis extending from injection site
GI: Indigestion, nausea, severe hepatic dysfunction, vomiting
RESP: Hyperventilation
SKIN: Extravasation
Other: Injection site infection, irritation, or pain; hypovolemia; severe metabolic acidosis (with large doses)

Nursing Considerations
•Before use, warm ammonium chloride solution to room temperature to dissolve crystals by placing infusion in warm water.
•During I.V. administration, keep sodium bicarbonate or sodium lactate nearby to treat overdose.
•Infuse ammonium chloride slowly to avoid I.V. site pain and irritation.
•WARNING Monitor for signs and symptoms of ammonia toxicity, including arrhythmias, such as bradycardia; coma; irregular breathing; pallor; retching; seizures; diaphoresis; and twitching.
•Monitor for signs of metabolic acidosis, such as increased respirations, increased serum pH, restlessness, and diaphoresis.
•Monitor serum bicarbonate level and results of urinalysis and renal and liver function tests as appropriate.

PATIENT TEACHING
•Tell patient to consume more potassium-rich food, such as bananas, oranges, cantaloupe, spinach, dried fruit, and potatoes, during ammonium chloride therapy.

amobarbital sodium
Amytal, Novamobarb (CAN)

Class, Category, and Schedule
Chemical: Barbiturate
Therapeutic: Anticonvulsant, sedative-hypnotic
Pregnancy category: D
Controlled substance: Schedule II

Indications and Dosages
➤ *To produce preanesthesia sedation*
CAPSULES, ELIXIR, TABLETS
Adults. 200 mg 1 to 2 hr before surgery.
Children. 2 to 6 mg/kg up to a maximum of 100 mg/dose.

➤ *To produce sedation*
CAPSULES, ELIXIR, TABLETS, I.V. OR I.M. INJECTION
Adults. 30 to 50 mg b.i.d. or t.i.d. and may range from 15 to 120 mg b.i.d or t.i.d. *Maximum I.V.:* 1,000 mg/dose. *Maximum I.M.:* 500 mg/dose.
Children over age 6. 2 mg/kg/day in four divided doses.

➤ *To treat insomnia*
CAPSULES, ELIXIR, TABLETS
Adults. 65 to 200 mg h.s. for up to 2 wk.

➤ *To induce a hypnotic state*
CAPSULES, ELIXIR, TABLETS, I.V. OR I.M. INJECTION
Adults. 65 to 200 mg/dose. *Maximum I.V.:* 1,000 mg/dose. *Maximum I.M.:* 500 mg/dose.
Children up to age 6. 2 to 3 mg/kg I.M. per dose.
➤ *To manage seizures*
I.V. OR I.M. INJECTION
Adults. *Usual:* 65 to 500 mg up to a maximum of 1,000 mg. The dosage for acute seizures is determined by response. Doses of 200 to 500 mg are typically required to control seizures.
Children age 6 and older. 65 to 500 mg I.V.
Children up to age 6. 3 to 5 mg/kg/dose.
WARNING Use I.V. route only when other routes aren't appropriate. For I.V. injection, use I.M. dose and inject slowly at a rate of 50 mg/min or less to prevent sudden respiratory depression, apnea, laryngospasm, or hypotension.

Route	Onset	Peak	Duration
P.O.*	60 min	Unknown	10 to 12 hr
I.V.	Unknown	Unknown	10 to 12 hr
I.M.	Unknown	Unknown	10 to 12 hr

Mechanism of Action
Nonselectively acts on the CNS to depress the sensory cortex, decrease motor activity, alter cerebellar function, and produce drowsiness, sedation, and hypnosis. Appears to reduce wakefulness and alertness by acting in the thalamus, where it depresses the reticular activating system and interferes with impulse transmission from the periphery to the cortex. Produces CNS depressant effects ranging from mild sedation and anxiety reduction to anesthesia and coma, depending on the dose, route, and individual patient's response.

Incompatibilities
Don't mix amobarbital in solution with other drugs.

Contraindications
Alcoholism, history of porphyria, history of sedative or barbiturate addiction, hypersensitivity to barbiturates, renal or hepatic dis-

_____
* For capsules, elixir, and tablets.

ease, severe respiratory disease, sleep apnea, suicidal tendency, uncontrolled pain

Interactions
DRUGS
acetaminophen: Increased blood acetaminophen level and risk of hepatotoxicity
antihistamines, CNS depressants, phenothiazines, tranquilizers: Increased CNS depression
beta blockers, carbamazepine, clonazepam, corticosteroids, digitoxin, doxycycline, estrogens, griseofulvin, metronidazole, oral anticoagulants, oral contraceptives, phenylbutazones, quinidine, theophyllines, tricyclic antidepressants: Decreased blood levels and effects of these drugs
chloramphenicol: Inhibited amobarbital metabolism; enhanced chloramphenicol metabolism
MAO inhibitors: Increased serum level and sedative effects of amobarbital
methoxyflurane: Increased nephrotoxicity
phenytoin: Altered effects of phenytoin
rifampin: Decreased serum level and effects of amobarbital
valproic acid: Increased amobarbital effects
ACTIVITIES
alcohol use: Increased serum level of amobarbital and additive CNS depressant effects

Adverse Reactions
CNS: Agitation, anxiety, ataxia, CNS depression, confusion, dizziness, hallucinations, hangover, headache, hyperkinesia, insomnia, nightmares, nervousness, paradoxical stimulation, permanent neurologic deficit (with injection near nerve), psychiatric disturbance, somnolence, syncope, vertigo
CV: Bradycardia, hypotension, shock
EENT: Laryngospasm
GI: Constipation, diarrhea, epigastric pain, nausea, vomiting
RESP: Apnea, bronchospasm, hypoventilation, respiratory depression
SKIN: Exfoliative dermatitis, rash, Stevens-Johnson syndrome, urticaria
Other: Angioedema, gangrene of arm or leg from accidental injection into artery, injection site tissue damage and necrosis, physical and psychological dependence, potentially fatal withdrawal syndrome, tolerance

Nursing Considerations
•Use amobarbital cautiously in patients with cardiac disease, debilitation, diabetes mellitus, fever, hyperthyroidism, severe anemia, shock, status asthmaticus, or uremia.

•Administer by deep I.M. injection, preferably in large muscle.
•During I.V. administration, closely monitor blood pressure, pulse, and respirations. Keep emergency equipment and drugs nearby in case respiratory depression occurs.
•**WARNING** Don't administer solution after 30 minutes of exposure to air. Solution quickly becomes unstable because amobarbital sodium hydrolyzes in solution.
•To prevent withdrawal symptoms, such as diaphoresis, insomnia, irritability, nightmares, and tremors, expect to taper amobarbital dosage gradually after long-term use, especially for epileptic patients.
•**WARNING** To prevent tissue damage and necrosis at I.M. injection site, don't administer more than 5 ml of this highly alkaline drug at any one site. Know that accidental arterial injection may cause gangrene of the arm or leg.
PATIENT TEACHING
•Advise patient to use caution when driving or performing tasks that require alertness.
•Instruct patient not to use alcohol or other CNS depressants (unless prescribed) because they increase amobarbital's effects.
•Warn patient not to stop taking drug abruptly because withdrawal symptoms can occur.
•Instruct patient to report severe dizziness, persistent drowsiness, rash, or skin lesions.
•Advise patient that amobarbital's effects, such as drowsiness, may become less pronounced after a few days and when drug is taken with food.

amoxapine
Asendin

Class and Category
Chemical: Dibenzoxazepine derivative
Therapeutic: Tricyclic antidepressant
Pregnancy category: C

Indications and Dosages
➤ *To relieve depression, including endogenous (long-term) depression and depression associated with anxiety and agitation*
TABLETS
Adults and children age 16 and older. *Initial:* 50 mg b.i.d. or t.i.d., increased to 100 mg

b.i.d. or t.i.d. by end of first wk, if tolerated. *Maintenance:* If 300-mg daily dose is ineffective after 2-wk trial period, dosage increased to a maximum of 400 mg/day in divided doses. Inpatients may receive up to a maximum of 600 mg/day in divided doses. When effective dose is achieved, a single dose may be given h.s., not to exceed 300 mg.

DOSAGE ADJUSTMENT For elderly patients: *Initial:* 25 mg b.i.d. or t.i.d., increased to 50 mg b.i.d. or t.i.d. by end of first wk. *Maintenance:* 100 to 150 mg/day in divided doses, carefully increased to 300 mg/day as tolerated. When effective dose is achieved, a single dose may be given h.s., not to exceed 300 mg.

Route	Onset	Peak	Duration
P.O.	2 to 3 wk	Unknown	Unknown

Mechanism of Action

Blocks serotonin and norepinephrine reuptake by adrenergic nerves. By doing this, it raises serotonin and norepinephrine levels at nerve synapses. This action may elevate mood and reduce depression.

Normally, when an impulse reaches adrenergic nerves, they release serotonin and norepinephrine from their storage sites. Some serotonin and norepinephrine reach receptor sites on target tissues. The majority is taken back into the nerves and stored by the reuptake mechanism.

Contraindications

Acute recovery phase after MI, hypersensitivity to amoxapine or its components, MAO inhibitor therapy within 14 days

Interactions

DRUGS

anticholinergics, epinephrine, norepinephrine: Increased effects of these drugs
barbiturates: Decreased serum amoxapine level
carbamazepine: Decreased serum amoxapine level; increased serum carbamazepine level, increasing its therapeutic and toxic effects
cimetidine, disulfiram, fluoxetine, fluvoxamine, haloperidol, H₂-receptor antagonists, methylphenidate, oral contraceptives, paroxetine, phenothiazines, sertraline: Increased serum amoxapine level

clonidine, guanethidine, other antihypertensives: Decreased antihypertensive effects
dicumarol: Increased anticoagulant effect of dicumarol
levodopa: Decreased levodopa absorption; agitation, hypertension, sinus tachycardia, sympathetic hyperactivity
MAO inhibitors: Possibly seizures and death
thyroid replacement drugs: Arrhythmias and increased antidepressant effects

ACTIVITIES

alcohol use: Increased CNS depression
smoking: Decreased amoxapine effects

Adverse Reactions

CNS: Agitation, anxiety, ataxia, chills, confusion, CVA, dizziness, drowsiness, excitement, extrapyramidal reactions, fatigue, fever, headache, insomnia, nervousness, nightmares, paresthesia, restlessness, sedation, seizures, syncope, tremor, weakness
CV: Atrial arrhythmias, heart block, heart failure, hypertension, hypotension, MI, palpitations, tachycardia
EENT: Blurred vision, dry mouth, increased salivation, nasal congestion, taste perversion, tinnitus
ENDO: Altered blood glucose level, elevated prolactin level, gynecomastia, syndrome of inappropriate ADH secretion
GI: Anorexia, constipation, diarrhea, elevated liver function test results, excessive appetite, flatulence, nausea, vomiting
GU: Impotence, libido changes, menstrual irregularities, testicular swelling, urinary hesitancy, urine retention
HEME: Agranulocytosis, leukopenia
SKIN: Diaphoresis, flushing, photosensitivity, pruritus, rash
Other: Weight gain or loss; withdrawal symptoms, such as headache, nausea, nightmares, and vertigo

Nursing Considerations

•WARNING Don't administer MAO inhibitors within 14 days of amoxapine therapy.
•Don't discontinue drug abruptly; otherwise, withdrawal symptoms can occur.

PATIENT TEACHING

•Advise patient to take amoxapine at bedtime if daytime sedation occurs.
•Instruct patient not to stop taking drug abruptly because withdrawal symptoms can occur.

- Encourage patient to avoid alcohol because it can potentiate amoxapine's effects.
- Tell patient to report dry mouth, difficulty urinating, palpitations, nausea, or dizziness.
- Instruct patient to take drug with food to prevent GI upset.
- Warn patient to avoid driving and other tasks that require alertness until the drug's effects are known.

amoxicillin and clavulanate potassium

Augmentin, Augmentin ES, Clavulin (CAN)

Class and Category

Chemical: Aminopenicillin, beta-lactamase inhibitor
Therapeutic: Antibiotic
Pregnancy category: B

Indications and Dosages

➤ *To treat otitis media, sinusitis, skin and soft-tissue infections, and UTIs caused by susceptible strains of gram-positive and gram-negative organisms*

ORAL SUSPENSION, TABLETS

Adults and children who weigh 40 kg (88 lb) or more. 500 mg q 12 hr or 250 mg q 8 hr.
Children age 12 wk and older who weigh less than 40 kg. 25 mg/kg/day in divided doses q 12 hr or 20 mg/kg/day in divided doses q 8 hr.
Children under age 12 wk. 30 mg/kg/day q 12 hr.

➤ *To treat respiratory tract infections and severe otitis media and sinusitis caused by susceptible strains of gram-positive and gram-negative organisms*

CHEWABLE TABLETS, ORAL SUSPENSION, TABLETS

Adults and children who weigh 40 kg or more. 875 mg q 12 hr or 500 mg q 8 hr.
Children age 12 wk and older who weigh less than 40 kg. 45 mg/kg/day in divided doses q 12 hr or 40 mg/kg q 8 hr.
Children under age 12 wk. 30 mg/kg/day in divided doses q 12 hr.

DOSAGE ADJUSTMENT For patients with renal failure and a GFR of 10 to 30 ml/min, dosage reduced to 250 or 500 mg q 12 hr, depending on the severity of the infection. For patients with a GFR less than 10 ml/min, dosage reduced to 250 to 500 mg q 24 hr, depending on the severity of the infection. For hemodialysis patients, dosage reduced to 250 or 500 mg q 24 hr with an additional dose provided during and at the end of dialysis.

➤ *To treat acute otitis media caused by beta-lactamase–producing strains of* Haemophilus influenzae, Moraxella catarrhalis, *and* Streptococcus pneumoniae *(including penicillin-resistant strains)*

EXTRA-STRENGTH ORAL SUSPENSION

Children. 90 mg/kg/day in divided doses b.i.d. for 10 days.

Route	Onset	Peak	Duration
P.O.	Unknown	Unknown	6 to 8 hr

Mechanism of Action

Kills bacteria by binding to and inactivating penicillin-binding proteins on the inner membrane of bacterial cell walls. Penicillin-binding proteins play a role in bacterial cell wall synthesis and cell division. When this type of penicillin binds to proteins, it weakens bacterial cell walls and causes lysis. Clavulanic acid inactivates bacterial beta-lactamase enzymes, thus protecting amoxicillin from degradation by these enzymes. This makes the drug effective against many bacteria that normally are resistant to amoxicillin.

Contraindications

History of amoxicillin and clavulanate–induced cholestatic jaundice or hepatic dysfunction; hypersensitivity to amoxicillin and clavulanate, its components, or penicillin; phenylketonuria (chewable tablets)

Interactions

DRUGS

aminoglycosides: Possibly inactivation of both drugs
chloramphenicol, erythromycins, sulfonamides, tetracyclines: Reduced bactericidal effect of amoxicillin
heparin, oral anticoagulants: Possibly increased risk of bleeding with large doses of amoxicillin and clavulanate
methotrexate: Increased risk of methotrexate toxicity
oral contraceptives with estrogen: Possibly reduced effectiveness of contraceptive
probenecid: Increased amoxicillin effects

Adverse Reactions
CNS: Agitation, anxiety, behavioral changes, confusion, dizziness, drowsiness, headache, insomnia, reversible hyperactivity
EENT: Black "hairy" tongue, glossitis, muco-cutaneous candidiasis, stomatitis
GI: Diarrhea, enterocolitis, gastritis, hemorrhagic pseudomembranous colitis, indigestion, nausea, vomiting
GU: Hematuria, interstitial nephritis, vaginal candidiasis
HEME: Agranulocytosis, anemia, eosinophilia, leukopenia, neutropenia, thrombocytopenia, thrombocytopenic purpura
SKIN: Erythema multiforme, exfoliative dermatitis, pruritus, rash, Stevens-Johnson syndrome, urticaria
Other: Allergic reaction, anaphylaxis, angioedema, serum sickness–like reaction (urticaria or rash, arthritis, arthralgia, myalgia, and fever)

Nursing Considerations
•For children under age 12 weeks, expect to use 125-mg/5-ml amoxicillin and clavulanate suspension because experience with 200-mg/5-ml suspension is limited.
•**WARNING** If allergic reaction occurs, discontinue drug immediately. Be prepared to give antihistamines and I.V. corticosteroids, as prescribed. If anaphylaxis occurs, expect to give epinephrine, oxygen, and I.V. corticosteroids immediately and to maintain a patent airway.
•Monitor patient closely for diarrhea, which may indicate pseudomembranous colitis. If diarrhea occurs, notify prescriber and expect to withhold amoxicillin and clavulanate. Expect to treat pseudomembranous colitis with fluids, electrolytes, protein, and an antibiotic effective against *Clostridium difficile.*
•Be aware that Augmentin 250-mg regular tablets should not be substituted for chewable tablets because they contain different amounts of clavulanic acid.
•For a child under 40 kg, expect to use 250-mg chewable tablets because the ratio of amoxicillin to clavulanic acid differs from that of Augmentin 250-mg regular tablets.
PATIENT TEACHING
•Tell patient to take amoxicillin/clavulanate with food to reduce GI upset.
•Instruct patient to refrigerate reconstituted suspension.

•Tell patient to chew or crush chewable tablets and not to swallow them whole.
•Teach patient to recognize and report adverse reactions and to seek emergency care if signs of anaphylaxis occur.
•Tell patient to notify prescriber if signs of infection worsen or don't improve after 72 hours of therapy.

amoxicillin trihydrate (amoxycillin)

Amoxil, Apo-Amoxi (CAN), Novamoxin (CAN), Nu-Amoxi (CAN), Polymox, Trimox, Wymox

Class and Category
Chemical: Aminopenicillin
Therapeutic: Antibiotic
Pregnancy category: B

Indications and Dosages
➤ *To treat ear, nose, throat, GU tract, skin, and soft-tissue infections caused by susceptible strains of gram-positive and gram-negative organisms*
CAPSULES, ORAL SUSPENSION, POWDER FOR RECONSTITUTION, TABLETS
Adults and children who weigh 20 kg (44 lb) or more. 250 mg q 8 hr; for severe infections, 500 mg q 8 hr or 875 mg q 12 hr.
Children who weigh less than 20 kg. 20 mg/kg/day in divided doses q 8 hr; for severe infections, 40 to 45 mg/kg/day in divided doses q 8 hr.
➤ *To treat lower respiratory tract infections caused by susceptible strains of gram-positive and gram-negative organisms*
CAPSULES, ORAL SUSPENSION, POWDER FOR RECONSTITUTION, TABLETS
Adults and children who weigh 20 kg or more. 875 mg q 12 hr; for severe infections, 500 mg q 8 hr.
Children who weigh less than 20 kg. 40 to 45 mg/kg/day in divided doses q 8 hr.
➤ *To treat gonorrhea and acute uncomplicated anogenital and urethral infections caused by susceptible strains of gram-positive and gram-negative organisms*
CAPSULES, ORAL SUSPENSION, POWDER FOR RECONSTITUTION, TABLETS
Adults and postpubertal children. 3 g as a single dose.

Prepubertal children age 2 and older. 50 mg/kg of amoxicillin plus 25 mg/kg of probenecid as a single dose.

➤ *To prevent bacterial endocarditis before dental, oral, or upper respiratory tract procedures*

CAPSULES, ORAL SUSPENSION, POWDER FOR RECONSTITUTION, TABLETS

Adults and children who weigh 20 kg or more. 2 g 1 hr before procedure.
Children who weigh less than 20 kg. 50 mg/kg 1 hr before procedure.

Route	Onset	Peak	Duration
P.O.	Unknown	Unknown	6 to 8 hr

Mechanism of Action

Kills bacteria by binding to and inactivating penicillin-binding proteins on the inner membrane of bacterial cell walls. Penicillin-binding proteins play a role in bacterial cell wall synthesis and cell division. When this type of penicillin binds to these proteins, it weakens bacterial cell walls and causes lysis.

Contraindications

Hypersensitivity to amoxicillin, its components, or penicillin

Interactions

DRUGS
chloramphenicol, erythromycins, sulfonamides, tetracyclines: Reduced bactericidal effect of amoxicillin
methotrexate: Increased risk of methotrexate toxicity
oral contraceptives with estrogen: Possibly reduced effectiveness of contraceptive
probenecid: Increased amoxicillin effects

Adverse Reactions

CNS: Agitation, anxiety, behavior changes, confusion, dizziness, insomnia, reversible hyperactivity, seizures
GI: Diarrhea, nausea, vomiting
HEME: Anemia, eosinophilia, granulocytosis, leukopenia, thrombocytopenia, thrombocytopenic purpura
SKIN: Erythema multiforme, erythematous maculopapular rash, Stevens-Johnson syndrome, toxic epidermal necrolysis, urticaria
Other: Allergic reaction, anaphylaxis

Nursing Considerations

• Use amoxicillin cautiously in patients with infectious mononucleosis and patients who are breast-feeding.
• **WARNING** If allergic reaction occurs, discontinue amoxicillin immediately. Be prepared to treat patient with antihistamines and I.V. corticosteroids, as prescribed. If anaphylaxis occurs, plan to administer epinephrine, oxygen, and I.V. corticosteroids immediately and to maintain a patent airway.
• Monitor closely for diarrhea, which may indicate pseudomembranous colitis. If diarrhea occurs, notify prescriber and expect to withhold amoxicillin. Expect to treat pseudomembranous colitis by discontinuing amoxicillin and administering fluids, electrolytes, protein, and an antibiotic that's effective against *Clostridium difficile*.
• Expect to initiate therapy before culture and sensitivity test results are known.
• For stubborn or severe infections, expect to administer a higher amoxicillin dosage for up to several weeks.
• To prevent acute rheumatic fever or glomerulonephritis, expect treatment to last at least 10 days for infections caused by hemolytic streptococci.

PATIENT TEACHING
• Tell patient that amoxicillin may be taken without regard to food.
• When amoxicillin suspension is prescribed for a child, instruct parents to place it directly on child's tongue to swallow. If this doesn't work, tell parents to mix dose of suspension with formula, milk, fruit juice, ginger ale, water, or cold drink and then have child drink all of it immediately.
• Instruct patient to refrigerate reconstituted suspension.
• Tell patient to shake amoxicillin suspension well before each dose.
• To prevent infection from recurring, urge patient to take amoxicillin for full length of time prescribed even if he feels better.
• Tell patient to chew or crush chewable amoxicillin tablets and not to swallow them whole.
• Teach patient to recognize and report adverse reactions and to seek emergency care if signs of anaphylaxis occur.
• Tell patient to notify prescriber if signs of infection worsen or don't improve after 72 hours of therapy.

amphetamine and dextroamphetamine
Adderall, Adderall XR

Class, Category, and Schedule
Chemical: Phenylisopropylamine
Therapeutic: CNS stimulant
Pregnancy category: C
Controlled substance: Schedule II

Indications and Dosages
➤ *To treat attention deficit hyperactivity disorder (ADHD)*

E.R. CAPSULES

Children age 6 and older. *Initial:* 5 or 10 mg q.d. Dosage increased by 5 or 10 mg/day q wk until desired response occurs. *Maximum:* 30 mg/day.

TABLETS

Children age 6 and older. *Initial:* 5 mg q.d. or b.i.d. Dosage increased by 5 mg/day q wk until desired response occurs. *Maximum:* 40 mg/day.

Children ages 3 to 6. *Initial:* 2.5 mg q.d. Dosage increased by 2.5 mg/day q wk until desired response occurs. *Maximum:* 40 mg/day.

➤ *To treat narcolepsy*

TABLETS

Adults and children age 12 and older. *Initial:* 10 mg q.d. Dosage increased by 10 mg/day q wk until desired response occurs. *Maximum:* 60 mg/day for adults.

Mechanism of Action
May produce its CNS stimulant effects by facilitating the release of norepinephrine at adrenergic nerve terminals and blocking its reuptake and by directly stimulating alpha and beta receptors in the peripheral nervous system. The drug also causes the release and blocks the reuptake of dopamine in limbic regions of the brain. The main action of the drug appears to be in the cerebral cortex and, possibly, the reticular activating system. Also, dextroamphetamine may stimulate inhibitory autoreceptors in the brain. These actions decrease drowsiness, fatigue, and motor restlessness and increase mental alertness. Peripheral actions include increased blood pressure, mild bronchodilation, and respiratory stimulation.

Children ages 6 to 12. *Initial:* 5 mg q.d. Dosage increased by 5 mg/day q wk until desired response occurs. *Maximum:* 40 mg/day.

Contraindications
Advanced arteriosclerosis; agitation; glaucoma; history of drug abuse; hypersensitivity to amphetamine, dextroamphetamine, or any of their components; hyperthyroidism; MAO inhibitor therapy within 14 days; moderate to severe hypertension; symptomatic CV disease

Interactions
DRUGS

anesthetics (inhaled): Increased risk of severe ventricular arrhythmias
antacids (calcium- and magnesium-containing), carbonic anhydrase inhibitors, citrates, sodium bicarbonate: Increased effects of amphetamine
antihypertensives, diuretics: Possibly decreased hypotensive effects
beta blockers: Increased risk of hypertension or excessive bradycardia, possibly heart block
CNS stimulants: Additive CNS stimulation
digoxin, levodopa: Possibly arrhythmias
ethosuximide, phenobarbital, phenytoin: Delayed intestinal absorption of these drugs
glutamic acid hydrochloride; urinary acidifiers, such as ammonium chloride and sodium acid phosphate: Increased excretion and decreased blood level and effects of amphetamine and dextroamphetamine
haloperidol, loxapine, molindone, phenothiazines, pimozide, thioxanthenes: Reduced antipsychotic effectiveness of these drugs, inhibited CNS stimulant effects of amphetamine and dextroamphetamine
MAO inhibitors: Potentiated effects of amphetamine, possibly hypertensive crisis
meperidine: Increased analgesia
metrizamide: Increased risk of seizures
norepinephrine: Possibly increased adrenergic effect of norepinephrine
propoxyphene: Increased CNS stimulation, risk of fatal seizures
sympathomimetics: Increased CV effects of both drugs
thyroid replacement drugs: Enhanced effects of both drugs
tricyclic antidepressants: Possibly increased CV effects

FOODS

ascorbic acid, fruit juices: Decreased absorption and effects of amphetamine and dextroamphetamine

A

Adverse Reactions
CNS: Depression, dizziness, drowsiness, fatigue, headache, insomnia, irritability, lightheadedness, psychoses, tremor
CV: Arrhythmias, hypertension, tachycardia
EENT: Blurred vision, dry mouth, taste perversion
GI: Abdominal pain, anorexia, constipation, diarrhea, nausea, vomiting
GU: Decreased libido
RESP: Dyspnea
SKIN: Diaphoresis
Other: Weight loss

Nursing Considerations
• Keep in mind that, when signs and symptoms of ADHD occur with acute stress reactions, treatment with amphetamines usually isn't indicated.
• **WARNING** If patient suddenly stops taking drug after long-term, high-dose therapy, assess him for withdrawal signs and symptoms, such as abdominal pain, depression, nausea, tremor, unusual fatigue, vomiting, and weakness. Anticipate restarting drug therapy and gradually tapering dosage, as prescribed.
• Monitor growth and development in children because drug may adversely affect growth.
• Administer first dose of tablet form when patient awakens and additional doses at 4- to 6-hour intervals. Administer E.R. capsule form when patient awakens.
• If patient currently takes divided doses of tablet form, know that he may be switched to E.R. capsule form at the same daily dose to be taken once in the morning.
• Assess patient for potential dependence, drug-seeking behavior, or drug tolerance. Be alert for signs and symptoms of long-term amphetamine abuse characterized by hyperactivity, irritability, marked insomnia, personality changes, and severe dermatoses.
• Assess patient with history of Tourette's syndrome or motor or vocal tics for exacerbation of these conditions during amphetamine therapy.
PATIENT TEACHING
• Advise patient to take amphetamine and dextroamphetamine with food or after a meal because anorexia may occur.
• Advise patient not to take drug with acidic fruit juice because it may decrease drug absorption.

• Tell patient or caregiver that E.R. capsules may be taken whole or opened and sprinkled on applesauce, then swallowed immediately without chewing.
• Urge patient to avoid potentially hazardous activities until he knows how drug affects him.
• Inform patient of abuse potential of drug, and stress the importance of not altering dosage unless prescribed.
• Inform parents or caregivers that child may be placed on drug-free weekend and holiday schedule, as prescribed, if signs and symptoms of ADHD are controlled.

amphetamine sulfate
Class, Category, and Schedule
Chemical: Sympathomimetic amine
Therapeutic: CNS stimulant
Pregnancy category: C
Controlled substance: Schedule II

Indications and Dosages
➤ *To treat attention deficit hyperactivity disorder (ADHD)*
TABLETS
Children age 6 and older. 5 mg q.d. or b.i.d., then increased by 5 mg/day at 1-wk intervals until desired response occurs. *Usual:* 0.1 to 0.5 mg/kg/day.
Children ages 3 to 5. 2.5 mg q.d., then increased by 2.5 mg/day at 1-wk intervals until desired response occurs. *Usual:* 0.1 to 0.5 mg/kg/day.
➤ *To treat narcolepsy*
TABLETS
Adults and children age 12 and older. *Initial:* 10 mg/day, then increased by 10 mg/day at 1-wk intervals until desired response occurs.
Children ages 6 to 12. 2.5 mg b.i.d., then increased by 5 mg/day at 1-wk intervals until desired response occurs or adult dosage is reached to a maximum of 60 mg/day.

Contraindications
Advanced arteriosclerosis, agitation (for narcolepsy treatment), glaucoma, history of drug abuse, hypersensitivity or idiosyncratic reaction to sympathomimetic amines, hyperthyroidism, MAO inhibitor therapy within 14 days, moderate to severe hypertension, symptomatic cardiovascular disease

Mechanism of Action
May produce its CNS stimulant effects by facilitating the release and blocking the reuptake of norepinephrine at the adrenergic nerve terminals and by direct stimulation of alpha and beta receptors in the peripheral nervous system. It also releases and blocks the reuptake of dopamine in limbic regions of the brain. The drug's main action appears to be in the cerebral cortex and, possibly, the reticular activating system. These actions cause decreased motor restlessness, increased alertness, and diminished drowsiness and fatigue. Its peripheral actions include increased blood pressure and mild bronchodilation and respiratory stimulation.

Interactions
DRUGS
adrenergic blockers: Inhibited adrenergic blockade
acetazolamide, alkalinizers (such as sodium bicarbonate), some thiazides: Increased blood level and effects of amphetamine
antihistamines: Possibly reduced sedation from antihistamine
antihypertensives: Possibly decreased antihypertensive effects
chlorpromazine: Inhibited CNS stimulant effects of amphetamine
ethosuximide: Possibly delayed ethosuximide absorption
GI acidifiers (such as ascorbic acid), reserpine: Decreased amphetamine absorption
guanethidine: Decreased antihypertensive effect and decreased amphetamine absorption
haloperidol: Decreased CNS stimulation
lithium carbonate: Possibly decreased anorectic and stimulant effects of amphetamine
MAO inhibitors: Potentiated effects of amphetamine; possibly hypertensive crisis
meperidine: Increased analgesia
methenamine: Increased urine excretion and decreased effects of amphetamine
norepinephrine: Possibly increased adrenergic effect of norepinephrine
phenobarbital, phenytoin: Synergistic anticonvulsant action
propoxyphene: Increased CNS stimulation, potentially fatal seizures

tricyclic antidepressants: Possibly enhanced antidepressant effects and decreased effects of amphetamine
urinary acidifiers (such as ammonium chloride and sodium acid phosphate): Increased amphetamine excretion and decreased amphetamine blood level and effects
Veratrum *alkaloids:* Decreased hypotensive effect
FOODS
acidic fruit juices: Decreased amphetamine absorption

Adverse Reactions
CNS: Anxiety, dizziness, dyskinesia, dysphoria, euphoria, exacerbation of motor and phonic tics and Tourette's syndrome, hallucinations, headache, insomnia, overstimulation, paranoia, psychotic episodes, restlessness, tremor
CV: Cardiomyopathy, hypertension, palpitations, tachycardia
EENT: Dry mouth, unpleasant taste
GI: Anorexia, constipation, diarrhea
GU: Impotence, libido changes
SKIN: Urticaria
Other: Weight loss

Nursing Considerations
•Keep in mind that when symptoms of ADHD occur with acute stress reactions, treatment with amphetamines usually isn't indicated.
•**WARNING** To prevent hypertensive crisis, don't administer amphetamine during or for up to 14 days after MAO therapy.
•Administer first dose when patient awakens and additional doses at 4- to 6-hour intervals.
•If patient experiences bothersome adverse reactions, such as insomnia and anorexia, expect to decrease dosage. To minimize insomnia, administer drug earlier in day.
•Be alert for signs of long-term amphetamine abuse, such as severe dermatoses, marked insomnia, irritability, hyperactivity, and personality changes. If patient suddenly stops drug after long-term, high-dose regimen, watch for extreme fatigue and depression.
PATIENT TEACHING
•Instruct breast-feeding patient to avoid breast-feeding during amphetamine therapy because drug is excreted in breast milk.
•Teach patient to take first dose on awakening and subsequent doses at 4- to 6-hour intervals. Tell him not to take last dose late in evening because insomnia may occur.

- Urge patient to avoid potentially hazardous activities until drug's effects are known.
- Advise patient not to take amphetamine with acidic fruit juice because it decreases drug absorption.
- Inform patient of drug's abuse potential and stress importance of not altering dosage unless prescribed.

amphotericin B

Amphocin, Fungizone Intravenous

amphotericin B cholesteryl sulfate complex

Amphotec

amphotericin B lipid complex

Abelcet

amphotericin B liposomal complex

AmBisome

Class and Category

Chemical: Amphoteric polyene macrolide
Therapeutic: Antifungal
Pregnancy category: B (I.V.); C (oral suspension)

Indications and Dosages

➤ *To treat severe fungal infections, using amphotericin B*

I.V. INFUSION

Adults and adolescents. *Initial:* 1-mg test dose in 20 ml of D_5W infused over 20 to 30 min; if test dose is tolerated, then 0.25 to 0.3 mg/kg/day prepared as a 0.1 mg/ml infusion, given over 2 to 6 hr. Increased in 5- to 10-mg increments up to 50 mg/day, based on patient tolerance and infection severity, not to exceed a total daily dose of 1.5 mg/kg. *Maximum:* 50 mg/day infused over 2 to 6 hr.
Children. *Initial:* 0.25 mg/kg/day in D_5W infused over 6 hr; then increased in 0.125- to 0.25-mg/kg increments daily or every other day as tolerated. *Maximum:* 1 mg/kg or 30 mg/m² of body surface daily.

➤ *To treat oral candidiasis, using amphotericin B*

ORAL SUSPENSION

Adults and children. 1 ml (100 mg) q.i.d. for 14 days.

➤ *To treat aspergillosis, using amphotericin B cholesteryl sulfate complex*

I.V. INFUSION

Adults and children. Test dose of 1.6 to 8.3 mg in 10 ml of D_5W infused over 15 to 30 min; if test dose is tolerated, then 3 to 4 mg/kg once daily infused at 1 mg/kg/hr.

➤ *To treat invasive amphotericin B-resistant fungal infections, using amphotericin B lipid complex*

I.V. INFUSION

Adults and children. 5 mg/kg/day infused at 2.5 mg/kg/hr.

➤ *To treat severe aspergillosis, candidiasis, or cryptococcosis, using amphotericin B liposomal complex*

I.V. INFUSION

Adults and children. 3 to 5 mg/kg/day infused over 2 hr. Infusion time may be decreased to 1 hr if tolerated or increased if patient experiences discomfort.

➤ *To treat leishmaniasis, using amphotericin B liposomal complex*

I.V. INFUSION

Immunocompetent adults and children. 3 mg/kg/day for days 1 through 5 and on days 14 and 21 infused over 2 hr. Infusion time may be decreased to 1 hr if tolerated or increased if patient experiences discomfort.
Immunocompromised adults and children. 4 mg/kg/day for days 1 through 5 and on days 10, 17, 24, 31, and 38 infused over 2 hr. Infusion time may be decreased to 1 hr if tolerated or increased if patient experiences discomfort.

➤ *To treat presumed fungal infections in patients with febrile neutropenia, using amphotericin B lipid complex*

I.V. INFUSION

Adults and children. 3 mg/kg/day infused over 2 hr. Infusion time may be decreased to 1 hr if tolerated or increased if patient experiences discomfort.

Route	Onset	Peak	Duration
I.V.	Immediate	Unknown	Unknown

Mechanism of Action

Binds to sterols in fungal cell plasma membranes, which changes membrane permeability and allows loss of potassium and small molecules from cells. This action results in cell impairment or death.

Incompatibilities
Don't reconstitute amphotericin B with diluents other than those recommended because solutions with sodium chloride or bacteriostatic agents (such as benzyl alcohol) may cause drug precipitation.

Contraindications
Hypersensitivity to amphotericin B or its components

Interactions
DRUGS
antineoplastics: Increased risk of bronchospasm, hypotension, and nephrotoxicity
corticosteroids, corticotropin: Increased risk of hypokalemia and subsequent cardiac dysfunction
cyclosporine, nephrotoxic drugs: Increased risk of nephrotoxicity
digitalis glycosides: Possibly hypokalemia and more severe digitalis toxicity
flucytosine: Possibly increased flucytosine toxicity
leukocyte transfusion: Possibly dyspnea, hypoxemia, and pulmonary infiltrates
skeletal muscle relaxants: Possibly hypokalemia and subsequent increased muscle relaxation
zidovudine: Possibly myelotoxicity and nephrotoxicity

Adverse Reactions
CNS: Fever, headache, shaking chills, tiredness, weakness
CV: Chest pain, hypotension, irregular heartbeat
EENT: Difficulty swallowing, pharyngitis
GI: Abdominal pain, anorexia, diarrhea, hepatic failure, indigestion, nausea, vomiting
GU: Decreased or increased urine output, impaired renal function
HEME: Anemia, leukopenia, thrombocytopenia, unusual bleeding or bruising
MS: Arthralgia, muscle spasms, myalgia
RESP: Apnea, dyspnea, hypoxia, pulmonary edema, tachypnea
SKIN: Flushing, jaundice, maculopapular rash, pruritus and redness especially around ears, urticaria
Other: Anaphylaxis, hypocalcemia, hypokalemia, hypomagnesemia, infusion site pain and thrombophlebitis

Nursing Considerations
•To prepare amphotericin B, add 10 ml of sterile water for injection without a bacteriostatic agent to vial containing 50 mg of amphotericin B. For I.V. infusion, dilute the solution containing 5 mg/ml to 0.1 mg/ml by adding 1 ml (5 mg) of solution to 49 ml of D_5W with a pH above 4.2.
•Before using D_5W to dilute amphotericin B solution, determine the injection's pH aseptically. If the pH is below 4.2, follow the manufacturer's instructions for buffering it.
•Because reconstituted amphotericin B is a colloidal suspension, avoid using an in-line membrane filter or use one with a mean pore diameter of more than 1 micron to prevent significant drug removal.
•To prepare amphotericin B cholesteryl sulfate complex, reconstitute it with sterile water for injection. Using a sterile syringe and a 20G needle, rapidly add 10 or 20 ml of sterile water for injection to a 50- or 100-mg vial, respectively, to obtain a solution containing 5 mg of amphotericin B per milliliter. Shake gently by hand, rotating vial until solids are dissolved; fluid may be clear or opalescent. For infusion, further dilute reconstituted solution to about 0.6 mg/ml. Don't filter the solution or use an in-line filter. Flush existing line with D_5W or use a separate line.
•To prepare amphotericin B lipid complex, shake vial gently until you see no yellow sediment. Using an 18G needle, withdraw prescribed dose from required number of vials into one or more 20-ml syringes. Replace needle with 5-micron filter needle that's supplied with each vial. Empty syringe contents into bag of D_5W so that final concentration is 1 mg/ml. Expect to use a concentration of 2 mg/ml for children and patients with cardiovascular disease. Before infusion, shake bag until contents are mixed thoroughly. Flush existing line with D_5W or use a separate line. Don't use an in-line filter. If infusion exceeds 2 hours, shake infusion bag every 2 hours.
•To prepare amphotericin B liposomal complex, add 12 ml of sterile water for injection (without a bacteriostatic agent) to each 50-mg vial to achieve a concentration of 4 mg amphotericin B per milliliter. Immediately shake vial vigorously for at least

A

30 seconds until all particles completely disperse. Withdraw prescribed dose of amphotericin B liposomal complex suspension. Then use a 5-micron filter to inject it into D_5W to provide a final concentration of 1 to 2 mg/ml. Expect to use a lower concentration (0.2 to 0.5 mg/ml) for infants and young children. Flush existing line with D_5W or use a separate line. You may use an in-line filter with a mean pore diameter of at least 1 micron.

• To help minimize fever and shaking chills, expect to administer an antipyretic, antihistamine, meperidine, or corticosteroid just before infusing amphotericin B.

• Before administering amphotericin B oral suspension, shake bottle well. Drop suspension directly on tongue with calibrated dropper. Then direct patient to swish suspension in mouth for as long as possible before swallowing. If drug must be swabbed on, use a nonabsorbent swab.

• Administer amphotericin B oral suspension between meals to permit prolonged contact with oral lesions.

• Assess I.V. insertion site regularly to detect extravasation of amphotericin B, which may cause severe local irritation. To minimize local thrombophlebitis, plan to add heparin to infusion or expect to administer amphotericin on alternate days, which also may help prevent anorexia. Alternate-day dose shouldn't exceed 1.5 mg/kg.

• Monitor renal function because of the risk of renal impairment. Plan to obtain serum creatinine level every other day while amphotericin B dosage is increasing and then at least twice weekly during therapy. If serum creatinine or BUN level increases significantly, expect to discontinue amphotericin B until renal function improves. Know that a cumulative dose of more than 4 g may cause irreversible renal dysfunction.

• Expect to monitor CBC and platelet count weekly throughout therapy to detect adverse hematologic effects. Also monitor serum calcium, magnesium, and potassium levels twice weekly to detect abnormalities.

• Use reconstituted amphotericin B within 24 hours if stored at room temperature or within 1 week if refrigerated. Use reconstituted amphotericin B cholesteryl sulfate

complex within 24 hours. Use amphotericin B lipid complex within 6 hours if stored at room temperature or within 48 hours if refrigerated. Use diluted amphotericin B liposomal complex within 24 hours if refrigerated, but begin infusion within 6 hours.

• Because reconstituted amphotericin B is a colloidal suspension, avoid using an in-line membrane filter or use one with a mean pore diameter of more than 1 micron to prevent significant drug removal.

PATIENT TEACHING
• Instruct patient to shake bottle of oral suspension well before each dose; to drop suspension directly on his tongue, using calibrated dropper; and then to swish suspension in his mouth for as long as possible before swallowing. If prescriber orders drug swabbing onto oral lesions, tell patient to use nonabsorbent swab. Instruct him to take drug four times a day—between meals and at bedtime.

• Tell patient to notify prescriber if he develops local irritation, if existing symptoms worsen or return, or if new symptoms arise.

ampicillin

Apo-Ampi (CAN), Novo-Ampicillin (CAN), Nu-Ampi (CAN), Omnipen

ampicillin sodium

Ampicin (CAN), Omnipen-N, Polycillin-N, Totacillin-N

ampicillin trihydrate

D-Amp, Omnipen, Penbritin (CAN), Polycillin, Principen-250, Principen-500, Totacillin

Class and Category
Chemical: Semisynthetic aminopenicillin
Therapeutic: Antibiotic
Pregnancy category: B

Indications and Dosages
➤ *To treat GI infections and genitourinary infections (other than gonorrhea) caused by susceptible strains of* Shigella, Salmonella typhi *and other species,* Escherichia coli, Proteus mirabilis, *and enterococci*

CAPSULES, ORAL SUSPENSION, I.V. INFUSION, I.M. INJECTION

Adults and children who weigh 20 kg (44 lb) or more. 500 mg P.O. q 6 hr or 250 to 500 mg I.V. or I.M. q 6 hr.

Children who weigh less than 20 kg. 50 to 100 mg/kg/day in divided doses P.O. q 6 hr or 12.5 mg/kg I.V. or I.M. q 6 hr.

➤ *To treat gonorrhea caused by susceptible strains of non-penicillinase-producing* Neisseria gonorrhoeae

CAPSULES, ORAL SUSPENSION

Adults and children. 3.5 g as a single dose with 1 g of probenecid.

I.V. INFUSION, I.M. INJECTION

Adults and children who weigh 45 kg (99 lb) or more. 500 mg q 6 hr.

Children who weigh less than 40 kg (88 lb). 50 mg/kg/day in divided doses q 6 to 8 hr.

➤ *To treat respiratory tract infections caused by susceptible strains of non-penicillinase–producing* Haemophilus influenzae, *staphylococci, and streptococci, including* Streptococcus pneumoniae

CAPSULES, ORAL SUSPENSION, I.V. INFUSION, I.M. INJECTION

Adults and children who weigh 40 kg or more. 250 to 500 mg I.V. or I.M. q 6 to 8 hr.

Adults and children who weigh 20 kg or more. 250 mg P.O. q 6 hr.

Children who weigh less than 40 kg. 25 to 50 mg/kg/day I.V. or I.M. in divided doses q 6 to 8 hr.

Children who weigh less than 20 kg. 50 mg/kg/day P.O. in divided doses q 6 or 8 hr or 12.5 mg/kg I.V. or I.M. q 6 hr.

➤ *To treat septicemia*

I.V. INFUSION, I.M. INJECTION

Adults. 8 to 14 g I.V. daily in divided doses q 3 to 4 hr for at least 3 days; then I.M.

Children. 150 to 200 mg/kg/day I.V. in divided doses q 3 to 4 hr for at least 3 days; then I.M.

➤ *To prevent bacterial endocarditis from dental, oral, or upper respiratory tract procedures*

I.V. INFUSION, I.M. INJECTION

Adults. 2 g within 30 min of procedure

Children. 50 mg/kg within 30 min of procedure

➤ *To treat bacterial meningitis caused by susceptible strains of* Neisseria meningitidis

I.V. INFUSION, I.M. INJECTION

Adults. 8 to 14 g/day or 150 to 200 mg/kg/day I.V. in equally divided doses q 3 to 4 hr for at least 3 days; then I.M. at same dosage and schedule.

Children. 100 to 200 mg/kg/day I.V. in equally divided doses q 3 to 4 hr for at least 3 days; then I.M. at same dosage and schedule.

➤ *To treat listeriosis*

I.V. INFUSION, I.M. INJECTION

Adults and children who weigh 20 kg or more. 50 mg/kg q 6 hr.

Children who weigh less than 20 kg. 12.5 mg/kg q 6 hr.

Route	Onset	Peak	Duration
I.V.	Immediate	Unknown	Unknown

Mechanism of Action

Inhibits bacterial cell wall synthesis. The rigid, cross-linked cell wall is assembled in several steps. Ampicillin exerts its effects on susceptible bacteria in the final stage of the cross-linking process by binding with and inactivating penicillin-binding proteins (enzymes responsible for linking the cell wall strands). This action causes bacterial cell lysis and death.

Incompatibilities

Don't mix ampicillin and any aminoglycoside in the same I.V. bag, bottle, or tubing; otherwise, both drugs will be inactivated. If patient must receive both drugs, administer them in separate sites at least 1 hour apart.

Contraindications

Hypersensitivity to any penicillin, infection caused by penicillinase-producing organism

Interactions
DRUGS

allopurinol: Increased risk of rash, particularly in hyperuricemic patient

aminoglycosides: Possibly inactivated action of aminoglycoside and ampicillin when given together

heparin, oral anticoagulants: Increased risk of bleeding

oral contraceptives: Possibly reduced contraceptive effectiveness and breakthrough bleeding

probenecid: Possibly increased serum ampicillin level and ampicillin toxicity

tetracyclines: Possibly impaired action of ampicillin

Adverse Reactions
CNS: Chills, fatigue, fever, headache, malaise
CV: Chest pain, edema, thrombophlebitis
EENT: Epistaxis, glossitis, laryngeal stridor, mucocutaneous candidiasis, stomatitis, throat tightness
GI: Abdominal distention, diarrhea, enterocolitis, flatulence, gastritis, nausea, pseudomembranous colitis, vomiting
GU: Dysuria, urine retention, vaginal candidiasis
HEME: Agranulocytosis, anemia, eosinophilia, leukopenia, thrombocytopenia, thrombocytopenic purpura
SKIN: Erythema multiforme; erythematous, mildly pruritic maculopapular rash or other types of rash; exfoliative dermatitis; pruritus; urticaria
Other: Anaphylaxis, facial edema, injection site pain

Nursing Considerations
•Expect to administer ampicillin for 48 to 72 hours after patient becomes asymptomatic. For streptococcal infection, expect to administer ampicillin for at least 10 days after cultures show streptococcal eradication to reduce risk of rheumatic fever or glomerulonephritis.
•To dilute ampicillin for I.M. use, add 1.2 ml of sterile water or bacteriostatic water for injection to each 125-mg vial, 1 ml of diluent to each 250-mg vial, 1.8 ml of diluent to each 500-mg vial, 3.5 ml of diluent to each 1-g vial, or 6.8 ml of diluent to each 2-g vial.
•To dilute ampicillin for intermittent I.V. infusion, add 5 ml of sterile water or bacteriostatic water for injection to each 125-, 250-, or 500-mg vial or at least 7.4 to 10 ml of diluent to each 1- or 2-g vial. Administer I.V. infusion in suitable diluent in a concentration of less than 30 mg/ml.
•**WARNING** Infuse I.V. solution over 3 to 5 minutes for each 125 or 500 mg or over 10 to 15 minutes for each 1 or 2 g. More rapid infusion may cause seizures.
•Monitor patient closely for anaphylaxis, which may be life-threatening. Patients at greatest risk are those with a history of multiple allergies, hypersensitivity to cephalosporins, or a history of asthma, hay fever, or urticaria.

•**WARNING** If ampicillin triggers an anaphylactic reaction, discontinue drug, notify prescriber immediately, and provide appropriate therapy. Anaphylaxis requires immediate treatment with epinephrine as well as airway management and administration of oxygen and I.V. corticosteroids, as needed.
•If long-term or high-dose ampicillin therapy is required, closely monitor results of renal and liver function tests and CBCs.
PATIENT TEACHING
•Tell patient to take oral ampicillin with 8 oz of water 30 minutes before or 2 hours after meals.
•Instruct patient to shake suspension well before each use, keep bottle tightly closed between uses, and discard unused portion after 14 days if refrigerated or 7 days if stored at room temperature.
•Teach patient to recognize signs of allergic reaction and, if they occur, to withhold next ampicillin dose and contact prescriber immediately.

ampicillin sodium and sulbactam sodium
Unasyn

Class and Category
Chemical: Aminopenicillin, beta-lactamase inhibitor
Therapeutic: Antibiotic
Pregnancy category: B

Indications and Dosages
➤ *To treat skin and soft-tissue infections caused by beta-lactamase–producing strains of* Staphylococcus aureus, Escherichia coli, Klebsiella *species (including* K. pneumoniae*),* Proteus mirabilis, Bacteroides fragilis, Enterobacter *species, and* Acinetobacter calcoaceticus; *intra-abdominal infections caused by beta-lactamase–producing strains of* E. coli, Klebsiella *species (including* K. pneumoniae*),* Bacteroides *species (including* B. fragilis*), and* Enterobacter *species; gynecologic infections caused by beta-lactamase–producing strains of* E. coli *and* Bacteroides *species (including* B. fragilis*)*

I.V. INFUSION, I.M. INJECTION

Adults and children age 12 and older who weigh 40 kg (88 lb) or more. 1.5 (1 g of ampicillin and 0.5 g of sulbactam) to 3 g (2 g of ampicillin and 1 g of sulbactam) q 6 hr, up to a maximum of 8 g of ampicillin and 4 g of sulbactam daily.

Children age 1 and older who weigh less than 40 kg. 300 mg/kg (200 mg of ampicillin and 100 mg of sulbactam) daily in divided doses q 6 hr.

DOSAGE ADJUSTMENT Dosing frequency reduced to q 6 to 8 hr for patients with creatinine clearance of 30 ml/min/1.73 m^2 or more. Dosing frequency reduced to q 12 hr for patients with creatinine clearance of 15 to 29 ml/min/1.73 m^2. Dosing frequency reduced to 1.5 to 3.0 g q 24 hr for patients with creatinine clearance of 5 to 14 ml/min/1.73 m^2.

Route	Onset	Peak	Duration
I.V.	Immediate	Unknown	Unknown

Mechanism of Action

Inhibits bacterial cell wall synthesis. The rigid, cross-linked cell wall is assembled in several steps. The drug exerts its effects on susceptible bacteria in the final stage of the cross-linking process by binding with and inactivating penicillin-binding proteins (enzymes responsible for linking the cell wall strands). This action causes bacterial cell lysis and death. When ampicillin is administered alone, beta-lactamases may degrade it, making it ineffective. When combined with sulbactam, degradation can't occur. So sulbactam extends ampicillin's bactericidal effects to beta-lactamase–producing bacteria.

Incompatibilities

Don't mix ampicillin sodium and sulbactam sodium in the same I.V. bag, bottle, or tubing with an aminoglycoside to prevent mutual inactivation. If patient must receive both drugs, administer them in separate sites at least 1 hour apart.

Contraindications

Hypersensitivity to ampicillin sodium and sulbactam sodium, its components, or any penicillin

Interactions

allopurinol: Increased risk of rash, particularly in hyperuricemic patient

aminoglycosides: Possibly inactivated action of both drugs when given together

heparin, oral anticoagulants: Increased risk of bleeding

oral contraceptives: Possibly reduced contraceptive effectiveness and breakthrough bleeding

probenecid: Possibly increased serum ampicillin level and ampicillin toxicity

tetracyclines: Possibly impaired action of ampicillin and sulbactam

Adverse Reactions

CNS: Chills, fatigue, fever, headache, malaise

CV: Chest pain, edema, thrombophlebitis

EENT: Black "hairy" tongue, epistaxis, glossitis, laryngeal stridor, mucocutaneous candidiasis, stomatitis, throat tightness

GI: Abdominal distention, diarrhea, enterocolitis, flatulence, gastritis, nausea, pseudomembranous colitis, vomiting

GU: Dysuria, urine retention, vaginal candidiasis

HEME: Agranulocytosis, anemia, eosinophilia, leukopenia, thrombocytopenia, thrombocytopenic purpura

SKIN: Erythema multiforme; erythematous, mildly pruritic maculopapular rash or other rash; exfoliative dermatitis; mucosal bleeding; pruritus; urticaria

Other: Anaphylaxis, facial edema, injection site pain

Nursing Considerations

•Avoid administering ampicillin sodium and sulbactam sodium to patients with mononucleosis because of the increased risk of rash.

•Administer I.V. dose by slow injection over 10 to 15 minutes or by infusion over 15 to 30 minutes in greater dilutions with 50 to 100 ml of a compatible diluent.

•Reconstitute drug for I.M. use with sterile water for injection or 0.5% or 2% lidocaine hydrochloride injection. For a 1.5-g vial, add 3.2 ml of diluent; for a 3.0-g vial, add 6.4 ml of diluent. Let solution stand until foaming dissipates. Inspect vial before withdrawing drug to ensure that dissolution has occurred.

A

After reconstituting solution, inject it within 1 hour.
•Administer by deep I.M. injection.
•Monitor closely for anaphylaxis, which may be life-threatening. Patients at greatest risk are those with a history of hypersensitivity to penicillin, multiple allergies, hypersensitivity to cephalosporins, or a history of asthma, hay fever, or urticaria.
•WARNING If drug triggers an anaphylactic reaction, discontinue drug, notify prescriber immediately, and provide appropriate therapy. Anaphylaxis requires immediate treatment with epinephrine as well as airway management and administration of oxygen and I.V. corticosteroids, as needed.
•Monitor closely for diarrhea, which may herald pseudomembranous colitis. If diarrhea occurs, notify prescriber. If pseudomembranous colitis is diagnosed, expect to discontinue drug and, possibly, administer fluids, electrolytes, protein, and antibiotic effective against *Clostridium difficile.*

PATIENT TEACHING
•Warn patient that I.M. injection of ampicillin and sulbactam is likely to cause discomfort.
•Instruct patient to report diarrhea or sudden or unusual symptoms to his prescriber immediately.

amyl nitrite

Class and Category
Chemical: Nitrite ester
Therapeutic: Antianginal
Pregnancy category: C

Indications and Dosages
➤ *To treat acute attacks of angina pectoris*
CRUSHABLE AMPULES
Adults. 1 ampule (0.18 or 0.3 ml) inhaled and repeated in 3 to 5 min, if needed.

Route	Onset	Peak	Duration
Inhalation	10 to 30 sec	Unknown	3 to 5 min

Contraindications
Hypersensitivity to amyl nitrite, its components, or nitrates

Mechanism of Action
After inhalation, is absorbed by pulmonary alveoli, which causes relaxation of vascular smooth-muscle cells, dilation of large coronary blood vessels, decreased systemic vascular resistance, decreased venous return to the heart, reduced afterload, decreased cardiac ouput, and subsequent relief of angina.

Interactions
DRUGS
aspirin: Increased serum level and action of amyl nitrite
calcium channel blockers: Possibly severe symptomatic hypotension
sildenafil: Increased risk of hypotension
sympathomimetics: Possibly decreased antianginal effects and severe hypotension and tachycardia
ACTIVITIES
alcohol use: Increased risk of severe hypotension and cardiovascular collapse

Adverse Reactions
CNS: Dizziness, headache, restlessness, syncope, weakness
CV: Orthostatic hypotension, tachycardia
GI: Fecal incontinence, nausea, vomiting
GU: Urinary incontinence
HEME: Hemolytic anemia, methemoglobinemia
SKIN: Face and neck flushing, pallor, rash

Nursing Considerations
•Use amyl nitrite cautiously in elderly patients and patients with cerebral hemorrhage, glaucoma, hyperthyroidism, recent head trauma or MI, or severe anemia.
•Monitor blood pressure during and after drug administration. Also monitor cardiac function periodically in patients who use amyl nitrite regularly.
•WARNING Discontinue drug and notify prescriber if you detect signs of overdose, such as bluish lips, fingernails, or palms; dizziness; fainting; extreme pressure in head; dyspnea; unusual tiredness or weakness; a weak or fast heartbeat; or increased methemoglobin level. Cyanosis may occur when methemoglobin level reaches 1.5 g/dl. More pronounced signs occur at 20 to 50 g/dl.
•Expect to treat overdose with high-flow oxygen and I.V. methylene blue. If hypoten-

sion is severe, place patient head down. If he needs a vasopressor, avoid epinephrine because it may cause severe hypotension.

PATIENT TEACHING
• Advise patient to store amyl nitrate in a tight container, protected from light.
• Tell patient to crush ampule between finger and thumb, hold it to nostrils, and inhale one to six times.
• Instruct patient to remain seated or supine during administration and to rise slowly afterward to prevent dizziness.
• Inform patient that relief usually occurs in 1 to 5 minutes. If pain continues, he should repeat dose. If pain continues after another 5 minutes, he should seek emergency help.
• Remind patient not to use more amyl nitrite than prescribed because of danger of overdose.
• WARNING Caution patient that drug is flammable and must be guarded from flames or heat.
• Inform patient that amyl nitrite commonly causes headaches. Tell him to notify prescriber if headache becomes severe or bothersome.

anagrelide hydrochloride

Agrylin

Class and Category
Chemical: Imidazo-quinazolinone
Therapeutic: Platelet count–reducing agent
Pregnancy category: C

Indications and Dosages
➤ *To treat essential thrombocythemia*
CAPSULES
Adults. 0.5 mg q.i.d. or 1 mg b.i.d. for 1 wk, then adjusted to the lowest effective dose (dose that maintains platelet count below 600,000/ml or within normal range). Dosage should not be increased by more than 0.5 mg/day in any one wk. *Maximum:* 10 mg/day or 2.5 mg in a single dose.

Route	Onset	Peak	Duration
P.O.	7 to 14 days	Unknown	Up to 4 days

Contraindications
Hypersensitivity to anagrelide

Mechanism of Action
May decrease megakaryocyte hypermaturation (large, overmature bone marrow cells from which platelets are formed), reducing the platelet count. At higher doses, may inhibit platelet aggregation.

Interactions
DRUGS
sucralfate: Possibly interference with anagrelide absorption

Adverse Reactions
CNS: Amnesia, asthenia, chills, confusion, CVA, depression, dizziness, fever, headache, insomnia, malaise, nervousness, paresthesia, seizures, somnolence, syncope, weakness
CV: Angina, arrhythmias, edema, heart failure, hypertension, MI, orthostatic hypotension, palpitations, tachycardia, vasodilation
EENT: Amoblyopia, diplopia, epistaxis, rhinitis, sinusitis, stomatitis, tinnitus, vision or visual field abnormality
GI: Abdominal pain, anorexia, constipation, diarrhea, elevated liver function test results, eructation, flatulence, gastric and duodenal ulceration, gastritis, GI hemorrhage, hepatotoxicity, indigestion, melena, nausea, pancreatitis, vomiting
GU: Dysuria, hematuria, renal failure
HEME: Anemia, hemorrhage, thrombocytopenia
MS: Arthralgia, back pain, leg cramps, myalgia, neck pain
RESP: Asthma, bronchitis, dyspnea, pneumonia
SKIN: Alopecia, ecchymosis, photosensitivity, pruritus, rash, urticaria
Other: Dehydration, flulike symptoms, generalized body pain, lymphadenoma

Nursing Considerations
• Use anagrelide cautiously in patients with heart disease because it may cause cardiovascular problems, such as heart failure. Use it cautiously in patients with renal insufficiency (with serum creatinine level of 2 mg/dl or more) or hepatic dysfunction (with liver function tests more than 1.5 times normal) because of the risk of nephrotoxicity and hepatotoxicity.
• To assess anagrelide effectiveness and prevent thrombocytopenia, expect to monitor platelet count every 2 days during first week

A

of therapy and then at least weekly until lowest effective dose is reached.
• While platelet count is being reduced (usually during first 2 weeks of treatment), monitor WBC count and hemoglobin, AST, ALT, creatinine, and BUN levels to detect abnormalities.
• Monitor blood pressure to detect orthostatic hypotension.

PATIENT TEACHING
• Stress importance of returning for laboratory tests, such as platelet counts, to monitor drug effectiveness and adjust its dosage.
• Tell patient to keep bottle tightly capped between uses and to protect drug from light to prevent degradation.

anakinra

Kineret

Class and Category
Chemical: Recombinant human interleukin-1 receptor antagonist
Therapeutic: Antirheumatic
Pregnancy category: B

Indications and Dosages
➤ *To reduce signs and symptoms of moderate to severe active rheumatoid arthritis in patients who have not responded to disease-modifying antirheumatics*

S.C. INJECTION
Adults. 100 mg/day.

Mechanism of Action
Inhibits the binding of interleukin-1 (IL-1) to the IL-1 type 1 receptor, thus blocking the biological activity of IL-1. T cells release IL-1, a mediator of the immune and inflammatory process, in response to inflammatory stimuli. IL-1 contributes to the inflammation, pain, and stiffness associated with rheumatoid arthritis.

Contraindications
Active infection; hypersensitivity to anakinra, its components, or *Escherichia coli*-derived proteins

Interactions
DRUGS
etanercept, infliximab, and other drugs that block tumor necrosis factor (TNF): Increased risk of serious infection

vaccines, live virus: Possibly decreased antibody response to vaccine, potential for infection with live virus

Adverse Reactions
CNS: Headache
EENT: Sinusitis
GI: Abdominal pain, diarrhea, nausea
HEME: Neutropenia
RESP: Upper respiratory tract infection
Other: Flulike symptoms; hypersensitivity reaction; injection site ecchymosis, erythema, inflammation, pain, and pruritus; serious infections

Nursing Considerations
• Obtain baseline neutrophil count before administration, as ordered. Expect to monitor neutrophil count every month for 3 months and then every 3 months for up to 1 year.
• Discard solution if it contains particles or is discolored. Use prefilled syringe and needles to administer drug. Don't shake syringe; allow time for solution to clear if it's foamy.
• Administer drug at approximately the same time each day.
• **WARNING** Be aware that anakinra is not recommended for patients with active infections. Monitor patient for signs and symptoms of infection, such as fever, chills, sore throat, and mouth sores, before and during therapy because drug increases the risk of infections, such as cellulitis, pneumonia, and bone and joint infections. Notify prescriber if such signs are present. Patients with asthma and those receiving etanercept or infliximab concurrently are at increased risk for serious infections. Expect anakinra to be discontinued if patient develops a serious infection.
• Be aware that live virus vaccines should not be given to patients receiving anakinra because drug decreases the immune response.
• Monitor patients with impaired renal function for signs of anakinra toxicity; they're at increased risk because drug is excreted primarily by the kidneys.
• Store anakinra at 2° to 8° C (36° to 46° F). Protect from freezing and light.

PATIENT TEACHING
• Teach patient proper injection technique if prescriber recommends self-administration of anakinra. Verify that patient understands the process and can correctly prepare and inject first few doses.

•Instruct patient to rotate injection sites among the thigh, stomach, and upper arms and to avoid areas that are tender, hard, red, or bruised. Advise him to make sure that each site is at least 1″ away from previous site.
•Urge patient to discard used needles and syringes in a puncture-resistant container and not to reuse them. Instruct him to return container to prescriber for proper disposal.
•Review with patient signs and symptoms of a possible allergic reaction, including rash and shortness of breath.
•Urge patient to immediately report signs of infection, such as cough, fever, chills, dyspnea, or headache, to prescriber.

anastrozole

Arimidex

Class and Category

Chemical: Non-steroidal selective aromatase inhibitor
Therapeutic: Antineoplastic
Pregnancy category: D

Indications and Dosages

➤ *To treat postmenopausal women with unknown or positive hormone receptor and locally advanced or metastatic breast cancer, and those with advanced breast cancer following disease progression after tamoxifen therapy*

TABLETS

Adult women. 1 mg q.d.

Contraindications

None known

Interactions

None

Adverse Reactions

CNS: Asthenia, depression, dizziness, headache, hypertonia, insomnia, lethargy, paresthesia
EENT: Dry mouth, pharyngitis
ENDO: Hot flashes, weight gain
CV: Chest pain, hypertension, peripheral edema, thromboembolic disease, vasodilation
GI: Abdominal or pelvic pain, anorexia, increased appetite, constipation, diarrhea, nausea, vomiting

Mechanism of Action

Anastrozole works to treat certain types of breast cancer in postmenopausal women by inhibiting the enzyme aromatase. Normally after menopause, estrogen is derived from androgens, such as androstenedione, produced by the adrenal glands. Anastrozole blocks aromatase, preventing the production of estrone and estradiol. In women with breast tumors that contain estrogen receptors, anastrozole prevents the stimulatory effects of estrogen on the tumors' growth.

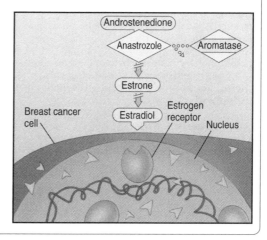

GU: Leukorrhea; vaginal bleeding, dryness, or hemorrhage
MS: Back or bone pain
RESP: Increased cough, dyspnea
SKIN: Rash, sweating
Other: Flulike syndrome, pain, tumor flare

Nursing Considerations
• Assess patient for signs and symptoms of thromboembolic events during anastrozole therapy, such as shortness of breath, leg pain, and change in mental status.
• Store drug in a tightly closed container at room temperature.
PATIENT TEACHING
• Advise patient to notify prescriber immediately about known or suspected pregnancy. Explain that anastrozole may be harmful to fetus and that the benefits versus risks to fetus will need to be evaluated.
• Inform patient about possible dizziness and lethargy, and advise her to avoid potentially hazardous activities until drug's CNS effects are known.
• Advise patient to notify prescriber if she experiences leg pain or calf swelling, which may indicate a blood clot.
• Urge patient taking anastrozole to comply with follow-up appointments.

anisindione

Miradon

Class and Category
Chemical: Indanedione derivative
Therapeutic: Anticoagulant
Pregnancy category: X

Indications and Dosages
➤ *To prevent and treat venous thrombosis, atrial fibrillation with embolization, and pulmonary embolism; and as an adjunct to treat coronary artery occlusion, usually in patients who can't tolerate coumarin anticoagulants*
TABLETS
Adults. *Initial:* 300 mg on day 1; then 200 mg on day 2, and 100 mg on day 3. *Maintenance:* 25 to 250 mg q.d.

Route	Onset	Peak	Duration
P.O.	In 6 hr	48 to 72 hr	1 to 3 days

Mechanism of Action
Prevents coagulation by interfering with liver's ability to synthesize vitamin K-dependent clotting factors, which results in the depletion of clotting factors II (prothrombin), VII, IX, and X. Normally, a stable fibrin clot is formed from a cascade of proteolytic reactions involving the interaction of several clotting factors, including those that are vitamin K-dependent. These clotting factors circulate in the blood in an inactive form and must be converted to an activated form before the next step in the clotting cascade can be stimulated. By depleting vitamin K-dependent clotting factors, anisindione interferes with the clotting cascade and prevents coagulation.

Contraindications
Ascorbic acid deficiency; blood dyscrasias; continuous small-intestine drainage tube; diverticulitis; emaciation; GI, GU, or respiratory tract bleeding; hemophilia; hemorrhagic tendency; history of warfarin-induced necrosis; hypersensitivity to anisindione or its components; leukemia; major recent surgery; malnutrition; pericardial effusion; pericarditis; polyarthritis; pregnancy; prostatectomy; recent spinal puncture, percutaneous invasive procedure, diagnostic testing, or intrauterine device insertion; recent or potential for CNS or eye surgery; severe renal or hepatic disease; severe uncontrolled diabetes; severe uncontrolled malignant hypertension; subacute bacterial endocarditis; thrombocytopenic purpura; visceral carcinomas; ulcerative colitis

Interactions
DRUGS
abciximab, acetaminophen, allopurinol, alteplase, amiodarone, amitriptyline, amoxapine, androgens, aspirin, beta blockers, cephalosporins, chloral hydrate, chloramphenicol, chlorpropamide, cimetidine, cisapride, clofibrate, clomipramine, corticosteroids, co-trimoxazole, cyclophosphamide, danazol, desipramine, dextrothyroxine, diclofenac, diflunisal, disulfiram, doxepin, erythromycin, etodolac, fluconazole, fluoxymesterone, fosphenytoin, gemfibrozil, glucagon, hydantoins, ifosfamide, influenza virus vaccines, imipramine, indomethacin, isoniazid, itraconazole, ketoconazole, ketorolac, lepirudin, loop diuretics, lovastatin, low–molecu-

lar-weight heparins, meclofenamate, mefenamic acid, methyltestosterone, metronidazole, miconazole, moricizine, nabumetone, naproxen, nalidixic acid, neomycin, nortriptyline, NSAIDs, omeprazole, oxandrolone, penicillins, phenylbutazones, phenytoin, piroxicam, propafenone, propoxyphene, protriptyline, quinidine, quinine, quinolones, reteplase, salicylates, stanazolol, streptokinase, sulfamethoxazole, sulfinpyrazone, sulindac, tamoxifen, testosterone, thioamines, thyroid hormones, tomentin, urokinase: Increased anticoagulant effects
aminoglutethimide, ascorbic acid, barbiturates, carbamazepine, cholestyramine, corticosteroids, dicloxacillin, estrogen, ethanol, ethchlorvynol, etretinate, glutethimide, griseofulvin, nafcillin, oral contraceptives, rifampin, spironolactone, sucralfate, thiazide diuretics, thiopurines, trazodone, vitamin K: Decreased anticoagulant effects
aminoglycosides, mineral oil, tetracycline, vitamin E: Interference with vitamin K, leading to increased anticoagulant effects

FOODS
enteral products and foods high in vitamin K, such as dark green leafy vegetables: Interference with anticoagulant effects

ACTIVITIES
alcohol use: Possibly increased or decreased anticoagulation

Adverse Reactions
CNS: Fever, headache
EENT: Blurred vision, mouth ulcers, pharyngitis
GI: Abdominal cramps, diarrhea, hepatic dysfunction, hepatitis, nausea, steatorrhea
GU: Albuminuria, anuria, priaprism, red-orange urine, renal tubular necrosis
HEME: Agranulocytosis, anemia, atypical mononuclear cells, eosinophilia, hemorrhage, leukocytosis, leukopenia, RBC aplasia, thrombocytopenia
SKIN: Alopecia, exfoliative dermatitis, jaundice, necrosis of the skin and tissues evidenced by gangrene and purple toes, urticaria

Nursing Considerations
•Watch for PT to become prolonged 6 hours after anisindione administration, although maximum therapeutic effects may take 48 to 72 hours to appear.
•**WARNING** Watch for signs of overanticoagulation, such as microscopic hematuria, excessive menstrual bleeding, melena, petechiae, and bleeding from superficial trauma, such as tooth brushing or shaving.
•Monitor INR, CBC, fecal occult blood test, and urinalysis results for signs of overanticoagulation.

PATIENT TEACHING
•Advise patient to avoid alcohol, salicylates, and drastic changes in his intake of vitamin K–rich food.
•Instruct patient to promptly report pregnancy to prescriber.
•Provide patient with a list of vitamin K–rich food. Advise him to eat consistent daily amounts of vitamin K.
•Counsel patient to consult prescriber before undergoing dental work or elective surgery.
•Urge patient to notify prescriber immediately if he develops unusual bleeding, bruising, red or red-orange urine, red or tarry black stools, diarrhea, bleeding from gums or nose, or excessive bleeding from minor cuts or scratches.

anistreplase

(anisoylated plasminogen-streptokinase activator complex)
Eminase

Class and Category
Chemical: p-Anisoylated derivative of the Lys-plasminogen-streptokinase activator complex
Therapeutic: Thrombolytic enzyme
Pregnancy category: C

Indications and Dosages
➤ To treat acute MI, lyse thrombi obstructing coronary arteries, reduce infarct size, improve ventricular function after acute MI, reduce mortality from acute MI
I.V. INFUSION
Adults. 30 U injected over 2 to 5 min.

Route	Onset	Peak	Duration
I.V.	Immediate	20 min to 2 hr	4 to 6 hr

Incompatibilities
Don't add other drugs to anistreplase solution or infuse other drugs through same I.V. line.

A

Mechanism of Action
Indirectly promotes the conversion of plasminogen to plasmin, an enzyme that breaks down fibrin clots, fibrinogen, and other plasma proteins, including procoagulant factors V and VIII.

Contraindications
Active internal bleeding, arteriovenous malformation or aneurysm, bleeding diathesis, history of CVA, hypersensitivity to anistreplase or streptokinase, intracranial neoplasm, intracranial or intraspinal surgery or trauma within past 2 months, severe uncontrolled hypertension

Interactions
DRUGS
aspirin, dipyridamole, and other drugs that alter platelet function; heparin; vitamin K antagonists: Possibly increased risk of bleeding if administered before anistreplase

Adverse Reactions
CNS: Dizziness, fever, headache, intracranial hemorrhage
CV: Ankle edema, arrhythmias (especially accelerated idioventricular rhythm, conduction disorders, premature ventricular beats, sinus bradycardia, ventricular fibrillation, ventricular tachycardia), hypotension, vasculitis
EENT: Epistaxis
GI: Abdominal pain or swelling, constipation, GI bleeding, nausea, vomiting
GU: Hematuria, proteinuria, vaginal bleeding
HEME: Bleeding tendency, eosinophilia, mild to severe hemorrhage
MS: Arthralgia, back pain, joint stiffness, myalgia
RESP: Bronchospasm, dyspnea, hemoptysis
SKIN: Flushing, pruritus, rash, urticaria
Other: Anaphylaxis (rare), angioedema

Nursing Considerations
• Use anistreplase cautiously in patients with acute pericarditis; cerebrovascular disease; hemorrhagic ophthalmic conditions; history of major surgery, GI or GU bleeding, or trauma within past 10 days; hypertension; mitral stenosis with atrial fibrillation; pregnancy; septic thrombophlebitis; severe hepatic or renal disease; or subacute bacterial endocarditis.

• Reconstitute anistreplase by slowly directing 5 ml of sterile water for injection USP or sodium chloride for injection against side of vial. Then gently roll vial to mix dry powder and fluid and minimize foaming. Don't shake vial. The resulting solution should be colorless to pale yellow and transparent.
• Before administering, inspect solution for particles and discoloration. If present, discard and reconstitute drug from a new vial. Then withdraw entire contents of vial. Don't dilute reconstituted solution further before administration or add it to I.V. fluid. Don't add other drugs to vial or syringe that contains anistreplase. Discard drug if it isn't administered within 30 minutes after reconstitution.
• For maximum effectiveness, expect to administer anistreplase as soon as possible after onset of MI symptoms.
• Closely monitor all puncture sites, such as catheter insertion and needle puncture sites, for bleeding.
• Don't give I.M. injections, and avoid handling patient unnecessarily during anistreplase therapy. Perform venipuncture only when necessary.
• If an arterial puncture is needed after anistreplase administration, use an arm vessel that allows easy manual compression. Apply a pressure dressing afterward and check puncture site frequently for bleeding.
• Use continuous cardiac monitoring because arrhythmias may occur during reperfusion. Keep antiarrhythmics on hand during anistreplase therapy, and manage arrhythmias according to facility policy.
• Keep epinephrine nearby to treat anaphylaxis.
• Know that anistreplase may be less effective if it's given more than 5 days after anistreplase or streptokinase administration. This occurs because patient may have developed antistreptokinase antibodies, which makes him more resistant to the drug and drug therapy less effective. Elevated serum antistreptokinase antibody levels and reduced drug effectiveness can persist for 5 days to 12 months.
• Closely monitor blood coagulation test results. The drug markedly decreases plasminogen and fibrinogen levels and increases thrombin time, APTT, and PT.

•Instruct patient to report adverse reactions immediately, especially bleeding, dizziness, and chest pain.

antithrombin III, human
(AT-III, heparin co-factor I)
ATnativ, Thrombate III

Class and Category
Chemical: Alpha$_2$-globulin
Therapeutic: Anticoagulant, antithrombotic
Pregnancy category: C

Indications and Dosages
➤ *To treat patients with hereditary anti-thrombin III (AT-III) deficiency who are undergoing surgery or obstetric procedures or who have thromboembolism*
I.V. INJECTION
Adults and children. *Initial:* Individualized dosage (based on weight, degree of AT-III deficiency, and desired level of AT-III to be achieved) sufficient to increase AT-III activity to 120% of normal, administered at 50 to 100 IU/min. *Maintenance:* Individualized dosage sufficient to keep AT-III activity at 80% or more of normal, administered q 24 hr, continued for 2 to 8 days, depending on the patient's condition and history and prescriber's judgment. A pregnant, immobilized, or postsurgical patient may need more prolonged therapy.

Route	Onset	Peak	Duration
I.V.	Immediate	Unknown	4 days

Mechanism of Action
Inhibits blood coagulation by inactivating thrombin; activated forms of factors IX, X, XI, and XII; and plasmin.

Contraindications
None known

Interactions
DRUGS
heparin: Enhanced anticoagulant effect

Adverse Reactions
CNS: Chills, dizziness, fever, light-headedness
CV: Chest pain or tightness, hypotension, vasodilation

EENT: Unpleasant taste
GI: Abdominal cramps, bowel fullness, nausea
GU: Diuresis
HEME: Hematoma
RESP: Dyspnea
SKIN: Oozing lesions, urticaria

Nursing Considerations
•Reconstitute AT-III with 10 ml of sterile water for injection (provided by manufacturer) or alternate solution, such as NS or D$_5$W injection. *Don't* shake vial during reconstitution. Let solution come to room temperature before administration. If desired, dilute reconstituted solution further, using same diluent.
•**WARNING** Don't use diluent that contains benzyl alcohol to reconstitute AT-III for a neonate. This can cause a fatal toxic syndrome with metabolic acidosis, CNS depression, respiratory problems, renal failure, hypotension, seizures, and intracranial hemorrhage.
•Don't refrigerate reconstituted solution. Use it within 3 hours; discard unused solution.
•Administer AT-III alone. Don't mix it with other drugs or solutions.
•If after 30 minutes the initial dose doesn't increase AT-III activity to 120% of normal, expect the prescriber to increase the dosage.
•If patient requires a dosage increase, monitor AT-III activity more frequently and expect to adjust dosage accordingly.
•To avoid bleeding, anticipate a reduction in heparin dosage during AT-III therapy.
•If mild adverse reactions occur, decrease infusion rate, as prescribed. If severe reactions occur, discontinue infusion, as prescribed, until they subside.
•Evaluate serum AT-III level twice daily until dosage is stabilized. After that, evaluate level once daily, immediately before a dose.
PATIENT TEACHING
•Inform patient that blood will be drawn periodically to guide AT-III dosage adjustments.

aprotinin
Trasylol

Class and Category
Chemical: Protease inhibitor
Therapeutic: Antifibrinolytic
Pregnancy category: B

Indications and Dosages

➤ *To reduce blood loss and the need for blood transfusion in patients undergoing repeat coronary artery bypass graft surgery and for those undergoing first-time surgery who are at high risk for bleeding or when blood transfusion is unavailable or unacceptable*

I.V. INFUSION

Adults. *High-dose regimen:* Test dose of 10,000 KIU (kallikrein inactivator units, 1 ml) 10 min before initial dose. If test dose is tolerated, 2,000,000 KIU (200 ml) given over 20 to 30 min followed by maintenance dosage of 500,000 KIU/hr (50 ml/hr). To the priming fluid of the cardiopulmonary bypass circuit (pump prime dose), 2,000,000 KIU (200 ml) is added. *Low-dose regimen:* Test dose of 10,000 KIU (1 ml) 10 min before initial dose. If test dose is tolerated, 1,000,000 KIU (100 ml) given over 20 to 30 min followed by maintenance dosage of 250,000 KIU/hr (25 ml/hr). Pump prime dose of 1,000,000 KIU (100 ml) is added to priming fluid.

Mechanism of Action

Reduces bleeding, possibly by affecting plasmin and kallikrein, which prevents fibrinolysis and may inhibit the early phase of the intrinsic clotting cascade. Aprotinin also increases the resistance of platelets to damage from elevated plasmin levels and mechanical injury during cardiopulmonary bypass.

Incompatibilities

Don't administer aprotinin with corticosteroids, heparin, tetracyclines, or nutrient solutions that contain amino acids or fat emulsions. Don't administer I.V. aprotinin through same I.V. line as any other drug; use a different I.V. line or catheter.

Contraindications

Hypersensitivity to aprotinin

Interactions

DRUGS

captopril: Reduced antihypertensive effect
fibrinolytics, such as anistreplase and streptokinase: Inhibited fibrinolysis
heparin: Prolonged activated clotting time

Adverse Reactions

CNS: Confusion, fever

CV: Arrhythmias, cardiac arrest, heart failure, hypertension, hypotension, increased CK level, MI, pericarditis, peripheral edema
ENDO: Hyperglycemia
GI: Diarrhea, elevated liver function test results, nausea, vomiting
GU: Renal failure, UTI
HEME: Leukocytosis, thrombocytopenia
RESP: Apnea, asthma, dyspnea, pleural effusion, pneumonia, pneumothorax
Other: Anaphylaxis, infection, sepsis, shock

Nursing Considerations

• Administer aprotinin cautiously to patient with multiple allergies or history of previous aprotinin treatments. Also use drug cautiously in patient undergoing deep hypothermic circulatory arrest, especially one over age 65.
• If aprotinin is cloudy or contains precipitate or particles, discard it and obtain a new vial.
• Use aprotinin immediately after opening vial. Discard unused portion.
• To reduce risk of anaphylaxis, expect to administer a H_1-receptor antagonist, such as diphenhydramine, shortly before giving a loading dose of aprotinin to patient who has received aprotinin previously.
• Give aprotinin through a central line.
• After anesthesia induction and before sternotomy, expect the initial aprotinin dose to be given with patient supine. Maintenance dosage is given by constant infusion until patient leaves operating room. Before cardiopulmonary bypass begins, the pump prime dose is added to priming fluid of cardiopulmonary bypass circuit by replacing an aliquot of priming fluid with aprotinin.
• If anaphylaxis occurs, discontinue aprotinin immediately and notify prescriber. Then administer oxygen and I.V. epinephrine, antihistamines, and corticosteroids, as prescribed, and maintain a patent airway.

PATIENT TEACHING

• Inform patient that he'll receive aprotinin during surgery and explain its purpose.

argatroban

Acova

Class and Category

Chemical: N2-substituted derivative of arginine
Therapeutic: Anticoagulant
Pregnancy category: B

Indications and Dosages

➤ *To prevent or treat thrombosis in patients with heparin-induced thrombocytopenia (HIT)*

I.V. INFUSION

Adults. 2 mcg/kg/min as a continuous infusion. *Maximum:* 10 mcg/kg/min.

DOSAGE ADJUSTMENT Dosage adjusted as prescribed to maintain a therapeutic activated partial thromboplastin time (APTT) of 1.5 to 3 times the initial baseline value, not to exceed 100 sec. Initial dosage reduced to 0.5 mcg/kg/min for patients with moderate hepatic impairment.

➤ *To prevent or treat thrombosis in patients with or at risk for HIT when undergoing percutaneous coronary interventions (PCI)*

I.V. INFUSION

Adults. *Initial:* 350 mcg/kg over 3 to 5 min followed by a continuous infusion of 25 mcg/kg/min.

DOSAGE ADJUSTMENT Dosage adjusted as prescribed to maintain therapeutic activated clotting time (ACT) between 300 and 450 sec. If ACT is less than 300 sec, give additional I.V. bolus dose of 150 mcg/kg and increase infusion to 30 mcg/kg/min; if ACT is greater than 450 sec, reduce dosage to 15 mcg/kg/min. For dissection, impending abrupt closure, thrombus formation during PCI, or inability to achieve or maintain ACT greater than 300 sec, administer additional bolus dose of 150 mcg/kg and increase infusion to 40 mcg/kg/min.

Route	Onset	Peak	Duration
I.V.	Immediate	3 to 4 hr	Unknown

Mechanism of Action

Forms a tight bond with thrombin, neutralizing this enzyme's actions, even when the enzyme is trapped within clots. Thrombin causes fibrinogen to convert to fibrin, which is essential for clot formation.

Contraindications

Active major bleeding, hypersensitivity to argatroban or its components

Interactions

DRUGS

alteplase, antineoplastic drugs, antiplatelets, antithymocyte globulin, heparin, NSAIDs, reteplase, salicylates, streptokinase, stron-

tium chloride Sr 89, warfarin: Increased risk of bleeding

porfimer: Possibly decreased efficacy of porfimer photodynamic therapy

Adverse Reactions

CNS: Cerebrovascular bleeding, fever, headache
CV: Atrial fibrillation, cardiac arrest, hypotension, unstable angina, ventricular tachycardia
GI: Abdominal pain, anorexia, diarrhea, elevated liver function test results, GI bleeding, nausea, vomiting
GU: Elevated BUN and serum creatinine levels, hematuria (microscopic), UTI
HEME: Hypoprothrombinemia
RESP: Cough, dyspnea, hemoptysis, pneumonia
SKIN: Bleeding at puncture site, rash
Other: Sepsis

Nursing Considerations

•**WARNING** Be aware that argatroban isn't recommended for PCI patients with significant hepatic disease or AST/ALT levels greater than or equal to three times the upper limits of normal.

•Reconstitute drug to 1 mg/ml before administration.

•Protect solution from direct sunlight.

•**WARNING** Monitor patients with thrombocytopenia or those receiving daily doses of salicylates greater than 6 g for signs and symptoms of bleeding because they're at increased risk of bleeding from hypoprothrombinemia.

•**WARNING** Expect to perform blood coagulation tests before and 2 hours after start of therapy because of the major risk of bleeding associated with argatroban. Be aware that coagulopathy must be ruled out before therapy is initiated. When giving drug to a patient undergoing PCI, expect to check ACT 5 to 10 minutes after each bolus and each infusion rate change and every 20 to 30 minutes during the PCI.

•Monitor the following patients for signs and symptoms of bleeding because they're at increased risk during argatroban therapy: females with active menstruation; patients with known vascular or organ abnormalities, such as severe uncontrolled hypertension, advanced renal disease, infective endocarditis, dissecting aortic aneurysm, diverticulitis, hemophilia, hepatic disease (especially if associated with a deficiency of vitamin K-dependent clotting factors), inflammatory bowel disease, or peptic ulcer disease; and those who have recently had a cerebrovascular accident, major surgery (including eye, brain, or spinal cord surgery), large vessel puncture or organ biopsy, lumbar puncture, spinal anesthesia, or major bleeding (including intracranial, GI, intraocular, retroperitoneal, or pulmonary bleeding).

•Whenever possible, avoid I.M. injections in patients receiving argatroban to decrease the risk of bleeding.

•Be aware that thrombin times may not be helpful for monitoring argatroban activity because all thrombin-dependent coagulation tests are affected by the drug.

•Expect drug dosage to be tapered before discontinuation to prevent the risk of rebound hypercoagulopathy; drug's effects last for only a short time once drug is discontinued.

PATIENT TEACHING

•Inform patient that argatroban is a blood thinner that is administered in the hospital by infusion into a vein. If he requires long-term anticoagulation, he'll be switched to another drug before discharge.

•Advise patient to immediately report unusual or unexplained bleeding, such as blood in urine, easy bruising, nosebleeds, tarry stools, and vaginal bleeding.

•Instruct patient to avoid injury while receiving argatroban. For example, suggest that he brush his teeth gently, using a soft-bristled toothbrush, and take special care when flossing.

aspirin

(acetylsalicylic acid, ASA)

Ancasal (CAN), Apo-As (CAN), Apo-ASEN (CAN), Arthrinol (CAN), Arthrisin (CAN), Aspergum, Aspirin, Atria S.R. (CAN), Bayer, Easprin, Ecotrin, Ecotrin Maximum Strength, 8-Hour Bayer Time Release, Empirin, Genprin, Maximum Bayer, Norwich Extra-Strength, Novasen (CAN), Sal-Adult (CAN), Sal-Infant (CAN), St. Joseph Children's, Supasa (CAN), Therapy Bayer, ZORprin

Class and Category

Chemical: Salicylate
Therapeutic: Antiplatelet, antipyretic, non-narcotic analgesic, NSAID
Pregnancy category: D

Indications and Dosages

➤ *To relieve mild pain or fever*

CHEWABLE TABLETS, CHEWING GUM, CONTROLLED-RELEASE TABLETS, ENTERIC-COATED TABLETS, SOLUTION, TABLETS, TIMED-RELEASE TABLETS, SUPPOSITORIES

Adults abd adolescents. 325 to 650 mg q 4 hr, p.r.n., or 500 mg q 3 hr, p.r.n., or 1,000 mg q 6 hr, p.r.n.

Children ages 2 to 14. 10 to 15 mg/kg/dose q 4 hr, p.r.n., up to 80 mg/kg/day.

➤ *To relieve mild to moderate pain from inflammation, as in rheumatoid arthritis and osteoarthritis*

CHEWABLE TABLETS, CHEWING GUM, CONTROLLED-RELEASE TABLETS, ENTERIC-COATED TABLETS, SOLUTION, TABLETS, TIMED-RELEASE TABLETS, SUPPOSITORIES

Adults and adolescents. 3.2 to 6 g/day in divided doses. *Maximum:* 6 g/day.

Children. 10 to 15 mg/kg/day, up to 80 mg/kg/day, in divided doses q 4 to 6 hr.

➤ *To treat juvenile rheumatoid arthritis*

CHEWABLE TABLETS, CHEWING GUM, CONTROLLED-RELEASE TABLETS, ENTERIC-COATED TABLETS, SOLUTION, TABLETS, TIMED-RELEASE TABLETS, SUPPOSITORIES

Children. 60 to 110 mg/kg/day in divided doses q 6 to 8 hr.

➤ *To treat acute rheumatic fever*

CHEWABLE TABLETS, CHEWING GUM, CONTROLLED-RELEASE TABLETS, ENTERIC-COATED TABLETS, SOLUTION, TABLETS, TIMED-RELEASE TABLETS, SUPPOSITORIES

Adults and adolescents. 5 to 8 g/day in divided doses.

Children. *Initial:* 100 mg/kg/day in divided doses for first 2 wk. *Maintenance:* 75 mg/kg/day in divided doses for next 4 to 6 wk.

➤ *To reduce the risk of recurrent transient ischemic attacks or CVA in men*

CHEWABLE TABLETS, CHEWING GUM, CONTROLLED-RELEASE TABLETS, ENTERIC-COATED TABLETS, SOLUTION, TABLETS, TIMED-RELEASE TABLETS, SUPPOSITORIES

Adults. 650 mg b.i.d. or 325 mg q.i.d.

➤ *To reduce severity of or prevent acute MI*

CHEWABLE TABLETS, CHEWING GUM, CONTROLLED-RELEASE TABLETS, ENTERIC-COATED TABLETS, SOLUTION, TABLETS, TIMED-RELEASE TABLETS, SUPPOSITORIES

Adults. *Initial:* 160 to 162.5 mg (one-half of a 325-mg tablet or two 80- or 81-mg tablets) as soon as MI is suspected. *Maintenance:* 160 to 162.5 mg/day for 30 days.

➤ *To reduce risk of MI in patients with previous MI or unstable angina*

CHEWABLE TABLETS, CHEWING GUM, CONTROLLED-RELEASE TABLETS, ENTERIC-COATED TABLETS, SOLUTION, TABLETS, TIMED-RELEASE TABLETS, SUPPOSITORIES

Adults. 325 mg/day.

Contraindications
Allergy to tartrazine dye, asthma, bleeding problems such as hemophilia, hypersensitivity to aspirin or its components, peptic ulcer disease

Interactions
DRUGS
ACE inhibitors: Decreased antihypertensive effect
activated charcoal: Decreased aspirin absorption
antacids, urine alkalinizers: Decreased aspirin effectiveness
anticoagulants: Increased risk of bleeding; prolonged bleeding time
carbonic anhydrase inhibitors: Salicylism
corticosteroids: Increased excretion and decreased blood level of aspirin
heparin: Increased risk of bleeding
methotrexate: Increased blood level and decreased excretion of methotrexate, causing toxicity
nizatidine: Increased blood aspirin level
NSAIDs: Possibly decreased blood NSAID level and increased risk of adverse GI effects
sulfonylureas: Possibly enhanced effect of sulfonylureas with large doses of aspirin
urine acidifiers, such as ammonium chloride and ascorbic acid: Decreased aspirin excretion
vancomycin: Increased risk of ototoxicity
ACTIVITIES
alcohol use: Increased risk of ulcers

Route	Peak	Onset	Duration
P.O. (chewable tablets)	Rapid	Unknown	1 to 4 hr
P.O. (controlled-release)	5 to 30 min	1 to 4 hr	4 to 6 hr
P.O. (enteric-coated)	5 to 30 min	Unknown	1 to 4 hr
P.O. (solution)	5 to 30 min	15 to 40 min	1 to 4 hr
P.O. (tablets)	15 to 30 min	1 to 2 hr	4 to 6 hr
P.O. (timed-release)	5 to 30 min	1 to 4 hr	4 to 6 hr
P.R.	Unknown	Unknown	4 to 6 hr

Mechanism of Action
Blocks the activity of cyclooxygenase, the enzyme necessary for prostaglandin synthesis. Prostaglandins, important mediators in the inflammatory response, cause local vasodilation with swelling and pain. With the blocking of cyclooxygenase and the inhibition of prostaglandins, inflammatory symptoms subside. Pain relief is also achieved by inhibiting prostaglandins because they play a role in pain transmission from the periphery to the spinal cord. Aspirin inhibits platelet aggregation by interfering with the production of thromboxane A_2, a substance that stimulates platelet aggregation. Aspirin acts on the heat-regulating center in the hypothalamus and causes peripheral vasodilation, diaphoresis, and heat loss.

Adverse Reactions
CNS: Confusion, CNS depression
EENT: Hearing loss, tinnitus
GI: Diarrhea, GI bleeding, heartburn, hepatotoxicity, nausea, stomach pain, vomiting
HEME: Decreased blood iron level, leukopenia, prolonged bleeding time, shortened life span of RBCs, thrombocytopenia
SKIN: Ecchymosis, rash, urticaria
Other: Angioedema, Reye's syndrome, salicylism (dizziness, tinnitus, difficulty hearing, vomiting, diarrhea, confusion, CNS depression, diaphoresis, headache, hyperventilation, and lassitude) with regular use of large doses

Nursing Considerations
•Don't crush timed-release or controlled-release aspirin tablets unless directed.
•Ask about tinnitus. This reaction usually occurs when blood aspirin level reaches or exceeds maximum for therapeutic effect.
PATIENT TEACHING
•WARNING Advise parents not to give aspirin to a child or adolescent with chickenpox or flu symptoms because of risk of Reye's syndrome (rare life-threatening reaction characterized by vomiting, lethargy, belligerence, delirium, and coma). Tell them to consult prescriber about alternative drugs.
•Instruct patient to take aspirin with food or after meals because it may cause GI upset if taken on an empty stomach.

•Advise patient with tartrazine allergy not to take aspirin.
•Tell patient to consult prescriber before taking aspirin with any prescription drug for blood disorder, diabetes, gout, or arthritis.
•Tell patient not to use aspirin if it has a strong vinegar-like odor.

aspirin and dipyridamole

Aggrenox

Class and Category
Chemical: Salicylate (aspirin), pyrimidine (dipyridamole)
Therapeutic: Platelet aggregation inhibitor
Pregnancy category: Not rated (aspirin D, dipyridamole B)

Indications and Dosages
➤ *To prevent the recurrence of thrombo-embolic CVA*
CAPSULES
Adults. *Initial:* One capsule (25 mg aspirin and 200 mg extended-release dipyridamole) b.i.d.

Route	Onset	Peak	Duration
P.O.	1 to 7.5 min*	Unknown	2 to 2.5 hr*

Mechanism of Action
Aspirin inhibits platelet aggregation by interfering with production of thromboxane A_2, a substance that stimulates platelet aggregation. Dipyridamole inhibits platelet uptake of adenosine, thus increasing the amount of adenosine in surrounding blood. The increased adenosine acts on platelet A_2 receptors, which stimulates the activity of intraplatelet adenylate cyclase. This action in turn increases the level of cyclic adenosine monophosphate in platelets, which decreases platelet activation and aggregation.

Contraindications
Allergy to NSAIDs or tartrazine dye; hypersensitivity to aspirin, dipyridamole, or their components

Interactions
DRUGS (ASPIRIN)
ACE inhibitors, beta blockers: Decreased antihypertensive effect

acetazolamide: Increased blood acetazolamide level and risk of toxicity
activated charcoal: Decreased aspirin absorption
antacids, urinary alkalinizers: Decreased aspirin effectiveness
carbonic anhydrase inhibitors: Salicylism
corticosteroids: Increased excretion and decreased blood level of aspirin
heparin: Increased risk of bleeding
methotrexate: Increased blood level and decreased excretion rate of methotrexate, causing toxicity
nizatidine: Increased blood aspirin level
NSAIDs: Possibly decreased blood NSAID level and increased risk of bleeding
oral anticoagulants: Increased risk of bleeding; prolonged bleeding time
phenytoin: Decreased blood phenytoin level
sulfonylureas: Possibly enhanced effect of sulfonylureas with large doses of aspirin
urinary acidifiers, such as ammonium chloride and ascorbic acid: Decreased aspirin excretion
valproic acid: Increased blood valproic acid level
vancomycin: Increased risk of ototoxicity
DRUGS (DIPYRIDAMOLE)
adenosine: Increased blood adenosine level; potentiated effects of adenosine
cefamandole, cefoperazone, cefotetan, plicamyin, valproic acid: Possibly hypoprothrombinemia and increased risk of bleeding
cholinesterase inhibitors: Possibly counteracted effects of these drugs and aggravation of myasthenia gravis
heparin, NSAIDs, thrombolytics: Possibly increased risk of bleeding
ACTIVITIES (ASPIRIN)
alcohol use: Increased risk of GI bleeding

Adverse Reactions
CNS: Amnesia, asthenia, headache, seizures, somnolence, syncope
EENT: Epistaxis
GI: Abdominal pain, anorexia, diarrhea, dyspepsia, esophageal irritation, GI bleeding, hemorrhoids, hepatic impairment, nausea, vomiting
HEME: Anemia
MS: Arthralgia, arthritis, back pain
SKIN: Purpura

Nursing Considerations
•Be aware that combination drug aspirin and dipyridamole isn't interchangeable with individual aspirin or dipyridamole tablets.

•**WARNING** Monitor patients with severe hepatic impairment for evidence of bleeding, such as easy bruising, tarry stools, and epistaxis. Monitor coagulation test results as appropriate, and notify prescriber immediately about significant changes. These patients already have an increased risk of bleeding, and platelet inhibition increases the risk further.
•Monitor liver function test results as appropriate if patient has hepatic impairment because dipyridamole may increase hepatic enzyme levels and cause hepatic failure.
•Monitor renal function test results, such as GFR, if patient has renal impairment. Because aspirin is excreted by the kidneys, it should be avoided in patients with a GFR below 10 ml/min. Otherwise, patient may develop aspirin toxicity.
•If patient consumes three or more alcoholic beverages daily or has hypoprothrombinemia, peptic ulcer disease, or vitamin K deficiency, monitor him for signs and symptoms of bleeding.
•If patient has coronary artery disease, assess him for chest pain and hypotension because of dipyridamole's vasodilatory effect.

PATIENT TEACHING
•Advise patient to swallow capsule whole and not to break, chew, or crush it.
•Instruct patient to take drug with a full glass of water and to not lie down for 15 to 30 minutes to prevent esophageal irritation.
•Warn patient to consult prescriber before taking any drug to treat pain, fever, or arthritis.
•Urge patient not to discontinue drug for any reason without first consulting prescriber.
•Advise patient to notify other health care providers that he takes aspirin and dipyridamole.

atenolol

Apo-Atenol (CAN), Novo-Atenol (CAN), Tenormin

Class and Category

Chemical: Beta-adrenergic blocker (beta$_1$ and at high doses beta$_2$)
Therapeutic: Antianginal, antihypertensive
Pregnancy category: D

Indications and Dosages

➤ *To treat angina pectoris and control hypertension*

TABLETS
Adults. 50 mg q.d. increased, p.r.n., after 1 to 2 wk to 100 mg/day.

➤ *To treat acute MI*
TABLETS, I.V. INFUSION
Adults. *Initial:* 5 mg I.V. over 5 min followed by 5 mg I.V. 10 min later. After an additional 10 min, 50 mg given and followed by another 50 mg in 12 hr. *Maintenance:* 50 mg P.O. b.i.d. or 100 mg P.O. q.d. for 6 to 9 days or until discharged from hospital.

DOSAGE ADJUSTMENT Dosage reduced to 50 mg/day P.O. for renally impaired patients and elderly, renally impaired patients with creatinine clearance of 15 to 35 ml/min/1.73 m^2. Dosage reduced to 25 mg/day P.O. for renally impaired patients and elderly, renally impaired patients with creatinine clearance of less than 15 ml/min/1.73 m^2.

Route	Onset	Peak	Duration
P.O.	1 hr	2 to 4 hr	24 hr
I.V.	Immediate	5 min	12 hr

Mechanism of Action

Inhibits stimulation of beta$_1$-receptor sites, located primarily in the heart, causing a decrease in cardiac excitability, cardiac output, and myocardial oxygen demand. Atenolol also acts to decrease the release of renin from the kidneys, aiding in reducing blood pressure. At high doses, it inhibits stimulation of beta$_2$ receptors in the lungs, which may cause bronchoconstriction.

Contraindications

Cardiogenic shock, heart block greater than first degree, hypersensitivity to beta blockers, overt heart failure, sinus bradycardia

Interactions

DRUGS
calcium channel blockers, such as verapamil and diltiazem: Possibly symptomatic bradycardia and conduction abnormalities
catecholamine-depleting drugs, such as reserpine: Additive antihypertensive effect
clonidine: Rebound hypertension

Adverse Reactions

CNS: Depression, disorientation, dizziness, drowsiness, emotional lability, fatigue, fever, lethargy, light-headedness, short-term memory loss, vertigo

CV: Arrhythmias, including bradycardia and heart block; cardiogenic shock; cold arms and legs; heart failure; mesenteric artery thrombosis; mitral insufficiency; myocardial reinfarction; orthostatic hypotension; Raynaud's phenomenon
EENT: Dry eyes, laryngospasm, pharyngitis
GI: Diarrhea, ischemic colitis, nausea
GU: Renal failure
HEME: Agranulocytosis
MS: Leg pain
RESP: Bronchospasm, dyspnea, pulmonary emboli, respiratory distress, wheezing
SKIN: Erythematous rash
Other: Allergic reaction

Nursing Considerations

• Use atenolol cautiously in patients with heart failure controlled by digitalis glycosides or diuretics. Use it cautiously in patients with conduction abnormalities or left ventricular dysfunction who are receiving verapamil or diltiazem, in those with arterial circulatory disorders, and in those with impaired renal function.
• Use atenolol cautiously in diabetic patients because it may mask tachycardia caused by hypoglycemia. Unlike other beta-adrenergic blockers, it doesn't mask other signs of hypoglycemia, cause hypoglycemia, or delay the return of blood glucose to a normal level.
• At first sign of heart failure, expect patient to receive a digitalis glycoside, a diuretic, or both and to be monitored closely. If failure continues, expect to discontinue atenolol.
• Closely monitor patient with hyperthyroidism because atenolol may mask some signs of thyrotoxicosis. Avoid abrupt withdrawal of atenolol, which may precipitate thyrotoxicosis.
• If patient also receives clonidine, expect to discontinue atenolol several days before gradually withdrawing clonidine. Then expect to restart atenolol therapy several days after clonidine has been discontinued.
• During I.V. atenolol therapy, monitor vital signs and cardiac rhythm closely.
• Discard parenteral mixture with atenolol if it isn't used within 48 hours.
• Stop atenolol therapy and notify prescriber if patient develops bradycardia, hypotension, or other serious adverse reaction.

PATIENT TEACHING
• Instruct patient *not* to stop taking atenolol abruptly. Otherwise, angina may worsen and an MI or arrhythmia may occur.
• While patient is being weaned from atenolol, tell him to perform minimal physical activity to prevent chest pain.
• Instruct patient to take a missed dose as soon as possible. However, if it's within 8 hours of the next scheduled dose, tell him to skip the missed dose and return to his regular schedule.
• Inform patient that atenolol may alter his blood glucose level and mask symptoms of hypoglycemia.
• Inform the patient that he may experience fatigue and reduced tolerance to exercise and that he should notify his prescriber if this interferes with his normal lifestyle.

atorvastatin calcium

Lipitor

Class and Category

Chemical: Synthetically derived fermentation product
Therapeutic: Antilipemic, HMG-CoA reductase inhibitor
Pregnancy category: X

Indications and Dosages

➤ *To control lipid levels as an adjunct to diet in primary (heterozygous familial and nonfamilial) hypercholesterolemia and mixed dyslipidemia*
TABLETS
Adults. *Initial:* 10 or 20 mg once daily, then increased according to lipid level. *Maintenance:* 10 to 80 mg once daily.
DOSAGE ADJUSTMENT Initial dose may be increased to 40 mg once daily for patients who require large reduction (more than 45%) of cholesterol levels.

➤ *To control lipid levels in homozygous familial hypercholesterolemia*
TABLETS
Adults. 10 to 80 mg/day.

Contraindications

Active hepatic disease, hypersensitivity to atorvastatin or its components, unexplained persistent elevation of serum transaminase level

Mechanism of Action

Reduces plasma cholesterol and lipoprotein levels by inhibiting HMG-CoA reductase and cholesterol synthesis in the liver and by increasing the number of low-density lipoprotein (LDL) receptors on liver cells to enhance LDL uptake and breakdown.

Interactions

DRUGS

antacid, colestipol: Possibly decreased plasma atorvastatin level

cyclosporine: Increased risk of severe myopathy or rhabdomyolysis

digoxin: Possibly increased serum digoxin level, causing toxicity

erythromycin: Increased serum atorvastatin level

nicotinic acid: Increased risk of severe myopathy or rhabdomyolysis

oral contraceptives, such as ethinyl estradiol and norethindrone: Increased hormone level

Adverse Reactions

CNS: Abnormal dreams, amnesia, emotional lability, facial paralysis, fever, headache, hyperkinesia, lack of coordination, malaise, paresthesia, peripheral neuropathy, somnolence, syncope, weakness

CV: Arrhythmias, elevated serum CK level, orthostatic hypotension, palpitations, phlebitis, vasodilation

EENT: Amblyopia, altered refraction, cheilitis, dry eyes, dry mouth, epistaxis, eye hemorrhage, gingival hemorrhage, glaucoma, glossitis, hearing loss, pharyngitis, sinusitis, stomatitis, taste loss or perversion, tinnitus

ENDO: Hyperglycemia or hypoglycemia

GI: Abdominal or biliary pain, anorexia, colitis, constipation, diarrhea, duodenal or stomach ulcers, dysphagia, eructation, esophagitis, flatulence, gastroenteritis, hepatitis, increased appetite, indigestion, melena, pancreatitis, rectal hemorrhage, tenesmus, vomiting

GU: Abnormal ejaculation; cystitis; decreased libido; dysuria; epididymitis; hematuria; impotence; nephritis; nocturia; renal calculi; urinary frequency, incontinence, or urgency; urine retention; vaginal hemorrhage

HEME: Anemia, thrombocytopenia

MS: Arthralgia, back pain, bursitis, gout, leg cramps, myalgia, myasthenia gravis, myositis, neck rigidity, tendon contracture, tenosynovitis, torticollis

RESP: Dyspnea, pneumonia

SKIN: Acne, alopecia, contact dermatitis, diaphoresis, dry skin, ecchymosis, eczema, jaundice, petechiae, photosensitivity, pruritus, rash, seborrhea, skin ulcers, urticaria

Other: Allergic reaction, facial or generalized edema, flulike symptoms, infection, lymphadenopathy, weight gain

Nursing Considerations

•Be aware that atorvastatin is used in patients with homozygous familial hypercholesterolemia as an adjunct to other lipid-lowering treatments or alone only if other treatments aren't available.

•Know that atorvastatin may be used with colestipol or cholestyramine for additive antilipemic effects.

•Know that liver function tests are performed before atorvastatin therapy, after 6 and 12 weeks of therapy, during each dosage increase, and every 6 months thereafter.

•Expect to measure lipid levels 2 to 4 weeks after initial atorvastatin dose, and adjust dosage as directed. Repeat this process periodically until lipid levels are within desired range.

PATIENT TEACHING

•Emphasize that atorvastatin is an adjunct to—not a substitute for—a low-cholesterol diet.

•Tell patient to take atorvastatin at the same time each day to maintain antilipemic effects.

•Instruct patient to take a missed dose as soon as possible. If it's almost time for his next dose, he should skip the missed dose. Tell him not to double the dose.

•Instruct patient to consult prescriber before taking OTC niacin preparations because of increased risk of rhabdomyolysis.

•Advise patient to notify prescriber immediately if he develops unexplained muscle pain, tenderness, or weakness, especially if accompanied by fatigue or fever.

•Be aware that drug therapy is expensive. Reinforce the benefits of therapy and encourage patient to comply if possible.

atovaquone

Mepron

Class and Category

Chemical: Hydroxy-1,4-naphthoquinone
Therapeutic: Antiprotozoal
Pregnancy category: C

Indications and Dosages

➤ *To prevent* Pneumocystis carinii *pneumonia in patients who can't tolerate co-trimoxazole*

SUSPENSION, TABLETS

Adults and adolescents. 750 mg (5 ml) b.i.d. with meals for 21 days.

➤ *To treat mild to moderate* P. carinii *pneumonia in patients who can't tolerate co-trimoxazole*

SUSPENSION, TABLETS

Adults and adolescents. 750 mg (5 ml) b.i.d. with meals for 21 days. *Maximum:* 1,500 mg/day.

Mechanism of Action

May destroy *P. carinii* by inhibiting the enzymes necessary for nucleic acid and adenosine triphosphate synthesis.

Contraindications

Hypersensitivity to atovaquone or its components

Interactions

DRUGS

rifabutin, rifampin: Possibly decreased plasma atovaquone level

Adverse Reactions

CNS: Fever, headache, insomnia
EENT: Rhinitis
GI: Abdominal pain, diarrhea, nausea, vomiting
HEME: Anemia
RESP: Cough, dyspnea
SKIN: Rash
Other: Allergic reaction

Nursing Considerations

• Monitor blood test results, as indicated, because atovaquone may decrease serum sodium and hemoglobin levels and neutro-phil count and may increase AST, ALT, alkaline phosphatase, and serum amylase levels.
• Crush atovaquone tablets, if needed, for ease of administration.
• Don't substitute atovaquone tablets and oral suspension; these drug forms aren't bioequivalent.

PATIENT TEACHING

• Instruct patient to take atovaquone with meals for maximum effectiveness.
• Instruct patient to take a missed dose as soon as possible. If it's almost time for the next dose, tell him to skip the missed dose. Advise him not to double the dose because this can cause adverse reactions.
• Tell patient to notify prescriber if his condition doesn't improve in a few days or if he develops signs of an allergic reaction, such as fever or rash.

atracurium besylate

Tracrium

Class and Category

Chemical: Biquaternary ammonium ester
Therapeutic: Skeletal muscle relaxant
Pregnancy category: C

Indications and Dosages

➤ *To facilitate endotracheal intubation and induce skeletal muscle relaxation for surgery or mechanical ventilation as adjunct to anesthesia*

I.V. INFUSION OR INJECTION

Adults and children age 2 or older. *Initial:* 0.4 to 0.5 mg/kg by I.V. bolus for nearly complete neuromuscular blockade. *Maintenance:* 0.08 to 0.10 mg/kg 20 to 45 min after initial dose during prolonged surgery. Maintenance doses may be given q 15 to 25 min for patients under balanced anesthesia. For patients undergoing extended surgical procedures, after an initial I.V. bolus, an infusion of 9 to 10 mcg/kg/min may be required to counteract the spontaneous return of neuromuscular function and thereafter 5 to 10 mcg/kg/min as a constant infusion.
Children ages 1 month to 2 years who are undergoing halothane anesthesia. *Initial:* 0.3 to 0.4 mg/kg. Frequent maintenance doses may be required.

Route	Onset	Peak	Duration
I.V.	2 to 2.5 min	3 to 5 min	35 to 70 min

Mechanism of Action
Inhibits nerve impulse transmission by competing with acetylcholine for cholinergic receptors on motor end plate.

Incompatibilities
Don't mix atracurium in same syringe or administer it through same I.V. needle as an alkaline solution, such as a barbiturate injection. Don't mix atracurium with lactated Ringer's injection.

Contraindications
Hypersensitivity to atracurium, its components, or benzyl alcohol

Interactions
aminoglycosides, enflurane, furosemide, halothane, isoflurane, lithium, magnesium salts, polymyxin antibiotics, procainamide, quinidine, thiazide diuretics: Possibly enhanced or prolonged atracurium effects
opioid analgesics: Possibly additive histamine release and increased risk and severity of bradycardia and hypotension

Adverse Reactions
CNS: Seizures
CV: Bradycardia, hypertension, hypotension, tachycardia
MS: Inadequate or prolonged neuromuscular blockade
RESP: Apnea, bronchospasm, dyspnea, laryngospasm, wheezing
SKIN: Flushing, rash, urticaria
Other: Anaphylaxis, injection site reaction

Nursing Considerations
•Use atracurium cautiously in patients with hypotension, and monitor blood pressure closely.
•Monitor closely for adverse reactions, especially those associated with histamine release. Be aware that atracurium is more likely than other neuromuscular blockers to cause skin flushing.
•Anticipate using lower doses for patients with neuromuscular disease, severe electrolyte disorders, or carcinomatosis because of risk of enhanced neuromuscular blockade and difficulties with reversal.

•Keep atropine nearby to treat atracurium-induced bradycardia.
•For I.V. infusion, dilute atracurium with NS, D_5W, or D_5NS. To prepare a solution that yields 200 mcg of atracurium per milliliter, add 2 ml of atracurium to 98 ml of diluent. To prepare a solution that yields 500 mcg per milliliter, add 5 ml of atracurium to 95 ml of diluent.
•Refrigerate solution or store at room temperature for up to 24 hours.
PATIENT TEACHING
•Explain atracurium's purpose and administration during anesthesia. Keep in mind that the patient can still hear.

atropine sulfate

Class and Category
Chemical: Belladonna alkaloid
Therapeutic: Anticholinergic, antimuscarinic
Pregnancy category: C

Indications and Dosages
➤ *To reduce respiratory tract secretions related to anesthesia*
TABLETS
Adults. 0.4 to 0.6 mg given preoperatively.
Children. 0.01 mg/kg up to total of 0.4 mg given preoperatively and repeated q 4 to 6 hr, p.r.n.
I.V., I.M., OR S.C. INJECTION
Adults. 0.4 to 0.6 mg given preoperatively.
Children. 0.01 mg/kg up to total of 0.4 mg given preoperatively and repeated q 4 to 6 hr, p.r.n.
➤ *To correct bradycardia*
I.V. INJECTION
Adults. 0.4 to 1 mg q 1 to 2 hr, p.r.n. Dosage may be increased up to 2 mg if needed.
Children. 0.01 to 0.03 mg/kg.
➤ *To treat cholinesterase inhibitor (such as neostigmine, pilocarpine, and methacholine) toxicity*
I.V. INJECTION
Adults. 2 to 4 mg. Then 2 mg q 5 to 10 min until muscarinic signs (bradycardia, vasodilation, and pupil dilation) disappear or signs of atropine intoxication develop.
I.V. OR I.M. INJECTION
Children. 1 mg. Then 0.5 to 1.0 mg q 5 to 10 min until muscarinic signs disappear or signs of atropine intoxication develop.

➤ *To treat mushroom (muscarine) toxicity*
I.V. OR I.M. INJECTION
Adults. 1 to 2 mg q hr until respiratory signs and symptoms (such as bronchoconstriction) subside.

➤ *To treat pesticide (organophosphate) toxicity*
I.V. OR I.M. INJECTION
Adults. 1 to 2 mg, repeated in 20 to 30 min as soon as cyanosis has cleared. Then dosage continued until definite improvement is maintained, possibly for 2 or more days.

Route	Onset	Peak	Duration
P.O.	30 to 120 min	1 to 2 hr	4 to 6 hr
I.V.	Immediate	2 to 4 min	Brief
I.M.	5 to 40 min	20 to 60 min	Brief
S.C.	Unknown	Unknown	Brief

Mechanism of Action
Inhibits acetylcholine's muscarinic action at the neuroeffector junctions of smooth muscles, cardiac muscles, exocrine glands, SA and AV nodes, and the urinary bladder. In small doses, atropine inhibits salivary and bronchial secretions and diaphoresis. In moderate doses, it increases impulse conduction through the AV node and increases heart rate. In large doses, it decreases GI and urinary tract motility and gastric acid secretion.

Contraindications
Angle-closure glaucoma, asthma, GI obstructive disease (achalasia, pyloric obstruction, pyloroduodenal stenosis), hepatic disease, hypersensitivity to atropine or its components, ileus, intestinal atony, myasthenia gravis, myocardial ischemia, obstructive uropathy, renal disease, severe ulcerative colitis, tachycardia, toxic megacolon, unstable cardiovascular status in acute hemorrhage

Interactions
DRUGS
adsorbent antidiarrheals, antacids: Decreased atropine absorption
amantadine, anticholinergics, antidyskinetics, glutethimide, meperidine, muscle relaxants, phenothiazines, tricyclic antidepressants and
other drugs with anticholinergic properties, including antiarrhythmics (disopyramide, procainamide, quinidine), antihistamines, buclizine, meclizine:* Increased atropine effects
antimyasthenics: Reduced intestinal motility
cyclopropane: Risk of ventricular arrhythmias
haloperidol: Decreased antipsychotic effect
ketoconazole: Decreased ketoconazole absorption
metoclopramide: Decreased effect on GI motility
opioid analgesics: Increased risk of ileus, severe constipation, and urine retention
potassium chloride, especially wax-matrix forms: Possibly GI ulcers
urinary alkalizers (calcium or magnesium antacids, carbonic anhydrase inhibitors, citrates, sodium bicarbonate): Delayed excretion and increased risk of adverse atropine effects

Adverse Reactions
CNS: CNS stimulation (with high doses), confusion, dizziness, drowsiness, headache, insomnia, nervousness, weakness
CV: Bradycardia (with low doses), palpitations, tachycardia (with high doses)
EENT: Altered taste, blurred vision, dry mouth, increased intraocular pressure, mydriasis, nasal congestion, photophobia
GI: Bloating, constipation, dysphagia, heartburn, ileus, nausea, vomiting
GU: Impotence, urinary hesitancy, urine retention
SKIN: Decreased sweating, flushing, urticaria
Other: Anaphylaxis

Nursing Considerations
•Avoid using high-dose atropine therapy in patients with ulcerative colitis because of risk of toxic megacolon or in patients with hiatal hernia and reflux esophagitis because of risk of esophagitis.
•**WARNING** Assess for symptoms of toxic doses of atropine, such as excitement, agitation, drowsiness, and confusion, which are likely to affect elderly patients even with low doses. If these symptoms occur, take safety precautions to prevent patient injury.
•Assess bowel and bladder elimination. Notify prescriber if diarrhea, constipation, urinary hesitancy, or urine retention develop.
PATIENT TEACHING
•Instruct patient to take atropine 30 to 60 minutes before meals.
•Advise patient to notify prescriber if he has persistent or severe diarrhea, constipation, or difficulty urinating.

auranofin

Ridaura

Class and Category
Chemical: Gold salt
Therapeutic: Anti-inflammatory
Pregnancy category: C

Indications and Dosages
➤ *To treat active rheumatoid arthritis that's unresponsive to NSAIDs*
CAPSULES
Adults. *Initial:* 6 mg q.d. or 3 mg b.i.d. *Maintenance:* Up to 9 mg/day after 3 mo of treatment, if needed.
Children age 6 and older. *Initial:* 0.1 mg/kg/day. *Maintenance:* 0.15 mg/kg/day. *Maximum:* 0.2 mg/kg/day.
DOSAGE ADJUSTMENT Drug discontinued if therapeutic response isn't adequate after 3 mo at 9 mg/day.

Route	Onset	Peak	Duration
P.O.	3 to 6 mo	1 to 2 hr	Up to 26 days

Mechanism of Action
Decreases rheumatoid factor and humoral antibody (immunoglobulin) levels. Although its exact anti-inflammatory action is unknown, the drug may suppress the increased phagocytic activity of macrophages and polymorphonuclear leukocytes that occurs with rheumatoid arthritis and thereby inhibits the release of the destructive enzymes that cause inflammation in joints.

Contraindications
Agranulocytosis, blood dyscrasias, bone marrow aplasia, colitis, eczema, exfoliative dermatitis, hepatic disease, history of gold or heavy metal toxicity, hypersensitivity to auranofin, marked hypertension, necrotizing enterocolitis, pulmonary fibrosis, recent radiation therapy, renal disease, severe debilitation, systemic lupus erythematosus, uncontrolled diabetes mellitus, uncontrolled heart failure, urticaria, youth (under age 6)

Interactions
DRUGS
phenytoin: Possibly increased phenytoin level

Adverse Reactions
CNS: Confusion, dizziness, EEG abnormalities, hallucinations, seizures
EENT: Gingivitis, glossitis, iritis or corneal ulcers from gold deposits in ocular tissue, metallic taste, stomatitis
GI: Abdominal cramps, anorexia, constipation, diarrhea, enterocolitis, flatulence, indigestion, melena, nausea, vomiting
GU: Hematuria, elevated BUN and serum creatinine levels, proteinuria, vaginitis
HEME: Agranulocytosis, aplastic anemia, eosinophilia, leukopenia, neutropenia, thrombocytopenia
RESP: Cough, dyspnea, fibrosis, interstitial pneumonitis
SKIN: Alopecia, dermatitis, exfoliative dermatitis, jaundice, photosensitivity, pruritus, rash, urticaria

Nursing Considerations
• Monitor blood and urine tests for signs of gold toxicity during auranofin therapy.
• **WARNING** Gold toxicity may occur during treatment or several months after its discontinuation. Toxicity, which usually occurs with a cumulative dose of 400 to 800 mg, may cause a decreased hemoglobin level, WBC count of less than 4,000/mm^3, granulocyte count of less than 1,500/mm^3, platelet count of less than 150,000/mm^3, severe diarrhea, stomatitis, hematuria, proteinuria, rash, and pruritus.
• Monitor fluid intake and output for signs of imbalance. If urine output decreases, assess BUN and serum creatinine levels for signs of renal impairment.
• Notify prescriber if you detect signs of allergic reaction, such as dermatitis, rash, and pruritus. The drug may need to be discontinued.
PATIENT TEACHING
• Advise patient that diarrhea commonly occurs, but that he should notify prescriber immediately if diarrhea becomes severe.
• Instruct patient to take drug exactly as prescribed and to return monthly for blood tests.
• Inform patient that drug may take 3 to 4 months to reach a therapeutic level.
• Advise patient to report skin problems, fatigue, or stomatitis, which may signal blood dyscrasias.
• Tell patient to notify prescriber if he sees blood in his stool or urine, he bruises easily, or his gums bleed.

azathioprine

Imuran

azathioprine sodium

Imuran

Class and Category

Chemical: Purine analogue
Therapeutic: Antimetabolite, immunosuppressant
Pregnancy category: D

Indications and Dosages

➤ *To prevent kidney transplant rejection*
TABLETS, I.V. INFUSION

Adults and children. *Initial:* 3 to 5 mg/kg/day P.O. or I.V. as a single dose on, or 1 to 3 days before, day of transplantation, followed by 3 to 5 mg/kg/day I.V. after surgery until P.O. dose is tolerated. *Maintenance:* 1 to 3 mg/kg/day P.O.

DOSAGE ADJUSTMENT Dosage reduced for patients with oliguria (such as from tubular necrosis) after transplantation because their drug or metabolite excretion may be delayed.

➤ *To treat refractory rheumatoid arthritis*
TABLETS

Adults. *Initial:* 1 mg/kg (50 to 100 mg) daily as a single dose or b.i.d. for 6 to 8 wk. *Maintenance:* If initial therapy doesn't produce therapeutic effects or serious adverse effects, dosage increased q 4 wk by 0.5 mg/kg up to 2.5 mg/kg. Optimal dosage is 2 to 2.5 mg/kg/day.

DOSAGE ADJUSTMENT Dosage reduced to 25% to 33% of usual dosage for patients who also take allopurinol.

Route	Onset	Peak	Duration
P.O., I.V.	4 to 8 wk	Unknown	Several days

Mechanism of Action

May prevent proliferation and differentiation of activated B and T cells by interfering with purine (protein) and nucleic acid (DNA and RNA) synthesis.

Contraindications

Hypersensitivity to azathioprine

Interactions

DRUGS

ACE inhibitors and drugs that affect bone marrow and cell development in bone marrow, such as co-trimoxazole: Possibly severe leukopenia

allopurinol: Possibly increased therapeutic and adverse effects of azathioprine
anticoagulants: Possibly decreased anticoagulant action
cyclosporine: Possibly decreased plasma cyclosporine level
methotrexate: Possibly increased plasma level of azathioprine's metabolite, 6-mercaptopurine, which can lead to cell death
nondepolarizing neuromuscular blockers: Possibly decreased or reversed action of neuromuscular blocker

Adverse Reactions

CNS: Fever, malaise
GI: Abdominal pain, diarrhea, hepatoxicity (elevated liver function test results), nausea, pancreatitis, steatorrhea, vomiting
HEME: Leukopenia, macrocytic anemia, pancytopenia, thrombocytopenia
MS: Arthralgia, myalgia
SKIN: Alopecia, rash
Other: Infection, lymphomas and other neoplasms

Nursing Considerations

•Before I.V. administration, add 20 ml of sterile water for injection to azathioprine vial and swirl it until clear solution forms. The resulting drug concentration is 100 mg and can be diluted further as prescribed. Calculate infusion rate based on final volume to be infused. Then administer over 30 to 60 minutes or as prescribed (from 5 minutes to 8 hours).

•Obtain results of baseline laboratory tests, including WBC, RBC, and platelet counts. Then expect to monitor results once a week during first month of therapy, twice a month during second and third months of therapy, and once a month or more frequently thereafter.

•Be aware that hematologic reactions typically are dose-related and may occur late in therapy, especially in patients with transplant rejection.

•WARNING If WBC count decreases rapidly or remains significantly and consistently low, expect to reduce dosage or discontinue use of azathioprine.

•Periodically monitor liver function test results to detect early signs of hepatotoxicity.

•If patient develops thrombocytopenia, take bleeding precautions, such as avoiding I.M. injections and venipunctures, applying ice to

areas of trauma, and checking I.V. infusion sites every 2 hours for bleeding.
• If patient also receives an oral anticoagulant, monitor his PT.
• Know that azathioprine therapy increases risk of viral, fungal, bacterial, and protozoal infections. Monitor for signs of infection, such as fever, chills, sore throat, and mouth sores. Expect to administer aggressive antibiotic, antiviral, or other drug therapy and reduce azathioprine dosage.
• Minimize the risk of infection. If patient has severe leukopenia, take neutropenic precautions, such as placing him in a private room and limiting visitors.
• Be aware that rheumatoid arthritis requires at least 12 weeks of azathioprine therapy. During this time, continue other pain-relief measures, such as rest, physical therapy, and other drugs, such as salicylates and corticosteroids.
• If oral azathioprine causes GI upset, administer it in divided doses or with meals.
• Plan to use lowest possible maintenance dosage for patient with rheumatoid arthritis. Expect to reduce dosage gradually in 0.5-mg/kg (about 25-mg) increments at 4-week intervals. Know that drug can be discontinued abruptly, but its effects may persist for several days.

PATIENT TEACHING
• Advise patient to take oral drug with food or meals to minimize GI upset.
• **WARNING** Teach patient to recognize and report signs of infection, such as sore throat and fever.
• Teach patient how to reduce the risk of bleeding and falling.

azelastine hydrochloride

Astelin

Class and Category
Chemical: Phthalazinone derivative
Therapeutic: Antihistamine, H_1-receptor antagonist
Pregnancy category: C

Indications and Dosages
➤ *To treat symptoms of seasonal rhinitis (rhinorrhea, sneezing, and nasal itching)*
NASAL SPRAY
Adults and children age 12 and older.
2 sprays in each nostril b.i.d.

Route	Onset	Peak	Duration
Nasal	In 3 hr	Unknown	12 hr

Mechanism of Action
Binds nonselectively to central and peripheral H_1 receptors, preventing histamine from reaching its site of action, which reduces or prevents most of histamine's physiologic effects. By blocking histamine at its site of action, azelastine inhibits respiratory, vascular, and GI smooth-muscle contraction; decreases capillary permeability, which reduces wheals, flares, and itching; and decreases salivary and lacrimal gland secretions.

Contraindications
Hypersensitivity to azelastine or its components

Interactions
DRUGS
cimetidine, ketoconazole: Possibly increased serum azelastine level
CNS depressants: Possibly increased sedative effects and reduced mental alertness
ACTIVITIES
alcohol use: Possibly increased sedative effects and reduced mental alertness

Adverse Reactions
CNS: Dizziness, fatigue, headache, somnolence
EENT: Bitter taste, dry mouth, epistaxis, nasal burning, paroxysmal sneezing, pharyngitis, rhinitis
GI: Nausea
Other: Weight gain

Nursing Considerations
• Assess for changes in alertness and take safety precautions, if needed.
PATIENT TEACHING
• Teach patient how to use azelastine nasal spray properly to achieve maximum therapeutic effects.
• Before patient's first use of nasal spray, instruct him to prime pump by placing his thumb on base and his index and middle fingers on shoulder area of bottle and then pressing thumb firmly and quickly against bottle four times or until fine mist appears.
• If patient hasn't used spray in more than 3 days, instruct him to reprime pump with two sprays or until fine mist appears.
• Advise patient to clear nostrils gently, if needed, before using spray.

•Teach patient to inhale deeply after each spray and then exhale through his mouth and tilt his head back so drug can spread over nasopharynx.

Advise patient to store bottle upright and tightly closed.

•**WARNING** Emphasize that patient must check with prescriber before taking any OTC drug, such as a cough syrup or cold remedy, because of risk of extreme CNS depression.

•Inform patient that decreased alertness may occur. Advise him to avoid activities that require alertness, such as driving or operating machinery, until drug's effects are known.

azithromycin

Zithromax

Class and Category

Chemical: Azalide (subclass of macrolide)
Therapeutic: Antibiotic
Pregnancy category: B

Indications and Dosages

➤ *To treat mild community-acquired pneumonia, otitis media, pharyngitis, tonsillitis, and uncomplicated skin and soft-tissue infections*

CAPSULES, ORAL SUSPENSION, TABLETS

Adults. 500 mg as a single dose on day 1, followed by 250 mg q.d. on days 2 through 5.

Children age 6 months or older with acute otitis media or community-acquired pneumonia. 10 mg/kg as a single dose (not to exceed 500 mg/day) on day 1, followed by 5 mg/kg (not to exceed 250 mg/day) q.d. on days 2 through 5. Alternatively for acute otitis media, 30 mg/kg of oral suspension as a single dose or 10 mg/kg q.d. for 3 days.

Children age 12 or older with pharyngitis or tonsillitis. 12 mg/kg (not to exceed 500 mg/day) as a single dose daily for 5 days.

➤ *To treat mild to moderate acute bacterial exacerbations of COPD*

CAPSULES, ORAL SUSPENSION, TABLETS

Adults. 500 mg q.d. for 3 days. Alternatively, 500 mg as single dose on day 1, followed by 250 mg q.d. on days 2 through 5.

➤ *To treat community-acquired pneumonia*

CAPSULES, ORAL SUSPENSION, TABLETS, I.V. INFUSION

Adults and children age 16 or older. 500 mg I.V. as a single dose daily for at least 2 days, followed by 500 mg P.O. as a single dose daily until patient completes 7 to 10 days of therapy.

➤ *To treat chancroid caused by* Haemophilus ducreyi; *gonococcal pharyngitis; urethritis, cervicitis, or other infections caused by* Chlamydia trachomatis

CAPSULES, ORAL SUSPENSION, TABLETS

Adults. 1 g as a one-time dose.

Children age 8 or older and children under age 8 who weigh 45 kg (99 lb) or more (with infections caused by *C. trachomatis***).** 1 g as a one-time dose.

➤ *To treat urethritis or cervicitis caused by* Neisseria gonorrhoeae

CAPSULES, ORAL SUSPENSION, TABLETS

Adults. 2 g as a one-time dose.

➤ *To prevent* Mycobacterium avium *complex in patients with advanced HIV infection*

CAPSULES, ORAL SUSPENSION, TABLETS, I.V. INFUSION

Adults. 1.2 g once weekly, as indicated.

➤ *To treat pelvic inflammatory disease*

CAPSULES, ORAL SUSPENSION, TABLETS, I.V. INFUSION

Adults. 500 mg I.V. as a single dose daily for 1 to 2 days, followed by 250 mg P.O. as a single dose daily until patient completes 7 days of therapy.

Route	Onset	Peak	Duration
P.O.	Varies	Unknown	Unknown

Mechanism of Action

Inhibits bacterial protein synthesis. Specifically, azithromycin binds to a ribosomal subunit of susceptible bacteria. This blocks peptide translocation, which inhibits RNA-dependent protein synthesis. Azithromycin concentrates in phagocytes, macrophages, and fibroblasts, which release it slowly and may help distribute it to infection sites.

Incompatibilities

Don't add I.V. substances, additives, or drugs to azithromycin I.V. solution, and don't infuse them through the same I.V. line as azithromycin.

Contraindications

Hypersensitivity to azithromycin, erythromycin, or other macrolide antibiotics

Interactions

DRUGS

antacids that contain aluminum or magnesium: Possibly decreased peak serum level of azithromycin, but extent of absorption is unchanged

carbamazepine, cyclosporine, phenytoin, terfenadine (drugs metabolized by P⁴⁵⁰ cytochrome system): Possibly increased serum levels of these drugs
digoxin: Possibly increased serum digoxin level
dihydroergotamine, ergotamine: Possibly severe peripheral vasospasm and abnormal sensations (acute ergot toxicity)
HMG-CoA reductase inhibitors: Increased risk of severe myopathy or rhabdomyolysis
pimozide: Possibly sudden death
theophylline: Possibly increased serum theophylline level
triazolam: Possibly decreased excretion and increased therapeutic effects of triazolam
warfarin: Possibly increased anticoagulant effects

FOODS
food: Dramatically increased absorption rate of azithromycin

Adverse Reactions

CNS: Dizziness, fatigue, headache, somnolence, vertigo
CV: Chest pain, elevated serum CK level, palpitations
EENT: Hearing loss, mucocutaneous candidiasis, tinnitus
ENDO: Hyperglycemia
GI: Abdominal pain, diarrhea, elevated liver function test results, nausea, pseudomembranous colitis, vomiting
GU: Elevated BUN and serum creatinine levels, nephritis, vaginal candidiasis
HEME: Leukopenia, neutropenia, thrombocytopenia
SKIN: Jaundice, photosensitivity, rash, Stevens-Johnson syndrome, toxic epidermal necrolysis, urticaria
Other: Allergic reaction, angioedema, elevated serum phosphorus level, hyperkalemia, I.V. site reaction (such as redness and pain), superinfection

Nursing Considerations

• Obtain culture and sensitivity test results, if possible, before starting therapy.
• Administer azithromycin capsules or suspension 1 hour before or 2 to 3 hours after food or meals. Give tablets without regard to food.
• **WARNING** Don't give azithromycin as an I.V. bolus or I.M. injection because this may cause a reaction at the infusion site, including erythema, pain, swelling, or tenderness. Instead,

infuse it over 60 minutes or longer, as prescribed. (Typical infusion rates are 1 mg/ml over 3 hours and 2 mg/ml over 1 hour.)
• If hepatic function is impaired, monitor liver function studies because azithromycin is eliminated mainly by the liver.
• Assess patient for signs of bacterial or fungal superinfection, which may occur with prolonged or repeated therapy. If superinfection occurs, expect to administer another antibiotic or antifungal.
• Monitor bowel elimination; if needed, obtain stool culture to rule out pseudomembranous colitis. If this adverse reaction occurs, expect to discontinue azithromycin and administer fluid, electrolytes, and antibiotics that are effective against *Clostridium difficile.*

PATIENT TEACHING
• Tell patient to take azithromycin capsules or suspension 1 hour before or 2 to 3 hours after food or meals. Instruct patient to take tablets without regard to food.
• **WARNING** Urge patient to contact prescriber before taking any OTC drugs, including antacids, to avoid interactions. If antacids are prescribed, instruct patient to take azithromycin 1 hour before or 2 to 3 hours after antacids.
• Teach patient to recognize and immediately report evidence of allergic reactions, such as rash, itching, hives, chest tightness, and difficulty breathing.
• Warn patient that abdominal pain and loose, watery stools may occur. If diarrhea persists or becomes severe, urge him to contact prescriber and replace fluids.
• Because azithromycin may destroy normal flora, teach patient to watch for and immediately report signs of superinfection, such as white patches in the mouth.

aztreonam

Azactam

Class and Category

Chemical: Monobactam
Therapeutic: Antibiotic
Pregnancy category: B

Indications and Dosages

➤ *To treat infections of the urinary tract, lower respiratory tract, skin, soft tissue, female reproductive tract; intra-abdominal infections; septicemia; and surgical*

A

abscesses caused by susceptible strains of gram-negative bacteria

I.V. INFUSION, I.V. OR I.M. INJECTION

Adults. 0.5 to 2.0 g q 8 to 12 hr up to a maximum of 8 g/day. For life-threatening systemic infection, 2 g q 6 to 8 hr up to a maximum of 8 g/day.

Children ages 9 months to 16 years. 30 mg/kg q 6 to 8 hr up to 120 mg/kg/day; 50 mg/kg q 4 to 6 hr (for *Pseudomonas aeruginosa* infection).

DOSAGE ADJUSTMENT For patients with impaired renal function and creatinine clearance between 10 and 30 ml/min/1.73 m^2, initial dose of 1 to 2 g followed by 50% of the usual dose at the usual interval. For patients with severe renal failure and creatinine clearance less than 10 ml/min/1.73 m^2, initial dose of 500 mg to 2 g followed by 25% of the usual dose every 6, 8, or 12 hr.

Route	Onset	Peak	Duration
I.V. infusion	Immediate	Immediate	Unknown
I.V. injection	Immediate	Immediate	Unknown
I.M.	Variable	60 min	Unknown

Mechanism of Action

Inhibits bacterial cell wall synthesis in susceptible aerobic gram-negative bacteria. These bacteria assemble rigid, cross-linked cell walls in several steps. Aztreonam affects final stage of cross-linking by inactivating penicillin-binding protein 3 (enzyme that links cell wall strands). This action causes bacterial cell lysis and death.

Incompatibilities

Don't mix aztreonam in same I.V. solution as cephradine, metronidazole, or nafcillin sodium. Don't mix it in same I.M. injection solution as local anesthetic.

Contraindications

Hypersensitivity to aztreonam or its components

Interactions

DRUGS

aminoglycosides (prolonged or high-dose therapy): Increased risk of nephrotoxicity and ototoxicity

cefoxitin, imipenem: Possibly antagonized action of aztreonam
furosemide, probenecid: Possibly increased serum aztreonam level

Adverse Reactions

CNS: Confusion, dizziness, fever, headache, insomnia, malaise, paresthesia, seizures, vertigo
CV: Chest pain, hypotension, transient ECG changes
EENT: Altered taste, diplopia, halitosis, mouth ulcers, mucocutaneous candidiasis, nasal congestion, sneezing, tinnitus, tongue numbness
GI: Abdominal cramps, diarrhea, elevated liver function test results, GI bleeding, hepatitis, nausea, pseudomembranous colitis, vomiting
GU: Breast tenderness, elevated serum creatinine level, vaginal candidiasis
HEME: Anemia, eosinophilia, increased PT and APTT, leukocytosis, neutropenia, pancytopenia, positive Coombs' test, thrombocytopenia, thrombocytosis
MS: Myalgia
RESP: Bronchospasm, dyspnea, wheezing
SKIN: Diaphoresis, erythema multiforme, exfoliative dermatitis, flushing, jaundice, petechiae, pruritus, purpura, rash, toxic epidermal necrolysis, urticaria
Other: Allergic reaction; injection site pain, phlebitis, swelling, or thrombophlebitis

Nursing Considerations

• Obtain culture and sensitivity test results, if possible, before initiating therapy. If patient is acutely ill, expect to begin therapy before results are available.
• Keep in mind that other antimicrobial drugs may be used with aztreonam in seriously ill patients at risk for gram-positive infection.
• Expect to use I.V. route for patients who need single doses over 1 g and those with life-threatening systemic infections, such as septicemia or peritonitis.
• To reconstitute aztreonam for I.V. bolus injection, use sterile water for injection.
• Immediately after adding diluent to vial, shake it vigorously to mix it properly. After obtaining correct dose, discard unused solution.
• Be aware that reconstituted solution may turn light pink on standing at room temperature. This doesn't affect drug potency.

•Administer I.V. bolus injection directly into I.V. tubing over 3 to 5 minutes.

•**WARNING** When preparing aztreonam for I.V. infusion, use at least 50 ml of appropriate infusion solution per gram of aztreonam. Then further dilute it in I.V. solution, such as NS, D_5W, D_5NS, LR, or Ringer's solution.

•Know that I.V. infusion may be administered over 20 to 60 minutes.

•Flush I.V. tubing with solution, such as NS, before and after administering I.V. infusion to reduce risk of incompatibilities.

•If prescribed, mix aztreonam in same I.V. solution with other antibiotics, such as clindamycin phosphate, gentamicin sulfate, tobramycin sulfate, cefazolin sodium, and ampicillin sodium, or mix it with cloxacillin sodium and vancomycin hydrochloride in peritoneal dialysis solution.

•Prepare solution for I.M. injection using sterile or bacteriostatic water or sodium chloride for injection. Administer injection deep into large muscle, such as in dorsogluteal or ventrogluteal area.

•Assess for signs of bacterial or fungal superinfection, which may occur with prolonged or repeated therapy. If superinfection occurs, treat it as prescribed.

•Monitor bowel elimination; if needed, obtain stool culture to rule out pseudomembranous colitis. If this adverse reaction occurs, expect to discontinue aztreonam and administer fluid, electrolytes, and antibiotics that are effective against *Clostridium difficile*.

PATIENT TEACHING

•Teach patient to recognize and immediately report signs of allergic reactions, such as rash, itching, hives, chest tightness, and difficulty breathing.

•Warn patient that abdominal pain and loose, watery stools may occur. If diarrhea persists or becomes severe, urge him to contact prescriber and replace fluids.

•Because aztreonam may destroy normal flora, teach patient to watch for and immediately report signs of superinfection, such as white patches in mouth.

B

bacampicillin hydrochloride

Penglobe (CAN), Spectrobid

Class and Category
Chemical: Aminopenicillin
Therapeutic: Antibiotic
Pregnancy category: B

Indications and Dosages
➤ *To treat upper respiratory tract infections (including otitis media) caused by* streptococci, pneumococci, non-penicillinase-producing staphylococci, *and* Haemophilus influenzae; *UTIs caused by* Escherichia coli, Proteus mirabilis, *and* Streptococcus faecalis; *skin and soft-tissue infections caused by streptococci and susceptible staphylococci*

TABLETS
Adults. 400 mg q 12 hr; 800 mg q 12 hr for severe infections and those caused by less susceptible organisms.
Children who weigh 25 kg (55 lb) or more. 25 mg/kg/day in divided doses q 12 hr; 50 mg/kg/day in divided doses q 12 hr for severe infections and those caused by less susceptible organisms.
➤ *To treat lower respiratory tract infections caused by streptococci, pneumococci, non-penicillinase-producing staphylococci, and* H. influenzae

TABLETS
Adults. 800 mg q 12 hr.
Children who weigh 25 kg or more. 50 mg/kg/day in divided doses q 12 hr.
➤ *To treat uncomplicated gonorrhea caused by* Neisseria gonorrhoeae

TABLETS
Adults. 1.6 g plus 1 g of probenecid as a single dose.

Route	Onset	Peak	Duration
P.O.	Variable	Unknown	12 hr

Contraindications
Cholestatic jaundice and hepatic dysfunction associated with amoxicillin and clavulanate potassium; hypersensitivity to penicillins, cephalosporins, imipenem and cilastatin, or beta-lactamase inhibitors, such as piperacillin and tazobactam

Mechanism of Action
Inhibits bacterial cell wall synthesis in susceptible bacteria. These bacteria assemble rigid, cross-linked cell walls in several steps. Bacampicillin, which undergoes hydrolysis to ampicillin, affects final stage of cross-linking by binding with and inactivating penicillin-binding protein (enzyme responsible for linking cell wall strands). This action inhibits bacterial cell wall synthesis and causes cell lysis and death.

Interactions
DRUGS
allopurinol: Increased risk of rash from bacampicillin use
beta-adrenergic blockers: Increased risk of anaphylaxis
disulfiram: Possibly disulfiram reaction when administered together
oral contraceptives: Possibly reduced effectiveness of oral contraceptives, contraceptive failure, and breakthrough bleeding
tetracyclines: Possibly impaired bactericidal effects of bacampicillin

Adverse Reactions
CNS: Anxiety, confusion, CVA, depression, fatigue, fever, hallucinations, lethargy, malaise, neuromuscular irritability, seizures, syncope
CV: Hypotension, palpitations, periarteritis nodosa, pulmonary hypertension, tachycardia, vascular collapse
EENT: Altered taste, black "hairy" tongue, blurred vision, glossitis, laryngospasm, mouth soreness, mucocutaneous candidiasis, stomatitis, taste disorders
GI: Abdominal cramps or pain, anorexia, diarrhea, enterocolitis, epigastric distress, elevated liver function test results, gastritis, nausea, pseudomembranous colitis, vomiting
GU: Elevated BUN and serum creatinine levels, hematuria, impotence, interstitial nephritis, neurogenic bladder, priapism, renal failure, vaginal candidiasis
HEME: Agranulocytosis, anemia, bone marrow depression, decreased hemoglobin level and hematocrit, eosinophilia, leukopenia, neutropenia, prolonged PT, thrombocytopenia, thrombocytopenic purpura

MS: Arthralgia, arthritis exacerbation
RESP: Bronchospasm
SKIN: Exfoliative dermatitis, rash, urticaria
Other: Allergic reaction, lymphadenopathy, serum sickness

Nursing Considerations

• Obtain culture and sensitivity test results, if possible, before initiating therapy. Be prepared to start bacampicillin therapy before results are available.
• Expect to continue treatment for at least 48 hours after symptoms resolve or culture detects no signs of infection.
• **WARNING** Expect to administer bacampicillin for 10 days to treat infection caused by group A beta-hemolytic streptococci to prevent development of acute rheumatic fever or acute glomerulonephritis.
• Assess for signs of bacterial or fungal superinfection, which may occur with prolonged or repeated therapy. If superinfection occurs, expect to administer another antibiotic or antifungal drug.
• Monitor bowel elimination; if needed, obtain stool culture to rule out pseudomembranous colitis. If this adverse reaction occurs, expect to discontinue bacampicillin and administer fluid, electrolytes, and antibiotics that are effective against *Clostridium difficile.*

PATIENT TEACHING
• Teach patient to recognize and immediately report signs of allergic reaction, including rash, itching, hives, chest tightness, and difficulty breathing.
• Warn patient that abdominal pain and loose, watery stools may occur. If diarrhea persists or becomes severe, urge him to contact prescriber and drink plenty of fluids.
• Because bacampicillin may destroy normal flora, teach patient to watch for and immediately report signs of superinfection, such as white patches in mouth and vaginal itching and discharge.

bacitracin

Baci-IM

Class and Category

Chemical: Bacillus subtilis derivative (polypeptide)
Therapeutic: Antibiotic
Pregnancy category: C

Indications and Dosages

➤ *To treat pneumonia and empyema caused by susceptible staphylococci*

I.M. INJECTION
Infants who weigh more than 2.5 kg (5.5 lb). 1,000 U/kg/day in two or three divided doses.
Infants who weigh less than 2.5 kg. 900 U/kg/day in two or three divided doses.

Route	Onset	Peak	Duration
I.M.	Rapid	Unknown	About 6 hr

Mechanism of Action

Interferes with bacterial cell wall synthesis by binding with isoprenyl pyrophosphate (a lipid-carrying molecule that transports substances out of bacterial cells to help build new cell walls), forming an unusable complex in bacterial cells. This weakens cell walls and causes lysis and death. Bacitracin is considered a bacteriostatic and bactericidal drug.

Incompatibilities

Don't dilute bacitracin with a solution that contains parabens.

Contraindications

Hypersensitivity or toxic reaction to bacitracin

Interactions

DRUGS
aminoglycosides: Increased risk of respiratory paralysis and renal dysfunction
nondepolarizing neuromuscular blockers: Possibly increased neuromuscular blockade

Adverse Reactions

GI: Nausea, vomiting
GU: Albuminuria, azotemia, cylindrical mucus casts in urine, nephrotoxicity
SKIN: Rash
Other: Injection site pain, superinfection

Nursing Considerations

• Obtain culture and sensitivity test results before therapy begins, if possible. However, be prepared to start bacitracin therapy before results are available.
• **WARNING** Use parenteral bacitracin for I.M. injection only.
• For an I.M. solution of 5,000 U/ml, reconstitute 50,000 U of bacitracin powder with

9.8 ml of sodium chloride for injection that contains 2% procaine hydrochloride.

• Administer I.M. injection into upper outer quadrant of buttocks, alternating right and left sides. To prevent pain at injection site, avoid multiple injections in same site.

• During therapy, compare daily results of renal function tests with baseline results, as appropriate.

• Assess urine output frequently (even hourly, if indicated), and replace fluids orally and parenterally to maintain adequate renal function.

• **WARNING** Because of increased risk of nephrotoxicity, avoid concurrent use of other nephrotoxic drugs, such as streptomycin, kanamycin, polymyxin B, and neomycin.

• Assess infant for signs of superinfection, especially white patches in mouth and perineal area. If superinfection develops, plan to treat it with appropriate antibiotics.

PATIENT TEACHING

• Advise parents that daily blood tests are needed to assess infant's renal function.

• Encourage parents to provide oral fluids to promote renal function. Teach them how to record infant's fluid intake.

• Instruct parents to report signs of superinfection, such as white patches in mouth or perineal area and bright red diaper rash.

baclofen

Apo-Baclofen (CAN), Lioresal, Lioresal Intrathecal, Novo-Baclofen (CAN)

Class and Category

Chemical: Gamma-aminobutyric acid (GABA) chlorophenyl derivative
Therapeutic: Skeletal muscle relaxant, spasmolytic
Pregnancy category: C

Indications and Dosages

➤ *To relieve symptoms of spasticity caused by multiple sclerosis (particularly flexor spasms and pain, clonus, and muscle rigidity) and spasticity from spinal cord injury or disease and brain injury*

TABLETS

Adults and children age 12 and older. 5 mg t.i.d. for 3 days, then 10 mg t.i.d. for 3 days, then 15 mg t.i.d. for 3 days, then 20 mg t.i.d.

for 3 days, then increased if needed up to 80 mg/day. Usual dosage ranges from 40 to 80 mg/day.

➤ *To relieve severe symptoms of spasticity of spinal cord origin when symptoms don't respond to oral drug or when oral drug causes severe adverse CNS effects*

INTRATHECAL BOLUS, INTRATHECAL INFUSION

Adults. *For screening before implantable pump insertion:* 50 mcg in 1 ml of sterile preservative-free sodium chloride for injection as bolus injection into intrathecal space over 1 min or more. After 4 to 8 hr, if symptoms don't improve as much as desired, second bolus of 75 mcg in 1.5 ml of sterile preservative-free sodium chloride for injection injected after 24 hr followed by third bolus of 100-mcg/2 ml dilution injected after another 24 hr, if needed.

After implantable pump insertion: Effective screening dose doubled and infused over 24 hr. Or effective screening dose (if it provided desired effects for more than 12 hr) infused over 24 hr.

For spasticity of spinal cord origin after implantable pump insertion: After first 24 hr, daily dose increased by 10% to 30% once every 24 hr until desired effects achieved.

For spasticity of cerebral origin after implantable pump insertion: Daily dose increased by 5% to 15% once every 24 hr until desired effects achieved.

For long-term maintenance therapy in spasticity of spinal cord origin: 12 to 2,003 mcg/day (usual dose 300 to 800 mcg/day). Lowest possible therapeutic dose should be used. If adverse effects occur, daily dose may be decreased by 10% to 20%. During periodic pump refills, daily dose may be increased by 10% up to 40% to control symptoms adequately.

For long-term maintenance therapy in spasticity of cerebral origin: 90 to 703 mcg/day (usual) but ranging from 22 to 1,400 mcg/day. If adverse effects occur, daily dose may be decreased by 10% to 20%. During periodic pump refills, daily dose may be increased by 5% to 20% to control symptoms adequately.

Children. *For screening before implantable pump insertion:* 1 ml of a 50-mcg/ml dilution or 1 ml of a 25-mcg/ml dilution (if child is very young) as bolus injection into intrathecal space over 1 min or more. After 4 to 8 hr, if symptoms don't improve as desired, second bolus of 75 mcg in 1.5 ml of sterile preservative-free sodium chloride for injection injected after 24 hr followed by third bolus of 100-mcg/2 ml dilution injected after another 24 hr, if needed.

After implantable pump insertion: Daily dose increased by 5% to 15% once every 24 hr until the desired effect is achieved.

For maintenance therapy: In children over age 12: 90 to 703 mcg/day (usual) but ranging from 22 to 1,400 mcg/day. In children under age 12: 274 mcg/day (average) but ranging from 24 to 1,199 mcg/day.

DOSAGE ADJUSTMENT Dosage reduced for patients with renal impairment because drug is excreted primarily unchanged by kidneys.

Route	Onset	Peak	Duration
P.O.	Hours to weeks	Unknown	Unknown
Intrathecal bolus injection	30 to 60 min	About 4 hr	4 to 8 hr
Intrathecal infusion	6 to 8 hr	24 to 48 hr	Unknown

Mechanism of Action

May inhibit transmission of monosynaptic and polysynaptic impulses, similar to effects of GABA. Baclofen may work in the spinal cord at the afferent spinal end of upper motor neurons, where it hyperpolarizes nerve fibers and inhibits impulse transmission. This reduces excess muscle activity caused by muscle hypertonia, spasms, and spasticity.

Contraindications

Hypersensitivity to baclofen; treatment of skeletal muscle spasm resulting from rheumatic disorders, CVA, cerebral palsy, or Parkinson's disease (oral form only)

Interactions

DRUGS

CNS depressants: Possibly increased CNS depression
epidural morphine: Possibly hypotension and dyspnea

ACTIVITIES

alcohol use: Possibly increased CNS depression

Adverse Reactions

CNS: Abnormal gait, anxiety, ataxia, chills, coma, confusion, CVA, depression, dizziness, drowsiness, dystonia, emotional lability, euphoria, excitement, fatigue, fever, hallucinations, headache, hypertonia, hypothermia, hypotonia, impaired concentration, insomnia, lack of coordination, lethargy, memory loss, paresthesia, personality disorder, seizures, somnolence, syncope, tremor, weakness
CV: Bradycardia, chest pain, chest tightness, deep vein thrombosis, hypertension, orthostatic hypotension, palpitations, peripheral edema
EENT: Amblyopia, blurred vision, diplopia, dry mouth, miosis, mydriasis, nasal congestion, nystagmus, photophobia, ptosis, rhinitis, slurred speech, strabismus, taste loss, tinnitus
ENDO: Hyperglycemia
GI: Abdominal pain, anorexia, constipation, dysphagia, elevated liver function test results, flatulence, ileus, indigestion, nausea, vomiting
GU: Albuminuria, bladder spasms, dysuria, enuresis, hematuria, impotence, renal failure, sexual dysfunction, urinary frequency, urinary incontinence, urine retention
HEME: Anemia
MS: Muscle twitching
RESP: Aspiration pneumonia, pulmonary embolism, respiratory depression
SKIN: Alopecia, diaphoresis, facial edema, flushing, pruritus, rash, urticaria, wound dehiscence
Other: Dehydration, infection at pump implantation site, weight loss

Nursing Considerations

•Expect to initiate baclofen therapy at a low dose and gradually increase it until desired effects are achieved.

•WARNING Before screening dose is administered, expect prescriber to ensure that patient is free of infection to prevent systemic infection from interfering with patient's response. Before implantable pump insertion, also expect prescriber to ensure that patient is free of infection to reduce risk of complications and interference with determining most appropriate dose.

•Use baclofen cautiously in patients with history of autonomic dysreflexia. Nociceptor stimulation may precipitate autonomic dysreflexia. Be aware that abrupt withdrawal of intrathecal infusion may produce symptoms similar to autonomic dysreflexia, high fever,

life-threatening complications such as multiple organ-system failure, and death.
•**WARNING** Never administer intrathecal form of baclofen by I.V., I.M., or S.C. route.
•Assess for signs of effectiveness, such as relief of spasms, pain, and muscle rigidity.
•Because CNS depression can occur, take safety precautions to help prevent injury. Also take precautions for patients who use spasticity to maintain locomotion or upright posture and balance. Relief of spasticity may increase risk of falls and injury.
•**WARNING** Because continuous intrathecal infusion increases risk of life-threatening CNS depression, keep emergency equipment nearby.
•Expect baclofen to be discontinued slowly; hallucinations and seizures may occur with abrupt withdrawal.

PATIENT TEACHING
•Teach patient how to care for and operate programmable implanted pump. Have her demonstrate all procedures.
•Advise patient not to stop taking baclofen abruptly. Stress the importance of keeping refill visits for intrathecal infusion.
•Instruct patient to avoid driving and other activities that require mental alertness, coordination, or physical dexterity until baclofen's effects are known.
•Urge patient to contact prescriber before taking OTC drugs, such as cough syrups and cold remedies, which may increase risk of sedation.
•Advise patient to notify prescriber if spasticity increases or baclofen is no longer effective.

balsalazide disodium

Colazal

Class and Category
Chemical: Prodrug of 5-aminosalicylic acid (5-ASA)
Therapeutic: Anti-inflammatory
Pregnancy category: B

Indications and Dosages
➤ *To treat mildly to moderately active ulcerative colitis*

CAPSULES
Adults. 2.25 g t.i.d. for 8 wk. *Maximum:* 6.75 g/day for 12 wk.

Contraindications
Hypersensitivity to balsalazide, salicylates, or their components

B

Mechanism of Action
After it has been metabolized to 5-ASA, balsalazide may reduce inflammation by inhibiting the enzyme cyclooxygenase and decreasing the production of arachidonic acid metabolites, which may be increased in patients with inflammatory bowel disease. Cyclooxygenase is needed to form prostaglandin from arachidonic acid. Prostaglandin mediates inflammatory activity and produces signs and symptoms of inflammation. By inhibiting prostaglandin synthesis, balsalazide may reduce signs and symptoms of inflammation in inflammatory bowel disease. Balsalazide also may reduce inflammation by interfering with leukotrine synthesis and by inhibiting the enzyme lipoxygenase. These substances also are involved in the inflammatory response.

Adverse Reactions
CNS: Headache
GI: Abdominal pain, diarrhea, nausea, vomiting
MS: Arthralgia
RESP: Respiratory tract infection

Nursing Considerations
•**WARNING** Monitor patients who are sensitive to sulfasalazine or olsalazine for possible cross-sensitivity to balsalazide.
•Monitor patients with pyloric stenosis for decreased or delayed drug effects due to prolonged gastric retention of balsalazide capsules.
•Monitor patient for possible exacerbation of colitis symptoms.

PATIENT TEACHING
•Inform patient that balsalazide is used to reduce bowel inflammation and pain associated with ulcerative colitis and to minimize recurring inflammation.
•Instruct patient to swallow capsules whole, with a full glass of water, and not to crush or chew them.
•Advise patient to notify prescriber of any other drugs she may be taking, including OTC drugs, nutritional supplements, and herbal products, because they may interact with balsalazide.
•Instruct patient to notify prescriber immediately if her colitis symptoms worsen.
•Inform patient that she can expect some im-

provement in symptoms in 3 to 21 days but that she may need up to 6 weeks of treatment before she achieves optimal results.

basiliximab

Simulect

Class and Category

Chemical: Chimeric (murine or human) monoclonal antibody
Therapeutic: Immunosuppressant
Pregnancy category: B

Indications and Dosages

➤ *To prevent acute kidney transplant rejection*

I.V. INFUSION OR INJECTION

Adults and adolescents over age 15. 20 mg within 2 hr before transplant, then 20 mg 4 days after transplant.
Children and adolescents ages 2 to 15. 12 mg/m² within 2 hr before transplant, then 12 mg/m² 4 days after transplant. *Maximum:* 20 mg/dose.

Route	Onset	Peak	Duration
I.V.	Unknown	Unknown	22 to 50 days

Mechanism of Action

Initiates immunosuppression by blocking interleukin-2 receptors located on the surface of activated T cells. Normally, interleukin-2 is released by stimulated T lymphocytes, causing activation and differentiation of other T lymphocytes responsible for cell-mediated immunity.

Incompatibilities

Don't add or infuse any other drugs simultaneously through same I.V. line.

Contraindications

Hypersensitivity to basiliximab or its components

Adverse Reactions

CNS: Asthenia, dizziness, fever, headache, insomnia, tremor
CV: Hypertension, peripheral edema
EENT: Oral candidiasis, pharyngitis, rhinitis
ENDO: Hyperglycemia
GI: Abdominal pain, constipation, diarrhea, indigestion, nausea, vomiting
GU: Dysuria, increased urinary nitrogen level, UTI
HEME: Anemia
MS: Back pain, leg pain
RESP: Cough, dyspnea, upper respiratory tract infection
SKIN: Acne
Other: Hypercholesterolemia, hyperkalemia, hyperuricemia, hypocalcemia, hypokalemia, hypophosphatemia, impaired wound healing, injection site reaction, metabolic acidosis, weight gain

Nursing Considerations

• To reconstitute basiliximab, add 5 ml of sterile water for injection to powder and shake vial gently to dissolve. Further dilute with NS or D_5W for infusion to a volume of 50 ml. Gently invert infusion bag to avoid foaming; don't shake. Drug should appear clear to opalescent and colorless.
• Administer reconstituted drug I.V. over 20 to 30 minutes or as a bolus dose directly through a central or peripheral I.V. line. Be aware that bolus dose may cause nausea, vomiting, and a localized injection site reaction, including pain.
• Expect drug to be given as adjunct to cyclosporine and corticosteroids.
• Don't store drug at room temperature for longer than 4 hours; don't refrigerate for longer than 24 hours.
• **WARNING** Be aware that patient may develop hypersensitivity reactions, including anaphylaxis, bronchospasm, dyspnea, hypotension, pruritus, rash, respiratory failure, sneezing, tachycardia, urticaria, and wheezing, on initial exposure or following reexposure after several months. Notify prescriber immediately if such reactions occur.

PATIENT TEACHING

• Inform patient that second dose of basiliximab will be given 4 days after transplant and that she may also receive cyclosporine and corticosteroid therapy.
• Inform patient that because of drug's immunosuppressant effects, she may experience slower wound healing and be more susceptible to upper respiratory tract infections.

beclomethasone dipropionate

Beclodisk (CAN), Beclovent Rotacaps (CAN), Beconase, Beconase AQ, Vancenase, Vanceril

Class and Category
Chemical: Synthetic glucocorticoid
Therapeutic: Antiasthmatic, anti-inflammatory
Pregnancy category: C

Indications and Dosages
➤ *To control and prevent symptoms in patients with chronic asthma and those who also require oral corticosteroids*

INHALATION AEROSOL (84 MCG)

Adults and children age 12 and older. *Initial:* 2 inhalations (168 mcg) b.i.d. For patients with severe asthma, 6 to 8 inhalations (504 to 672 mcg) daily with dosage reduced based on patient response. *Maximum:* 10 inhalations (840 mcg) daily.
Children ages 6 to 12. *Initial:* 2 inhalations (168 mcg) b.i.d. *Maximum:* 5 inhalations (420 mcg) daily.

INHALATION AEROSOL (42 MCG)

Adults and children age 12 and older. *Initial:* 2 inhalations (84 mcg) t.i.d. or q.i.d. or 4 inhalations (168 mcg) b.i.d. For patients with severe asthma, 12 to 16 (504 to 672 mcg) inhalations daily with dosage reduced based on patient response. *Maximum:* 20 inhalations (840 mcg) daily.
Children ages 6 to 12. *Initial:* 1 or 2 inhalations (42 mcg or 84 mcg) t.i.d. or q.i.d. or 4 inhalations (168 mcg) b.i.d. with dosage reduced based on patient response. *Maximum:* 10 inhalations (420 mcg) daily.

➤ *To relieve symptoms of seasonal or perennial allergic and nonallergic (vasomotor) rhinitis and prevent nasal polyps from recurring after surgical removal*

NASAL INHALATION AEROSOL

Adults and children age 12 and older. *Initial:* 1 inhalation (42 mcg) in each nostril b.i.d. to q.i.d. for total dose of 168 to 336 mcg/day. *Maintenance:* 1 inhalation (42 mcg) in each nostril t.i.d. for total dose of 252 mcg/day.
Children ages 6 to 12. 1 inhalation (42 mcg) in each nostril t.i.d. for total dose of 252 mcg/day.

NASAL SPRAY

Adults and children age 12 and older. 1 or 2 inhalations (42 or 84 mcg) in each nostril b.i.d. for total dose of 168 or 336 mcg/day.

Contraindications
Hypersensitivity to beclomethasone's ingredients, infrequent oral corticosteroid treatment, primary treatment of status asthmaticus or other acute asthma attack, relief of acute bronchospasm or of asthma controlled by bronchodilators or other nonsteroidal drugs, treatment of nonasthmatic bronchitis

Mechanism of Action
May decrease number and activity of cells involved in the inflammatory response of asthma, allergies, and rhinitis, such as mast cells, eosinophils, basophils, lymphocytes, macrophages, and neutrophils. Also may inhibit production or secretion of chemical mediators, such as histamine, eicosanoids, leukotrienes, and cytokines. May produce direct smooth-muscle cell relaxation and decrease airway hyperresponsiveness.

Adverse Reactions
CNS: Depression, fatigue, fever, headache, insomnia, light-headedness
CV: Chest pain, tachycardia
EENT: Cataracts, dry mouth, dysphonia, earache, epistaxis, glaucoma, hoarseness, lacrimation, nasal congestion, nose and throat dryness and irritation, oral candidiasis, pharyngitis, rhinorrhea, sinusitis, sneezing, unpleasant smell and taste
ENDO: Adrenal insufficiency, cushingoid symptoms
GI: Diarrhea, indigestion, nausea, rectal hemorrhage
GU: Dysmenorrhea, UTI
MS: Arthralgia
RESP: Bronchitis, bronchospasm, chest congestion, cough, pulmonary infiltrates, upper respiratory tract infection, wheezing
SKIN: Acne, eczema, pruritus, rash, skin discoloration, urticaria
Other: Angioedema, flulike symptoms, lymphadenopathy, weight gain

Nursing Considerations
•If patient also receives an oral corticosteroid, expect to taper its dosage slowly (by decreasing the daily dosage or using the drug every other day) about 1 week after beclomethasone therapy begins. Expect dosage reductions of more than 2.5 mg/day.
•WARNING When gradually switching patient from an oral corticosteroid to inhaled beclomethasone, assess her for signs of life-threatening adrenal insufficiency, such as fatigue, lassitude, weakness, nausea, vomiting, and hypotension, during transition period and when exposed to trauma, surgery, infection, or other stressor. If signs occur, notify prescriber immediately.

• Expect to resume oral corticosteroid during a stressful period or severe asthma attack.

• Because beclomethasone may be absorbed systemically, monitor for signs of adrenal insufficiency during periods of stress.

• If patient experiences an acute asthma attack or increased wheezing after administering beclomethasone, administer a fast-acting bronchodilator, as prescribed. Expect to discontinue beclomethasone and begin alternative therapy.

• Assess for cushingoid symptoms, such as moon face, weight gain, acne, and centralized obesity, which may result from long-term use and systemic absorption of beclomethasone.

• Use beclomethasone cautiously in patients with pulmonary tuberculosis, ocular herpes simplex, or untreated systemic fungal, bacterial, parasitic, or viral infection.

• Assess for signs of candidiasis, such as thick white plaques or coating on tongue and sides of mouth. If present, notify prescriber and expect to reduce drug dose or frequency or discontinue beclomethasone. Also anticipate treatment with antifungal drug.

• When administering beclomethasone nasal spray, periodically assess nasal discharge for color or consistency changes, which may indicate infection. Notify prescriber if significant changes occur.

PATIENT TEACHING

• Advise patient not to abruptly stop taking beclomethasone because adrenal insufficiency may occur. Urge her to notify prescriber if she develops signs of adrenal insufficiency, such as nausea, fatigue, anorexia, dyspnea, hypotension, fever, malaise, dizziness, and fainting.

• Before patient uses nasal spray for first time, instruct her to prime the pump by placing her thumb on its base and index and middle fingers on its shoulder area and then pressing her thumb firmly and quickly against bottle several times or until fine mist appears. Before patient uses nasal inhalation canister for first time, instruct her to shake it and check that it's working properly by spraying it once in the air while looking for fine mist.

• Teach patient to inhale deeply after each nasal spray or inhalation, exhaling through mouth and tilting head back to let drug spread over the nasopharynx.

• Teach patient how to properly use oral inhalation aerosol, shaking canister well before using. If patient has difficulty using device and coordinating inhalation with it, suggest using a spacer device. Before patient uses canister for first time, instruct her to check that it's working properly by spraying it once in the air while looking for fine mist.

• If two inhalations are prescribed, advise patient to wait at least 1 minute between inhalations.

• If patient uses an inhaled bronchodilator with beclomethasone oral inhalation, instruct her to use bronchodilator first, wait 5 minutes, and then use beclomethasone.

• **WARNING** Warn patient that beclomethasone isn't intended to relieve acute bronchospasm. Urge patient to notify prescriber if asthma symptoms don't respond to bronchodilator therapy.

• Advise patient to wear medical identification that states need for supplemental oral corticosteroids during stress or severe asthma attack. Inform patient that prescriber may order high-dose oral corticosteroid therapy for these situations.

• **WARNING** Caution patient to avoid exposure to chickenpox and measles because beclomethasone may cause immunosuppression. If she's exposed to these disorders, urge her to notify prescriber immediately.

belladonna alkaloids

Class and Category

Chemical: Tertiary amine
Therapeutic: GI anticholinergic
Pregnancy category: C

Indications and Dosages

➤ *To treat peptic ulcer disease, functional digestive disorders (including spastic, mucous, and ulcerative colitis), diarrhea, diverticulitis, pancreatitis, dysmenorrhea, nocturnal enuresis, idiopathic and postencephalitic parkinsonism, motion sickness, and nausea and vomiting of pregnancy*

TABLETS

Adults. 0.25 to 0.5 mg t.i.d.
Children over age 6. 0.125 to 0.25 mg t.i.d.

TINCTURE

Adults. 0.6 to 1 ml t.i.d. or q.i.d.
Children. 0.03 ml/kg (0.8 ml/m^2) t.i.d.

Route	Onset	Peak	Duration
P.O.	1 to 2 hr	Unknown	4 hr

Mechanism of Action
Inhibits acetylcholine's muscarinic actions at postganglionic parasympathetic receptor sites, including smooth muscles, secretory glands, and CNS. These actions relax smooth muscles and diminish GI, GU, and biliary tract secretions.

Contraindications
Hepatic disease, hypersensitivity to anticholinergic drugs or scopolamine, ileus, myasthenia gravis, myocardial ischemia, narrow-angle glaucoma, obstructive condition of GI or GU tract, renal disease, severe ulcerative colitis, tachycardia, toxic megacolon, unstable cardiovascular status in acute hemorrhage

Interactions
DRUGS
amantadine: Increased adverse anticholinergic effects
atenolol, digoxin: Possibly increased therapeutic and adverse effects of these drugs
phenothiazines: Possibly decreased phenothiazine effectiveness and increased adverse effects of belladonna alkaloids
tricyclic antidepressants: Possibly increased adverse anticholinergic effects

Adverse Reactions
CNS: CNS stimulation (with high doses), confusion, dizziness, drowsiness, headache, insomnia, nervousness, weakness
CV: Bradycardia, palpitations, tachycardia
EENT: Altered taste, blurred vision, dry mouth, increased intraocular pressure, mydriasis, nasal congestion, photophobia
GI: Bloating, constipation, dysphagia, heartburn, ileus, nausea, vomiting
GU: Impotence, urinary hesitancy, urine retention
SKIN: Decreased sweating, flushing, urticaria
Other: Anaphylaxis

Nursing Considerations
•Avoid using high doses of belladonna alkaloids in patients with ulcerative colitis because they may inhibit intestinal motility and precipitate or aggravate toxic megacolon. Also avoid using high doses in patients with hiatal hernia and reflux esophagitis because they may aggravate esophagitis.
•Use belladonna alkaloids cautiously in patients with allergies, arrhythmias, asthma, autonomic neuropathy, coronary artery disease, debilitating chronic lung disease, heart failure, hypertension, hyperthyroidism, and prostatic hypertrophy.
•Administer drug 30 to 60 minutes before patient eats.
•**WARNING** Monitor for excitement, agitation, drowsiness, and confusion in elderly patients even with small doses. Elderly patients are more sensitive to the effects of the drug and are more likely to develop these adverse reactions. If they develop, the dosage may need to be decreased.
•Take safety precautions to protect patient from injury from falling.
PATIENT TEACHING
•Instruct patient to take belladonna alkaloids 30 to 60 minutes before eating.
•Tell patient to notify prescriber if she has persistent or severe diarrhea, constipation, or difficulty urinating.
•Caution patient to avoid driving and similar activities until the effects of belladonna alkaloids are known.
•**WARNING** Urge patient to avoid extremely hot or humid conditions because heatstroke may occur.

benazepril hydrochloride
Lotensin

Class and Category
Chemical: Ethylester of benazeprilat
Therapeutic: Antihypertensive
Pregnancy category: C (D in second and third trimesters)

Indications and Dosages
➤ *To control hypertension alone or with a thiazide diuretic*
TABLETS
Adults who don't receive a diuretic. *Initial:* 10 mg/day. *Maintenance:* 20 to 40 mg/day as a single dose or in two divided doses.
Adults who receive a diuretic. 5 mg/day.
DOSAGE ADJUSTMENT Initial dosage of 5 mg q.d. for patients with impaired renal function and creatinine clearance of less than 30 ml/min/1.73 m^2, then increased gradually until blood pressure is controlled or dosage reaches maximum of 40 mg/day.

Route	Onset	Peak	Duration
P.O.	1 hr	2 to 4 hr	24 hr

Mechanism of Action

May reduce blood pressure by affecting renin-angiotensin-aldosterone system. By inhibiting ACE, benazepril:

•prevents conversion of angiotensin I to angiotensin II, a potent vasoconstrictor that also stimulates adrenal cortex to secrete aldosterone.

•may inhibit renal and vascular production of angiotensin II.

•decreases serum angiotensin II level and increases serum renin activity. This decreases aldosterone secretion, slightly increasing serum potassium level and fluid loss.

•decreases vascular tone and blood pressure.

•inhibits aldosterone release, which reduces sodium and water reabsorption and increases their excretion, further reducing blood pressure.

Contraindications

Hypersensitivity to benazepril or other ACE inhibitor

Interactions

DRUGS

antacids: Possibly decreased bioavailability of benazepril, requiring administration of drugs separated by 2 hours

capsaicin: Possibly induction or exacerbation of ACE cough caused by benazepril

digoxin: Increased serum digoxin level

diuretics: Possibly excessive hypotension

indomethacin: Reduced hypotensive effects of benazepril

lithium: Increased serum lithium level and risk of lithium toxicity

phenothiazines: Possibly increased therapeutic and adverse effects of benazepril

potassium preparations, potassium-sparing diuretics: Possibly increased serum potassium level

Adverse Reactions

CNS: Anxiety, asthenia, dizziness, drowsiness, fatigue, headache, hypertonia, insomnia, nervousness, paresthesia, sleep disturbance, somnolence, syncope, weakness

CV: Angina, ECG changes, hypotension, orthostatic hypotension, palpitations, peripheral edema

EENT: Sinusitis

ENDO: Hyperglycemia

GI: Abdominal pain, constipation, elevated liver function test results, gastritis, melena, nausea, pancreatitis, vomiting

GU: Decreased libido, elevated BUN and serum creatinine levels, impotence, nephrotic syndrome, proteinuria, renal insufficiency, UTI

HEME: Agranulocytosis, decreased hemoglobin level, leukopenia, neutropenia, thrombocytopenia

MS: Arthralgia, arthritis, myalgia

RESP: ACE cough, asthma, bronchitis, bronchospasm, dyspnea

SKIN: Dermatitis, diaphoresis, flushing, photosensitivity, pruritus, rash

Other: Angioedema, hyperkalemia, hyponatremia

Nursing Considerations

•Evaluate blood pressure with patient lying down, sitting, and standing before initiating benazepril therapy and then every 4 to 8 hours, as appropriate, to monitor drug's effectiveness.

•Monitor urine output and BUN and serum creatinine levels, as appropriate, before therapy begins.

•**WARNING** Be alert for angioedema, especially after first dose of benazepril. If angioedema extends to larynx and patient exhibits laryngeal stridor or signs of airway obstruction, prepare to give epinephrine S.C. immediately, as prescribed, and discontinue benazepril.

•Monitor WBC count periodically to detect neutropenia and agranulocytosis.

•Monitor serum potassium and other electrolyte levels to detect electrolyte imbalances.

•To prevent injury caused by orthostatic hypotension, take safety precautions, such as having patient change position slowly and sit on edge of bed before arising.

PATIENT TEACHING

•Teach patient how to monitor blood pressure, if appropriate, and how to recognize signs of hypertension and hypotension.

•**WARNING** Strongly urge patient to contact prescriber before using any OTC salt substitutes, which may contain potassium, or potassium supplements. These substances increase the risk of hyperkalemia.

•Inform patient that a persistent dry cough may develop and may not subside unless benazepril is discontinued. If cough becomes bothersome or interferes with her sleep or activities, instruct her to notify prescriber.

•**WARNING** Instruct patient to contact prescriber immediately if she experiences signs of angioedema, such as swelling of the face, eyes, lips, or tongue.
•Caution patient to avoid sudden position changes and to rise slowly from a seated or reclining position to minimize orthostatic hypotension.
•**WARNING** Advise patient to stop benazepril and notify prescriber as soon as possible if she experiences syncope.

benzonatate

Benzonatate Softgels, Tessalon Perles

Class and Category
Chemical: Para-aminobenzoic acid (tetracaine-like)
Therapeutic: Nonnarcotic antitussive
Pregnancy category: C

Indications and Dosages
➤ *To relieve cough*
CAPSULES
Adults and children over age 10. 100 mg t.i.d. up to 600 mg/day.

Route	Onset	Peak	Duration
P.O.	15 to 20 min	Unknown	3 to 8 hr

Mechanism of Action
Anesthetizes stretch receptors in respiratory tract, lung tissue, and pleura, interfering with their activity and reducing cough reflex at its source. In usual doses, benzonatate doesn't inhibit respiratory center.

Contraindications
Hypersensitivity to benzonatate or related compounds

Adverse Reactions
CNS: Confusion, hallucinations, headache, mild dizziness, sedation
CV: Cardiogenic shock, chest numbness
EENT: Burning eyes, laryngospasm, nasal congestion
GI: Constipation, GI upset, nausea
RESP: Bronchospasm
SKIN: Pruritus, rash

Nursing Considerations
•Assess type and frequency of cough. Don't attempt to suppress cough with benzonatate if cough has therapeutic benefit, such as to move secretions and improve airflow.
•**WARNING** Don't break or crush capsules or let patient chew or dissolve them in her mouth. This may cause benzonatate's release in patient's mouth, which can anesthetize her mouth and throat, placing her at risk for choking. Also don't let patient suck or chew the capsule to prevent severe hypersensitivity reaction.
PATIENT TEACHING
•Instruct patient to swallow capsules whole and not to chew, suck, or open them.
•Warn patient that mild dizziness and sedation may occur. Teach her to take safety measures, and encourage her to avoid activities that require mental alertness until benzonatate's effects are known.

benzquinamide hydrochloride

Emete-Con

Class and Category
Chemical: Benzoquinolizine amide
Therapeutic: Antiemetic
Pregnancy category: Not rated

Indications and Dosages
➤ *To treat nausea and vomiting related to anesthesia or surgery*
I.V. OR I.M. INJECTION
Adults. 50 mg or 0.5 to 1 mg/kg I.M., repeated in 1 hr, then q 3 to 4 hr, p.r.n. Or 25 mg or 0.2 to 0.4 mg/kg by slow infusion (1 ml every 0.5 to 1 min) as a single dose. Then, I.M. doses begin.

➤ *To prevent nausea and vomiting related to anesthesia and surgery*
I.M. INJECTION
Adults. 50 mg or 0.5 to 1 mg/kg 15 min before emergence from anesthesia.

Route	Onset	Peak	Duration
I.V., I.M.	15 min	Unknown	Unknown

Mechanism of Action
Exhibits antiemetic, antihistaminic, mild cholinergic, and sedative effects by unknown mechanism.

Contraindications
Hypersensitivity to benzquinamide or its components

Interactions
DRUGS
vasopressors: Increased hypertensive effects

Adverse Reactions
CNS: Chills, dizziness, drowsiness, excitement, fatigue, fever, headache, insomnia, nervousness, restlessness, tremor, weakness
CV: Atrial fibrillation, hypertension, hypotension, premature atrial or ventricular contractions
EENT: Blurred vision, dry mouth, increased salivation
GI: Anorexia, hiccups, nausea
MS: Muscle twitching
SKIN: Diaphoresis, flushing, rash, urticaria

Nursing Considerations
•**WARNING** Avoid I.V. route in patients with cardiovascular disease because sudden blood pressure increases and transient arrhythmias may occur. Use I.V. route only for patients without cardiovascular disease who aren't receiving a preanesthetic or cardiovascular drug.
•Administer benzquinamide I.M. into large, well-developed muscle. Avoid using deltoid muscle unless it's well developed.
•Take safety precautions to reduce the risk of injury from CNS depression.
PATIENT TEACHING
•Advise patient to stay in bed and call for assistance to reduce risk of injury.
•Tell patient to report whether nausea and vomiting have been relieved.

benztropine mesylate

Apo-Benztropine (CAN), Cogentin, PMS Benztropine (CAN)

Class and Category
Chemical: Tertiary amine
Therapeutic: Antiparkinsonian, central-acting anticholinergic
Pregnancy category: C

Indications and Dosages
➤ *As adjunct, to treat all forms of Parkinson's disease*

TABLETS, I.M. OR I.V. INJECTION
Adults with Parkinson's disease. 1 to 2 mg/day (usual dose) with a range of 0.5 to 6.0 mg/day.
Adults with idiopathic Parkinson's disease. *Initial:* 0.5 to 1.0 mg h.s. *Maximum:* 4 to 6 mg/day.
Adults with postencephalitic Parkinson's disease. 2 mg/day in one or more doses; may begin with 0.5 mg h.s. and increase as needed.
➤ *To control extrapyramidal symptoms (except tardive dyskinesia) caused by phenothiazines and other neuroleptic drugs*
TABLETS, I.M. OR I.V. INJECTION
Adults. 1 to 4 mg q.d. or b.i.d.
➤ *To treat acute dystonic reactions*
TABLETS, I.M. OR I.V. INJECTION
Adults. *Initial:* 1 to 2 ml (1 to 2 mg total dose) I.V. or I.M. *Maintenance:* 1 to 2 mg P.O. b.i.d. to prevent recurrence.

Route	Onset	Peak	Duration
P.O.	1 to 2 hr	Unknown	24 hr
I.V., I.M	15 min	Unknown	24 hr

Mechanism of Action
Blocks acetylcholine's action at cholinergic receptor sites. This restores the brain's normal dopamine and acetylcholine balance, which relaxes muscle movement and decreases drooling, rigidity, and tremor. Benztropine also may inhibit dopamine reuptake and storage, which prolongs dopamine's action.

Contraindications
Achalasia, bladder neck obstruction, glaucoma, hypersensitivity to benztropine mesylate or its components, megacolon, myasthenia gravis, prostatic hypertrophy, pyloric or duodenal obstruction, stenosing peptic ulcer

Interactions
DRUGS
amantadine: Possibly increased adverse anticholinergic effects
digoxin: Possibly increased serum digoxin level
haloperidol: Possibly increased schizophrenic symptoms, decreased serum haloperidol level, and development of tardive dyskinesia

levodopa: Possibly decreased levodopa effectiveness

phenothiazines: Possibly reduced phenothiazine effects and increased psychiatric symptoms

Adverse Reactions

CNS: Agitation, confusion, delirium, delusions, depression, disorientation, dizziness, drowsiness, euphoria, excitement, fever, hallucinations, headache, light-headedness, listlessness, memory loss, nervousness, paranoia, psychosis, weakness
CV: Hypotension, mild bradycardia, orthostatic hypotension, palpitations, tachycardia
EENT: Blurred vision, diplopia, dry mouth, increased intraocular pressure, mydriasis, narrow-angle glaucoma, suppurative parotitis
GI: Constipation, duodenal ulcer, epigastric distress, ileus, nausea, vomiting
GU: Dysuria, urinary hesitancy, urine retention
MS: Muscle spasms, muscle weakness
SKIN: Decreased sweating, dermatoses, flushing, rash, urticaria

Nursing Considerations

•Expect to administer I.V. or I.M. benztropine when patient needs more rapid response than oral drug can provide. Be aware that I.M. route is commonly used because it provides effects in about the same time as I.V. route. Watch for improvement a few minutes after administration. If Parkinsonian symptoms reappear, expect to repeat dose.
•Know that therapy generally begins with a low dose followed by gradual increases of 0.5 mg every 5 or 6 days because benztropine has a cumulative action.
•Assess muscle rigidity and tremor as a baseline. Then monitor them frequently for improvement, which indicates benztropine's effectiveness.
•Administer drug before or after meals based on patient's need and response. If patient has increased salivary secretions, expect to administer benztropine after meals. If patient has dry mouth, plan to give drug before meals unless nausea develops.
•WARNING When administering benztropine to patient with drug-induced extrapyramidal reactions, be alert for exacerbation of psychiatric symptoms.
•Know that high-dose benztropine therapy may cause weakness and inability to move specific muscle groups. If this occurs, expect to reduce benztropine dosage.

PATIENT TEACHING
•Warn patient that benztropine has a cumulative effect, increasing risk of adverse reactions and overdose.
•Caution patient to avoid driving and similar activities until benztropine's effects are known because drug may cause blurred vision, dizziness, or drowsiness.
•WARNING Because benztropine decreases sweating, urge patient to avoid extremely hot or humid conditions to reduce risk of heatstroke and severe hyperthermia. This is especially important for elderly patients and those who abuse alcohol or have chronic illness or CNS disease.
•Stress need for periodic eye examinations and intraocular pressure measurements because benztropine may cause narrow-angle glaucoma and increase intraocular pressure.

bepridil hydrochloride

Vascor

Class and Category

Chemical: Calcium channel blocker, diarylammopropylamine derivative
Therapeutic: Antianginal
Pregnancy category: C

Indications and Dosages

➤ *To treat chronic stable angina in patients who don't respond to or can't tolerate other antianginal drugs*

TABLETS
Adults. *Initial:* 200 mg/day for 10 days followed by dosage increases, depending on patient's response (ability to perform daily activities, length of QT interval, heart rate, and frequency and severity of angina attacks). *Maintenance:* 300 to 400 mg/day (maximum).

Route	Onset	Peak	Duration
P.O.	Unknown	8 days	Unknown

Contraindications

Congenital prolonged QT interval, history of serious ventricular arrhythmias, hypersensitivity to bepridil, hypotension (systolic pressure below 90 mm Hg), sick sinus syndrome and second- or third-degree AV block unless artificial pacemaker in place, uncompensated cardiac insufficiency, use of other drugs that prolong QT interval

---

Mechanism of Action
Inhibits calcium movement into coronary and vascular smooth-muscle cells by blocking slow calcium channels in their membranes. This decreases intracellular calcium level, which inhibits smooth-muscle cell contractions and causes:
• relaxation of coronary and vascular smooth muscles, decreased peripheral vascular resistance, and reduced systolic and diastolic blood pressure, which decrease myocardial oxygen demand
• depression of impulse formation (automaticity) and conduction velocity.
Bepridil also inhibits fast inward sodium channels, reducing speed and degree of action potential and increasing its duration in cardiac muscle.

Interactions
DRUGS
antiarrhythmics, such as quinidine and procainamide, with actions similar to bepridil's: Exaggerated and prolonged QT interval
beta blockers: Possibly increased depression of myocardial contractility and AV conduction
digoxin: Possibly increased serum digoxin level
fentanyl: Severe hypotension and increased need for fluid
nitrates: Additive hypotensive effect
tricyclic antidepressants: Exaggerated and prolonged QT interval

Adverse Reactions
CNS: Amnesia, anxiety, asthenia, depression, dizziness, drowsiness, fever, hallucinations, headache, insomnia, nervousness, paranoia, paresthesia, psychosis, syncope, tremor, vertigo
CV: Edema, hypertension, palpitations, premature ventricular contractions, prolonged QT interval, sinus bradycardia or tachycardia, torsades de pointes, vasodilation, ventricular fibrillation, ventricular tachycardia
EENT: Altered taste, blurred vision, dry mouth, pharyngitis, rhinitis, tinnitus
GI: Abdominal cramps or discomfort, anorexia, appetite increase, constipation, diarrhea, flatulence, gastritis, nausea
GU: Decreased libido, impotence

HEME: Agranulocytosis, leukopenia, neutropenia
MS: Arthritis, myalgia
RESP: Cough, dyspnea, respiratory tract infection
SKIN: Dermatitis, diaphoresis, rash
Other: Flulike symptoms

Nursing Considerations
• Use bepridil cautiously in patients with heart failure because it can induce new arrhythmias and may worsen heart failure.
• Because bepridil is metabolized by the liver and its metabolites are excreted in urine, monitor results of liver function studies as well as BUN and serum electrolyte and creatinine levels as appropriate.
• Assess heart rate and rhythm to obtain baseline. Then monitor frequently during therapy. Also, monitor serial 12-lead ECG tracings. Be aware that bepridil can induce new arrhythmias, including ventricular tachycardia and fibrillation (which are more difficult to convert), torsades de pointes, and prolonged QT intervals.
• **WARNING** Be alert for QT intervals that exceed 0.52 second. If this occurs, expect to reduce bepridil dose or discontinue drug.
• Monitor WBC count to detect agranulocytosis, which may require drug discontinuation.
• **WARNING** Be aware that bepridil shouldn't be discontinued abruptly. Instead, gradually taper its dosage as prescribed to prevent increased frequency and duration of chest pain as increased calcium moves into cells, causing coronary artery spasm.
• Monitor blood pressure frequently if patient also receives nitrates or beta blockers. Assess for hypotension.
• Monitor serum electrolyte levels. Especially note decreased potassium level, which may exacerbate existing arrhythmias or induce new ones.

PATIENT TEACHING
• Advise patient to avoid driving and other activities that require alertness and coordination until bepridil's CNS effects are known.

betamethasone
Celestone

betamethasone acetate-betamethasone sodium phosphate
Celestone Soluspan

betamethasone sodium phosphate

Betnesol (CAN), Celestone Phosphate, Selestoject

Class and Category

Chemical: Synthetic glucocorticoid
Therapeutic: Anti-inflammatory
Pregnancy category: C

Indications and Dosages

➤ *To treat conditions with severe inflammation and conditions requiring immunosuppression*

SYRUP, TABLETS (BETAMETHASONE)
Adults. 0.6 to 7.2 mg/day.

I.M. INJECTION (BETAMETHASONE ACETATE-BETAMETHASONE SODIUM PHOSPHATE)
Adults. 0.5 to 9 mg I.M. daily, or ⅓ to ½ of P.O. dose q 12 hr.

I.M OR I.V. INJECTION (BETAMETHASONE SODIUM PHOSPHATE)
Adults. *Initial:* Variable (given in emergency situations or when oral therapy isn't possible). *Maximum:* 9 mg/day.

➤ *To treat bursitis, gouty arthritis, osteoarthritis, periostitis of cuboid, peritendinitis, rheumatoid arthritis, skin lesions, tenosynovitis*

INTRA-ARTICULAR, INTRABURSAL, OR INTRADERMAL INJECTION (BETAMETHASONE ACETATE-BETAMETHASONE SODIUM PHOSPHATE)
Adults with bursitis, peritendinitis, or tenosynovitis. 1 ml by intrabursal or intra-articular injection. Three or four injections given q 1 to 2 wk.
Adults with osteoarthritis or rheumatoid arthritis. 0.5 to 2 ml, depending on joint size.
Adults with foot bursitis. 0.25 to 0.5 ml q 3 to 7 days.
Adults with foot tenosynovitis or periostitis of cuboid. 0.5 ml q 3 to 7 days.
Adults with acute gouty arthritis. 0.5 to 1 ml q 3 to 7 days.
Adults with skin lesions. 0.2 ml/cm² intradermally, up to 1 ml weekly.
DOSAGE ADJUSTMENT Dosage reduced for elderly patients and accompanied by periodic monitoring of blood pressure and blood glucose and electrolyte levels.

Contraindications

Idiopathic thrombocytopenic purpura (I.M. injection), live virus vaccination, systemic fungal infection

Route	Onset	Peak	Duration
P.O.	Unknown	1 to 2 hr	3.25 days
I.V., I.M. (sodium phosphate)	Rapid	Unknown	Unknown
I.M. (acetate-sodium phosphate)	1 to 3 hr	Unknown	1 wk
Other (acetate-sodium phosphate)	Unknown	Unknown	1 to 2 wk*

Mechanism of Action

Binds to intracellular glucocorticoid receptors and suppresses inflammatory and immune responses by:
• inhibiting neutrophil and monocyte accumulation at inflammation site and suppressing their phagocytic and bactericidal activity
• stabilizing lysosomal membranes
• suppressing antigen response of macrophages and helper T cells
• inhibiting synthesis of inflammatory response mediators, such as cytokines, interleukins, and prostaglandins.

Interactions

DRUGS
anticholinesterase drugs: Possibly antagonized anticholinesterase effects in myasthenia gravis
barbiturates: Possibly decreased effects of betamethasone
cyclosporine: Possibly increased risk of cyclosporine toxicity
digitalis glycosides: Possibly increased risk of digitalis toxicity
estrogens: Possibly decreased excretion of betamethasone
hydantoins, rifampin: Possibly increased excretion and decreased therapeutic effects of betamethasone
isoniazid: Possibly decreased serum isoniazid level

---

* For intra-arterial or intrasynovial injection; 1 week for intralesional injection in soft tissue.

ketoconazole: Possibly decreased excretion of betamethasone

oral anticoagulants: Possibly increased or decreased action of anticoagulants, requiring adjusted anticoagulant dosage

oral contraceptives: Possibly increased half-life and concentration and decreased excretion of betamethasone

potassium-wasting diuretics: Increased risk of hypokalemia

salicylates: Possibly decreased serum level and therapeutic effects of salicylates

somatrem: Possibly inhibition of somatrem's growth-promoting effects

theophyllines: Possibly changes in both drugs' effects

Adverse Reactions

CNS: Fatigue, headache, increased intracranial pressure with papilledema, insomnia, malaise, neuritis, paresthesia, seizures, steroid psychosis, syncope, vertigo

CV: Arrhythmias, ECG changes, fat embolism, heart failure, hypertension, thromboembolism, thrombophlebitis

EENT: Cataracts, exophthalmos, glaucoma, increased intraocular pressure

ENDO: Cushingoid symptoms (buffalo hump, central obesity, decreased carbohydrate tolerance, fat pad enlargement, moon face), fluid retention, growth suppression in children, hyperglycemia, masked signs of infection, negative nitrogen balance, secondary adrenocortical and pituitary unresponsiveness (in times of stress)

GI: Abdominal distention, increased appetite, nausea, pancreatitis, peptic ulcer possibly with perforation, ulcerative esophagitis, vomiting

GU: Amenorrhea, glycosuria, menstrual irregularities

HEME: Leukocytosis

MS: Aseptic necrosis of femoral and humeral heads, loss of muscle mass, muscle weakness, osteoporosis, spontaneous pathologic and vertebral compression fractures, tendon rupture

SKIN: Acneiform lesions, allergic dermatitis, ecchymosis, facial erythema, hirsutism, impaired wound healing, increased sweating, petechiae, lupuslike lesions, purpura, subcutaneous fat atrophy, thin and fragile skin, urticaria

Other: Angioedema, hypocalcemia, hypokalemia, sodium retention, suppressed reaction to skin tests, weight gain

Nursing Considerations

• Expect prescriber to order baseline ophthalmologic examination before initiating therapy because prolonged betamethasone use may lead to increased intraocular pressure, glaucoma, and subsequent optic nerve damage. Use betamethasone cautiously in patients with ocular herpes simplex because corneal perforation may occur.

• Assess for signs of infection before administering betamethasone because drug may mask those signs. Because drug may cause immunosuppression, new infection may develop during therapy. If so, expect to administer appropriate antibiotic.

• Review serum electrolyte levels, as ordered, before initiating therapy. Monitor these levels frequently during therapy to detect imbalances. Sodium and water retention and potassium and calcium depletion may occur with high-dose betamethasone therapy. If so, expect to restrict sodium intake and provide potassium and calcium supplements.

• Because betamethasone is linked to peptic ulcer formation, expect to administer it with an antacid or H_2-receptor blocker.

• **WARNING** Monitor ECG tracings for arrhythmias, and evaluate patient for anaphylactic reactions, such as angioedema and seizures, which have been associated with rapid I.V. administration of high-dose corticosteroids.

• **WARNING** During long-term betamethasone therapy, assess for signs of adrenal suppression and insufficiency (fatigue, hypotension, lassitude, nausea, vomiting, and weakness) when patient is exposed to stress. If she exhibits these signs, notify prescriber at once.

• Watch for signs of steroid psychosis, such as delirium, clouded sensorium, euphoria, insomnia, mood swings, personality changes, and severe depression, which may develop 15 to 30 days after therapy begins. Be prepared to discontinue therapy. If this isn't possible, expect to administer psychotropic drugs.

• Rotate I.M. injection sites. To prevent muscle atrophy, avoid S.C. injection, injection in deltoid site, and repeated I.M. injections into same site.

• Administer oral betamethasone before 9 a.m., if appropriate, to mimic body's natural release of corticosteroids.

• After intra-articular injection, assess joint

for marked increase in pain, local swelling, and more restricted movement. If patient also develops fever and malaise, suspect septic arthritis and notify prescriber immediately. Expect to assist with joint fluid aspiration to confirm septic arthritis.
•Monitor patient for cushingoid signs and symptoms, such as moon face, buffalo hump, central obesity, striae, acne, ecchymosis, and weight gain. Notify prescriber if you detect these symptoms.
•Expect to slowly taper oral betamethasone dosage to prevent adrenal insufficiency.

PATIENT TEACHING
•Instruct patient to take betamethasone with food if GI upset occurs.
•Reinforce signs of adrenal insufficiency and possible need for dosage increases during stress. Advise patient to notify prescriber immediately if signs of insufficiency occur or if she's exposed to stress.
•Instruct patient to avoid exposure to infections because drug can cause immunosuppression. Also teach patient to recognize and immediately report signs of infection.
•After intra-articular injection, advise patient not to overuse joint and to continue other treatments such as physical therapy.

betaxolol hydrochloride

Kerlone

Class and Category
Chemical: Selective beta$_1$-adrenergic blocker
Therapeutic: Antihypertensive
Pregnancy category: C

Indications and Dosages
➤ *To treat hypertension alone or with other antihypertensives*

TABLETS
Adults. *Initial:* 10 mg/day. If no response in 7 to 14 days, then 20 mg/day.
DOSAGE ADJUSTMENT For elderly patients and patients who have renal failure or are undergoing hemodialysis, initial dosage reduced to 5 mg/day. If desired response isn't achieved, dosage increased by 5-mg increments q 2 wk up to 20 mg/day.

Route	Onset	Peak	Duration
P.O.	Unknown	3 to 4 hr	Unknown

Mechanism of Action
Inhibits stimulation of beta$_1$-adrenergic receptor sites, primarily in the heart. This decreases myocardial excitability, cardiac output, and myocardial oxygen demand. It also decreases renin release from the kidneys, which helps reduce blood pressure.

Contraindications
Cardiogenic shock, heart failure unless caused by tachyarrhythmia or overt heart failure, hypersensitivity to betaxolol, second- or third-degree heart block, sinus bradycardia

Interactions
DRUGS
aluminum salts, barbiturates, calcium salts, cholestyramine, colestipol, NSAIDs, penicillins, rifampin, salicylates, sulfinpyrazone: Decreased therapeutic and adverse effects of betaxolol
beta blockers: Increased risk of additive systemic beta blockade
calcium channel blockers: Possibly increased therapeutic and adverse effects of betaxolol
ciprofloxacin, other quinolones: Possibly increased bioavailability of betaxolol, increasing the drug's pharmacologic effect
clonidine: Possibly severe hypertension when both drugs (or just clonidine) are simultaneously withdrawn
epinephrine: Possibly severe hypertension followed by bradycardia
ergot alkaloids: Possibly peripheral ischemia and gangrene
flecainide: Possibly increased therapeutic and adverse effects of both drugs
lidocaine: Possibly increased risk of lidocaine toxicity
nondepolarizing neuromuscular blockers: Possibly increased or decreased neuromuscular blockade
oral contraceptives: Possibly increased bioavailability and plasma level of betaxolol, increasing the drug's pharmacologic effect
prazosin: Possibly increased orthostatic hypotension
quinidine: Possibly increased effects of betaxolol
sulfonylureas: Possibly masking of hypoglycemic symptoms

Adverse Reactions

CNS: Amnesia, anxiety, behavior changes, confusion, CVA, depression, dizziness, emotional lability, fatigue, fever, hallucinations, headache, insomnia, lethargy, malaise, mood changes, nightmares, paresthesia, peripheral neuropathy, sedation, syncope, tremor, vertigo
CV: Arrhythmias, including asystole, bradycardia, heart block, and torsades de pointes; cardiogenic shock; chest pain; claudication; heart failure; hypercholesterolemia; hyperlipidemia; hypotension; mitral insufficiency; MI; orthostatic hypotension; peripheral vascular insufficiency; Raynaud's phenomenon; renal and mesenteric artery thrombosis
EENT: Altered taste, blurred vision, burning eyes, conjunctivitis, dry eyes, dry mouth, earache, eye irritation, eye pain or pressure, increased salivation, laryngospasm, mouth ulcers, nasal stuffiness, pharyngitis, ptosis, rhinitis, sinusitis, tinnitus
ENDO: Breast pain (in women), hyperglycemia, hypoglycemia
GI: Acute pancreatitis, anorexia, bloating, constipation, diarrhea, elevated liver function test results, epigastric pain, flatulence, gastritis, heartburn, hepatomegaly, increased appetite, indigestion, nausea, vomiting
GU: Decreased libido, dysuria, impotence, nocturia, Peyronie's disease, prostatitis, renal colic, renal failure, urinary frequency, urine retention, UTI
HEME: Agranulocytosis, eosinophilia, leukopenia, thrombocytopenia
MS: Arthralgia, arthritis, gout, muscle spasms or twitching, myalgia, neck pain, tendinitis
RESP: Bronchial obstruction, bronchitis, bronchospasm, cough, pulmonary embolus, respiratory distress, upper respiratory tract infection, wheezing
SKIN: Acne, diaphoresis, dry skin, eczema, erythema, exfoliative dermatitis, flushing, increased pigmentation, pallor, photophobia, pruritus, rash
Other: Acidosis, facial edema, hyperkalemia, hyperuricemia, lymphadenopathy, positive ANA titer, weight gain

Nursing Considerations

• Use betaxolol cautiously in patients with peripheral vascular disease. Assess color, temperature, and pulses of patient's arms and legs and ask about numbness or tingling and pain.
• Check blood pressure with patient lying, sitting, and standing before starting betaxolol therapy and periodically throughout day to detect changes.
• Review renal function test results before and during therapy.
• Closely monitor diabetic patient's blood glucose level for hypoglycemia because betaxolol may mask tachycardia, but not dizziness and diaphoresis. Be aware that betaxolol may mask tachycardia and blood pressure changes associated with hyperthyroidism.
• **WARNING** Avoid abrupt withdrawal of betaxolol, which can exacerbate or precipitate thyroid storm. Instead, expect to withdraw drug gradually and monitor patient closely.
• Expect to discontinue betaxolol over 2 weeks to prevent MI, ventricular arrhythmias, and, possibly, death from catecholamine hypersensitivity caused by beta blocker therapy.
• If systolic pressure falls below 90 mm Hg, expect to discontinue drug and prepare for hemodynamic monitoring.
• Take safety precautions to prevent injury from falls caused by orthostatic hypotension.

PATIENT TEACHING
• Teach patient how to check her blood pressure, if appropriate. Also discuss signs and symptoms of hypertension and hypotension.
• Advise patient to avoid sudden position changes and to rise slowly from a sitting or lying position to minimize the effects of orthostatic hypotension.
• Advise patient to avoid driving and activities that require mental alertness until drug's CNS effects are known.
• Counsel patient to consult prescriber before using an OTC product, such as a cold remedy or nasal decongestant.

bethanechol chloride

Duvoid, PMS-Bethanechol chloride (CAN), Urabeth, Urecholine

Class and Category

Chemical: Synthetic choline ester
Therapeutic: Cholinergic, parasympathomimetic
Pregnancy category: C

Indications and Dosages

➤ *To treat postoperative and postpartal urine retention and retention caused by neurogenic atony of bladder*

TABLETS

Adults. 10 to 50 mg t.i.d. or q.i.d. *To determine minimum effective dose:* 5 to 10 mg repeated q hr until response is obtained or maximum of 50 mg is reached.

S.C. INJECTION

Adults. 2.5 to 5.0 mg t.i.d. or q.i.d. *To determine minimum effective dose:* 2.5 mg repeated q 15 to 30 min until response is obtained or maximum of four doses is reached. Minimum effective dose may be repeated t.i.d. or q.i.d., p.r.n.

Route	Onset	Peak	Duration
P.O.	30 to 90 min	60 min	6 hr
S.C.	5 to 15 min	15 to 30 min	2 hr

Mechanism of Action

Acts directly on muscarinic receptors of parasympathetic nervous system, increasing detrusor muscle tone in bladder and allowing contraction of sufficient strength to initiate voiding. Similar to natural neurotransmitter acetylcholine, bethanechol also stimulates gastric motility, increases gastric tone, and enhances peristalsis.

Contraindications

Acute inflammatory lesions of GI tract, AV conduction defects, bronchial asthma, coronary artery disease, epilepsy, hypersensitivity to bethanecol or its components, hypertension, hyperthyroidism, hypotension, marked vagotonia, mechanical obstruction of GI or GU tract, Parkinson's disease, peptic ulcer disease, peritonitis, pronounced bradycardia, questionable integrity of GI or GU mucosa, spastic GI disorders, vasomotor instability

Interactions

DRUGS

cholinergic drugs: Possibly increased effects of bethanechol
ganglionic blockers: Possibly severe hypotension, usually first manifested by severe adverse GI reactions
procainamide, quinidine: Possibly decreased effects of bethanechol

Adverse Reactions

CNS: Headache, malaise
CV: Hypotension with reflex tachycardia, vasomotor response
EENT: Excessive salivation, lacrimation, miosis

GI: Abdominal cramps, colicky pain, diarrhea, eructation, nausea, vomiting
GU: Urinary urgency
RESP: Asthma attack, bronchoconstriction

Nursing Considerations

• Assess urine elimination before initiating bethanechol therapy.

• **WARNING** Be aware that patient must have functioning urinary sphincter because a sphincter that doesn't relax when bladder contracts can push urine up into renal pelvis and cause reflux infection.

• Administer oral bethanechol 1 hour before or 2 hours after meals to reduce risk of nausea and vomiting.

• **WARNING** Don't administer bethanechol I.M. or I.V. because of risk of cholinergic overstimulation, which can cause abdominal cramps, bloody diarrhea, hypotension, shock, or sudden cardiac arrest. Always keep atropine nearby during S.C. administration.

PATIENT TEACHING

• Advise patient to take bethanechol on an empty stomach 1 hour before or 2 hours after meals to reduce risk of nausea and vomiting.

biperiden hydrochloride

Akineton

biperiden lactate

Akineton Lactate

Class and Category

Chemical: Tertiary amine
Therapeutic: Anticholinergic, antidyskinetic
Pregnancy category: C

Indications and Dosages

➤ *As adjunct to treat all forms of Parkinson's disease*

TABLETS

Adults. 2 mg t.i.d. or q.i.d up to 16 mg/day.

➤ *To control extrapyramidal symptoms (except tardive dyskinesia) caused by phenothiazines and other neuroleptic drugs*

TABLETS

Adults. 2 mg q.d. to t.i.d.

I.V. OR I.M. INJECTION

Adults. 2 mg repeated q 30 min until symptoms resolve or maximum of four consecutive doses in 24 hr is reached.

B

Route	Onset	Peak	Duration
I.V.	15 min	Unknown	1 to 8 hr
I.M.	10 to 30 min	Unknown	Unknown

Mechanism of Action

Blocks acetylcholine's action at cholinergic receptor sites. This action restores the brain's normal dopamine and acetylcholine balance, which relaxes muscle movement and decreases rigidity and tremors. Biperiden also may inhibit dopamine reuptake and storage, which prolongs dopamine's action.

Contraindications

Achalasia, bladder neck obstruction, hypersensitivity to biperiden, myasthenia gravis, narrow-angle glaucoma, prostatic hypertrophy, pyloric or duodenal obstruction, stenosing peptic ulcer, toxic megacolon

Interactions

DRUGS

amantadine: Possibly increased adverse anticholinergic effects
digoxin: Possibly increased serum digoxin level
haloperidol: Possibly increased schizophrenic symptoms, decreased serum haloperidol level, and development of tardive dyskinesia
levodopa: Possibly decreased levodopa effectiveness
phenothiazines: Possibly reduced phenothiazine effects and increased psychiatric symptoms

Adverse Reactions

CNS: Agitation, confusion, delirium, delusions, depression, disorientation, dizziness, drowsiness, euphoria, excitement, fever, hallucinations, headache, light-headedness, listlessness, memory loss, nervousness, paranoia, psychosis, weakness
CV: Hypotension, mild bradycardia, orthostatic hypotension, palpitations, tachycardia
EENT: Blurred vision, diplopia, dry mouth, increased intraocular pressure, mydriasis, narrow-angle glaucoma, suppurative parotitis
GI: Constipation, duodenal ulcer, epigastric distress, ileus, nausea, vomiting
GU: Dysuria, urinary hesitancy, urine retention
MS: Muscle spasms, muscle weakness
SKIN: Decreased sweating, dermatosis, flushing, rash, urticaria

Nursing Considerations

•Expect to administer I.V. or I.M. biperiden when patient needs more rapid response than oral drug can provide.
•Assess muscle rigidity and tremor as baseline. Then monitor them frequently for improvement, which indicates biperiden's effectiveness.
•WARNING When administering biperiden to patient with drug-induced extrapyramidal reactions, be alert for exacerbation of psychiatric symptoms.

PATIENT TEACHING

•Caution patient to avoid driving and other activities that require alertness until biperiden's CNS effects are known.
•WARNING Because biperiden decreases sweating, urge patient to avoid extremely hot and humid conditions to reduce risk of heatstroke and severe hyperthermia. This is especially important for elderly patients and those who abuse alcohol or have chronic illness or CNS disease.
•Stress need for periodic eye examinations and intraocular pressure measurements because biperiden may cause narrow-angle glaucoma and increase intraocular pressure.

bisoprolol fumarate

Zebeta

Class and Category

Chemical: Selective beta$_1$-adrenergic blocker
Therapeutic: Antihypertensive
Pregnancy category: C

Indications and Dosages

➤ *To treat hypertension, alone or with other antihypertensives*

TABLETS

Adults. 5 mg q.d., increased to 10 to 20 mg q.d. if blood pressure doesn't respond to lower dosage.

DOSAGE ADJUSTMENT Dosage reduced to 2.5 mg q.d. initially and increased gradually for patients with impaired renal function and creatinine clearance of less than 40 ml/min/1.73 m^2 or with impaired hepatic function, such as from cirrhosis or hepatitis.

Contraindications

Cardiogenic shock, heart failure unless caused by tachyarrhythmia, overt heart failure, second- or third-degree heart block, sinus bradycardia

Mechanism of Action
Inhibits stimulation of beta$_1$-receptors primarily in the heart, which decreases cardiac excitability, cardiac output, and myocardial oxygen demand. Bisoprolol also decreases renin release from kidneys, which helps reduce blood pressure.

Interactions
DRUGS
aluminum salts, barbiturates, calcium salts, cholestyramine, colestipol, NSAIDs, penicillins, rifampin, salicylates, sulfinpyrazone: Possibly decreased therapeutic and adverse effects of bisoprolol
calcium channel blockers: Possibly increased therapeutic and adverse effects of bisoprolol
ciprofloxacin, quinolones: Possibly increased bioavailability of bisoprolol
clonidine: Possibly severe hypertension caused by withdrawal of clonidine or both drugs
epinephrine: Possibly hypertension followed by bradycardia
ergot alkaloids: Possibly peripheral ischemia and gangrene
flecainide: Possibly increased therapeutic and adverse effects of either drug
lidocaine: Possibly increased risk of lidocaine toxicity
oral contraceptives: Possibly increased bioavailability and plasma level of bisoprolol
prazosin: Possibly increased orthostatic hypotension
quinidine: Possibly increased effects of bisoprolol
sulfonylureas: Possibly masking of hypoglycemic symptoms

Adverse Reactions
CNS: Anxiety, confusion, depression, dizziness, emotional lability, fatigue, fever, hallucinations, headache, insomnia, malaise, nightmares, paresthesia, tremor, vertigo
CV: Bradycardia, heart block, and other arrhythmias; chest pain; claudication; cold arms and legs; edema; heart failure; hypercholesterolemia; hyperlipidemia; hypotension; MI; orthostatic hypotension; palpitations; peripheral vascular insufficiency; renal and mesenteric artery thrombosis
EENT: Altered taste, blurred vision, dry mouth, eye pain or pressure, increased sali-
vation, laryngospasm, pharyngitis, rhinitis, sinusitis, tinnitus
GI: Constipation, diarrhea, epigastric pain, gastritis, indigestion, ischemic colitis, nausea, vomiting
GU: Cystitis, decreased libido, impotence, Peyronie's disease, renal colic
HEME: Agranulocytosis, eosinophilia, leukopenia, thrombocytopenia, thrombocytopenic purpura
MS: Arthralgia, gout, muscle twitching, neck pain
RESP: Asthma, bronchitis, bronchospasm, cough, dyspnea, respiratory distress, upper respiratory tract infection
SKIN: Alopecia, diaphoresis, eczema, exfoliative dermatitis, flushing, pruritus, rash
Other: Angioedema, hyperkalemia, hyperuricemia, weight gain

Nursing Considerations
• Use bisoprolol cautiously in patients with peripheral vascular disease because reduced cardiac output can precipitate or aggravate symptoms of arterial insufficiency. Assess arms and legs for changes in color, temperature, and pulses; ask about numbness, tingling, and pain.
• Measure blood pressure with patient lying, sitting, and standing before initiating bisoprolol therapy and then every 4 to 8 hours, as appropriate, to evaluate drug effectiveness.
• If patient has diabetes, monitor closely for signs of hypoglycemia, which may be masked by bisoprolol.
• If patient has hyperthyroidism, monitor for signs of continued hyperthyroidism, such as tachycardia and hypertension, which may be masked by bisoprolol.
• **WARNING** Keep in mind that abrupt withdrawal of bisoprolol may exacerbate or precipitate thyroid storm. During drug withdrawal, monitor patient closely.
• Expect to discontinue bisoprolol over 1 to 2 weeks to prevent MI, ventricular arrhythmias, and, possibly, death from catecholamine hypersensitivity caused by beta blocker therapy.
• If systolic blood pressure falls below 90 mm Hg, expect to discontinue drug. Prepare for hemodynamic monitoring, if needed.
• **WARNING** If patient is scheduled for surgery with general anesthesia, expect to discontinue bisoprolol about 48 hours beforehand to reduce risk of excessive myocardial depression during anesthesia.

PATIENT TEACHING
• Teach patient how to monitor her blood pressure, if appropriate, and to recognize signs of hypertension and hypotension.
• Instruct patient to avoid sudden position changes and to rise slowly from a sitting or lying position to minimize the effects of orthostatic hypotension.
• Advise patient to avoid driving and other activities that require mental alertness until bisoprolol's CNS effects are known.
• Instruct patient to contact prescriber before using any OTC product, such as a cold remedy or nasal decongestant.

bitolterol mesylate

Tornalate

Class and Category
Chemical: Acid ester of colterol
Therapeutic: Bronchodilator, sympathomimetic
Pregnancy category: C

Indications and Dosages
➤ *To prevent and treat asthma and other conditions associated with reversible bronchospasm, such as emphysema and chronic bronchitis*
INTERMITTENT AEROSOL SOLUTION
Adults and children age 12 and older. 1 mg of bitolterol diluted in 0.5 ml of NS and inhaled over 10 to 15 min t.i.d. *Maximum:* 8 mg/day.
CONTINUOUS AEROSOL SOLUTION
Adults and children age 12 and older. 2.5 mg of bitolterol diluted in 1.25 ml of NS and inhaled over 10 to 15 min t.i.d. *Maximum:* 14 mg/day.
METERED-DOSE INHALER
Adults and children age 12 and older. *To treat acute bronchospasm:* 2 inhalations over 1 to 3 min followed by a third inhalation, if needed.
To prevent bronchospasm: 2 inhalations q 8 hr not to exceed 3 inhalations q 6 hr or 2 inhalations q 4 hr.

Route	Onset	Peak	Duration
Aerosol, inhalation	In 2 to 3 min	30 to 60 min	6 to 8 hr
Metered-dose inhalation	3 to 5 min	30 min to 2 hr	4 to 8 hr

Mechanism of Action
Is hydrolyzed to active agent colterol (a long-acting agent that primarily affects beta$_2$-adrenergic receptors). Then it attaches to beta$_2$ receptors on bronchial cell membranes. This action stimulates the intracellular enzyme adenylate cyclase to convert adenosine triphosphate to cAMP. An increased intracellular level of cAMP relaxes bronchial smooth-muscle cells, stabilizes mast cells, and inhibits histamine release.

Incompatibilities
Don't mix bitolterol in inhalation solution with cromolyn sodium or acetylcysteine.

Contraindications
Hypersensitivity to bitolterol or its ingredients

Interactions
DRUGS
beta blockers: Possibly inhibition of bronchodilating effect of bitolterol
epinephrine, other sympathomimetic drugs: Possibly additive effects of either drug
MAO inhibitors, tricyclic antidepressants: Possibly potentiation of bitolterol's action on cardiovascular system

Adverse Reactions
CNS: Dizziness, fatigue, headache, hyperkinesia, insomnia, light-headedness, nervousness, paresthesia, somnolence, tremor, vertigo
CV: Chest pain, hypertension, irregular pulse, palpitations, tachycardia, transient ECG changes
EENT: Mouth and throat irritation, rhinitis
GI: Elevated liver function test results, nausea
HEME: Decreased hemoglobin level, hematocrit, and WBC count
RESP: Bronchospasm, cough

Nursing Considerations
• Assess respiratory rate, rhythm, and depth and breath sounds before, during, and after bitolterol therapy. Expect improved air movement and improvement in abnormal breath sounds.
• Because beta-adrenergic bronchodilators can significantly increase blood pressure and pulse rate, monitor blood pressure and pulse rate frequently.

•Expect therapy to begin with lowest effective dose because higher doses or more frequent use may reduce drug effectiveness and cause paradoxical reactions or overdose.

PATIENT TEACHING

•Teach patient how to properly use and care for aerosol nebulizer or metered-dose inhaler. Before patient uses aerosol nebulizer, advise her to look for slight bubbling in solution-filled chamber and fine mist when nebulizer is turned on. Before patient uses inhaler for first time, instruct her to check that it's working properly by spraying it once in the air and looking for fine mist.

•Teach patient to mix nebulizer solution immediately before each use. After treatment, instruct patient to clean nebulizer and solution chamber according to manufacturer's recommendations.

•WARNING Advise patient not to use more than the recommended dosage of bitolterol because of the risk of death associated with excessive use of sympathomimetic drugs.

•If two or three metered-dose inhalations are prescribed, tell patient to wait 1 to 3 minutes between inhalations.

bivalirudin

Angiomax

Class and Category

Chemical: Hirudin analogue
Therapeutic: Anticoagulant
Pregnancy category: B

Indications and Dosages

➤ *As adjunct to provide anticoagulation and to prevent thrombosis in patients with unstable angina who are undergoing percutaneous transluminal coronary angioplasty*

I.V. INFUSION

Adults. *Initial:* Immediately before angioplasty, 1-mg/kg bolus, then 2.5 mg/kg/hr for 4 hr by continuous infusion, followed by 0.2 mg/kg/hr for up to 20 hr.

DOSAGE ADJUSTMENT Dosage possibly reduced by 20% for patients with moderate renal impairment (glomerular filtration rate [GFR] of 30 to 59 ml/min), by 60% for patients with severe renal impairment (GFR of 10 to 29 ml/min), and by 90% for dialysis-dependent patients.

Route	Onset	Peak	Duration
I.V.	Immediate	Unknown	1 hr after end of infusion

Mechanism of Action

Selectively binds to thrombin, including thrombin trapped in established clots. Without thrombin, fibrinogen can't convert to fibrin and clots can't form.

Incompatibilities

Don't mix any other drugs in same I.V. line before or during bivalirudin administration. Mixing with alteplase, amiodarone, amphotericin B, chlorpromazine HCL, diazepam, prochlorperazine edisylate, reteplase, streptokinase, and vancomycin HCL can result in haze, particulate formation, or precipitation.

Contraindications

Active major bleeding, hypersensitivity to bivalirudin or its components

Interactions

DRUGS

alteplase, antineoplastic drugs, antithymocyte globulin, heparin, NSAIDs, platelet inhibitors, reteplase, streptokinase, strontium chloride Sr 89, warfarin: Additive risk of bleeding
porfimer: Possibly decreased efficacy of porfimer photodynamic therapy
salicylates: Increased risk of hypoprothrombinemia and bleeding

Adverse Reactions

CNS: Headache, intracranial hemorrhage
CV: Hypotension
EENT: Bleeding from mouth, epistaxis
GI: Abdominal cramps, diarrhea, GI or retroperitoneal bleeding, nausea, vomiting
GU: Hematuria, vaginal bleeding
MS: Back pain
RESP: Hemoptysis, hemothorax
SKIN: Ecchymosis
Other: Injection site bleeding, hematoma, or pain

Nursing Considerations

•To reconstitute bivalirudin, add 5 ml of sterile water for injection to each 250-mg vial and swirl gently until dissolved. For initial infusion, further dilute each reconstituted vial in 50 ml of D_5W or NS to a final concentration of 5 mg/ml.

•For subsequent low-rate infusion, further

dilute reconstituted drug in 500 ml of D_5W or NS to a final concentration of 0.5 mg/ml.
•Expect to give patient 300 to 325 mg of aspirin P.O. daily, as prescribed, during bivalirudin therapy.
•**WARNING** Expect to monitor blood coagulation tests before and regularly during therapy because bleeding is a major risk associated with bivalirudin use.
•**WARNING** Monitor patient frequently for signs and symptoms of bleeding because no specific antidote for bivalirudin is available. If life-threatening bleeding occurs, notify prescriber immediately, discontinue drug therapy, and prepare to monitor APTT and other coagulation tests as ordered. Be aware that blood transfusions may be necessary. Patients with an increased risk of bleeding include females with active menstruation; patients with known vascular or organ abnormalities, such as severe uncontrolled hypertension, advanced renal disease, infective endocarditis, dissecting aortic aneurysm, diverticulitis, hemophilia, hepatic disease (especially if due to a deficiency in vitamin K–dependent clotting factors), inflammatory bowel disease, or peptic ulcer disease; and those who have recently had a CVA, major surgery (including eye, brain, or spinal cord surgery), large vessel or lumbar puncture, organ biopsy, spinal anesthesia, or major bleeding (including intracranial, GI, intraocular, retroperitoneal, or pulmonary bleeding).
•If possible, avoid I.M. injections of any kind to decrease the risk of bleeding.
•Discard any unused portion of drug.

PATIENT TEACHING
•Inform patient that bivalirudin is a blood thinner used only in the hospital setting.
•Instruct patient to check her skin for bruising or red spots and to immediately report back or stomach pain, difficulty breathing, dizziness or fainting, and unusual bleeding, such as black or tarry stools, blood in urine, coughing up blood, heavy menstrual bleeding, or nosebleeds. Drug may need to be discontinued.
•Urge patient to avoid injury while receiving bivalirudin—for example, by brushing her teeth gently, using a soft-bristled toothbrush.
•Caution patient not to take anti-inflammatory drugs, such as ibuprofen, naproxen, ketoprofen, aspirin, and aspirin-like products, or other blood thinners, such as warfarin, while receiving bivalirudin unless prescriber instructs her to do so.

bosentan

Tracleer

Class and Category

Chemical: Endothelin receptor antagonist, pyrimidine derivative
Therapeutic: Antihypertensive
Pregnancy category: X

Indications and Dosages

➤ *To treat pulmonary arterial hypertension in patients with World Health Organization class III or IV symptoms, to improve exercise ability, and to slow worsening of clinical condition*

TABLETS
Adults. *Initial:* 62.5 mg b.i.d. in the morning and evening for 4 wk. *Maintenance:* 125 mg b.i.d. in the morning and evening.
DOSAGE ADJUSTMENT For adults who weigh less than 40 kg (88 lb), maintenance dosage decreased to 62.5 mg b.i.d. in the morning and evening.

Contraindications

Hypersensitivity to bosentan or its components, concurrent use of cyclosporine or glyburide, pregnancy

Interactions

DRUGS
atorvastatin, lovastatin, simvastatin: Decreased blood level and efficacy of these drugs
cyclosporine: Markedly increased blood bosentan level
glyburide: Elevated liver enzyme levels and possibly increased glucose level; possibly decreased blood level of both drugs (and of other oral antidiabetic drugs metabolized by CYP2C9 or CYP3A4)
hormonal contraceptives (oral, injectable, implantable): Possibly decreased contraceptive effects
ketoconazole and other CYP3A4 inhibitors: Increased blood level and possibly effects of bosentan
warfarin: Increased elimination and decreased blood level of warfarin

Adverse Reactions

CNS: Fatigue, headache
CV: Edema, hypotension, palpitations
EENT: Nasopharyngitis
GI: Elevated liver function test results, hepatic injury, indigestion

Mechanism of Action

Bosentan is an endothelin receptor antagonist that inhibits the effects of endothelin (ET), a potent vasoconstrictor. ET, a neurohormone produced by endothelial cells that line blood vessels, normally increases during times of cardiovascular stress. Patients with pulmonary arterial hypertension have an abnormal increase in the blood ET level.

ET binds with its receptors, ET_A and ET_B, which are located on endothelial and vascular smooth-muscle cells. When ET binds with these receptors, it causes vasoconstriction, as shown below left, and such long-term effects as fibrosis and hypertrophy. By binding to ET_A and ET_B receptors, as shown below right, bosentan blocks the vasoconstrictive effects of ET, causing pulmonary artery vasodilation and decreased pulmonary artery pressure. As a result, the patient experiences increased exercise tolerance and decreased breathlessness.

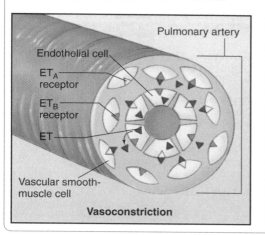

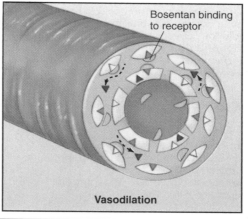

HEME: Decreased hemoglobin level and hematocrit
SKIN: Flushing, pruritus

Nursing Considerations

•Before administering bosentan, obtain baseline hemoglobin level and liver function test results, as ordered.
•WARNING Because bosentan use may cause major birth defects, make sure that female patient of childbearing age has undergone a pregnancy test and isn't pregnant before administering drug.
•WARNING Be aware that bosentan may put patient at risk for serious hepatic injury. Assess patient for signs and symptoms of hepatic dysfunction, including jaundice, nausea, vomiting, fever, abdominal pain, and fatigue. Monitor liver function test results every month, as ordered.
•Expect dosage to be adjusted or drug discontinued if liver function test results become elevated. Expect treatment to be stopped if bilirubin level increases to twice the upper limit of normal (or higher) or if clinical symptoms occur in conjunction with liver function test elevations. Bosentan probably won't be prescribed for patients with moderate to severe hepatic dysfunction or for those with liver function test levels higher than three times the upper limit of normal.
•Monitor hemoglobin level 1 and 3 months after initiation of therapy and every 3 months thereafter, as ordered.
•Monitor patient's response to drug, and evaluate her activity tolerance.

PATIENT TEACHING
•WARNING Because major birth defects are associated with bosentan, caution female patient of childbearing age to have a urine or serum pregnancy test monthly during bosentan therapy to verify that she isn't pregnant. Advise her to notify prescriber immediately

if she experiences a late or missed menstrual period. Instruct patient to use a reliable non-hormonal method of contraception because bosentan may decrease the effectiveness of hormonal contraceptives.

• Urge patient to immediately report signs or symptoms of hepatic dysfunction, including yellow skin or eyes, fever, nausea, vomiting, fatigue, and abdominal pain.

• Stress the importance of keeping appointments for follow-up testing so that drug's effects can be evaluated.

• Inform patient that bosentan is dispensed only by a special access program set up by the drug's manufacturer and is not available from a commercial pharmacy. Advise her to allow for delivery time when refilling prescription so that she doesn't run out of drug. Instruct her to review the medication guide that comes with each renewed prescription.

bretylium tosylate

Bretylate (CAN), Bretylol

Class and Category

Chemical: Bromobenzyl quaternary ammonium compound
Therapeutic: Class III antiarrhythmic
Pregnancy category: C

Indications and Dosages

➤ *To prevent and treat ventricular fibrillation and treat life-threatening ventricular arrhythmias that don't respond to first-line antiarrhythmics, such as lidocaine*

I.V. INFUSION, I.V. OR I.M. INJECTION

Adults with immediate life-threatening ventricular arrhythmias. *Initial:* 5 mg/kg undiluted by rapid I.V. injection; if ventricular fibrillation persists, 10 mg/kg repeated as often as needed. *Continuous suppression:* 1 to 2 mg/min or 5 to 10 mg/kg of diluted I.V. solution infused over at least 8 min q 6 hr.

Adults with other ventricular arrhythmias. *Initial:* 5 to 10 mg/kg of diluted I.V. solution infused over at least 8 min, repeated q 1 to 2 hr if arrhythmia continues; or 5 to 10 mg/kg undiluted I.M. injection, repeated q 1 to 2 hr if arrhythmia continues. *Maintenance:* 5 to 10 mg/kg diluted I.V. solution infused over at least 8 q 6 hours, 1 to 2 mg/min infused continuously, or 5 to 10 mg/kg undiluted I.M. injection q 6 to 8 hr.

DOSAGE ADJUSTMENT Interval between dosages increased for patients with impaired renal function because bretylium is excreted primarily by kidneys.

Children with acute ventricular fibrillation. 5 mg/kg I.V. given over 8 to 10 min, followed by 10 mg/kg q 15 to 30 min up to total dose of 30 mg/kg. *Maintenance:* 5 to 10 mg/kg q 6 hr.

Children with other ventricular arrhythmias. 5 to 10 mg/kg q 6 hr.

Route	Onset	Peak	Duration
I.V.	5 to 10 min*	6 to 9 hr	6 to 24 hr
I.M.	20 to 60 min*	6 to 9 hr	6 to 24 hr

Contraindications

Digitalis toxicity, hypersensitivity to bretylium

Interactions

DRUGS

catecholamines, such as dopamine and norepinephrine: Increased vasopressor effects of catecholamines
digoxin: Possibly worsening of digitalis toxicity

Adverse Reactions

CNS: Anxiety, confusion, dizziness, emotional lability, fever, lethargy, light-headedness, paranoid psychosis, syncope, vertigo
CV: Angina, arrhythmias (including bradycardia and more frequent PVCs), hypotension, orthostatic hypotension, transient hypertension
EENT: Mild conjunctivitis, nasal stuffiness
GI: Abdominal pain, diarrhea, hiccups, nausea, vomiting
GU: Renal impairment
RESP: Dyspnea
SKIN: Diaphoresis, erythematous macular rash, flushing
Other: Pain at I.V. or I.M. injection site

Nursing Considerations

• **WARNING** Use bretylium cautiously in patients with severe aortic stenosis or pulmonary hypertension because hypotension may occur.

---

* For suppression of ventricular fibrillation; 20 to 120 min for suppression of ventricular tachycardia.

Mechanism of Action

Bretylium prolongs the repolarization phase of the action potential and lengthens the effective refractory period, which helps terminate reentry arrhythmias. The drug also acts on adrenergic nerve terminals. Initially, it causes early release of norepinephrine, which increases the heart rate and blood pressure. Then it blocks the release of norepinephrine, as shown here. This reduces the heart rate and blood pressure. Bretylium also increases the ventricular threshold, making the ventricular myocardium less responsive to ectopic impulses and preventing ventricular fibrillation.

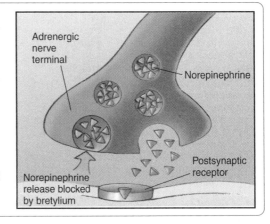

• For I.V. infusion, dilute bretylium and administer at 1 to 2 mg/min.

• Dilute bretylium in compatible I.V. solution, such as D_5W, D_5NS, D_5LR, NS, 5% sodium bicarbonate, 20% mannitol, 1/6 molar sodium lactate, LR, calcium chloride in D_5W, and potassium chloride in D_5W.

• **WARNING** Be aware that patient may experience hypotension while supine. Have patient remain supine until tolerance develops. If her supine systolic blood pressure falls below 75 mm Hg, expect to administer dopamine or norepinephrine and monitor her blood pressure closely because vasopressor effects are increased when these drugs are given together.

• Be alert for transient hypertension and increased frequency of arrhythmias because bretylium initially triggers release of norepinephrine. Monitor patient's ECG tracings and blood pressure continuously and notify prescriber of changes.

• Monitor serum bretylium level. Notify prescriber if level falls outside therapeutic range of 0.5 to 1.5 mcg/ml.

PATIENT TEACHING

• Advise patient to immediately report chest pain or pressure, pain at I.V. site, or rash.

• Warn patient that she may feel dizzy or lightheaded even when lying down. Instruct her to remain supine and ask for assistance when attempting to move or sit up. Tell her that this sensation usually subsides in a few days.

bromocriptine mesylate

Alti-Bromocriptine (CAN), Apo-Bromocriptine (CAN), Parlodel, Parlodel SnapTabs

Class and Category

Chemical: Ergot alkaloid derivative
Therapeutic: Antidyskinetic, antihyperprolactinemic, dopamine-receptor agonist, growth hormone suppressant, infertility therapy adjunct
Pregnancy category: B

Indications and Dosages

➤ *To treat amenorrhea, galactorrhea, male hypogonadism, and infertility from hyperprolactinemia*

CAPSULES, TABLETS

Adults. *Initial:* 1.25 to 2.5 mg q h.s. with snack. Increased by 2.5 mg q 3 to 7 days as needed to a total daily dose of 5 to 7.5 mg given in divided doses with snacks. *Maintenance:* 2.5 mg b.i.d. or t.i.d. with meals.

➤ *To treat prolactin-secreting adenoma*

CAPSULES, TABLETS

Adults and children age 15 and older. *Initial:* 1.25 mg b.i.d. or t.i.d. with meals. Increased gradually over several weeks, if needed, to 10 to 20 mg/day in divided doses with meals. Some patients may need higher doses. *Maintenance:* 2.5 to 20 mg/day in divided doses with meals.

➤ *To treat Parkinson's disease*

CAPSULES, TABLETS

Adults. *Initial:* 1.25 mg q h.s. with snack or b.i.d. with meals. Increased by 2.5 mg q 14 to 28 days, if needed. *Maintenance:* 2.5 to 40 mg/day in divided doses with meals.

➤ *To treat acromegaly*

CAPSULES, TABLETS

Adults and children age 15 and older. *Initial:* 1.25 to 2.5 mg q h.s. with snack for 3 days. Then increased by 1.25 to 2.5 mg q 3 to 7 days, if needed, up to 30 mg/day. *Maintenance:* Usually 10 to 30 mg/day h.s. with snack or in divided doses with meals.

Route	Onset	Peak	Duration
P.O.*	2 hr	8 hr	24 hr
P.O.†	30 to 90 min	2 hr	Unknown
P.O.‡	1 to 2 hr	4 to 8 wk	4 to 8 hr

Mechanism of Action

Inhibits the release of prolactin and growth hormone from the anterior pituitary gland, thus restoring testicular or ovarian function and suppressing lactation. The drug decreases dopamine turnover in the CNS, depleting dopamine or blocking dopamine receptors in the brain. This alleviates dyskinesia.

Contraindications

Hypersensitivity to bromocriptine, other ergot alkaloids, or their components; severe ischemic heart disease or peripheral vascular disease

Interactions

DRUGS

antihypertensives: Increased hypotensive effects

clarithromycin, erythromycin, troleandomycin: Increased risk of bromocriptine toxicity

ergot alkaloids or derivatives: Increased risk of hypertension

haloperidol, loxapine, MAO inhibitors, methyldopa, metoclopramide, molindone, pheno-

thiazines, pimozide, reserpine, risperidone, thioxanthenes: Increased serum prolactin level, decreased bromocriptine effectiveness

levodopa: Additive effects requiring reduced levodopa dose

ritonavir: Increased blood bromocriptine level

ACTIVITIES

alcohol use: Possibly disulfiram-like reaction

Adverse Reactions

CNS: Dizziness, drowsiness, fatigue, headache, light-headedness, syncope

CV: Hypertension, hypotension, orthostatic hypotension, Raynaud's phenomenon

EENT: Dry mouth, nasal congestion

GI: Abdominal cramps, anorexia, constipation, diarrhea, GI bleeding, indigestion, nausea, vomiting

Nursing Considerations

• Use bromocriptine cautiously if patient has a history of psychosis or cardiovascular disease, especially after MI with residual arrhythmia.

• Expect to perform a pregnancy test every 4 weeks during the amenorrheic period. Once menses resume, test whenever a period is missed, as ordered.

• Plan to withhold bromocriptine if patient becomes pregnant.

• If a rapidly expanding adenoma requires continued therapy, monitor closely for hypertensive crisis.

• Be aware that bromocriptine shouldn't be given post partum if patient has a history of coronary artery disease or other severe cardiovascular problem unless risk of withdrawing drug is greater than risk of use. If so, monitor closely for signs and symptoms of cardiovascular dysfunction, such as chest pain.

• Expect to give bromocriptine with levodopa if patient is being treated for Parkinson's disease.

• Assess for hypotension (when therapy starts) and hypertension (typically during second week). Monitor blood pressure frequently if patient takes other drugs with hypertensive effects.

• If patient has a history of peptic ulcer or GI bleeding, monitor for signs and symptoms of new bleeding.

• Take safety precautions, such as keeping the bed in low position with side rails up, because bromocriptine can cause dizziness, drowsiness, light-headedness, and syncope.

---

* For amenorrhea, galactorrhea, male hypogonadism, infertility from hyperprolactinemia, and prolactin-secreting adenoma.

† For Parkinson's disease.

‡ For acromegaly.

PATIENT TEACHING

•Tell patient to take each dose with a meal, milk, or a snack to minimize nausea.
•Caution patient about possible dizziness, drowsiness, and light-headedness.
•Advise patient to avoid sudden position changes to minimize the effects of orthostatic hypotension.
•Warn patient to avoid alcohol while taking bromocriptine because it may cause disulfiram-like reactions, such as chest pain, confusion, a fast or pounding heartbeat, facial flushing, diaphoresis, nausea, vomiting, a throbbing headache, blurred vision, and severe weakness.
•Tell patient to take a missed dose as soon as she remembers it, unless it's almost time for the next dose. In that case, tell her to wait until the next scheduled dose. Warn her not to double the dose. Advise her to contact prescriber if she misses more than one dose.
•Urge patient to notify prescriber if adverse reactions, such as an unremitting headache, nausea, vomiting, or other signs of CNS toxicity, develop.
•Tell patient who takes large doses of bromocriptine to schedule regular dental checkups because the drug can decrease salivary flow, which may encourage dental caries, periodontal disease, oral candidiasis, and discomfort.
•Tell patient with acromegaly to keep her fingers warm to prevent cold-sensitive digital vasospasm.

budesonide

Pulmicort Respules, Pulmicort Turbuhaler, Rhinocort, Rhinocort Aqua, Rhinocort Turbuhaler (CAN)

Class and Category

Chemical: Glucocorticoid
Therapeutic: Antiasthmatic, anti-inflammatory
Pregnancy category: C, B (Pulmicort Turbuhaler only)

Indications and Dosages

➤ *To manage symptoms of seasonal or perennial allergic rhinitis*

NASAL AEROSOL

Adults and children over age 6. 64 mcg in each nostril b.i.d. or 128 mcg in each nostril q.d. *Maximum:* 256 mcg/day. *Maintenance:* Lowest dosage that controls symptoms.

NASAL POWDER

Adults and children over age 6. 200 mcg in each nostril q.d. *Maximum:* 800 mcg/day (adults and adolescents); 400 mcg/day (children). *Maintenance:* Lowest dosage that controls symptoms.

NASAL SUSPENSION

Adults and children over age 6. 32 mcg in each nostril q.d. *Maximum:* 256 mcg/day (adults and adolescents); 128 mcg/day (children). *Maintenance:* Lowest dosage that controls symptoms.

➤ *To manage symptoms of perennial non-allergic rhinitis*

NASAL AEROSOL

Adults and adolescents. 64 mcg in each nostril b.i.d. or 128 mcg in each nostril q.d. *Maximum:* 256 mcg/day. *Maintenance:* Lowest dosage that controls symptoms.

NASAL POWDER

Adults and adolescents. 200 mcg in each nostril q.d. *Maximum:* 800 mcg/day. *Maintenance:* Lowest dosage that controls symptoms.

➤ *To provide maintenance therapy in chronic bronchial asthma*

ORAL INHALATION

Adults previously on bronchodilators alone. 1 or 2 inhalations (200 to 400 mcg) b.i.d. *Maximum:* 800 mcg/day.
Adults previously on inhaled corticosteroids. 1 or 2 inhalations (200 to 400 mcg) b.i.d. *Maximum:* 800 mcg b.i.d. as needed and tolerated.
Adults previously on systemic corticosteroids. 2 to 4 inhalations (400 to 800 mcg) b.i.d. *Maximum:* 1,600 mcg/day.
Children age 6 and older. 1 inhalation (200 mcg) b.i.d. *Maximum:* 400 mcg b.i.d. as needed and tolerated.

NEBULIZED INHALATION (PULMICORT RESPULES)

Children ages 1 to 8 previously on bronchodilators alone. 0.25 mg b.i.d. or 0.5 mg q.d. inhaled by jet nebulizer. *Maximum:* 0.5 mg/day.
Children ages 1 to 8 previously on inhaled steroids. 0.25 mg b.i.d. or 0.5 mg q.d. inhaled by jet nebulizer. *Maximum:* 1 mg/day.
Children ages 1 to 8 previously on systemic corticosteroids. 0.5 mg b.i.d. or 1 mg q.d. inhaled by jet nebulizer. *Maximum:* 1 mg/day.

Contraindications

Hypersensitivity to budesonide or its components; recent septal ulcers, nasal surgery, or nasal trauma (for nasal spray); status asthmaticus or other acute asthma episodes (for oral inhalation)

Route	Onset	Peak	Duration
Nasal aerosol	10 hr to 3 days	3 days to 3 wk	Unknown
Nasal powder or suspension, oral inhalation	In 4 wk	Unknown	Unknown
Nebulized inhalation	2 to 8 days	4 to 6 wk	Unknown

Mechanism of Action

Inhibits the activity of cells and mediators active in the inflammatory response, possibly by decreasing influx of inflammatory cells into nasal passages or bronchial walls. As a result, nasal or airway inflammation decreases. Oral inhalation form also inhibits mucus secretion in airways, decreasing the amount and viscosity of sputum.

Interactions

DRUGS

ketoconazole: Possibly increased blood budesonide level

Adverse Reactions

CNS: Asthenia, headache
EENT: Bad taste, dry mouth, epistaxis, nasal irritation, oral candidiasis, pharyngitis, rhinitis, sinusitis
ENDO: Growth suppression in children
GI: Indigestion, nausea
MS: Arthralgia
RESP: Increased cough, respiratory tract infection

Nursing Considerations

• Use budesonide cautiously if patient has tubercular infection; untreated fungal, bacterial, or systemic viral infection; or ocular herpes simplex.
• Closely monitor a child's growth pattern; budesonide may stunt growth.
• WARNING Assess patient who switches from a systemic corticosteroid to inhaled budesonide for signs of adrenal insufficiency (fatigue, lassitude, weakness, nausea, vomiting, and hypotension), which may be life-threat-

ening. Hypothalamic-pituitary-adrenal axis function may take several months to recover after systemic corticosteroids are discontinued. Abrupt withdrawal of budesonide also may precipitate adrenal insufficiency.
• Administer Respules by a jet nebulizer connected to an air compressor.

PATIENT TEACHING

• Instruct patient who uses nasal spray to shake container before each use. Instruct her to blow her nose, tilt her head slightly forward, and insert tube into a nostril, pointing toward inner corner of eye, away from nasal septum. Tell her to hold the other nostril closed and spray while inhaling gently. Then have her repeat the procedure in the other nostril.
• Instruct patient to prime oral inhaler before using it for first time by holding canister upright with mouthpiece on top and then twisting base of device fully to the right and then fully to the left until it clicks. Teach patient to load each subsequent dose just before use in the same manner. After loading a dose, caution patient not to shake device or blow into it. Instruct patient to turn her head away from device and exhale. Then have her hold device upright, place her lips around mouthpiece, and inhale deeply. The device will discharge a dose. Tell patient to remove her lips from mouthpiece to exhale.
• Caution patient not to use an oral inhaler with a spacer device.
• Instruct patient not to use budesonide as a rescue inhaler.
• Instruct patient to contact prescriber if symptoms persist or have worsened after 3 weeks.
• Inform parents of small children using nebulized Respules that improvement may begin within 2 to 8 days but that full effect may not be evident for 4 to 6 weeks.
• Caution patient to avoid exposure to chickenpox and measles and, if exposed, to contact prescriber immediately.

bumetanide

Bumex

Class and Category

Chemical: Sulfonamide derivative
Therapeutic: Loop diuretic
Pregnancy category: C

Indications and Dosages

➤ *To treat edema caused by heart failure, hepatic disease, and renal disease, including nephrotic syndrome*

TABLETS

Adults. 0.5 to 2 mg q.d., increased as needed, with a second or third dose q 4 to 5 hr or 0.5 to 2 mg q.o.d. or q.d. for 3 or 4 days each week. *Maximum:* 10 mg/day.

I.V. INFUSION, I.V. OR I.M. INJECTION

Adults. 0.5 to 1 mg over 1 to 2 min q.d., increased p.r.n. with a second or third dose q 2 to 3 hr. *Maximum:* 10 mg/day.

DOSAGE ADJUSTMENT Continuous infusion (12 mg over 12 hr) may be more effective and less toxic than intermittent infusion in patients with severe chronic renal insufficiency.

Route	Onset	Peak	Duration
P.O.	30 to 60 min	1 to 2 hr	4 to 6 hr
I.V.	In min	15 to 30 min	3.5 to 4 hr

Mechanism of Action

Inhibits the reabsorption of sodium, chloride, and water in the ascending limb of the loop of Henle, which promotes their excretion and reduces fluid volume.

Contraindications

Anuria, hepatic coma, hypersensitivity to bumetanide or its components, severe electrolyte depletion

Interactions

DRUGS

aminoglycosides: Increased risk of ototoxicity
antihypertensives: Increased antihypertensive effect
indomethacin: Slowed increase in urine and sodium excretion, inhibited plasma renin activity
lithium: Reduced lithium renal clearance, increased risk of lithium toxicity
probenecid: Reduced sodium excretion

Adverse Reactions

CNS: Dizziness, encephalopathy, headache
CV: Hypotension
EENT: Ototoxicity
ENDO: Hyperglycemia
GI: Nausea
GU: Azotemia, elevated serum creatinine level

MS: Muscle spasms
Other: Hyperuricemia, hypocalcemia, hypochloremia, hypokalemia, hyponatremia, hypovolemia

Nursing Considerations

•WARNING Know that a patient who is hypersensitive to sulfonamides may be hypersensitive to bumetanide. Monitor such a patient closely when starting therapy.

•Expect to use the parenteral route for patients with impaired GI absorption or in whom the oral route isn't practical. Switch to the oral route, as prescribed, as soon as possible.

•Discard unused parenteral solution 24 hours after preparation.

•Assess fluid and electrolyte balance closely because bumetanide is a potent diuretic (40 to 60 times more potent than furosemide). Monitor fluid intake and output once every 8 hours, evaluate serum electrolyte levels when ordered, and assess for imbalances.

•WARNING Be aware that high-dose or too-frequent administration can cause profound diuresis and water and electrolyte depletion, especially in elderly patients.

•Monitor serum potassium level regularly to check for hypokalemia, especially if patient takes a digitalis glycoside for heart failure or has hepatic cirrhosis, ascites, aldosteronism, potassium-losing nephropathy, diarrhea, or a history of ventricular arrhythmias.

•Assess for signs of ototoxicity, such as tinnitus, daily. Rarely, bumetanide may cause ototoxicity, especially with I.V. administration, high doses, and increased frequency of dosing in a patient with renal impairment.

•Monitor results of renal function tests during bumetanide therapy to detect adverse reactions.

PATIENT TEACHING

•Advise patient to avoid potentially hazardous activities until drug's CNS effects are known.

•Stress the importance of monitoring fluid intake and output and watching for signs and symptoms of electrolyte imbalances, such as dizziness, headache, and muscle spasms.

•Review adverse reactions. If they develop, tell patient to notify prescriber if they're severe or persistent.

•Review potassium-rich foods, and encourage patient to include them in her daily diet.

B

•Encourage patient to return for appropriate follow-up care, especially if she's receiving bumetanide for a chronic condition.
•Tell diabetic patient to monitor blood glucose level regularly and to notify prescriber if hyperglycemia persistently occurs.

buprenorphine hydrochloride

Buprenex

Class, Category, and Schedule

Chemical: Opioid, thebaine derivative
Therapeutic: Narcotic analgesic
Pregnancy category: C
Controlled substance: Schedule V

Indications and Dosages

➤ *To control moderate to severe pain*
I.V OR I.M. INJECTION
Adults and children age 12 and older. 0.3 mg q 6 hr or more, p.r.n. A second 0.3-mg dose given 30 to 60 min after first dose, if needed.
DOSAGE ADJUSTMENT In patients not at high risk for opioid toxicity, I.M. dose increased to 0.6 mg or frequency increased to q 4 hr, if needed, depending on pain severity and patient response. I.V. or I.M. dose reduced by half in elderly or debilitated patients and in those who have respiratory disease or also use another CNS depressant.
Children ages 2 to 12. 0.002 to 0.006 mg/kg q 4 to 6 hr, p.r.n.

Route	Onset	Peak	Duration
I.V.	Under 15 min	Under 1 hr	6 to 10 hr*
I.M.	15 min	1 hr	6 to 10 hr*

Mechanism of Action

May bind with CNS receptors to alter the perception of and emotional response to pain. Buprenorphine may act by displacing narcotic agonists from their binding sites and competitively inhibiting their actions.

Incompatibilities

Don't administer I.V. buprenorphine through the same I.V. line as diazepam or lorazepam.

---

* 4 to 5 hr in children ages 2 to 12.

Contraindications

Hypersensitivity to buprenorphine or its components

Interactions

DRUGS
CNS depressants, MAO inhibitors: Additive hypotensive and respiratory and CNS depressant effects of these drugs
narcotic analgesics: Reduced therapeutic effects if buprenorphine is given before another narcotic analgesic

Adverse Reactions

CNS: Dizziness, headache, sedation, vertigo
CV: Bradycardia, hypertension, hypotension
EENT: Miosis
GI: Nausea, vomiting
RESP: Hypoventilation
SKIN: Diaphoresis
Other: Injection site pain, redness, and swelling

Nursing Considerations

•Use buprenorphine cautiously in patients with severe hepatic or renal impairment, myxedema, hypothyroidism, adrenal insufficiency, CNS depression, coma, toxic psychosis, prostatic hypertrophy, urethral stricture, acute alcoholism, alcohol withdrawal syndrome, kyphoscoliosis, or biliary tract dysfunction. Also use cautiously in patients who receive a drug that decreases hepatic clearance, are known drug abusers, or have been addicted to narcotics.
•Because buprenorphine can increase CSF pressure, use cautiously in patients with head injury, intracranial lesions, or other conditions that could increase CSF pressure.
•Administer I.V. form over at least 2 minutes.
•Inspect injection site for local reactions; don't use the same site twice.
•Frequently monitor vital signs and response to drug and take safety precautions, especially after giving first dose.
•In a physically dependent patient, assess for withdrawal symptoms, which reach peak intensity about 15 days after abrupt withdrawal. Symptoms resemble those of morphine withdrawal (body aches, diaphoresis, diarrhea, nausea, tremor, vomiting), are mild to moderate, and may persist for 1 to 2 weeks.
PATIENT TEACHING
•Advise patient to avoid potentially hazardous activities until drug's CNS effects are known.

bupropion hydrochloride
Wellbutrin, Wellbutrin SR, Zyban

Class and Category
Chemical: Aminoketone derivative
Therapeutic: Antidepressant, smoking cessation adjunct
Pregnancy category: B

Indications and Dosages
➤ *To treat depression*
E.R. TABLETS
Adults. *Initial:* 150 mg q.d. in the morning for 3 days, then 150 mg b.i.d., and after several weeks 200 mg b.i.d., as needed and tolerated. *Maximum:* 400 mg/day or 200 mg/dose.
TABLETS
Adults. *Initial:* 100 mg b.i.d., increased after 3 or more days to 100 mg t.i.d., as needed. *Maximum:* 450 mg/day or 150 mg/dose.

➤ *To aid in smoking cessation*
E.R. TABLETS
Adults. *Initial:* 150 mg q.d. for 3 days and then 150 mg b.i.d. for 7 to 12 wk. *Maximum:* 300 mg/day or 150 mg/dose.

Route	Onset	Peak	Duration
P.O.	1 to 3 wk	Unknown	Unknown

Mechanism of Action
May inhibit norepinephrine, serotonin, and dopamine uptake by neurons. Such inhibition significantly relieves signs and symptoms of depression, improving the patient's sense of well-being and mood.

Contraindications
Anorexia, bulimia, concurrent treatment with another form of bupropion or an MAO inhibitor, hypersensitivity to bupropion or its components, seizure disorder

Interactions
DRUGS
carbamazepine, cimetidine, phenobarbital, phenytoin: Increased bupropion metabolism
clozapine, fluoxetine, haloperidol, lithium, loxapine, maprotiline, molindone, phenothiazines, thioxanthenes, trazodone, tricyclic antidepressants: Increased risk of major motor seizures
levodopa: Increased adverse reactions to bupropion

MAO inhibitors: Increased risk of acute bupropion toxicity
nicotine: Possibly increased blood pressure
warfarin: Possible risk of altered PT and INR with a risk of hemorrhagic or thrombotic complications
ACTIVITIES
alcohol use, recreational drug abuse: Lowered seizure threshold

Adverse Reactions
CNS: Agitation, anxiety, asthenia, CNS stimulation, confusion, decreased concentration or memory, delusions, dizziness, euphoria, fever, general or migraine headache, hallucinations, hot flashes, insomnia, irritability, nervousness, paranoia, paresthesia, seizures, somnolence, syncope, tremor
CV: Chest pain, palpitations
EENT: Altered taste, amblyopia, blurred vision, dry mouth, pharyngitis, sinusitis, tinnitus
GI: Abdominal pain, anorexia, constipation, diarrhea, dysphagia, nausea, vomiting
GU: Urinary frequency and urgency, UTI, vaginal hemorrhage
MS: Arthralgia, arthritis, muscle twitching, myalgia
RESP: Cough
SKIN: Diaphoresis, flushing, pruritus, rash, urticaria
Other: Generalized pain, infection, weight loss

Nursing Considerations
•Be aware that bupropion shouldn't be started within 14 days of stopping an MAO inhibitor.
•To reduce the risk of seizures, allow at least 4 hours between doses of tablets and 8 hours between doses of E.R. tablets.
•Although a nicotine transdermal system may be used with bupropion to treat nicotine dependence, the combination may cause hypertension. Monitor blood pressure frequently.
•Because of increased risk of seizures, take seizure precautions, especially in patients addicted to narcotics, alcohol, cocaine, or stimulants and in those with head trauma or CNS tumors or who take an antidiabetic drug.
•If patient has left ventricular dysfunction, monitor closely for ventricular arrhythmias, conduction disorders, hypertension, and vital sign changes.

PATIENT TEACHING
•Advise patient who uses bupropion for smoking cessation to take it for 7 or more days before stopping smoking. Encourage her to join a smoking cessation support program.
•Tell patient to swallow E.R. tablets whole and not to crush, break, or chew them.
•Tell patient to take bupropion with food to minimize GI distress.
•Advise patient to take the last dose early in the evening to avoid insomnia.
•Advise patient to avoid potentially hazardous activities until drug's CNS effects are known.
•Instruct patient to minimize or avoid alcohol because it can lower the seizure threshold when combined with bupropion.
•Tell patient to skip a missed dose and resume the regular dosing schedule but not to double-dose.
•To reduce the risk of seizures from drug interactions, tell patient to inform all prescribers that she takes bupropion.
•Tell patient to report bothersome or severe adverse reactions to prescriber.

buspirone hydrochloride

BuSpar, BuSpar DIVIDOSE, Bustab (CAN)

Class and Category
Chemical: Azaspirodecanedione
Therapeutic: Antianxiety
Pregnancy category: B

Indications and Dosages
➤ *To manage anxiety*
TABLETS
Adults. *Initial:* 5 mg t.i.d. or 7.5 mg b.i.d. increased by 5 mg/day at 2- to 3-day intervals until desired response occurs. *Maintenance:* 20 to 30 mg/day (usual therapeutic range). *Maximum:* 60 mg/day.

Route	Onset	Peak	Duration
P.O.	1 to 4 wk	3 to 6 wk	Unknown

Mechanism of Action
May act as a partial agonist at serotonin 5-hydroxytryptamine$_{1A}$ receptors in the brain, producing antianxiety effects.

Contraindications
Hypersensitivity to buspirone or its components

Interactions
DRUGS
diltiazem, erythromycin, itraconazole, nefazodone, verapamil: Increased blood level and adverse effects of buspirone
haloperidol: Increased blood haloperidol level
hepatic enzyme CYP3A4 inducers, such as dexamethasone and certain anticonvulsants (phenytoin, phenobarbital, carbamazepine): Possibly increased rate of buspirone metabolism
hepatic enzyme CYP3A4 inhibitors, such as ketoconazole and ritonavir: Possibly inhibited buspirone metabolism and increased blood level
MAO inhibitors: Increased risk of hypertension
nefazadone: Increased risk of adverse CNS effects
rifampin: Decreased blood buspirone level and pharmacodynamic effects
FOODS
food: Possibly decreased buspirone clearance
grapefruit juice: Increased blood buspirone level

Adverse Reactions
CNS: Anger, confusion, decreased concentration, depression, dizziness, dream disturbances, drowsiness, excitement, fatigue, headache, hostility, insomnia, lack of coordination, light-headedness, nervousness, paresthesia, tremor, weakness
CV: Chest pain, palpitations, tachycardia
EENT: Blurred vision, dry mouth, nasal congestion, pharyngitis, tinnitus
GI: Abdominal or gastric distress, constipation, diarrhea, nausea, vomiting
MS: Myalgia
SKIN: Diaphoresis, rash

Nursing Considerations
•Use buspirone cautiously in patients with hepatic or renal impairment.
•Institute safety precautions because of possible adverse CNS reactions. Expect to administer a lower dose when given with nefazodone to avoid increased CNS effects.
PATIENT TEACHING
•Advise patient to take buspirone consistently, either always with or always without food.
•Caution patient to avoid drinking large amounts of grapefruit juice.
•Inform patient that 1 to 2 weeks of therapy may be needed before she notices drug's antianxiety effect.
•Stress the importance of not taking more buspirone than prescribed.

•Advise patient to avoid potentially hazardous activities until drug's CNS effects are known.

butabarbital sodium

Busodium, Butalan, Butisol, Sarisol No. 2

Class, Category, and Schedule
Chemical: Barbiturate
Therapeutic: Sedative-hypnotic
Pregnancy category: D
Controlled substance: Schedule III

Indications and Dosages
➤ *To provide daytime sedation*
ELIXIR, TABLETS
Adults. 15 to 30 mg t.i.d. or q.i.d.
➤ *To treat insomnia*
ELIXIR, TABLETS
Adults. 50 to 100 mg q h.s.
➤ *To provide preoperative sedation*
ELIXIR, TABLETS
Adults. 50 to 100 mg 60 to 90 min before surgery.
Children. 2 to 6 mg/kg. *Maximum:* 100 mg/dose.
DOSAGE ADJUSTMENT Dosage reduced in patients with impaired renal or hepatic function and in elderly or debilitated patients because they may be more sensitive to drug.

Route	Onset	Peak	Duration
P.O.	45 to 60 min	Unknown	6 to 8 hr

Mechanism of Action
Inhibits the upward conduction of nerve impulses in the brain's reticular formation, which disrupts impulse transmission to the cortex. As a result, butabarbital depresses the CNS and produces drowsiness, sedation, and hypnosis.

Contraindications
History of addiction to sedative or hypnotic drug, hypersensitivity to butabarbital or its components, porphyria, severe hepatic or respiratory disease

Interactions
DRUGS
acetaminophen: Increased risk of hepatotoxicity (with large doses of or long-term therapy with butabarbital)

activated charcoal: Reduced butabarbital absorption
carbamazepine: Decreased blood carbamazepine level
chloramphenicol, corticosteroids, digitalis glycosides: Increased metabolism and decreased effects of these drugs
clonazepam: Increased clearance and reduced efficacy of clonazepam
CNS depressants, including OTC sedatives and hypnotics: Additive CNS depression
doxycycline: Shortened half-life and decreased effects of doxycycline
fenoprofen: Reduced bioavailability and effects of fenoprofen
griseofulvin: Reduced griseofulvin absorption
hydantoins, such as phenytoin: Unpredictable effects on barbiturate metabolism
MAO inhibitors: Prolonged barbiturate effects
meperidine: Prolonged CNS depressant effects of meperidine
methadone: Reduced methadone actions
methoxyflurane: Increased risk of nephrotoxicity
metronidazole: Decreased antimicrobial effect of metronidazole
oral anticoagulants: Decreased anticoagulant effect
oral contraceptives with estrogen: Decreased contraceptive effect
phenylbutazone: Reduced elimination half-life of phenylbutazone
rifampin: Decreased butabarbital effectiveness
sodium valproate, valproic acid: Decreased butabarbital metabolism and increased adverse CNS effects
theophylline: Decreased blood level and effects of theophylline
ACTIVITIES
alcohol use: Additive CNS depression

Adverse Reactions
CNS: Agitation, anxiety, ataxia, clumsiness, CNS depression, confusion, depression, dizziness, drowsiness, fever, hallucinations, headache, hyperkinesia, insomnia, irritability, nervousness, nightmares, psychiatric disturbance, somnolence, syncope
CV: Hypertension
EENT: Laryngospasm
GI: Constipation, hepatic dysfunction, nausea, vomiting
MS: Rickets

RESP: Apnea, bronchospasm, respiratory depression
SKIN: Exfoliative dermatitis, Stevens-Johnson syndrome
Other: Drug tolerance, physical and psychological dependence

Nursing Considerations
•Use butabarbital cautiously, if at all, in patients with depression, suicidal tendency, history of drug abuse, or hepatic dysfunction. Don't administer drug to patients with premonitory signs of hepatic coma.
•Expect to give drug for no more than 2 weeks to treat insomnia because, like all barbiturates, it loses effectiveness for sleep induction and sleep maintenance after 2 weeks.
•Monitor butabarbital intake closely during long-term use because tolerance and psychological and physical dependence may develop.
•Avoid abrupt withdrawal of butabarbital to prevent withdrawal symptoms.
•Monitor elderly and debilitated patients closely because drug may cause marked excitement, depression, and confusion in these patients.
•If patient in pain receives butabarbital, monitor closely for paradoxical excitement.
•If pregnant woman took butabarbital during last trimester, monitor infant for withdrawal symptoms.
PATIENT TEACHING
•Stress the importance of taking butabarbital exactly as prescribed because it can be addictive. Warn against increasing the dose or decreasing the dosage interval without consulting prescriber.
•Tell patient to avoid alcohol and OTC sedatives and hypnotics during butabarbital therapy because of additive CNS effects.
•Advise patient to avoid potentially hazardous activities until drug's CNS effects are known.
•Advise female patient not to rely on oral contraceptives during butabarbital therapy.

butorphanol tartrate
Stadol, Stadol NS

Class, Category, and Schedule
Chemical: Opioid
Therapeutic: Anesthesia adjunct, narcotic analgesic
Pregnancy category: C
Controlled substance: Schedule II

Indications and Dosages
➤ *To manage pain*
I.V. INJECTION
Adults. 0.5 to 2 mg (usually 1 mg) q 3 to 4 hr, p.r.n.
I.M. INJECTION
Adults. 1 to 4 mg (usually 2 mg) q 3 to 4 hr, p.r.n. *Maximum:* 4 mg/single dose.
NASAL INHALATION
Adults. 1 spray (1 mg) in one nostril. Dose repeated after 60 to 90 min; two-dose sequence repeated q 3 to 4 hr, p.r.n. For severe pain, 2 sprays (one in each nostril) q 3 to 4 hr, p.r.n.
DOSAGE ADJUSTMENT Dose reduced to 1 spray in one nostril for elderly patients and those with impaired hepatic or renal function; dose repeated after 90 to 120 min; two-dose sequence repeated q 6 hr or more, p.r.n.
➤ *As adjunct to provide preoperative anesthesia*
I.V. OR I.M. INJECTION
Adults. Individualized. *Average:* 2 mg 60 to 90 min before surgery.
➤ *As adjunct to provide anesthesia*
I.V. INJECTION
Adults. Individualized. *Average:* 1 to 4 mg and then supplemental doses of 0.5 to 1 mg, p.r.n. Total usually required during surgery is 60 to 180 mcg/kg.
DOSAGE ADJUSTMENT Parenteral doses reduced by half for elderly patients and those with impaired hepatic or renal function.

Route	Onset	Peak	Duration
I.V.	2 to 3 min	30 min	2 to 4 hr
I.M.	10 to 30 min	30 to 60 min	3 to 4 hr
Inhalation	In 15 min	1 to 2 hr	4 to 5 hr

Mechanism of Action
Binds with specific CNS receptors to alter the perception of and emotional response to pain.

Contraindications
Hypersensitivity to butorphanol or its components (including the preservative benzethonium chloride)

Interactions
DRUGS
CNS depressants: Additive CNS depression

nasal vasoconstrictors, such as oxymetazo-line: Decreased absorption rate and delayed onset of butorphanol

ACTIVITIES

alcohol use: Additive CNS depression

Adverse Reactions

CNS: Anxiety, confusion, difficulty performing purposeful movements, difficulty speaking, dizziness, euphoria, floating feeling, headache, insomnia (with nasal form), lethargy, nervousness, paresthesia, sensation of heat, somnolence, syncope, tremor, vertigo

CV: Chest pain, hypotension, palpitations, tachycardia, vasodilation

EENT: Blurred vision, dry mouth, ear pain, epistaxis, nasal congestion or irritation (with nasal form), pharyngitis, rhinitis, sinus congestion, sinusitis, tinnitus, unpleasant taste

GI: Anorexia, constipation, epigastric pain, nausea, vomiting

RESP: Apnea, bronchitis, cough, dyspnea, respiratory depression, shallow breathing, upper respiratory tract infection

SKIN: Clammy skin, pruritus

Nursing Considerations

• Use butorphanol cautiously, if at all, in patients with depression, suicidal tendency, history of drug abuse, or hepatic or renal dysfunction.

• Because drug can raise CSF pressure, use it cautiously, if at all, in patients with head injury. Because it can increase cardiac workload, use with extreme caution in patients with acute MI, ventricular dysfunction, or coronary insufficiency.

• Be aware that butorphanol has a high potential for abuse.

• Monitor patient after first dose of nasal form because hypotension and syncope may occur.

• Take safety precautions because butorphanol causes CNS depression.

• Assess respiratory status closely because drug causes respiratory depression.

• Frequently monitor blood pressure after giving drug. If severe hypertension develops (rare), stop drug at once and notify prescriber. If patient isn't narcotic-dependent, expect to administer naloxone to reverse butorphanol's effects.

PATIENT TEACHING

• Stress the importance of taking butorphanol exactly as prescribed because it can be addictive. Warn patient not to increase the dose or decrease the dosage interval without consulting prescriber.

• Advise patient to avoid potentially hazardous activities until drug's CNS effects are known.

• Tell patient to avoid alcohol and other CNS depressants, including OTC drugs, while taking butorphanol because of additive adverse CNS reactions.

• Teach patient how to use nasal form properly. After blowing the nose to clear the nostrils, pull the clear cover from the pump unit and remove the protective clip from its neck. Prime the pump unit by placing the nozzle between the first and second fingers with the thumb on the bottom of the bottle. Then pump the sprayer unit firmly and quickly until a fine spray appears (7 or 8 strokes). Insert the spray tip about 1 cm ($1/3''$) into one nostril, pointing the tip toward the back of the nose. Close the other nostril with one finger and tilt the head slightly forward. Then pump the sprayer firmly and quickly by pushing down on the pump unit's finger grips and against the thumb at the bottom of the bottle. Sniff gently with the mouth closed. After spraying, remove the pump from the nose, tilt the head back, and sniff gently for a few more seconds. Then replace the protective clip and clear cover.

cabergoline

Dostinex

Class and Category
Chemical: Ergot alkaloid derivative
Therapeutic: Antihyperprolactinemic
Pregnancy category: B

Indications and Dosages
➤ *To treat idiopathic or adenoma-induced hyperprolactinemic disorders*
TABLETS
Adults. 0.25 mg twice a week. Increased by 0.25 mg/wk at 4-wk intervals, if needed, up to 1 mg twice a week.

Route	Onset	Peak	Duration
P.O.	Unknown	48 hr	Up to 14 days

Mechanism of Action
Binds with dopamine$_2$ receptors to block prolactin synthesis and secretion by the anterior pituitary gland, thereby reducing the serum prolactin level.

Contraindications
Hypersensitivity to cabergoline, ergot derivatives, or their components; uncontrolled hypertension

Interactions
DRUGS
antihypertensives: Increased risk of hypotension
dopamine antagonists (butyrophenones, metoclopramide, phenothiazines, or thioxanthenes): Decreased cabergoline effectiveness

Adverse Reactions
CNS: Asthenia, depression, fatigue, headache, nervousness, paresthesia, somnolence, vertigo
CV: Orthostatic hypotension
EENT: Dry mouth
ENDO: Breast pain
GI: Abdominal pain, constipation, diarrhea, flatulence, indigestion, nausea, vomiting
GU: Dysmenorrhea, increased libido

Nursing Considerations
•Before each dose increase, check serum prolactin level to assess cabergoline's effectiveness.
•If patient has moderate to severe hepatic impairment, monitor closely for adverse reactions because of decreased cabergoline metabolism.
•**WARNING** If you detect signs of overdose, such as syncope, hallucinations, light-headedness, tachycardia, and nasal congestion, notify prescriber and treat as ordered.
PATIENT TEACHING
•Urge patient to read and follow printed information that explains how to use cabergoline for maximum therapeutic results.
•Advise patient to take drug with meals to help decrease GI distress.
•Tell patient to take a missed dose as soon as possible within 1 to 2 days. If the missed dose isn't remembered until it's time for the next dose, instruct him to double the dose if the drug is generally well tolerated and doesn't cause nausea. If the drug isn't well tolerated, instruct him to consult prescriber before taking the missed dose.
•Instruct patient to change positions slowly to avoid the effects of orthostatic hypotension. Tell him to notify prescriber if such effects occur.
•Encourage patient to keep regular appointments to monitor drug effectiveness.
•Advise patient that drug therapy will end when serum prolactin level is normal for 6 months. Explain that he'll need periodic monitoring of the level to determine whether therapy should resume.
•Tell female patient to notify prescriber and discuss possible drug discontinuation if pregnancy occurs or is suspected during therapy or if she plans to become pregnant during therapy.

calcifediol

Calderol

Class and Category
Chemical: Sterol derivative, vitamin D analogue
Therapeutic: Antihypocalcemic
Pregnancy category: C

Indications and Dosages
➤ *To treat metabolic bone disease or hypocalcemia in patients receiving renal dialysis*

CAPSULES

Adults and children age 10 and older. 300 to 350 mcg/wk given in divided doses q.d. or q.o.d. Increased at 4-wk intervals, p.r.n. Most patients respond to 50 to 100 mcg q.d. or 100 to 200 mcg q.o.d.

Children ages 2 to 10. 0.05 mg q.d.

Children up to age 2. 0.02 to 0.05 mg q.d.

DOSAGE ADJUSTMENT Dosage decreased as low as 20 mcg q.o.d. in patients with normal serum calcium level.

Route	Onset	Peak	Duration
P.O.	Unknown	Unknown	15 to 20 days

Mechanism of Action
Is converted to calcitriol in the kidneys and then binds to specific receptors in the intestinal mucosa to increase calcium absorption from the intestines. Calcifediol may also regulate calcium ion transfer from bone to blood and stimulate calcium reabsorption in the distal renal tubules, making more calcium available in the body.

Contraindications
Abnormal sensitivity to vitamin D's effects, decreased renal function, hypercalcemia, hyperphosphatemia, hypervitaminosis, malabsorption syndrome, vitamin D toxicity

Interactions
DRUGS

aluminum-containing antacids: Increased blood aluminum level, especially in patients with chronic renal failure

barbiturates, corticosteroids, hydantoin anticonvulsants, primidone: Decreased effects of vitamin D

calcitonin, etidronate, gallium nitrate, pamidronate, plicamycin: Decreased effects of these drugs

calcium (high doses), thiazide diuretics: Increased risk of hypercalcemia

cholestyramine, colestipol, mineral oil: Decreased vitamin D absorption

digitalis glycosides: Increased risk of arrhythmias from hypercalcemia

magnesium-containing antacids: Hypermagnesemia, especially in chronic renal failure

phosphorous-containing drugs: Increased risk of hyperphosphatemia

verapamil: Increased risk of atrial fibrillation

vitamin D derivatives, such as calcitriol, dihydrotachysterol, ergocalciferol: Increased risk of vitamin D toxicity

Adverse Reactions
None with usual dosages

Nursing Considerations
• Use calcifediol cautiously in patients with sarcoidosis or other granulomatous disease because of increased sensitivity to effects of vitamin D.

• If hypercalcemia develops, expect to discontinue therapy. Calcium level usually returns to normal in 2 to 4 weeks. To manage acute hypercalcemia, administer I.V. NS and, possibly, a loop diuretic as prescribed to enhance diuresis or prepare for dialysis with a calcium-free dialysate if needed. Be aware that chronic hypercalcemia may lead to diffuse vascular calcification, nephrocalcinosis, and other soft-tissue calcification.

• If patient receives high-dose or long-term calcifediol therapy, be alert for vitamin D toxicity. Early signs and symptoms include bone pain, constipation, dry mouth, headache, metallic taste, myalgia, nausea, somnolence, vomiting, and weakness. Late signs and symptoms include albuminuria, anorexia, arrhythmias, azotemia, conjunctivitis (calcific), decreased libido, elevated AST and ALT levels, elevated BUN level, generalized vascular calcification, hypercholesterolemia, hypertension, hyperthermia, irritability, mild acidosis, nephrocalcinosis, nocturia, pancreatitis, photophobia, polydipsia, polyuria, pruritus, rhinorrhea, and weight loss.

PATIENT TEACHING

• Instruct patient to swallow capsule whole and not to crush or chew it.

• Advise patient to consult prescriber before taking OTC drugs.

• Instruct patient to store drug tightly capped in a cool, dry place away from direct light.

• Encourage patient to eat a balanced diet that includes foods high in vitamin D and calcium. Calcifediol is most effective when patient follows a high-calcium diet.

• If patient takes vitamin supplements, warn him not to exceed recommended daily allowances.

C

•Tell patient to avoid calcium-, magnesium-, and phosphate-containing laxatives and antacids; mineral oil; and vitamin D preparations because they may increase the risk of calcifediol's toxic effects.
•Advise patient to notify prescriber immediately if signs of toxicity, such as headache, irritability, nausea, photophobia, vomiting, weakness, and weight loss, develop.
•Stress the importance of follow-up care, including laboratory tests to evaluate progress and identify signs of toxicity early.

calcitonin, human

Cibacalcin

calcitonin, salmon

Calcimar, Miacalcin

Class and Category

Chemical: Polypeptide hormone
Therapeutic: Antihypercalcemic, bone resorption inhibitor, osteoporosis therapy adjunct
Pregnancy category: C

Indications and Dosages

➤ *To treat hypercalcemic emergency*
I.M. OR S.C. INJECTION
Adults. *Initial:* 4 IU/kg q 12 hr. Increased after 1 or 2 days, if needed, to 8 IU/kg q 12 hr. *Maximum:* 8 IU/kg q 6 hr.

➤ *To treat postmenopausal osteoporosis*
I.M. OR S.C. INJECTION (CALCITONIN, SALMON)
Adults. *Initial:* 100 IU q.d., q.o.d., or 3 times/ wk. *Maximum:* 100 IU q.d.
NASAL SPRAY
Adults. 200 IU (1 spray) q.d., alternating nostrils.

➤ *To treat Paget's disease of the bone*
I.M. OR S.C INJECTION (CALCITONIN, SALMON)
Adults. *Initial:* 100 IU q.d. *Maintenance:* 50 to 100 IU q.d. or q.o.d. *Maximum:* 100 IU q.d.
S.C. INJECTION (CALCITONIN, HUMAN)
Adults. 0.5 mg/day, 0.5 mg 2 or 3 times/wk, or 0.25 mg/day.

Route	Onset	Peak	Duration
I.M., S.C.	In 15 min*	2 hr†	6 to 8 hr†

---

* For hypercalcemia; 6 to 24 mo for Paget's disease.
† For hypercalcemia; unknown for other indications.

Mechanism of Action

Directly inhibits bone resorption. Besides reducing the serum calcium level, this action slows bone metabolism (a major factor in the development of Paget's disease) and calcium loss from the bone (a major factor in the development of osteoporosis).

Contraindications

Hypersensitivity to calcitonin, human; calcitonin, salmon; or their components

Adverse Reactions

CNS: Agitation, anxiety, CVA, dizziness, headache, insomnia, neuralgia, paresthesia, vertigo
CV: Bundle-branch block, hypertension, MI, palpitations, peripheral edema, tachycardia, thrombophlebitis
EENT: Blurred vision; dry mouth; earache; epistaxis; eye pain; hearing loss; nasal irritation, lesions, or redness; pharyngitis; rhinitis; salty taste; sinusitis; taste perversion; tinnitus; vitreous floaters
ENDO: Goiter, hyperthyroidism
GI: Anorexia, cholelithiasis, epigastric discomfort, flatulence, gastritis, hepatitis, increased appetite, nausea, thirst, vomiting
GU: Hematuria, nocturia, pyelonephritis, renal calculi
HEME: Anemia
MS: Arthritis, arthrosis, back pain, joint stiffness, polymyalgia rheumatica
RESP: Bronchitis, cough, dyspnea, pneumonia, upper respiratory tract infection
SKIN: Alopecia, diaphoresis, eczema, flushing of face or hands, pruritus of earlobes, rash, ulceration
Other: Antibody formation, feverish sensation, injection site inflammation, lymphadenopathy, mild tetanic symptoms

Nursing Considerations

•If sensitivity to calcitonin, human; calcitonin, salmon; or their components is suspected, expect to perform a skin test before administration. Prepare a mixture of 10 IU/ ml by withdrawing 0.05 ml of 200-IU solution in a tuberculin syringe and filling the syringe to 1 ml with sodium chloride for injection. Mix well, discard 0.9 ml, and inject 0.1 ml intradermally on the inner forearm. Observe the site for 15 minutes after injection. If you detect signs of sensitivity, such as more than mild erythema or a wheal, notify prescriber.

•If patient receives calcitonin for hypercalcemia, monitor serum calcium level. During first several doses, keep parenteral calcium available in case the calcium level is inadvertently overcorrected.

•If the calcitonin dose exceeds 2 ml, expect to use I.M. route and multiple injection sites.

•For patient receiving calcitonin for postmenopausal osteoporosis, also expect to administer 1.5 g of supplemental calcium carbonate and at least 400 U of vitamin D daily. Plan to provide a balanced diet that includes foods high in calcium and vitamin D.

•Assess for nausea, especially with the first dose. Nausea tends to decrease or disappear with continued use.

•If patient with Paget's disease relapses after treatment, check for antibody formation, as ordered.

PATIENT TEACHING

•Tell patient to refrigerate injection or unopened nasal spray container.

•Teach patient how to self-administer injections.

•If patient has postmenopausal osteoporosis, teach her about dietary needs, including foods rich in calcium and vitamin D.

•For a nasal spray user, explain how to activate the nasal pump by holding the bottle upright and depressing two white side arms toward the bottle six times. When the bottle emits a faint spray, the pump is activated. Tell patient to store the activated nasal pump upright at room temperature and to discard it after 30 days.

•Tell patient to place the nozzle firmly into a nostril while holding the head upright and then to depress the pump toward the bottle.

•Remind patient that he doesn't need to reactivate the pump before each daily dose.

•Instruct patient to report nasal symptoms, such as redness, lesions, sinusitis, and rhinitis, to prescriber.

calcitriol

(1,25-dihydroxycholecalciferol)

Calcijex, Rocaltrol

Class and Category

Chemical: Sterol derivative, vitamin D analogue

Therapeutic: Antihypocalcemic, antihypoparathyroid

Pregnancy category: C

Indications and Dosages

➤ *To treat hypocalcemia in dialysis patients*

CAPSULES, ORAL SOLUTION

Adults. *Initial:* 0.25 mcg q.d. Increased by 0.25 mcg/day q 4 to 8 wk, if needed to achieve normal serum calcium level. *Maintenance:* 0.5 to 3 mcg q.d.

➤ *To treat hypocalcemia in predialysis patients*

CAPSULES, ORAL SOLUTION

Adults and children age 3 and older. *Initial:* 0.25 mcg q.d. Increased after 4 to 8 wk, if needed, to 0.5 mcg q.d.

ORAL SOLUTION

Children up to age 3. 10 to 15 ng/kg/day.

➤ *To treat hypoparathyroidism*

TABLETS

Adults and children age 6 and older. *Initial:* 0.25 mcg q.d. in the morning. Increased q 2 to 4 wk, if needed to achieve normal serum calcium level. *Usual:* 0.5 to 2 mcg q.d.

Children ages 1 to 5. 0.25 to 0.75 mcg q.d in the morning.

I.V. INJECTION

Adults. *Initial:* 1 to 2 mcg 3 times/wk given q.o.d. Each dose increased 0.5 to 1 mcg at 2- to 4-wk intervals, if needed.

Route	Onset	Peak	Duration
P.O.	2 to 6 hr	10 hr	3 to 5 days

Mechanism of Action

Binds to specific receptors of the intestinal mucosa to increase calcium absorption from the intestines. It also may regulate calcium ion transfer from bone to blood and stimulate calcium reabsorption in the distal renal tubules, making more calcium available in the body.

Contraindications

Hypercalcemia, vitamin D toxicity

Interactions

DRUGS

cholestyramine: Decreased calcitriol absorption

digitalis glycosides: Possibly arrhythmias

ketoconazole: Decreased blood calcitriol level
magnesium-containing antacids (I.V. form): Hypermagnesemia
mineral oil: Decreased blood calcitriol level (with prolonged use of mineral oil)
phenobarbital, phenytoin: Decreased synthesis and blood level of calcitriol
thiazide diuretics: Hypercalcemia

Adverse Reactions
None with usual dosages

Nursing Considerations
• Make sure patient has adequate calcium intake.
• Store drug at room temperature and protect from heat and direct light.
• If patient receives high-dose or long-term calcitriol therapy, be alert for vitamin D toxicity. Early signs and symptoms include bone pain, constipation, dry mouth, headache, metallic taste, myalgia, nausea, somnolence, vomiting, and weakness. Late signs and symptoms include albuminuria, anorexia, arrhythmias, azotemia, conjunctivitis (calcific), decreased libido, elevated AST and ALT levels, elevated BUN level, generalized vascular calcification, hypercholesterolemia, hypertension, hyperthermia, irritability, mild acidosis, nephrocalcinosis, nocturia, pancreatitis, photophobia, polydipsia, polyuria, pruritus, rhinorrhea, and weight loss.

PATIENT TEACHING
• Warn patient not to take other forms of vitamin D while taking calcitriol.
• Instruct patient to take a missed dose as soon as possible.
• Advise patient to notify prescriber immediately if signs of toxicity, such as headache, irritability, nausea, photophobia, vomiting, weakness, and weight loss, develop.

calcium acetate

PhosLo

calcium carbonate

Apo-Cal (CAN), Calci-Mix, Calsan (CAN), Liqui-Cal, Liquid Cal-600, Titralac

calcium chloride

Calciject (CAN)

calcium citrate

Citracal, Citracal Liquitabs

calcium glubionate

Calcionate, Calcium-Sandoz (CAN), Neo-Calglucon

calcium gluceptate

Calcium Stanley (CAN)

calcium gluconate

calcium lactate

Class and Category
Chemical: Elemental cation
Therapeutic: Antacid, antihypermagnesemic, antihyperphosphatemic, antihypocalcemic, calcium replacement, cardiotonic
Pregnancy category: C (Not rated for calcium carbonate, citrate, and lactate)

Indications and Dosages
➤ *To treat hyperphosphatemia*
TABLETS (CALCIUM ACETATE)
Adults. *Initial:* 2 tabs (338 mg elemental calcium, 1,334 mg calcium acetate) t.i.d. with meals. Dosage increased to reduce serum phosphorous level below 6 mg/dl as long as hypercalcemia doesn't develop. *Maintenance:* 3 or 4 tabs t.i.d. with each meal.

➤ *To prevent hypocalcemia*
CAPSULES, ORAL SUSPENSION, TABLETS (CALCIUM CARBONATE); EFFERVESCENT TABLETS, TABLETS (CALCIUM CITRATE); SYRUP (CALCIUM GLUBIONATE); TABLETS (CALCIUM GLUCONATE OR LACTATE)
Adults and children over age 10. 800 to 1,200 mg/day.
Pregnant and breast-feeding women. 1,200 mg/day.
Children ages 4 to 10. 800 mg/day.
Children up to age 4. 400 to 800 mg/day.

➤ *To provide antacid effects*
CHEWABLE TABLETS, ORAL SUSPENSION, TABLETS (CALCIUM CARBONATE)
Adults and children age 12 and older. 350 to 1,500 mg 1 hr p.c. and h.s., p.r.n.

➤ *To replace calcium in hypocalcemia*
I.V. INFUSION (CALCIUM CHLORIDE)
Adults. 0.5 to 1 g q 1 to 3 days, infused at less than 1 ml/min.
Children. 25 mg/kg given over several minutes.
I.V. OR I.M. INJECTION (CALCIUM GLUCEPTATE)
Adults and children. 0.44 to 1.1 g I.M. or 1.1 to 4.4 g I.V. at a rate not to exceed 2 ml (36 mg)/min.

I.V. INJECTION (CALCIUM GLUCONATE)

Adults. 970 mg given slowly, repeated if needed until tetany is controlled.

Children. 200 to 500 mg as a single dose given slowly, repeated if needed until tetany is controlled.

➤ *As adjunct to treat magnesium intoxication*

I.V. INJECTION (CALCIUM CHLORIDE)

Adults. 500 mg promptly and repeated p.r.n., based on response.

➤ *As adjunct in cardiac resuscitation*

I.V. INJECTION (CALCIUM CHLORIDE)

Adults. 0.5 to 1 g.
Children. 0.2 ml/kg.

➤ *As adjunct in exchange transfusion*

I.V. INJECTION (CALCIUM GLUCONATE)

Adults. 1.35 mEq with each 100 ml of citrated blood exchanged.

Neonates. 0.45 mEq after each 100 ml of citrated blood exchanged.

I.V. INJECTION (CALCIUM GLUCEPTATE)

Neonates. 110 mg after each 100 ml of citrated blood exchanged.

Mechanism of Action

Increases levels of intracellular and extracellular calcium, which is needed to maintain homeostasis, especially in the nervous and musculoskeletal systems. Also plays a role in normal cardiac and renal function, respiration, coagulation, and cell membrane and capillary permeability. Helps regulate the release and storage of neurotransmitters and hormones. Oral forms also neutralize or buffer stomach acid to relieve discomfort cause by hyperacidity.

Incompatibilities

To avoid precipitation, don't administer I.V. calcium chloride, gluceptate, or gluconate through the same I.V. line as bicarbonates, carbonates, phosphates, sulfates, or tartrates.

Contraindications

Hypercalcemia, hypersensitivity to calcium salts or their components, hypophosphatemia, renal calculi

Interactions
DRUGS

aluminum-containing antacids: Enhanced aluminum absorption with calcium citrate use
atenolol: Decreased blood atenolol level and beta blockade
calcitonin: Possibly antagonized effects of calcitonin in hypercalcemia treatment
calcium supplements, magnesium-containing preparations: Increased serum calcium or magnesium level, especially in patients with impaired renal function
cellulose sodium phosphate: Decreased effectiveness of cellulose sodium phosphate in preventing hypercalciuria
digitalis glycosides: Increased risk of arrhythmias
estrogens, oral contraceptives (estrogen-containing): Increased calcium absorption
etidronate: Decreased etidronate absorption
fluoroquinolones: Reduced fluoroquinolone absorption by calcium carbonate
gallium nitrate: Antagonized effects of gallium nitrate
iron salts: Decreased gastric absorption of iron
magnesium sulfate (parenteral): Neutralized effects of magnesium by parenteral calcium salts
neuromuscular blockers (except succinylcholine): Possibly reversal of neuromuscular blockade by parenteral calcium salts; enhanced or prolonged neuromuscular blockade induced by tubocurarine
norfloxacin: Decreased norfloxacin bioavailability
phenytoin: Decreased bioavailability of phenytoin and calcium
potassium phosphates, potassium and sodium phosphates: Increased risk of calcium deposition in soft tissue
sodium bicarbonate: Possibly milk-alkali syndrome
sodium fluoride: Reduced fluoride and calcium absorption
sodium polystyrene sulfonate: Possibly metabolic alkalosis if patient has renal impairment
tetracyclines: Decreased tetracycline absorption and blood level, leading to decreased anti-infective response
thiazide diuretics: Possibly hypercalcemia
verapamil: Reversed verapamil effects
vitamin A (more than 25,000 U/day): Possibly stimulation of bone loss, decreased ef-

fects of calcium supplementation, and hypercalcemia
vitamin D (high doses): Excessively increased calcium absorption
FOODS
caffeine, high-fiber food: Possibly decreased calcium absorption
ACTIVITIES
alcohol use (excessive), smoking: Possibly decreased calcium absorption

Adverse Reactions
CNS: Paresthesia (parenteral form)
CV: Hypotension, irregular heartbeat (parenteral form)
GI: Nausea or vomiting (parenteral form)
SKIN: Diaphoresis, flushing, or sensation of warmth (parenteral form)
Other: Hypercalcemia; injection site burning, pain, rash, or redness (parenteral form)

Nursing Considerations
•Store calcium at room temperature and protect from heat, moisture, and direct light. Don't freeze.
•Warm solution to room temperature before parenteral administration.
•Maintain patient in a recumbent position for 30 minutes after parenteral administration to prevent dizziness from hypotension.
•Administer I.V. calcium through an infusing I.V. solution, using a small-bore needle inserted into a large vein to minimize irritation. Give calcium slowly to prevent excess calcium from reaching the heart and causing adverse cardiovascular reactions. Adverse reactions often result from too-rapid administration. If ECG tracings are abnormal or patient reports injection site discomfort, expect to temporarily discontinue administration.
•Assess regularly for extravasation because calcium causes necrosis. If infiltration occurs, discontinue I.V. calcium and notify prescriber immediately.
•Divide I.M. calcium glucoptate dose of 5 ml or more in half and inject in gluteal region.
•Regularly monitor serum calcium level and evaluate therapeutic response by assessing for Chvostek's and Trousseau's signs, which shouldn't appear.
•Be aware that calcium chloride injection contains three times as much calcium per milliliter as calcium gluconate injection.

PATIENT TEACHING
•If chewable tablets are prescribed, urge patient to chew them thoroughly before swallowing and to drink a glass of water afterward.
•If suspension is prescribed, tell patient to shake bottle well before each use.
•If calcium citrate effervescent tablets are prescribed, tell patient to dissolve them in water and drink immediately.
•Instruct patient to take calcium carbonate tablets 1 to 2 hours after meals, calcium glubionate syrup before meals (diluted in water or fruit juice, if desired, for an infant or a child), and other calcium supplements with meals.
•Tell patient to store calcium at room temperature away from heat, moisture, and direct light. Warn against freezing the suspension or syrup.
•Instruct patient to avoid taking calcium within 2 hours of taking another oral drug because of risk of interactions.
•Advise patient to consult prescriber before taking OTC drugs because of risk of interactions.
•Tell patient to avoid excessive use of tobacco and excessive consumption of alcoholic beverages, caffeine-containing products, and high-fiber foods because these substances may decrease calcium absorption.

candesartan cilexetil

Atacand

Class and Category
Chemical: Angiotensin II receptor antagonist
Therapeutic: Antihypertensive
Pregnancy category: C (first trimester), D (later trimesters)

Indications and Dosages
➤ *To manage, or as adjunct in managing, hypertension*
TABLETS
Adults. *Initial:* 16 mg q.d. *Maintenance:* 8 to 32 mg q.d. or 4 to 16 mg q 12 hr. *Maximum:* 32 mg/day.

Route	Onset	Peak	Duration
P.O.	In 2 wk	In 4 to 5 wk	Unknown

Mechanism of Action
Selectively blocks binding of the potent vasoconstrictor angiotensin (AT) II to AT_1 (a subtype of angiotensin II) receptor sites in many tissues, including vascular smooth muscle and adrenal glands. This inhibits the vasoconstrictive and aldosterone-secreting effects of angiotensin II, which reduces blood pressure.

Contraindications
Hypersensitivity to candesartan or its components

Interactions
DRUGS
diuretics, other antihypertensives: Possibly increased risk of hypotension

Adverse Reactions
CNS: Dizziness, headache
EENT: Pharyngitis, rhinitis
GI: Elevated liver function test results
GU: Elevated BUN and serum creatinine levels
MS: Back pain
RESP: Upper respiratory tract infection

Nursing Considerations
•If patient has known or suspected hypovolemia, expect to provide treatment, such as I.V. normal saline solution, as prescribed, to correct this condition before beginning candesartan therapy.
•Monitor for increased BUN and serum creatinine levels, especially in patients with heart failure or impaired renal function, because drug may cause acute renal failure. If increases are significant or persistent, notify prescriber immediately.
•If blood pressure is not controlled with candesartan alone, expect to administer a diuretic, such as hydrochlorothiazide, as prescribed.
•**WARNING** If patient receives a diuretic or another antihypertensive during candesartan therapy, monitor his blood pressure frequently because he has an added risk of developing hypotension.
•If patient experiences hypotension, expect to discontinue drug temporarily. Immediately place patient in supine position and prepare to administer I.V. normal saline solution, as prescribed. Expect to resume drug therapy after blood pressure stabilizes.

•If patient also receives a diuretic, provide adequate hydration, as appropriate, to help prevent hypovolemia. Also, monitor patient for signs and symptoms of hypovolemia, such as hypotension with dizziness and fainting.
•Monitor patient's CBC for possible decreases in hemoglobin and hematocrit. If decreases are significant or persistent, notify prescriber immediately.

PATIENT TEACHING
•Advise patient that full effects of candesartan may not occur for 4 to 5 weeks.
•Explain the importance of regular exercise, proper diet, and other lifestyle choices in controlling hypertension.
•Advise female patient to notify prescriber immediately about known or suspected pregnancy. Explain that if she becomes pregnant, prescriber may replace candesartan with another antihypertensive that is safe to use during pregnancy.

capreomycin sulfate
Capastat

Class and Category
Chemical: Polypeptide antibiotic isolated from *Streptomyces capreolus*
Therapeutic: Antitubercular
Pregnancy category: C

Indications and Dosages
➤ *As adjunct to treat pulmonary tuberculosis caused by* Mycobacterium tuberculosis *in which primary drugs have been ineffective or can't be used because of toxicity*
I.V. INFUSION, I.M. INJECTION
Adults. 1 g q.d. for 60 to 120 days followed by 1 g 2 or 3 times/wk for 12 to 24 mo. *Maximum:* 20 mg/kg/day.

Mechanism of Action
May interfere with lipid and nucleic acid biosynthesis in actively growing tubercle bacilli.

Contraindications
Hypersensitivity to capreomycin or its components

Interactions
DRUGS
aminoglycosides (parenteral): Increased risk of ototoxicity, nephrotoxicity, and neuromuscular blockade
nephrotoxic drugs, such as amphotericin B: Increased risk of nephrotoxicity
nondepolarizing neuromuscular blockers: Enhanced neuromuscular blockade
ototoxic drugs, such as quinidine: Increased risk of ototoxicity
polymyxins (parenteral): Increased risk of nephrotoxicity and neuromuscular blockade

Adverse Reactions
CNS: Dizziness, vertigo
EENT: Ototoxicity
GI: Elevated liver function test results
GU: Nephrotoxicity
HEME: Leukocytosis, leukopenia
SKIN: Maculopapular rash, sterile abscess, urticaria
Other: Injection site pain, induration, and bleeding

Nursing Considerations
• Use capreomycin cautiously in patients with renal insufficiency, impaired hearing, or a history of hypersensitivity, especially to other drugs.
• To reconstitute drug for I.V. injection, add 100 ml of NS. Administer over 60 minutes.
• To reconstitute drug for I.M. injection, add 2 ml of sodium chloride for injection or sterile water for injection to each 1-g vial. Allow 2 to 3 minutes for complete dissolution.
• Administer I.M. injection deeply into a large muscle mass, such as the gluteus maximus.
• Observe injection site for excessive bleeding or sterile abscess.
• Monitor results of renal function tests to detect nephrotoxicity.
• Ensure that patient receives audiometric testing and vestibular function assessments regularly.
• Closely monitor for urticaria and maculopapular rash.
PATIENT TEACHING
• Advise patient to alert nurse or prescriber if injection site bleeds excessively.
• Warn patient to contact prescriber immediately if hearing ability declines or tinnitus develops.

• Explain the need for frequent laboratory tests to monitor renal function.
• Tell patient that tuberculosis therapy lasts for 12 to 24 months.
• Explain that noncompliance may decrease the effectiveness and increase the length of treatment.

captopril

Capoten

Class and Category
Chemical: ACE inhibitor
Therapeutic: Antihypertensive
Pregnancy category: C (first trimester), D (later trimesters)

Indications and Dosages
➤ *To control hypertension*
TABLETS
Adults and adolescents. *Initial:* 25 mg b.i.d. or t.i.d. Increased to 50 mg b.i.d. or t.i.d. after 1 to 2 wk, if needed. If blood pressure isn't well controlled at this dosage and with the addition of a diuretic, dosage increased to 100 mg b.i.d. or t.i.d. and then, if needed, to 150 mg b.i.d. or t.i.d. while continuing diuretic. *Maximum:* 450 mg/day.
➤ *To control accelerated or malignant hypertension when temporary discontinuation of current antihypertensive therapy isn't practical or when prompt titration of blood pressure is needed*
TABLETS
Adults and adolescents. *Initial:* 25 mg b.i.d. or t.i.d while continuing diuretic but discontinuing current antihypertensive drug. Increased q 24 hr as needed until satisfactory response is obtained or maximum dosage is reached. *Maximum:* 450 mg/day.
➤ *To treat heart failure that's unresponsive to conventional therapy*
TABLETS
Adults and adolescents. *Initial:* 25 mg b.i.d. or t.i.d. Increased to 50 mg b.i.d. or t.i.d., as needed. After 14 days, increased to 100 mg t.i.d. and then to 150 mg t.i.d., if needed. *Maximum:* 450 mg/day.
➤ *To treat left-sided heart failure after MI*
TABLETS
Adults and adolescents. *Initial:* 6.25 mg as a single dose starting 3 days after MI and then 12.5 mg t.i.d. Increased to 25 mg t.i.d. for sev-

eral days and then increased again to maintenance dosage. *Maintenance:* 50 mg t.i.d.

➤ *To treat diabetic nephropathy*

TABLETS

Adults and adolescents. 25 mg t.i.d.

DOSAGE ADJUSTMENT Starting dosage reduced to 6.25 mg b.i.d. or t.i.d. if patient with hypertension also has heart failure, is undergoing dialysis, or is being vigorously treated with diuretics that result in hyponatremia or hypovolemia.

Route	Onset	Peak	Duration
P.O.	15 to 60 min	60 to 90 min	6 to 12 hr

Mechanism of Action

May reduce blood pressure by affecting the renin-angiotensin-aldosterone system. By inhibiting ACE, captopril:
• prevents conversion of angiotensin I to angiotensin II, a potent vasoconstrictor that also stimulates the adrenal cortex to secrete aldosterone. Inhibition of aldosterone release reduces sodium and water reabsorption and increases their excretion, reducing blood pressure.
• may inhibit renal and vascular production of angiotensin II.
• decreases serum angiotensin II level and increases serum renin activity. This decreases aldosterone secretion, slightly increasing serum potassium level and fluid loss.
• decreases vascular tone and blood pressure.

Contraindications

Hypersensitivity to captopril, other ACE inhibitors, or their components

Interactions

DRUGS

allopurinol: Increased risk of hypersensitivity reactions, including Stevens-Johnson syndrome, skin eruptions, fever, arthralgia
antacids: Possibly impaired captopril absorption
capsaicin: Possibly initiation or worsening of cough caused by ACE inhibitor
cyclosporine, potassium-containing drugs, potassium-sparing diuretics, potassium supplements: Increased risk of hyperkalemia
digoxin: Increased blood digoxin level

diuretics; hypotension-producing drugs, such as hydralazine: Additive hypotensive effects
lithium: Increased risk of lithium toxicity
NSAIDs: Decreased antihypertensive response to ACE inhibition
probenecid: Increased blood level and decreased total clearance of captopril

ACTIVITIES

alcohol use: Additive hypotensive effects

Adverse Reactions

CNS: Fever
CV: Chest pain, hypotension, orthostatic hypotension, palpitations, tachycardia
EENT: Loss of taste
GU: Dysuria, impotence, nephrotic syndrome, nocturia, oliguria, polyuria, proteinuria, urinary frequency
HEME: Eosinophilia
MS: Arthralgia
RESP: Cough
SKIN: Photosensitivity, pruritus, rash
Other: Hyperkalemia, hyponatremia, positive ANA titer

Nursing Considerations

• Closely monitor blood pressure, especially when therapy begins and with dosage increases. Keep patient supine if hypotension occurs.
• Monitor results of renal function tests for signs of nephrotic syndrome, such as proteinuria and increased BUN level and serum creatinine level. Also monitor for renal symptoms, such as oliguria, polyuria, and urinary frequency.

PATIENT TEACHING

• Instruct patient to take captopril 1 hour before meals.
• Tell patient to rise slowly from sitting or lying position to minimize effects of orthostatic hypotension.
• Tell patient to avoid sunlight or to wear sunscreen in direct sunlight because photosensitivity may occur.
• Warn patient not to stop taking drug abruptly.
• Advise patient not to use salt substitutes that contain potassium and to consult prescriber before increasing dietary potassium intake to avoid increasing the risk of hyperkalemia.

carbamazepine

Apo-Carbamazepine (CAN), Atretol, Carbatrol, Epitol, Novo-Carbamaz (CAN), Tegretol, Tegretol-XR

Mechanism of Action

Normally, sodium moves into a neuronal cell by passing through a gated sodium channel in the cell membrane. Carbamazepine may prevent or halt seizures by closing or blocking sodium channels, as shown, thus preventing sodium from entering the cell. Keeping sodium out of the cell may slow nerve impulse transmission, thus slowing the rate at which neurons fire.

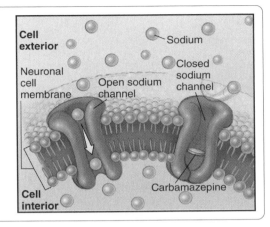

Class and Category

Chemical: Tricyclic iminostilbene derivative
Therapeutic: Analgesic, anticonvulsant
Pregnancy category: C

Indications and Dosages

➤ *To treat epilepsy*

E.R. CAPSULES, E.R. TABLETS

Adults and children age 12 and older. *Initial:* 200 mg b.i.d. Increased weekly by 200 mg/day, if needed. *Maximum:* 1,600 mg/day in adults, 1,200 mg/day in children age 16 and older, and 1,000 mg/day in children ages 12 to 16.
Children ages 6 to 12. *Initial:* 100 mg b.i.d. Increased weekly by 100 mg/day, if needed. *Maximum:* 1,000 mg/day.

ORAL SUSPENSION

Adults and children age 12 and older. *Initial:* 100 mg q.i.d. Increased weekly by 200 mg/day, if needed, given in divided doses t.i.d or q.i.d. *Maximum:* 1,600 mg/day in adults, 1,200 mg/day in children age 16 and older, and 1,000 mg/day in children ages 12 to 16.
Children ages 6 to 12. *Initial:* 50 mg q.i.d. Increased weekly by 100 mg/day, if needed, given in divided doses t.i.d or q.i.d. *Maximum:* 1,000 mg/day.
Children up to age 6. *Initial:* 10 to 20 mg/kg/day in divided doses q.i.d. *Maximum:* 35 mg/kg/day.

TABLETS

Adults and children age 12 and older. *Initial:* 200 mg b.i.d. Increased weekly by 200 mg/day, if needed, given in divided doses t.i.d. or q.i.d. *Maximum:* 1,600 mg/day in adults,

1,200 mg/day in children age 16 and older, and 1,000 mg/day in children ages 12 to 16.
Children ages 6 to 12. *Initial:* 100 mg b.i.d. Increased weekly by 100 mg/day, if needed, given in divided doses t.i.d. or q.i.d. *Maximum:* 1,000 mg/day.
Children up to age 6. *Initial:* 10 to 20 mg/kg in divided doses b.i.d. or t.i.d. Increased weekly, if needed, divided and given t.i.d. or q.i.d. *Maximum:* 35/kg/day.

➤ *To relieve pain in trigeminal neuralgia*

E.R. CAPSULES, E.R. TABLETS, TABLETS

Adults. *Initial:* 100 mg b.i.d. Increased by up to 200 mg/day, if needed, in increments of 100 mg q 12 hr. *Maintenance:* 400 to 800 mg/day. *Maximum:* 1,200 mg/day.

ORAL SUSPENSION (100 MG/5 ML)

Adults. 50 mg q.i.d. Increased by up to 200 mg/day, if needed, in increments of 50 mg q.i.d. *Maintenance:* 400 to 800 mg/day. *Maximum:* 1,200 mg/day.

Route	Onset	Peak	Duration
P.O. (all forms)	In 1 mo*	Unknown	Unknown

Contraindications

History of bone marrow depression; hypersensitivity to carbamazepine, tricyclic com-

---

*For anticonvulsant use; 8 to 72 hr for use in trigeminal neuralgia.

pounds, or their components; MAO inhibitor therapy

Interactions

DRUGS

acetaminophen (long-term use): Increased metabolism, leading to acetaminophen-induced hepatotoxicity or decreased acetaminophen effectiveness
bupropion, cyclosporine, haloperidol: Decreased blood levels of these drugs
cimetidine, clarithromycin, danazol, diltiazem, erythromycin, fluoxetine, fluvoxamine, itraconazole, ketoconazole, niacinamide, nicotinamide, propoxyphene, troleandomycin, verapamil: Increased blood carbamazepine level
cisplatin, doxorubicin, phenytoin, rifampin, theophylline: Decreased blood carbamazepine level
doxycycline: Decreased doxycycline half-life
felbamate: Decreased blood level of felbamate or carbamazepine
felodipine: Decreased felodipine effects
isoniazid: Increased risk of carbamazepine toxicity and isoniazid hepatotoxicity
lamotrigine, phenobarbital, primidone, tricyclic antidepressants, valproic acid: Decreased blood levels of these drugs, increased blood level of carbamazepine
lithium: Increased risk of CNS toxicity
oral anticoagulants: Increased metabolism and decreased effectiveness of anticoagulant
oral contraceptives: Decreased contraceptive effectiveness
nondepolarizing neuromuscular blockers: Possibly reduced duration or decreased effectiveness of neuromuscular blocker

Adverse Reactions

CNS: Chills, confusion, dizziness, drowsiness, fatigue, fever, headache, syncope, talkativeness, unsteadiness, visual hallucinations
CV: Arrhythmias, including AV block; edema; heart failure; hypertension; hypotension; thromboembolism; thrombophlebitis; worsened coronary artery disease
EENT: Blurred vision, conjunctivitis, dry mouth, glossitis, nystagmus, oculomotor disturbances, stomatitis, tinnitus, transient diplopia
ENDO: Syndrome of inappropriate ADH secretion, water intoxication
GI: Abdominal pain, anorexia, constipation, diarrhea, dyspepsia, elevated liver function

test results, hepatitis, nausea, pancreatitis, vomiting
GU: Acute urine retention, albuminuria, azotemia, glycosuria, impotence, oliguria, renal failure, urinary frequency
HEME: Acute intermittent porphyria, agranulocytosis, aplastic anemia, bone marrow depression, eosinophilia, leukocytosis, leukopenia, pancytopenia, thrombocytopenia
MS: Arthralgia, leg cramps, myalgia
RESP: Pulmonary hypersensitivity (dyspnea, fever, pneumonia, or pneumonitis)
SKIN: Aggravation of disseminated lupus erythematosus, alopecia, altered skin pigmentation, diaphoresis, erythema multiforme, erythema nodosum, exfoliative dermatitis, jaundice, Lyell's syndrome, photosensitivity reactions, pruritic and erythematous rash, purpura, Stevens-Johnson syndrome, urticaria
Other: Adenopathy, lymphadenopathy

Nursing Considerations

• Use carbamazepine cautiously in patients with impaired hepatic function because it's mainly metabolized in the liver. Monitor results of liver function tests, as directed.
• Monitor closely for adverse reactions because many are serious.
• Periodically monitor blood carbamazepine level to assess for therapeutic and toxic levels; a blood level of 6 to 12 mcg/ml is optimal for anticonvulsant effects.
• **WARNING** Monitor WBC and platelet counts monthly for first 2 months. Decreased counts may indicate bone marrow depression.

PATIENT TEACHING

• Tell patient to take carbamazepine with food (except oral suspension, which shouldn't be taken with other liquid drugs or diluents).
• Warn patient about possible dizziness, blurred vision, and unsteadiness.
• Inform patient that the coating of E.R. tablets isn't absorbed and may appear in stool.
• Advise patient not to crush or chew E.R. capsules or tablets. If he can't swallow capsules whole, have him open them and sprinkle contents on food.
• Instruct patient to wear sunscreen and protective clothing to prevent photosensitivity reactions.
• Tell patient to notify prescriber of unusual bleeding or bruising, fever, rash, or mouth ulcers.
• Warn female patient that drug decreases oral

contraceptive effectiveness and urge her to use another form of contraception. Because drug may cause fetal abnormalities, urge her to notify prescriber if pregnancy is suspected or occurs.

carbenicillin indanyl sodium

Geocillin, Geopen, Pyopen (CAN)

Class and Category

Chemical: Carboxypenicillin
Therapeutic: Antibiotic
Pregnancy category: B

Indications and Dosages

➤ *To treat acute and chronic infections of the upper and lower urinary tract and asymptomatic bacteriuria caused by susceptible strains of* Escherichia coli, Morganella morganii, Proteus mirabilis, Proteus vulgaris, *and* Providencia rettgeri

TABLETS

Adults. 382 or 764 mg (1 or 2 tabs) q.i.d.

➤ *To treat acute and chronic infections of the upper and lower urinary tract and asymptomatic bacteriuria caused by susceptible strains of* Enterobacter *sp.,* Enterococcus *sp., and* Pseudomonas *sp.*

TABLETS

Adults: 764 mg (2 tabs) q.i.d.

➤ *To treat prostatitis caused by susceptible strains of* E. coli, Enterobacter *sp.,* Enterococcus *sp., and* P. mirabilis

TABLETS

Adults: 764 mg (2 tabs) q.i.d.

Mechanism of Action

Is bactericidal to susceptible organisms by inhibiting the biosynthesis of cell wall mucopeptides, especially when target cells are actively multiplying.

Contraindications

Hypersensitivity to carbenicillin, penicillin, or their components

Interactions

DRUGS

probenecid: Increased and prolonged blood level of carbenicillin indanyl sodium and increased risk of toxicity

Adverse Reactions

EENT: Altered taste, glossitis
GI: Diarrhea, flatulence, mildly elevated AST level, nausea, vomiting
SKIN: Pruritus, rash, urticaria
Other: Anaphylaxis

Nursing Considerations

•If patient has never taken penicillin, monitor for signs of hypersensitivity, such as urticaria and laryngeal edema.

PATIENT TEACHING

•Advise patient to take carbenicillin indanyl sodium on empty stomach 1 hour before or 2 hours after meals.
•Instruct patient to take drug at even intervals around the clock, if possible.
•Encourage patient to drink plenty of fluids unless he's on a fluid restriction.
•Instruct patient to complete the full course of therapy.
•Tell patient to notify prescriber immediately if a rash, itching, or difficulty breathing develops, especially if he hasn't taken penicillin before.

carbidopa-levodopa

Apo-Levocarb (CAN), Atamet, Sinemet, Sinemet CR

Class and Category

Chemical: Hydralazine analogue of levodopa (carbidopa), levorotatory isomer of dihydroxyphenylalanine (levodopa)
Therapeutic: Antidyskinetic
Pregnancy category: C

Indications and Dosages

➤ *To relieve symptoms of Parkinson's disease*

E.R. TABLETS

Adults who aren't currently taking levodopa. *Initial:* 1 tab of 25 mg carbidopa/100 mg levodopa b.i.d. or 1 tab of 50 mg carbidopa/200 mg levodopa b.i.d. with doses spaced at least 6 hr apart. Dose increased or decreased q 3 days or more, if needed, based on response. *Maintenance:* 400 to 1,600 mg levodopa/day in divided doses q 4 to 8 hr. *Maximum:* 2,400 mg levodopa/day.
Adults who currently take levodopa regardless of dose. 1 tab of 25 mg carbidopa/100 mg levodopa b.i.d. or 1 tab of 50 mg carbidopa/200 mg levodopa b.i.d. at least 12 hr after

levodopa is discontinued. *Maximum:* 2,400 mg levodopa/day.

Adults who currently take conventional carbidopa/levodopa. If patient takes 300 to 400 mg of levodopa in combination product, regimen switched to 1 E.R. tab (200 mg levodopa) b.i.d. given 4 to 8 hr apart; if patient takes 500 to 600 mg of levodopa in combination product, regimen switched to 1 E.R. tab (300 mg levodopa) b.i.d. or t.i.d. given 4 to 8 hr apart; if patient takes 700 to 800 mg of levodopa in combination product, regimen switched to 4 E.R. tabs (800 mg levodopa)/day divided into three doses and given 4 to 8 hr apart. *Maximum:* 2,400 mg levodopa/day.

TABLETS

Adults who aren't currently taking levodopa. *Initial:* 1 tab of 25 mg carbidopa/100 mg levodopa t.i.d., or 1 tab of 10 mg carbidopa/100 mg levodopa t.i.d. or q.i.d. Increased by 1 tab q.d. or q.o.d., if needed, up to maximum dosage. *Maximum:* 200 mg carbidopa/2,000 mg levodopa/day.

Adults who currently take more than 1,500 mg of levodopa. 1 tab of 25 mg carbidopa/250 mg levodopa t.i.d. or q.i.d. at least 12 hr after levodopa is discontinued. *Maximum:* 200 mg carbidopa/2,000 mg levodopa/day.

Adults who currently take less than 1,500 mg of levodopa. 1 tab of 25 mg carbidopa/100 mg levodopa t.i.d. or q.i.d. or 1 tab of 10 mg carbidopa/100 mg levodopa t.i.d. or q.i.d. at least 12 hr after levodopa is discontinued. *Maximum:* 200 mg carbidopa/2,000 mg levodopa/day.

Mechanism of Action

Carbidopa inhibits peripheral distribution of levodopa, making more levodopa available for transport to the brain. In extracerebral tissues, levodopa is converted to dopamine. Then it's transported to the CNS, where it replenishes depleted dopamine stores, which are thought to cause Parkinson's disease, thus helping to improve muscle control and normalize body movements.

Contraindications

Angle-closure glaucoma; concurrent MAO inhibitor therapy; history of melanoma; hypersensitivity to carbidopa, levodopa, or their components; suspicious undiagnosed skin lesions

Interactions
DRUGS

antihypertensives: Increased risk of symptomatic orthostatic hypotension
benzodiazepines, droperidol, haloperidol, hydantoin anticonvulsants, loxapine, metoclopramide, metyrosine, molindone, papaverine, phenothiazines, rauwolfia alkaloids, thioxanthenes: Decreased carbidopa-levodopa effects
bromocriptine: Additive carbidopa-levodopa effects
iron salts: Decreased absorption, blood level, and effectiveness of levodopa
MAO inhibitors: Increased risk of severe orthostatic hypotension
methyldopa: Altered antiparkinsonian effects of levodopa, additive toxic CNS effects
pyridoxine: Reversed levodopa effects
tricyclic antidepressants: Increased risk of adverse reactions to carbidopa-levodopa
FOODS
high-protein food: Possibly delayed or reduced drug absorption

Adverse Reactions

CNS: Anxiety, confusion, depression, headache, insomnia, mood or mental changes, nervousness, neuroleptic malignant syndrome, nightmares, tiredness, uncontrolled movements, weakness
CV: Arrhythmias, orthostatic hypotension
EENT: Blurred vision, darkened saliva, dry mouth, eyelid spasm, ptosis
GI: Anorexia, constipation, diarrhea, nausea, vomiting
GU: Darkened urine, dysuria
MS: Muscle twitching
SKIN: Darkened sweat, flushing

Nursing Considerations
•Use carbidopa-levodopa cautiously in patients with history of psychoses because drug can cause mental disturbances. Carefully monitor all patients for depression and suicidal tendencies.
•Administer cautiously to patients with severe cardiovascular or pulmonary disease; bronchial asthma; renal, hepatic, or endocrine disease; history of MI and residual atrial, nodal, or ventricular arrhythmias; or history of peptic ulcer. Monitor closely, especially when therapy begins and dosage is adjusted.
•**WARNING** Avoid giving carbidopa-levodopa within 2 weeks of an MAO inhibitor because

doing so could cause sudden, extremely high blood pressure.

•Assess for neuroleptic malignant syndrome during dose reduction or drug discontinuation, especially in patient who also receives a neuroleptic drug. This uncommon syndrome is life-threatening and causes altered level of consciousness, autonomic dysfunction, diaphoresis, fever, high or low blood pressure, involuntary movement, muscle rigidity, tachycardia, and tachypnea. If these signs and symptoms occur, notify prescriber immediately.

PATIENT TEACHING

•If patient can't swallow E.R. tablet whole, tell him to break it in half for swallowing but not to crush or chew it.

•Remind patient that he may need to take drug for several weeks or months before full effects occur.

•Stress importance of taking carbidopa-levodopa regularly and in exact dose prescribed. Altering the dose or dosing interval may increase the risk of adverse reactions or decrease drug effectiveness.

•Tell patient to notify prescriber if involuntary movements appear or worsen during therapy because dose may need to be adjusted.

•Inform patient who is switching from regular to E.R. tablets that the onset of effect may be delayed for up to 1 hour after the first morning dose, compared with the effect usually obtained from the regular tablet. If this delay poses a problem, tell patient to notify prescriber.

carisoprodol

Soma, Vanadom

Class and Category

Chemical: Dicarbamate
Therapeutic: Skeletal muscle relaxant
Pregnancy category: Not rated

Indications and Dosages

➤ *As adjunct to relieve acute musculo-skeletal pain and stiffness*

TABLETS

Adults and children over age 12. 350 mg t.i.d. and h.s.

Children ages 5 to 12. 6.25 mg/kg t.i.d. and h.s.

Route	Onset	Peak	Duration
P.O.	30 min	Unknown	4 to 6 hr

Mechanism of Action

Blocks interneuronal activity in the descending reticular formation and spinal cord, producing muscle relaxation and sedation.

Contraindications

Hypersensitivity to carisoprodol or its components, intermittent porphyria

Interactions

DRUGS

CNS depressants, psychotropic drugs: Additive CNS depression

ACTIVITIES

alcohol use: Additive CNS depression

Adverse Reactions

CNS: Agitation, ataxia, depression, dizziness, drowsiness, fever, headache, insomnia, irritability, syncope, tremor, vertigo
CV: Orthostatic hypotension, tachycardia
EENT: Diplopia, transient vision loss
GI: Epigastric discomfort, hiccups, nausea, vomiting
HEME: Eosinophilia
SKIN: Erythema multiforme, facial flushing, pruritus, rash

Nursing Considerations

•Use carisoprodol cautiously in patients with history of drug addiction.

•Closely monitor for hypersensitivity or idiosyncratic reactions, which usually occur before the fourth dose in patients who have had no previous contact with drug.

•Provide rest and other pain-relief measures.

•To avoid mild withdrawal symptoms, expect to taper therapy as prescribed, rather than stopping it abruptly.

PATIENT TEACHING

•Tell patient to take carisoprodol with meals if GI distress occurs.

•Warn patient about possible dizziness, drowsiness, syncope, and vertigo.

•Inform patient that abruptly stopping drug can cause headache, insomnia, nausea, and other adverse reactions.

•Instruct patient to avoid alcohol and other CNS depressants while taking drug.

•Inform patient that saliva, urine, and sweat may appear darker (red, brown, or black). Reassure him that this discoloration is harmless but may stain garments.
•Tell patient to store drug in a tightly capped container at room temperature.
•Tell patient not to store drug in the bathroom, near the kitchen sink, or in other damp places. Heat and moisture may break it down.

carteolol hydrochloride

Cartrol

Class and Category
Chemical: Beta-adrenergic blocker
Therapeutic: Antihypertensive
Pregnancy category: C

Indications and Dosages
➤ *To control hypertension*
TABLETS
Adults. *Initial:* 2.5 mg q.d. If response is inadequate, dosage increased to 5 mg and then 10 mg q.d., p.r.n. *Maintenance:* 2.5 or 5 mg q.d.
DOSAGE ADJUSTMENT Dosage interval increased to q 48 hr for patients with creatinine clearance of 20 to 60 ml/min/1.73 m^2 or to q 72 hr for patients with creatinine clearance below 20 ml/min/1.73 m^2.

Route	Onset	Peak	Duration
P.O.	Unknown	1 to 3 hr	Unknown

Mechanism of Action
May reduce blood pressure by competing with beta-adrenergic receptor agonists, which helps reduce cardiac output, decrease sympathetic outflow to peripheral blood vessels, and inhibit renin release by the kidneys.

Contraindications
Asthma, bradycardia (less than 45 beats/min), cardiogenic shock, hypersensitivity to carteolol or its components, second- or third-degree heart block

Interactions
DRUGS
allergen immunotherapy, allergenic extracts for skin testing: Increased risk of serious systemic reaction or anaphylaxis

catecholamine-depleting drugs, such as reserpine: Additive effects, increased risk of hypotension and bradycardia
clonidine: Increased risk of tachycardia and hypertension after clonidine discontinuation
diltiazem, nifedipine, verapamil: Potentiated effects of carteolol
general anesthetics: Exaggeration of hypotension
NSAIDs: Reduced antihypertensive effect of carteolol
oral antidiabetic drugs: Reduced symptomatic responses to hypoglycemia
sympathomimetics with alpha- and beta-adrenergic effects, such as pseudoephedrine: Possibly hypertension and excessive bradycardia or heart block

Adverse Reactions
CNS: Fatigue, insomnia, lassitude, paresthesia, tiredness, weakness
CV: Chest pain, heart failure, peripheral edema
EENT: Dry mouth, nasal congestion, pharyngitis
GI: Abdominal pain, diarrhea, flatulence, nausea
MS: Arthralgia, back pain, leg pain, muscle spasms
SKIN: Rash

Nursing Considerations
•WARNING Be aware that abrupt cessation of carteolol in patients with angina may cause angina exacerbation or MI; abrupt cessation in patients with hyperthyroidism may cause thyroid storm.
•Carefully monitor blood glucose level in diabetic patient because carteolol can mask hypoglycemic symptoms. It also can interfere with endogenous insulin release in response to hyperglycemia, requiring dosage adjustment of oral antidiabetic drug.

PATIENT TEACHING
•Advise patient to follow dosing schedule even if he feels better and not to discontinue therapy abruptly.
•Instruct patient to report signs of heart failure, such as fatigue, difficulty breathing, cough, and unusually fast heartbeat, to prescriber.
•Tell diabetic patient to frequently monitor his blood glucose level.
•Advise patient to consult prescriber before taking OTC preparations, such as nasal de-

congestants and cold preparations that contain sympathomimetics, because of the risk of serious drug interactions.

carvedilol

Coreg

Class and Category
Chemical: Nonselective beta-adrenergic blocker with alpha$_1$-adrenergic blocking activity
Therapeutic: Antihypertensive, heart failure treatment adjunct
Pregnancy category: C

Indications and Dosages
➤ *To control hypertension*
TABLETS
Adults. 6.25 mg b.i.d. for 7 to 14 days, if tolerated. Then dosage increased to 12.5 mg b.i.d. for 7 to 14 days, and up to 25 mg, if tolerated and needed. *Maximum:* 50 mg/day.
➤ *As adjunct to treat mild to severe heart failure of ischemic or cardiomyopathic origin*
TABLETS
Adults. 3.125 mg b.i.d. for 2 wk, then increased to 6.25, 12.5, and 25 mg b.i.d. at successive 2-wk intervals, as tolerated. *Maximum (for patients with mild to moderate heart failure):* 50 mg b.i.d. if patient weighs more than 85 kg (187 lb).

Route	Onset	Peak	Duration
P.O.	In 30 min	1.5 to 7 hr	Unknown

Mechanism of Action
Reduces cardiac output and tachycardia, causes vasodilation, and decreases peripheral vascular resistance, which in turn reduces blood pressure and cardiac workload. When administered for at least 4 weeks, carvedilol reduces plasma renin activity.

Contraindications
Asthma or related bronchospastic conditions; cardiogenic shock; hypersensitivity to carvedilol or its components; decompensated heart failure that requires I.V. inotropics; and second- or third-degree AV block, severe bradycardia, or sick sinus syndrome unless pacemaker is in place

Interactions
DRUGS
calcium channel blockers, especially diltiazem and verapamil: Abnormal cardiac conduction and, possibly, increased adverse effects of calcium channel blockers
catecholamine-depleting drugs, such as reserpine and MAO inhibitors: Additive effects, increased risk of hypotension and bradycardia
cimetidine: Increased blood carvedilol level
clonidine: Risk of tachycardia and hypertension when clonidine is discontinued
cyclosporine, digoxin: Increased blood levels of these drugs
oral antidiabetic drugs: Increased risk of hypoglycemia
rifampin: Decreased blood carvedilol level

Adverse Reactions
CNS: Dizziness, fatigue, hypoesthesia, insomnia, light-headedness, malaise, somnolence, syncope, vertigo
CV: Bradycardia, edema, hypertriglyceridemia, orthostatic hypotension
EENT: Dry eyes, periodontitis, pharyngitis, rhinitis
ENDO: Hypoglycemia
GI: Abdominal pain, diarrhea, elevated liver function test results, melena, nausea
GU: UTI
HEME: Thrombocytopenia, unusual bleeding or bruising
MS: Back pain
RESP: Dyspnea
SKIN: Jaundice, pruritus
Other: Anaphylaxis, fluid overload, hyperuricemia, hyponatremia, hypovolemia, viral infection

Nursing Considerations
•Use carvedilol cautiously in patients with peripheral vascular disease because it may aggravate symptoms of arterial insufficiency. Also use drug cautiously in patients with diabetes mellitus because it may mask some signs of hypoglycemia, such as tachycardia, and may delay recovery.
•WARNING Avoid abrupt cessation of carvedilol in patients with angina because angina exacerbation or MI may occur and in patients with hyperthyroidism because thyroid storm may occur.
•For a patient with heart failure, expect to use drug with digoxin, a diuretic, and an ACE inhibitor.

PATIENT TEACHING
• Tell patient to take carvedilol with food to minimize adverse GI reactions.
• Advise patient to follow dosing schedule even if he feels better and not to discontinue therapy abruptly.
• Warn patient that drug may cause orthostatic hypotension, light-headedness, and dizziness; advise him to take safety precautions.
• Tell patient with heart failure to notify prescriber if he gains 5 lb or more in 2 days or if shortness of breath increases. These changes may signal worsening heart failure.
• Tell patient to notify prescriber if he feels dizzy or faint. These symptoms may require a dosage adjustment.
• Advise diabetic patient to frequently monitor his blood glucose level.
• If patient wears contact lenses, mention that drug may cause dry eyes.

caspofungin acetate

Cancidas

Class and Category
Chemical: Echinocandins
Therapeutic: Antifungal
Pregnancy category: C

Indications and Dosages
➤ *To treat invasive aspergillosis in patients who are refractory to or intolerant of other therapies*

I.V. INFUSION
Adults. *Initial:* 70 mg on day 1, followed by 50 mg q.d. *Maximum:* 70 mg/day.
DOSAGE ADJUSTMENT Dosage reduced to 35 mg q.d. after initial 70-mg loading dose for patients with moderate hepatic insufficiency.

Incompatibilities
Don't mix or infuse caspofungin with other drugs. Don't admix with diluents containing dextrose.

Contraindications
Hypersensitivity to caspofungin acetate or its components

Interactions
DRUGS
carbamazepine, dexamethasone, efavirenz, nelfinavir, nevirapine, phenytoin, rifampin: Possibly decreased blood caspofungin level
cyclosporine: Transient increases in ALT and AST levels
tacrolimus: Possibly decreased blood tacrolimus level

Mechanism of Action
Caspofungin acetate interferes with fungal cell membrane synthesis by inhibiting the synthesis of β (1,3)-D-glucan. A polypeptide, β (1,3)-D-glucan is the essential component of the fungal cell membrane that makes it rigid and protective. Without it, fungal cells rupture and die. This mechanism of action is most effective against susceptible filamentous fungi, such as *Aspergillus*.

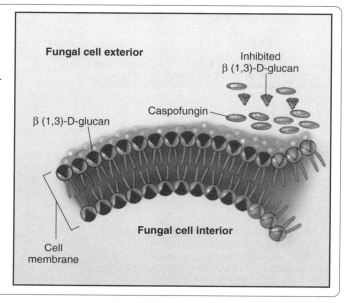

Adverse Reactions

CNS: Fever
CV: Edema
GI: Nausea, vomiting
RESP: Dyspnea, stridor
SKIN: Flushing, rash, pruritus, sensation of warmth
Other: Facial edema, infusion site reaction

Nursing Considerations

•Be aware that caspofungin acetate should not be given to a patient also receiving the antirejection drug cyclosporine unless the prescriber determines that the potential benefit outweighs the potential risk of liver damage to patient.
•To prepare the 70-mg loading dose, allow vial of drug to reach room temperature. To reconstitute, add 10.5 ml of NS to vial. Further dilute for administration by transferring 10 ml of reconstituted drug to 250 ml of NS.
•To prepare the 70-mg loading dose from two 50-mg vials, add 10.5 ml of NS to each vial; then transfer 14 ml of prepared solution to 250 ml of NS.
•To prepare the daily 50-mg infusion, allow vial of drug to reach room temperature. To reconstitute, add 10.5 ml of NS to vial. Further dilute for administration by transferring only 10 ml of reconstituted drug to 250 ml of NS.
•To prepare the daily 50-mg infusion at reduced volume, add 10 ml of reconstituted drug to 100 ml of NS.
•To prepare a 35-mg daily dose for patients with moderate hepatic insufficiency, reconstitute 50-mg vial with 10.5 ml of NS. Further dilute for administration by transferring only 7 ml of reconstituted drug to 250 ml of NS or, if medically necessary, to 100 ml of NS.
•When preparing powder for reconstitution, mix gently until you obtain a clear solution. Don't use if solution is cloudy or contains precipitate. Discard any unused solution after 24 hours.
•Infuse drug slowly over approximately 1 hour.
•Expect to increase daily dose to 70 mg, as prescribed, for patients who are receiving carbamazepine, dexamethasone, efavirenz, nelfinavir, nevirapine, phenytoin, or rifampin and who are not responding clinically.
•Monitor skin for flushing, and frequently assess patient for unexplained temperature elevation.

•Assess for airway patency if patient develops excessive facial edema or respiratory stridor. Be prepared to intervene with emergency airway management if complete obstruction occurs.

PATIENT TEACHING
•Inform patient that he may experience sensations of warmth during caspofungin infusion. Advise him to notify prescriber if sensation becomes intolerable.
•Urge patient to notify prescriber immediately if he has difficulty talking, swallowing, or breathing during drug administration.

cefaclor

Apo-Cefaclor (CAN), Ceclor, Ceclor CD

Class and Category

Chemical: Second-generation cephalosporin, 7-aminocephalosporanic acid
Therapeutic: Antibiotic
Pregnancy category: B

Indications and Dosages

➤ *To treat otitis media caused by* Haemophilus influenzae, *staphylococci,* Streptococcus pneumoniae, *and* Streptococcus pyogenes; *lower respiratory tract infections, including pneumonia caused by* H. influenzae, S. pneumoniae, *and* S. pyogenes; *pharyngitis and tonsillitis caused by* S. pyogenes; *UTIs, including cystitis and pyelonephritis, caused by* Escherichia coli, Klebsiella *sp.,* Proteus mirabilis, *and coagulase-negative staphylococci; and skin and soft-tissue infections caused by* S. pyogenes *and* Staphylococcus aureus

CAPSULES
Adults and adolescents. 250 mg q 8 hr. For severe infections, such as pneumonia, or those caused by less susceptible organisms, 500 mg q 8 hr. *Maximum:* 4 g/day.
ORAL SUSPENSION
Adults and adolescents. 250 mg q 8 hr. For severe infections, such as pneumonia, or those caused by less susceptible organisms, 500 mg q 8 hr. *Maximum:* 4 g/day.
Children. 20 mg/kg/day in divided doses q 8 hr. For serious infections, such as otitis media, and infections caused by less susceptible organisms, 40 mg/kg/day in divided doses q 8 hr. For otitis media and pharyn-

gitis, total daily dosage divided and administered q 12 hr, if needed. *Maximum:* 1 g/day.

➤ *To treat acute bacterial infection in patients with chronic bronchitis or secondary bacterial infection in patients with acute bronchitis (not caused by* H. influenzae*)*

E.R. TABLETS
Adults and adolescents age 16 and older. 500 mg q 12 hr for 7 days.

➤ *To treat pharyngitis and tonsillitis (not caused by* H. influenzae*)*

E.R. TABLETS
Adults and adolescents age 16 and older. 375 mg q 12 hr for 10 days.

➤ *To treat uncomplicated skin and soft-tissue infections caused by* S. aureus

E.R. TABLETS
Adults and adolescents age 16 and older. 375 mg q 12 hr for 7 to 10 days.

Mechanism of Action
Interferes with bacterial cell wall synthesis by inhibiting the final step in the cross-linking of peptidoglycan strands. Peptidoglycan makes cell membranes rigid and protective. Without it, bacterial cells rupture and die.

Contraindications
Hypersensitivity to cephalosporins or their components

Interactions
DRUGS
aminoglycosides, loop diuretics: Increased risk of nephrotoxicity
antacids: Decreased plasma level of cefaclor E.R. tablets
oral anticoagulants: Increased anticoagulant effect

Adverse Reactions
CNS: Chills, fever, headache, seizures
CV: Edema
EENT: Hearing loss
GI: Abdominal cramps, diarrhea, elevated liver function test results, hepatic failure, hepatomegaly, nausea, oral candidiasis, pseudomembranous colitis, vomiting
GU: Elevated BUN level, nephrotoxicity, renal failure, vaginal candidiasis

HEME: Eosinophilia, hemolytic anemia, hypoprothrombinemia, neutropenia, thrombocytopenia, unusual bleeding
MS: Arthralgia
RESP: Dyspnea
SKIN: Ecchymosis, erythema, erythema multiforme, pruritus, rash, Stevens-Johnson syndrome
Other: Anaphylaxis, superinfection

Nursing Considerations
• Use cefaclor cautiously in patients with impaired renal function or a history of GI disease, particularly colitis. Also use drug cautiously in patients who are hypersensitive to penicillin because cross-sensitivity has occurred in about 10% of such patients.
• If possible, obtain culture and sensitivity test results, as ordered, before giving drug.
• Monitor BUN and serum creatinine levels for early signs of nephrotoxicity. Also monitor fluid intake and output; decreasing urine output may indicate nephrotoxicity.
• Be aware that an allergic reaction may occur a few days after therapy starts.
• Assess bowel pattern daily; severe diarrhea may indicate pseudomembranous colitis.
• Assess for signs of superinfection, such as perineal itching, fever, malaise, redness, pain, swelling, drainage, rash, diarrhea, and cough or sputum changes.
PATIENT TEACHING
• Instruct patient to complete the prescribed course of therapy, even if he feels better.
• Tell patient to swallow E.R. tablets whole and not to crush, break, or chew them.
• Advise patient to take E.R. tablets with food to enhance absorption.
• Tell patient to shake oral suspension well before measuring and to use a liquid-measuring device to ensure accurate dosage.
• Instruct patient to refrigerate oral suspension and to discard unused portion after 14 days.
• Tell patient to immediately report severe diarrhea to prescriber.
• Inform patient that yogurt and buttermilk can help maintain intestinal flora and decrease diarrhea.
• Teach patient to recognize and report signs of superinfection, such as perineal itching and loose, foul-smelling stools.

cefadroxil
Duricef

Class and Category

Chemical: First-generation cephalosporin, 7-aminocephalosporanic acid
Therapeutic: Antibiotic
Pregnancy category: B

Indications and Dosages

➤ *To treat UTIs caused by* Escherichia coli, Klebsiella *sp., and* Proteus mirabilis

CAPSULES, TABLETS
Adults. For uncomplicated lower UTIs, 1 to 2 g q.d. or in divided doses q 12 hr. For all other UTIs, 2 g q 12 hr.

ORAL SUSPENSION
Adults. For uncomplicated lower UTIs, 1 to 2 g q.d. or in divided doses q 12 hr. For all other UTIs, 2 g q 12 hr.
Children. 30 mg/kg/day in divided doses q 12 hr. *Maximum:* Adult dosage.

➤ *To treat skin and soft-tissue infections caused by staphylococci or streptococci*

CAPSULES, TABLETS
Adults. 1 g q.d. or 500 mg q 12 hr.

ORAL SUSPENSION
Adults. 1 g q.d. or 500 mg q 12 hr.
Children. 30 mg/kg/day in divided doses q 12 hr. *Maximum:* Adult dosage.

➤ *To treat pharyngitis and tonsillitis caused by group A beta-hemolytic streptococci*

CAPSULES, TABLETS
Adults. 1 g q.d. or 500 mg b.i.d for 10 days.

ORAL SUSPENSION
Adults. 1 g q.d. or 500 mg b.i.d. for 10 days.
Children. 30 mg/kg/day in divided doses q 12 hr for 10 days. *Maximum:* 1 g q.d. or 500 mg b.i.d. for 10 days.

DOSAGE ADJUSTMENT Initial dose of 1 g followed by maintenance dosage of 0.5 g q 12 hr for patients with creatinine clearance of 25 to 50 ml/min/1.73 m^2; 0.5 g q 24 hr for patients with creatinine clearance of 10 to 25 ml/min/1.73 m^2; and 0.5 g q 36 hr for those with creatinine clearance of 0 to 10 ml/min/1.73 m^2.

Mechanism of Action

Interferes with bacterial cell wall synthesis by inhibiting the final step in the cross-linking of peptidoglycan strands. Peptidoglycan makes cell membranes rigid and protective. Without it, bacterial cells rupture and die.

Contraindications

Hypersensitivity to cephalosporins or their components

Interactions

DRUGS
aminoglycosides, loop diuretics: Increased toxicity of these drugs

Adverse Reactions

CNS: Chills, fever, headache, seizures
CV: Edema
EENT: Hearing loss
GI: Abdominal cramps, diarrhea, elevated liver function test results, hepatic failure, hepatomegaly, nausea, oral candidiasis, pseudomembranous colitis, vomiting
GU: Elevated BUN level, nephrotoxicity, renal failure, vaginal candidiasis
HEME: Eosinophilia, hemolytic anemia, hypoprothrombinemia, neutropenia, thrombocytopenia, unusual bleeding
MS: Arthralgia
RESP: Dyspnea
SKIN: Ecchymosis, erythema, erythema multiforme, pruritus, rash, Stevens-Johnson syndrome
Other: Anaphylaxis, superinfection

Nursing Considerations

•Use cefadroxil cautiously in patients with impaired renal function or a history of GI disease, particularly colitis. Also use drug cautiously in patients who are hypersensitive to penicillin because cross-sensitivity has occurred in about 10% of such patients.
•If possible, obtain culture and sensitivity test results, as ordered, before giving drug.
•Be aware that an allergic reaction may occur a few days after therapy starts.
•Monitor BUN and serum creatinine levels for early signs of nephrotoxicity. Also monitor fluid intake and output; decreasing urine output may indicate nephrotoxicity.
•Assess bowel pattern daily; severe diarrhea may indicate pseudomembranous colitis.
•Assess for signs of superinfection, such as perineal itching, fever, malaise, redness, pain, swelling, drainage, rash, diarrhea, and cough or sputum changes.

PATIENT TEACHING
•Instruct patient to complete the prescribed course of therapy.
•Tell patient to shake oral suspension

well before measuring and to use a liquid-measuring device to ensure accurate dosage.
• Instruct patient to refrigerate oral suspension and to discard unused portion after 14 days.
• Urge patient to immediately report severe diarrhea to prescriber.
• Inform patient that yogurt and buttermilk can help maintain intestinal flora and decrease diarrhea.
• Teach patient to recognize and report signs of superinfection, such as furry tongue, perineal itching, and loose, foul-smelling stools.

cefamandole nafate

Mandol

Class and Category
Chemical: Second-generation cephalosporin, 7-aminocephalosporanic acid
Therapeutic: Antibiotic
Pregnancy category: B

Indications and Dosages
➤ *To treat lower respiratory tract infections, including pneumonia, caused by beta-hemolytic streptococci,* Haemophilus influenzae, Klebsiella *sp.,* Proteus mirabilis, Staphylococcus aureus, *and* Streptococcus pneumoniae; *peritonitis caused by* Enterobacter sp. *and* Escherichia coli; *septicemia caused by* E. coli, H. influenzae, Klebsiella *sp.,* S. aureus, S. pneumoniae, *and* Streptococcus pyogenes; *and bone and joint infections caused by* S. aureus

I.V. INFUSION, I.V. OR I.M. INJECTION
Adults. 0.5 to 1 g q 4 to 8 hr. For uncomplicated pneumonia, 0.5 g q 6 hr. For severe infections, 1 g q 4 to 6 hr. For life-threatening infections or infections caused by less susceptible organisms, 2 g q 4 hr. *Maximum:* 12 g/day.
Children. 50 to 100 mg/kg/day in equally divided doses q 4 to 8 hr. For severe infections, 150 mg/kg/day. *Maximum:* Maximum adult dosage.

➤ *To treat soft-tissue infections caused by* E. coli, Enterobacter *sp.,* H. influenzae, P. mirabilis, S. aureus, *and* S. pyogenes

I.V. INFUSION, I.V. OR I.M. INJECTION
Adults. 500 mg q 6 hr.
Children. 50 to 100 mg/kg/day in equally divided doses q 4 to 8 hr. For severe infections,

150 mg/kg/day. *Maximum:* Maximum adult dosage.

➤ *To treat UTIs caused by* E. coli, Enterobacter *sp., group D streptococci,* Klebsiella *sp.,* Proteus *sp., and* Staphylococcus epidermidis

I.V. INFUSION, I.V. OR I.M. INJECTION
Adults. 500 to 1,000 mg q 8 hr.
Children. 50 to 100 mg/kg/day in equally divided doses q 4 to 8 hr. For severe infections, 150 mg/kg/day. *Maximum:* Maximum adult dosage.

➤ *To provide surgical prophylaxis*
I.V. INFUSION, I.V. OR I.M. INJECTION
Adults. 1 to 2 g 30 to 60 min before surgery followed by 1 to 2 g q 6 hr for 24 to 48 hr (or for 72 hr for prosthetic arthroplasty).
Children age 3 months or older. 50 to 100 mg/kg/day in divided doses with first dose given 30 to 60 min before surgery and then q 6 hr for 24 to 48 hr.

DOSAGE ADJUSTMENT After initial dose of 1 to 2 g, dosage reduced for patients with creatinine clearance of 50 to 80 ml/min/1.73 m^2 to 1.5 g q 4 hr or 2 g q 6 hr for life-threatening infections and 0.75 to 1.5 g q 6 hr for less severe infections; for those with creatinine clearance of 25 to 50 ml/min/1.73 m^2, dosage reduced to 1.5 g q 6 hr or 2 g q 8 hr for life-threatening infections and 0.75 to 1.5 g q 8 hr for less severe infections; for those with creatinine clearance of 10 to 25 ml/min/1.73 m^2, dosage reduced to 1 g q 6 hr or 1.25 g q 8 hr for life-threatening infections and 0.5 to 1 g q 8 hr for less severe infections; for those with creatinine clearance of 2 to 10 ml/min/1.73 m^2, dosage reduced to 0.67 g q 8 hr or 1 g q 12 hr for life-threatening infections and 0.5 to 0.75 g q 12 hr for less severe infections; and for those with creatinine clearance of less than 2 ml/min/1.73 m^2, dosage reduced to 0.5 g q 8 hr or 0.75 g q 12 hr for life-threatening infections and 0.25 to 0.5 g q 12 hr for less severe infections.

Mechanism of Action
Interferes with bacterial cell wall synthesis by inhibiting the final step in the cross-linking of peptidoglycan strands. Peptidoglycan makes cell membranes rigid and protective. Without it, bacterial cells rupture and die.

Incompatibilities

To prevent mutual inactivation, don't mix cefamandole with aminoglycosides. Also don't mix drug with Ringer's injection or lactated Ringer's injection.

Contraindications

Hypersensitivity to cephalosporins or their components

Interactions

DRUGS

aminoglycosides, loop diuretics: Increased risk of nephrotoxicity
oral anticoagulants, other drugs that affect blood clotting: Increased anticoagulant effect

ACTIVITIES

alcohol use: Disulfiram-like reaction from acetaldehyde accumulation

Adverse Reactions

CNS: Chills, fever, headache, seizures
CV: Edema
EENT: Hearing loss
GI: Abdominal cramps, diarrhea, elevated liver function test results, hepatic failure, hepatomegaly, nausea, oral candidiasis, pseudomembranous colitis, vomiting
GU: Elevated BUN level, nephrotoxicity, renal failure, vaginal candidiasis
HEME: Eosinophilia, hemolytic anemia, hypoprothrombinemia, neutropenia, thrombocytopenia, unusual bleeding
MS: Arthralgia
RESP: Dyspnea
SKIN: Ecchymosis, erythema, erythema multiforme, pruritus, rash, Stevens-Johnson syndrome
Other: Anaphylaxis; injection site pain, redness, and swelling; superinfection

Nursing Considerations

• Use cefamandole cautiously in patients who are hypersensitive to penicillin because cross-sensitivity has occurred in about 10% of such patients.
• Also use drug cautiously in patients with a history of bleeding disorders. Monitor PT and bleeding time, as ordered. Assess for ecchymosis, bleeding, pharyngitis, and arthralgia, which may indicate a blood dyscrasia. Be prepared to administer vitamin K, if ordered, to treat hypoprothrombinemia.
• If possible, obtain culture and sensitivity test results, as ordered, before giving drug.

• For direct intermittent I.V. injection, dilute each gram of drug with 10 ml of sterile water for injection, D_5W, or sodium chloride for injection. Slowly inject solution over 3 to 5 minutes through tubing of a flowing compatible I.V. solution.
• For continuous I.V. infusion, dilute each gram of drug with 10 ml of sterile water for injection and add to compatible I.V. solution, such as NS. (See manufacturer's guidelines for complete listing.)
• For I.M. injection, dilute each gram of drug with 3 ml of sterile water for injection, bacteriostatic water for injection, or bacteriostatic sodium chloride for injection. Shake well until dissolved. To minimize pain, administer by deep injection into a large muscle mass, such as gluteus maximus.
• Store reconstituted cefamandole for up to 24 hours at room temperature or 96 hours under refrigeration.
• Monitor BUN and serum creatinine levels for early signs of nephrotoxicity. Also monitor fluid intake and output; decreasing urine output may indicate nephrotoxicity.
• Be aware that an allergic reaction may occur a few days after therapy starts.
• Assess bowel pattern daily; severe diarrhea may indicate pseudomembranous colitis.
• Assess for signs of superinfection, such as perineal itching, fever, malaise, redness, rash, diarrhea, and cough or sputum changes.

PATIENT TEACHING

• Advise patient to immediately report severe diarrhea to prescriber.
• Inform patient that I.M. injection may be painful.

cefazolin sodium

Ancef, Kefzol

Class and Category

Chemical: First-generation cephalosporin, 7-aminocephalosporanic acid
Therapeutic: Antibiotic
Pregnancy category: B

Indications and Dosages

➤ *To treat respiratory tract infections caused by group A beta-hemolytic streptococci,* Haemophilus influenzae, Klebsiella *sp.,* Staphylococcus aureus, *and* Streptococcus pneumoniae; *skin and soft-*

tissue infections caused by S. aureus, *group A beta-hemolytic and other strains of streptococci; biliary tract infections caused by* Escherichia coli, Klebsiella *sp.,* Proteus mirabilis, S. aureus, *and various strains of streptococci; bone and joint infections caused by* S. aureus; *genital infections, such as epididymitis and prostatitis, caused by* E. coli, Klebsiella *sp.,* P. mirabilis, *and some strains of enterococci; septicemia caused by* E. coli, Klebsiella *sp.,* P. mirabilis, S. aureus, *and* S. pneumoniae; *and endocarditis caused by group A beta-hemolytic streptococci and* S. aureus

I.V. INFUSION, I.V. OR I.M. INJECTION

Adults. For mild infections, 250 to 500 mg q 8 hr; for moderate to severe infections, 500 to 1,000 mg q 6 to 8 hr; and for severe life-threatening infections, 1,000 to 1,500 mg q 6 hr. *Maximum:* 6 g/day.

Children: For mild to moderate infections, 25 to 50 mg/kg/day divided equally and given t.i.d. or q.i.d.; for severe infections, 100 mg/kg/day divided equally and given t.i.d. or q.i.d.

➤ *To treat pneumococcal pneumonia*

I.V. INFUSION, I.V. OR I.M. INJECTION

Adults. 500 mg q 12 hr.

➤ *To treat acute uncomplicated UTIs caused by* E. coli, Klebsiella *sp.,* P. mirabilis, *and some strains of* Enterobacter *and* Enterococcus

I.V. INFUSION, I.V. OR I.M. INJECTION

Adults. 1 g q 12 hr.

➤ *To provide surgical prophylaxis*

I.V. INFUSION, I.V. OR I.M. INJECTION

Adults. 1 g 30 to 60 min before surgery, 0.5 to 1 g during surgery if procedure lasts 2 hr or longer, then 0.5 to 1 g q 6 to 8 hr for 24 hr after surgery.

DOSAGE ADJUSTMENT After initial loading dose appropriate to infection's severity, dosage interval restricted to at least 8 hr for adults with creatinine clearance of 35 to 54 ml/min/1.73 m^2; dosage reduced by 50% and given q 12 hr for adults with creatinine clearance of 11 to 34 ml/min/1.73 m^2; and dosage reduced by 50% and given q 18 to 24 hr for adults with creatinine clearance of 10 ml/min/1.73 m^2 or less. Dosage reduced to 60% and given q 12 hr for children with creatinine clearance of 40 to 70 ml/min/1.73 m^2; dosage reduced to 25% and given q 12 hr for children with creatinine clearance of 20 to 40 ml/min/1.73 m^2; and dosage reduced to 10% and given q 24 hr for children with creatinine clearance of 5 to 20 ml/min/1.73 m^2.

Mechanism of Action

Interferes with bacterial cell wall synthesis by inhibiting the final step in the cross-linking of peptidoglycan strands. Peptidoglycan makes cell membranes rigid and protective. Without it, bacterial cells rupture and die.

Incompatibilities

To prevent mutual inactivation, don't mix cefazolin with aminoglycosides. Also avoid mixing cefazolin with other drugs, including pentamidine isethionate.

Contraindications

Hypersensitivity to cephalosporins or their components

Interactions

DRUGS

aminoglycosides, loop diuretics: Additive nephrotoxicity

probenecid: Increased and prolonged plasma cefazolin level

Adverse Reactions

CNS: Chills, fever, headache, seizures

CV: Edema

EENT: Hearing loss

GI: Abdominal cramps, diarrhea, elevated liver function test results, hepatic failure, hepatomegaly, nausea, oral candidiasis, pseudomembranous colitis, vomiting

GU: Elevated BUN level, nephrotoxicity, renal failure, vaginal candidiasis

HEME: Eosinophilia, hemolytic anemia, hypoprothrombinemia, neutropenia, thrombocytopenia, unusual bleeding

MS: Arthralgia

RESP: Dyspnea

SKIN: Ecchymosis, erythema, erythema multiforme, pruritus, rash, Stevens-Johnson syndrome

Other: Anaphylaxis; injection site pain, redness, and swelling; superinfection

Nursing Considerations

•Use cefazolin cautiously in patients with impaired renal function or a history of GI disease, particularly colitis. Also use drug cautiously in patients who are hypersensitive to penicillin because cross-sensitivity has occurred in 10% of such patients.

•If possible, obtain culture and sensitivity test results, as ordered, before giving drug.

•Reconstitute 500-mg vial of drug with 2 ml of sterile water for injection (or 1-g vial with 2.5 ml). Shake well until dissolved.

•For direct I.V. injection, further dilute reconstituted solution with at least 5 ml of sterile water for injection. Inject slowly over 3 to 5 minutes through tubing of a flowing compatible I.V. solution.

•For intermittent I.V. infusion, reconstitute 500 to 1,000 mg in 50 to 100 ml of NS, D_5W, $D_{10}W$, D_5LR, $D_5/0.2NS$, $D_5/0.45NS$, D_5NS, LR injection, 5% or 10% invert sugar in sterile water for injection, 5% sodium bicarbonate (Ancef), or Ringer's injection.

•Administer I.M injection deep into large muscle mass, such as the gluteus maximus.

•Store reconstituted cefazolin for up to 24 hours at room temperature or 10 days under refrigeration.

•Monitor I.V. site for irritation, phlebitis, and extravasation.

•Monitor BUN and serum creatinine levels for early signs of nephrotoxicity. Also monitor fluid intake and output; decreasing urine output may indicate nephrotoxicity.

•Be aware that an allergic reaction may occur a few days after therapy starts.

•Assess bowel pattern daily; severe diarrhea may indicate pseudomembranous colitis.

•Assess for signs of superinfection, such as perineal itching, fever, malaise, redness, pain, swelling, drainage, rash, diarrhea, and cough or sputum changes.

•Assess for pharyngitis, ecchymosis, bleeding, and arthralgia; they may indicate a blood dyscrasia.

PATIENT TEACHING

•Instruct patient to complete the prescribed course of therapy.

•Reassure patient that I.M. injection doesn't typically cause pain.

•Tell patient to immediately report severe diarrhea to prescriber.

cefdinir

Omnicef

Class and Category

Chemical: Cephalosporin
Therapeutic: Antibiotic
Pregnancy category: B

Indications and Dosages

➤ *To treat community-acquired pneumonia caused by* Haemophilus influenzae *(including beta-lactamase–producing strains),* Haemophilus parainfluenzae *(including beta-lactamase–producing strains),* Streptococcus pneumoniae *(penicillin-susceptible strains only), and* Moraxella catarrhalis *(including beta-lactamase–producing strains)*

CAPSULES

Adults and adolescents. 300 mg q 12 hr for 10 days. *Maximum:* 600 mg/day.

➤ *To treat pharyngitis or tonsillitis caused by* Streptococcus pyogenes *and acute exacerbations of chronic bronchitis caused by* H. influenzae *(including beta-lactamase–producing strains),* H. parainfluenzae *(including beta-lactamase–producing strains),* S. pneumoniae *(penicillin-susceptible strains only), and* M. catarrhalis *(including beta-lactamase–producing strains)*

CAPSULES

Adults and adolescents. 300 mg q 12 hr for 5 to 10 days or 600 mg q 24 hr for 10 days. *Maximum:* 600 mg/day.

ORAL SUSPENSION

Children ages 6 months to 12 years. 7 mg/kg q 12 hr for 5 to 10 days or 14 mg/kg q 24 hr for 10 days (for pharyngitis or tonsillitis).

➤ *To treat acute maxillary sinusitis caused by* H. influenzae *(including beta-lactamase–producing strains),* S. pneumoniae *(penicillin-susceptible strains only), and* M. catarrhalis *(including beta-lactamase–producing strains)*

CAPSULES

Adults and adolescents. 300 mg q 12 hr or 600 mg q 24 hr for 10 days. *Maximum:* 600 mg/day.

ORAL SUSPENSION

Children ages 6 months to 12 years. 7 mg/kg q 12 hr or 14 mg/kg q 24 hr for 10 days.

➤ *To treat uncomplicated skin and soft-tissue infections caused by* Staphylococcus aureus *(including beta-lactamase-producing strains) and* Streptococcus pyogenes

CAPSULES
Adults and adolescents. 300 mg q 12 hr for 10 days. *Maximum:* 600 mg/day.

ORAL SUSPENSION
Children ages 6 months to 12 years. 7 mg/kg q 12 hr for 10 days.

➤ *To treat acute bacterial otitis media caused by* H. influenzae *(including beta-lactamase–producing strains),* S. pneumoniae *(penicillin-susceptible strains only), and* M. catarrhalis *(including beta-lactamase–producing strains)*

ORAL SUSPENSION
Children ages 6 months to 12 years. 7 mg/kg q 12 hr for 5 to 10 days or 14 mg/kg q 24 hr for 10 days.

DOSAGE ADJUSTMENT For adults with creatinine clearance of less than 30 ml/min/1.73 m², expect to reduce dosage to 300 mg q.d.; for children with creatinine clearance of less than 30 ml/min/1.73 m², dosage is 7 mg/kg (up to 300 mg) q.d. For patients undergoing intermittent hemodialysis, dosage is 300 mg or 7 mg/kg q.o.d., beginning at the end of each hemodialysis session, as prescribed.

Mechanism of Action
Interferes with bacterial cell wall synthesis by inhibiting the final step in the cross-linking of peptidoglycan strands. Peptidoglycan makes cell membranes rigid and protective. Without it, bacterial cells rupture and die. Because cefdinir is not degraded by some bacterial beta-lactamase enzymes, it is effective against many organisms that are resistant to both penicillins and some cephalosporins.

Contraindications
Hypersensitivity to cefdinir, other cephalosporins, or their components

Interactions
DRUGS
aluminum- or magnesium-containing antacids: Decreased cefdinir absorption if given within 2 hours of antacid

iron salts: Reduced cefdinir absorption if given within 2 hours of iron
probenecid: Increased blood level and prolonged half-life of cefdinir

Adverse Reactions
CNS: Asthenia, dizziness, drowsiness, headache, insomnia, somnolence
EENT: Dry mouth, pharyngitis, rhinitis
GI: Abdominal pain, anorexia, constipation, diarrhea, flatulence, indigestion, nausea, pseudomembranous colitis, stool discoloration, vomiting
GU: Leukorrhea, vaginal candidiasis, vaginitis
HEME: Leukopenia
SKIN: Pruritus, rash

Nursing Considerations
•To reconstitute powder for oral suspension, tap bottle to loosen powder. Add water to obtain dilution of 125 mg/5 ml of suspension. Shake well before each administration. Discard any unused portion after 10 days. Keep suspension bottle tightly closed and store it at room temperature.
•Administer antacids that contain aluminum or magnesium and iron salts at least 2 hours before or after cefdinir because they may interfere with cefdinir absorption.
•Monitor patient who is allergic to penicillin for signs and symptoms of a hypersensitivity reaction, ranging from a mild rash to fatal anaphylaxis, because cross-sensitivity can occur.
•Monitor patient with a chronic GI condition, such as colitis, for signs and symptoms of a drug-related exacerbation.
•Because all cephalosporins have the potential to cause bleeding, monitor elderly patients and patients with a preexisting coagulopathy, including vitamin K deficiency, for elevated PT or APTT.
•Assess bowel pattern daily; severe diarrhea may indicate pseudomembranous colitis. Notify prescriber immediately if you detect signs or symptoms of this adverse reaction.
•Assess for other signs of superinfection, including perineal itching; loose, foul-smelling stools; and vaginal drainage.

PATIENT TEACHING
•Advise patient taking cefdinir oral suspension to shake bottle well before use and to use a liquid-measuring device to ensure accurate dosage.
•Inform patient that tablet coating may cause stools to become a reddish color.

•Instruct patient to complete entire course of therapy, even if he feels better.
•Inform patient with history of colitis that drug may exacerbate the condition; urge him to notify prescriber immediately if symptoms develop.
•Inform patient with diabetes mellitus that oral suspension contains 2.86 g of sucrose per teaspoon; advise him to monitor his blood glucose levels as appropriate.
•Teach patient to recognize and report signs of superinfection, such as perineal itching; loose, foul-smelling stools; and vaginal drainage.
•Inform patient that yogurt and buttermilk can help prevent superinfection and may decrease diarrhea.

cefditoren pivoxil

Spectracef

Class and Category
Chemical: Cephalosporin
Therapeutic: Antibiotic
Pregnancy category: B

Indications and Dosages
➤ *To treat mild to moderate acute bacterial exacerbation of chronic bronchitis caused by* Haemophilus influenzae *(including beta-lactamase–producing strains),* Haemophilus parainfluenzae *(including beta-lactamase–producing strains),* Streptococcus pneumoniae *(penicillin-susceptible strains), or* Moraxella catarrhalis *(including beta-lactamase–producing strains)*

TABLETS
Adults and children age 12 and older. 400 mg b.i.d. for 10 days.
➤ *To treat mild to moderate pharyngitis and tonsillitis caused by* Streptococcus pyogenes

TABLETS
Adults and children age 12 and older. 200 mg b.i.d. for 10 days.
➤ *To treat mild to moderate uncomplicated skin and soft-tissue infections caused by* Staphylococcus aureus *(including beta-lactamase–producing strains) or* S. pyogenes

TABLETS
Adults and children age 12 and older. 200 mg b.i.d. for 10 days.

DOSAGE ADJUSTMENT For patients with moderate renal impairment (creatinine clearance of 30 to 49 ml/min/1.73 m^2), maximum dosage reduced to 200 mg b.i.d. For patients with severe renal impairment (creatinine clearance less than 30 ml/min/1.73 m^2), maximum dosage reduced to 200 mg q.d.

Mechanism of Action
Interferes with bacterial cell wall synthesis by inhibiting the final step in the cross-linking of peptidoglycan strands. Peptidoglycan makes the cell membrane rigid and protective. Without it, bacterial cells rupture and die. This mechanism of action is most effective against bacteria that divide rapidly, including many gram-positive and gram-negative bacteria. Cefditoren isn't inactivated by beta lactamase produced by some bacteria.

Contraindications
Carnitine deficiency or inborn metabolic disorder that causes carnitine deficiency; hypersensitivity to cephalosporins or their components

Interactions
DRUGS
aluminum- and magnesium-containing antacids, H$_2$-receptor antagonists: Reduced cefditoren absorption
probenecid: Increased and prolonged blood cefditoren level
FOODS
food: Increased cefditoren absorption

Adverse Reactions
CNS: Headache, hyperactivity, hypertonia, seizures
GI: Abdominal pain, diarrhea, dyspepsia, hepatic dysfunction, nausea, pseudomembranous colitis, vomiting
GU: Renal dysfunction, toxic nephropathy
HEME: Aplastic anemia, hemolytic anemia, hemorrhage
SKIN: Erythema multiforme, Stevens-Johnson syndrome, toxic epidermal necrolysis
Other: Allergic reaction, anaphylaxis, carnitine deficiency, drug fever, serum sickness–like reaction, superinfection

Nursing Considerations
•**WARNING** Before instituting cefditoren therapy, determine if patient is hypersensitive to

milk protein because cefditoren contains sodium caseinate, a milk protein. Be aware that drug should not be given to patient with this hypersensitivity. Also determine if patient has had a hypersensitivity reaction to cefditoren or other cephalosporins (because drug is contraindicated in these patients) or to penicillin (because cross-sensitivity has occurred in 10% of patients).

•Expect that cefditoren shouldn't be used for prolonged treatment because of the risk of carnitine deficiency during therapy that lasts several months.

•If possible, obtain culture and sensitivity test results, as ordered, before giving cefditoren.

•Assess patient for signs and symptoms of *Clostridium difficile* infection and pseudomembranous colitis, such as profuse, watery diarrhea. For mild cases, expect to discontinue drug. For moderate to severe cases, expect to also administer fluids and electrolytes, protein supplementation, and an antibacterial drug effective against *C. difficile* colitis, as prescribed.

•If an allergic reaction occurs, expect to discontinue drug, as prescribed. For serious acute hypersensitivity reactions, expect to also administer epinephrine, oxygen, I.V. fluids, I.V. antihistamines, I.V. corticosteroids, and I.V. vasopressors, as prescribed.

•Monitor BUN and serum creatinine levels to detect early signs of renal dysfunction. Also monitor fluid intake and output.

PATIENT TEACHING

•Urge patient to complete prescribed course of therapy.

•Instruct patient to take cefditoren with meals to enhance drug absorption.

•Advise patient not to take cefditoren with aluminum- or magnesium-containing antacids or other drugs used to reduce stomach acids because these drugs may interfere with cefditoren absorption.

•Explain that yogurt and buttermilk help maintain normal intestinal flora and can decrease diarrhea during therapy.

•Instruct patient to immediately report severe diarrhea to prescriber.

cefepime hydrochloride

Maxipime

Class and Category

Chemical: Fourth-generation cephalosporin, 7-aminocephalosporanic acid

Therapeutic: Antibiotic
Pregnancy category: B

Indications and Dosages

➤ *To treat mild to moderate UTIs caused by* Escherichia coli, Klebsiella pneumoniae, *and* Proteus mirabilis

I.V. INFUSION, I.M. INJECTION (ONLY FOR UTI CAUSED BY E. COLI)

Adults and children age 12 and older. 500 to 1,000 mg q 12 hr for 7 to 10 days.

➤ *To treat severe UTIs caused by* E. coli *or* K. pneumoniae, *moderate to severe skin and soft-tissue infections caused by* Staphylococcus aureus *or* Streptococcus pyogenes

I.V. INFUSION

Adults and children age 12 and older. 2 g q 12 hr for 10 days.

➤ *To treat moderate to severe pneumonia caused by* Enterobacter sp., K. pneumoniae, Pseudomonas aeruginosa, *or* Streptococcus pneumoniae

I.V. INFUSION

Adults and children age 12 and older. 1 to 2 g q 12 hr for 10 days.

➤ *To treat febrile neutropenia*

I.V. INFUSION

Adults and children age 12 and older. 2 g q 8 hr for 7 days or until neutropenia resolves.

➤ *To treat complicated intra-abdominal infections (together with metronidazole) caused by alpha-hemolytic streptococci,* Bacteroides fragilis, E. coli, Enterobacter *sp.,* K. pneumoniae, *or* P. aeruginosa

I.V. INFUSION

Adults and children age 12 and older. 2 g q 12 hr for 7 to 10 days.

DOSAGE ADJUSTMENT Dosing interval increased from 12 to 24 hr and from 8 to 12 hr for patients with creatinine clearance of 30 to 60 ml/min/1.73 m^2; dosing interval increased from 8 or 12 hr to 24 hr and dose decreased from 2 g q 12 hr to 1 g q 24 hr (all other doses remain unchanged) for patients with creatinine clearance of 11 to 29 ml/min/1.73 m^2; dosage decreased from 500 mg q 12 hr to 250 mg q 24 hr, from 1,000 mg q 12 hr to 250 mg q 24 hr, from 2,000 mg q 12 hr to 500 mg q 24 hr, and from 2 g q 8 hr to 1 g q 24 hr if creatinine clearance is less than 11 ml/min/1.73 m^2.

Mechanism of Action
Interferes with bacterial cell wall synthesis by inhibiting the final step in the cross-linking of peptidoglycan strands. Peptidoglycan makes cell membranes rigid and protective. Without it, bacterial cells rupture and die.

Incompatibilities
Don't add cefepime to solutions that contain ampicillin in a concentration of more than 40 mg/ml. Don't add drug to solutions that contain aminophylline, gentamycin, metronidazole, netilmicin sulfate, tobramycin, or vancomycin.

Contraindications
Hypersensitivity to cephalosporins or their components

Interactions
DRUGS
aminoglycosides, loop diuretics: Increased risk of renal failure in patients with renal disease

Adverse Reactions
CNS: Chills, fever, headache, seizures
CV: Edema
EENT: Hearing loss
GI: Abdominal cramps, diarrhea, elevated liver function test results, hepatic failure, hepatomegaly, nausea, oral candidiasis, pseudomembranous colitis, vomiting
GU: Elevated BUN level, nephrotoxicity, renal failure, vaginal candidiasis
HEME: Eosinophilia, hemolytic anemia, hypoprothrombinemia, neutropenia, thrombocytopenia, unusual bleeding
MS: Arthralgia
RESP: Dyspnea
SKIN: Ecchymosis, erythema, erythema multiforme, pruritus, rash, Stevens-Johnson syndrome
Other: Anaphylaxis; injection site pain, redness, and swelling; superinfection

Nursing Considerations
•Use cefepime cautiously in patients with impaired renal function or a history of GI disease, particularly colitis. Also use drug cautiously in patients who are hypersensitive to penicillin because cross-sensitivity has occurred in 10% of such patients.

•If possible, obtain culture and sensitivity test results, as ordered, before giving drug.
•For I.V. infusion, reconstitute according to manufacturer's guidelines. Administer over 30 minutes.
•For I.M. injection, reconstitute 500-mg vial of drug with 1.3 ml of diluent, such as sterile water for injection (or 1-g vial with 2.4 ml of diluent). See manufacturer's guidelines for complete list of appropriate diluents.
•Monitor BUN and serum creatinine levels for early signs of nephrotoxicity. Also monitor fluid intake and output; decreasing urine output may indicate nephrotoxicity.
•Be aware that an allergic reaction may occur a few days after therapy starts.
•Assess bowel pattern daily; severe diarrhea may indicate pseudomembranous colitis.
•Assess for signs of superinfection, such as perineal itching, fever, malaise, redness, pain, swelling, drainage, rash, diarrhea, and cough or sputum changes.
•Assess for pharyngitis, ecchymosis, bleeding, and arthralgia; they may indicate a blood dyscrasia.
PATIENT TEACHING
•Tell patient to immediately report severe diarrhea to prescriber.

cefixime

Suprax

Class and Category
Chemical: Third-generation cephalosporin, 7-aminocephalosporanic acid
Therapeutic: Antibiotic
Pregnancy category: B

Indications and Dosages
➤ *To treat uncomplicated UTIs caused by* Escherichia coli *and* Proteus mirabilis; *otitis media caused by* Haemophilus influenzae, Moraxella catarrhalis, *and* Streptococcus pyogenes; *pharyngitis and tonsillitis caused by* S. pyogenes; *acute bronchitis and acute exacerbations of chronic bronchitis caused by* H. influenzae *and* Streptococcus pneumoniae

ORAL SUSPENSION
Children. 8 mg/kg q.d. or 4 mg/kg q 12 hr.
TABLETS
Adults and children over 50 kg (110 lb) or age 12. 400 mg q.d. or 200 mg q 12 hr.

➤ *To treat uncomplicated gonorrhea caused by* Neisseria gonorrhoeae

TABLETS

Adults and children over 50 kg or age 12. 400 mg q.d.

DOSAGE ADJUSTMENT Dosage reduced to 75% for patients who have creatinine clearance of 21 to 60 ml/min/1.73 m^2 or receive hemodialysis. Dosage reduced to 50% for patients who have creatinine clearance of 20 ml/min/ 1.73 m^2 or less.

Mechanism of Action

Interferes with bacterial cell wall synthesis by inhibiting the final step in the cross-linking of peptidoglycan strands. Peptidoglycan makes cell membranes rigid and protective. Without it, bacterial cells rupture and die.

Contraindications

Hypersensitivity to cephalosporins or their components

Interactions

DRUGS

aminoglycosides, loop diuretics: Increased risk of nephrotoxicity
carbamazepine: Increased blood carbamazepine level

Adverse Reactions

CNS: Chills, fever, headache, seizures
CV: Edema
EENT: Hearing loss
GI: Abdominal cramps, diarrhea, elevated liver function test results, hepatic failure, hepatomegaly, nausea, oral candidiasis, pseudomembranous colitis, vomiting
GU: Elevated BUN level, nephrotoxicity, renal failure, vaginal candidiasis
HEME: Eosinophilia, hemolytic anemia, hypoprothrombinemia, neutropenia, thrombocytopenia, unusual bleeding
MS: Arthralgia
RESP: Dyspnea
SKIN: Ecchymosis, erythema, erythema multiforme, pruritus, rash, Stevens-Johnson syndrome
Other: Anaphylaxis, superinfection

Nursing Considerations

•Use cefixime cautiously in patients with impaired renal function or a history of GI disease, especially colitis. Also use drug cautiously in patients who are hypersensitive to penicillin because cross-sensitivity has occurred in 10% of such patients.
•If possible, obtain culture and sensitivity test results, as ordered, before giving drug.
•Be aware that tablets shouldn't be substituted for oral suspension to treat otitis media because cefixime suspension produces a higher peak blood level than do tablets when administered at the same dose.
•Monitor BUN and serum creatinine levels to detect early signs of nephrotoxicity. Also monitor fluid intake and output; decreasing urine output may indicate nephrotoxicity.
•Be aware that an allergic reaction may occur a few days after therapy starts.
•Assess bowel pattern daily; severe diarrhea may indicate pseudomembranous colitis.
•Assess for signs of superinfection, such as perineal itching, fever, malaise, redness, pain, swelling, drainage, rash, diarrhea, and cough or sputum changes.
•Assess for pharyngitis, ecchymosis, bleeding, and arthralgia; they may indicate a blood dyscrasia.

PATIENT TEACHING

•Instruct patient to complete the prescribed course of therapy.
•Advise patient to shake oral suspension well before pouring dose and to use a liquid-measuring device to obtain an accurate dose.
•Instruct patient to store oral suspension at room temperature and to discard unused portion after 14 days.
•Tell patient to immediately report severe diarrhea to prescriber.
•Inform patient that yogurt and buttermilk can help maintain intestinal flora and decrease diarrhea.
•Teach patient to recognize and report signs of superinfection, such as furry tongue, perineal itching, and loose, foul-smelling stools.

cefmetazole sodium

Zefazone

Class and Category

Chemical: Second-generation cephalosporin, 7-aminocephalosporanic acid
Therapeutic: Antibiotic
Pregnancy category: B

Indications and Dosages

➤ *To treat UTIs caused by* Escherichia coli; *lower respiratory tract infections, such as bronchitis and pneumonia, caused by* E. coli, Haemophilus influenzae, Staphylococcus aureus, *and* Streptococcus pneumoniae; *skin and soft-tissue infections caused by* Bacteroides fragilis, Bacteroides melaninogenicus, E. coli, Klebsiella oxytoca, Klebsiella pneumoniae, Morganella morganii, Proteus mirabilis, Proteus vulgaris, S. aureus, Staphylococcus epidermidis, Streptococcus agalactiae, *and* Streptococcus pyogenes; *intra-abdominal infections caused by* B. fragilis, Clostridium perfringens, E. coli, K. oxytoca, *and* K. pneumoniae

I.V. INFUSION

Adults. 2 g q 6 to 12 hr for 5 to 14 days. DOSAGE ADJUSTMENT Dosage reduced to 1 to 2 g q 12 hr for patients with creatinine clearance of 50 to 90 ml/min/1.73 m^2; 1 to 2 g q 16 hr for patients with creatinine clearance of 30 to 49 ml/min/1.73 m^2; 1 to 2 g q 24 hr for patients with creatinine clearance of 10 to 29 ml/min/1.73 m^2; and 1 to 2 g q 48 hr for patients with creatinine clearance of less than 10 ml/min/1.73 m^2.

➤ *To provide surgical prophylaxis for vaginal hysterectomy*

I.V. INFUSION

Adults. 2 g as a single dose 30 to 90 min before surgery or 1 g 30 to 90 min before surgery and repeated 8 and 16 hr later.

➤ *To provide surgical prophylaxis for abdominal hysterectomy and for high-risk cholecystectomy*

I.V. INFUSION

Adults. 1 g 30 to 90 min before surgery and repeated 8 and 16 hr later.

➤ *To provide surgical prophylaxis for cesarean section*

I.V. INFUSION

Adults. 2 g as a single dose after cord is clamped or 1 g after cord is clamped and then repeated 8 and 16 hr later.

➤ *To provide surgical prophylaxis for colorectal surgery*

I.V. INFUSION

Adults. 2 g as a single dose 30 to 90 min before surgery or 2 g 30 to 90 min before surgery and repeated 8 and 16 hr later.

Contraindications

Hypersensitivity to cephalosporins or their components

Mechanism of Action

Interferes with bacterial cell wall synthesis by inhibiting the final step in the cross-linking of peptidoglycan strands. Peptidoglycan makes cell membranes rigid and protective. Without it, bacterial cells rupture and die.

Interactions

DRUGS

aminoglycosides, loop diuretics: Increased risk of nephrotoxicity
anticoagulants: Possibly increased anticoagulant effect
probenecid: Increased and prolonged blood cefmetazole level

ACTIVITIES

alcohol use: Possibly disulfiram-like reaction

Adverse Reactions

CNS: Chills, fever, headache, seizures
CV: Edema
EENT: Hearing loss
GI: Abdominal cramps, diarrhea, elevated liver function test results, hepatic failure, hepatomegaly, nausea, oral candidiasis, pseudomembranous colitis, vomiting
GU: Elevated BUN level, nephrotoxicity, renal failure, vaginal candidiasis
HEME: Eosinophilia, hemolytic anemia, hypoprothrombinemia, neutropenia, thrombocytopenia, unusual bleeding
MS: Arthralgia
RESP: Dyspnea
SKIN: Ecchymosis, erythema, erythema multiforme, pruritus, rash, Stevens-Johnson syndrome
Other: Anaphylaxis; injection site pain, redness, and swelling; superinfection

Nursing Considerations

• Use cefmetazole cautiously in patients who are hypersensitive to penicillin; cross-sensitivity has occurred in 10% of such patients.
• If possible, obtain culture and sensitivity test results, as ordered, before giving drug.
• Reconstitute drug with sterile or bacteriostatic water for injection or sodium chloride for injection.
• Dilute primary solution as needed to 1 to 20 mg/ml in D$_5$W, NS, LR, or 1% lidocaine solution without epinephrine.
• Store reconstituted solution for up to 24 hours at room temperature or 7 days under refrigeration.

•Monitor BUN and serum creatinine levels and fluid intake and output to detect early signs of nephrotoxicity.
•Assess bowel pattern daily; severe diarrhea may indicate pseudomembranous colitis.
•Assess for signs of superinfection, such as perineal itching, fever, malaise, redness, rash, diarrhea, and cough or sputum changes.
•Assess for pharyngitis, bleeding, and arthralgia, which may indicate blood dyscrasia. Monitor PT and bleeding time, as ordered.

PATIENT TEACHING
•Advise patient to immediately report severe diarrhea to prescriber.
•Instruct patient to avoid alcohol during therapy and for at least 3 days after last dose.

cefonicid sodium

Monocid

Class and Category
Chemical: Second-generation cephalosporin, 7-aminocephalosporanic acid
Therapeutic: Antibiotic
Pregnancy category: B

Indications and Dosages
➤ *To treat lower respiratory tract infections caused by* Escherichia coli, Haemophilus influenzae, Klebsiella pneumoniae, *and* Streptococcus pneumoniae; *UTIs caused by* E. coli, K. pneumoniae, Morganella morganii, Proteus mirabilis, Proteus vulgaris, *and* Providencia rettgeri; *skin and soft-tissue infections caused by* Staphylococcus aureus, Staphylococcus epidermidis, Streptococcus agalactiae, *and* Streptococcus pyogenes; *septicemia caused by* E. coli *and* S. pneumoniae; *and bone and joint infections caused by* S. aureus

I.V. INFUSION, I.V. OR I.M. INJECTION
Adults. For mild to moderate infections, 1 g q 24 hr. For severe or life-threatening infections, 2 g q 24 hr.
➤ *To treat uncomplicated UTIs*
I.V. INFUSION, I.V. OR I.M. INJECTION
Adults. 500 mg q 24 hr.
DOSAGE ADJUSTMENT Initial dose reduced to 75 mg/kg I.V. or I.M. in patients with impaired renal function. Then dosage reduced to 10 to 25 mg/kg q 24 hr if creatinine clearance ranges from 60 to 79 ml/min/1.73 m^2; 8 to 20 mg/kg q 24 hr if creatinine clearance ranges from 40 to 59 ml/min/1.73 m^2; 4 to 15

mg/kg q 24 hr if creatinine clearance ranges from 20 to 39 ml/min/1.73 m^2; 4 to 15 mg/kg q 48 hr if creatinine clearance ranges from 10 to 19 ml/min/1.73 m^2; 4 to 15 mg/kg q 3 to 5 days if creatinine clearance ranges from 5 to 9 ml/minute/1.73 m^2; and 3 to 4 mg/kg q 3 to 5 days if creatinine clearance is less than 5 ml/min/1.73 m^2.
➤ *To provide surgical prophylaxis*
I.V. INFUSION, I.V. OR I.M. INJECTION
Adults. 1 g 60 min before surgery. Dose repeated once daily, if needed, for 2 days after prosthetic arthroplasty or open-heart surgery.

Mechanism of Action
Interferes with bacterial cell wall synthesis by inhibiting the final step in the cross-linking of peptidoglycan strands. Peptidoglycan makes cell membranes rigid and protective. Without it, bacterial cells rupture and die.

Incompatibilities
To prevent mutual inactivation, don't mix cefonicid with aminoglycosides.

Contraindications
Hypersensitivity to cephalosporins or their components

Interactions
DRUGS
aminoglycosides, loop diuretics: Increased risk of nephrotoxicity

Adverse Reactions
CNS: Chills, fever, headache, seizures
CV: Edema
EENT: Hearing loss
GI: Abdominal cramps, diarrhea, elevated liver function test results, hepatic failure, hepatomegaly, nausea, oral candidiasis, pseudomembranous colitis, vomiting
GU: Elevated BUN level, nephrotoxicity, renal failure, vaginal candidiasis
HEME: Eosinophilia, hemolytic anemia, hypoprothrombinemia, neutropenia, thrombocytopenia, unusual bleeding
MS: Arthralgia
RESP: Dyspnea
SKIN: Ecchymosis, erythema, erythema multiforme, pruritus, rash, Stevens-Johnson syndrome
Other: Anaphylaxis; injection site pain, redness, and swelling; superinfection

Nursing Considerations
•Use cefonicid cautiously in patients with impaired renal function. Also use drug cautiously in patients who are hypersensitive to penicillin because cross-sensitivity has occurred in about 10% of such patients.
•If possible, obtain culture and sensitivity test results, as ordered, before giving drug.
•Reconstitute each 500-mg vial of drug with 2 ml of sterile water for injection (or each 1-g vial with 2.5 ml).
•For I.V. infusion, dilute further in 50 to 100 ml of compatible solution, such as D_5W, $D_{10}W$, $D_5/0.2NS$, $D_5/0.45NS$, or D_5NS.
•Administer I.V. injection slowly over 3 to 5 minutes through tubing of a flowing compatible I.V. solution.
•For I.M. dose larger than 1 g, divide dose in half and give into large muscle mass, such as the gluteus maximus, at two different sites.
•Store reconstituted solution at room temperature for 24 hours or under refrigeration for 72 hours.
•Monitor BUN and serum creatinine levels to detect early signs of nephrotoxicity. Also monitor fluid intake and output; decreasing urine output may indicate nephrotoxicity.
•Assess bowel pattern daily; severe diarrhea may indicate pseudomembranous colitis.
•Assess for signs of superinfection, such as perineal itching, fever, malaise, redness, pain, swelling, drainage, rash, diarrhea, and cough or sputum changes.
•Assess for pharyngitis, ecchymosis, bleeding, and arthralgia; they may indicate a blood dyscrasia.

PATIENT TEACHING
•Warn patient that I.M. injection may be painful.
•Tell patient to immediately report severe diarrhea to prescriber.

cefoperazone sodium

Cefobid

Class and Category
Chemical: Third-generation cephalosporin, 7-aminocephalosporanic acid
Therapeutic: Antibiotic
Pregnancy category: B

Indications and Dosages
➤ *To treat respiratory tract infections caused by* Enterobacter *sp.,* Escherichia coli, Haemophilus influenzae, Klebsiella pneumoniae, Proteus mirabilis, Pseudomonas aeruginosa, Staphylococcus aureus, Streptococcus pneumoniae, Streptococcus pyogenes, *and other streptococci (excluding enterococci); UTIs caused by* E. coli *and* P. aeruginosa; *uncomplicated gonorrhea caused by* Neisseria gonorrhoeae; *gynecologic infections caused by anaerobic gram-positive cocci,* Bacteroides *sp.,* Clostridium *sp.,* E. coli, Staphylococcus epidermidis, *and* Streptococcus agalactiae; *bacterial septicemia caused by* E. coli, Klebsiella *sp.,* S. aureus, Serratia marcescens, *and streptococci; skin and soft-tissue infections caused by* P. aeruginosa, S. aureus, *and* S. pyogenes; *and intra-abdominal infections caused by anaerobic gram-negative bacilli,* E. coli, *and* P. aeruginosa

I.V. INFUSION, I.M. INJECTION
Adults. 1 to 2 g q 12 hr. For severe infections or those caused by less sensitive organisms, 6 to 12 g/day divided into equal doses and given b.i.d., t.i.d., or q.i.d. *Maximum:* 12 g/day.

Mechanism of Action
Interferes with bacterial cell wall synthesis by inhibiting the final step in the cross-linking of peptidoglycan strands. Peptidoglycan makes cell membranes rigid and protective. Without it, bacterial cells rupture and die.

Incompatibilities
To prevent mutual inactivation, don't mix cefoperazone with aminoglycosides. Also avoid mixing cefoperazone with other drugs, including pentamidine isethionate.

Contraindications
Hypersensitivity to cephalosporins or their components

Interactions
DRUGS
aminoglycosides, loop diuretics: Increased risk of nephrotoxicity
oral anticoagulants, other drugs that affect blood clotting: Increased anticoagulant effect
ACTIVITIES
alcohol use: Disulfiram-like reaction

Adverse Reactions
CNS: Chills, fever, headache, seizures
CV: Edema
EENT: Hearing loss

GI: Abdominal cramps, diarrhea, elevated liver function test results, hepatic failure, hepatomegaly, nausea, oral candidiasis, pseudomembranous colitis, vomiting
GU: Elevated BUN level, nephrotoxicity, renal failure, vaginal candidiasis
HEME: Eosinophilia, hemolytic anemia, hypoprothrombinemia, neutropenia, thrombocytopenia, unusual bleeding
MS: Arthralgia
RESP: Dyspnea
SKIN: Ecchymosis, erythema, erythema multiforme, pruritus, rash, Stevens-Johnson syndrome
Other: Anaphylaxis; injection site pain, redness, and swelling; superinfection

Nursing Considerations

•Use cefoperazone cautiously in patients with a history of bleeding problems, GI disease (especially colitis), or severely impaired hepatic or renal function. Also use drug cautiously in patients who are hypersensitive to penicillin because cross-sensitivity has occurred in 10% of such patients.
•If possible, obtain culture and sensitivity test results, as ordered, before giving drug.
•For I.V. use, reconstitute drug with required amount of diluent, and then further dilute in compatible solution, such as D_5W, D_5LR, $D_5.2NS$, D_5NS, $D_{10}W$, LR injection, NS, Normosol M and D_5W, or Normosol R. (See manufacturer's guidelines for details.)
•Administer I.V. drug as intermittent infusion over 15 to 30 minutes or as continuous infusion. Direct bolus injection isn't recommended.
•For I.M. injection, reconstitute drug with bacteriostatic water for injection (that contains benzyl alcohol or parabens) or sterile water for injection.
•After reconstitution, let foam dissipate and inspect the solution to ensure complete dissolution.
•Store reconstituted solution at room temperature for 24 hours.
•Monitor BUN and serum creatinine levels to detect early signs of nephrotoxicity. Also monitor fluid intake and output; decreasing urine output may indicate nephrotoxicity.
•Assess bowel pattern daily; severe diarrhea may indicate pseudomembranous colitis.
•Assess for pharyngitis, ecchymosis, bleeding, and arthralgia; they may indicate a blood dyscrasia.
•Assess for signs of superinfection, such as perineal itching, fever, malaise, redness, pain,

swelling, drainage, rash, diarrhea, and cough or sputum changes.
PATIENT TEACHING
•Advise patient to avoid alcohol during therapy and for at least 3 days after taking the last dose.
•Warn patient that I.M. injection may cause pain.
•Tell patient to immediately report severe diarrhea to prescriber.

cefotaxime sodium

Claforan

Class and Category

Chemical: Third-generation cephalosporin, 7-aminocephalosporanic acid
Therapeutic: Antibiotic
Pregnancy category: B

Indications and Dosages

➤ *To provide perioperative prophylaxis*
I.V. INFUSION, I.V. OR I.M. INJECTION
Adults and children who weigh more than 50 kg (110 lb). 1 g 30 to 90 min before surgery.
➤ *To provide perioperative prophylaxis related to cesarean section*
I.V. INFUSION, I.V. OR I.M. INJECTION
Adults. 1 g as soon as cord is clamped, then 1 g q 6 hr for up to two doses.
➤ *To treat gonococcal urethritis and cervicitis in men and women*
I.M. INJECTION
Adults who weigh more than 50 kg. 500 mg as a single dose.
➤ *To treat rectal gonorrhea in women*
I.M. INJECTION
Adults who weigh more than 50 kg. 500 mg as a single dose.
➤ *To treat rectal gonorrhea in men*
I.M. INJECTION
Adults who weigh more than 50 kg. 1 g as a single dose.
➤ *To treat disseminated gonorrhea*
I.V. INFUSION OR INJECTION
Adults and children who weigh more than 50 kg. 1 g q 8 hr.
➤ *To treat uncomplicated infections caused by susceptible organisms*
I.V. INFUSION, I.V. OR I.M. INJECTION
Adults and children who weigh more than 50 kg. 1 g q 12 hr.

Children ages 1 month to 12 years who weigh less than 50 kg. 50 to 180 mg/kg/day in four to six divided doses.
Children ages 1 to 4 weeks. 50 mg/kg I.V. q 8 hr.
Children age 1 week and younger. 50 mg/kg I.V. q 12 hr.

➤ *To treat moderate to severe infections caused by susceptible organisms*

I.V. INFUSION, I.V. OR I.M. INJECTION
Adults and children who weigh more than 50 kg. 1 to 2 g q 8 hr.
Children ages 1 month to 12 years who weigh less than 50 kg. 50 to 180 mg/kg/day in four to six divided doses. For more serious infections, including meningitis, higher dosages are used.
Children ages 1 to 4 weeks. 50 mg/kg I.V. q 8 hr.
Children age 1 week and younger. 50 mg/kg I.V. q 12 hr.

➤ *To treat septicemia and other infections that commonly require antibiotics in higher doses than those used to treat moderate to severe infections*

I.V. INFUSION OR INJECTION
Adults and children who weigh more than 50 kg. 2 g q 6 to 8 hr.

➤ *To treat life-threatening infections caused by susceptible organisms*

I.V. INFUSION OR INJECTION
Adults and children who weigh more than 50 kg. 2 g q 4 hr. *Maximum:* 12 g/day.
Children ages 1 month to 12 years who weigh less than 50 kg. 50 to 180 mg/kg/day in four to six divided doses.
Children ages 1 to 4 weeks. 50 mg/kg q 8 hr.
Children age 1 week and younger. 50 mg/kg q 12 hr.
DOSAGE ADJUSTMENT Dosage reduced by 50% for patients with estimated creatinine clearance below 20 ml/min/1.73 m^2.

Mechanism of Action
Interferes with bacterial cell wall synthesis by inhibiting the final step in the cross-linking of peptidoglycan strands. Peptidoglycan makes cell membranes rigid and protective. Without it, bacterial cells rupture and die.

Incompatibilities
To prevent mutual inactivation, don't mix cefotaxime with aminoglycosides. Also avoid mixing cefotaxime with other drugs, including pentamidine isethionate.

Contraindications
Hypersensitivity to cephalosporins or their components

Interactions
DRUGS
aminoglycosides, loop diuretics: Increased risk of nephrotoxicity
probenecid: Increased and prolonged blood cefotaxime level

Adverse Reactions
CNS: Chills, fever, headache, seizures
CV: Edema
EENT: Hearing loss
GI: Abdominal cramps, diarrhea, elevated liver function test results, hepatic failure, hepatomegaly, nausea, oral candidiasis, pseudomembranous colitis, vomiting
GU: Elevated BUN level, nephrotoxicity, renal failure, vaginal candidiasis
HEME: Eosinophilia, hemolytic anemia, hypoprothrombinemia, neutropenia, thrombocytopenia, unusual bleeding
MS: Arthralgia
RESP: Dyspnea
SKIN: Ecchymosis, erythema, erythema multiforme, pruritus, rash, Stevens-Johnson syndrome, toxic epidermal necrolysis
Other: Anaphylaxis; injection site pain, redness, and swelling; superinfection

Nursing Considerations
• Use cefotaxime cautiously in patients with impaired renal function or a history of GI disease, especially colitis. Also use drug cautiously in patients who are hypersensitive to penicillin because cross-sensitivity has occurred in 10% of such patients.
• If possible, obtain culture and sensitivity test results, as ordered, before giving drug.
• For I.V. use, reconstitute each 0.5-, 1-, or 2-g vial with 10 ml of sterile water for injection. Shake to dissolve.
• For intermittent I.V. infusion, further dilute in 50 to 100 ml of D$_5$W or NS.
• For I.M. use, reconstitute each 500-mg vial with 2 ml of sterile water for injection or bacteriostatic water for injection; each 1-g vial with 3 ml of diluent; and each 2-g vial with 5 ml of diluent. Shake to dissolve.

•**WARNING** When preparing drug for administration to a neonate, don't use diluents that contain benzyl alcohol because they have been linked to a fatal toxic syndrome.
•Administer cefotaxime by I.V. injection slowly over 3 to 5 minutes through tubing of a flowing compatible I.V. solution. Temporarily stop other solutions being given through same I.V. site.
•Discard unused portion after 24 hours when stored at room temperature or after 5 days when refrigerated.
•Protect cefotaxime powder and solution from light and heat.
•Monitor I.V. sites for signs of phlebitis or extravasation. Rotate I.V. sites every 72 hours.
•Monitor BUN and serum creatinine levels and fluid intake and output for signs of nephrotoxicity.
•Be aware that an allergic reaction may occur a few days after therapy starts.
•Assess bowel pattern daily; severe diarrhea may indicate pseudomembranous colitis.
•Assess for pharyngitis, ecchymosis, bleeding, and arthralgia, which may indicate a blood dyscrasia. Monitor PT and bleeding time, as ordered.

PATIENT TEACHING
•Caution patient that I.M. injection may be painful.
•Instruct patient to immediately report severe diarrhea to prescriber.

cefotetan disodium

Cefotan

Class and Category

Chemical: Second-generation cephalosporin, 7-aminocephalosporanic acid
Therapeutic: Antibiotic
Pregnancy category: B

Indications and Dosages

➤ *To provide surgical prophylaxis*
I.V. INJECTION
Adults. 1 to 2 g 30 to 60 min before surgery or, in cesarean section, as soon as cord is clamped.
➤ *To treat lower respiratory tract infections caused by* Escherichia coli, Haemophilus influenzae, Klebsiella *sp.,* Proteus mirabilis, Serratia marcescens, Staphylococcus aureus, *and* Streptococcus pneumoniae; *gynecologic infections caused by* Bacteroides *sp. (excluding* B.

distasonis, B. ovatus, *and* B. thetaiotaomicron*),* E. coli, Fusobacterium *sp., gram-positive anaerobic cocci,* Neisseria gonorrhoeae, P. mirabilis, S. aureus, Staphylococcus epidermidis, *and* Streptococcus *sp. (excluding enterococci); intra-abdominal infections caused by* Bacteroides *sp. (excluding* B. distasonis, B. ovatus, *and* B. thetaiotaomicron*),* Clostridium *sp.,* E. coli, Klebsiella *sp., and* Streptococcus *sp. (excluding enterococci); and bone and joint infections caused by* S. aureus

I.V. INFUSION, I.V. OR I.M. INJECTION
Adults. For mild to moderate infections, 1 to 2 g q 12 hr.
I.V. INFUSION OR INJECTION
Adults. For severe infections, 2 g q 12 hr; for life-threatening infections, 3 g q 12 hr.
➤ *To treat UTIs caused by* E. coli, Klebsiella *sp., and* Proteus *sp.*
I.V. INFUSION, I.V. OR I.M. INJECTION
Adults. 0.5 to 2 g q 12 hr or 1 to 2 g q 24 hr.
➤ *To treat skin and soft-tissue infections caused by* E. coli, Klebsiella pneumoniae, Peptostreptococcus *sp.,* S. aureus, S. epidermidis, Streptococcus pyogenes, *and* Streptococcus *sp. (excluding enterococci)*
I.V. INFUSION, I.V. OR I.M. INJECTION
Adults. For mild to moderate infections due to *K. pneumoniae,* 1 or 2 g q 12 hr. For mild to moderate infections caused by other organisms, 1 g I.M. or I.V. q 12 hr or 2 g I.V. q 24 hr; for severe infections, 2 g I.V. q 12 hr.
DOSAGE ADJUSTMENT Dosing interval reduced to 24 hr in patients with creatinine clearance of 10 to 30 ml/min/1.73 m^2 and to 48 hr in patients with creatinine clearance below 10 ml/min/1.73 m^2.

Mechanism of Action

Interferes with bacterial cell wall synthesis by inhibiting the final step in the cross-linking of peptidoglycan strands. Peptidoglycan makes cell membranes rigid and protective. Without it, bacterial cells rupture and die.

Incompatibilities

To prevent mutual inactivation, don't mix cefotetan with aminoglycosides.

Contraindications

Hypersensitivity to cephalosporins or their components

Interactions

DRUGS

aminoglycosides, loop diuretics: Increased risk of nephrotoxicity
oral anticoagulants, other drugs that affect blood clotting: Enhanced anticoagulant effect
probenecid: Increased and prolonged blood cefotetan level

ACTIVITIES

alcohol use: Disulfiram-like reaction

Adverse Reactions

CNS: Chills, fever, headache, seizures
CV: Edema
EENT: Hearing loss
GI: Abdominal cramps, diarrhea, elevated liver function test results, hepatic failure, hepatomegaly, nausea, oral candidiasis, pseudomembranous colitis, vomiting
GU: Elevated BUN level, nephrotoxicity, renal failure, vaginal candidiasis
HEME: Eosinophilia, hemolytic anemia, hypoprothrombinemia, neutropenia, thrombocytopenia, unusual bleeding
MS: Arthralgia
RESP: Dyspnea
SKIN: Ecchymosis, erythema, erythema multiforme, pruritus, rash, Stevens-Johnson syndrome
Other: Anaphylaxis; injection site pain, redness, and swelling; superinfection

Nursing Considerations

• Use cefotetan cautiously in patients with impaired renal function or a history of GI disease, especially colitis. Also use drug cautiously in patients who are hypersensitive to penicillin because cross-sensitivity has occurred in 10% of such patients.
• If possible, obtain culture and sensitivity test results, as ordered, before giving drug.
• For I.V. use, reconstitute each 1-g vial of drug with 10 ml of sterile water for injection. For each 2-g vial, use 10 to 20 ml of diluent. For I.V. infusion, further dilute solution in 50 to 100 ml of D_5W or NS.
• For direct I.V. injection, administer drug slowly over 3 to 5 minutes through tubing of a flowing compatible I.V. solution.
• For I.M. use, reconstitute each 1-g vial of drug with 2 ml of sterile or bacteriostatic water for injection, or sodium chloride for injection. For a 2-g vial, use 3 ml of diluent.
• Monitor I.V. site for signs of phlebitis and extravasation; rotate sites every 72 hours.
• Protect reconstituted solution from light

and store for up to 24 hours at room temperature or 96 hours under refrigeration.
• Be aware than an allergic reaction may occur a few days after therapy starts.
• Monitor BUN and serum creatinine levels and fluid intake and output for signs of nephrotoxicity.
• If patient receives long-term therapy, monitor CBC and serum AST, ALT, bilirubin, LD, and alkaline phosphatase levels.
• Assess bowel pattern daily; severe diarrhea may indicate pseudomembranous colitis.
• Assess for pharyngitis, ecchymosis, bleeding, and arthralgia, which may indicate a blood dyscrasia. Monitor PT and bleeding time, as ordered. Be prepared to administer vitamin K, if ordered, to treat hypoprothrombinemia.

PATIENT TEACHING

• Warn patient that I.M. injection may be painful.
• Tell patient to immediately report severe diarrhea to prescriber.
• Urge patient to avoid alcohol during cefotetan therapy and for at least 3 days after taking last dose.

cefoxitin sodium

Mefoxin

Class and Category

Chemical: Second-generation cephalosporin, 7-aminocephalosporanic acid
Therapeutic: Antibiotic
Pregnancy category: B

Indications and Dosages

➤ *To provide surgical prophylaxis*

I.V. INFUSION OR INJECTION

Adults. 2 g 30 to 60 min before surgery and then 2 g q 6 hr after first dose for up to 24 hr.
Children age 3 months or older. 30 to 40 mg/kg 30 to 60 min before surgery and then q 6 hr after first dose for up to 24 hr.
➤ *To provide surgical prophylaxis for cesarean section*

I.V. INFUSION OR INJECTION

Adults. 2 g as a single dose as soon as cord is clamped or 2 g as soon as cord is clamped followed by 2 g 4 and 8 hr after initial dose.
➤ *To provide surgical prophylaxis for transurethral prostatectomy*

I.V. INFUSION OR INJECTION

Adults. 1 g 30 to 60 min before surgery and then 1 g q 8 hr for up to 5 days.

➤ *To treat infections, including septicemia,*
gynecologic infections, intra-abdominal
infections, UTIs, and infections of the
lower respiratory tract, skin, soft tissue,
bones, and joints caused by anaerobes
(including Bacteroides *sp.,* Clostridium
sp., Fusobacterium *sp.,* Peptococcus
niger, *and* Peptostreptococcus *sp.),*
gram-negative organisms (including
Escherichia coli, Haemophilus influenzae *[also ampicillin-resistant strains],*
Klebsiella, *and* Proteus *sp.), and gram-*
positive organisms (including Staphylococcus aureus *[penicillinase- and non-*
penicillinase-producing strains], Staphylococcus epidermidis, Streptococcus
agalactiae, Streptococcus pneumoniae,
and Streptococcus pyogenes*)*

I.V. INFUSION OR INJECTION
Adults. For uncomplicated infections, 1 g q 6
to 8 hr; for moderate to severe infections, 1 g
q 4 hr or 2 g q 6 to 8 hr; for infections that
commonly require high-dose antibiotics (such
as gas gangrene), 2 g q 4 hr or 3 g q 6 hr.
Children age 3 months or older. 80 to 160
mg/kg/day in equal doses and given q 4 to 6
hr (with higher dosages used for more severe
infections). *Maximum:* 12 g/day.

➤ *To treat uncomplicated gonorrhea*
I.M. INJECTION
Adults. 2 g as a single dose along with 1 g
oral probenecid concurrently or within
30 min of cefoxitin.
DOSAGE ADJUSTMENT Dosage reduced to 1 to
2 g q 8 to 12 hr in patients with creatinine
clearance of 30 to 50 ml/min/1.73 m^2; 1 to
2 g q 12 to 24 hr in patients with creatinine
clearance of 10 to 29 ml/min/1.73 m^2; 0.5 to
1 g q 12 to 24 hr in patients with creatinine
clearance of 5 to 9 ml/min/1.73 m^2; and 0.5
to 1 g q 24 to 48 hr in patients with creatinine clearance of less than 5 ml/min/1.73 m^2.

Mechanism of Action
Interferes with bacterial cell wall synthesis
by inhibiting the final step in the cross-linking of peptidoglycan strands. Peptidoglycan
makes cell membranes rigid and protective.
Without it, bacterial cells rupture and die.

Incompatibilities
To prevent mutual inactivation, don't mix
cefoxitin with aminoglycosides. Also avoid
mixing cefoxitin with other drugs, including
pentamidine isethionate.

Contraindications
Hypersensitivity to cephalosporins or their
components

Interactions
DRUGS
aminoglycosides, loop diuretics: Increased
risk of nephrotoxicity

Adverse Reactions
CNS: Chills, fever, headache, seizures
CV: Edema
EENT: Hearing loss
GI: Abdominal cramps, diarrhea, elevated
liver function test results, hepatic failure, he-
patomegaly, nausea, oral candidiasis, pseudo-
membranous colitis, vomiting
GU: Elevated BUN level, nephrotoxicity,
renal failure, vaginal candidiasis
HEME: Eosinophilia, hemolytic anemia, hy-
poprothrombinemia, neutropenia, thrombo-
cytopenia, unusual bleeding
MS: Arthralgia
RESP: Dyspnea
SKIN: Ecchymosis, erythema, erythema multi-
forme, pruritus, rash, Stevens-Johnson syndrome
Other: Anaphylaxis; injection site pain, redness, and swelling; superinfection

Nursing Considerations
• Use cefoxitin cautiously in patients who are
hypersensitive to penicillin because cross-
sensitivity has occurred in 10% of such
patients.
• If possible, obtain culture and sensitivity
test results, as ordered, before giving drug.
• For I.V. use, reconstitute 1 g with 10 ml of
sterile water for injection or 2 g with 10 to
20 ml of diluent.
• For I.V. injection, administer slowly over 3
to 5 minutes through tubing of a flowing
compatible I.V. solution.
• For intermittent infusion, further dilute
with 50 to 100 ml of D$_5$W or NS.
• For continuous high-dose infusion, add
cefoxitin to I.V. solutions of D$_5$W, NS, or D$_5$NS.
• For I.M. use, reconstitute each 1 g with
2 ml of sterile water for injection.
• Discard unused drug after 24 hours if
stored at room temperature or after 1 week if
refrigerated.
• Be aware that powder or solution may
darken during storage, a change that doesn't
reflect altered potency.
• Be aware that an allergic reaction may
occur a few days after therapy starts.

• Monitor BUN and serum creatinine levels for early signs of nephrotoxicity. Also monitor fluid intake and output; decreasing urine output may indicate nephrotoxicity.
• Assess bowel pattern daily; severe diarrhea may indicate pseudomembranous colitis.
• Assess for pharyngitis, ecchymosis, bleeding, and arthralgia; they may indicate a blood dyscrasia.

PATIENT TEACHING
• Tell patient to immediately report severe diarrhea to prescriber.

cefpodoxime proxetil

Vantin

Class and Category

Chemical: Third-generation cephalosporin, 7-aminocephalosporanic acid
Therapeutic: Antibiotic
Pregnancy category: B

Indications and Dosages

➤ *To treat acute community-acquired pneumonia caused by* Haemophilus influenzae *or* Streptococcus pneumoniae

ORAL SUSPENSION, TABLETS
Adults and adolescents over age 13. 200 mg q 12 hr for 14 days.

➤ *To treat acute bacterial exacerbation of chronic bronchitis caused by* H. influenzae, Moraxella catarrhalis, *or* S. pneumoniae

TABLETS
Adults and adolescents over age 13. 200 mg q 12 hr for 10 days.

➤ *To treat uncomplicated gonorrhea in men and women and rectal gonococcal infections in women caused by* Neisseria gonorrhoeae

ORAL SUSPENSION, TABLETS
Adults. 200 mg as a single dose.

➤ *To treat uncomplicated UTIs caused by* Escherichia coli, Klebsiella pneumoniae, Proteus mirabilis, *or* Staphylococcus saprophyticus

ORAL SUSPENSION, TABLETS
Adults. 100 mg q 12 hr for 7 days.

➤ *To treat skin and soft-tissue infections caused by* Staphylococcus aureus *or* Staphylococcus pyogenes

ORAL SUSPENSION, TABLETS
Adults and adolescents over age 13. 400 mg q 12 hr for 7 to 14 days.

➤ *To treat acute otitis media caused by* H. influenzae, M. catarrhalis, *or* S. pneumoniae

ORAL SUSPENSION, TABLETS
Children ages 5 months through 12 years. 5 mg/kg q 12 hr (*Maximum:* 200 mg/dose) or 10 mg/kg q 24 hr (*Maximum:* 400 mg/dose) for 10 days.

➤ *To treat pharyngitis and tonsillitis caused by* S. pyogenes

ORAL SUSPENSION, TABLETS
Adults and adolescents over age 13. 100 mg q 12 hr for 5 to 10 days.
Children ages 2 months through 12 years. 5 mg/kg q 12 hr for 5 to 10 days. *Maximum:* 100 mg/dose.

DOSAGE ADJUSTMENT Dosing interval increased to 24 hr in patients with creatinine clearance of less than 30 ml/min/1.73 m^2.

Mechanism of Action

Interferes with bacterial cell wall synthesis by inhibiting the final step in the cross-linking of peptidoglycan strands. Peptidoglycan makes cell membranes rigid and protective. Without it, bacterial cells rupture and die.

Contraindications

Hypersensitivity to cephalosporins or their components

Interactions

DRUGS
aminoglycosides, loop diuretics: Increased risk of nephrotoxicity
antacids, H$_2$-receptor antagonists: Reduced bioavailability and blood level of cefpodoxime
oral anticholinergics: Delayed peak blood level of cefpodoxime
probenecid: Possibly increased and prolonged blood cefpodoxime level

Adverse Reactions

CNS: Chills, fever, headache, seizures
CV: Edema
EENT: Hearing loss
GI: Abdominal cramps, diarrhea, elevated liver function test results, hepatic failure, hepatomegaly, nausea, oral candidiasis, pseudomembranous colitis, vomiting
GU: Elevated BUN level, nephrotoxicity, renal failure, vaginal candidiasis
HEME: Eosinophilia, hemolytic anemia, hypoprothrombinemia, neutropenia, thrombocytopenia, unusual bleeding
MS: Arthralgia
RESP: Dyspnea

SKIN: Ecchymosis, erythema, erythema multiforme, pruritus, rash, Stevens-Johnson syndrome
Other: Anaphylaxis, superinfection

Nursing Considerations
• Use cefpodoxime cautiously in patients who have impaired renal function or are receiving potent diuretics. Also use drug cautiously in patients who are hypersensitive to penicillin because cross-sensitivity has occurred in 10% of such patients.
• If possible, obtain culture and sensitivity test results, as ordered, before giving drug.
• Assess bowel pattern daily; severe diarrhea may indicate pseudomembranous colitis.
• Be aware that an allergic reaction may occur a few days after therapy starts.

PATIENT TEACHING
• Urge patient to complete the prescribed course of therapy.
• Tell patient to take tablets with food to enhance absorption.
• Advise patient to refrigerate oral suspension and discard after 14 days.
• Instruct patient to shake oral suspension bottle well before pouring dose and to use a liquid-measuring device to ensure accurate doses.
• Inform patient that yogurt and buttermilk can help maintain intestinal flora and decrease diarrhea.
• Warn patient not to take an antacid within 2 hours before or after taking cefpodoxime.
• Tell patient to immediately report severe diarrhea to prescriber.

cefprozil

Cefzil

Class and Category
Chemical: Second-generation cephalosporin, 7-aminocephalosporanic acid
Therapeutic: Antibiotic
Pregnancy category: B

Indications and Dosages
➤ *To treat secondary bacterial infections in patients with acute bronchitis and acute bacterial exacerbations of acute bronchitis caused by* Haemophilus influenzae, Moraxella catarrhalis, *and* Streptococcus pneumoniae
ORAL SUSPENSION, TABLETS
Adults and adolescents. 500 mg q 12 hr for 10 days.

➤ *To treat uncomplicated skin and soft-tissue infections caused by* Staphylococcus aureus *and* Streptococcus pyogenes
ORAL SUSPENSION, TABLETS
Adults and adolescents. 250 mg q 12 hr or 500 mg q 12 to 24 hr for 10 days.
Children ages 2 to 12. 20 mg/kg q 24 hr for 10 days.
➤ *To treat pharyngitis and tonsillitis caused by* S. pyogenes
ORAL SUSPENSION, TABLETS
Adults and adolescents. 500 mg q 24 hr for 10 days.
Children ages 2 to 12. 7.5 mg/kg q 12 hr for 10 days.
➤ *To treat otitis media caused by* H. influenzae, M. catarrhalis, *and* S. pneumoniae
ORAL SUSPENSION, TABLETS
Children ages 6 months to 12 years. 15 mg/kg q 12 hr for 10 days.
➤ *To treat acute sinusitis caused by* H. influenzae, M. catarrhalis, *and* S. pneumoniae
ORAL SUSPENSION, TABLETS
Adults and adolescents. 250 to 500 mg q 12 hr for 10 days.
Children ages 6 months to 12 years. 7.5 or 15 mg/kg q 12 hr for 10 days.
DOSAGE ADJUSTMENT Dosage reduced by half and given at usual intervals in patients with creatinine clearance of less than 30 ml/min/ 1.73 m².

Mechanism of Action
Interferes with bacterial cell wall synthesis by inhibiting the final step in the cross-linking of peptidoglycan strands. Peptidoglycan makes the cell membrane rigid and protective. Without it, bacterial cells rupture and die.

Contraindications
Hypersensitivity to cephalosporins or their components

Interactions
DRUGS
aminoglycosides, loop diuretics: Increased risk of nephrotoxicity
probenecid: Increased blood cefprozil level

Adverse Reactions
CNS: Chills, fever, headache, seizures
CV: Edema
EENT: Hearing loss

GI: Abdominal cramps, diarrhea, elevated liver function test results, hepatic failure, hepatomegaly, nausea, oral candidiasis, pseudomembranous colitis, vomiting
GU: Elevated BUN level, nephrotoxicity, renal failure, vaginal candidiasis
HEME: Eosinophilia, hemolytic anemia, hypoprothrombinemia, neutropenia, thrombocytopenia, unusual bleeding
MS: Arthralgia
RESP: Dyspnea
SKIN: Ecchymosis, erythema, erythema multiforme, pruritus, rash, Stevens-Johnson syndrome
Other: Anaphylaxis, superinfection

Nursing Considerations

• Use cefprozil cautiously in patients with impaired renal function or a history of GI disease, especially colitis. Also use drug cautiously in patients who are hypersensitive to penicillin because cross-sensitivity has occurred in 10% of such patients.
• If possible, obtain culture and sensitivity test results, as ordered, before giving drug.
• **WARNING** Don't administer oral suspension to patients with phenylketonuria because it contains phenylalanine 28 mg/5 ml.
• Monitor BUN and serum creatinine levels to detect early signs of nephrotoxicity. Also monitor fluid intake and output; decreasing urine output may indicate nephrotoxicity.
• Be aware that an allergic reaction may occur a few days after therapy starts.
• Assess bowel pattern daily; severe diarrhea may indicate pseudomembranous colitis.

PATIENT TEACHING
• Urge patient to complete the prescribed course of therapy.
• Tell patient to refrigerate oral suspension and discard after 14 days.
• Instruct patient to shake oral suspension bottle well before pouring and to use a liquid-measuring device to ensure accurate doses.
• Inform patient that yogurt and buttermilk can help maintain intestinal flora and decrease diarrhea.
• Tell patient to immediately report severe diarrhea to prescriber.

ceftazidime

Ceptaz, Fortaz, Tazicef, Tazidime

Class and Category

Chemical: Third-generation cephalosporin, 7-aminocephalosporanic acid
Therapeutic: Antibiotic
Pregnancy category: B

Indications and Dosages

➤ *To treat infections caused by gram-negative organisms (including* Acinetobacter, Citrobacter, Enterobacter, Escherichia coli, Haemophilus influenzae, Klebsiella, Neisseria, Proteus mirabilis, Proteus vulgaris, Pseudomonas aeruginosa, Salmonella, Serratia, *and* Shigella), *gram-positive organisms (including* Streptococcus agalactiae, Streptococcus pneumoniae, *and* Streptococcus pyogenes *[group B streptococci]), as well as* Staphylococcus aureus *(penicillinase- and non-penicillinase-producing strains)*

I.V. INFUSION, I.M. INJECTION
Adults and children age 12 and older. 1 g q 8 to 12 hr.
I.V. INFUSION
Children ages 1 month to 12 years. 30 to 50 mg/kg q 8 hr.
Neonates up to age 1 month. 30 mg/kg q 12 hr. *Maximum:* 6 g/day.
➤ *To treat uncomplicated UTIs*
I.V. INFUSION, I.M. INJECTION
Adults and children age 12 and older. 250 mg q 12 hr.
➤ *To treat complicated UTIs*
I.V. INFUSION, I.M. INJECTION
Adults and children age 12 and older. 500 mg q 8 to 12 hr.
➤ *To treat uncomplicated pneumonia and mild skin and soft-tissue infections*
I.V. INFUSION, I.M. INJECTION
Adults and children age 12 and older. 0.5 to 1 g q 8 hr.
➤ *To treat bone and joint infections*
I.V. INFUSION
Adults and children age 12 and older. 2 g q 12 hr.
➤ *To treat serious gynecologic and intra-abdominal infections, meningitis, and life-threatening infections, especially in immunocompromised patients*
I.V. INFUSION
Adults and children age 12 and older. 2 g q 8 hr.
➤ *To treat pseudomonal lung infection in patients with cystic fibrosis and normal renal function*

I.V. INFUSION

Adults and children age 1 month and older. 30 to 50 mg/kg q 8 hr. *Maximum:* 6 g/day.
Neonates up to age 1 month. 30 mg/kg q 12 hr.

DOSAGE ADJUSTMENT Dosage reduced to 1 g q 12 hr if creatinine clearance is 31 to 50 ml/min/1.73 m^2; to 1 g q 24 hr if creatinine clearance is 16 to 30 ml/min/1.73 m^2; to 0.5 g q 24 hr if creatinine clearance is 6 to 15 ml/min/1.73 m^2; and to 0.5 g q 48 hr if creatinine clearance is less than 6 ml/min/1.73 m^2.

Mechanism of Action

Interferes with bacterial cell wall synthesis by inhibiting the final step in the cross-linking of peptidoglycan strands. Peptidoglycan makes the cell membrane rigid and protective. Without it, bacterial cells rupture and die.

Incompatibilities

Don't mix ceftazidime with aminoglycosides to prevent mutual inactivation. Vancomycin is physically incompatible with ceftazidime and a precipitate may form; I.V. line must be flushed between administration of these two drugs if given through same tubing. Also avoid mixing ceftazidime with other drugs, including pentamidine isethionate.

Contraindications

Hypersensitivity to cephalosporins or their components

Interactions

DRUGS

aminoglycosides, loop diuretics: Increased risk of nephrotoxicity

Adverse Reactions

CNS: Chills, fever, headache, seizures
CV: Edema
EENT: Hearing loss
GI: Abdominal cramps, diarrhea, elevated liver function test results, hepatic failure, hepatomegaly, nausea, oral candidiasis, pseudomembranous colitis, vomiting
GU: Elevated BUN level, nephrotoxicity, renal failure, vaginal candidiasis
HEME: Eosinophilia, hemolytic anemia, hypoprothrombinemia, neutropenia, thrombocytopenia, unusual bleeding
MS: Arthralgia
RESP: Dyspnea
SKIN: Ecchymosis, erythema, erythema multiforme, pruritus, rash, Stevens-Johnson syndrome
Other: Anaphylaxis; injection site pain, redness, and swelling; superinfection

Nursing Considerations

• Use ceftazidime cautiously in patients who are hypersensitive to penicillin because cross-sensitivity has occurred in 10% of such patients. Watch for allergic reactions a few days after therapy starts.
• Be aware that use of ceftazidime L-arginine formulation (Ceptaz) is not recommended for children under age 12.
• If possible, obtain culture and sensitivity test results, as ordered, before giving drug.
• Protect ceftazidime powder and reconstituted drug from heat and light; both tend to darken during storage.
• If pharmacy delivers frozen solution, thaw it at room temperature, not in water bath or microwave. Store thawed solution for up to 12 hours at room temperature or 7 days in refrigerator; don't refreeze.
• WARNING When preparing drug for administration to neonates or immature infants, don't use diluents containing benzyl alcohol because they have been linked to a fatal toxic syndrome characterized by CNS, respiratory, circulatory, and renal impairment and metabolic acidosis.
• For I.V. bolus, reconstitute 1 to 2 g with 10 ml sterile water for injection, D_5W, or sodium chloride for injection. Shake to dissolve. Administer I.V. injection slowly over 3 to 5 minutes through tubing of a flowing compatible I.V. fluid.
• For intermittent infusion, further dilute in 50 to 100 ml of D_5W or NS. Avoid using sodium bicarbonate injection as a diluent because drug is least stable in it. During ceftazidime administration, temporarily stop other solutions being given at the same I.V. site.
• For I.M. use, reconstitute each gram with 3 ml sterile water for injection or bacteriostatic water for injection.
• Administer I.M. injection deep into large muscle mass, such as gluteus maximus.
• Rotate I.V. sites every 72 hours. Assess for phlebitis and extravasation.
• Assess bowel pattern daily; severe diarrhea may indicate pseudomembranous colitis.
• Monitor CBC, hematocrit, and serum AST, ALT, bilirubin, LD, and alkaline phosphatase levels during long-term therapy.
• Assess for perineal itching, fever, malaise, redness, swelling, rash, and change in cough or sputum; they may indicate a superinfection.

•Assess for pharyngitis, ecchymosis, bleeding, and arthralgia, which may indicate a blood dyscrasia. Monitor PT and bleeding time, as ordered.

PATIENT TEACHING
•Advise patient to immediately report to prescriber severe diarrhea or signs of blood dyscrasia or superinfection.

ceftibuten

Cedax

Class and Category
Chemical: Third-generation cephalosporin, 7-aminocephalosporanic acid
Therapeutic: Antibiotic
Pregnancy category: B

Indications and Dosages
➤ *To treat acute bacterial exacerbations of chronic bronchitis caused by* Haemophilus influenzae, Moraxella catarrhalis, *or* Streptococcus pneumoniae; *pharyngitis and tonsillitis caused by* Streptococcus pyogenes; *and acute bacterial otitis media caused* by H. influenzae, M. catarrhalis, *or* S. pneumoniae

CAPSULES, ORAL SUSPENSION
Adults and children age 12 and older. 400 mg q.d. for 10 days.
➤ *To treat pharyngitis and tonsillitis caused by* S. pyogenes *and acute bacterial otitis media caused* by H. influenzae, M. catarrhalis, *or* S. pneumoniae

ORAL SUSPENSION
Children under age 12. 9 mg/kg q.d. for 10 days. *Maximum:* 400 mg/day.

DOSAGE ADJUSTMENT Dosage reduced to 4.5 mg/kg or 200 mg q 24 hr if creatinine clearance is 30 to 49 ml/min/1.73 m²; to 2.25 mg/kg or 100 mg q 24 hr if creatinine clearance is 5 to 29 ml/min/1.73 m².

Mechanism of Action
Interferes with bacterial cell wall synthesis by inhibiting the final step in the cross-linking of peptidoglycan strands. Peptidoglycan makes the cell membrane rigid and protective. Without it, bacterial cells rupture and die.

Contraindications
Hypersensitivity to cephalosporins or their components

Interactions
DRUGS
aminoglycosides, loop diuretics: Increased risk of nephrotoxicity

Adverse Reactions
CNS: Chills, fever, headache, seizures
CV: Edema
EENT: Hearing loss
GI: Abdominal cramps, diarrhea, elevated liver function test results, hepatic failure, hepatomegaly, nausea, oral candidiasis, pseudomembranous colitis, vomiting
GU: Elevated BUN level, nephrotoxicity, renal failure, vaginal candidiasis
HEME: Eosinophilia, hemolytic anemia, hypoprothrombinemia, neutropenia, thrombocytopenia, unusual bleeding
MS: Arthralgia
RESP: Dyspnea
SKIN: Ecchymosis, erythema, erythema multiforme, pruritus, rash, Stevens-Johnson syndrome
Other: Anaphylaxis, superinfection

Nursing Considerations
•Use ceftibuten cautiously in patients who are hypersensitive to penicillins because cross-sensitivity has occurred in up to 10% of such patients.
•If possible, obtain culture and sensitivity test results, as ordered, before giving drug.
•Store oral suspension in refrigerator, and shake well before using. Discard unused suspension after 14 days.
•Monitor BUN and serum creatinine levels to detect early signs of nephrotoxicity. Also, monitor fluid intake and output; decreasing urine output may indicate nephrotoxicity.
•Be aware that an allergic reaction may occur a few days after therapy starts.
•Assess bowel pattern daily; severe diarrhea may indicate pseudomembranous colitis.
•Assess for perineal itching, fever, malaise, redness, swelling, rash, and change in cough or sputum; they may indicate a superinfection.
•Assess for pharyngitis, ecchymosis, bleeding, and arthralgia; they may indicate a blood dyscrasia.

PATIENT TEACHING
•Urge patient to complete the drug therapy.
•Instruct patient to take drug on an empty stomach at least 2 hours before or 1 hour after meals.
•Inform patient that unflavored oral suspension has a bitter taste. Suggest that he ask that a flavor be added when prescription is filled.

• Advise patient that yogurt and buttermilk can help maintain intestinal flora and decrease diarrhea during therapy.
• Tell patient to immediately report hypersensitivity reactions, severe diarrhea, and evidence of blood dyscrasia or superinfection to prescriber.

ceftizoxime sodium

Cefizox

Class and Category
Chemical: Third-generation cephalosporin, 7-aminocephalosporanic acid
Therapeutic: Antibiotic
Pregnancy category: B

Indications and Dosages
➤ *To treat mild to moderate infections of the lower respiratory tract, skin, soft tissue, bones, and joints; septicemia; meningitis; and intra-abdominal infections caused by anaerobes (such as* Bacteroides *sp.,* Peptococcus, *and* Peptostreptococcus*), gram-negative organisms (including* Escherichia coli, Haemophilus influenzae, Klebsiella, *and* Proteus mirabilis*), and gram-positive organisms (including* Enterobacter *sp.,* Serratia *sp.,* Staphylococcus aureus, Staphylococcus epidermidis, Streptococcus agalactiae, Streptococcus pneumoniae, *and* Streptococcus pyogenes*)*

I.V. INFUSION, I.V. OR I.M. INJECTION
Adults and children age 12 and older. 1 to 2 g q 8 to 12 hr.

➤ *To treat severe or refractory infections of the type listed above*
I.V. INFUSION OR INJECTION
Adults and children age 12 and older. 1 g q 8 hr or 2 g q 8 to 12 hr.

➤ *To treat life-threatening infections of the type listed above*
I.V. INFUSION OR INJECTION
Adults and children age 12 and older. 3 to 4 g q 8 hr or, if required, up to 2 g q 4 hr.

➤ *To treat bacterial infections in children*
I.V. INFUSION, I.V. OR I.M. INJECTION
Children age 6 months and older. 50 mg/kg q 6 to 8 hr.

➤ *To treat uncomplicated UTIs*
I.V. INFUSION, I.V. OR I.M. INJECTION
Adults. 500 mg q 12 hr.

➤ *To treat pelvic inflammatory disease*
I.V. INFUSION OR INJECTION
Adults. 2 g q 8 hr.

➤ *To treat uncomplicated gonococcal infections*
I.M. INJECTION
Adults. 1 g as a single dose.
DOSAGE ADJUSTMENT Dosage reduced to 0.5 g q 8 hr for less severe infections and 0.75 to 1.5 g q 8 hr for life-threatening infections if creatinine clearance is 50 to 79 ml/min/1.73 m^2; to 0.25 to 0.5 g q 12 hr for less severe infections and 0.5 to 1 g q 12 for life-threatening infections if creatinine clearance is 5 to 49 ml/min/1.73 m^2; and to 0.5 g q 48 hr or 0.25 g q 24 hr for less severe infections and 0.5 to 1 g q 48 hr or 0.5 g q 24 hr for life-threatening infections if creatinine clearance is 4 ml/min/1.73 m^2 or less.

Mechanism of Action
Interferes with bacterial cell wall synthesis by inhibiting the final step in the cross-linking of peptidoglycan strands. Peptidoglycan makes the cell membrane rigid and protective. Without it, bacterial cells rupture and die.

Contraindications
Hypersensitivity to cephalosporins or their components

Interactions
DRUGS
aminoglycosides, loop diuretics: Increased risk of nephrotoxicity

Adverse Reactions
CNS: Chills, fever, headache, seizures
CV: Edema
EENT: Hearing loss
GI: Abdominal cramps, diarrhea, elevated liver function test results, hepatic failure, hepatomegaly, nausea, oral candidiasis, pseudomembranous colitis, vomiting
GU: Elevated BUN level, nephrotoxicity, renal failure, vaginal candidiasis
HEME: Eosinophilia, hemolytic anemia, hypoprothrombinemia, neutropenia, thrombocytopenia, unusual bleeding
MS: Arthralgia
RESP: Dyspnea
SKIN: Ecchymosis, erythema, erythema multiforme, pruritus, rash, Stevens-Johnson syndrome

Other: Anaphylaxis; injection site pain, redness, and swelling; superinfection

Nursing Considerations

•Use ceftizoxime cautiously in patients who are hypersensitive to penicillin because cross-sensitivity has occurred in 10% of such patients.
•If possible, obtain culture and sensitivity test results, as ordered, before giving drug.
•For I.V. administration, reconstitute with sterile water for injection as follows: for 500-mg vial, add 5 ml; for 1-g vial, add 10 ml; and for 2-g vial, add 20 ml. Shake well. Dilute reconstituted solution further with 50 to 100 ml of a compatible solution, such as NS or D₅W, before administration. Administer I.V. injection slowly over 3 to 5 minutes through tubing of a flowing compatible I.V. fluid.
•For I.M. administration, reconstitute with sterile water for injection as follows: for 500-mg vial, add 1.5 ml; for 1-g vial, add 3 ml; and for 2-g vial, add 6 ml. Shake well. Divide 2-g doses and administer in different sites. Inject deeply in large muscle mass, such as the gluteus maximus.
•Reconstituted drug may be stored for 24 hours at room temperature or 96 hours if refrigerated.
•Assess I.V. site for extravasation and phlebitis.
•Monitor BUN and serum creatinine levels to detect early signs of nephrotoxicity. Also, monitor fluid intake and output; decreasing urine output may indicate nephrotoxicity.
•Assess bowel pattern daily; severe diarrhea may indicate pseudomembranous colitis.
•Monitor for allergic reactions a few days after therapy starts.
•Assess CBC, hematocrit, and serum AST, ALT, bilirubin, LD, and alkaline phosphatase levels during long-term therapy.
•Assess for pharyngitis, ecchymosis, bleeding, and arthralgia; they may indicate a blood dyscrasia.

PATIENT TEACHING
•Advise patient to immediately report severe diarrhea or evidence of blood dyscrasia to prescriber.

ceftriaxone sodium

Rocephin

Class and Category

Chemical: Third-generation cephalosporin, 7-aminocephalosporanic acid
Therapeutic: Antibiotic
Pregnancy category: B

Indications and Dosages

➤ *To treat infections of the lower respiratory tract, skin, soft tissue, urinary tract, bones, and joints; sinusitis; intra-abdominal infections; and septicemia caused by anaerobes (including* Bacteroides bivius, Bacteroides fragilis, Bacteroides melaninogenicus, *and* Peptostreptococcus *sp.), gram-negative organisms (including* Citrobacter *sp.,* Enterobacter aerogenes, Escherichia coli, Haemophilus influenzae, Klebsiella *sp.,* Neisseria *sp.,* Proteus mirabilis, Proteus vulgaris, Providencia *sp.,* Salmonella *sp.,* Serratia marcescens, Shigella, *and some strains of* Pseudomonas aeruginosa*), and gram-positive organisms (including* Staphylococcus aureus, Streptococcus pneumoniae, *and* Streptococcus pyogenes*)*

I.V. INFUSION, I.M. INJECTION
Adults. 1 to 2 g q.d. or in equally divided doses b.i.d. *Maximum:* 4 g/day.
Children. 50 to 75 mg/kg/day in divided doses q 12 hr. *Maximum:* 2 g/day.

➤ *To treat meningitis*
I.V. INFUSION
Children. *Initial:* 100 mg/kg on first day, then 100 mg/kg q.d. or in divided doses q 12 hr for 7 to 14 days. *Maximum:* 4 g/day.

➤ *To treat acute bacterial otitis media*
I.M. INJECTION
Children. 50 mg/kg as a single dose. *Maximum:* 1 g.

➤ *To treat chancroid (*Haemophilus ducreyi *infection) and uncomplicated gonorrhea*
I.M. INJECTION
Adults. 250 mg as a single dose.

➤ *To treat gonococcal conjunctivitis*
I.M. INJECTION
Adults. 1 g as a single dose.

➤ *To treat disseminated gonococcal infection and pelvic inflammatory disease*
I.V. INFUSION, I.M. INJECTION
Adults: 1 g q 24 hr.

➤ *To treat gonococcal meningitis and endocarditis*
I.V. INFUSION
Adults. 1 to 2 g q 12 hr for 10 to 14 days (meningitis) or for 4 wk or longer (endocarditis).

➤ *To provide surgical prophylaxis*
I.V. INFUSION
Adults. 1 g 30 min to 2 hr before surgery.

Mechanism of Action
Interferes with bacterial cell wall synthesis by inhibiting the final step in the cross-linking of peptidoglycan strands. Peptidoglycan makes the cell membrane rigid and protective. Without it, bacterial cells rupture and die.

Incompatibilities
Don't admix ceftriaxone with pentamidine isethionate, labetalol, or other antibiotics, such as aminoglycosides, because of potential for incompatibility, such as substantial mutual inactivation.

Contraindications
Hypersensitivity to cephalosporins or their components

Interactions
DRUGS
aminoglycosides, loop diuretics: Increased risk of nephrotoxicity

Adverse Reactions
CNS: Chills, fever, headache, seizures
CV: Edema
EENT: Hearing loss
GI: Abdominal cramps, diarrhea, elevated liver function test results, hepatic failure, hepatomegaly, nausea, oral candidiasis, pseudolithiasis, pseudomembranous colitis, vomiting
GU: Elevated BUN level, nephrotoxicity, renal failure, vaginal candidiasis
HEME: Eosinophilia, hemolytic anemia, hypoprothrombinemia, neutropenia, thrombocytopenia, unusual bleeding
MS: Arthralgia
RESP: Dyspnea
SKIN: Ecchymosis, erythema, erythema multiforme, pruritus, rash, Stevens-Johnson syndrome
Other: Anaphylaxis; injection site pain, redness, and swelling; superinfection

Nursing Considerations
•Use ceftriaxone cautiously in patients who are hypersensitive to penicillins because cross-sensitivity has occurred in about 10% of such patients.
•If possible, obtain culture and sensitivity results, as ordered, before giving drug.
•Protect powder from light before reconstitution.
•For I.V. administration, reconstitute with an appropriate diluent, such as sterile water for injection or sodium chloride for injection, as

follows: 250-mg vial, add 2.4 ml; 500-mg vial, add 4.8 ml; 1-g vial, add 9.6 ml; and 2-g vial, add 19.2 ml to yield a concentration of 100 mg/ml. For piggyback bottles, reconstitute with 10 ml of diluent indicated above for 1-g bottle and 20 ml for 2-g bottle. After reconstitution, further dilute to 50 to 100 ml with diluent indicated above and administer as an infusion over 30 minutes.
•For I.M. administration, reconstitute with an appropriate diluent, such as sterile water for injection or sodium chloride for injection, as follows: 250-mg vial, add 0.9 ml; 500-mg vial, add 1.8 ml; 1-g vial, add 3.6 ml; and 2-g vial, add 7.2 ml to make a 250 mg/ml concentration. Shake well. Inject deeply in large muscle mass, such as the gluteus maximus.
•Monitor BUN and serum creatinine levels to detect early signs of nephrotoxicity. Also, monitor fluid intake and output; decreasing urine output may indicate nephrotoxicity.
•Monitor for allergic reactions a few days after therapy starts.
•Assess CBC, hematocrit, and serum AST, ALT, bilirubin, LD, and alkaline phosphatase levels during long-term therapy.
•Assess bowel pattern daily; severe diarrhea may indicate pseudomembranous colitis.
•Assess for perineal itching, fever, malaise, redness, swelling, rash, and change in cough or sputum; they may indicate a superinfection.
•Assess for pharyngitis, ecchymosis, bleeding, and arthralgia; they may indicate a blood dyscrasia.
PATIENT TEACHING
•Tell patient to immediately report severe diarrhea or evidence of blood dyscrasia or superinfection to prescriber.

cefuroxime axetil
Ceftin

cefuroxime sodium
Kefurox, Zinacef

Class and Category
Chemical: Second-generation cephalosporin, 7-aminocephalosporanic acid
Therapeutic: Antibiotic
Pregnancy category: B

Indications and Dosages
➤ *To treat pharyngitis and tonsillitis*
ORAL SUSPENSION
Children ages 3 months to 12 years. 10 mg/

kg/day in equally divided doses b.i.d. for 10 days. *Maximum:* 500 mg/day.

TABLETS

Adults and children age 13 and over. 250 mg b.i.d. for 10 days.

Children under age 13 who can swallow tablets. 125 mg b.i.d. for 10 days.

➤ *To treat acute otitis media*

ORAL SUSPENSION

Children ages 3 months to 12 years. 30 mg/kg/day in equally divided doses b.i.d. for 10 days. *Maximum:* 1,000 mg/day.

TABLETS

Children under age 13 who can swallow tablets. 250 mg b.i.d. for 10 days.

➤ *To treat impetigo*

ORAL SUSPENSION

Children ages 3 months to 12 years. 30 mg/kg/day in equally divided doses b.i.d. for 10 days. *Maximum:* 1,000 mg/day.

➤ *To treat acute bacterial maxillary sinusitis*

ORAL SUSPENSION

Children ages 3 months to 12 years. 30 mg/kg/day in equally divided doses b.i.d. for 10 days. *Maximum:* 1,000 mg/day.

TABLETS

Adults and children age 13 and older and children under age 13 who can swallow tablets. 250 mg b.i.d. for 10 days.

➤ *To treat acute bacterial exacerbations of chronic bronchitis and uncomplicated skin and soft-tissue infections*

TABLETS

Adults and children age 13 and older. 250 to 500 mg b.i.d. for 10 days.

I.V. INFUSION, I.V. OR I.M. INJECTION

Adults. 750 mg q 8 hr.

➤ *To treat secondary bacterial infection in patients with acute bronchitis*

Adults and children age 13 and older. 250 to 500 mg b.i.d. for 5 to 10 days.

➤ *To treat early Lyme disease*

TABLETS

Adults and children age 13 and older. 500 mg b.i.d. for 20 days.

➤ *To treat uncomplicated UTIs*

TABLETS

Adults. 125 to 250 mg b.i.d. for 7 to 10 days.

I.V. INFUSION, I.V. OR I.M. INJECTION

Adults. 750 mg q 8 hr.

➤ *To treat uncomplicated gonorrhea*

TABLETS

Adults. 1 g as a single dose.

I.M. INJECTION

Adults. 1.5 g as a single dose divided equally and injected into two different sites; given with oral probenecid 1 g.

➤ *To treat disseminated gonococcal infection and uncomplicated pneumonia*

I.V. INFUSION, I.V. OR I.M. INJECTION

Adults. 750 mg q 8 hr.

➤ *To treat bone and joint infections*

I.V. INFUSION, I.V. OR I.M. INJECTION

Adults. 1.5 g q 8 hr.

Children over age 3 months. 50 to 150 mg/kg/day in divided doses q 8 hr. *Maximum:* Adult dose.

➤ *To treat bacterial meningitis*

I.V. INFUSION

Adults. 1.5 to 3 g q 8 hr.

Children over age 1 month. 50 to 80 mg/kg q 6 to 8 hr.

Neonates up to age 1 month. 33.3 to 50 mg/kg q 8 to 12 hr.

➤ *To treat moderate infections other than those listed above*

I.V. INFUSION, I.V. OR I.M. INJECTION

Adults. 750 mg q 8 hr for 5 to 10 days.

I.V. INFUSION OR INJECTION

Children over age 3 months. 50 mg/kg/day in equally divided doses q 6 to 8 hr.

➤ *To treat severe or complicated infections other than those listed above*

I.V. INFUSION OR INJECTION

Adults. 1.5 g q 8 hr.

Children over age 3 months. 100 mg/kg/day in equally divided doses q 6 to 8 hr.

➤ *To treat life-threatening infections other than those listed above*

I.V. INFUSION OR INJECTION

Adults. 1.5 g q 6 hr.

➤ *To provide perioperative prophylaxis*

I.V. INFUSION OR INJECTION

Adults. 1.5 g 30 to 60 min before surgery (at induction of anesthesia for open-heart surgery), and then 0.75 g q 8 hr thereafter (1.5 g q 12 hr for total of 6 g with open-heart surgery).

DOSAGE ADJUSTMENT Parenteral dosage reduced to 0.75 g q 12 hr if creatinine clearance is 10 to 20 ml/min/1.73 m² or 0.75 g q 24 hr if creatinine clearance is less than 10 ml/min/1.73 m².

Mechanism of Action

Interferes with bacterial cell wall synthesis by inhibiting the final step in the cross-linking of peptidoglycan strands. Peptidoglycan makes the cell membrane rigid and protective. Without it, bacterial cells rupture and die.

Incompatibilities

Don't admix parenteral cefuroxime with other antibiotics, such as aminoglycosides, because of potential for incompatibility, such as substantial mutual inactivation. If they're administered concurrently, don't mix them in the same I.V. bag or bottle.

Contraindications

Hypersensitivity to cephalosporins or their components

Interactions

DRUGS

aminoglycosides, loop diuretics: Increased risk of nephrotoxicity
antacids, H$_2$-receptor antagonists, omeprazole: Decreased cefuroxime axetil absorption
probenecid: Increased and prolonged blood cefuroxime level

Adverse Reactions

CNS: Chills, fever, headache, seizures
CV: Edema
EENT: Hearing loss, oral candidiasis
GI: Abdominal cramps, diarrhea, elevated liver function test results, hepatic failure, hepatomegaly, nausea, pseudomembranous colitis, vomiting
GU: Elevated BUN level, nephrotoxicity, renal failure, vaginal candidiasis
HEME: Eosinophilia, hemolytic anemia, hypoprothrombinemia, neutropenia, thrombocytopenia, unusual bleeding
MS: Arthralgia
RESP: Dyspnea
SKIN: Ecchymosis, erythema, erythema multiforme, pruritus, rash, Stevens-Johnson syndrome
Other: Anaphylaxis; injection site edema, pain, and redness; superinfection

Nursing Considerations

• Use cefuroxime cautiously in patients hypersensitive to penicillin because cross-sensitivity has occurred in 10% of such patients.
• If possible, obtain culture and sensitivity results, as ordered, before giving drug.
• Give oral form with food to decrease GI distress, as needed.
• Remember that oral forms—tablets and suspension—aren't bioequivalent.
• For I.V. use, reconstitute following manufacturer's instructions according to type of preparation available. Solution ranges in color from light yellow to amber.
• For I.M. use, add 3 or 3.6 ml of sterile water for injection to each 750-mg vial to yield 220 mg/ml.
• If using a container of frozen parenteral solution, thaw at room temperature or under refrigeration before administration; make sure all ice crystals have melted. Don't force thawing by microwave irradiation.
• Store reconstituted parenteral drug for up to 24 hours at room temperature or 96 hours in refrigerator. (Thawed solutions may be stable for 24 hours at room temperature or 28 days if refrigerated.) Store reconstituted oral suspension in refrigerator or at room temperature for up to 10 days.
• Administer I.V. injection over 3 to 5 minutes through tubing of a flowing compatible I.V. fluid.
• Monitor I.V. site for extravasation and phlebitis.
• Monitor BUN and serum creatinine levels and fluid intake and output to detect signs of nephrotoxicity.
• Monitor patient for allergic reactions a few days after therapy starts.
• Assess bowel pattern daily; severe diarrhea may indicate pseudomembranous colitis.
• Assess patient for pharyngitis, ecchymosis, bleeding, and arthralgia, which may indicate a blood dyscrasia.
• Monitor PT and bleeding time, as ordered. Be prepared to administer vitamin K, if ordered, to treat hypothrombinemia.

PATIENT TEACHING

• Instruct patient to shake oral suspension well before measuring each dose and to use a liquid-measuring device for each dose.
• Advise patient using single-dose packets of oral suspension to empty the contents of one packet into a glass and add at least 10 ml (2 tsp) of cold water; apple, grape, or orange juice; or lemonade. Tell him to stir well and consume entire mixture at once.
• Inform patient that yogurt and buttermilk help maintain intestinal flora and can decrease diarrhea during therapy.
• Instruct patient to immediately report to prescriber severe diarrhea or evidence of blood dyscrasia.

celecoxib

Celebrex

Class and Category

Chemical: Diaryl-substituted pyrazole derivative

Therapeutic: Anti-inflammatory, antirheumatic
Pregnancy category: C

Indications and Dosages
➤ *To relieve pain from osteoarthritis*
CAPSULES
Adults. 200 mg q.d. or 100 mg b.i.d.
➤ *To relieve pain from rheumatoid arthritis*
CAPSULES
Adults. 100 to 200 mg b.i.d.
➤ *As adjunct to reduce adenomatous colorectal polyps in patients with familial adenomatous polyposis*
CAPSULES
Adults. 400 mg b.i.d.
➤ *To manage acute pain, to treat primary dysmenorrhea*
CAPSULES
Adults. 400 mg, followed by 200 mg if needed, on 1st day. On subsequent days, 200 mg b.i.d. as needed.
DOSAGE ADJUSTMENT Daily dosage reduced for patients with hepatic impairment. For patients weighing less than 50 kg (110 lb), expect to begin therapy with lowest recommended dose.

Mechanism of Action
Selectively inhibits the enzymatic activity of cyclooxygenase-2 (COX-2), the enzyme needed to convert arachidonic acid to prostaglandin. Prostaglandins are responsible for mediating the inflammatory response and causing local vasodilation, swelling, and pain. Prostaglandins also play a role in peripheral pain transmission to the spinal cord. By inhibiting COX-2 activity and prostaglandin production, this NSAID reduces inflammatory symptoms and relieves pain. Celecoxib's mechanism of action in reducing the number of colorectal polyps is unknown.

Contraindications
Allergic reaction (such as anaphylaxis or angioedema) to aspirin, other NSAIDs, or sulfonamide derivatives or history of aspirin-induced nasal polyps with bronchospasm; hypersensitivity to celecoxib or its components

Interactions
DRUGS
ACE inhibitors: Decreased antihypertensive effect of ACE inhibitors, increased risk of renal failure

aspirin: Increased risk of GI ulceration and other GI complications
fluconazole: Increased blood celecoxib level
furosemide, thiazide diuretics: Reduced diuretic effects of these drugs, increased risk of renal failure
lithium: Possibly elevated blood lithium level
warfarin: Possibly increased PT and risk of bleeding

Adverse Reactions
CNS: Dizziness, headache, insomnia
CV: Peripheral edema
EENT: Pharyngitis, rhinitis, sinusitis
GI: Abdominal pain, diarrhea, elevated liver function test results, flatulence, indigestion, nausea, vomiting
MS: Back pain
RESP: Upper respiratory tract infection
SKIN: Rash

Nursing Considerations
•Be aware that serious GI tract ulceration and bleeding can occur without warning or symptoms. To minimize the risk of these complications, administer celecoxib with food.
•WARNING In patient who has bone marrow suppression or is receiving antineoplastic drug therapy, monitor laboratory results (including WBC) and assess for signs and symptoms of infection because celecoxib has anti-inflammatory and antipyretic actions that may mask signs and symptoms, such as fever and pain.
•Monitor patient—especially if he's elderly or receiving long-term celecoxib therapy—for less common but serious adverse GI reactions, including anorexia, constipation, diverticulitis, dysphagia, esophagitis, gastritis, gastroenteritis, gastroesophageal reflux disease, hemorrhoids, hiatal hernia, melena, stomatitis, and vomiting.
•Monitor liver function test results because in rare cases, elevations may progress to severe hepatic reactions, including fatal hepatitis, liver necrosis, and hepatic failure.
•Monitor intake and output, especially in patients with edema, heart failure, or hypertension, because drug may cause fluid retention.
•Monitor BUN and serum creatinine levels in patients with heart failure because drug may cause renal failure.
•Monitor CBC for decreases in hemoglobin and hematocrit because drug may worsen preexisting anemia.

PATIENT TEACHING
•Instruct patient to swallow celecoxib capsules whole with a full glass of water and to take drug with food or milk to prevent stomach upset.
•Advise patient to notify prescriber if pain continues or is poorly controlled.
•Urge patient to avoid smoking and alcohol use during celecoxib therapy because these activities may increase the risk of adverse GI reactions.
•Instruct patient to notify prescriber immediately if he notices black, tarry stools or vomits coffee-ground material.

cephalexin hydrochloride
Keftab

cephalexin monohydrate
Apo-Cephalex (CAN), Keflex, Novo-Lexin (CAN), Nu-Cephalex (CAN), PMS-Cephalexin (CAN)

Class and Category
Chemical: First-generation cephalosporin, 7-aminocephalosporanic acid
Therapeutic: Antibiotic
Pregnancy category: B

Indications and Dosages
➤ *To treat streptococcal tonsillitis, pharyngitis, and skin and soft-tissue infections*
CAPSULES, ORAL SUSPENSION, TABLETS
Adults and adolescents age 15 and older. 500 mg q 12 hr. *Maximum:* 4 g/day.

Children ages 2 to 15. 25 to 50 mg/kg/day divided into two equal doses and given q 12 hr. If infection is severe, dose may be doubled.
➤ *To treat mild to moderate respiratory tract, skin, soft-tissue, bone, and GU infections caused by susceptible organisms other than streptococci*
CAPSULES, ORAL SUSPENSION, TABLETS
Adults. 250 mg q 6 hr.
ORAL SUSPENSION
Children. 25 to 50 mg/kg/day in equally divided doses b.i.d. or q.i.d.
➤ *To treat severe respiratory tract, soft-tissue, bone, and GU infections*
CAPSULES, ORAL SUSPENSION, TABLETS
Adults. 0.5 to 1 g q 6 hr. *Maximum:* 4 g/day.
Children. 50 to 100 mg/kg/day in equally divided doses q.i.d.
➤ *To treat otitis media*
ORAL SUSPENSION
Children. 75 to 100 mg/kg/day in equally divided doses q.i.d.
➤ *To treat uncomplicated cystitis*
CAPSULES, ORAL SUSPENSION, TABLETS
Adults and adolescents age 15 and older. 500 mg q 12 hr.

Contraindications
Hypersensitivity to cephalosporins or their components

Interactions
DRUGS
aminoglycosides, loop diuretics: Increased risk of nephrotoxicity

Mechanism of Action
Like all cephalosporins, cephalexin interferes with bacterial cell wall synthesis by inhibiting the final step in the cross-linking of peptidoglycan strands. Peptidoglycan makes the cell membrane rigid and protective. Without it, bacterial cells rupture and die. This mechanism of action is most effective against bacteria that divide rapidly, including many gram-positive and gram-negative bacteria.

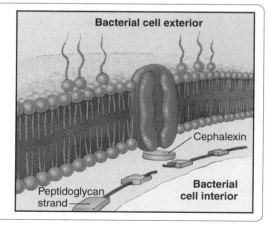

probenecid: Increased and prolonged blood cephalexin level

Adverse Reactions
CNS: Chills, fever, headache, seizures
CV: Edema
EENT: Hearing loss
GI: Abdominal cramps, diarrhea, elevated liver function test results, hepatic failure, hepatomegaly, nausea, oral candidiasis, pseudomembranous colitis, vomiting
GU: Elevated BUN level, nephrotoxicity, renal failure, vaginal candidiasis
HEME: Eosinophilia, hemolytic anemia, hypoprothrombinemia, neutropenia, thrombocytopenia, unusual bleeding
MS: Arthralgia
RESP: Dyspnea
SKIN: Ecchymosis, erythema, erythema multiforme, pruritus, rash, Stevens-Johnson syndrome
Other: Anaphylaxis, superinfection

Nursing Considerations
•Use cephalexin cautiously in patients who are hypersensitive to penicillin because cross-sensitivity has occurred in 10% of such patients.
•If possible, obtain culture and sensitivity test results, as ordered, before giving drug.
•Monitor BUN and serum creatinine levels to detect early signs of nephrotoxicity. Also, monitor fluid intake and output; decreasing urine output may indicate nephrotoxicity.
•Monitor for allergic reactions a few days after therapy starts.
•Assess CBC, hematocrit, and serum AST, ALT, bilirubin, LD, and alkaline phosphatase levels during long-term therapy.
•Assess bowel pattern daily; severe diarrhea may indicate pseudomembranous colitis.
•Assess for pharyngitis, ecchymosis, bleeding, and arthralgia; they may indicate a blood dyscrasia.

PATIENT TEACHING
•Advise patient to complete prescribed course of therapy.
•Instruct patient to shake oral suspension well before measuring each dose and to use a liquid-measuring device to ensure accurate dosing.
•Tell patient that yogurt and buttermilk can help maintain intestinal flora and decrease diarrhea during therapy.
•Instruct patient to immediately report severe diarrhea to prescriber.

cephapirin sodium
Cefadyl

Class and Category
Chemical: First-generation cephalosporin, 7-aminocephalosporanic acid
Therapeutic: Antibiotic
Pregnancy category: B

Indications and Dosages
➤ *To treat respiratory tract infections, skin and soft-tissue infections, UTIs, septicemia, endocarditis, and osteomyelitis caused by gram-negative organisms (including* Escherichia coli, Haemophilus influenzae, Klebsiella *sp., and* Proteus mirabilis*) and gram-positive organisms (including group A beta-hemolytic streptococci,* Streptococcus pneumoniae, *and staphylococci, including coagulase-positive, coagulase-negative, and penicillinase-producing strains but not methicillin-resistant* Staphylococcus aureus*)*

I.V. INFUSION, I.V. OR I.M. INJECTION
Adults. 0.5 to 1 g q 4 to 6 hr. *Maximum:* 12 g/day. For serious infections, higher doses are given by I.V. route.
Children older than age 3 months. 40 to 80 mg/kg/day divided into four equal doses and given q 6 hr. *Maximum:* 12 g/day.

➤ *To provide surgical prophylaxis*
I.V. INFUSION, I.V. OR I.M. INJECTION
Adults. 1 to 2 g 30 to 60 min before surgery, 1 to 2 g during long procedure, and 1 to 2 g q 6 hr after surgery for 24 hr.
DOSAGE ADJUSTMENT For open-heart surgery or prosthetic arthroplasty, prophylaxis continued 3 to 5 days after procedure, if needed.

Mechanism of Action
Interferes with bacterial cell wall synthesis by inhibiting the final step in the cross-linking of peptidoglycan strands. Peptidoglycan makes the cell membrane rigid and protective. Without it, bacterial cells rupture and die.

Contraindications
Hypersensitivity to cephalosporins or their components

Interactions
DRUGS
aminoglycosides, loop diuretics: Increased risk of nephrotoxicity

probenecid: Increased and prolonged blood cephapirin level

Adverse Reactions
CNS: Chills, fever, headache, seizures
CV: Edema
EENT: Hearing loss
GI: Abdominal cramps, diarrhea, elevated liver function test results, hepatic failure, hepatomegaly, nausea, oral candidiasis, pseudomembranous colitis, vomiting
GU: Elevated BUN level, nephrotoxicity, renal failure, vaginal candidiasis
HEME: Eosinophilia, hemolytic anemia, hypoprothrombinemia, neutropenia, thrombocytopenia, unusual bleeding
MS: Arthralgia
RESP: Dyspnea
SKIN: Ecchymosis, erythema, erythema multiforme, pruritus, rash, Stevens-Johnson syndrome
Other: Anaphylaxis; injection site pain, redness, and swelling; superinfection

Nursing Considerations
• Use cephapirin cautiously in patients who are hypersensitive to penicillins because cross-sensitivity has occurred in about 10% of such patients.
• If possible, obtain culture and sensitivity test results, as ordered, before giving drug.
• For I.V. injection, reconstitute 1 g with 10 ml or more of appropriate diluent, such as sterile water for injection. Administer I.V. injection slowly over 3 to 5 minutes through tubing of a flowing compatible I.V. fluid.
• For I.V. infusion, dilute further in 50 ml of D_5W or NS and infuse over 15 to 30 minutes. Stop primary I.V. solution during cephapirin administration.
• For I.M. injection, reconstitute 1-g vial with 2 ml of sterile water for injection or bacteriostatic water for injection. Inject deeply into large muscle mass, such as the gluteus maximus.
• Store reconstituted drug for up to 24 hours at room temperature or 10 days in refrigerator.
• Don't give a cloudy solution.
• Assess I.V. site for extravasation and phlebitis.
• Monitor BUN and serum creatinine levels to detect early signs of nephrotoxicity. Also, monitor fluid intake and output; decreasing urine output may indicate nephrotoxicity.
• Monitor for allergic reactions a few days after therapy starts.

• Assess CBC, hematocrit, and serum AST, ALT, bilirubin, LD, and alkaline phosphatase levels during long-term therapy.
• Assess bowel pattern daily; severe diarrhea may indicate pseudomembranous colitis.
• Assess for pharyngitis, ecchymosis, bleeding, and arthralgia; they may indicate a blood dyscrasia.
• Assess for furry tongue, perineal itching, and loose, foul-smelling stool; they may indicate superinfection.

PATIENT TEACHING
• Instruct patient to immediately report severe diarrhea or evidence of blood dyscrasia or superinfection to prescriber.

cephradine
Velosef

Class and Category
Chemical: First-generation cephalosporin, 7-aminocephalosporanic acid
Therapeutic: Antibiotic
Pregnancy category: B

Indications and Dosages
➤ *To treat respiratory tract infections (other than lobar pneumonia) and skin and soft-tissue infections*
CAPSULES, ORAL SUSPENSION
Adults. 250 mg q 6 hr or 500 mg q 12 hr. *Maximum:* 4 g/day.
ORAL SUSPENSION
Children age 9 months and older. 25 to 50 mg/kg/day in equally divided doses q 6 or 12 hr. *Maximum:* 4 g/day.
➤ *To treat lobar pneumonia*
CAPSULES, ORAL SUSPENSION
Adults. 0.5 g q 6 hr or 1 g q 12 hr. *Maximum:* 4 g/day.
ORAL SUSPENSION
Children age 9 months and older. 25 to 50 mg/kg/day in equally divided doses q 6 or 12 hr. *Maximum:* 4 g/day.
➤ *To treat uncomplicated UTIs*
CAPSULES, ORAL SUSPENSION
Adults. 500 mg q 12 hr. For more serious infections, 500 mg q 6 hr or 1,000 mg q 12 hr. *Maximum:* 4 g/day.
➤ *To treat otitis media caused by* Haemophilus influenzae
ORAL SUSPENSION
Children. 75 to 100 mg/kg/day in equally divided doses q 6 to 12 hr. *Maximum:* 4 g/day.

DOSAGE ADJUSTMENT Dosage reduced to 500 mg q 6 hr if creatinine clearance exceeds 20 ml/min/1.73 m^2; 250 mg q 6 hr if creatinine clearance is 5 to 20 ml/min/1.73 m^2; and 250 mg q 12 hr if creatinine clearance is less than 5 ml/min/1.73 m^2.

Mechanism of Action
Interferes with bacterial cell wall synthesis by inhibiting the final step in the cross-linking of peptidoglycan strands. Peptidoglycan makes the cell membrane rigid and protective. Without it, bacterial cells rupture and die.

Contraindications
Hypersensitivity to cephalosporins or their components

Interactions
DRUGS
aminoglycosides, loop diuretics: Increased risk of nephrotoxicity
probenecid: Increased and prolonged blood cephradine level

Adverse Reactions
CNS: Chills, fever, headache, seizures
CV: Edema
EENT: Hearing loss, oral candidiasis
GI: Abdominal cramps, diarrhea, elevated liver function test results, hepatic failure, hepatomegaly, nausea, pseudomembranous colitis, vomiting
GU: Elevated BUN level, nephrotoxicity, renal failure, vaginal candidiasis
HEME: Eosinophilia, hemolytic anemia, hypoprothrombinemia, neutropenia, thrombocytopenia, unusual bleeding
MS: Arthralgia
RESP: Dyspnea
SKIN: Ecchymosis, erythema, erythema multiforme, pruritus, rash, Stevens-Johnson syndrome
Other: Anaphylaxis, superinfection

Nursing Considerations
• If possible, obtain culture and sensitivity test results, as ordered, before giving drug.
• Monitor patients who are hypersensitive to penicillin for signs and symptoms of a hypersensitivity reaction because cross-sensitivity has occurred in 10% of such patients.
• Store oral suspension for 7 days at room temperature or for 14 days if refrigerated.

• Monitor BUN and serum creatinine levels to detect early signs of nephrotoxicity. Also monitor fluid intake and output; decreasing urine output may indicate nephrotoxicity.
• Monitor patient for allergic reactions a few days after therapy starts. If patient develops hypersensitivity, be prepared to discontinue the drug and administer antihistamines, corticosteroids, and vasopressors, as ordered. Also prepare to administer oxygen, maintain an open airway, and assist with endotracheal intubation, as appropriate.
• Assess CBC, hematocrit, and serum AST, ALT, bilirubin, LD, and alkaline phosphatase levels during long-term therapy.
• Assess bowel pattern daily; severe diarrhea may indicate pseudomembranous colitis. Obtain a stool specimen to test for *Clostridium difficile.* Keep in mind that this serious adverse reaction can occur during therapy or up to several weeks after therapy is discontinued. Also avoid giving antiperistaltic antidiarrheals, such as atropine and diphenoxylate or loperamide, because they may delay elimination of toxins from the bowel and cause damage to the colon from toxin retention. Mild cases may respond after drug is discontinued. For moderate or severe cases, be prepared to administer fluid, electrolyte, and protein replacement as ordered.
• If patient has a history of GI disease, especially ulcerative colitis, regional enteritis, or antibiotic-associated colitis, assess him frequently for diarrhea because he is at risk for pseudomembranous colitis.
• Assess for pharyngitis, ecchymosis, bleeding, and arthralgia; these may indicate a blood dyscrasia.
• If patient has a seizure, notify prescriber immediately and expect to discontinue drug. Institute seizure precautions according to facility policy.
PATIENT TEACHING
• If patient develops GI distress, advise him to take cephradine with food.
• Advise patient to complete prescribed course of therapy.
• Explain that patient should avoid missing doses and that he should take the drug at evenly spaced intervals. If patient misses a dose, instruct him to take the dose as soon as possible unless it's almost time for the next dose. Emphasize that he shouldn't double the dose.

•Tell patient that yogurt and buttermilk help maintain intestinal flora and can decrease diarrhea during therapy.
•Instruct patient to immediately report to prescriber severe diarrhea or evidence of blood dyscrasia or superinfection. Warn patient not to take any OTC antidiarrheals before consulting prescriber.
•Advise patient to notify prescriber if symptoms don't improve within a few days.

cevimeline hydrochloride

Evoxac

Class and Category

Chemical: Quinuclidine derivative of acetylcholine
Therapeutic: Cholinergic enhancer, dry mouth reliever
Pregnancy category: C

Indications and Dosages

➤ *To treat dry mouth associated with Sjögren's syndrome*
CAPSULES
Adults. 30 mg t.i.d. *Maximum:* 90 mg/day.

Mechanism of Action

As a cholinergic agonist, binds to and activates muscarinic receptors of the parasympathetic nervous system and increases secretions of the exocrine glands, such as salivary glands.

Contraindications

Acute iritis, angle-closure glaucoma, hypersensitivity to cevimeline or its components, uncontrolled asthma

Interactions

DRUGS

amiodarone, cimetidine, clarithromycin, diltiazem, erythromycin, fluconazole, haloperidol, itraconazole, ketoconazole, metoclopramide, mibefradil, nefazodone, propafenone, quinidine, ritonavir, selective serotonin reuptake inhibitors, thioridazine, tricyclic antidepressants, troleandomycin, verapamil: Possibly inhibited metabolism and increased blood level of cevimeline
anticholinergics: Decreased effectiveness of anticholinergics

antimuscarinics: Altered effects of antimuscarinics and decreased therapeutic action of cevimeline
beta blockers: Possibly cardiac conduction disturbances
parasympathomimetics: Additive effects of either drug

Adverse Reactions

CNS: Depression, fatigue, fever, hypoesthesia, insomnia, migraine headache, tremor
CV: Edema, palpitations
EENT: Abnormal vision, conjunctivitis, dry mouth, earache, epistaxis, excessive salivation, eye pain, rhinitis, salivary gland pain
GI: Abdominal pain, anorexia, constipation, eructation, heartburn, hiccups, nausea, vomiting
HEME: Anemia
MS: Arthralgia, leg cramps, myalgia
RESP: Cough, dyspnea
SKIN: Diaphoresis, pruritus
Other: Flulike symptoms, hot flashes

Nursing Considerations

•Administer cevimeline on an empty stomach because food may decrease rate and extent of drug absorption and thus delay peak blood concentrations.
•Assess patient with a pulmonary disorder for wheezing and increased respiratory secretions because drug may cause increased bronchiolar smooth-muscle contractions, airway resistance, and respiratory secretions.
•Monitor patient with known or suspected gallbladder disease for abdominal pain or other signs and symptoms that may indicate biliary obstruction, cholecystitis, or cholangitis; each of these conditions may be precipitated by cevimeline.
PATIENT TEACHING
•Instruct patient to take cevimeline on an empty stomach.
•Inform patient that drug may cause vision changes; advise him to avoid driving at night or performing potentially hazardous activities until drug's adverse effects are known.
•Urge patient to drink plenty of fluids during hot weather and while exercising because drug may cause excessive sweating and dehydration.

chloral hydrate

Aquachloral Supprettes, Novo-Chlorhydrate (CAN), PMS-Chloral Hydrate (CAN)

Class, Category, and Schedule
Chemical: Chloral derivative
Therapeutic: Sedative-hypnotic
Pregnancy category: C
Controlled substance: Schedule IV

Indications and Dosages
➤ *To prevent or suppress alcohol withdrawal symptoms, act as an adjunct to opioids and analgesics to control postoperative pain*
CAPSULES, SYRUP, SUPPOSITORIES
Adults. 250 mg t.i.d. p.c. *Maximum:* 2,000 mg.
➤ *To produce nocturnal sedation*
CAPSULES, SYRUP, SUPPOSITORIES
Adults. 0.5 to 1 g 30 min before bedtime. *Maximum:* 2 g.
➤ *To produce preoperative sedation*
CAPSULES, SYRUP, SUPPOSITORIES
Adults. 0.5 to 1 g 30 min before surgery.
➤ *To provide sedation before dental or medical procedure*
SYRUP, SUPPOSITORIES
Children. 25 mg/kg up to 500 mg/single dose; up to 75 mg/kg for dental procedure supplemented by nitrous oxide.

Route	Onset	Peak	Duration
P.O.	30 min to 1 hr	Unknown	4 to 8 hr
P.R.	Unknown	Unknown	4 to 8 hr

Mechanism of Action
Produces CNS depression by an unknown mechanism involving trichloroethanol, the drug's active metabolite.

Contraindications
Gastritis; hypersensitivity or idiosyncrasy to chloral hydrate or its components; severe cardiac, hepatic, or renal disease

Interactions
DRUGS
CNS depressants: Increased CNS effects of chloral hydrate
furosemide (I.V.): Increased incidence of adverse effects when administered after chloral hydrate
phenytoin: Increased excretion and subsequent decreased effectiveness of phenytoin
warfarin: Transient increase in anticoagulant effect

ACTIVITIES
alcohol use: Increased CNS effects of chloral hydrate

Adverse Reactions
CNS: Ataxia, disorientation, hangover, incoherence, paranoia, somnolence
GI: Gastric irritation, nausea, vomiting
SKIN: Rash, urticaria
Other: Drug dependence

Nursing Considerations
•Administer with full glass of water or juice to minimize GI distress from chloral hydrate capsules. Dilute syrup in a half-glass of water, ginger ale, or fruit juice.
•WARNING Monitor carefully for hypersensitivity reaction in patients with a history of tartrazine sensitivity.
•Suspect physical or psychological dependence if withdrawal of chloral hydrate produces confusion, hallucinations, nausea, nervousness, restlessness, stomach pain, tremor, unusual excitement, or vomiting.
PATIENT TEACHING
•Advise patient to take capsules with a full glass of water or juice or to mix syrup in a half-glass of water, ginger ale, or fruit juice.
•Advise patient to avoid hazardous activities until drug's CNS effects are known.
•Caution patient that drug may be habit-forming. Advise taking it exactly as prescribed and not to stop taking it abruptly because withdrawal symptoms could occur.
•Instruct patient to notify prescriber at once about stomach pains or tarry stools.

chloramphenicol
Chloromycetin, Novochlorocap (CAN)

chloramphenicol palmitate
Chloromycetin

chloramphenicol sodium succinate
Chloromycetin

Class and Category
Chemical: Dichloroacetic acid derivative
Therapeutic: Antibiotic
Pregnancy category: Not rated

Indications and Dosages
➤ *To treat serious infections for which less potentially dangerous drugs are ineffective or contraindicated*

I.V. INFUSION

Adults. 12.5 mg/kg q 6 hr. *Maximum:* 4 g/day.

Children. 50 to 75 mg/kg/day in divided doses q 6 hr.

Full-term infants age 2 weeks and older. 12.5 mg/kg q 6 hr or 25 mg/kg q 12 hr.

Preterm and full-term infants up to age 2 weeks. 6.25 mg/kg q 6 hr.

➤ *To treat bacteremia or meningitis*

I.V. INFUSION

Children. 50 to 100 mg/kg/day in divided doses q 6 hr.

DOSAGE ADJUSTMENT Dosage limited to 25 mg/kg/day for infants and children with immature metabolic processes.

Mechanism of Action

Produces a bacteriostatic effect on susceptible organisms by inhibiting protein synthesis, thereby preventing amino acids from being transferred to growing polypetide chains.

Contraindications

Hypersensitivity to chloramphenicol or its components

Interactions

DRUGS

alfentanil: Prolonged alfentanil effect
barbiturates: Increased blood barbiturate level; decreased blood chloramphenicol level
blood-dyscrasia–causing drugs (such as captopril and cephalosporins), bone marrow depressants (including colchicine and methotrexate): Increased bone marrow depression
chlorpropamide, tolbutamide: Increased hypoglycemic effects
clindamycin, erythromycin, lincomycin: Decreased antibacterial effects of these drugs
cyclophosphamide: Decreased or delayed activation of cyclophosphamide, increased bone marrow depression
hepatic enzyme inducers (including rifampin): Decreased blood chloramphenicol level
hydantoins: Increased blood hydantoin level, possibly resulting in toxicity; increased or decreased blood chloramphenicol level
iron salts: Increased serum iron level
oral anticoagulants: Enhanced anticoagulant action

oral contraceptives containing estrogen: Decreased contraceptive effect with prolonged chloramphenicol use
penicillins: Decreased penicillin activity; synergistic effects with treatment of certain microorganisms
vitamin B$_{12}$: Antagonized hematopoietic response to vitamin B$_{12}$

Adverse Reactions

CNS: Confusion, delirium, depression, fever, headache, peripheral neuropathy
CV: Gray syndrome in neonates
EENT: Optic neuritis
GI: Diarrhea, nausea, vomiting
HEME: Aplastic anemia, bone marrow depression, granulocytopenia, hypoplastic anemia, leukopenia, reticulocytopenia, thrombocytopenia
SKIN: Rash
Other: Anaphylaxis, angioedema

Nursing Considerations

•As appropriate and ordered, obtain specimen for culture and sensitivity testing before beginning chloramphenicol therapy.
•Keep in mind that chloramphenicol should never be used to treat minor infections or for prophylaxis because of the many serious toxicities associated with its use.
•Be aware that repeated courses of therapy should be avoided because of the risk of serious adverse reactions.
•For I.V. use, prepare a 10% solution by adding 10 ml of sterile water for injection or D$_5$W to each 1-g vial. Administer over at least 1 minute.
•Know that diluted I.V. solution is stable for 24 to 48 hours when stored at room temperature or refrigerated. Don't use if cloudy.
•Assess patient for fever, sore throat, tiredness, unusual bleeding, or ecchymosis; these may indicate a blood dyscrasia.
•Perform neurologic assessments regularly, looking for signs and symptoms of peripheral neuropathy.
•WARNING If early signs of gray syndrome appear (failure to eat, pallor, cyanosis, abdominal distention, irregular respirations, and vasomotor collapse), notify prescriber and be prepared to stop drug immediately.
•Monitor blood chloramphenicol level as appropriate. Keep in mind that therapeutic peak levels are 10 to 20 mcg/ml and trough levels are 5 to 10 mcg/ml.

•Monitor CBC and platelet and reticulocyte counts as ordered to detect signs of blood dyscrasia. Notify prescriber immediately about abnormal results.

PATIENT TEACHING

•Instruct patient to immediately report to prescriber signs of blood dyscrasia.

•**WARNING** Tell patient to stay alert for signs of potentially fatal, irreversible bone marrow depression that leads to aplastic anemia and is characterized by fever, pallor, pharyngitis, severe fatigue and weakness, and unusual bleeding or bruising. Bone marrow depression may occur weeks to months after therapy stops. Stress the importance of follow-up care.

chlordiazepoxide hydrochloride

Apo-Chlordiazepoxide (CAN), Librium, Novo-Poxide (CAN)

Class, Category, and Schedule

Chemical: Benzodiazepine
Therapeutic: Antianxiety
Pregnancy category: Not rated
Controlled substance: Schedule IV

Indications and Dosages

➤ *To provide short-term management of mild anxiety*

CAPSULES, TABLETS

Adults. 5 to 10 mg t.i.d. or q.i.d.

Children over age 6. 5 mg b.i.d. to q.i.d. increased as needed to 10 mg b.i.d. or t.i.d., or 0.5 mg/kg/day in equally divided doses q 6 to 8 hr.

➤ *To provide short-term management of severe anxiety*

CAPSULES, TABLETS

Adults. 20 to 25 mg t.i.d. or q.i.d.

I.V. OR I.M. INJECTION

Adults. *Initial:* 50 to 100 mg. Then, 25 to 50 mg t.i.d. or q.i.d., p.r.n. *Maximum:* 300 mg/day.

I.M. INJECTION

Children age 12 and older. 0.5 mg/kg/day in equally divided doses q 6 to 8 hr.

➤ *To provide short-term treatment of acute alcohol withdrawal*

CAPSULES, TABLETS, I.V. OR I.M. INJECTION

Adults. *Initial:* 50 to 100 mg, usually given I.V. or I.M. Repeated in 2 to 4 hr followed by individualized oral dosage if needed to control symptoms. *Maximum:* 300 mg/day.

➤ *To provide perioperative relaxation and reduce apprehension and anxiety*

CAPSULES, TABLETS, I.M. INJECTION

Adults. 5 to 10 mg P.O. t.i.d. or q.i.d. several days before surgery; 50 to 100 mg I.M. 1 hr before surgery.

DOSAGE ADJUSTMENT Dosage reduced to 5 mg P.O. b.i.d. to q.i.d., p.r.n., for elderly or debilitated patients.

Mechanism of Action

May potentiate the effects of gamma-aminobutyric acid (GABA) and other inhibitory neurotransmitters by binding to specific benzodiazepine receptors in the limbic and cortical areas of the CNS. By binding to these receptors, chlordiazepoxide increases GABA's inhibitory effects and blocks cortical and limbic arousal, which helps control emotional behavior. It also helps relieve symptoms of alcohol withdrawal by causing CNS depression.

Contraindications

Hypersensitivity to chlordiazepoxide or its components

Interactions

DRUGS

antacids: Altered rate of chlordiazepoxide absorption

cimetidine, disulfiram, fluoxetine, isoniazid, ketoconazole, metoprolol, oral contraceptives, propoxyphene, propranolol, valproic acid: Increased blood chlordiazepoxide level

CNS depressants: Increased CNS effects

digoxin: Increased blood digoxin level and risk of digitalis toxicity

levodopa: Decreased efficacy of levodopa's antiparkinsonian effects

neuromuscular blockers: Potentiated, counteracted, or diminished effects of neuromuscular blockers

phenytoin: Possibly increased phenytoin toxicity

probenecid: Shortened onset of action or prolonged effect of chlordiazepoxide

rifampin: Decreased chlordiazepoxide effect

theophyllines: Antagonized sedative effects of chlordiazepoxide

ACTIVITIES

alcohol use: Increased CNS effects

Adverse Reactions

CNS: Ataxia, confusion, depression, drowsiness

CV: ECG changes, hypotension, tachycardia

GI: Hepatic dysfunction
HEME: Agranulocytosis
SKIN: Jaundice
Other: Injection site pain, redness, and swelling

Nursing Considerations

•Use chlordiazepoxide cautiously in patients with renal or hepatic impairment or porphyria.
•**WARNING** Be aware that prolonged use of therapeutic doses can lead to dependence.
•For I.V. use, reconstitute ampule contents with 5 ml of sterile water for injection or sodium chloride for injection. Agitate gently until completely dissolved. Give slowly over 1 minute.
•For I.M. use, reconstitute only with diluent provided by manufacturer.
•**WARNING** Don't use supplied diluent to prepare drug for I.V. use because air bubbles form on the surface.
•Don't give opalescent or hazy solution.
•Observe for signs of phlebitis or thrombophlebitis after I.V. administration.
•Monitor liver function test results during therapy.
•If patient is a hyperactive, aggressive child or has a history of psychiatric disorders, monitor for paradoxical reactions, such as excitement, stimulation, and acute rage, during first 2 weeks of therapy.

PATIENT TEACHING

•Warn patient about possible drowsiness.
•Advise patient to avoid other CNS depressants during therapy.
•Warn patient not to take antacids with drug.

chlorothiazide

Diuril

chlorothiazide sodium

Diuril

Class and Category

Chemical: Sulfonamide derivative
Therapeutic: Antihypertensive, diuretic
Pregnancy category: B

Indications and Dosages

➤ *To treat hypertension*
ORAL SUSPENSION, TABLETS
Adults. 250 to 1,000 mg/day in a single dose or divided doses b.i.d. *Maximum:* 2,000 mg/day in divided doses.

Children age 6 months and older. 10 to 20 mg/kg/day in a single dose or divided doses b.i.d. *Maximum:* 1,000 mg/day for children ages 2 to 12; 375 mg/day for children ages 6 months to 2 years.
Children under age 6 months. Up to 30 mg/kg/day in divided doses given b.i.d.
➤ *To produce diuresis*
ORAL SUSPENSION, TABLETS
Adults. 250 mg q 6 to 12 hr. Administered on an intermittent schedule, if needed, such as alternate days or 3 to 5 days/wk.
Children age 6 months and older. 10 to 20 mg/kg/day in a single dose or divided doses b.i.d. *Maximum:* 1,000 mg/day for children ages 2 to 12; 375 mg/day for children ages 6 months to 2 years.
Children under age 6 months. Up to 33 mg/kg/day in divided doses b.i.d.
I.V. INFUSION OR INJECTION
Adults. 250 mg q 6 to 12 hr.

Route	Onset	Peak	Duration
P.O.	2 hr	4 hr	6 to 12 hr
I.V.	15 min	4 hr	6 to 12 hr

Mechanism of Action

May promote sodium, chloride, and water excretion by inhibiting sodium reabsorption in the kidneys' distal tubules. Initially, chlorothiazide may decrease extracellular fluid volume, plasma volume, and cardiac output, which helps explain how it reduces blood pressure. It also may dilate arteries directly, which helps reduce peripheral vascular resistance and blood pressure. After several weeks, extracellular fluid and plasma volume and cardiac output return to normal, but peripheral vascular resistance remains decreased.

Contraindications

Anuria; hepatic coma; hypersensitivity to chlorothiazide or its components, sulfonamides, or related thiazide diuretics; renal failure

Interactions

DRUGS

allopurinol: Increased risk of allopurinol hypersensitivity
amiodarone: Increased risk of arrhythmias from hypokalemia

amphotericin B, glucocorticoids: Intensified electrolyte depletion
anesthetics: Potentiated effects of anesthetics
anticholinergics: Increased chlorothiazide absorption
anticoagulants, methenamines, sulfonylureas: Decreased effects of these drugs
antihypertensives: Increased antihypertensive effect
antineoplastics: Prolonged antineoplastic-induced leukopenia
calcium: Possibly increased blood calcium level
cholestyramine, colestipol: Decreased chlorothiazide absorption
diazoxide: Hyperglycemia, hypotension
digitalis glycosides: Increased risk of digitalis-induced arrhythmias
dopamine: Increased diuretic effect of both drugs
lithium: Increased risk of lithium toxicity
loop diuretics: Synergistic effects, resulting in profound diuresis and serious electrolyte imbalances
methyldopa: Potential development of hemolytic anemia
neuromuscular blockers: Increased neuromuscular blockade
NSAIDs: Possibly reduced diuretic effect of chlorothiazide
sympathomimetics: Possibly inhibited antihypertensive effect of chlorothiazide
vitamin D: Enhanced vitamin D action

Adverse Reactions

CNS: Dizziness, headache, paresthesia, restlessness, vertigo, weakness
CV: Orthostatic hypotension
ENDO: Hyperglycemia
GI: Abdominal cramps, anorexia, constipation, diarrhea, gastric irritation, nausea, pancreatitis, vomiting
GU: Glycosuria, hematuria (I.V. form), impotence, interstitial nephritis, renal dysfunction or failure
HEME: Agranulocytosis, aplastic anemia, hemolytic anemia, leukopenia, thrombocytopenia
MS: Muscle spasms
SKIN: Jaundice, photosensitivity, purpura, rash, urticaria
Other: Anaphylactic reactions, hypercalcemia, hyperuricemia, hypochloremic alkalosis, hypokalemia, hypomagnesemia, hyponatremia, hypovolemia

Nursing Considerations

• Don't give parenteral form of chlorothiazide by I.M. or S.C. route.

• For I.V. administration, reconstitute with at least 18 ml of sterile water for injection. Discard unused solution after 24 hours. Reconstituted solution is compatible with dextrose solution or NS for infusion.
• Monitor I.V. site closely. Extravasation must be avoided. If it occurs, stop drug administration and notify prescriber immediately.
• Weigh patient daily to assess fluid loss and drug effectiveness. Also, check blood pressure often if used to treat hypertension; antihypertensive effect may not appear for days.
• Monitor for electrolyte imbalances.

PATIENT TEACHING
• Tell patient to take chlorothiazide early in the day to avoid nocturia and to take it with food or milk if GI distress occurs.
• Encourage patient to eat a high-potassium diet.
• Instruct patient to rise slowly to minimize effects of orthostatic hypotension.
• Urge patient to weigh himself at least weekly and to notify prescriber if weight rises or falls by 5 lb (2.25 kg) or more in 2 days.
• Tell patient to immediately notify prescriber if any of these signs and symptoms occur: weakness, cramps, nausea, vomiting, restlessness, excessive thirst, drowsiness, tiredness, increased heart rate, diarrhea, sudden joint pain, or dizziness.
• If patient has diabetes mellitus, instruct him to monitor his blood glucose level frequently. Oral antidiabetic drug dosage may need to be increased.
• Tell patient to avoid prolonged exposure to sun, use sunscreen, and wear protective clothing.
• Advise patient to consult prescriber or pharmacist before using alcohol and such OTC drugs as those used for appetite control, colds, cough, hay fever, and sinus problems.

chlorphenesin carbamate

Maolate

Class and Category

Chemical: Chemically related to mephenesin
Therapeutic: Skeletal muscle relaxant
Pregnancy category: Not rated

Indications and Dosages

➤ *As adjunct to relieve pain in acute musculoskeletal conditions*

TABLETS
Adults: 800 mg t.i.d. until desired effect occurs. *Maintenance:* 400 mg q.i.d or less, p.r.n.

Mechanism of Action
May act on the CNS, rather than directly on skeletal muscle, producing a sedative effect that aids in muscle relaxation.

Contraindications
Hypersensitivity to chlorphenesin or its components

Interactions
DRUGS
CNS depressants: Increased adverse CNS effects
ACTIVITIES
alcohol use: Increased adverse CNS effects

Adverse Reactions
CNS: Confusion, dizziness, drowsiness, headache, insomnia, nervousness, paradoxical stimulation
EENT: Diplopia, transient vision loss
GI: Epigastric discomfort, nausea
Other: Anaphylaxis, drug-induced fever

Nursing Considerations
•**WARNING** Use chlorphenesin carbamate cautiously in patients who are hypersensitive to aspirin; drug contains tartrazine, which may cause similar hypersensitivity.
•Expect drug therapy to last for no more than 8 weeks because safety beyond this point is unknown.
•Provide rest and other pain-relief measures.
PATIENT TEACHING
•Because of possible reduced alertness, advise patient to avoid potentially hazardous activities until drug's CNS effects are known.
•Instruct patient to notify prescriber if these symptoms occur: confusion, dizziness, drowsiness, insomnia, nervousness, or paradoxical stimulation.
•Tell patient to immediately notify prescriber if he develops a fever or any signs or symptoms of an allergic reaction, such as rash, hives, itching, facial swelling, or difficulty breathing.

chlorpromazine

Largactil (CAN), Thorazine

chlorpromazine hydrochloride

Chlorpromanyl (CAN), Novo-Chlorpromazine (CAN), Thorazine, Thorazine Spansule

Class and Category
Chemical: Propylamine derivative of phenothiazine
Therapeutic: Antiemetic, antipsychotic, tranquilizer
Pregnancy category: Not rated

Indications and Dosages
➤ *To manage symptoms of psychotic disorders or control manic manifestations of manic-depression in outpatients*
E.R. CAPSULES
Adults. 30 to 300 mg q.d. to t.i.d. with dosage adjusted as needed. *Maximum:* 1 g/day.
ORAL CONCENTRATE, SYRUP, TABLETS
Adults. 10 mg t.i.d. or q.i.d., or 25 mg b.i.d. or t.i.d. After 1 or 2 days, dose increased by 20 to 50 mg semiweekly until patient is calm. After 2 wk of calmness, dosage gradually reduced to maintenance level of 200 to 800 mg/day in equally divided doses.
➤ *To control acutely disturbed or manic hospitalized patients*
I.M. INJECTION
Adults. 25 mg. Repeated 25 to 50 mg in 1 hr, if needed. Increased gradually over several days up to 400 mg q 4 to 6 hr for severe cases until behavior is controlled. Then, regimen switched to oral form and outpatient dosage.
➤ *To treat severe behavioral problems in children*
ORAL CONCENTRATE, SYRUP, TABLETS
Children ages 6 months to 12 years. 0.55 mg/kg q 4 to 6 hr, p.r.n.
SUPPOSITORIES
Children ages 6 months to 12 years. 1 mg/kg q 6 to 8 hr, p.r.n.
I.M. INJECTION
Children ages 6 months to 12 years. 0.55 mg/kg q 6 to 8 hr. *Maximum:* 75 mg/day for children ages 5 to 12 years or weighing 50 to 100 lb (23 to 45 kg), except in unmanageable cases; 40 mg/day for children up to age 5 years or weighing up to 50 lb.
➤ *To treat nausea and vomiting*
ORAL CONCENTRATE, SYRUP, TABLETS
Adults and adolescents. 10 to 25 mg q 4 to 6 hr, p.r.n.
Children ages 6 months to 12 years. 0.55 mg/kg q 4 to 6 hr, p.r.n.
I.M. INJECTION
Adults. 25 mg. If no hypotension occurs, 25 to 50 mg q 3 to 4 hr, p.r.n., until vomiting stops; then drug switched to oral form.

Children age 6 months and older. 0.55 mg/kg q 6 to 8 hr, p.r.n. *Maximum:* 75 mg/day for children ages 5 to 12 years or weighing 50 to 100 lb; 40 mg/day for children up to age 5 years or weighing up to 50 lb.

SUPPOSITORIES

Adults and adolescents. 50 to 100 mg q 6 to 8 hr, p.r.n.

Children ages 6 months to 12 years. 1 mg/kg q 6 to 8 hr, p.r.n.

➤ *To provide intraoperative control of nausea and vomiting*

I.V. INJECTION

Adults. 25 mg diluted to 1 mg/ml with sodium chloride for injection and given at a rate not to exceed 2 mg q 2 min. *Maximum:* 25 mg.

Children age 6 months and older. 0.275 mg/kg diluted to at least 1 mg/ml with sodium chloride for injection and given at a rate not to exceed 1 mg q 2 min. *Maximum:* 75 mg/day for children ages 5 to 12 years or weighing 50 to 100 lb; 40 mg/day for children up to age 5 years or weighing up to 50 lb.

I.M. INJECTION

Adults. 12.5 mg. Repeated in 30 min if needed and no hypotension occurs.

Children age 6 months and older. 0.275 mg/kg. Repeated in 30 min if needed and tolerated.

➤ *To treat intractable hiccups*

TABLETS

Adults. 25 to 50 mg t.i.d. or q.i.d. If hiccups last longer than 2 days, route switched to I.M., as prescribed.

I.V. INFUSION

Adults. 25 to 50 mg diluted in 500 to 1,000 ml of NS and administered at a rate of 1 mg/min with patient in supine position.

I.M. INJECTION

Adults. 25 to 50 mg given only if oral route is ineffective. If symptoms persist, route switched to I.V., as prescribed.

➤ *To provide preoperative relaxation*

ORAL CONCENTRATE, SYRUP, TABLETS

Adults and adolescents. 25 to 50 mg 2 to 3 hr before surgery.

Children ages 6 months to 12 years. 0.55 mg/kg 2 to 3 hr before surgery.

I.M. INJECTION

Adults. 12.5 to 25 mg 1 to 2 hr before surgery.

Children age 6 months and older. 0.55 mg/kg 1 to 2 hr before surgery.

➤ *To treat acute intermittent porphyria*

ORAL CONCENTRATE, SYRUP, TABLETS

Adults and adolescents. 25 to 50 mg t.i.d. or q.i.d.

I.M. INJECTION

Adults. 25 mg t.i.d. or q.i.d. until oral route is possible.

➤ *To treat tetanus (usually as adjunct with barbiturates)*

I.V. INFUSION

Adults. 25 to 50 mg diluted to at least 1 mg/ml and given at a rate not to exceed 1 mg/min.

Children age 6 months and older. 0.55 mg/kg q 6 to 8 hr, diluted to at least 1 mg/ml and given at a rate not to exceed 1 mg/2 min. *Maximum:* 75 mg/day for children ages 5 to 12 years or weighing 50 to 100 lb; 40 mg/day for children up to age 5 years or weighing up to 50 lb.

I.M. INJECTION

Adults. 25 to 50 mg t.i.d. or q.i.d.

Children age 6 months and older. 0.55 mg/kg q 6 to 8 hr. *Maximum:* 75 mg/day for children ages 5 to 12 years or weighing 50 to 100 lb; 40 mg/day for children up to age 5 years or weighing up to 50 lb.

DOSAGE ADJUSTMENT Dosage possibly reduced for patients with hepatic dysfunction. Dosage reduced to one-third to one-half the normal adult dosage for elderly or debilitated patients.

Mechanism of Action

Depresses areas of the brain that control activity and aggression, including the cerebral cortex, hypothalamus, and limbic system, by an unknown mechanism. Drug prevents nausea and vomiting by inhibiting or blocking dopamine receptors in the medullary chemoreceptor trigger zone and peripherally by blocking the vagus nerve in the GI tract. It may relieve anxiety by causing indirect reduction in arousal and increased filtering of internal stimuli to the reticular activating system in the brain stem.

Incompatibilities

Don't mix chlorpromazine with thiopental, atropine, or solutions that don't have a pH of 4 to 5 because a precipitate will form. Don't mix chlorpromazine injection with other drugs in a syringe.

Contraindications

Comatose states; hypersensitivity to chlorpromazine, phenothiazines, or their components; use of large amounts of CNS depressants

Interactions
DRUGS
amphetamines: Decreased amphetamine effectiveness, decreased antipsychotic effectiveness of chlorpromazine
antacids (aluminum hydroxide or magnesium trisilicate gel): Decreased chlorpromazine absorption and effectiveness
barbiturates: Decreased plasma level and, possibly, effectiveness of chlorpromazine
CNS depressants: Prolonged and intensified CNS depression
metrizamide: Possibly lowered seizure threshold
oral anticoagulants: Decreased anticoagulant effect
phenytoin: Interference with phenytoin metabolism, increased risk of phenytoin toxicity
propranolol: Increased plasma levels of both drugs
thiazide diuretics: Possibly increased orthostatic hypotension
ACTIVITIES
alcohol use: Prolonged and intensified CNS depression

Adverse Reactions
CNS: Drowsiness, extrapyramidal reactions (such as dystonia, fever, motor restlessness, pseudoparkinsonism, and tardive dyskinesia), neuroleptic malignant syndrome, seizures
CV: ECG changes, such as nonspecific, usually reversible Q- and T-wave changes; orthostatic hypotension; tachycardia
EENT: Blurred vision, dry mouth, nasal congestion, ocular changes (fine particle deposits in lens and cornea) with long-term therapy
ENDO: Gynecomastia, hyperglycemia, hypoglycemia, lactation, moderate breast engorgement
GI: Constipation, ileus, nausea
GU: Amenorrhea, ejaculation disorders, impotence, priapism, urine retention
HEME: Agranulocytosis, aplastic anemia, eosinophilia, hemolytic anemia, leukopenia, pancytopenia, thrombocytopenic purpura
SKIN: Exfoliative dermatitis, jaundice, photosensitivity, tissue necrosis, urticaria

Nursing Considerations
•Don't open or crush E.R. capsules.
•Use chlorpromazine cautiously in patients (especially children) with chronic respiratory disorders (such as severe asthma or emphysema) or acute respiratory tract infections because drug has CNS depressant effect. Also use cautiously in patients with cardiovascular, hepatic, or renal disease because of increased risk of developing hypotension, heart failure, and arrhythmias.
•Because of chlorpromazine's anticholinergic effects, use it cautiously in patients with glaucoma. Also use it cautiously in those who are exposed to extreme heat or organophosphorus insecticides and those receiving atropine or related drugs.
•Protect concentrate from light. Refrigeration isn't required.
•Dilute concentrate in at least 60 ml of diluent just before giving it. Use tomato or fruit juice, milk, simple syrup, orange syrup, a carbonated beverage, coffee, tea, water, or semisolid food, such as pudding and soup.
•Protect parenteral solution from light. Solution should be clear and colorless to pale yellow. Discard markedly discolored solution.
•Don't inject drug by S.C. route because it can cause severe tissue necrosis.
•Wear gloves when working with liquid or injectable form because parenteral solution may cause contact dermatitis.
•For I.V. injection, dilute chlorpromazine with sodium chloride for injection to a concentration that yields 1 mg/ml before administration.
•Give I.M. injection slowly and deep into upper outer quadrant of buttocks, such as in the gluteus maximus. To minimize hypotensive effects, keep patient lying flat and monitor blood pressure for 30 minutes after injection.
•**WARNING** Stay alert for possible suppressed cough reflex, which increases the risk of the patient's aspirating vomitus.
•Monitor for increased sensitivity to drug's CNS effects if patient has a history of hepatic encephalopathy from cirrhosis.
•**WARNING** If neuroleptic malignant syndrome (hyperpyrexia, muscle rigidity, altered mental status, autonomic instability) develops, notify prescriber immediately and expect to discontinue drug and begin intensive medical treatment. Monitor carefully for recurrence if patient resumes antipsychotic therapy.
PATIENT TEACHING
•Instruct patient to swallow E.R. capsules whole and not to crush, break, or chew them.
•Tell patient not to take drug within 2 hours of taking an antacid. Allow him to take drug with food or a full glass of milk or water.

•If patient takes the suppository form, instruct him to chill the suppository, moisten it with cold water, and insert it well inside the rectum.
•Tell patient to store oral concentrate at room temperature and away from light. Instruct him to measure it with the dropper provided and to dilute it in 4 oz of fluid just before use.
•Because of possible drowsiness, dizziness, and blurred vision (especially during the first few days of therapy), advise the patient to avoid potentially hazardous activities until drug's CNS effects are known.
•Tell patient to avoid alcohol because of possible additive effects and hypotension.
•Advise patient, especially if elderly, to rise slowly from a supine or seated position to avoid dizziness, light-headedness, and fainting.
•Tell patient to inform doctors and dentists that he's taking chlorpromazine before he undergoes surgery, medical tests, or dental work.
•Explain that drug may reduce the body's response to heat and cold; tell patient to avoid temperature extremes, as in a sauna, hot tub, or very cold or hot shower. Remind patient to dress warmly in cold weather.
•Warn patient not to take OTC drugs for a cold or an allergy; they can increase the risk of heatstroke and other unwanted effects.
•Inform patient that drug increases sensitivity to sunlight; tell him to stay out of the sun as much as possible or to protect his skin from exposure.
•If patient reports dry mouth, suggest sugarless chewing gum, hard candy, and fluids.
•Urge patient to report sudden sore throat or other signs of infection.

chlorpropamide

Apo-Chlorpropamide (CAN), Diabinese, Novo-Propamide (CAN)

Class and Category
Chemical: Sulfonylurea
Therapeutic: Antidiabetic
Pregnancy category: C

Indications and Dosages
➤ *As adjunct to manage non–insulin-dependent diabetes in patients for whom diet alone fails to lower blood glucose level*

TABLETS
Adults. *Initial:* 250 mg q.d. for 5 to 7 days. After therapy begins, dosage may be adjusted

up or down by increments of 50 to 125 mg at intervals of 3 to 5 days to obtain optimal control. *Maintenance:* 100 to 500 mg q.d. *Maximum:* 750 mg q.d.

DOSAGE ADJUSTMENT Dosage reduced to one-half usual insulin dose during first few days of chlorpropamide therapy if patient takes more than 40 U of insulin daily. Insulin dose can be further reduced, depending on response. If patient takes an oral antidiabetic drug or less than 40 U of insulin daily, therapy may be stopped abruptly when chlorpropamide starts.

Dosage reduced to one-half usual dose if patient has mild renal failure because metabolites and unchanged drug are excreted in urine. To avoid hypoglycemic reactions, initial dosage reduced to 100 to 125 mg q.d. for elderly, debilitated, or malnourished patients and patients with impaired hepatic function.

Route	Onset	Peak	Duration
P.O.	1 hr	3 to 6 hr	24 to 72 hr

Mechanism of Action
Lowers blood glucose level by stimulating release of insulin from the pancreas in patients who have functioning beta cells. It also may increase insulin sensitivity in target tissues, which may result in a decrease in liver breakdown of glycogen to glucose or the liver's production of new glucose.

Contraindications
Diabetic ketoacidosis (with or without coma), hypersensitivity to chlorpropamide or its components

Interactions
DRUGS
androgens, anticoagulants, azole antifungals, chloramphenicol, clofibrate, fenfluramine, fluconazole, gemfibrozil, H₂-receptor antagonists, magnesium salts, MAO inhibitors, methyldopa, probenecid, salicylates, sulfinpyrazone, sulfonamides, tricyclic antidepressants, urinary acidifiers: Increased hypoglycemic effect
barbiturates: Prolonged barbiturate action
beta blockers, calcium channel blockers, cholestyramine, corticosteroids, diazoxide, estrogens, hydantoins, isoniazid, nicotinic

acid, oral contraceptives, phenothiazines, rifampin, sympathomimetics, thiazide diuretics, thyroid drugs, urinary alkalizers: Decreased hypoglycemic effect
digitalis glycosides: Increased blood digitalis level
oral miconazole: Risk of severe hypoglycemia
ACTIVITIES
alcohol use: Disulfiram-like reaction

Adverse Reactions
ENDO: Hypoglycemia
GI: Anorexia, diarrhea, hunger, nausea, vomiting
SKIN: Maculopapular eruptions, photosensitivity, pruritus, urticaria
Other: Disulfiram-like reaction

Nursing Considerations
•Use chlorpropamide cautiously in patients with renal or hepatic dysfunction; in elderly, debilitated, or malnourished patients; and in those with adrenal or pituitary insufficiency because of increased susceptibility to drug's hypoglycemic action.
•Monitor blood glucose level frequently during initiation of therapy and during dosage adjustment or changes in patient's life, such as stress and illness. Hypoglycemia may be difficult to recognize in elderly patients and those who take beta-adrenergic blockers.
•Assess for hypoglycemia—the most common adverse reaction to chlorpropamide—especially in patients whose caloric intake is deficient, who have just engaged in strenuous or prolonged exercise, who have ingested alcohol, and who receive more than one glucose-lowering drug.
•Treat hypoglycemia promptly by administering 15 g of simple carbohydrate, such as 4 oz of orange juice or soda or 8 oz of milk. Repeat in 15 minutes, if needed. Because of chlorpropamide's long half-life, careful monitoring and frequent feedings are required for 3 to 5 days after a hypoglycemic episode. If episode is severe, hospitalization and I.V. glucose may be needed.
•Monitor patients receiving long-term chlorpropamide therapy for secondary failure. Secondary failure causes loss of blood glucose control despite adherence to prescribed drug therapy and diet and exercise guidelines. If it occurs, therapy should be discontinued and a different antidiabetic drug substituted.

PATIENT TEACHING
•Instruct patient to store chlorpropamide in a sealed container, away from heat and light.
•Tell patient to take drug with breakfast.
•Stress that drug works with diet and exercise to help control blood glucose level and isn't a substitute for them.
•Tell patient to monitor blood glucose level as instructed.
•Instruct patient not to skip meals or exercise excessively.
•Teach patient how to recognize and treat hypoglycemia. Tell him to report frequent or severe hypoglycemia to prescriber.
•Tell patient to take a missed dose as soon as he remembers it unless it's almost time for the next scheduled dose.
•Urge patient to carry identification showing that he has diabetes and listing his drugs.
•Advise the patient to protect his skin from the sun.
•Instruct the patient to report a fever, sore throat, dark yellow or brown urine, yellow skin and eyes, bleeding, and bruising.

chlorthalidone

Apo-Chlorthalidone (CAN), Hygroton, Novo-Thalidone (CAN), Thalitone, Uridon (CAN)

Class and Category
Chemical: Phthalimidine derivative of benzenesulfonamide (thiazide-like diuretic)
Therapeutic: Antihypertensive, diuretic
Pregnancy category: B

Indications and Dosages
➤ *To reduce edema caused by heart failure, hepatic cirrhosis, corticosteroid or estrogen therapy, or renal dysfunction*
TABLETS
Adults. *Initial:* 50 to 100 mg (Thalitone, 30 to 60 mg) q.d., 100 mg (Thalitone, 60 mg) q.o.d., or 150 to 200 mg (Thalitone, 90 to 120 mg) q.d. or q.o.d. *Maintenance:* Individualized; may be lower than initial dosage.

➤ *To treat hypertension*
TABLETS
Adults. *Initial:* 25 mg q.d. (Thalitone, 15 mg q.d.). If response is insufficient, dosage increased to 50 mg q.d. (Thalitone, 30 to 50 mg q.d.). If additional control is required, dosage increased to 100 mg q.d. (except Thalitone) or a second antihypertensive added. *Mainte-*

nance: Individualized; may be lower than initial dosage.

Route	Onset	Peak	Duration
P.O.	2 to 3 hr	2 to 6 hr	24 to 72 hr

Mechanism of Action

May promote sodium, chloride, and water excretion by inhibiting sodium reabsorption in the kidneys' distal tubules. Initially, chlorthalidone may decrease extracellular fluid volume, plasma volume, and cardiac output, which helps explain how it reduces blood pressure. It also may dilate arteries directly, which helps reduce peripheral vascular resistance and blood pressure. After several weeks, extracellular fluid and plasma volume and cardiac output return to normal, but peripheral vascular resistance remains decreased.

Contraindications

Anuria; hypersensitivity to chlorthalidone, other sulfonamides, or their components; renal decompensation

Interactions

DRUGS

allopurinol: Increased risk of allopurinol hypersensitivity

amphotericin B, glucocorticoids: Intensified electrolyte depletion

anesthetics: Potentiated effects of anesthetics

anticholinergics: Increased chlorthalidone absorption

antidiabetics, methenamines, oral anticoagulants, sulfonylureas: Decreased effects of these drugs

antihypertensives: Potentiated action of antihypertensives and chlorthalidone

antineoplastics: Prolonged antineoplastic-induced leukopenia

cholestyramine, colestipol: Decreased chlorthalidone absorption

diazoxide: Increased risk of hyperglycemia and hypotension

digitalis glycosides: Increased risk of digitalis-induced arrhythmias

lithium: Decreased renal lithium clearance and increased risk of lithium toxicity

loop diuretics: Increased synergistic effects, resulting in profound diuresis and serious electrolyte imbalances

methyldopa: Potential development of hemolytic anemia

neuromuscular blockers: Increased neuromuscular blockade

NSAIDs: Possibly reduced diuretic effect of chlorthalidone

vitamin D: Enhanced vitamin D action

Adverse Reactions

CNS: Dizziness, headache, insomnia, light-headedness, paresthesia, restlessness, vertigo, weakness

CV: Orthostatic hypotension, vasculitis

EENT: Yellow vision

ENDO: Hyperglycemia

GI: Abdominal cramps or pain, anorexia, bloating, constipation, diarrhea, gastric irritation, nausea, pancreatitis, vomiting

GU: Decreased libido, impotence

HEME: Agranulocytosis, aplastic anemia, hypoplastic anemia, leukopenia, thrombocytopenia

MS: Gout attacks, muscle spasms

SKIN: Cutaneous vasculitis, exfoliative dermatitis, jaundice, necrotizing vasculitis, photosensitivity, purpura, rash, urticaria

Other: Hyperuricemia

Nursing Considerations

•Use chlorthalidone cautiously in patients with impaired hepatic function or progressive hepatic disease because minor changes in fluid and electrolyte balance may cause hepatic coma.

•Assess BUN, serum electrolyte and uric acid, and blood glucose levels before therapy and periodically throughout therapy. Monitor for signs of fluid and electrolyte imbalance.

•**WARNING** Monitor renal function periodically to detect cumulative drug effects, which may cause azotemia in patients with impaired renal function.

PATIENT TEACHING

•Stress the importance of taking chlorthalidone even when feeling well.

•Tell patient to store drug at room temperature in tightly closed container.

•Tell patient to take drug in the morning with food or milk.

•Encourage patient to eat high-potassium foods, such as bananas, apricots, grapefruits, tomato juice, and orange juice.

•To minimize effects of orthostatic hypotension, instruct patient to rise slowly from a seated or lying position.

C

•Advise patient to check blood pressure regularly.
•Instruct patient to report signs of low potassium, such as muscle weakness and fatigue.
•Advise patient to protect his skin from the sun.
•Urge patient to immediately report sudden joint pain to prescriber because drug can cause sudden gout attacks.
•Instruct patient to take a missed dose as soon as he remembers it. If he misses one day in an every-other-day schedule, tell him to take the dose on the off day and then resume usual dosing schedule. Warn against taking double or extra doses.

chlorzoxazone

EZE-DS, Paraflex, Parafon Forte DSC, Relaxazone, Remular, Remular-S, Strifon Forte DSC

Class and Category
Chemical: Benzoxazole derivative
Therapeutic: Skeletal muscle relaxant
Pregnancy category: C

Indications and Dosages
➤ *As adjunct to relieve acute musculo-skeletal pain and stiffness*
TABLETS
Adults. 250 to 750 mg t.i.d. or q.i.d., usually 500 mg t.i.d. or q.i.d., increased or decreased according to patient response.

Route	Onset	Peak	Duration
P.O.	In 1 hr	Unknown	3 to 4 hr

Mechanism of Action
Reduces muscle spasm by inhibiting multisynaptic reflex arcs at the level of the spinal cord and subcortical areas of the brain that are active in producing and maintaining skeletal muscle spasm.

Contraindications
Hypersensitivity or known intolerance to chlorzoxazone or any of its components

Interactions
DRUGS
CNS depressants: Additive CNS depression
ACTIVITIES
alcohol use: Additive CNS depression

Adverse Reactions
CNS: Dizziness, drowsiness, headache, light-headedness, malaise, paradoxical stimulation
GI: Abdominal cramps or pain, constipation, diarrhea, GI bleeding, heartburn, hepatotoxicity, nausea, vomiting
GU: Urine discoloration
HEME: Agranulocytosis, anemia
SKIN: Allergic dermatitis, ecchymosis, petechiae
Other: Anaphylaxis, angioedema

Nursing Considerations
•If necessary, crush chlorzoxazone tablets and mix with food or liquid for easier swallowing.
•Assess patients, especially those with a history of allergies, for signs and symptoms of hypersensitivity, such as rash, hives, and itching.
•**WARNING** Monitor patient for signs of hepatotoxicity, including fever, rash, jaundice, and darkened urine. Notify prescriber immediately and expect to discontinue drug if any of these signs or symptoms occur. Monitor patient for abnormal liver function test results, such as elevated AST, ALT, alkaline phosphatase, and bilirubin levels.
•Provide rest and other pain-relief measures.
•Institute safety measures to prevent falls or injury (such as raising bed rails and assisting with ambulation) until drug's full CNS effects are known.
PATIENT TEACHING
•Advise patient to take a missed dose of chlorzoxazone as soon as possible unless it's almost time for the next dose.
•Advise patient to avoid potentially hazardous activities until drug's CNS effects are known.
•Instruct patient to avoid alcohol and other CNS depressants during chlorzoxazone therapy.
•Inform patient that, in rare instances, urine may turn orange or reddish purple during therapy.
•Advise patient to store drug in a tightly capped container at room temperature.

cholestyramine

Questran, Questran Light

Class and Category
Chemical: Quaternary ammonium anion exchange resin

Therapeutic: Antihyperlipidemic, antipruritic (cholestasis)
Pregnancy category: Not rated

Indications and Dosages

➤ *As adjunct to reduce serum cholesterol level in patients with primary hypercholesterolemia, to relieve pruritus associated with partial biliary obstruction*

ORAL SUSPENSION

Adults. *Initial:* 4 g q.d. or b.i.d. before meals. *Maintenance:* 8 to 24 g equally divided and given 2 to 6 times a day. *Maximum:* 24 g/day when used as antihyperlipidemic drug and 16 g/day when used as antipruritic drug.

Route	Onset	Peak	Duration
P.O.	In 1 to 2 wk*	Unknown	2 to 4 wk†

Mechanism of Action

Increases bile acid excretion in the feces. The resulting decreased bile acid level increases the activity of the enzyme that regulates cholesterol synthesis in the liver. As a result, the liver increases its cholesterol synthesis to produce more bile acids. However, the liver's synthesis of cholesterol typically can't match the amount needed to synthesize bile acids, which reduces the cholesterol level. Also, a decreased cholesterol level causes liver cells to increase their uptake of LDLs, which further reduces the cholesterol level. Cholestyramine may relieve pruritus by decreasing the body's bile acid level. This reduces the amount of excess bile acids that are deposited in the dermis and that typically cause pruritus in patients with cholestasis.

Contraindications

Complete biliary obstruction (when bile isn't excreted into intestine), hypersensitivity to cholestyramine or its components

Interactions

DRUGS

chenodiol, digitalis glycosides, fat-soluble vitamins, folic acid, gemfibrozil, penicillin G

(oral), phenylbutazone, propranolol (oral), tetracyclines (oral), thiazide diuretics (oral), thyroid hormones, ursodiol, vancomycin (oral): Decreased absorption and effects of these drugs
oral anticoagulants: Decreased or increased anticoagulant effect

Adverse Reactions

CNS: Headache, dizziness
GI: Bloating, constipation, diarrhea, epigastric pain, eructation, fecal impaction, flatulence, indigestion, nausea, vomiting

Nursing Considerations

•Store cholestyramine at room temperature.
•Don't administer dry powder without mixing it in a beverage because it may cause esophageal distress.
•**WARNING** Be aware that long-term use may increase bleeding tendency from hyperprothrombinemia caused by vitamin K deficiency. If this occurs, patient will require treatment with vitamin K₁.
•Monitor for deficiencies of fat-soluble vitamins, such as A and D. If long-term therapy prevents absorption of these vitamins, expect to provide supplementation.

PATIENT TEACHING

•Urge patient to follow a low-fat, low-cholesterol diet and regular exercise program.
•Tell patient to take drug before meals.
•Instruct patient to mix dry powder as follows: Place the amount of powder equal to his dosage in any beverage and stir vigorously. Then, vigorously stir an additional 2 to 4 oz of beverage into the mixture. After drinking the mixture, rinse the glass with more liquid, and swallow that liquid to make sure all the drug is taken. Explain that the drug also can be mixed in thin soups or moist, pulpy fruits, such applesauce and crushed pineapple.
•Tell patient to drink plenty of fluids and increase bulk in his diet to minimize constipation; remind him to notify prescriber if constipation, nausea, or other adverse GI reactions develop.
•Explain that the serum cholesterol level will need to be measured frequently during the first few months of therapy and periodically thereafter.
•Advise patient to take other drugs at least 1 hour before or 4 to 6 hours after cholestyramine to avoid interference with their absorption.

---

* For hypercholesterolemia; in 1 to 3 wk for pruritus.
† For hypercholesterolemia; 1 to 2 wk for pruritus.

•Tell patient to take a missed dose as soon as he remembers but not to take double or extra doses.

choline and magnesium salicylates

Tricosal, Trilisate

Class and Category
Chemical: Salicylate
Therapeutic: Analgesic, anti-inflammatory, antipyretic
Pregnancy category: C (first trimester), Not rated (later trimesters)

Indications and Dosages
➤ *To treat osteoarthritis, rheumatoid arthritis, and acute painful shoulder*
LIQUID, TABLETS
Adults. 1,500 mg b.i.d. or 3,000 mg h.s.
Children who weigh more than 37 kg (81 lb). 2,250 mg/day in equally divided doses b.i.d.
Children who weigh 37 kg or less. 50 mg/kg/day in equally divided doses b.i.d.
➤ *To treat mild to moderate pain, to reduce fever*
LIQUID, TABLETS
Adults. 2,000 to 3,000 mg/day in equally divided doses b.i.d.
DOSAGE ADJUSTMENT Dosage reduced to 750 mg t.i.d. for elderly patients.

Route	Onset	Peak	Duration
P.O.	Unknown	Several wk*	Unknown

Mechanism of Action
Block the activity of cyclooxygenase, the enzyme needed for prostaglandin synthesis. As mediators in the inflammatory process, prostaglandins cause local vasodilation with swelling and pain. They also play a role in pain transmission from the periphery to the spinal cord. By blocking cyclooxygenase and inhibiting prostaglandins, this NSAID decreases inflammatory symptoms and relieves pain. It acts on the heat-regulating center in the hypothalamus and causes peripheral vasodilation, sweating, and heat loss.

* For rheumatoid arthritis.

Contraindications
Hypersensitivity to nonacetylated salicylates

Interactions
DRUGS
antacids: Increased clearance and decreased blood level of salicylate
carbonic anhydrase inhibitors, phenytoin, valproic acid: Decreased blood levels and therapeutic effects of these drugs
corticosteroids: Decreased blood salicylate level, increased salicylate dosage requirements
insulin, sulfonylureas: Increased hypoglycemic response
methotrexate: Increased therapeutic and toxic effects of methotrexate, especially when given in chemotherapeutic doses
oral anticoagulants: Increased blood level of unbound anticoagulant and risk of bleeding
salicylate-containing products: Increased plasma salicylate level, possibly to toxic level
uricosuric drugs: Decreased uricosuric drug efficacy

Adverse Reactions
CNS: Dizziness, drowsiness, headache, lethargy, light-headedness
EENT: Hearing loss, tinnitus
GI: Constipation, diarrhea, epigastric pain, heartburn, indigestion, nausea, vomiting
HEME: Easy bruising, unusual bleeding

Nursing Considerations
•Use choline and magnesium salicylates cautiously in patients with gastritis, hepatic or renal dysfunction, or peptic ulcer disease.
•Don't give salicylates to children and adolescents with chickenpox or influenza symptoms because of the risk of Reye's syndrome.
•WARNING During high-dose or long-term therapy, monitor for signs of salicylate intoxication, such as headache, dizziness, tinnitus, hearing loss, confusion, drowsiness, diaphoresis, vomiting, diarrhea, and hyperventilation. CNS disturbance, electrolyte imbalance, respiratory acidosis, hyperthermia, and dehydration also may occur. If intoxication occurs, prepare to induce vomiting, administer gastric lavage, and give activated charcoal, as ordered. In extreme cases, prepare patient for peritoneal dialysis or hemodialysis.
PATIENT TEACHING
•Tell patient to store drug at room temperature, away from heat and light, and not in bathroom.

- Instruct patient to take drug with food or after meals and to swallow tablets with a full glass of water.
- Tell patient to take a missed dose as soon as he remembers but to avoid double-dosing.
- Advise patient that optimal effects may not occur for 2 to 3 weeks.
- Teach patient to recognize and immediately report signs of salicylate toxicity.
- Explain that drug is closely related to aspirin. Advise against taking aspirin-containing OTC remedies during therapy.

choline salicylate

Arthropan

Class and Category
Chemical: Salicylate
Therapeutic: Analgesic, anti-inflammatory, antipyretic
Pregnancy category: C (first trimester), Not rated (later trimesters)

Indications and Dosages
➤ *To treat mild to moderate pain, to reduce fever*
LIQUID
Adults and adolescents. 435 to 870 mg q 4 hr, p.r.n. *Maximum:* 5,325 mg/day.
Children ages 11 to 12. 435 to 652.5 mg q 4 hr, p.r.n. *Maximum:* Five doses/day.
Children ages 9 to 11. 435 to 543.8 mg q 4 hr, p.r.n. *Maximum:* Five doses/day.
Children ages 6 to 9. 435 mg q 4 hr, p.r.n. *Maximum:* Five doses/day.
Children ages 4 to 6. 326.5 mg q 4 hr, p.r.n. *Maximum:* Five doses/day.
Children ages 2 to 4. 217.5 mg q 4 hr, p.r.n. *Maximum:* Five doses/day.
Children up to age 2. Individualized dosage. *Maximum:* Five doses/day.
➤ *To treat rheumatoid arthritis*
LIQUID
Adults and adolescents. 870 to 1,740 mg up to four times/day.
Children age 12 and younger. 107 to 133 mg/kg/day in divided doses.

Route	Onset	Peak	Duration
P.O.	Unknown	Several wk*	Unknown

* For rheumatoid arthritis.

Mechanism of Action
Blocks the activity of cyclooxygenase, the enzyme needed for prostaglandin synthesis. As mediators in the inflammatory process, prostaglandins cause local vasodilation with swelling and pain. They also play a role in pain transmission from the periphery to the spinal cord. By blocking cyclooxygenase and inhibiting prostaglandins, this NSAID decreases inflammatory symptoms and relieves pain. It acts on the heat-regulating center in the hypothalamus and causes peripheral vasodilation, sweating, and heat loss.

Contraindications
Hypersensitivity to nonacetylated salicylates

Interactions
DRUGS
antacids: Increased clearance and decreased blood level of salicylate
carbonic anhydrase inhibitors, phenytoin, valproic acid: Decreased blood levels and therapeutic effects of these drugs
corticosteroids: Decreased blood salicylate level, increased salicylate dosage requirements
insulin, sulfonylureas: Increased hypoglycemic response
methotrexate: Increased therapeutic and toxic effects of methotrexate, especially when given in chemotherapeutic doses
oral anticoagulants: Increased blood level of unbound anticoagulant and risk of bleeding
salicylate-containing products: Increased plasma salicylate level, possibly to toxic level
uricosuric drugs: Decreased uricosuric drug efficacy

Adverse Reactions
CNS: Confusion, dizziness, drowsiness, hallucinations, headache, light-headedness
CV: Tachycardia
EENT: Hearing loss, tinnitus
GI: Constipation, diarrhea, epigastric pain, heartburn, indigestion, nausea, vomiting
HEME: Easy bruising, unusual bleeding

Nursing Considerations
- Use choline salicylate cautiously in patients with renal impairment.
- Don't give salicylates to children and adolescents with chickenpox or influenza symptoms because of the risk of Reye's syndrome.

•WARNING During high-dose or long-term therapy, monitor for signs of salicylate intoxication, such as headache, dizziness, tinnitus, hearing loss, confusion, drowsiness, diaphoresis, vomiting, diarrhea, and hyperventilation. CNS disturbance, electrolyte imbalance, respiratory acidosis, hyperthermia, and dehydration also may occur. If intoxication occurs, prepare to induce vomiting, administer gastric lavage, and give activated charcoal, as ordered. In extreme cases, prepare patient for peritoneal dialysis or hemodialysis.

PATIENT TEACHING

•Tell patient to store drug at room temperature, away from heat and light, and not in bathroom.

•Instruct patient to take drug with full glass of water or with food.

•Tell patient to take a missed dose as soon as he remembers but to avoid double-dosing.

•If patient has arthritis, advise him that optimal drug effects may not occur for 2 to 3 weeks.

•Teach patient to recognize and immediately report signs of salicylate toxicity.

•Explain that drug is closely related to aspirin. Advise against taking aspirin-containing OTC remedies during therapy.

cilostazol

Pletal

Class and Category

Chemical: Quinolinone derivative
Therapeutic: Phosphodiesterase III inhibitor, platelet aggregation inhibitor
Pregnancy category: C

Indications and Dosages

➤ *To reduce symptoms of intermittent claudication*

TABLETS

Adults. 100 mg b.i.d. taken at least 30 min before or 2 hr after breakfast and dinner.

Mechanism of Action

May inhibit phosphodiesterase, decreasing phosphodiesterase activity and suppressing cAMP degradation. This action increases cAMP in platelets and blood vessels, which inhibits platelet aggregation and causes vasodilation. This in turn relieves symptoms of claudication.

Contraindications

Heart failure, hypersensitivity to cilostazol or its components

Interactions

DRUGS

diltiazem, erythromycin, itraconazole, ketoconazole, omeprazole: Increased plasma cilostazol level

FOODS

grapefruit juice: Increased risk of adverse reactions

high-fat foods: Faster cilostazol absorption and increased risk of adverse reactions

ACTIVITIES

smoking: Decreased cilostazol effects by about 20%

Adverse Reactions

CNS: Dizziness, headache
CV: Palpitations, peripheral edema, tachycardia
EENT: Pharyngitis, rhinitis
ENDO: Diabetes mellitus, hyperglycemia
GI: Abdominal pain, abnormal stool, diarrhea, flatulence, indigestion
MS: Back pain, myalgia
RESP: Cough
Other: Infection

Nursing Considerations

•Monitor vital signs and cardiovascular status closely because cilostazol may cause cardiovascular lesions, which could lead to problems, such as endocardial hemorrhage.

•Monitor blood glucose level to detect hyperglycemia. Also assess for signs of type 2 diabetes mellitus, such as polyuria, polydipsia, polyphagia, and fatigue.

PATIENT TEACHING

•Instruct patient to take cilostazol on an empty stomach because high-fat foods can increase the risk of adverse reactions.

•Warn patent to avoid grapefruit juice during therapy because it can increase the risk of adverse reactions.

•Urge patient not to smoke because it decreases drug's effects.

•Explain that assessment of drug effectiveness is based on ability to walk increased distances. Stress that drug effects won't appear until 2 to 4 weeks after therapy starts and that full effects may take up to 12 weeks.

cimetidine

Apo-Cimetidine (CAN), Gen-Cimetidine (CAN), Novo-Cimetine (CAN), Nu-Cimet (CAN), PMS-Cimetidine (CAN), Tagamet, Tagamet HB

cimetidine hydrochloride

Novo-Cimetine (CAN), Tagamet

Class and Category

Chemical: Imidazole derivative
Therapeutic: Antiulcer agent, gastric acid secretion inhibitor, H_2-receptor antagonist
Pregnancy category: B

Indications and Dosages

➤ *To treat and prevent recurrence of duodenal ulcer*

ORAL SOLUTION, TABLETS

Adults and adolescents. *Initial:* 800 mg h.s., 300 mg q.i.d. with meals and h.s., or 400 to 600 mg in morning and h.s. for 4 to 6 wk. *Maintenance:* 400 mg h.s.
Children. 20 to 40 mg/kg/day in divided doses q.i.d. with meals and h.s.

I.V. OR I.M. INJECTION

Adults. *Initial:* 300 mg q 6 to 8 hr. Dosage increased, if needed, by increasing frequency. *Maximum:* 2,400 mg/day.

➤ *To treat active, benign gastric ulcer*

ORAL SOLUTION, TABLETS

Adults and adolescents. 800 mg h.s., 300 mg q.i.d. with meals and h.s., or 600 mg b.i.d. in morning and h.s., or 800 mg h.s. for up to 8 wk.
Children. 20 to 40 mg/kg/day in divided doses q.i.d. with meals and h.s.

I.V. OR I.M. INJECTION

Adults and adolescents. *Initial:* 300 mg q 6 to 8 hr. Dosage increased, if needed, by increasing frequency. *Maximum:* 2,400 mg/day.

➤ *To manage gastroesophageal reflux disease*

ORAL SOLUTION, TABLETS

Adults and adolescents. 1,600 mg/day in divided doses (800 mg b.i.d or 400 mg q.i.d.) for up to 12 wk.
Children. 40 to 80 mg/kg/day in divided doses q.i.d.

➤ *To treat pathological hypersecretory conditions, such as Zollinger-Ellison syndrome*

ORAL SOLUTION, TABLETS

Adults and adolescents. 300 mg q.i.d. with meals and h.s. Given more often, if needed. *Maximum:* 2,400 mg/day.

I.V. OR I.M. INJECTION

Adults and adolescents. *Initial:* 300 mg q 6 to 8 hr. Dosage increased, if needed, by increasing frequency. *Maximum:* 2,400 mg/day.

➤ *To treat heartburn and acid indigestion*

ORAL SOLUTION, TABLETS

Adults and adolescents. *Initial:* 200 mg with water at onset of symptoms. *Maximum:* 400 mg q 24 hr for no more than 2 wk unless prescribed.

DOSAGE ADJUSTMENT Oral dosage for all indications reduced to 300 mg q 12 hr (and increased to q 8 hr with caution, if needed) for patients with renal impairment.

➤ *To prevent stress-related upper GI bleeding during hospitalization*

I.V. INFUSION

Adults. 50 mg/hr by continuous infusion for 7 days.

Route	Onset	Peak	Duration
P.O.	Unknown	1 to 2 hr	4 to 5 hr
I.V., I.M.	Unknown	Unknown	4 to 5 hr

Mechanism of Action

Blocks histamine's action at H_2-receptor sites on the stomach's parietal cells. This action reduces gastric fluid volume and acidity. Cimetidine also decreases the amount of gastric acid that's secreted in response to food, caffeine, insulin, betazole, or pentagastrin.

Incompatibilities

Don't mix cimetidine with aminophylline or barbiturates in I.V. solution. Don't mix drug with pentobarbital sodium in the same syringe.

Contraindications

Hypersensitivity to cimetidine or its components

Interactions
DRUGS

antacids, anticholinergics, metoclopramide: Decreased cimetidine absorption
benzodiazepines, calcium channel blockers, carbamazepine, chloroquine, labetalol, lidocaine, metoprolol, metronidazole, moricizine, pentoxifylline, phenytoin, propafenone, propranolol, quinidine, quinine, sulfonylureas, tacrine, theophyllines, triamterene, tricyclic antidepressants, valproic acid, warfarin: Re-

duced metabolism and increased blood levels and effects of these drugs, possibly toxicity from these drugs

carmustine: Increased carmustine myelotoxicity

digoxin, fluconazole: Possibly decreased blood levels of these drugs

ferrous salts, indomethacin, ketoconazole, tetracyclines: Decreased effects of these drugs

flecainide: Increased flecainide effects

fluorouracil: Increased blood fluorouracil level after long-term cimetidine use

ketoconazole: Decreased blood ketoconazole level

narcotic analgesics: Increased toxic effects of narcotic analgesics

oral anticoagulants: Increased anticoagulant effect

procainamide: Increased blood procainamide level

succinylcholine: Increased neuromuscular blockade

tocainide: Decreased tocainide effects

FOODS

caffeine: Reduced metabolism and increased blood level and effects of caffeine

ACTIVITIES

alcohol use: Possibly increased blood alcohol level

Adverse Reactions

CNS: Confusion, dizziness, hallucinations, headache, peripheral neuropathy, somnolence
ENDO: Mild gynecomastia if used longer than 1 month
GI: Mild and transient diarrhea
GU: Impotence, transiently elevated serum creatinine level
SKIN: Rash
Other: Pain at I.M. injection site

Nursing Considerations

•**WARNING** Be aware that rapid administration of cimetidine can increase patient's risk of developing arrhythmias and hypotension.
•For I.V. injection, dilute cimetidine in NS to a total volume of 20 ml. Inject drug over 5 minutes or more.
•For intermittent I.V. infusion, dilute drug in at least 50 ml of D_5W or other compatible I.V. solution. Infuse over 15 to 20 minutes.
•For I.M. injection, don't dilute drug.
•Be especially alert for confusion in elderly or debilitated patients who receive cimetidine.

PATIENT TEACHING
•Tell patient to use a liquid-measuring device to ensure accurate measurement of oral solution.
•Advise patient to avoid alcohol while taking cimetidine to prevent interactions.
•Instruct patient to avoid taking antacids within 1 hour of taking cimetidine.
•Warn patient that cigarette smoking increases gastric acid secretion and can worsen gastric disease.
•Caution patient not to take drug for more than 14 days, unless prescribed.

cinoxacin

Cinobac

Class and Category

Chemical: Quinolone derivative
Therapeutic: Antibiotic
Pregnancy category: B

Indications and Dosages

➤ *To treat UTIs caused by* Enterobacter *sp.,* Escherichia coli, Klebsiella *sp.,* Proteus mirabilis, *and* Proteus vulgaris

CAPSULES

Adults. 1 g/day in divided doses b.i.d. to q.i.d. for 7 to 14 days.

DOSAGE ADJUSTMENT After initial dose of 500 mg, dosage reduced to 250 mg t.i.d. if creatinine clearance is 50 to 80 ml/min/1.73 m^2, 250 mg b.i.d. if creatinine clearance is 20 to 50 ml/min/1.73 m^2, and 250 mg q.d. if creatinine clearance is less than 20 ml/min/1.73 m^2.

➤ *To prevent UTIs in women with a history of chronic UTIs*

CAPSULES

Adults. 250 mg h.s. for up to 5 mo.

Mechanism of Action

Inhibits the enzyme DNA gyrase, which is responsible for the unwinding and supercoiling of bacterial DNA before it replicates. By inhibiting this enzyme, cinoxacin causes bacterial cells to die.

Contraindications

Hypersensitivity to cinoxacin, other quinolones, or their components

Interactions

DRUGS

probenecid: Increased blood cinoxacin level

Adverse Reactions

CNS: Dizziness, headache
CV: Edema
EENT: Altered taste
GI: Abdominal cramps, anorexia, diarrhea, elevated liver function test results, nausea, vomiting
GU: Perineal burning
HEME: Eosinophilia
SKIN: Angioedema, photosensitivity, pruritus, rash, urticaria

Nursing Considerations

•Obtain results of urine culture and sensitivity test before administering first dose of cinoxacin.
•Review results of liver function tests, as indicated, during treatment.
•Administer drug with food, if needed; food decreases peak blood level but doesn't change total absorption.

PATIENT TEACHING

•Stress the importance of completing the full course of therapy, even if patient feels better before it's finished.
•Tell patient to take drug with food, if needed, to avoid GI distress.
•Instruct patient to drink 2 to 3 L of fluid daily unless contraindicated.
•Instruct patient to avoid direct sunlight, use sunscreen, and wear protective clothing. If photosensitivity occurs, tell patient to notify prescriber.
•Advise patient to immediately report a rash, severe adverse GI reactions, or edema.
•Advise patient to take safety precautions if he experiences dizziness.

ciprofloxacin

Cipro, Cipro I.V.

Class and Category

Chemical: Fluoroquinolone derivative
Therapeutic: Antibiotic
Pregnancy category: C

Indications and Dosages

➤ *To prevent inhalation anthrax after exposure or to treat inhalation anthrax*

ORAL SUSPENSION, TABLETS

Adults and adolescents. 500 mg q 12 hr for 60 days.
Children. 15 mg/kg q 12 hr for 60 days. *Maximum:* 500 mg/dose.

I.V. INFUSION

Adults and adolescents. 400 mg q 12 hr for 60 days.
Children. 10 mg/kg q 12 hr for 60 days. *Maximum:* 400 mg/dose or 800 mg/day.

➤ *To treat acute sinusitis caused by gram-negative organisms (including* Campylobacter jejuni, Citrobacter diversus, Citrobacter freundii, Enterobacter cloacae, Escherichia coli, Haemophilus influenzae, Haemophilus parainfluenzae, Klebsiella pneumoniae, Morganella morganii, Neisseria gonorrhoeae, Proteus mirabilis, Proteus vulgaris, Providencia rettgeri, Providencia stuartii, Pseudomonas aeruginosa, Serratia marcescens, Shigella flexneri, *and* Shigella sonnei*) and gram-positive organisms (including* Enterococcus faecalis, Staphylococcus aureus, Staphylococcus epidermidis, *and* Streptococcus pneumoniae*)*

ORAL SUSPENSION, TABLETS

Adults. 500 mg q 12 hr for 10 days.

I.V. INFUSION

Adults. For mild to moderate infections, 400 mg q 12 hr.

➤ *To treat bone and joint infections caused by susceptible organisms listed above*

ORAL SUSPENSION, TABLETS

Adults. For mild to moderate infections, 500 mg q 12 hr for 4 to 6 wk. For severe or complicated infections, 750 mg q 12 hr for 4 to 6 wk.

I.V. INFUSION

Adults. For mild to moderate infections, 400 mg q 12 hr for 4 to 6 wk. For severe or complicated infections, 400 mg q 8 hr.

➤ *To treat skin and soft-tissue infections caused by susceptible organisms listed above*

ORAL SUSPENSION, TABLETS

Adults. For mild to moderate infections, 500 mg q 12 hr for 7 to 14 days. For severe or complicated infections, 750 mg q 12 hr for 7 to 14 days.

I.V. INFUSION

Adults. For mild to moderate infections, 400 mg q 12 hr. For severe or complicated infections, 400 mg q 8 hr.

➤ *To treat chronic bacterial prostatitis caused by susceptible organisms listed above*

ORAL SUSPENSION, TABLETS

Adults. 500 mg q 12 hr for 28 days.

I.V. INFUSION
Adults. 400 mg q 12 hr.
➤ *To treat infectious diarrhea caused by susceptible organisms listed above*
ORAL SUSPENSION, TABLETS
Adults. 500 mg q 12 hr for 5 to 7 days.
➤ *To treat UTIs caused by susceptible organisms listed above*
ORAL SUSPENSION, TABLETS
Adults. For acute uncomplicated infections, 100 mg q 12 hr for 3 days. For mild to moderate infections, 250 mg q 12 hr for 7 to 14 days. For severe or complicated infections, 500 mg q 12 hr for 7 to 14 days.
I.V. INFUSION
Adults. For mild to moderate infections, 200 mg q 12 hr. For severe or complicated infections, 400 mg q 12 hr.
➤ *To treat lower respiratory tract infections caused by susceptible organisms listed above*
ORAL SUSPENSION, TABLETS
Adults. For mild to moderate infections, 500 mg q 12 hr for 7 to 14 days. For severe or complicated infections, 750 mg q 12 hr for 7 to 14 days.
I.V. INFUSION
Adults. For mild to moderate infections, 400 mg q 12 hr. For severe or complicated infections, 400 mg q 8 hr.
➤ *To treat intra-abdominal infections caused by susceptible organisms listed above*
I.V. INFUSION
Adults. 400 mg q 8 hr along with parenteral metronidazole.
➤ *To treat mild to severe nosocomial pneumonia caused by susceptible organisms listed above*
I.V. INFUSION
Adults. 400 mg q 8 hr.
➤ *To treat typhoid fever caused by* Salmonella typhi *or infectious diarrhea caused by* C. jejuni, E. coli, S. flexneri, *or* S. sonnei
ORAL SUSPENSION, TABLETS
Adults. 500 mg q 12 hr for 10 days.
➤ *To treat uncomplicated urethral or cervical gonococcal infections caused by* N. gonorrhoeae
ORAL SUSPENSION, TABLETS
Adults. 250 mg as a single dose.
DOSAGE ADJUSTMENT Dosage reduced to 250 to 500 mg q 12 hr in patients with creatinine

clearance of 30 to 50 ml/min/1.73 m²; and to 250 to 500 mg P.O. or 200 to 400 mg I.V. q 18 hr in patients with creatinine clearance of 5 to 29 ml/min/1.73 m².

Mechanism of Action
Inhibits the enzyme DNA gyrase, which is responsible for the unwinding and supercoiling of bacterial DNA before it replicates. By inhibiting this enzyme, ciprofloxacin causes bacterial cells to die.

Incompatibilities
Don't administer parenteral ciprofloxacin with aminophylline, amoxicillin, cefepime, clindamycin, dexamethasone, floxacillin, furosemide, heparin, or phenytoin.

Contraindications
Hypersensitivity to ciprofloxacin, quinolones, or their components

Interactions
DRUGS
antacids, iron supplements, sucralfate, zinc- or iron-containing multivitamins: Decreased ciprofloxacin absorption
cyclosporine: Elevated serum creatinine and cyclosporine levels
glyburide: Severe hypoglycemia
oral anticoagulants: Enhanced anticoagulant effects
phenytoin: Increased or decreased blood phenytoin level
probenecid: Increased blood level of ciprofloxacin and, possibly, toxicity
theophylline: Increased blood level, half-life, and risk of adverse effects of theophylline
FOODS
caffeine: Increased caffeine effects
dairy products: Delayed drug absorption

Adverse Reactions
CNS: Confusion, headache, restlessness, seizures
CV: Orthostatic hypotension
EENT: Oral candidiasis
GI: Abdominal pain, constipation, diarrhea, elevated liver function test results, flatulence, indigestion, nausea, pseudomembranous colitis, vomiting
GU: Crystalluria, hematuria, increased serum creatinine level, nephrotoxicity, renal calculi, vaginal candidiasis

SKIN: Exfoliative dermatitis, photosensitivity, rash, Stevens-Johnson syndrome, toxic epidermal necrolysis

Nursing Considerations
• Obtain culture and sensitivity test results, as ordered, before giving ciprofloxacin.
• Use drug cautiously in patients with CNS disorders, such as cerebral arteriosclerosis and seizure disorder.
• Dilute I.V. ciprofloxacin concentrate to 1 to 2 mg/ml using D_5W or sodium chloride for injection. Don't dilute solutions that come from the manufacturer in D_5W before I.V. infusion. Infuse slowly over 1 hour.
• Store reconstituted solution for up to 14 days at room temperature or under refrigeration.
• Don't administer oral suspension through a feeding tube.
• Be aware that patient should be well hydrated during therapy to help prevent nephrotoxicity.
PATIENT TEACHING
• Urge patient to complete the prescribed course of therapy, even if he feels better before it's finished.
• Tell patient not to take drug with dairy products or calcium fortified juices alone.
• Advise patient to take ciprofloxacin 2 hours before or 6 hours after taking antacids, iron supplements, or multivitamins that contain iron or zinc. Tell patient to shake oral suspension for 15 seconds and to not chew microcapsules.
• Encourage patient to drink plenty of fluids during therapy to help prevent crystalluria.
• Instruct patient to notify prescriber immediately at first sign of allergy, such as rash.
• Advise patient to use safety measures until drug's CNS effects are known.

citalopram hydrobromide

Celexa

Class and Category
Chemical: Racemic, bicyclic phthalate derivative
Therapeutic: Antidepressant
Pregnancy category: C

Indications and Dosages
➤ *To treat depression*
ORAL SOLUTION, TABLETS
Adults. *Initial:* 20 mg q.d. Daily dosage increased by 20 mg at weekly intervals, as prescribed. *Usual:* 40 mg q.d. *Maximum:* 60 mg/day.

DOSAGE ADJUSTMENT For elderly patients, maximum dosage is 40 mg/day.

Route	Onset	Peak	Duration
P.O.	1 to 4 wk	Unknown	Unknown

Mechanism of Action
Blocks serotonin reuptake by adrenergic nerves, which normally release this neurotransmitter from their storage sites when activated by a nerve impulse. This blocked reuptake increases serotonin levels at nerve synapses, which may elevate mood and reduce depression.

Contraindications
Hypersensitivity to citalopram or its components, use within 14 days of MAO inhibitor therapy

Interactions
DRUGS
amitriptyline, bromocriptine, buspirone, clomipramine, dextromethorphan, fluoxetine, fluvoxamine, furazolidone, imipramine, levodopa, lithium, meperidine, naratriptan, nefazodone, paroxetine, pentazocine, phenelzine, procarbazine, selegiline, sertraline, sibutramine, sumatriptan, tramadol, tranylcypromine, trazodone, venlafaxine, zolmitriptan: Possibly enhanced serotonergic effects of citalopram, resulting in agitation, confusion, diaphoresis, diarrhea, fever, hyperreflexia, hypomania, incoordination, myoclonus, shivering, or tremor
carbamazepine: Possibly increased clearance of citalopram
cimetidine: Possibly increased blood citalopram level
desipramine, metoprolol: Increased blood levels of these drugs
furazolidone, procarbazine, selegiline: Possibly hyperthermia, rigidity, myoclonus, and extreme agitation progressing to delirium and coma
itraconazole, ketoconazole, macrolide antibiotics, omeprazole: Possibly decreased clearance of citalopram
warfarin: Possibly increased PT

Adverse Reactions
CNS: Agitation, anxiety, asthenia, dizziness, drowsiness, fatigue, fever, insomnia, tremor
EENT: Blurred vision, dry mouth, rhinitis, sinusitis

GI: Abdominal pain, anorexia, diarrhea, indigestion, nausea, vomiting
GU: Anorgasmia, decreased libido, dysmenorrhea, ejaculation disorders, impotence
MS: Arthralgia, myalgia
RESP: Upper respiratory tract infection
SKIN: Diaphoresis
Other: Weight gain or loss

Nursing Considerations

•**WARNING** Whenever citalopram dosage is increased, monitor for possible serotonin syndrome, characterized by agitation, confusion, diaphoresis, diarrhea, fever, hyperactive reflexes, poor coordination, restlessness, shaking, shivering, talking or acting with uncontrolled excitement, tremor, and twitching.

•Be aware that effective antidepressant therapy may transform depression into mania in predisposed individuals. If your patient develops symptoms of mania, notify prescriber immediately and expect to discontinue drug.

•During initial drug therapy, monitor patient for suicidal ideation and institute suicide precautions as appropriate, according to facility policy.

•Monitor patient with hepatic disease for increased adverse reactions because drug is extensively metabolized in the liver.

•Monitor elderly patients and those taking diuretics for signs suggesting syndrome of inappropriate secretion of antidiuretic hormone, including hyponatremia and increased serum and urine osmolarity.

•Monitor patient for changes in mental status because citalopram may impair judgment, thinking, and motor skills. Be prepared to institute safety precautions.

PATIENT TEACHING

•Inform patient that citalopram's full effects may take up to 4 weeks to occur.

•Advise patient to avoid potentially hazardous activities, such as driving, until drug's CNS effects are known.

•Advise patient not to self-medicate for coughs, colds, or allergies without consulting prescriber because some ingredients in these preparations can increase the risk of adverse reactions.

clarithromycin

Biaxin, Biaxin XL, Biaxin XL-PAK

Class and Category

Chemical: Macrolide derivative

Therapeutic: Antibiotic
Pregnancy category: C

Indications and Dosages

➤ *To treat pharyngitis and tonsillitis caused by* Streptococcus pyogenes
ORAL SUSPENSION, TABLETS
Adults and adolescents. 250 mg q 12 hr for 10 days.
Children. 15 mg/kg/day in divided doses q 12 hr for 10 days.

➤ *To treat acute maxillary sinusitis caused by* Haemophilus influenzae, Moraxella catarrhalis, *or* Streptococcus pneumoniae
ORAL SUSPENSION, TABLETS
Adults and adolescents. 500 mg q 12 hr for 14 days.
Children. 15 mg/kg/day in divided doses q 12 hr for 10 days.
EXTENDED-RELEASE TABLETS
Adults and adolescents. 1,000 mg q 24 hr for 14 days.

➤ *To treat acute exacerbations of chronic bronchitis caused by* H. influenzae, M. catarrhalis, *or* S. pneumoniae
ORAL SUSPENSION, TABLETS
Adults and adolescents. 250 to 500 mg q 12 hr for 7 to 14 days.
Children. 15 mg/kg/day in divided doses q 12 hr for 10 days.
EXTENDED-RELEASE TABLETS
Adults and adolescents. 1,000 mg q 24 hr for 7 days.

➤ *To treat uncomplicated skin and soft-tissue infections caused by* Staphylococcus aureus *or* S. pyogenes
ORAL SUSPENSION, TABLETS
Adults and adolescents. 250 mg q 12 hr for 7 to 14 days.
Children. 15 mg/kg/day in divided doses q 12 hr for 10 days.

➤ *To treat pneumonia caused by* Chlamydia pneumoniae, Mycoplasma pneumoniae, *or* S. pneumoniae
ORAL SUSPENSION, TABLETS
Adults and adolescents. 250 mg q 12 hr for 7 to 14 days.
Children. 15 mg/kg/day in divided doses q 12 hr for 10 days.

➤ *To treat pneumonia caused by* H. influenzae
ORAL SUSPENSION, TABLETS
Adults and adolescents. 250 mg q 12 hr for 7 days.
Children. 15 mg/kg/day in divided doses q 12 hr for 10 days.

➤ *To treat acute otitis media caused by* H. influenzae, M. catarrhalis, *or* S. pneumoniae

ORAL SUSPENSION, TABLETS

Children. 15 mg/kg/day in divided doses q 12 hr for 10 days.

➤ *To treat active duodenal ulcer caused by* Helicobacter pylori

ORAL SUSPENSION, TABLETS

Adults and adolescents. 500 mg q 8 hr for 14 days with omeprazole 40 mg q.d. in the morning. Then, omeprazole continued at 20 mg q.d. in the morning for days 15 through 28. Alternatively, 500 mg q 12 hr for 14 days with lansoprazole 30 mg and amoxicillin 1 g q 12 hr for 14 days.

➤ *To prevent or treat* Mycobacterium avium *complex in patients with HIV infection*

ORAL SUSPENSION, TABLETS

Adults and adolescents. 500 mg q 12 hr for 7 to 14 days.

Children. 7.5 mg/kg q 12 hr. *Maximum:* 500 mg b.i.d.

Mechanism of Action

Inhibits RNA-dependent protein synthesis in many types of aerobic, anaerobic, gram-positive, and gram-negative bacteria. By binding with the 50S ribosomal subunit of the bacterial 70S ribosome, clarithromycin causes bacterial cells to die.

Contraindications

Concurrent therapy with astemizole, cisapride, pimozide, or terfenadine; hypersensitivity to clarithromycin, erythromycin, or any macrolide antibiotic

Interactions

DRUGS

astemizole: Possibly prolonged QT interval or torsades de pointes

carbamazepine, other drugs metabolized by cytochrome P450 enzyme system: Increased blood levels of these drugs

cisapride, disopyramide, pimozide, quinidine, terfenadine: Increased risk of arrhythmias

digoxin: Increased serum digoxin level

dihydroergotamine, ergotamine: Risk of acute ergot toxicity

lovastatin, simvastatin: Risk of rhabdomyolysis

oral anticoagulants: Potentiated anticoagulant effects

rifabutin, rifampin: Decreased blood clarithromycin level by more than 50%

sildenafil: Possible prolonged blood sildenafil level

theophylline: Increased blood theophylline level

zidovudine: Decreased blood zidovudine level

Adverse Reactions

CNS: Anxiety, confusion, dizziness, fatigue, headache, insomnia, somnolence, vertigo

CV: Ventricular arrhythmias

EENT: Altered taste

GI: Abdominal pain, diarrhea, indigestion, nausea, pseudomembranous colitis

GU: Elevated BUN level

SKIN: Pruritus, rash, urticaria

Other: Superinfection

Nursing Considerations

•Expect to obtain a specimen for culture and sensitivity tests before giving first dose of clarithromycin.

•Use clarithromycin cautiously in patients with renal impairment.

PATIENT TEACHING

•Caution patient not to crush or chew extended-release tablets.

•Advise patient to take drug with food if GI distress occurs.

•Tell patient to report severe or watery diarrhea, severe nausea, rash, or itching.

clidinium bromide

Quarzan

Class and Category

Chemical: Synthetic quaternary ammonium derivative

Therapeutic: Anticholinergic

Pregnancy category: Not rated

Indications and Dosages

➤ *As adjunct to treat peptic ulcers*

CAPSULES

Adults. 2.5 to 5 mg t.i.d. or q.i.d. 30 to 60 min before meals and h.s.

DOSAGE ADJUSTMENT Dosage limited to 2.5 mg t.i.d. before meals for elderly or debilitated patients.

Route	Onset	Peak	Duration
P.O.	1 hr	Unknown	Up to 3 hr

Contraindications

Angle-closure glaucoma, benign bladder neck obstruction, hypersensitivity to clidinium bromide or its components, ileus, intestinal atony (elderly or debilitated patients), intestinal obstruction, myasthenia gravis, myocardial ischemia, ocular adhesions between lens and iris, prostatic hypertrophy, renal disease, severe ulcerative colitis, tachycardia, toxic megacolon, unstable cardiovascular status in acute hemorrhage

Mechanism of Action

Inhibits acetylcholine's muscarinic actions at postganglionic parasympathetic receptor sites, including smooth muscles, secretory glands, and the CNS. These actions relax smooth muscles and diminish GI, GU, and biliary tract secretions.

Interactions

DRUGS

amantadine: Increased risk of clidinium adverse effects
atenolol: Increased atenolol effects
CNS depressants: Increased clidinium effects
phenothiazines: Decreased antipsychotic effectiveness
tricyclic antidepressants: Increased clidinium adverse effects

ACTIVITIES

alcohol use: Increased clidinium effects

Adverse Reactions

CNS: Confusion, dizziness, drowsiness, excitement, fever, headache, insomnia, memory loss, nervousness, weakness
CV: Palpitations, tachycardia
EENT: Blurred vision, cycloplegia, dry mouth, increased intraocular pressure, loss of taste, mydriasis, nasal congestion, pharyngitis, photophobia
GI: Bloating, constipation, dysphagia, heartburn, ileus, nausea, vomiting
GU: Impotence, urinary hesitancy, urine retention
SKIN: Decreased sweating, flushing, rash, urticaria

Nursing Considerations

• Avoid high doses of clidinium in patients with ulcerative colitis because drug may inhibit intestinal motility and precipitate or aggravate toxic megacolon. Also avoid high doses in patients with hiatal hernia or reflux esophagitis because drug may aggravate esophagitis.
• Use clidinium cautiously in patients with heart failure, arrhythmias, hypertension, auto-

nomic neuropathy, hyperthyroidism, allergies, asthma, and debilitating chronic lung disease.
• **WARNING** Monitor for excitement, agitation, drowsiness, and confusion in elderly patients, even with small doses, because they're more sensitive to clidinium's effects. If these reactions occur, notify prescriber and expect to decrease dosage.
• Take safety precautions to protect patient from injury from falling.

PATIENT TEACHING

• Instruct patient to take clidinium exactly as prescribed and not to stop taking it suddenly because it can cause withdrawal symptoms, such as vomiting, diaphoresis, and dizziness.
• Advise patient to take drug 30 to 60 minutes before meals.
• Tell patient not to store capsules in the bathroom, near the kitchen sink, or in other damp places.
• Teach patient how to prevent or relieve constipation and dry mouth.
• Instruct patient to avoid alcohol and other CNS depressants because they increase the drug's effects.
• Instruct patient to report constipation, vision changes, sore throat, difficulty urinating, and palpitations.

clindamycin hydrochloride

Cleocin, Dalacin C

clindamycin palmitate hydrochloride

Cleocin Pediatric, Dalacin C Flavored Granules (CAN)

clindamycin phosphate

Cleocin, Dalacin C Phosphate (CAN)

Class and Category

Chemical: Lincosamide
Therapeutic: Antibacterial and antiprotozoal antibiotic
Pregnancy category: B

Indications and Dosages

➤ *To treat serious respiratory tract infections caused by anaerobes such as occur with anaerobic pneumonitis, empyema, and lung abscess and those caused by pneumococci, staphylococci, and strepto-*

cocci; serious skin and soft-tissue infections caused by anaerobes, staphylococci, and streptococci; septicemia caused by anaerobes; intra-abdominal infections caused by anaerobes such as occur with intra-abdominal abscess and peritonitis; infections of the female pelvis and genital tract caused by anaerobes such as occur with endometritis, nongonococcal tubo-ovarian abscess, pelvic cellulitis, and postsurgical vaginal cuff infection; bone and joint infections caused by Staphylococcus aureus; as adjunct therapy in chronic bone and joint infections

CAPSULES, ORAL SOLUTION

Adults and adolescents. For serious infections, 150 to 300 mg q 6 hr; for severe infections, 300 to 450 mg q 6 hr.

Children. For serious infections, 8 to 16 mg/kg/day in equally divided doses t.i.d. or q.i.d.; for severe infections, 16 to 20 mg/kg/day in equally divided doses t.i.d. or q.i.d.

I.V. INFUSION, I.M. INJECTION

Adults and adolescents age 16 and older. For serious infections, 600 to 1,200 mg/day in equally divided doses b.i.d. to q.i.d.; for severe infections, 1,200 to 2,700 mg/day in equally divided doses b.i.d. to q.i.d.; for life-threatening infections, 4,800 mg/day in equally divided doses b.i.d. to q.i.d.

Children ages 1 month to 16 years. 20 to 40 mg/kg/day in equally divided doses t.i.d. or q.i.d., depending on severity of infection.

Neonates less than age 1 month. 15 to 20 mg/kg/day in equally divided doses t.i.d. or q.i.d., depending on severity of infection.

➤ To treat vaginal infections caused by Gardnerella or Haemophilus

VAGINAL CREAM

Nonpregnant adults. 100 mg (1 applicatorful) into vaginia q.d., preferably h.s., for 3 to 7 consecutive days.

Pregnant adults in second or third trimester. 100 mg (1 applicatorful) into vaginia q.d., preferably h.s., for 7 consecutive days.

Mechanism of Action

Inhibits protein synthesis in susceptible bacteria by binding to the 50S subunits of bacterial ribosomes and preventing peptide bond formation, which causes bacterial cells to die.

Incompatibilities

To prevent physical incompatibility, don't administer with aminophylline, ampicillin, barbiturates, calcium gluconate, magnesium sulfate, or phenytoin.

Contraindications

Hypersensitivity to clindamycin or lincomycin

Interactions

DRUGS

erythromycin: Possibly blocked access of clindamycin to its site of action
kaolin-pectin antidiarrheals: Decreased absorption of oral clindamycin
neuromuscular blockers: Increased neuromuscular blockade

Adverse Reactions

CNS: Fatigue, headache
CV: Hypotension, thrombophlebitis (after I.V. injection)
EENT: Glossitis, metallic or unpleasant taste (with high I.V. doses), stomatitis
GI: Abdominal pain, diarrhea, esophagitis, nausea, pseudomembranous colitis, vomiting
GU: Cervicitis, vaginitis, and vulvar irritation (with vaginal form)
HEME: Agranulocytosis, eosinophilia, leukopenia, neutropenia, thrombocytopenic purpura
SKIN: Pruritus, rash, urticaria
Other: Anaphylaxis; induration, pain, or sterile abscess after injection; superinfection

Nursing Considerations

•Expect to obtain a specimen for culture and sensitivity testing before giving first dose.
•Use clindamycin cautiously in patients who have a history of asthma, significant allergies, or GI disease; in those with renal or hepatic dysfunction; and in elderly or atopic patients.
•WARNING Don't give 75- and 150-mg capsules to tartrazine-sensitive patients.
•Store oral solution for up to 2 weeks at room temperature or reconstituted parenteral solution for up to 24 hours at room temperature.
•Administer I.V. dose by infusion only; don't give bolus dose. Dilute 300 mg of clindamycin in 50 ml of diluent and administer over 10 minutes. Dilute 600 mg of clindamycin in 100 ml of diluent and administer over 20 minutes. Dilute 900 mg of clindamycin in 100 ml of diluent and administer over 30 minutes.
•WARNING Don't use diluents that contain benzyl alcohol when clindamycin is to be ad-

ministered to neonates because a fatal toxic syndrome may occur.

•Give I.M. injection deep into large muscle mass, such as the gluteus maximus. Rotate injection sites, and avoid giving more than 600 mg by I.M. injection.

•Check I.V. site frequently for phlebitis and irritation.

•Monitor results of liver function tests, CBC, and platelet counts during prolonged therapy.

•Observe patient for signs of superinfection, such as vaginal itching and sore mouth, and signs of pseudomembranous colitis, which may occur 2 to 9 days after therapy begins.

PATIENT TEACHING

•Tell patient to complete the prescribed course of therapy, even if he feels better before it's finished.

•Instruct patient to take oral clindamycin with at least 8 oz of water to prevent esophageal irritation.

•Advise patient to take oral drug with food, if needed, to reduce GI distress.

•Tell patient not to refrigerate reconstituted oral solution because it may become thick and difficult to pour and to discard unused drug after 14 days.

•Warn patient not to rely on latex or rubber condoms and diaphragms for 72 hours after vaginal treatment because mineral oil in the vaginal cream may weaken these items.

•Explain that engaging in intercourse after using vaginal cream can increase irritation.

•Inform patient that I.M. injection may be painful.

•Tell patient to immediately report symptoms of colitis (severe diarrhea and abdominal cramps), an inflamed mouth or vagina, and rash or lesions.

clofibrate

Abitrate, Atromid-S, Claripex (CAN), Novofibrate (CAN)

Class and Category

Chemical: Aryloxyisobutyric acid derivative
Therapeutic: Antihyperlipidemic
Pregnancy category: C

Indications and Dosages

➤ *To treat primary hyperlipidemia (type III) that doesn't respond to diet and type IV and type V hyperlipidemia that don't respond to diet in patients at risk for abdominal pain and pancreatitis*

CAPSULES

Adults. 1.5 to 2 g/day in divided doses b.i.d. to q.i.d.

Route	Onset	Peak	Duration
P.O.	2 to 5 days	3 wk	3 wk

Mechanism of Action

Increases the amount of cholesterol that's secreted into bile and of bile that's excreted in the feces. Clofibrate also may increase the activity of lipoprotein lipase, which degrades VLDLs.

Contraindications

Hepatic dysfunction, hypersensitivity to clofibrate, lactation, peptic ulcer, pregnancy, primary biliary cirrhosis, renal dysfunction

Interactions

DRUGS

chenodiol, ursodiol: Counteracted effectiveness of these drugs

dantrolene: Decreased plasma protein binding of dantrolene

furosemide: Increased furosemide and clofibrate effects

insulin, sulfonylureas: Increased antidiabetic effect

oral anticoagulants: Increased bleeding tendency

oral contraceptives: Decreased effectiveness of clofibrate

phenytoin: Displacement of phenytoin from binding site

probenecid: Increased clofibrate effects

rifampin: Decreased clofibrate effects

Adverse Reactions

CNS: Dizziness, drowsiness, fatigue, headache, weakness

CV: Angina, edema, phlebitis

EENT: Stomatitis

GI: Abdominal pain, bloating, diarrhea, flatulence, nausea, vomiting

GU: Decreased libido, decreased urine output, impotence, proteinuria

HEME: Eosinophilia

MS: Arthralgia, myalgia

SKIN: Alopecia, dry skin and hair, pruritus, rash, urticaria

Other: Weight gain

Nursing Considerations
- Obtain baseline CBC, liver and renal function studies, and cholesterol profile, as ordered.
- Use clofibrate cautiously in patients with a history of hepatic disease or jaundice and in those with peptic ulcer disease.

PATIENT TEACHING
- Tell patient to take clofibrate with milk or food to reduce GI distress.
- Tell patient that repeated laboratory tests will be needed to evaluate serum cholesterol and triglyceride levels.
- Stress the importance of diet, exercise, and weight loss to control cholesterol.
- Instruct patient to report chest pain, severe adverse GI reactions, decreased urine output, ankle or leg swelling, and unusual weight gain.
- If patient takes an anticoagulant, instruct him to watch carefully for abnormal bleeding.
- If patient takes antidiabetic drugs, instruct him to stay alert for signs of hypoglycemia from interactions with these drugs.
- Advise women of childbearing age to use contraception during and for several months after therapy because of clofibrate's teratogenic effects.

clomipramine hydrochloride

Anafranil

Class and Category
Chemical: Dibenzazepine derivative
Therapeutic: Antiobsessional tricyclic antidepressant
Pregnancy category: C

Indications and Dosages
➤ *To treat obsessive-compulsive disorder*

CAPSULES, TABLETS
Adults. *Initial:* 25 mg q.d. Gradually increased to 100 mg/day given in divided doses during first 2 wk and then to maximum of 250 mg/day in divided doses over next few weeks. Total daily dose may be given h.s. when maximum dose is reached.
Children age 10 and older. *Initial:* 25 mg q.d. Gradually increased to 3 mg/kg/day or 100 mg/day, whichever is less, given in divided doses during first 2 wk and then to maximum of 3 mg/kg/day or 200 mg/day, whichever is less. Total daily dose may be given h.s. when maximum dose is reached.

Route	Onset	Peak	Duration
P.O.	Unknown	2 to 4 wk	Unknown

Mechanism of Action
May inhibit neuronal reuptake of norepinephrine and serotonin, which may be a factor in normalizing neurotransmission in obsessive-compulsive behavior.

Contraindications
Acute recovery period after MI, hypersensitivity to clomipramine or its components, use of an MAO inhibitor within 14 days

Interactions
DRUGS
anticholinergics: Increased anticholinergic effects
barbiturates: Decreased blood level and effects of clomipramine; additive CNS depression
bupropion, cimetidine, haloperidol, H_2-receptor antagonists, selective serotonin reuptake inhibitors, valproic acid: Increased plasma concentration and therapeutic and adverse effects of clomipramine
carbamazepine: Decreased blood clomipramine level; increased blood carbamazepine level
CNS depressants: Increased CNS depression
clonidine: Severely increased blood pressure and risk of hypertensive crisis
dicumarol: Increased anticoagulant effect
grepafloxacin, quinolones, sparfloxacin: Increased risk of life-threatening arrhythmias
guanethidine: Antagonized antihypertensive effect of guanethidine
levodopa: Delayed absorption and decreased bioavailability of levodopa
MAO inhibitors: Increased risk of seizures, coma, or death
rifamycins: Decreased blood clomipramine level
sympathomimetics: Possibly potentiated cardiovascular effects
thyroid drugs: Increased effects of thyroid drugs and clomipramine
ACTIVITIES
alcohol use: Increased CNS depression

Adverse Reactions
CNS: Anxiety, confusion, depersonalization, depression, dizziness, drowsiness, emotional lability, fatigue, headache, insomnia, panic

reaction, paresthesia, somnolence, syncope, tremor, unusual dreams, yawning
CV: Orthostatic hypotension, palpitations, tachycardia
EENT: Blurred vision, dry mouth, epistaxis, pharyngitis, rhinitis, sinusitis, unpleasant taste
GI: Abdominal pain, anorexia, constipation, diarrhea, flatulence, increased appetite, indigestion, nausea, vomiting
GU: Dysmenorrhea, ejaculation failure, impotence, urinary hesitancy, urine retention
RESP: Bronchospasm
SKIN: Abnormal skin odor, acne, dermatitis, dry skin, photosensitivity, rash, urticaria
Other: Weight gain

Nursing Considerations
•Be aware that stopping clomipramine abruptly may cause withdrawal symptoms and worsen disorder.
•**WARNING** Don't give drug within 14 days of an MAO inhibitor to avoid possible seizures, coma, or death.

PATIENT TEACHING
•Tell patient not to use alcohol, barbiturates, or other CNS depressants; clomipramine increases their effects.
•Inform male patients about risk of sexual dysfunction while taking drug.
•Caution patient about possible drowsiness, especially during initial dosage adjustment.
•Warn patient not to stop taking drug abruptly.
•Instruct patient to take a missed dose as soon as he remembers unless it's almost time for the next scheduled dose, in which case he should skip the missed dose. Warn against double-dosing.
•Teach patient how to prevent photosensitivity reactions.
•Tell patient to report dry mouth, difficulty urinating, sedation, dizziness, and mental changes.

clonazepam

Apo-Clonazepam (CAN), Clonapam (CAN), Gen-Clonazepam (CAN), Klonopin, Rivotril (CAN)

Class, Category, and Schedule
Chemical: Benzodiazepine
Therapeutic: Anticonvulsant
Pregnancy category: D
Controlled substance: Schedule IV

Indications and Dosages
➤ *To treat Lennox-Gastaut syndrome (type of absence seizure disorder) and akinetic and myoclonic seizures*
TABLETS
Adults and children over age 10. 1.5 mg/day in divided doses t.i.d. Increased by 0.5 to 1 mg q 3 days, if needed, until seizures are controlled. *Maximum:* 20 mg/day.
Children age 10 and under or weighing less than 30 kg (66 lb). 0.01 to 0.03 mg/kg/day in divided doses b.i.d. or t.i.d. Increased by 0.25 to 0.5 mg every third day up to maintenance dosage. *Maintenance:* 0.1 to 0.2 mg/kg/day, preferably in three equal doses, or if unequal, with largest dose given h.s. *Maximum:* 0.05 mg/kg/day.
➤ *To treat panic disorder*
TABLETS
Adults. *Initial:* 0.25 mg b.i.d. Increased, if needed, to 1 mg/day after 3 days. If more than 1 mg/day is required, dosage increased in increments of 0.125 to 0.25 mg b.i.d. q 3 days until panic disorder is controlled or adverse reactions make further increases undesirable. This maintenance dosage may be given as a single dose h.s. *Maximum:* 4 mg/day.

Mechanism of Action
Prevents seizures by potentiating the effects of gamma-aminobutyric acid, which is an inhibitory neurotransmitter. Suppresses the spread of seizure activity caused by seizure-producing foci in the cortex, thalamus, and limbic structures.

Contraindications
Acute narrow-angle glaucoma, hepatic disease, hypersensitivity to benzodiazepines or their components

Interactions
DRUGS
antianxiety drugs, barbiturates, MAO inhibitors, narcotics, phenothiazines, tricyclic antidepressants: Increased CNS depression
ACTIVITIES
alcohol use: Increased CNS depression

Adverse Reactions
CNS: Ataxia, confusion, depression, dizziness, drowsiness, emotional lability, fatigue, headache, memory loss, nervousness, reduced intellectual ability
CV: Palpitations

EENT: Blurred vision, eyelid spasm, increased salivation, loss of taste, pharyngitis, rhinitis, sinusitis
GI: Abdominal pain, anorexia, constipation
GU: Difficult ejaculation, dysmenorrhea, dysuria, enuresis, impotence, nocturia, urine retention, UTI
HEME: Anemia, eosinophilia, leukopenia, thrombocytopenia
MS: Dysarthria, myalgia
RESP: Bronchitis, cough
Other: Allergic reaction

Nursing Considerations
•Use clonazepam cautiously in patients with renal failure, mixed seizure disorder (because drug can increase the risk of generalized tonic-clonic seizures), or respiratory disease and troublesome secretions (because clonaz-epam increases salivation) and in elderly pa-tients (because they're more sensitive to drug's CNS effects).
•Monitor blood drug level, CBC, and liver function test results during long-term or high-dose therapy, as ordered.
•WARNING Don't stop drug abruptly; expect to taper dosage gradually to avoid withdrawal symptoms and seizures.

PATIENT TEACHING
•Instruct patient to take drug exactly as pre-scribed. Explain that stopping drug abruptly can cause seizures and withdrawal symptoms.
•Advise patient to avoid alcohol and sleep-inducing drugs during therapy. Instruct him to consult prescriber before taking any OTC drugs.
•Urge patient to carry medical identification indicating his seizure disorder and drug therapy.
•Warn patient about possible drowsiness.
•Instruct patient to report severe dizziness, persistent drowsiness, palpitations, difficulty urinating, seizure activity, and other disrup-tive adverse reactions.
•Suggest that parents monitor child's perfor-mance in school because clonazepam can cause drowsiness or inattentiveness.

clonidine
Catapres-TTS

clonidine hydrochloride
Catapres, Dixarit (CAN), Duraclon

Class and Category
Chemical: Imidazoline derivative
Therapeutic: Analgesic, antihypertensive
Pregnancy category: C

Indications and Dosages
➤ *To manage hypertension*

TABLETS
Adults. *Initial:* 0.1 mg b.i.d. Dosage in-creased by 0.1 mg/wk to produce desired re-sponse. *Maintenance:* 0.2 to 0.6 mg/day in di-vided doses b.i.d. or t.i.d. *Maximum:* 2.4 mg/day.

TRANSDERMAL PATCH
Adults. *Initial:* 0.1-mg patch applied to hair-less area of intact skin on upper arm or torso q 7 days. After 1 to 2 wk, if blood pressure isn't controlled, two 0.1-mg patches or one 0.2-mg patch applied to skin. Dosage ad-justed, as needed, q 7 days. *Maximum:* Two 0.3-mg patches worn at same time.

➤ *To treat severe hypertension*
TABLETS
Adults. 0.2 mg, then 0.1 mg q 1 hr until dia-stolic blood pressure reaches acceptable range or 0.8 mg have been administered.
DOSAGE ADJUSTMENT Dosage individualized for patients with renal failure.

➤ *As adjunct to relieve severe pain (in cancer patients) that isn't adequately re-lieved by opioid analgesics alone*
CONTINUOUS EPIDURAL INFUSION
Adults. *Initial:* 30 mcg/hr. Titrated up or down, if needed, depending on comfort. *Maximum:* 40 mcg/hr.
Children old enough to tolerate placement and management of epidural catheter. *Initial:* 0.5 mcg/kg/hr. Then, titrated to achieve comfort.

Route	Onset	Peak	Duration
P.O.	30 to 60 min	2 to 4 hr	8 hr
Trans-dermal	2 to 3 days	Unknown	7 days

Contraindications
Anticoagulant therapy (epidural infusion); bleeding diathesis; hypersensitivity to cloni-dine or its components, including compo-nents of the transdermal patch adhesive; in-jection site infection (epidural infusion)

Mechanism of Action

Stimulates peripheral alpha-adrenergic receptors in the CNS to produce transient vasoconstriction and then stimulates central alpha-adrenergic receptors in the brain stem to reduce peripheral vascular resistance, heart rate, and systolic and diastolic blood pressure. May produce analgesia by preventing transmission of pain signals to the brain at presynaptic and postjunctional alpha$_2$-adrenoreceptors in the spinal cord. With epidural administration, clonidine produces analgesia in body areas innervated by the spinal cord segments in which the drug concentrates.

Interactions

DRUGS

barbiturates, other CNS depressants: Increased depressant effects of these drugs
beta blockers, calcium channel blockers, digoxin: Additive effects, such as bradycardia and AV block; increased risk of exacerbated hypertensive response when clonidine is withdrawn (beta blockers only)
diuretics, other antihypertensive drugs: Increased hypotensive effect
epidural local anesthetics: Prolonged effects of epidural local anesthetics when used with epidural clonidine
levodopa: Decreased levodopa effectiveness
prazosin, tricyclic antidepressants: Decreased antihypertensive effect of clonidine

ACTIVITIES

alcohol use: Enhanced CNS depressant effects of alcohol

Adverse Reactions

CNS: Agitation, depression, dizziness, drowsiness, fatigue, headache, malaise, nervousness, sedation, weakness
CV: Chest pain, orthostatic hypotension
EENT: Blurred vision, burning eyes, dry eyes and mouth
GI: Constipation, mildly elevated liver function test results, nausea, vomiting
GU: Decreased libido, impotence, nocturia
SKIN: Rash
Other: Weight gain, withdrawal symptoms

Nursing Considerations

• Use clonidine cautiously in elderly patients, who may be more sensitive to its hypotensive effect.

• Monitor blood pressure and heart rate frequently during clonidine therapy.
• Expect transdermal clonidine to take 2 to 3 days to lower blood pressure.
• Be aware that stopping drug abruptly can elevate serum catecholamine levels and cause such withdrawal symptoms as nervousness, agitation, headache, confusion, tremor, and rebound hypertension.
• Expect hypertension to return within 48 hours after drug is discontinued.

PATIENT TEACHING

• Advise patient to take drug exactly as prescribed and not to stop taking it abruptly because withdrawal symptoms and severe hypertension may occur.
• Instruct patient to consult prescriber if dry mouth or drowsiness becomes a problem during oral clonidine therapy. To minimize these effects, prescriber may suggest taking most of dosage at bedtime.
• If a transdermal patch loosens during the 7-day application period, tell patient to place the adhesive overlay directly over the patch to ensure adhesion.
• Tell patient to rotate transdermal application sites.
• Instruct patient to remove the patch and place a fresh patch on another site if skin irritation, redness, or rash develops at the patch site.
• Advise patient to fold used transdermal patch in half with the adhesive sides together and discard it out of the reach of children.
• Because of possible sedation, advise patient to avoid potentially hazardous activities until drug's CNS effects are known.
• Advise male patients about possibly decreased libido.
• Instruct patient to report urine retention, vision changes, excessive drowsiness, rash, chest pain, and dizziness with position changes. As needed, tell patient to rise slowly to avoid hypotensive effects.

clopidogrel bisulfate

Plavix

Class and Category

Chemical: Thienopyridine derivative
Therapeutic: Platelet aggregation inhibitor
Pregnancy category: B

Indications and Dosages

➤ *To reduce atherosclerotic events, such as CVA and MI, in patients with atherosclerosis documented by recent CVA, MI, or peripheral artery disease*

TABLETS

Adults. 75 mg q.d.

➤ *To reduce atherosclerotic events, such as CVA and MI, in patients with acute coronary syndrome (unstable angina or non-Q-wave MI)*

TABLETS

Adults. *Loading dose:* 300 mg. *Maintenance:* 75 mg q.d.

Route	Onset	Peak	Duration
P.O.	2 hr	3 to 7 days*	5 days

Mechanism of Action

Binds to adenosine diphosphate (ADP) receptors on the surface of activated platelets. This action blocks ADP, which deactivates nearby glycoprotein IIb/IIIa receptors and prevents fibrinogen from attaching to receptors. Without fibrinogen, platelets can't aggregate and form thrombi.

Contraindications

Active pathological bleeding, including peptic ulcer and intracranial hemorrhage; hypersensitivity to clopidogrel or its components

Interactions

DRUGS

fluvastatin, phenytoin, tamoxifen, tolbutamide, torsemide: Interference with metabolism of these drugs

NSAIDs: Increased risk of GI bleeding, interference with NSAID metabolism

warfarin: Prolonged bleeding time, interference with warfarin metabolism

Adverse Reactions

CNS: Depression, dizziness, fatigue, headache

CV: Chest pain, edema, hypercholesterolemia, hypertension

EENT: Epistaxis, rhinitis

GI: Abdominal pain, diarrhea, indigestion, nausea

GU: UTI

---

* With repeated doses.

HEME: Prolonged bleeding time, thrombocytopenic purpura

MS: Arthralgia, back pain

RESP: Bronchitis, cough, dyspnea

SKIN: Pruritus, purpura, rash

Other: Flulike symptoms

Nursing Considerations

•Use clopidogrel cautiously in patients with severe hepatic disease and in those at risk for increased bleeding from trauma, surgery, or conditions that produce a tendency to bleed (such as peptic ulcer disease).

•Expect to administer aspirin in combination with clopidogrel to patient who has acute coronary syndrome.

•WARNING Expect to discontinue therapy 7 days before surgery because drug prolongs bleeding time.

PATIENT TEACHING

•Discourage the use of NSAIDs, including OTC preparations, during clopidogrel therapy because of potential for bleeding.

•Caution patient that bleeding may continue for longer than usual. Instruct him to notify prescriber about unusual bleeding or bruising.

•Instruct patient to inform his health care providers about his clopidogrel therapy.

clorazepate dipotassium

Apo-Clorazepate (CAN), Novo-Clopate (CAN), Tranxene (CAN), Tranxene-SD, Tranxene-SD Half Strength

Class, Category, and Schedule

Chemical: Benzodiazepine

Therapeutic: Alcohol withdrawal adjunct, antianxiety, anticonvulsant

Pregnancy category: Not rated

Controlled substance: Schedule IV

Indications and Dosages

➤ *To relieve anxiety symptoms*

CAPSULES, TABLETS

Adults and adolescents. *Initial:* 15 mg h.s. or 7.5 to 15 mg b.i.d. Dosage adjusted, as needed, to 15 to 60 mg/day in divided doses b.i.d. to q.i.d. *Maximum:* 90 mg/day.

E.R. TABLETS

Adults and adolescents. 11.25 mg q.d. as substitute for capsules or tablets in patients who were stabilized on 3.75 mg t.i.d. of those forms; 22.5 mg q.d. as substitute for capsules or tablets in patients who were stabilized on 7.5 mg t.i.d. of those forms.

➤ *To relieve symptoms of acute alcohol withdrawal*

CAPSULES, TABLETS

Adults. *Initial:* 30 mg followed by 15 mg b.i.d. to q.i.d. on day 1 of therapy; 15 mg three to six times on day 2; 7.5 to 15 mg t.i.d. on day 3; 7.5 mg b.i.d. to q.i.d. on day 4; and thereafter, 3.75 mg b.i.d. to q.i.d. *Maximum:* 90 mg/day.

➤ *As adjunct to treat partial seizure disorder*

CAPSULES, TABLETS

Adults and adolescents. *Initial:* Up to 7.5 mg t.i.d. Increased, if needed, by up to 7.5 mg/wk. *Maximum:* 90 mg/day.

Children ages 9 to 12. *Initial:* 7.5 mg b.i.d. Increased, if needed, by up to 7.5 mg/wk. *Maximum:* 60 mg/day.

E.R. TABLETS

Adults and adolescents. 11.25 mg q.d. as substitute for capsules or tablets in patients who were stabilized on 3.75 mg t.i.d. of those forms; 22.5 mg q.d. as substitute for capsules or tablets in patients who were stabilized on 7.5 mg t.i.d. of those forms.

DOSAGE ADJUSTMENT Initial dosage reduced to 3.75 to 15 mg/day to treat anxiety in elderly patients.

Mechanism of Action

Potentiates the action of gamma-aminobutyric acid (GABA) and other inhibitory neurotransmitters by binding to specific benzodiazepine receptor sites in the limbic and cortical areas of the CNS. GABA inhibits excitatory stimulation, which helps control emotional behavior and suppresses the spread of seizure activity caused by seizure-producing foci in the cortex, thalamus, and limbic structures. The drug also helps relieve symptoms of alcohol withdrawal by depressing the CNS.

Contraindications

Hypersensitivity to chlorazepate dipotassium or its components, narrow-angle glaucoma

Interactions

DRUGS

barbiturates, MAO inhibitors, narcotics, other antidepressants, phenothiazines: Potentiated effects of clorazepate

cimetidine, disulfiram, fluoxetine, isoniazid, ketoconazole, metoprolol, oral contraceptives, propoxyphene, propranolol, valproic acid: Increased blood clorazepate level

clozapine: Possibly increased risk of shock

ACTIVITIES

alcohol use: Potentiated effects of clorazepate

Adverse Reactions

CNS: Anxiety, ataxia, confusion, depression, dizziness, drowsiness, fatigue, headache, insomnia, irritability, nervousness, psychosis, slurred speech, tremor

CV: Hypotension

EENT: Blurred vision, diplopia, dry mouth

GI: Anorexia, constipation, diarrhea, elevated liver function test results, nausea, vomiting

GU: Elevated BUN and serum creatinine levels, incontinence, libido changes, menstrual irregularities, urine retention

HEME: Decreased hematocrit

SKIN: Rash

Other: Drug dependence

Nursing Considerations

•**WARNING** Be aware that prolonged use of therapeutic doses can lead to dependence.

•Monitor liver function test results during therapy.

PATIENT TEACHING

•Tell patient to take clorazepate with food if GI distress occurs.

•Advise patient to avoid alcohol and other CNS depressants while taking drug.

•Because of possible drowsiness, advise patient to avoid potentially hazardous activities until drug's CNS effects are known.

cloxacillin sodium

Apo-Cloxi (CAN), Cloxapen, Novo-Cloxin (CAN), Nu-Cloxi (CAN), Orbenin (CAN), Tegopen

Class and Category

Chemical: Penicillinase-resistant isoxazolyl penicillin derivative
Therapeutic: Antibiotic
Pregnancy category: B

Indications and Dosages

➤ *To treat mild to moderate upper respiratory tract infections or localized skin and soft-tissue infections caused by penicillinase-producing staphylococci*

CAPSULES, ORAL SOLUTION, I.V. INFUSION, I.V. OR I.M. INJECTION

Adults and children who weigh 20 kg (44 lb) or more. 250 mg q 6 hr. *Maximum:* 6 g/day.

Children and infants who weigh less than 20 kg.
50 mg/kg/day in equally divided doses q 6 hr.

➤ *To treat severe lower respiratory tract infections or disseminated infections caused by penicillinase-producing staphylococci*

CAPSULES, ORAL SOLUTION, I.V. INFUSION, I.V. OR I.M. INJECTION

Adults and children who weigh 20 kg or more. 500 mg q 6 hr. *Maximum:* 6 g/day.
Infants and children who weigh less than 20 kg. 100 mg/kg/day in equally divided doses q 6 hr.

Mechanism of Action

Inhibits bacterial cell wall synthesis in susceptible bacteria. These bacteria assemble rigid, cross-linked cell walls in several steps. Cloxacillin affects the final stage of cross-linking by binding with and inactivating penicillin-binding protein, the enzyme responsible for linking cell wall strands. This action inhibits bacterial cell wall synthesis and causes cell lysis and death.

Incompatibilities

Don't mix cloxacillin with aminoglycosides because of risk of substantial mutual inactivation.

Contraindications

Hypersensitivity to cloxacillin, penicillin, or their components

Interactions

DRUGS

chloramphenicol, erythromycins, sulfonamides, tetracyclines: Decreased cloxacillin effects
hepatotoxic drugs, such as fluconazole: Increased risk of hepatotoxicity
methotrexate: Increased blood methotrexate level and risk of toxicity
probenecid: Increased and prolonged blood cloxacillin level

Adverse Reactions

CNS: Headache
EENT: Glossitis, oral candidiasis
GI: Abdominal pain, diarrhea, elevated liver function test results, nausea, pseudomembranous colitis, vomiting
GU: Hematuria, vaginal candidiasis
MS: Muscle twitching
SKIN: Pruritus, rash, urticaria
Other: Anaphylaxis

Nursing Considerations

•Use cloxacillin cautiously in patients who are hypersensitive to cephalosporins; allergic reaction may be delayed. Also use cautiously in patients with hypertension because drug is relatively high in sodium.
•For I.V. injection, reconstitute 250-mg vial with 4.9 ml of sterile water for injection, 500-mg vial with 4.8 ml, and 2,000-mg vial with 6.8 ml. Shake to dissolve.
•If giving by direct I.V. injection, administer over 2 to 4 minutes through the tubing of a compatible infusing I.V. solution. If giving by intermittent I.V. infusion, further dilute with a suitable diluent (see manufacturer's package insert) and administer over 30 to 40 minutes.
•For I.M. injection, reconstitute 250-mg vial with 1.9 ml of sterile water for injection and 500-mg vial with 1.7 ml of sterile water. Shake to dissolve.
•Be aware that parenteral solutions are stable for 24 hours at room temperature and for 72 hours if refrigerated.

PATIENT TEACHING

•Tell patient to complete prescribed course of therapy, even if he feels better before it's finished.
•Instruct patient to take oral cloxacillin 1 to 2 hours before meals.
•Tell patient to take oral form with a full glass of water only, not with fruit juice or a carbonated beverage.
•Instruct patient taking oral solution to refrigerate container and to discard unused portion after 14 days. Also instruct him to use a liquid-measuring device when measuring the dose.
•Advise patient to notify prescriber if an allergic reaction occurs.

clozapine

Clozaril

Class and Category

Chemical: Dibenzodiazepine derivative
Therapeutic: Antipsychotic
Pregnancy category: B

Indications and Dosages

➤ *To treat severe schizophrenia that fails to respond to standard drug treatment*

TABLETS

Adults. *Initial:* 12.5 mg q.d. or b.i.d. Increased by 25 to 50 mg/day to 300 to 450 mg/day by the end of 2 wk. Subsequent dosage adjustments shouldn't exceed 100 mg once or twice per wk. *Maximum:* 900 mg/day.

Route	Onset	Peak	Duration
P.O.	1 to 6 hr	Unknown	4 to 12 hr

Mechanism of Action
May produce antipsychotic effects by interfering with dopamine binding to dopamine—especially D_4—receptors in the limbic region of the brain and by antagonizing adrenergic, cholinergic, histaminic, and serotoninergic receptors.

Contraindications
Angle-closure glaucoma, coma, history of clozapine-induced agranulocytosis or severe granulocytopenia, hypersensitivity to clozapine or its components, myeloproliferative disorders, severe CNS depression, uncontrolled epilepsy, WBC count below 3,500/mm^3

Interactions
DRUGS
anticholinergics: Potentiated anticholinergic effects
benzodiazepines, psychotropics: Additive hypotensive effects; increased risk of cardiopulmonary collapse
bone marrow depressants: Potentiated myelosuppressive effects
carbamazepine, phenytoin: Decreased blood clozapine level
cimetidine, erythromycin: Increased blood clozapine level
CNS depressants: Increased CNS depression
digoxin, warfarin: Increased serum concentrations of digoxin and warfarin; displacement of clozapine from its binding site
lithium: Increased risk of seizures, confusion, neuroleptic malignant syndrome, and dyskinesia
selective serotonin reuptake inhibitors: Markedly increased blood clozapine level; increased risk of adverse effects and leukocytosis
ACTIVITIES
alcohol use: Increased CNS depression

Adverse Reactions
CNS: Agitation, akinesia, anxiety, ataxia, confusion, depression, dizziness, drowsiness, fatigue, fever, headache, hyperkinesia, hypokinesia, insomnia, lethargy, myoclonic jerks, neuroleptic malignant syndrome, nightmares, restlessness, rigidity, sedation, seizures, sleep disturbance, slurred speech, syncope, tardive dyskinesia, tremor, vertigo, weakness
CV: Cardiac arrest, chest pain, deep vein thrombosis, ECG changes, hypertension, hypotension, myocarditis, orthostatic hypotension, tachycardia
EENT: Blurred vision, dry mouth, increased nasal congestion, increased salivation, pharyngitis, tongue numbness or soreness
ENDO: Ketoacidosis, severe hyperglycemia
GI: Abdominal discomfort, anorexia, constipation, diarrhea, elevated liver function test results, heartburn, nausea, vomiting
GU: Abnormal ejaculation; urinary frequency, urgency, and incontinence; urine retention
HEME: Agranulocytosis, eosinophilia, leukopenia, neutropenia
MS: Back or leg pain, muscle spasm or weakness, myalgia
RESP: Dyspnea, respiratory arrest
SKIN: Rash
Other: Weight gain

Nursing Considerations
•Use clozapine cautiously in patients with hepatic, renal, or cardiovascular disease.
•WARNING Be aware that clozapine rarely may cause severe or life-threatening adverse reactions, such as agranulocytosis, myocarditis (especially in first month of treatment), respiratory or cardiac arrest, deep vein thrombosis, severe hyperglycemia that leads to ketoacidosis in nondiabetic patients, and neuroleptic malignant syndrome. It also rarely may produce tardive dyskinesia and seizures. Monitor patient closely throughout drug therapy and take safety and infection-control precautions.
•If patient's WBC count falls below 3,500/mm^3 or granulocyte count falls below 1,500/mm^3, expect to discontinue therapy temporarily. Monitor for flulike symptoms or other evidence of infection. If no infection develops, WBC count exceeds 3,000/mm^3, and granulocyte count is 1,500/mm^3 or more, plan to resume therapy. Monitor WBC count and differential twice weekly until WBC count returns to 3,500/mm^3.
•WARNING Stay alert for blood dyscrasias for up to 4 weeks after treatment ends.
•Monitor temperature. A transient temperature elevation above 100.4° F (38° C) may

occur, most often within the first 3 weeks of therapy.

PATIENT TEACHING

- Tell patient that he'll receive only a 1-week supply at a time.
- Inform patient that he'll need weekly blood tests to check for blood dyscrasias. Teach him how to recognize their signs and symptoms (including fatigue, fever, sore throat, and weakness) and urge him to report them to his prescriber if they occur.
- Instruct patient to take safety precautions and avoid potentially hazardous activities until clozapine's CNS effects are known.
- Advise patient to get up slowly from a lying or sitting position to minimize effects of orthostatic hypotension.
- Stress the importance of notifying prescriber if patient stops taking clozapine for more than 2 days. Tell him not to restart drug on his own because dosage will need to be changed.
- Tell patient to consult prescriber before using alcohol or taking OTC drugs.
- Advise female patients of childbearing age to notify prescriber as soon as pregnancy occurs or is suspected.

codeine phosphate

codeine sulfate

Class, Category, and Schedule

Chemical: Phenanthrene derivative
Therapeutic: Antitussive, narcotic analgesic
Pregnancy category: C
Controlled substance: Schedule II

Indications and Dosages

➤ *To treat mild to moderate pain*

ORAL SOLUTION, TABLETS, I.M. OR S.C. INJECTION

Adults. 15 to 60 mg q 4 hr, p.r.n. *Usual:* 30 mg/dose.

Children age 1 year or older. 0.5 mg/kg q 4 to 6 hr, p.r.n.

I.V. INJECTION

Adults. 15 to 60 mg q 4 hr. *Usual:* 30 mg/dose.

➤ *To treat cough induced by chemical or mechanical irritation of the respiratory system*

ORAL SOLUTION, TABLETS

Adults and adolescents. 10 to 20 mg q 4 to 6 hr. *Maximum:* 120 mg/day.

Children ages 6 to 12. 5 to 10 mg q 4 to 6 hr. *Maximum:* 60 mg/day.

Children ages 2 to 6. 2.5 to 5 mg q 4 to 6 hr. *Maximum:* 30 mg/day.

Route	Onset	Peak	Duration
P.O.	30 to 45 min	1 to 2 hr	4 hr*
I.M.	10 to 30 min	30 to 60 min	4 hr*
S.C.	10 to 30 min	Unknown	4 hr*

Mechanism of Action

May produce analgesia through partial metabolism to morphine. The drug binds with mu, delta, and kappa receptors in the spinal cord and with mu_1 and $kappa_3$ receptors at higher levels in the CNS, altering the perception of—and emotional response to—pain. By binding with these receptors, the drug decreases intracellular cAMP, which inhibits adenylate cyclase activity. This action prevents the release of pain neurotransmitters, such as substance P and dopamine. Codeine also suppresses cough by directly acting on opiate receptors in the medulla's cough center.

Contraindications

Hypersensitivity to codeine, other narcotics, or their components; significant respiratory depression

Interactions

DRUGS

anticholinergics, paregoric: Increased risk of severe constipation
antihypertensives, diuretics: Potentiated hypotensive effects
buprenorphine: Decreased effectiveness of codeine
CNS depressants: Additive CNS effects
hydroxyzine: Increased codeine analgesic effect; increased CNS depressant and hypotensive effects
MAO inhibitors: Increased risk of unpredictable, severe, and sometimes fatal reactions
metoclopramide: Antagonized effect of metoclopramide on GI motility
naloxone: Antagonized codeine analgesic effect

---

* For pain; 4 to 6 hr for cough.

naltrexone: Precipitated withdrawal symptoms in codeine-dependent patients
neuromuscular blockers: Additive respiratory depressant effects
other opioids: Additive CNS and respiratory depressant effects and hypotensive effects
ACTIVITIES
alcohol use: Additive CNS effects

Adverse Reactions
CNS: Coma, delirium, depression, disorientation, dizziness, drowsiness, euphoria, hallucinations, headache, lack of coordination, lethargy, light-headedness, mental and physical impairment, mood changes, restlessness, sedation, seizures, tremor
CV: Bradycardia, heart block, hypertension, orthostatic hypotension, palpitations, tachycardia
EENT: Altered taste, blurred vision, diplopia, dry mouth, laryngeal edema, laryngospasm, miosis
GI: Abdominal cramps and pain, anorexia, constipation, flatulence, gastroesophageal reflux, ileus, indigestion, nausea, vomiting
GU: Decreased libido, difficult ejaculation, dysuria, impotence, oliguria, ureteral spasm, urinary incontinence, urine retention
MS: Muscle rigidity
RESP: Apnea, bronchoconstriction, bronchospasm, depressed cough reflex, respiratory depression
SKIN: Diaphoresis, flushing, pallor, pruritus, rash, urticaria
Other: Anaphylaxis, facial edema, physical and psychological dependence

Nursing Considerations
• Evaluate for therapeutic response, including decreased pain, cough, and facial grimacing.
• Take safety precautions, if needed.
• Monitor respiratory depth, effort, and rate. Notify prescriber immediately if respiratory rate drops below 10 breaths/min.
• Assess urine output; decreasing output may signal urine retention.
• WARNING Assess patient for evidence of physical and psychological dependence.
• Rotate sites when administering codeine S.C. Local tissue irritation, pain, and induration may occur with repeated injection into the same site.
PATIENT TEACHING
• Advise patient to avoid alcohol or other CNS depressants while taking codeine.

• To minimize nausea, suggest that patient take drug with food.
• Advise patient to avoid potentially hazardous activities until drug's CNS effects are known.
• Caution patient to get up slowly from a sitting or lying position.
• To prevent constipation, encourage patient to consume plenty of fluids and high-fiber foods, if not contraindicated by another condition.
• Instruct patient to take codeine exactly as prescribed and not to adjust dose or frequency without consulting prescriber.
• Advise patient to notify prescriber if he becomes short of breath or has difficulty breathing.

colchicine

Class and Category
Chemical: Colchicum alkaloid derivative
Therapeutic: Antigout, anti-inflammatory
Pregnancy category: C (oral form), D (parenteral forms)

Indications and Dosages
➤ *To prevent gouty arthritis attacks*
TABLETS
Adults. 0.5 to 0.6 mg q.d. Dosage increased to 0.5 to 0.6 mg b.i.d. or t.i.d., if needed.
I.V. INFUSION OR INJECTION
Adults. 0.5 to 1 mg q.d. or b.i.d. *Maximum:* 4 mg/day.
➤ *To prevent gouty arthritis attacks before, during, and after surgery*
TABLETS
Adults. 0.5 to 0.6 mg t.i.d. for 3 days before and 3 days after surgery.
➤ *To treat acute gouty arthritis*
TABLETS
Adults. *Initial:* 0.5 to 1.2 mg; then 0.5 to 0.6 mg q 1 to 2 hr, or 1 to 1.2 mg q 2 hr until pain decreases or adverse reactions occur. *Maximum:* 6 mg/day.
I.V. INFUSION OR INJECTION
Adults. 2 mg over 2 to 5 min; then 0.5 mg q 6 hr or 1 mg q 6 to 12 hr until pain decreases. *Maximum:* 4 mg/day.
DOSAGE ADJUSTMENT For elderly patients, maximum I.V. dosage reduced to 2 mg/24 hr; maximum oral dosage reduced to 2 mg/24 hr. After initial course of I.V. therapy, elderly patient should receive no form of colchicine for 21 days.

Route	Onset	Peak	Duration
P.O.	In 12 hr	In 24 to 48 hr	Unknown
I.V.	In 6 to 12 hr	Unknown	Unknown

Contraindications

Blood dyscrasias; hypersensitivity to colchicine or its components; serious cardiac, GI, hepatic, or renal disorders

Incompatibilities

Don't combine colchicine with bacteriostatic agents, any solution or injection that contains D_5W, and any other solution that may change colchicine's pH because precipitation may occur.

Interactions

DRUGS

anticoagulants, such as heparin; platelet aggregation inhibitors, such as aspirin; thrombolytics, such as alteplase: Possibly significantly increased risk of GI ulceration or hemorrhage
antineoplastics: Possibly increased serum uric acid level and decreased therapeutic effectiveness of colchicine
cyclosporine: Increased blood cyclosporine level
NSAIDs, such as phenylbutazone: Possibly increased risk of bone marrow depression, GI bleeding, leukopenia, or thrombocytopenia

vitamin B_{12}: Possibly impaired absorption of and increased dosage requirements for vitamin B_{12}

ACTIVITIES

alcohol use: Increased risk of adverse GI effects

Adverse Reactions

CNS: Peripheral neuropathy
CV: Arrhythmias (I.V. form)
GI: Abdominal pain, anorexia, diarrhea, nausea, vomiting
HEME: Agranulocytosis, aplastic anemia, thrombocytopenia
MS: Myopathy
SKIN: Alopecia, rash
Other: Injection site pain and tenderness, median nerve neuritis in affected arm, and skin and soft-tissue necrosis if extravasation occurs (I.V. form)

Nursing Considerations

•**WARNING** Avoid S.C. or I.M. administration of colchicine because these routes may cause tissue necrosis and sloughing. To prevent extravasation, ensure that the I.V. catheter is patent and correctly positioned before administering drug. Throughout therapy, check I.V. injection site frequently for pain, tenderness, and skin peeling. Consult prescriber about switching to oral form as soon as possible.
•**WARNING** To reduce the risk of toxicity, avoid giving colchicine by any route within 7 days after a full I.V. course (4 mg). Expect to wait 3 days after oral therapy before be-

Mechanism of Action

In gouty arthritis, leukocytes phagocytose urate crystals in affected joints, a process that releases chemotactic factors, degradation enzymes, and other inflammatory substances. Colchicine helps stop this process, probably by disrupting microtubules within leukocytes. Normally, microtubules contribute to cell structure and movement. When colchicine binds to tubulin (the protein from which microtubules are made), the microtubule falls apart, as shown. This process disrupts cell function and prevents leukocytes from invading joints and producing inflammation.

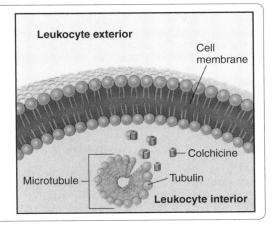

Leukocyte exterior
Cell membrane
Colchicine
Microtubule
Tubulin
Leukocyte interior

ginning second oral course. Be aware that elderly or debilitated patients and those with a history of cardiac disease or impaired renal or hepatic function are at increased risk for cumulative toxicity.
•Dilute I.V. form with 10 to 20 ml of NS. Alternatively, administer colchicine into a large vein through an I.V. line with NS infusion.
•Administer I.V. form over 2 to 5 minutes.
•Expect to monitor CBC and platelet and reticulocyte counts at baseline and every 3 months after therapy starts.
•Notify prescriber immediately and expect to stop therapy if patient develops signs or symptoms of colchicine toxicity, such as abdominal pain, diarrhea, nausea, or vomiting.
PATIENT TEACHING
•Instruct patient to return for blood tests every 3 months, as ordered, while taking colchicine.
•Explain that gouty arthritis pain and swelling typically subside in 24 to 48 hours after therapy begins.
•Advise patient to notify prescriber immediately if abdominal pain, diarrhea, nausea, or vomiting occurs.

colesevelam hydrochloride

Welchol

Class and Category
Chemical: Nonabsorbed hydrogel polymer
Therapeutic: Bile acid sequestrant
Pregnancy category: B

Indications and Dosages
➤ *As adjunct to diet and exercise to reduce elevated low-density-lipoprotein (LDL) cholesterol levels in patients with primary hypercholesterolemia*
TABLETS
Adults. *Initial:* 1.9 g b.i.d. *Usual:* 3.8 g/day. *Maximum:* 4.5 g/day.

Contraindications
Bowel obstruction, cholelithiasis or complete biliary obstruction, hypersensitivity to colesevelam or its components

Interactions
DRUGS
sustained-release verapamil: Possibly decreased blood level of sustained-release verapamil

Mechanism of Action
Binds with bile acids in the intestines, preventing their absorption and forming an insoluble complex that's excreted in feces. This action decreases the amount of bile acids returning through the entero-hepatic circulation to the liver. As a result, the liver must convert more cholesterol to bile acids, which increases the liver's demand for cholesterol. This, in turn, causes an increase in the production and activity of the hepatic enzyme hydroxymethyl-glutaryl-coenzyme A (HMG-CoA) reductase, which is necessary for cholesterol production. However, the liver's synthesis of cholesterol typically can't match the amount needed to synthesize bile acids. Because the cholesterol levels can't be sustained, LDLs, lipoproteins composed mostly of cholesterol, are increasingly removed from the blood, thereby decreasing the blood LDL level.

Adverse Reactions
CNS: Asthenia
EENT: Pharyngitis
GI: Constipation, indigestion
MS: Myalgia

Nursing Considerations
•Because colesevelam may decrease or delay absorption of other drugs, administer it separately if possible.
•Ensure that patient drinks enough fluids when taking drug.
•**WARNING** Monitor patients with preexisting constipation, who are at increased risk for developing fecal impaction.
•Monitor frequency of bowel movements and consistency of stools in patients with coronary artery disease or hemorrhoids because constipation may aggravate these conditions.
PATIENT TEACHING
•Instruct patient to take colesevelam with meals and to drink plenty of liquids when taking drug.
•Advise patient to protect tablets from moisture.
•Caution patient not to change prescribed dosage or stop taking drug abruptly because significant increases in serum lipid levels may result.
•Remind patient that drug therapy doesn't reduce the importance of making dietary changes.

•Encourage patient to keep regularly scheduled appointments for follow-up blood tests.

colestipol hydrochloride

Colestid

Class and Category
Chemical: Diethylenetriamine and 1-chloro-2,3-epoxypropane copolymer, high-molecular-weight anion exchange resin
Therapeutic: Antihyperlipidemic
Pregnancy category: Not rated

Indications and Dosages
➤ *To treat primary hypercholesterolemia*
GRANULES
Adults. 15 to 30 g/day in divided doses b.i.d. to q.i.d., a.c. and h.s.
TABLETS
Adults. *Initial:* 2 g q.d. or in divided doses b.i.d., increased q 1 to 2 mo in 2-g increments q.d. or b.i.d. *Maximum:* 16 g/day.

Mechanism of Action
Combines with bile acids in the intestine, preventing their absorption and forming an insoluble complex that's excreted in feces. Loss of bile acids increases hepatic production of cholesterol to form new bile acids and increases oxidation of cholesterol to bile acids. The depletion of cholesterol increases hepatic LDL receptor activity, which removes LDLs from the blood.

Contraindications
Complete biliary obstruction, hypersensitivity to colestipol or its components

Interactions
DRUGS
chenodiol, ursodiol: Possibly reduced therapeutic effects of colestipol
digitalis glycosides: Possibly increased risk of digitalis toxicity when colestipol is discontinued
furosemide, sulfonylureas, thyroid hormones: Decreased absorption and therapeutic effects of these drugs
oral anticoagulants: Possibly increased or decreased anticoagulant effect
penicillin G, propranolol, tetracyclines (oral), thiazide diuretics: Decreased absorption of these drugs

vancomycin (oral): Possibly markedly decreased antibacterial action of vancomycin
vitamins (fat-soluble): Possibly interference with vitamin absorption

Adverse Reactions
CNS: Headache
GI: Abdominal distention and pain, constipation, diarrhea, eructation, esophageal reaction, fecal impaction, heartburn, nausea, vomiting

Nursing Considerations
•Mix colestipol granules with at least 90 ml of fluid before administration to prevent accidental inhalation or esophageal distress.
•Because colestipol may interact with various drugs, administer it on a separate schedule from other drugs when possible.
•Ensure that patient has adequate fluid intake, and obtain an order for a stool softener or laxative to prevent constipation. To prevent impaction, expect to decrease dosage or discontinue drug if constipation occurs or worsens.
•Expect to discontinue drug if no response occurs after 3 months.
•Monitor serum cholesterol level as appropriate, usually at baseline, 4 to 6 weeks after starting therapy, and then every 3 months. Expect to reduce monitoring frequency to every 4 months if response is adequate.
•Be aware that HDL and serum triglyceride levels may increase or remain unchanged during colestipol therapy.
•Keep in mind that adverse GI reactions are more common in patients over age 60.
PATIENT TEACHING
•To help minimize adverse GI reactions, advise patient to mix granules thoroughly in fluid so that they're completely wet before drinking.
•Remind patient that drug therapy doesn't reduce the importance of dietary changes.
•Caution patient not to increase or decrease the prescribed dosage or to suddenly stop taking drug. Inform him that abrupt discontinuation may significantly increase serum lipid levels.
•Instruct patient to keep appointments for follow-up blood tests.
•Teach patient how to prevent constipation, and advise him to contact prescriber if constipation occurs or worsens.

cortisone acetate

Cortisone Acetate-ICN (CAN), Cortone (CAN), Cortone Acetate

Class and Category

Chemical: Glucocorticoid
Therapeutic: Anti-inflammatory, corticosteroid replacement, immunosuppressant
Pregnancy category: Not rated

Indications and Dosages

➤ *To treat allergic and inflammatory disorders, collagen disorders, congenital adrenal hyperplasia, dermatologic disorders, edema (from systemic lupus erythematosus or nephrotic syndrome), GI disorders, hematologic disorders, multiple sclerosis (acute exacerbations), neoplastic diseases, primary or secondary adrenocortical insufficiency, respiratory disorders, rheumatic disorders, trichinosis with myocardial or neurologic involvement, tuberculous meningitis*

TABLETS

Adults and adolescents. *Initial:* 25 to 300 mg before 9 a.m. q.d. *Maintenance:* Dosage adjusted based on patient response.
Children. 2.5 to 10 mg/kg/day before 9 a.m. For adrenocortical insufficiency, 0.7 mg/kg/day before 9 a.m.

I.M. INJECTION

Adults and adolescents. *Initial:* 25 to 300 mg q.d. *Maintenance:* Dosage adjusted based on patient response.
Children. 0.83 to 5 mg/kg q 12 to 24 hr. For adrenocortical insufficiency, 0.7 mg/kg q.d. or q third day, or 0.23 to 0.35 mg/kg q.d.

Route	Onset	Peak	Duration
P.O.	Rapid	2 hr	1.25 to 1.5 days
I.M.	Slow	20 to 48 hr	1.25 to 1.5 days

Contraindications

Hypersensitivity to cortisone or its components, idiopathic thrombocytopenic purpura (parenteral form), live-virus vaccine administration, systemic fungal infection

Interactions

DRUGS

anticholinesterases: Possibly antagonized anticholinesterase effects in myasthenia gravis

barbiturates: Decreased cortisone effectiveness, increased cortisol clearance
digitalis glycosides: Increased risk of digitalis toxicity
estrogens, oral contraceptives: Increased therapeutic effects and risk of toxicity of cortisone
hydantoins, rifampin: Increased metabolism and decreased effects of cortisone
isoniazid: Decreased blood isoniazid level
neuromuscular blockers: Possibly enhanced blockade of neuromuscular blockers, leading to increased or prolonged respiratory depression or apnea
oral anticoagulants: Possibly obstructed anticoagulant effects
potassium-wasting diuretics: Possibly hypokalemia
salicylates: Decreased effectiveness and blood level of salicylates
somatrem: Decreased growth-promoting effect

Mechanism of Action

Binds to intracellular glucocorticoid receptors and suppresses the inflammatory and immune responses by:
• inhibiting neutrophil and monocyte accumulation at the inflammation site and suppressing their phagocytic and bactericidal activity
• stabilizing lysosomal membranes
• suppressing the antigen response of macrophages and helper T cells
• inhibiting the synthesis of cellular mediators of the inflammatory response, such as cytokines, interleukins, and prostaglandins.

Adverse Reactions

CNS: Ataxia, behavior changes, depression, dizziness, euphoria, fatigue, headache, increased ICP with papilledema, insomnia, lassitude, malaise, mood swings, paresthesia, seizures, steroid psychosis, syncope, vertigo
CV: Arrhythmias (from hypokalemia), fat embolism, heart failure, hypertension, hypotension, thromboembolism, thrombophlebitis
EENT: Exophthalmos, glaucoma, increased intraocular pressure, nystagmus, posterior subcapsular cataracts
ENDO: Adrenal insufficiency during stress, Cushing's syndrome, diabetes mellitus, growth suppression in children, hyperglyce-

mia, negative nitrogen balance from protein catabolism

GI: Abdominal distention, hiccups, increased appetite, nausea, pancreatitis, peptic ulcer, ulcerative esophagitis, vomiting

GU: Glycosuria, menstrual irregularities, perineal burning or tingling

HEME: Leukocytosis

MS: Arthralgia; aseptic necrosis of femoral and humeral heads; compression fractures; muscle atrophy, weakness, and twitching; myalgia; osteoporosis; spontaneous fractures; steroid myopathy; tendon rupture

SKIN: Acne, diaphoresis, ecchymosis, erythema, hirsutism, hyperpigmentation, hypopigmentation, necrotizing vasculitis, petechiae, purpura, rash, scarring, sterile abscesses, striae, subcutaneous fat atrophy, thin fragile skin, urticaria

Other: Anaphylaxis, hypocalcemia, hypokalemia, hypokalemic alkalosis, impaired wound healing, masking of signs of infection, metabolic alkalosis, suppressed skin test reactions, weight gain

Nursing Considerations

•Use cortisone cautiously in patients with ocular herpes simplex because corneal perforation may occur.

•Expect prescriber to order baseline ophthalmologic examination before beginning therapy because prolonged use of cortisone may result in glaucoma, increased intraocular pressure, and subsequent damage to optic nerves.

•Assess for signs and symptoms of infection before giving cortisone because drug may mask them. Be aware that new infections may develop during therapy because of risk of immunosuppression. If a new infection develops, expect to administer appropriate antibiotics.

•Obtain serum electrolyte levels before beginning therapy, as ordered, and monitor results frequently during therapy to detect electrolyte imbalances. Increased calcium excretion, potassium depletion, and sodium and water retention may occur with large doses of cortisone. Anticipate the need for potassium and calcium supplementation and sodium restriction, if indicated.

•Keep in mind that prescriber will order lowest effective dose.

•To avoid peptic ulcer formation from corti-

sone, expect patient to receive concurrent antacid or histamine-blocker therapy.

•**WARNING** Be aware that live-virus vaccines shouldn't be given during cortisone therapy because patient may become immunosuppressed from cortisone and develop the viral infection.

•**WARNING** Assess for adrenal suppression or insufficiency (fatigue, hypotension, lassitude, nausea, vomiting, and weakness) in patient exposed to stress or receiving prolonged cortisone therapy. Notify prescriber immediately if patient exhibits signs or symptoms of this life-threatening adverse reaction.

•Monitor for signs of steroid psychosis (confusion, delirium, euphoria, insomnia, mood swings, personality changes, and severe depression), which may develop 15 to 30 days after beginning therapy. Be prepared to discontinue therapy if such signs occur. If discontinuation isn't possible, expect to administer psychotropic drugs.

•Monitor for cushingoid symptoms, such as acne, buffalo hump, central obesity, ecchymosis, moon face, striae, and weight gain. Notify prescriber at once if such symptoms occur.

•Expect to taper oral cortisone dosage slowly to prevent withdrawal syndrome (abdominal or back pain, anorexia, dizziness, fever, headache, and syncope).

PATIENT TEACHING

•Instruct patient to take oral cortisone exactly as prescribed, every morning before 9 a.m. Advise him to take it with food if GI distress occurs.

•Caution patient not to stop taking drug abruptly because doing so may lead to adrenal insufficiency, withdrawal syndrome, or both.

•Inform patient about signs and symptoms of adrenal insufficiency and need for possible dosage increases during stressful periods. Advise him to notify prescriber immediately if such signs or symptoms develop or if he's exposed to stress.

•Caution patient to avoid exposure to people with infections because cortisone can cause immunosuppression. Also teach him to recognize and immediately report signs and symptoms of infection.

•Teach patient to recognize and report adverse reactions to cortisone, including Cushing's syndrome.

• Encourage patient receiving long-term cortisone therapy to carry medical identification that records it.

• Advise patient to have regular eye examinations.

• Urge him to keep follow-up appointments with prescriber, which may include laboratory tests, to evaluate effects of therapy.

co-trimoxazole

(sulfamethoxazole and trimethoprim)

Apo-Sulfatrim (CAN), Bactrim, Bactrim-DS, Bactrim Pediatric, Cofatrim Forte, Cotrim, Cotrim DS, Cotrim Pediatric, Novo-Trimel (CAN), Nu-Cotrimox (CAN), Roubac (CAN), Septra, Septra DS, Septra Pediatric, Sulfatrim, Sulfatrim DS, Sulfatrim S/S, Sulfatrim Suspension

Class and Category

Chemical: Sulfonamide derivative (sulfamethoxazole), dihydrofolic acid analogue (trimethoprim)
Therapeutic: Antibiotic
Pregnancy category: C

Indications and Dosages

➤ *To treat acute otitis media, shigellosis, UTIs, and other infections caused by gram-negative organisms (including* Enterobacter *sp.,* Escherichia coli, Haemophilus ducreyi, Haemophilus influenzae, *indole-positive* Proteus *sp.,* Klebsiella pneumoniae, Neisseria gonorrhoeae, Proteus mirabilis, Providencia *sp.,* Salmonella *sp.,* Serratia *sp., and* Shigella *sp.) and gram-positive organisms (including group A beta-hemolytic streptococci,* Nocardia *sp.,* Staphylococcus aureus, *and* Streptococcus pneumoniae)

ORAL SUSPENSION, TABLETS

Adults. 800 mg of sulfamethoxazole (SMZ) and 160 mg of trimethoprim (TMP) q 12 hr for 10 to 14 days (5 days for shigellosis).

Children age 2 months and older. 40 mg/kg of SMZ and 8 mg/kg of TMP/day in two divided doses q 12 hr for 10 days (5 days for shigellosis).

DOSAGE ADJUSTMENT Dosage reduced by one-half if creatinine clearance is 15 to 30 ml/

min/1.73 m². Drug avoided if creatinine clearance is less than 15 ml/min/1.73 m².

I.V. INFUSION

Adults and children over age 2 months. 40 to 50 mg/kg of SMZ and 8 to 10 mg/kg of TMP daily in divided doses q 6, 8, or 12 hr for up to 5 days for shigellosis and 14 days for UTIs.

➤ *To treat acute exacerbation of chronic bronchitis*

ORAL SUSPENSION, TABLETS

Adults. 800 mg of SMZ and 160 mg of TMP q 12 hr for 14 days.

➤ *To treat traveler's diarrhea*

ORAL SUSPENSION, TABLETS

Adults. 800 mg of SMZ and 160 mg of TMP q 12 hr for 5 days.

➤ *To prevent* Pneumocystis carinii *pneumonia*

ORAL SUSPENSION, TABLETS

Adults. 800 mg of SMZ and 160 mg of TMP q 24 hr.

Children. 750 mg/m² of SMZ and 150 mg/m² of TMP/day in two divided doses on 3 consecutive days/wk. *Maximum:* 1,600 mg of SMZ and 320 mg of TMP/day.

➤ *To treat* P. carinii *pneumonia*

ORAL SUSPENSION, TABLETS

Adults. 100 mg/kg of SMZ and 15 to 20 mg/kg of TMP/day in divided doses q 6 hr for 14 to 21 days.

I.V. INFUSION

Adults and children over age 2 months. 75 to 100 mg/kg of SMZ and 15 to 20 mg/kg of TMP/day in three or four divided doses q 6 to 8 hr for up to 14 days.

Mechanism of Action

Blocks two consecutive steps in the formation of essential nucleic acids and proteins in susceptible organisms. Sulfamethoxazole inhibits synthesis of dehydrofolic acid (a nucleic acid) by competing with para-aminobenzoic acid. Trimethoprim inhibits the action of the enzyme dihydrofolate reductase, thus blocking production of tetrahydrofolic acid.

Incompatibilities

Don't mix co-trimoxazole with other drugs or solutions.

Contraindications
Age less than 2 months; hypersensitivity to sulfamethoxazole, sulfonamides, trimethoprim, or their components; megaloblastic anemia caused by folate deficiency

Interactions
DRUGS
cyclosporine: Decreased blood level and therapeutic effectiveness of cyclosporine, increased risk of nephrotoxicity
dapsone: Possibly increased blood levels of co-trimoxazole and dapsone
diuretics: Increased risk of thrombocytopenic purpura in elderly patients
methotrexate: Increased blood methotrexate level and risk of methotrexate toxicity
oral anticoagulants: Increased anticoagulant effects
phenytoin: Possibly decreased hepatic clearance and prolonged half-life of phenytoin
sulfonylureas: Possibly increased hypoglycemic effects of sulfonylureas
zidovudine: Possibly increased blood zidovudine level

Adverse Reactions
CNS: Anxiety, aseptic meningitis, ataxia, chills, depression, fatigue, hallucinations, headache, insomnia, seizures, vertigo
EENT: Glossitis, stomatitis
GI: Abdominal pain, anorexia, diarrhea, hepatitis, nausea, pancreatitis, pseudomembranous enterocolitis, vomiting
GU: Crystalluria, renal failure, toxic nephrosis
HEME: Agranulocytosis, eosinophilia, hemolytic anemia, leukopenia, methemoglobinemia, neutropenia, thrombocytopenia
RESP: Cough, dyspnea
SKIN: Dermatitis, erythema, photosensitivity, rash, Stevens-Johnson syndrome, toxic epidermal necrolysis, urticaria
Other: Anaphylaxis, injection site inflammation and pain

Nursing Considerations
•Expect to obtain culture and sensitivity test results before beginning co-trimoxazole therapy, as ordered.
•For I.V. infusion, dilute each 5 ml of co-trimoxazole with 75 to 125 ml of D_5W before administration.
•When administering drug to neonates, don't mix it with solutions that contain benzyl alcohol because this preservative has been linked to a fatal toxic syndrome characterized by CNS, respiratory, circulatory, and renal impairment and metabolic acidosis.
•Infuse slowly over 60 to 90 minutes.
•Monitor bowel pattern daily; severe diarrhea may indicate pseudomembranous enterocolitis.
•Assess for evidence of blood dyscrasia, including bleeding, ecchymosis, and joint pain.
PATIENT TEACHING
•To minimize photosensitivity, advise patient to avoid direct sunlight and to use sunscreen when outdoors.
•Instruct patient to notify prescriber immediately if rash, severe diarrhea, or other serious adverse reactions occur.
•Inform patient that yogurt and buttermilk can help minimize diarrhea during therapy.

cromolyn sodium
(disodium cromoglycate, sodium cromoglycate)
Apo-Cromolyn (CAN), Gastrocrom, Intal, Intal Syncroner (CAN), Nalcrom (CAN), Nasalcrom, Novo-cromolyn (CAN)

Class and Category
Chemical: Disodium chromoglycate
Therapeutic: Antiasthmatic, anti-inflammatory
Pregnancy category: B

Indications and Dosages
➤ *To prevent bronchial asthma attacks*
AEROSOL (METERED-DOSE INHALER)
Adults and children over age 5. 2 metered sprays (1.6 to 2 mg) q 4 to 6 hr. *Maximum:* 16 sprays (12.8 to 16 mg)/day.

CAPSULES FOR INHALATION
Adults and children over age 2. 1 capsule (20 mg) q 4 to 6 hr. *Maximum:* 8 capsules (160 mg)/day.

SOLUTION FOR NEBULIZATION
Adults and children over age 2. 20 mg q 4 to 6 hr. *Maximum:* 160 mg/day.

➤ *To prevent bronchospasm caused by environmental exposure or exercise*
AEROSOL (METERED-DOSE INHALER)
Adults and children over age 5. 2 metered sprays (1.6 to 2 mg) as a single dose at least 10 to 15 min (no longer than 1 hr) before exposure or exercise. *Maximum:* 16 sprays (12.8 to 16 mg)/day.

CAPSULES FOR INHALATION

Adults and children over age 2. 1 capsule (20 mg) as a single dose inhaled at least 10 to 15 min (no longer than 1 hr) before exposure or exercise. *Maximum:* 8 capsules (160 mg)/day.

SOLUTION FOR NEBULIZATION

Adults and children over age 2. *Initial:* 20 mg inhaled 10 to 15 min (no longer than 1 hr) before exposure or exercise. Repeated p.r.n. during prolonged exercise. *Maximum:* 160 mg/day.

➤ *To treat allergic rhinitis*

NASAL SOLUTION

Adults and children over age 2. 1 spray (5.2 mg) in each nostril at regular intervals t.i.d. or q.i.d. *Maximum:* 1 spray (5.2 mg) in each nostril 6 times/day.

➤ *To prevent systemic mastocytosis*

CAPSULES, ORAL CONCENTRATE

Adults and adolescents. 200 mg q.i.d., 30 min before meals and h.s.

Children ages 2 to 12. 100 mg q.i.d., 30 min before meals and h.s. *Maximum:* 40 mg/kg/day.

Children under age 2. 5 mg/kg q.i.d. *Maximum:* 40 mg/kg/day.

Route	Onset	Peak	Duration
Aerosol	In minutes	Unknown	Up to 2 hr
Nasal solution	In 1 wk	1 to 4 wk	Unknown
Nebulizer solution	In minutes	Unknown	3 to 6 hr

Contraindications

Arrhythmias, coronary artery disease (aerosol); hypersensitivity to cromolyn or its components, status asthmaticus (all forms); nasal polyps (nasal solution)

Adverse Reactions

CNS: Dizziness, headache, neuritis
EENT: Burning eyes, hoarseness, laryngeal edema, nasal congestion, and swollen parotid glands (all forms); increased sneezing, nasal stinging, and throat irritation (nasal solution); taste perversion (aerosol)
GI: Anorexia, diarrhea (capsules and oral concentrate), nausea, vomiting
GU: Dysuria, urinary frequency
MS: Arthralgia, joint swelling
RESP: Cough, wheezing
SKIN: Rash, urticaria

Nursing Considerations

•WARNING Be aware that cromolyn sodium shouldn't be used to relieve acute asthma attack or severe bronchospasm; it should be used only for prevention.
•Don't give drug through handheld nebulizer. Instead, administer via power-operated nebulizer with a face mask or mouthpiece.
•Evaluate patient for effective inhalation; patient must be able to inhale adequately for nebulizer solution to be effective.
•Thoroughly mix oral concentrate or capsule contents into half a glass of hot water (not fruit juice, milk, or food), and let cool before administering.

Mechanism of Action

In asthma, inflammation results when antigen reexposure causes mast cells to degranulate and release histamine and chemical mediators. Cromolyn helps reduce inflammation by preventing mast cells from degranulating. After exposure to an antigen, mast cells become sensitized to it, and immunoglobulin E (IgE) antibodies appear on their surfaces. When the antigen returns, it attaches to IgE antibodies (1) and triggers events that lead to degranulation (2). By preventing granules from opening on the cells' surfaces (3), cromolyn blocks the release of histamine and chemical mediators.

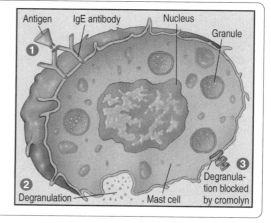

•Give drug at regular intervals to maximize effectiveness.

PATIENT TEACHING
•Teach patient how to use power-operated nebulizer; warn against using handheld nebulizer.
•Advise patient to use cromolyn sodium 10 to 15 minutes before exercising or exposing himself to precipitating factors.
•Instruct patient to thoroughly mix oral concentrate with hot water (not fruit juice, milk, or food) and let it cool before drinking.
•Inform patient that nasal spray may cause minor nasal irritation.
•Explain that cromolyn may take up to 1 month to achieve its full therapeutic effects.

crotamiton

Eurax

Class and Category
Chemical: Synthetic chloroformate salt
Therapeutic: Antipruritic, scabicide
Pregnancy category: C

Indications and Dosages
➤ *To treat scabies*
CREAM, LOTION
Adults. 30 to 60 g (thin layer) massaged into skin from chin down and repeated in 24 hr. Applied p.r.n. to skin folds, creases, and areas of intense pruritus for up to 48 hr.
➤ *To relieve pruritus caused by scabies*
CREAM, LOTION
Adults. 30 to 60 g (thin layer) massaged gently into affected areas until drug is completely absorbed. Repeated p.r.n.

Mechanism of Action
Exerts a toxic effect on *Sarcoptes scabiei* by an unknown mechanism.

Contraindications
Abrasions, application to mucous membranes, breaks in skin, hypersensitivity to crotamiton or its components, inflammation

Adverse Reactions
SKIN: Contact dermatitis, irritation, pruritus, rash

Nursing Considerations
•Expect pruritus to continue for 4 to 6 weeks after treatment.

PATIENT TEACHING
•Advise patient to shake lotion bottle well before applying.
•Warn him to keep drug away from eyes, nose, mouth, and inflamed skin.
•Advise patient to use a topical corticosteroid for dermatitis and an antihistamine for pruritus, as prescribed.
•Instruct patient to change clothing and bed linens the morning after final application and to take a cleansing bath 48 hours after final application.
•Inform patient that pruritus may continue for 4 to 6 weeks after treatment.
•Advise patient to notify prescriber if skin irritation or rash occurs.

cyclizine hydrochloride

Marezine

cyclizine lactate

Marzine (CAN)

Class and Category
Chemical: Piperazine derivative
Therapeutic: Anticholinergic, antiemetic
Pregnancy category: B

Indications and Dosages
➤ *To prevent postoperative vomiting*
I.M. INJECTION
Adults and adolescents. 50 mg 15 to 30 min before surgery ends, then q 4 to 6 hr, p.r.n., during first few postoperative days.
Children ages 6 to 12. 25 mg 15 to 30 min before surgery ends, then t.i.d., p.r.n., during first few postoperative days.
Children up to age 6. 12.5 mg 15 to 30 min before surgery ends, then t.i.d., p.r.n., during first few postoperative days.
➤ *To prevent and treat motion sickness*
TABLETS
Adults and adolescents. 50 mg 30 min before travel, then q 4 to 6 hr, p.r.n. *Maximum:* 200 mg/day.
Children ages 6 to 12. 25 mg 30 min before travel, then q 6 to 8 hr, p.r.n. *Maximum:* 75 mg/day.
I.M. INJECTION
Adults and adolescents. 50 mg q 4 to 6 hr, p.r.n.
Children. 1 mg/kg t.i.d., p.r.n.

Route	Onset	Peak	Duration
P.O., I.M.	30 to 60 min	Unknown	4 to 6 hr

Mechanism of Action
May act centrally on the vomiting center by blocking chemoreceptor trigger zones. Cyclizine also may reduce the sensitivity of the labyrinthine apparatus in the inner ear.

Contraindications
Hypersensitivity to cyclizine or its components, shock

Interactions
DRUGS
anticholinergics: Possibly potentiated anticholinergic effects
apomorphine: Possibly decreased emetic response of apomorphine
CNS depressants: Possibly potentiated CNS depression
ACTIVITIES
alcohol use: Possibly potentiated CNS depression

Adverse Reactions
CNS: Dizziness, drowsiness, euphoria, excitation, hallucinations, insomnia, nervousness, restlessness, seizures (in children), vertigo
CV: Hypotension, palpitations, tachycardia
EENT: Blurred vision; diplopia; dry mouth, nose, and throat; tinnitus
GI: Anorexia, constipation, diarrhea, nausea, vomiting
GU: Urinary frequency and hesitancy, urine retention
SKIN: Jaundice, rash, urticaria

Nursing Considerations
•Help patient with ambulation and take safety precautions to prevent injury from falls if drowsiness or dizziness occurs.
•Don't schedule skin tests using allergens until at least 5 days after cyclizine therapy stops because drug may interfere with test results.
PATIENT TEACHING
•Urge patient to avoid alcohol and other CNS depressants during cyclizine therapy.
•Advise patient to ask for help with ambulation if he feels drowsy or dizzy.

cyclobenzaprine hydrochloride
Flexeril

Class and Category
Chemical: Tricyclic amine salt
Therapeutic: Skeletal muscle relaxant
Pregnancy category: B

Indications and Dosages
➤ *As adjunct to treat muscle spasm or musculoskeletal pain*
TABLETS
Adults and adolescents. *Initial:* 20 to 40 mg/day in divided doses b.i.d. to q.i.d. *Usual:* 10 mg t.i.d. *Maximum:* 60 mg/day for 3 wk.

Route	Onset	Peak	Duration
P.O.	1 hr	1 to 2 wk	12 to 24 hr

Mechanism of Action
Acts in the brain stem to reduce or abolish tonic muscle hyperactivity. Because cyclobenzaprine doesn't act at the neuromuscular junction or directly on skeletal muscle, it relieves muscle spasm without disrupting muscle function.

Contraindications
Acute recovery phase of MI; age less than 12; arrhythmias, including heart block and other conduction disturbances; heart failure; hypersensitivity to cyclobenzaprine or its components; hyperthyroidism; MAO inhibitor use within 14 days

Interactions
DRUGS
anticholinergics, antidyskinetics: Possibly potentiated anticholinergic effects of these drugs
CNS depressants, tricyclic antidepressants: Possibly additive CNS depressant effects of these drugs, increased risk of adverse effects of antidepressants and cyclobenzaprine
guanadrel, guanethidine: Possibly decreased or blocked antihypertensive effects of these drugs
MAO inhibitors: Possibly hyperpyretic crisis, severe seizures, and death
ACTIVITIES
alcohol use: Possibly additive CNS depression

Adverse Reactions
CNS: Asthenia, confusion, depression, dizziness, drowsiness, fatigue, fever, headache, insomnia, irritability, nervousness, paresthesia, seizures, tremor, weakness

CV: Arrhythmias, including tachycardia; orthostatic hypotension; palpitations; vasodilation
EENT: Blurred vision, diplopia, dry mouth, transient vision loss, unpleasant taste
GI: Constipation, hiccups, indigestion, nausea, vomiting
GU: Libido changes, urinary frequency, urine retention
SKIN: Diaphoresis, facial flushing, pruritus, rash

Nursing Considerations
• Use cyclobenzaprine cautiously in patients with history of low seizure threshold.
• Keep in mind that elderly patients shouldn't receive drug, if possible, because of its anticholinergic effects.
• To prevent injury from falls, take safety precautions if patient experiences confusion, dizziness, or weakness.
PATIENT TEACHING
• Urge patient to avoid alcohol and other CNS depressants during therapy.
• Inform patient about possible lack of alertness and dexterity.
• Advise patient to ask for assistance with walking, driving, or potentially hazardous activities if he experiences dizziness or weakness.

cycloserine

Seromycin

Class and Category
Chemical: D-alanine analogue, *Streptomyces garyphalus* or *Streptomyces orchidaceus* derivative
Therapeutic: Antitubercular
Pregnancy category: C

Indications and Dosages
➤ *To treat tuberculosis along with other antitubercular drugs after failure of primary drugs, including ethambutol, isoniazid, pyrazinamide, rifampin, and streptomycin*
CAPSULES
Adults and adolescents. 250 mg q 12 hr for 2 wk, then q 6 to 8 hr for 2 wk. Dosage increased gradually to maintain blood cycloserine level below 30 mcg/ml. *Maximum:* 1 g/day.
Children. 10 to 20 mg/kg/day in divided doses q 12 hr. *Maximum:* 1 g/day.

Mechanism of Action
Inhibits bacterial cell wall synthesis in gram-positive organisms, including *Mycobacterium tuberculosis*. In the early stages of bacterial cell wall synthesis, cycloserine inhibits two enzymes that help form peptidoglycan, which is needed to make the cell membrane rigid and protective.

Contraindications
Chronic alcoholism, depression, hypersensitivity to cycloserine or its components, psychosis, renal disease, seizure disorder, severe anxiety

Interactions
DRUGS
ethionamide: Possibly increased risk of seizures
isoniazid: Possibly increased risk of adverse CNS effects
phenytoin: Possibly increased blood phenytoin level
pyridoxine: Possibly anemia or peripheral neuritis
ACTIVITIES
alcohol use: Possibly increased risk of seizures

Adverse Reactions
CNS: Aggression, anxiety, coma, confusion, depression, dizziness, drowsiness, headache, irritability, lethargy, memory loss, nervousness, nightmares, psychosis, restlessness, seizures, suicidal tendencies, tremor, vertigo
CV: Heart failure
HEME: Leukocytosis, megaloblastic anemia
MS: Dysarthria, hyperreflexia
SKIN: Dermatitis, photosensitivity
Other: Folic acid deficiency, vitamin B_{12} deficiency

Nursing Considerations
• Monitor blood cycloserine level, as appropriate. Blood level should be maintained at 25 to 30 mcg/ml.
• Monitor mental status, mood, and affect for aggression or depression.
• Monitor CBC to detect blood dyscrasias.
• To prevent injury from falls, take safety precautions if adverse CNS reactions, such as dizziness or drowsiness, develop.
PATIENT TEACHING
• Urge patient to avoid alcohol while taking cycloserine.

•Instruct patient to seek help immediately if he has suicidal thoughts.
•Advise patient to avoid driving and to ask for assistance with walking or hazardous activities if he develops adverse CNS reactions, such as dizziness and drowsiness.
•Advise patient to contact prescriber if he notices no improvement after 2 to 3 weeks.
•Emphasize the importance of complying with drug therapy because effective treatment may take years to complete.

cyclosporine
(cyclosporin A)
Neoral, Sandimmune, SangCya

Class and Category
Chemical: *Tolypocladium inflatum* Gams- or *Cylindrocarpon lucidum* Booth-derived polypeptide
Therapeutic: Antipsoriatic, antirheumatic, immunosuppressant
Pregnancy category: C

Indications and Dosages
➤ *To prevent or treat organ rejection in kidney, liver, and heart allogenic transplantation*
CAPSULES, MODIFIED CAPSULES, MODIFIED ORAL SOLUTION, ORAL SOLUTION
Adults and children. *Initial:* 12 to 15 mg/kg/day in divided doses q 12 hr beginning 4 to 12 hr before surgery and continuing for 1 to 2 wk postoperatively. Then, dosage reduced by 5%/wk to maintenance dose. *Maintenance:* 5 to 10 mg/kg/day in divided doses q 12 hr.
I.V. INFUSION
Adults. 2 to 6 mg/kg/day beginning 4 to 12 hr before surgery and continuing postoperatively until patient can tolerate oral form.
➤ *To treat severe rheumatoid arthritis*
MODIFIED CAPSULES, MODIFIED ORAL SOLUTION
Adults. 2.5 mg/kg/day in divided doses q 12 hr, increased by 0.5 to 0.75 mg/kg/day after 8 wk and again after 12 wk. *Maximum:* 4 mg/kg/day.
➤ *To treat psoriasis*
MODIFIED CAPSULES, MODIFIED ORAL SOLUTION
Adults. *Initial:* 2.5 mg/kg/day in divided doses b.i.d., increased by 0.5 mg/kg/day after 4 wk. Then dosage increased q 2 wk, if needed. *Maximum:* 4 mg/kg/day.

Mechanism of Action
Causes immunosuppression by inhibiting the proliferation of T lymphocytes, the production and release of lymphokines, and the release of interleukin-2.

Contraindications
Abnormal renal function, neoplastic diseases, and uncontrolled hypertension in patients with psoriasis or rheumatoid arthritis (modified capsules and oral solution); hypersensitivity to cyclosporine, its components, or polyoxyethylated castor oil (I.V. infusion)

Interactions
DRUGS
aminoglycosides, amphotericin B: Increased risk of nephrotoxicity
amiodarone, calcium channel blockers, chloroquine, clarithromycin, erythromycin, itraconazole, ketoconazole, miconazole, oral contraceptives, verapamil: Increased blood cyclosporine level and risk of nephrotoxicity
anabolic steroids, androgens: Increased blood cyclosporine level and risk of toxicity
carbamazepine, phenytoin, rifabutin, rifampin: Decreased blood cyclosporine level and therapeutic response
colchicine: Increased risk of adverse GI, hepatic, neuromuscular, and renal effects; increased blood cyclosporine level
corticosteroids: Increased risk of cyclosporine toxicity
co-trimoxazole, sulfonamides: Decreased blood cyclosporine level, increased risk of nephrotoxicity
digoxin: Increased blood digoxin level and risk of digitalis toxicity
etoposide: Decreased renal clearance of etoposide, increased risk of etoposide toxicity
foscarnet: Increased risk of renal failure
HMG-CoA reductase inhibitors: Risk of irreversible myopathy and rhabdomyolysis
imipenem-cilastatin: Increased risk of CNS toxicity
metoclopramide: Increased cyclosporine bioavailability and risk of toxicity
NSAIDs: Increased risk of cyclosporine nephrotoxicity
probucol: Possibly decreased blood level and effects of cyclosporine
quinupristin and dalfopristin: Increased blood cyclosporine level

terbinafine: Increased metabolism and decreased blood level of cyclosporine
vaccines (killed or live virus): Possibly suppressed immune response and increase adverse effects of vaccine

FOODS

grapefruit juice: Increased risk of nephrotoxicity (with oral drug)

Adverse Reactions

CNS: Confusion, headache, paresthesia, seizures, tremor
CV: Chest pain, hypertension
EENT: Gingival hyperplasia, oral candidiasis
ENDO: Gynecomastia
GI: Diarrhea, nausea, pancreatitis, vomiting
GU: Albuminuria, hematuria, proteinuria, renal failure
HEME: Anemia, leukopenia, thrombocytopenia
SKIN: Acne, flushing, hirsutism, rash
Other: Anaphylaxis, hyperkalemia, hypomagnesemia, lymphoma

Nursing Considerations

•Be aware that cyclosporine capsules and oral solution aren't interchangeable with modified capsules and modified oral solution. Modified forms have greater bioavailability than nonmodified forms.
•Prepare I.V. infusion by diluting each milliliter of concentrate in 20 to 100 ml of NS or D_5W. Use glass containers because of possible leaching of diethylhexyphthalate from polyvinyl chloride bags into cyclosporine solution.
•Administer I.V. infusion over 2 to 6 hr. If needed, the drug may be infused over 24 hr.
•WARNING Closely monitor for anaphylaxis at least during first 30 minutes of I.V. administration. Make sure emergency equipment and drugs are immediately available.
•WARNING Be aware that rapid I.V. infusion may cause acute nephrotoxicity.
•Don't draw blood to measure cyclosporine level through same I.V. tubing used to administer drug, even if line was flushed after administration. Blood level may be falsely elevated.
•Discard diluted solution after 24 hours.
•Be aware that oral solution contains alcohol and shouldn't be administered to patient who drinks heavily or has a history of alcohol dependence.
•Don't add water to oral solution because it will alter drug's effectiveness.

•Avoid giving oral forms of cyclosporine with grapefruit juice, which may raise trough level, increasing risk of nephrotoxicity.
•Monitor blood pressure, especially in patients with a history of hypertension, because drug can exacerbate this condition.
•Monitor results of hepatic and renal function tests, as ordered, to detect signs of decreased function.
•Be aware that cyclosporine use may result in increased serum cholesterol levels.
•Be aware St. John's Wort may decrease blood cyclosporine levels.
•Store capsules at 77° F (25° C) and in prepackaged foil wrap to protect them from light.
•Expect 50% of patients treated for psoriasis to relapse about 4 months after therapy stops.

PATIENT TEACHING

•Instruct patient to take drug at same time each day and in same relation to type and timing of food intake to help increase compliance and maintain steady blood level.
•Advise patient to mix oral solution in a glass—not plastic—container with milk, chocolate milk, orange juice, or apple juice to improve flavor. Also advise him to avoid grapefruit juice because it alters drug metabolism.
•Instruct patient to use accompanying syringe supplied by manufacturer to ensure accurate measurement of oral solution dose and to wipe syringe—not rinse it—after use to prevent cloudiness.
•Advise patient not to stop taking drug without consulting prescriber.
•Instruct patient not to receive virus vaccines during therapy. Urge him to avoid people who have received such vaccines or to wear a protective mask when he's around them.
•Caution patient to avoid contact with people who have infections during therapy because cyclosporine causes immunosuppression.
•Urge patient to maintain good dental hygiene because of risk of gingival hyperplasia.
•Advise patient to discard oral solution after it has been opened for 2 months.
•Inform patient with rheumatoid arthritis that drug effects may not appear for 4 to 6 weeks.

daclizumab

(dacliximab)

Zenapax

Class and Category

Chemical: Monoclonal antibody
Therapeutic: Immunosuppressant
Pregnancy category: C

Indications and Dosages

➤ *To prevent acute organ rejection after kidney transplantation*

I.V. INFUSION

Adults and children. 1 mg/kg given in five doses: dose 1 given no more than 24 hr before transplantation; doses 2 through 5, at 14-day intervals.

Mechanism of Action

Inhibits interleukin-2–mediated activation of lymphocytes, which prevents WBCs from attacking the transplanted kidney. Daclizumab also reduces the body's infection-fighting ability.

Contraindications

Hypersensitivity to daclizumab or its components

Interactions

None known.

Adverse Reactions

CNS: Anxiety, chills, depression, dizziness, fatigue, fever, headache, insomnia, prickly sensation, tremor, weakness
CV: Chest pain, edema, hypertension, hypotension, tachycardia, thrombosis
EENT: Blurred vision, pharyngitis, rhinitis
ENDO: Hyperglycemia
GI: Abdominal distention and pain, constipation, diarrhea, flatulence, gastritis, heartburn, hemorrhoids, indigestion, nausea, vomiting
GU: Dysuria, hematuria, hydronephrosis, oliguria, renal insufficiency, renal tubular necrosis, urine retention
HEME: Bleeding

MS: Arthralgia, back pain, leg cramps, myalgia
RESP: Atelectasis, cough, crackles, dyspnea, hypoxia, lung congestion, pleural effusion, pulmonary edema
SKIN: Acne, diaphoresis, hirsutism, impaired wound healing, night sweats, pruritus, rash
Other: Dehydration, fluid overload, injection site pain and redness, lymphocele

Nursing Considerations

• Dilute calculated dose of daclizumab in 50 ml of NS. Gently invert bag to mix; to prevent foaming, don't shake it.
• Use room temperature solution within 4 hours; if it isn't administered within that time, refrigerate it for up to 24 hours and then discard unused solution.
• Because daclizumab's compatibility with other drugs isn't known, don't add or simultaneously infuse other drugs through same I.V. line.
• Monitor blood glucose level for increases during therapy.
• **WARNING** Although daclizumab seldom causes severe hypersensitivity reactions, keep drugs to treat such a reaction nearby for immediate use.

PATIENT TEACHING

• Urge patient to complete the course of therapy and return for scheduled follow-up visits.

dalteparin sodium

(tedelparin)

Fragmin

Class and Category

Chemical: Low-molecular-weight heparin
Therapeutic: Anticoagulant, antithrombotic
Pregnancy category: B

Indications and Dosages

➤ *To prevent ischemic complications in patients who receive aspirin as part of treatment for unstable angina and non–Q wave MI*

S.C. INJECTION

Adults. 120 IU/kg q 12 hr with aspirin therapy (75 to 165 mg/day) until patient is stable, usually 5 to 8 days. *Maximum:* 10,000 IU/dose.

➤ *To prevent blood clots in patients undergoing hip replacement surgery*

S.C. INJECTION

Adults. *Initial:* 2,500 IU 1 to 2 hr before surgery, repeated in 8 to 12 hr and again 8 to 12 hr later. *Maintenance:* 5,000 IU q morning for 5 to 10 days postoperatively or until patient is fully ambulatory. *Alternate:* 5,000 IU the evening before surgery followed by 5,000 IU q.d. (starting the next evening) for 5 to 10 days or until patient is fully ambulatory.

➤ *To prevent blood clots in patients undergoing abdominal surgery who are at risk for thromboembolic complications*

S.C. INJECTION

Adults. 2,500 IU q.d., beginning 1 to 2 hr before surgery and repeated for 5 to 10 days. For patients at high risk (presence of cancer), 5,000 IU the evening before surgery, repeated q.d. for 5 to 10 days; or 2,500 IU 1 to 2 hr before surgery followed by 2,500 IU 12 hr later and then 5,000 IU q.d. for 5 to 10 days.

Mechanism of Action

Binds to and accelerates the activity of antithrombin III, thus inhibiting thrombin and blocking the formation of fibrin clots.

Contraindications

Active major bleeding; hypersensitivity to low-molecular-weight heparins, heparin, or pork products; thrombocytopenia associated with positive laboratory tests for antiplatelet antibodies in the presence of dalteparin

Interactions

DRUGS

NSAIDs, oral anticoagulants, platelet aggregation inhibitors, thrombolytics: Possibly increased risk of hemorrhage

Adverse Reactions

HEME: Hemorrhage, thrombocytopenia
Other: Injection site hematoma and pain

Nursing Considerations

• Use dalteparin with extreme caution in patients with a history of heparin-induced thrombocytopenia; those at increased risk for hemorrhage (such as those who use a platelet inhibitor or have bacterial endocarditis, bleeding disorders, active ulcerative GI disease, uncontrolled hypertension, or hemorrhagic CVA); and those who have recently had brain, eye, or spinal surgery.

• Use drug cautiously in patients with bleeding diathesis, diabetic retinopathy, platelet defects, recent GI bleeding, severe hepatic or renal insufficiency, or thrombocytopenia.

• Before administering first dose, inform Jewish patients that drug comes from porcine intestinal mucosa.

• Be aware that risk factors for thromboembolic events include age over 40, cancer, history of deep vein thrombosis or pulmonary embolism, obesity, and planned use of anesthesia for more than 30 minutes.

• Don't mix dalteparin with other injections or infusions because incompatibilities are unknown.

• Don't give drug by I.M. or I.V. injection.

• With the patient seated or supine, administer drug deep into S.C. tissue in U-shaped area around navel, upper outer thigh, or upper outer quadrant of buttocks. If using area around navel or on thigh, lift skin fold with thumb and forefinger while giving injection. Insert entire length of needle at a 45- to 90-degree angle. Rotate sites daily.

• Be aware that routine coagulation tests and subsequent dosage adjustments usually aren't required.

PATIENT TEACHING

• If therapy must continue at home, teach patient or caregiver how to administer S.C. injections. Advise which injection sites to use and how to rotate sites daily. Instruct her to discard drug if it's discolored or contains particles. Review safe handling and disposal of syringes and needles.

• Teach patient to store drug at room temperature, away from moisture and heat.

• Urge patient to report adverse reactions, especially bleeding, and to seek help immediately if signs of thromboembolism, such as severe dyspnea from pulmonary embolism or neurologic deficits from cerebral embolism, develop.

• Stress the importance of follow-up visits.

danaparoid sodium

Orgaran

Class and Category

Chemical: Glycosaminoglycan heparinoid, low-molecular-weight heparin
Therapeutic: Anticoagulant, antithrombotic
Pregnancy category: B

Indications and Dosages
➤ *To prevent deep vein thrombosis after hip replacement surgery*
S.C. INJECTION
Adults. 750 anti-factor Xa U b.i.d. (first dose 1 to 4 hr preoperatively; second dose no sooner than 2 hr after surgery) for 7 to 14 days, as indicated.

Mechanism of Action
Inhibits thrombin generation in coagulation pathway, thus preventing fibrin formation and clotting.

Contraindications
Active major bleeding (including hemorrhagic CVA); hypersensitivity to low-molecular-weight heparins, heparin, or pork products; severe hemorrhagic disorders, such as hemophilia and thrombocytopenic purpura; sulfite sensitivity; type II thrombocytopenia associated with positive laboratory tests for antiplatelet antibodies in the presence of danaparoid

Interactions
DRUGS
NSAIDs, oral anticoagulants, platelet aggregation inhibitors: Possibly increased risk of bleeding

Adverse Reactions
CNS: Asthenia, dizziness, fever, headache, insomnia
CV: Chest pain, edema
GI: Abdominal pain, constipation, nausea, vomiting
GU: Urine retention, UTI
HEME: Anemia, excessive bleeding
MS: Arthralgia, myalgia
SKIN: Pruritus, rash
Other: Anaphylaxis, injection site pain

Nursing Considerations
•Use danaparoid with extreme caution in patients who are at increased risk for hemorrhage (such as those with severe uncontrolled hypertension, acute bacterial endocarditis, bleeding disorders, active ulcerative GI disease, severe renal dysfunction, or nonhemorrhagic CVA); those with a postoperative indwelling epidural catheter; and those who have recently had brain, eye, or spinal surgery.
•Don't give drug by I.M. or I.V. injection.

•Administer drug with patient lying down. Use a 25G or 26G needle to minimize tissue trauma. Select site on left or right anterolateral or posterolateral abdominal wall. Hold skin fold gently between thumb and forefinger, and insert entire length of needle deep into S.C. tissue at a 45- to 90-degree angle. Don't pinch or rub site afterward. Rotate sites.
•Expect to monitor results of CBCs and fecal occult blood tests during therapy. Typical coagulation tests, such as PT, APTT, clotting time, whole blood clotting time, and thrombin time, aren't useful for monitoring danaparoid's anticoagulant effect.
PATIENT TEACHING
•Before administering first dose, inform Jewish patients that drug comes from porcine intestinal mucosa.
•If therapy must continue at home, teach patient or caregiver how to administer S.C. injections. Review appropriate injection sites, and instruct her to rotate them daily. Also instruct her to discard drug if it's discolored or contains particles. Review safe handling and disposal of syringes and needles.
•Teach patient to store drug at room temperature, away from moisture and heat.
•Instruct patient to consult prescriber before using aspirin, ibuprofen, indomethacin, ketoprofen, naproxen, and other NSAIDs because they may increase the risk of bleeding.
•Advise patient to stop taking drug and seek help immediately if she experiences severe dizziness, fever, rash, wheezing, or prolonged or unexplained bleeding and pain at the injection site.

dantrolene sodium
Dantrium, Dantrium Intravenous

Class and Category
Chemical: Hydantoin derivative, imidazolidinedione sodium salt
Therapeutic: Antispastic, malignant hyperthermia therapy adjunct
Pregnancy category: C (parenteral), Not rated (oral)

Indications and Dosages
➤ *To treat chronic spastic conditions caused by severe chronic disorders, such as cerebral palsy, CVA, multiple sclerosis, and spinal cord injury*

CAPSULES
Adults and adolescents. *Initial:* 25 mg q.d. for 7 days. Then dosage increased to 25 mg/day q 4 to 7 days until desired response occurs or dosage reaches 100 mg q.i.d. *Maximum:* 400 mg/day.
Children. *Initial:* 0.5 mg/kg b.i.d. for 7 days. Then increased by 0.5 mg/kg/day q 4 to 7 days until desired response occurs or dosage reaches 3 mg/kg q.i.d. *Maximum:* 400 mg/day.
➤ *To prevent malignant hyperthermia before surgery*
CAPSULES
Adults and children. 4 to 8 mg/kg/day in divided doses t.i.d. or q.i.d. 1 or 2 days before surgery, with last dose given 3 to 4 hr before surgery.
I.V. INFUSION
Adults and children. *Initial:* 2.5 mg/kg 60 to 75 min before anesthesia and infused over 1 hr. Additional individualized doses given as needed during surgery.
➤ *To treat malignant hyperthermic crisis*
I.V. INJECTION
Adults and adolescents. *Initial:* 1 mg/kg by rapid bolus repeated as needed until symptoms subside or cumulative dose of 10 mg/kg has been reached. Dose repeated if symptoms reappear.
➤ *To treat postmalignant hyperthermic crisis*
CAPSULES
Adults and children. 4 to 8 mg/kg/day in divided doses q.i.d. for 1 to 3 days.
I.V. INJECTION
Adults and children: *Initial:* Individualized dosage beginning with 1 mg/kg or more as needed if oral therapy can't be used. *Maximum:* 10 mg/kg total dose.

Route	Onset	Peak	Duration
P.O.	1 wk*	Unknown	Unknown

Incompatibilities
Don't administer parenteral dantrolene with acidic solutions, including D₅W and NS.

Contraindications
For oral drug only: Active hepatic disease (such as cirrhosis and hepatitis), conditions in which spasticity helps maintain upright posture and improve balance or function, skeletal muscle spasms caused by rheumatic disorders

* For spasticity; unknown for malignant hyperthermia.

Mechanism of Action
Acts directly on skeletal muscle to reduce the force of reflex muscle contraction. This in turn reduces hyperreflexia, spasticity, involuntary movements, and clonus, probably by preventing calcium release from the sarcoplasmic reticulum of skeletal muscle cells. Blocked calcium release also inhibits the activation of acute catabolism associated with malignant hyperthermic crisis syndrome.

Interactions
DRUGS
calcium channel blockers (especially verapamil): Possibly hyperkalemia, life-threatening arrhythmias, shock
hepatotoxic drugs: Increased risk of hepatotoxicity with long-term oral dantrolene use
sedatives: Possibly profound sedation
ACTIVITIES
alcohol use: Possibly increased CNS depression

Adverse Reactions
CNS: Chills, confusion, depression, dizziness, drowsiness, fatigue, fever, headache, insomnia, light-headedness, malaise, nervousness, seizures, slurred speech or other speech problems, weakness
CV: Heart failure (I.V.), labile blood pressure, pericarditis, phlebitis, tachycardia
EENT: Abnormal vision, altered taste, diplopia, lacrimation
GI: Abdominal cramps, anorexia, constipation, diarrhea, dysphagia, gastric irritation, GI bleeding, hepatitis, hepatotoxicity
GU: Crystalluria, dysuria, erectile dysfunction, hematuria, nocturia, urinary frequency, urinary incontinence, urine retention
MS: Backache, myalgia
RESP: Feeling of suffocation, pleural effusion
SKIN: Acne, diaphoresis, eczematoid eruption, erythema (I.V.), extravasation with tissue damage, hirsutism, pruritus, rash, urticaria

Nursing Considerations
• Use dantrolene cautiously in patients with impaired pulmonary function, especially those with COPD, and in those with severe cardiac or hepatic dysfunction.
• Reconstitute drug with 60 ml of sterile water for injection. Shake vial until clear. Store reconstituted solution at room temperature, protected from direct sunlight. Discard after 6 hours.
• To prevent precipitation, transfer reconsti-

tuted drug to a plastic I.V. bag, rather than a glass bottle, for infusion.
•Because drug has a high pH, infuse into a central vein, if possible, to avoid tissue damage from extravasation.
•Monitor blood pressure and heart rate frequently during drug administration to detect tachycardia and blood pressure changes.
•Notify prescriber if persistent diarrhea develops with oral therapy; drug may need to be stopped.
•Monitor results of liver function tests—especially ALT, AST, alkaline phosphatase, and total bilirubin levels—to detect hepatotoxicity. Expect to stop drug after 45 days if benefits aren't sufficient because the risk of hepatotoxicity increases with dose and time, especially for women and patients over age 35.

PATIENT TEACHING
•Advise patient to take dantrolene with food if gastric irritation develops.
•Inform patient that drug may weaken muscles used for walking and climbing stairs.
•Warn patient about drug's sedating effects. Caution her to avoid sedatives, unless prescribed, and other sedating substances, such as alcohol.
•Advise patient to notify prescriber if yellow skin or sclerae, itching, anorexia, or fatigue develop.
•Advise patient that if she misses a dose, she should wait until the next scheduled dose if more than 2 hours have passed since the missed dose. Instruct her not to double-dose.
•Caution patient not to stop taking drug without consulting prescriber. Gradual dosage reduction may be required, especially after long-term use.

darbepoetin alfa

Aranesp

Class and Category
Chemical: 165-amino acid glycoprotein identical to human erythropoietin
Therapeutic: Antianemic
Pregnancy category: C

Indications and Dosages
➤ *To treat anemia from chronic renal failure*
I.V. OR S.C. INJECTION
Adults. *Initial:* 0.45 mcg/kg as a single dose q wk. *Maintenance:* Dosage individualized and increased once a month to maintain a hemoglobin level not to exceed 12 g/dl.

DOSAGE ADJUSTMENT Dosage reduced by about 25% if hemoglobin level increases and approaches 12 g/dl. If hemoglobin level continues to increase, doses temporarily withheld until hemoglobin level begins to decrease; then therapy is restarted at a dose about 25% below previous dose. Dosage reduced by about 25% if hemoglobin level increases by more than 1.0 g/dl in a 2-week period. Dosage increased by about 25% of previous dose if hemoglobin level increases less than 1 g/dl over 4 weeks but only if serum ferritin level is 100 mcg/L or greater and serum transferrin saturation is 20% or greater. Further increases made at 4-week intervals until specified hemoglobin level is obtained.

DOSAGE ADJUSTMENT For conversion from epoetin alfa to darbepoetin alfa, dosage administered q wk for patient who previously received epoetin alfa 2 to 3 times/wk and once every 2 wk for patient who previously received epoetin alfa once/wk. For patients being converted from epoetin alfa, 6.25 mcg/wk darbepoetin alfa given q wk for patients who received < 2,500 units/wk of epoetin alfa; 12.5 mcg/wk darbepoetin alfa given q wk for patients who received 2,500 to 4,999 units/wk of epoetin alfa; 25 mcg/wk darbepoetin alfa given q wk for patients who received 5,000 to 10,999 units/wk of epoetin alfa; 40 mcg/wk darbepoetin alfa given q wk for patients who received 11,000 to 17,999 units/wk of epoetin alfa; 60 mcg/wk darbepoetin alfa given q wk for patients who received 18,000 to 33,999 units/wk of epoetin alfa; 100 mcg/wk darbepoetin alfa given q wk for patients who received 34,000 to 89,999 units/wk of epoetin alfa; 200 mcg/wk darbepoetin alfa given q wk for patients who received 90,000 or more units/wk of epoetin alfa.

➤ *To treat chemotherapy-induced anemia in patients with nonmyeloid malignancies*
S.C. INJECTION
Adults. *Initial:* 2.25 mcg/kg as a single dose q wk. *Maintenance:* Dosage individualized to maintain a target hemoglobin level.
DOSAGE ADJUSTMENT Dosage increased up to 4.5 mcg/kg if there is less than 1.0 g/dl increase in hemoglobin after 6 wk of therapy. If hemoglobin level increases by more than 1.0 g/dl over 2 wk or if hemoglobin exceeds 12 g/dl, dosage reduced by approximately 25%. If hemoglobin exceeds 13 g/dl, doses temporarily withheld until hemoglobin falls

to 12 g/dl. Then therapy is restarted at a dose about 25% less than last dose given.

Route	Onset	Peak	Duration
I.V., S.C.	In 2 to 6 wk	Unknown	Unknown

Mechanism of Action
Stimulates the release of reticulocytes from the bone marrow into the bloodstream, where they develop into mature RBCs.

Incompatibilities
Don't mix darbepoetin alfa with any other drug.

Contraindications
Hypersensitivity to human albumin or products made from mammal cells; uncontrolled hypertension

Interactions
DRUGS
None known

Adverse Reactions
CNS: Asthenia, dizziness, fatigue, fever, headache, seizures
CV: Arrhythmias, cardiac arrest, chest pain, congestive heart failure, hypertension, hypotension, peripheral edema, vascular access hemorrhage, vascular access thrombosis
GI: Abdominal pain, constipation, diarrhea, nausea, vomiting
MS: Arthralgia, back pain, limb pain, myalgia
RESP: Bronchitis, cough, dyspnea, upper respiratory tract infection
SKIN: Rash, urticaria
Other: Fluid overload, infection, flulike symptoms, injection site pain, sepsis

Nursing Considerations
• Before starting therapy, expect to correct folic acid or vitamin B_{12} deficiencies because these conditions may interfere with drug's effectiveness.
• To ensure effective drug response, expect to obtain serum ferritin level and serum transferrin saturation before beginning and during therapy, as ordered. If serum ferritin level is less than 100 mcg/l or serum transferrin saturation is less than 20%, expect to begin supplemental iron therapy.
• Don't shake vial during preparation to avoid denaturing drug and rendering it biologically inactive.
• Discard drug if you see particulate matter or discoloration.
• Don't dilute drug before giving it.
• Discard unused portion of drug because it contains no preservatives.
• Monitor blood pressure frequently during therapy for hypertension. Expect to reduce dosage or withhold drug if blood pressure is poorly controlled with antihypertensive and dietary measures.
• Monitor hemoglobin level weekly, as ordered, until hemoglobin stabilizes and maintenance dosage has been achieved. Thereafter, monitor hemoglobin level regularly, as ordered. After each dosage adjustment, expect to monitor hemoglobin level weekly for 4 weeks until hemoglobin level stabilizes in response to dosage change.
• **WARNING** Be aware that the risk of cardiac arrest, seizures, CVA, exacerbations of hypertension, congestive heart failure, vascular thrombosis, vascular ischemia, vascular infarction, acute myocardial infarction, and fluid overload with peripheral edema increases if hemoglobin level increases more than about 1 g/dl during any 2-week period. Expect to decrease darbepoetin dosage if this occurs.
• Institute seizure precautions according to facility policy.
• For patients with chronic renal failure who aren't receiving dialysis, expect to administer doses lower than those given to patients receiving dialysis. Also, monitor renal function test results and fluid and electrolyte balance in these patients for signs of deteriorating renal function.
• Store drug at 2° to 8° C (36° to 46° F). Don't freeze, and protect from light.

PATIENT TEACHING
• Advise patient that the risk of seizures is highest during the first 90 days of drug therapy. Discourage her from engaging in hazardous activities during this time.
• Stress the importance of complying with the dosage regimen and keeping follow-up medical and laboratory appointments.
• Advise patient to follow up with her prescriber for blood pressure monitoring.
• Encourage patient to eat iron-rich foods.
• If patient will self-administer darbepoetin, teach her and her caregiver the proper administration technique.
• Caution patient and her caregiver not to reuse needles, syringes, or drug product.

Thoroughly instruct them in proper needle and syringe disposal using a puncture-resistant container.
• Review possible adverse reactions, and urge patient to notify prescriber if she experiences chest pain, headache, rash, seizures, shortness of breath, or swelling.

demeclocycline hydrochloride

Declomycin

Class and Category
Chemical: Tetracycline derivative
Therapeutic: Antibiotic
Pregnancy category: D

Indications and Dosages
➤ *To treat Rocky Mountain spotted fever, typhus infections, Q fever, and rickettsialpox and tick fevers caused by Rickettsieae; psittacosis (ornithosis), lymphogranuloma venereum, granuloma inguinale, and* Mycoplasma pneumoniae *or* Borrelia recurrentis *infections; infections caused by gram-negative organisms, such as* Bacteroides *sp.,* Bartonella bacilliformis, Brucella *sp.,* Campylobacter fetus, Francisella tularensis, Haemophilus ducreyi, Vibrio cholerae, *and* Yersinia pestis*; infections caused by susceptible strains of* Acinetobacter calcoaceticus, Enterobacter aerogenes, Escherichia coli, Haemophilus influenzae *(respiratory tract infections),* Herellea *sp.,* Klebsiella *sp. (respiratory tract infections and UTIs), and* Shigella *sp.; infections caused by susceptible strains of* Staphylococcus aureus *(skin and soft-tissue infections) and* Streptococcus *sp.; infections caused by* Actinomyces *sp.,* Bacillus anthracis, Clostridium *sp.,* Fusobacterium fusiforme, Listeria monocytogenes, Treponema pallidum, *and* Treponema pertenue*; and acute intestinal amebiasis*

CAPSULES, TABLETS
Adults and adolescents. 150 mg q 6 hr or 300 mg q 12 hr.
Children ages 8 to 12. 6 to 12 mg/kg/day in divided doses q 6 to 12 hr.

➤ *To treat gonorrhea*
CAPSULES, TABLETS
Adults and adolescents. 600 mg followed by 300 mg q 12 hr for 4 days for total dose of 3,000 mg.

> ### Mechanism of Action
> Binds with ribosomal subunits of susceptible bacteria and alters the cytoplasmic membrane, inhibiting bacterial protein synthesis and rendering the organism ineffective.

Contraindications
Hypersensitivity to demeclocycline or other tetracyclines

Interactions
DRUGS
antacids, calcium supplements, cholestyramine, choline, colestipol, iron supplements, magnesium-containing laxatives, magnesium salicylate, sodium bicarbonate: Decreased demeclocycline absorption
digoxin: Possibly increased blood digoxin level and risk of digitalis toxicity
methoxyflurane: Increased nephrotoxic effect
oral anticoagulants: Increased anticoagulant effects
oral contraceptives: Decreased contraceptive effectiveness
penicillins: Decreased bactericidal action of penicillins
vitamin A: Possibly benign intracranial hypertension
FOODS
milk, other dairy products: Decreased drug absorption

Adverse Reactions
CNS: Dizziness
EENT: Tinnitus, vision changes
GI: Abdominal cramps, diarrhea, nausea, pseudomembranous colitis, vomiting
GU: Elevated BUN level, nephrogenic diabetes insipidus
HEME: Eosinophilia, hemolytic anemia, neutropenia, thrombocytopenia
SKIN: Photosensitivity, pruritus, rash, urticaria
Other: Anaphylaxis, angioedema

Nursing Considerations
• Monitor results of renal and liver function tests during demeclocycline therapy, as indicated.

D

•**WARNING** Watch for development of nephrogenic diabetes insipidus during long-term therapy.

PATIENT TEACHING
•Stress the importance of completing prescribed therapy, even if symptoms improve.
•Advise patient not to take demeclocycline within 3 hours of taking other drugs or dairy products because they may decrease its absorption.
•Instruct patient to avoid taking antacids while taking demeclocycline because of impaired absorption.
•Advise patient to avoid direct sunlight, use sunscreen, and wear protective clothing outdoors; among tetracyclines, demeclocycline causes the most photosensitivity.
•Urge patient to notify prescriber immediately if edema, rash, or severe GI problems develop.

desipramine hydrochloride

Norpramin, Pertofrane (CAN)

Class and Category
Chemical: Dibenzazepine derivative
Therapeutic: Antidepressant
Pregnancy category: C

Indications and Dosages
➤ *To treat depression*
TABLETS
Adults. *Initial:* 100 to 200 mg/day as a single dose or in divided doses. Increased gradually to 300 mg/day, if needed. *Maximum:* 300 mg/day.
Adolescents. *Initial:* 25 to 50 mg/day in divided doses. Increased gradually, if needed. *Maximum:* 100 mg/day.
Children ages 6 to 12. *Initial:* 10 to 30 mg/day, or 1 to 5 mg/kg, in divided doses.
DOSAGE ADJUSTMENT Initial dosage decreased to 25 to 50 mg/day in divided doses for elderly patients, then increased gradually if needed to maximum of 150 mg/day.

Route	Onset	Peak	Duration
P.O.	2 to 3 wk	Unknown	Unknown

Contraindications
Acute recovery phase of MI; hypersensitivity to desipramine, other tricyclic antidepres-

sants, or their components; MAO inhibitor therapy within 14 days

Mechanism of Action
Blocks serotonin and norepinephrine reuptake by adrenergic nerves, which normally release these neurotransmitters from their storage sites when activated by a nerve impulse. By blocking reuptake, this tricyclic antidepressant increases serotonin and norepinephrine levels at nerve synapses, which may elevate mood and reduce depression.

Interactions
DRUGS
activated charcoal: Prevention of desipramine absorption, reduced therapeutic effects
barbiturates: Decreased blood desipramine level, increased CNS depression
bupropion, haloperidol, H₂-receptor antagonists, valproic acid: Increased blood level and adverse effects of desipramine
carbamazepine: Increased blood carbamazepine level, decreased blood desipramine level
cimetidine: Increased blood desipramine level and anticholinergic effects (dry mouth, urine retention, blurred vision)
clonidine: Increased risk of hypertensive crisis
dicumarol: Increased anticoagulant effect
grepafloxacin, quinolones, sparfloxacin: Increased risk of arrhythmias, including torsades de pointes
guanethidine: Antagonized antihypertensive effect of guanethidine
levodopa: Delayed levodopa absorption, increased risk of hypotension
MAO inhibitors: Increased risk of life-threatening adverse effects, such as hyperpyretic or hypertensive crisis and severe seizures
phenothiazines: Increased blood desipramine level, possibly inhibited phenothiazine metabolism, increased risk of neuroleptic malignant syndrome
quinidine: Increased blood quinidine level
rifamycins: Decreased desipramine effects
selective serotonin-reuptake inhibitors: Increased desipramine effects
sympathomimetics: Possibly arrhythmias, possibly increased or decreased vasopressor effects of sympathomimetics
ACTIVITIES
alcohol use: Possibly increased CNS depression, respiratory depression, hypotension, and effects of alcohol

Adverse Reactions

CNS: Agitation, akathisia, anxiety, ataxia, confusion, CVA, delusions, disorientation, dizziness, drowsiness, exacerbation of psychosis, extrapyramidal reactions, fatigue, headache, hypomania, insomnia, lack of coordination, nervousness, nightmares, paresthesia, peripheral neuropathy, restlessness, seizures, sleep disturbance, tremor, weakness
CV: Arrhythmias, including heart block; hypertension; hypotension; palpitations
EENT: Black tongue, blurred vision, dry mouth, mydriasis, stomatitis, taste perversion, tinnitus
ENDO: Breast enlargement and galactorrhea (in women), gynecomastia (in men), hyperglycemia, hypoglycemia, syndrome of inappropriate ADH secretion
GI: Abdominal cramps, anorexia, constipation, diarrhea, elevated liver function test results, elevated pancreatic enzyme levels, epigastric distress, hepatitis, ileus, increased appetite, nausea, vomiting
GU: Acute renal failure, impotence, libido changes, nocturia, painful ejaculation, testicular swelling, urinary frequency and hesitancy, urine retention
HEME: Agranulocytosis, eosinophilia, thrombocytopenia
SKIN: Acne, alopecia, dermatitis, diaphoresis, dry skin, flushing, petechiae, photosensitivity, pruritus, purpura, rash, urticaria
Other: Angioedema, drug fever, weight gain

Nursing Considerations

• Use desipramine with extreme caution in patients with cardiovascular disease, glaucoma, seizure disorder, thyroid disease, or urine retention.
• WARNING Expect drug to produce sedation and, possibly, lower seizure threshold. Take safety and seizure precautions, according to facility protocol.
• Monitor blood glucose level frequently.
• Be prepared to obtain blood sample for leukocyte and differential counts from patients in whom fever develops during therapy.
• Expect to discontinue drug as soon as possible before elective surgery because of its possible adverse cardiovascular effects.

PATIENT TEACHING

• Advise patient to use sunscreen when outdoors and to avoid sunlamps and tanning beds.
• Instruct patient to notify prescriber immediately about a fast and pounding heartbeat, fainting, severe agitation or restlessness, and strange behavior or thoughts.
• Caution patient not to stop drug abruptly; doing so may cause dizziness, headache, hyperthermia, irritability, malaise, nausea, sleep disturbances, and vomiting.
• Advise patient not to drink alcoholic beverages because of increased risk of adverse CNS reactions.
• Advise patient to avoid potentially hazardous activities until drug's CNS effects are known.
• Advise diabetic patient to monitor her blood glucose level frequently.

D

desmopressin acetate

DDAVP Injection, DDAVP Nasal Spray, DDAVP Rhinal Tube, DDAVP Rhinyle Nasal Solution (CAN), DDAVP Tablets, Octostim (CAN), Stimate, Stimate Nasal Spray

Class and Category

Chemical: Synthetic ADH analogue
Therapeutic: Antidiuretic, antihemorrhagic
Pregnancy category: B

Indications and Dosages

➤ *To manage primary nocturnal enuresis*
TABLETS
Adults and children age 6 and older. *Initial:* 0.2 mg h.s., increased as needed. *Maximum:* 0.6 mg/day.
NASAL SOLUTION
Adults and children age 6 and older. 10 mcg in each nostril h.s. for 4 to 8 wk. Reduced to 10 mcg in only one nostril h.s. if response is adequate to 10 mcg in each nostril, or increased to 20 mcg in each nostril h.s. if response is inadequate to 10 mcg in each nostril daily.
➤ *To control symptoms of central diabetes insipidus*
TABLETS
Adults and children age 6 and older. *Initial:* 0.05 mg b.i.d., increased as needed. *Usual:* 0.1 to 0.8 mg in divided doses b.i.d. or t.i.d. *Maximum:* 1.2 mg/day.
I.V. INFUSION, I.M. OR S.C. INJECTION
Adults. 2 to 4 mcg/day in divided doses b.i.d. Dosage adjusted as needed.
NASAL SOLUTION
Adults and adolescents. 0.1 to 0.4 ml/day (10 to 40 mcg/day) as a single dose or in divided doses b.i.d. or t.i.d. Dosage adjusted as

needed. If daily dose is divided, each dose adjusted separately.

Children ages 3 months to 12 years. 0.25 mcg/kg/day as a single dose or in divided doses b.i.d. Dosage adjusted as needed. If daily dose is divided, each dose adjusted separately.

➤ *To prevent or manage bleeding episodes in hemophilia A or mild to moderate type I von Willebrand's disease*

I.V. INFUSION
Adults and children who weigh more than 10 kg (22 lb). 0.3 mcg/kg diluted in 50 ml of NS and infused over 15 to 30 min. If used preoperatively, dose is given 30 min before procedure.

Children who weigh 10 kg or less. 0.3 mcg/kg diluted in 10 ml of NS and infused over 15 to 30 min. If used preoperatively, dose is given 30 min before procedure.

NASAL SOLUTION (STIMATE NASAL SPRAY)
Adults and children who weigh more than 50 kg (110 lb). 150 mcg in each nostril. If used preoperatively, dose is given 2 hr before procedure.

Adults and children who weigh 50 kg or less. 150 mcg in one nostril. If used preoperatively, dose is given 2 hr before procedure.

Route	Onset	Peak	Duration
P.O.	1 hr*	4 to 7 hr*	8 to 12 hr*
I.V.	15 to 30 min†	30 to 60 min†	3 hr‡
Nasal	In 1 hr*	1 to 5 hr*	8 to 20 hr*

Contraindications
Hypersensitivity to desmopressin or its components

Interactions
DRUGS
carbamazepine, chlorpropamide, clofibrate: Possibly potentiated antidiuretic effect of desmopressin
demeclocycline, lithium: Possibly decreased antidiuretic effect of desmopressin
vasopressor drugs: Possibly potentiated vasopressor effect of desmopressin

---

* For antidiuretic effect.
† For antihemorrhagic effect.
‡ For von Willebrand's disease; 4 to 20 hr for mild hemophilia A.

Mechanism of Action
Exerts an antidiuretic effect similar to that of vasopressin by increasing cellular permeability of renal collecting ducts and distal tubules, thereby enhancing water reabsorption. This action results in reduced urine flow and increased osmolality. As an antihemorrhagic, desmopressin increases the blood concentration of clotting factor VIII (antihemophilic factor) and the activity of von Willebrand's factor (factor VII$_{VWF}$). Drug also may increase platelet aggregation and adhesion at injury sites by exerting a direct effect on blood vessel walls.

Adverse Reactions
CNS: Asthenia, chills, dizziness, headache
CV: Hypertension (with high doses), transient hypotension
EENT: Conjunctivitis, epistaxis, lacrimation, nasal congestion (nasal form), ocular edema, pharyngitis, rhinitis
GI: Nausea
GU: Vulvar pain (parenteral form)
SKIN: Flushing
Other: Injection site pain and redness; water intoxication

Nursing Considerations
•Use desmopressin cautiously in patients with conditions associated with fluid and electrolyte imbalance, such as cystic fibrosis; such patients are prone to hyponatremia.
•Be aware that nasal cavity scarring, edema, and other abnormalities may cause erratic absorption and require the use of a different administration route.
•Monitor blood pressure frequently during therapy.

PATIENT TEACHING
•To prevent hyponatremia and water intoxication in a child or an elderly patient, instruct family to restrict fluids as prescribed.
•Instruct patient to refrigerate nasal solution.
•Teach patient to prime nasal spray pump (only once) and spray dose into one or both nostrils, as prescribed, while inhaling briskly. Instruct her to clean tip of sprayer with hot water and dry it with clean tissue. Advise her to keep track of doses given and to discard bottle after 50 doses.

•Instruct patient who uses Stimate Nasal Spray to prime pump before first use by pressing down four times. Advise her to discard pump after 25 or 50 doses, depending on bottle, because delivery of an accurate dose can't be assured.

•Teach patient who uses nasal tube delivery system to draw prescribed amount of solution into calibrated flexible plastic tube, insert one end of tube into a nostril and the other end into her mouth, and gently blow into tube to deposit solution deep into nasal cavity. Caution her not to let drug drain into her mouth.

•Teach patient or caregiver how to administer S.C. injection, if appropriate.

•Urge patient to notify prescriber if adverse reactions occur.

dexamethasone

Decadron, Decadron Elixir, Deronil (CAN), Dexamethasone Intensol, Dexasone (CAN), Dexone, Hexadrol, Oradexon (CAN)

dexamethasone acetate

Cortastat LA, Dalalone D.P., Dalalone L.A., Decadron-LA, Decaject L.A., Dexacen LA-8, Dexacorten-LA, Dexasone L.A., Dexone LA, Solurex LA

dexamethasone sodium phosphate

Cortastat, Dalalone, Decadrol, Decadron Phosphate, Decadron Respihaler, Decaject, Dexacen-4, Dexacorten, Dexacort Turbinaire, Dexasone, Dexone, Hexadrol Phosphate, Primethasone, Solurex

Class and Category

Chemical: Synthetic adrenocortical steroid
Therapeutic: Anti-inflammatory, diagnostic aid, immunosuppressant
Pregnancy category: C

Indications and Dosages

➤ *To treat endocrine disorders, such as congenital adrenal hyperplasia, hypercalcemia associated with cancer, and nonsuppurative thyroiditis; acute episodes or exacerbations of rheumatic disorders; collagen diseases, such as systemic lupus erythematosus and acute rheumatic carditis; severe dermatologic diseases; severe allergic conditions, such as seasonal or perennial allergic rhinitis, bronchial asthma, laryngeal edema, serum sickness, and drug hypersensitivity reactions; respiratory diseases, such as symptomatic sarcoidosis, Löffler's syndrome, berylliosis, fulminating or disseminated pulmonary tuberculosis, and aspiration pneumonitis; hematologic disorders, such as idiopathic thrombocytopenic purpura and secondary thrombocytopenia in adults, autoimmune hemolytic anemia, aplastic crisis, and congenital hypoplastic anemia; tuberculous meningitis and trichinosis with neurologic or myocardial involvement*

➤ *To manage leukemias and lymphomas in adults and acute leukemia in children; to induce diuresis or remission of proteinuria in idiopathic nephrotic syndrome without uremia or nephrotic syndrome caused by systemic lupus erythematosus*

➤ *To provide palliative therapy during acute exacerbations of GI diseases, such as ulcerative colitis and regional enteritis*

ELIXIR, ORAL SOLUTION, TABLETS, I.V. OR I.M. INJECTION
Adults. Highly individualized dosage based on severity of disorder. *Usual:* 0.75 to 9 mg/day as a single dose or in divided doses.
ELIXIR, ORAL SOLUTION, TABLETS
Children. Highly individualized dosage based on severity of disorder. *Usual:* 83.3 to 333.3 mcg/kg/day in divided doses t.i.d. or q.i.d.
I.M. INJECTION
Children. Highly individualized dosage based on severity of disorder. *Usual:* 27.76 to 166.65 mcg/kg q 12 to 24 hr.

➤ *To manage adrenocortical insufficiency*
ELIXIR, ORAL SOLUTION, TABLETS, I.V. OR I.M. INJECTION
Adults. 0.5 to 9 mg/day as a single dose or in divided doses.
ELIXIR, ORAL SOLUTION, TABLETS
Children. 23.3 mcg/kg/day in divided doses t.i.d.
I.M. INJECTION
Children. 23.3 mcg/kg/day in divided doses t.i.d. given q third day; alternatively, 7.76 to 11.65 mcg/kg/day.

➤ *To test for Cushing's syndrome*
ELIXIR, ORAL SOLUTION, TABLETS
Adults. 0.5 mg q 6 hr for 48 hr followed by collection of 24-hr urine specimen to determine 17-hydroxycorticosteroid level. Alterna-

D

tively, 1 mg at 11 p.m. followed by plasma cortisol test performed at 8 a.m. the next day.

➤ *To distinguish Cushing's syndrome related to pituitary corticotropin excess from Cushing's syndrome related to other causes*

ELIXIR, ORAL SOLUTION, TABLETS

Adults. 2 mg q 6 hr for 48 hr followed by collection of 24-hr urine specimen to determine 17-hydroxycorticosteroid level.

➤ *To decrease cerebral edema*

ELIXIR, ORAL SOLUTION, TABLETS

Adults. 2 mg q 8 to 12 hr as maintenance after parenteral form has controlled initial symptoms.

I.V. OR I.M. INJECTION

Adults. 10 mg I.V. followed by 4 mg I.M. q 6 hr. Decreased after 2 to 4 days, if needed, gradually tapering off over 5 to 7 days unless inoperable or recurring brain tumor is present. If such a tumor is present, dosage gradually decreased after 2 to 4 days to maintenance dosage of 2 mg I.M. q 8 to 12 hr and switched to P.O. regimen as soon as possible.

➤ *To treat unresponsive shock*

I.V. INFUSION AND INJECTION

Adults. 20 mg as a single dose followed by 3 mg/kg over 24 hr as a continuous infusion; 40 mg as a single dose followed by 40 mg q 2 to 6 hr, as needed; or 1 mg/kg as a single dose. All regimens used for no more than 3 days.

➤ *To decrease localized inflammation*

INTRA-ARTICULAR INJECTION

Adults. 2 to 4 mg for large joint; 0.8 to 1 mg for small joint; 2 to 3 mg for bursae; 0.4 to 1 mg for tendon sheaths.

SOFT-TISSUE INJECTION

Adults. 2 to 6 mg; 1 to 2 mg for ganglia.

INTRALESIONAL INJECTION

Adults. 0.8 to 1.6 mg/injection site.

➤ *To decrease inflammation in allergic conditions or nasal polyps (except in sinuses)*

NASAL AEROSOL

Adults and children age 12 and older. 2 sprays (0.2 mg) in each nostril b.i.d. or t.i.d. *Maximum:* 12 sprays (1.2 mg)/day.

Children ages 6 to 12. 1 or 2 sprays (0.1 to 0.2 mg) in each nostril b.i.d. *Maximum:* 8 sprays (0.8 mg)/day.

Mechanism of Action

Binds to intracellular glucocorticoid receptors and suppresses inflammatory and immune responses by:
- inhibiting neutrophil and monocyte accumulation at inflammation site and suppressing their phagocytic and bactericidal activity
- stabilizing lysosomal membranes
- suppressing antigen response of macrophages and helper T cells
- inhibiting synthesis of inflammatory response mediators, such as cytokines, interleukins, and prostaglandins.

Contraindications

Administration of live virus vaccine to patient or family member, hypersensitivity to dexamethasone or its components (including sulfites), idiopathic thrombocytopenic purpura (I.M. use), systemic fungal infections

Interactions

DRUGS

aminoglutethimide, antacids, barbiturates, hydantoins, mitotane, rifampin: Decreased dexamethasone effectiveness

amphotericin B (parenteral), carbonic anhydrase inhibitors: Risk of hypokalemia

anticholinesterases: Decreased anticholinesterase effectiveness in myasthenia gravis

digoxin: Increased risk of digitalis toxicity related to hypokalemia

ephedrine: Decreased half-life and increased clearance of dexamethasone

estrogens, ketoconazole: Decreased dexamethasone clearance

isoniazid: Decreased blood isoniazid level

neuromuscular blockers: Possibly potentiated or counteracted neuromuscular blockade

oral anticoagulants: Altered coagulation times, requiring reduced anticoagulant dosage

oral contraceptives: Increased half-life and concentration of dexamethasone

potassium-wasting diuretics: Increased potassium loss and risk of hypokalemia

salicylates: Decreased blood level and effectiveness of salicylates

somatrem: Possibly inhibition of somatrem's growth-promoting effect

theophyllines: Altered effects of either drug

toxoids, vaccines: Decreased antibody response

ACTIVITIES
alcohol use: Increased risk of GI bleeding

Adverse Reactions

CNS: Depression, euphoria, fever, headache, increased ICP, insomnia, light-headedness, malaise, neuritis, paresthesia, psychosis, seizures, syncope, tiredness, vertigo, weakness
CV: Arrhythmias, edema, fat embolism, heart failure, hypercholesterolemia, hyperlipidemia, hypertension, myocardial rupture, thromboembolism, thrombophlebitis
EENT: Cataracts, glaucoma, vision changes (all forms); epistaxis, loss of smell and taste, nasal burning and dryness, oral candidiasis, perforated nasal septum, pharyngitis, rebound nasal congestion, rhinorrhea, sneezing (nasal aerosol)
ENDO: Cushingoid symptoms, decreased iodine uptake, growth suppression in children, hyperglycemia, menstrual irregularities
GI: Abdominal distention, bloody stools, heartburn, increased appetite, indigestion, melena, nausea, pancreatitis, peptic ulcer with possible perforation, ulcerative esophagitis, vomiting
GU: Glycosuria, increased or decreased number and motility of spermatozoa, perineal irritation, urinary frequency
HEME: Leukocytosis, leukopenia
MS: Muscle atrophy, spasms, or weakness; myalgia; osteonecrosis and tendon rupture (intra-articular injection); osteoporosis; pathologic fracture of long bones; vertebral compression fracture
RESP: Bronchospasm
SKIN: Acne, allergic dermatitis, diaphoresis, ecchymosis, erythema, hirsutism, necrotizing vasculitis, petechiae, subcutaneous fat atrophy, striae, thin and fragile skin, urticaria
Other: Aggravated or masked signs of infection, anaphylaxis, angioedema, hypernatremia, hypocalcemia, hypokalemia, hypokalemic alkalosis, impaired wound healing, metabolic acidosis, sodium and fluid retention, suppressed skin test reaction, weight gain

Nursing Considerations

• Give once-daily dose of dexamethasone in the morning to coincide with the body's natural cortisol secretion.
• Give oral drug with food to decrease GI distress.
• Be aware that dosage forms with a concentration of 24 mg/ml are for I.V. use only.

• Shake I.M. solution before injecting deep into large muscle mass.
• **WARNING** Avoid S.C. injection; it may cause atrophy and sterile abscess.
• Inject undiluted I.V. dose directly into I.V. tubing of infusing compatible solution over 30 seconds or less, as prescribed.
• **WARNING** Don't give acetate form by I.V. injection.
• Shake nasal aerosol container well, and hold it upright about 6″ (15 cm) from area being treated. Keep spray out of patient's eyes, and advise her not to inhale it.
• Expect to taper drug rather than stopping it abruptly; prolonged use can cause adrenal suppression.
• Monitor fluid intake and output and daily weight, and assess for crackles, dyspnea, peripheral edema, and steady weight gain.
• Periodically evaluate growth if patient is a child.
• Test stool for occult blood.
• Monitor results of hematology studies as well as blood glucose and serum electrolyte, cholesterol, and lipid levels. Dexamethasone may cause hyperglycemia, hypernatremia, hypocalcemia, hypokalemia, or leukopenia; may increase serum cholesterol and lipid levels; and may decrease iodine uptake by the thyroid.
• Assess for evidence of osteoporosis, Cushing's syndrome, and other systemic effects during long-term use.
• Monitor neonate for signs of hypoadrenocorticism if mother received dexamethasone during pregnancy. Be aware that some preparations also contain benzyl alcohol, which may cause a fatal toxic syndrome in neonates and immature infants.
• Assess for hypersensitivity reactions after giving acetate or sodium phosphate form; both may contain bisulfites or parabens, inactive ingredients to which some people are allergic.

PATIENT TEACHING
• Instruct patient not to store drug in damp or hot places and to protect liquid form from freezing.
• Instruct patient to take once-daily oral dose in the morning with food to help prevent GI distress.
• Caution patient to avoid alcoholic beverages during therapy because they increase the risk of GI bleeding.

•Advise patient to follow a low-sodium, high-potassium, high-protein diet, if prescribed, to help minimize weight gain (common with this drug). Instruct her to inform prescriber if she's on a special diet.

•Instruct patient not to stop using drug abruptly.

•Advise patient to notify prescriber if condition recurs or worsens after dosage is reduced or therapy stops.

•Urge patient to have regular eye examinations during long-term use.

•Advise patient receiving long-term therapy to carry medical identification and to notify all health care providers that she takes dexamethasone.

•Instruct patient (especially a child) to avoid close contact with anyone who has chickenpox or measles and to notify prescriber immediately if exposure occurs.

•Advise patient and family members to avoid live virus vaccinations, such as oral polio vaccine, during therapy unless prescriber approves.

•Inform diabetic patient that drug may affect her blood glucose level.

•If drug is injected into a joint, instruct patient not to put excess pressure on joint and to notify prescriber if it becomes red or swollen.

•Advise patient to notify prescriber about anorexia, depression, light-headedness, malaise, muscle pain, nausea, vomiting, and signs of early hyperadrenocorticism (abdominal distention, amenorrhea, easy bruising, extreme weakness, facial hair, increased appetite, moon face, weight gain). Inform patient and family about possible changes in appearance.

•Instruct patient to notify prescriber about illness, surgery, or changes in stress level.

dexchlorpheniramine maleate

Dexchlor, Polaramine, Polaramine Repetabs

Class and Category

Chemical: Propylamine derivative
Therapeutic: Antihistamine
Pregnancy category: B

Indications and Dosages

➤ *To treat allergic conjunctivitis; transfusion reaction; dermographism; mild, uncomplicated allergic skin reactions, such* *as urticaria and angioedema; perennial and seasonal allergic rhinitis; and vasomotor rhinitis and as adjunct to treat anaphylaxis*

E.R. TABLETS

Adults and adolescents. 4 to 6 mg/day h.s. or q 8 to 10 hr, p.r.n.

SYRUP, TABLETS

Adults and adolescents. 2 mg q 4 to 6 hr, p.r.n.
Children ages 6 to 12. 1 mg q 4 to 6 hr or 150 mcg/kg in divided doses q.i.d., p.r.n.
Children ages 2 to 6. 0.5 mg q 4 to 6 hr, p.r.n.

Route	Onset	Peak	Duration
P.O.	15 to 60 min*	Unknown*	4 to 8 hr*

Mechanism of Action

Binds to central and peripheral H_1 receptors, competing with histamine for these sites and preventing histamine from reaching its site of action. By blocking histamine, dexchlorpheniramine:

•inhibits respiratory, vascular, and GI smooth-muscle contraction, which prevents wheezing

•decreases capillary permeability, which reduces wheals, flares, and itching

•decreases salivary and lacrimal gland secretions, which prevents sneezing, itching, watery eyes, and increased nasal secretions.

Contraindications

Benign prostatic hyperplasia; bladder neck obstruction; hypersensitivity to dexchlorpheniramine or other antihistamines; lower respiratory tract disorders, such as asthma; MAO inhibitor therapy within 14 days; narrow-angle glaucoma; pyloroduodenal obstruction; stenosing peptic ulcer

Interactions

DRUGS

anticholinergics: Potentiated anticholinergic effects
CNS depressants: Increased CNS depression
MAO inhibitors: Possibly severe hypotension and prolonged and intensified anticholinergic and sedative effects of dexchlorpheniramine

---

* For syrup and tablets; unknown for E.R. tablets.

ACTIVITIES
alcohol use: Increased CNS depression

Adverse Reactions

CNS: Ataxia, confusion, dizziness, drowsiness, euphoria, excitement, headache, insomnia, irritability, nervousness, neuritis, nightmares, paresthesia, restlessness, vertigo, weakness
CV: Hypotension, palpitations, tachycardia
EENT: Acute labyrinthitis, blurred vision, dry mouth, tinnitus, vision changes
GI: Anorexia, constipation, diarrhea, indigestion, nausea, vomiting
GU: Urinary hesitancy, urine retention
RESP: Tenacious mucus
SKIN: Diaphoresis, photosensitivity, rash

Nursing Considerations

• Use dexchlorpheniramine cautiously in elderly patients and those with cardiovascular disease, hyperthyroidism, increased intraocular pressure, prostatic hypertrophy, or renal disease.
• Monitor for adverse reactions, especially in elderly patients and children.
• Assess for signs of overdose, including clumsiness; drowsiness; dry mouth, nose, or throat; dyspnea; flushed or red face; hallucinations; insomnia; light-headedness; seizures; and unsteadiness.

PATIENT TEACHING
• Inform patient that drug provides temporary relief of symptoms.
• Advise patient to take drug with food, water, or milk to reduce GI irritation. Inform her that she can crush regular (not E.R.) tablets and mix with food or fluid.
• If patient takes E.R. tablets, instruct her not to break, crush, or chew them before swallowing.
• Advise patient to take a missed dose as soon as possible unless almost time for the next dose.
• Because drug may cause drowsiness, caution patient to avoid potentially hazardous activities until its CNS effects are known.
• Instruct her to avoid prolonged sun exposure and to use a sunscreen.
• Suggest that patient use sugarless candy or gum, ice chips, or saliva substitute to relieve dry mouth. If dryness lasts longer than 2 weeks, advise her to notify prescriber.
• Caution patient to avoid alcohol and CNS depressants, such as sedatives, tranquilizers, and sleeping pills, while taking dexchlorpheniramine.

• If patient takes high doses of aspirin, urge her to inform prescriber because antihistamines may mask adverse reactions to aspirin overdose, such as tinnitus.
• Inform patient that drug needs to be discontinued 3 to 4 days before skin tests for allergies are performed.

dexmethylphenidate hydrochloride

Focalin

Class, Category, and Schedule

Chemical: d-*threo*-enantiomer of methylphenidate
Therapeutic: CNS stimulant
Pregnancy category: C
Controlled substance: Schedule II

Indications and Dosages

➤ *To treat attention deficit hyperactivity disorder (ADHD)*

TABLETS

Adults and children age 6 and older who are new to methylphenidate. 2.5 mg b.i.d. at least 4 hr apart, increased in weekly increments of 2.5 to 5 mg. *Maximum:* 10 mg b.i.d.

Adults and children age 6 and older who are currently using methylphenidate. One-half of racemic methylphenidate dosage. *Maximum:* 10 mg b.i.d. at least 4 hr apart.

DOSAGE ADJUSTMENT Drug discontinued if no improvement is noted within 1 month after appropriate dosage adjustments. Dosage decreased or drug discontinued if paradoxical aggravation of symptoms or adverse reactions occurs.

Mechanism of Action

May block the reuptake of norepinephrine and dopamine into the presynaptic neurons in the cerebral cortex, which increases the availability of norepinephrine and dopamine in the extraneuronal space.

Contraindications

Family history or diagnosis of Tourette syndrome; glaucoma; hypersensitivity to dexmethylphenidate, methylphenidate, or their components; marked anxiety, tension, and agitation; motor tics; use within 14 days of MAO inhibitor therapy

Interactions
DRUGS
anticonvulsants, oral anticoagulants, antide-pressants (tricyclic and selective serotonin reuptake inhibitors): Possibly decreased metabolism of these drugs
antihypertensives: Decreased therapeutic effect of these drugs
dopamine and other vasopressors: Increased therapeutic effect of these drugs
MAO inhibitors: Increased adverse effects, risk of hypertensive crisis

Adverse Reactions
CNS: Cerebral arteritis or occlusion, dizziness, drowsiness, dyskinesia, fever, headache, insomnia, motor or vocal tics, nervousness, seizures, Tourette syndrome, toxic psychosis
CV: Angina, arrhythmias, hypertension, hypotension, increased or decreased pulse rate, palpitations, tachycardia
GI: Abdominal pain, anorexia, nausea
HEME: Thrombocytopenic purpura
MS: Arthralgia
SKIN: Erythema multiforme, exfoliative dermatitis, necrotizing vasculitis, rash, urticaria
Other: Weight loss (with prolonged therapy)

Nursing Considerations
•WARNING Be aware that dexmethylphenidate may induce CNS stimulation and psychosis and may worsen behavior disturbances and thought disorders. Use drug cautiously in children with psychosis. Be aware that withdrawal symptoms may occur with long-term use.
•Monitor patient's blood pressure and pulse rate to detect hypertension and signs of excessive stimulation. Notify prescriber if you detect such signs.
•Be aware that dexmethylphenidate shouldn't be used to treat severe depression or to prevent or treat normal fatigue.
•WARNING Monitor patient for signs of physical or psychological dependence. Use drug cautiously in patients with a history of drug abuse, including alcoholism.
•Monitor CBC, differential, and platelet counts, as ordered, during prolonged therapy.
•Expect to discontinue drug if seizures occur. Drug may lower seizure threshold, especially in patients with a history of seizures or EEG abnormalities.
•Monitor children on long-term therapy for signs of growth suppression, which has been noted during long-term use of stimulants.

•Be aware that dosage adjustment may be prescribed for drugs that may be affected by dexmethylphenidate, such as anticoagulants and antihypertensives.
PATIENT TEACHING
•Advise patient to notify prescriber if she experiences excessive nervousness, fever, insomnia, palpitations, rash, or nausea during dexmethylphenidate therapy.
•Caution patient with seizure disorder that drug may cause seizures.
•Advise patient to protect drug from light and moisture.
•Teach patient (or parent) how to monitor for improved symptoms of ADHD, such as decreased impulsiveness and increased attention. Stress the importance of continued follow-up care, and suggest participation in an ADHD program.

dexrazoxane

Zinecard

Class and Category
Chemical: Piperazinedione
Therapeutic: Cardioprotective agent, chelating agent
Pregnancy category: C

Indications and Dosages
➤ *To prevent or reduce severity of cardio-myopathy associated with doxorubicin therapy in women with metastatic breast cancer*
I.V. INJECTION
Adults. *Initial:* 500 mg/m^2 for every 50 mg/m^2 of doxorubicin q 3 wk.

Mechanism of Action
Rapidly enters cardiac cells and acts as an intracellular heavy metal chelator. In cardiac tissues, anthracyclines, such as doxorubicin, form complexes with iron or copper, resulting in damage to cardiac cell membranes and mitochondria. Dexrazoxane combines with intracellular iron and protects against anthracycline-induced free radical damage to the myocardium. It also prevents the conversion of ferrous ions back to ferric ions for use by free radicals.

Incompatibilities
Don't mix dexrazoxane in same I.V. line with other drugs.

Contraindications

Hypersensitivity to dexrazoxane or its components; use with chemotherapy regimens that do not contain anthracycline such as daunorubicin, doxorubicin, epirubicin, idarubicin, or mitoxantrone

Interactions

bone marrow depressants: Possibly enhanced bone marrow depression

Adverse Reactions

HEME: Myelosuppression including granulocytopenia, leukopenia, or thrombocytopenia
Other: Injection site pain

Nursing Considerations

•**WARNING** Use gloves when preparing reconstituted solution. If dexrazoxane powder or solution comes in contact with your skin or mucosa, immediately and thoroughly wash with soap and water.
•Reconstitute drug by mixing with 25 or 50 ml of 0.167 molar sodium lactate, supplied by the manufacturer, to produce a final concentration of 10 mg/ml. Administer reconstituted solution by slow I.V. push, or further dilute with either NS or D₅W to a concentration of 1.3 to 5 mg/ml, as prescribed, for rapid I.V. infusion.
•Be aware that dexrazoxane may interfere with tumor response to doxorubicin, especially in patients receiving drug at beginning of fluorouracil-doxorubicin-cyclophosphamide (FAC) therapy.
•Monitor patient with preexisting immunosuppression or decreased bone marrow reserves resulting from prior chemotherapy or radiation therapy to prevent worsening of her condition. Notify prescriber if condition deteriorates.
PATIENT TEACHING
•Inform patient that dexrazoxane is used to protect the heart from damage caused by myelosuppression and that she'll be given the drug by a health care professional in the hospital or clinic before receiving chemotherapy.
•Inform patient that dexrazoxane and chemotherapy may make her feel generally unwell, but urge her to continue treatment unless prescriber tells her to stop.
•Instruct patient to report to prescriber such symptoms as fever, chills, sore throat, mouth sores, unusual bleeding or bruising, unusual tiredness or weakness, pain at injection site, and vomiting because these symptoms may require a change in dosage or discontinuation of drug.

•Inform patient that drug may exacerbate symptoms of bone marrow suppression caused by anthracycline chemotherapy, including increased risk of infection.
•Teach patient importance of avoiding injury and infection during dexrazoxane therapy. For example, advise her to use a soft-bristled toothbrush to prevent damage to teeth and gums; to avoid people with colds, the flu, or bronchitis; and to avoid anyone who has recently had oral polio vaccine because of the increased risk of infection from live virus.

dextrose

(d-glucose)

B-D Glucose, Glutose, Insta-Glucose, Insulin Reaction

glucose

2.5% Dextrose Injection, 5% Dextrose Injection, 10% Dextrose Injection, 20% Dextrose Injection, 25% Dextrose Injection, 50% Dextrose Injection, 60% Dextrose Injection, 70% Dextrose Injection

Class and Category

Chemical: Monosaccharide
Therapeutic: Antihypoglycemic, nutritional supplement
Pregnancy category: C

Indications and Dosages

➤ *To treat insulin-induced hypoglycemia*
CHEWABLE TABLETS, ORAL GEL
Adults and children. *Initial:* 10 to 20 g. Repeated in 10 to 20 min, if needed, based on blood glucose level.
I.V. INFUSION OR INJECTION
Adults and children. *Initial:* 20 to 50 ml of 50% solution given at 3 ml/min. *Maintenance:* 10% to 15% solution by continuous infusion until blood glucose level reaches therapeutic range.
Infants and neonates. 2 ml/kg of 10% to 25% solution until blood glucose level reaches therapeutic range.
➤ *To replace calories*
I.V. INFUSION
Adults and children. Individualized dosage of 2.5%, 5%, or 10% solution, based on need for fluids or calories and given through peripheral I.V. line. Or a 10% to 70% solution given through a large central vein, if needed,

typically mixed with amino acids or other solutions.

Route	Onset	Peak	Duration
P.O.	10 to 20 min	40 min	Unknown
I.V.	2 to 3 min	Unknown	Unknown

Mechanism of Action
Prevents protein and nitrogen loss, promotes glycogen deposition, prevents or decreases ketosis, and, in large amounts, acts as an osmotic diuretic. Dextrose is readily metabolized and undergoes oxidation to carbon dioxide and water. The oral form—glucose—is absorbed directly into the bloodstream from the intestines and is distributed and used (or stored in the liver).

Incompatibilities
Don't give dextrose through same infusion set as blood or blood products because pseudoagglutination of RBCs may occur.

Contraindications
For all solutions: Diabetic coma with excessively elevated blood glucose level
For concentrated solutions: Anuria, alcohol withdrawal syndrome in dehydrated patient, glucose-galactose malabsorption syndrome, hepatic coma, intracranial or intraspinal hemorrhage, overhydration

Interactions
DRUGS
corticosteroids, corticotropin: Increased risk of fluid and electrolyte imbalance if dextrose solution contains sodium ions

Adverse Reactions
CNS: Confusion, fever
GU: Glycosuria
Other: Dehydration; hyperosmolar coma; hypervolemia; hypovolemia; injection site extravasation with tissue necrosis, infection, phlebitis, and venous thrombosis

Nursing Considerations
•Give highly concentrated dextrose solution by central venous catheter—not by S.C. or I.M. route.
•Assess infusion site regularly for signs of infiltration, such as pain, redness, and swelling.
•Monitor blood glucose and electrolyte levels, as appropriate.

•Assess for glucosuria by using a urine reagent strip or collecting a urine sample and reviewing urinalysis results.
•When discontinuing a concentrated solution, expect to give a 5% to 10% dextrose infusion to avoid rebound hypoglycemia.
•Monitor for signs of hypervolemia, such as jugular vein distention and crackles.
PATIENT TEACHING
•Advise patient to swallow oral dextrose because it isn't absorbed from the buccal cavity.
•Instruct patient to monitor her blood glucose level as directed.
•Stress the importance of reporting discomfort, pain, or signs of infection at I.V. site.

dezocine
Dalgan

Class and Category
Chemical: Aminotetralin, synthetic opioid
Therapeutic: Analgesic
Pregnancy category: C

Indications and Dosages
➤ *To relieve pain*
I.V. INJECTION
Adult. *Initial:* 5 mg followed by 2.5 to 10 mg q 2 to 4 hr, p.r.n. *Maximum:* 120 mg/day.
I.M. INJECTION
Adult. *Initial:* 10 mg followed by 5 to 20 mg q 3 to 6 hr, p.r.n. *Maximum:* 20 mg/dose, 120 mg/day.

Route	Onset	Peak	Duration
I.V.	In 15 min	30 min	2 to 4 hr
I.M.	In 30 min	1 to 2 hr	2 to 4 hr

Mechanism of Action
Binds with opioid receptors at many CNS sites. This affects the perception of and emotional response to pain.

Contraindications
Hypersensitivity to dezocine or its components

Interactions
DRUGS
CNS depressants, general anesthetics, hypnotics, sedatives, tranquilizers: Increased CNS depressant effects

opioids: Possibly decreased therapeutic effects of opioid and withdrawal symptoms in patient receiving long-term opioid therapy

ACTIVITIES

alcohol use: Increased CNS depressant effects

Adverse Reactions

CNS: Dizziness, sedation, vertigo
GI: Nausea, vomiting
Other: Injection site redness and swelling

Nursing Considerations

• Use dezocine cautiously and in low doses in elderly patients and those with common bile duct, hepatic, renal, or respiratory disease.
• Discard solution if it contains precipitate.
• Frequently monitor blood pressure and pulse and respiratory rates after giving first dose, especially if given by I.V. route.
• **WARNING** Avoid administering dezocine to a patient who is opioid-dependent. Doing so may precipitate withdrawal symptoms because drug can antagonize opioid effects.
• Assess for pain relief and document findings frequently.

PATIENT TEACHING

• Instruct patient to notify prescriber if pain isn't relieved within 1 hour.
• Advise patient to avoid potentially hazardous activities until drug's CNS effects are known.

diazepam

Apo-Diazepam (CAN), Diastat, Diazepam Intensol, Dizac, Novo-Dipam (CAN), Valium, Vivol (CAN)

Class, Category, and Schedule

Chemical: Benzodiazepine
Therapeutic: Anticonvulsant, anxiolytic, sedative-hypnotic, skeletal muscle relaxant
Pregnancy category: D
Controlled substance: Schedule IV

Indications and Dosages

➤ *To relieve anxiety*

ORAL SOLUTION, TABLETS

Adults. 2 to 10 mg b.i.d. to q.i.d.

DOSAGE ADJUSTMENT Dosage reduced to 2 to 2.5 mg q.d. or b.i.d. and increased gradually as needed and tolerated for elderly or debilitated patients.

Children age 6 months and older. *Initial:* 1 to 2.5 mg t.i.d. or q.i.d. Increased gradually as needed and tolerated.

I.V. OR I.M. INJECTION

Adults. 2 to 5 mg q 3 to 4 hr, p.r.n., for moderate anxiety; 5 to 10 mg q 3 to 4 hr, p.r.n., for severe anxiety.

Children. Individualized dosage. *Maximum:* 0.25 mg/kg given over 3 min and repeated after 15 to 30 min if needed and after another 15 to 30 min if needed.

➤ *To treat symptoms of acute alcohol withdrawal*

ORAL SOLUTION, TABLETS

Adults. 10 mg t.i.d. or q.i.d. during first 24 hr. Then 5 mg t.i.d. or q.i.d., if needed.

I.V. OR I.M. INJECTION

Adults. 10 mg and then 5 to 10 mg in 3 to 4 hr, if needed.

➤ *To provide muscle relaxation, sedation*

ORAL SOLUTION, TABLETS

Adults. 2 to 10 mg t.i.d. or q.i.d.

DOSAGE ADJUSTMENT Dosage reduced to 2 to 2.5 mg q.d. or b.i.d. and increased gradually as needed and tolerated for elderly or debilitated patients.

Children age 6 months and older. *Initial:* 1 to 2.5 mg t.i.d. or q.i.d. Increased gradually as needed and tolerated.

I.V. OR I.M. INJECTION

Adults. 5 to 10 mg and then 5 to 10 mg in 3 to 4 hr, if needed.

DOSAGE ADJUSTMENT Dosage reduced to 2 to 5 mg/dose and increased as needed and tolerated for debilitated patients.

➤ *To treat seizures*

ORAL SOLUTION, TABLETS

Adults. 2 to 10 mg b.i.d. to q.i.d.

DOSAGE ADJUSTMENT Dosage reduced to 2 to 2.5 mg q.d. or b.i.d. and increased gradually as needed and tolerated for elderly or debilitated patients.

Children age 6 months and older. *Initial:* 1 to 2.5 mg t.i.d. or q.i.d. Increased gradually as needed and tolerated.

➤ *To treat status epilepticus and severe recurrent seizures*

I.V. INJECTION

Adults. 5 to 10 mg repeated q 10 to 15 min, as needed, up to a cumulative dose of 30 mg. Regimen repeated, if needed, in 2 to 4 hr. (Use I.M. route if I.V. access is impossible.)

Children age 5 and older. 1 mg repeated q 2 to 5 min, as needed, up to a cumulative dose of 10 mg. Regimen repeated, if needed, in 2 to 4 hr.

D

Children ages 1 month to 5 years. 0.2 to 0.5 mg repeated q 2 to 5 min, as needed, up to a cumulative dose of 5 mg. Regimen repeated, if needed, in 2 to 4 hr.

RECTAL GEL

Adults and adolescents. 0.2 mg/kg rounded up to next available unit dose (or rounded down for elderly or debilitated patient). Repeated in 4 to 12 hr, if needed.

Children ages 6 to 12. 0.3 mg/kg rounded up to next available unit dose. Repeated in 4 to 12 hr, if needed.

Children ages 2 to 6. 0.5 mg/kg rounded up to next available unit dose. Repeated in 4 to 12 hr, if needed.

➤ *To provide preoperative sedation*

I.V. OR I.M. INJECTION

Adults. 5 to 10 mg 30 min before surgery.

➤ *To reduce anxiety before cardioversion*

I.V. INJECTION

Adults. 5 to 15 mg 5 to 10 min before procedure.

➤ *To reduce anxiety before endoscopic procedures*

I.V. INJECTION

Adults. Up to 20 mg titrated to desired sedation and administered immediately before procedure.

I.M. INJECTION

Adults. 5 to 10 mg 30 min before procedure.

➤ *To treat tetanus*

I.V. OR I.M. INJECTION

Adults and children age 5 and older. *Initial:* 5 to 10 mg repeated q 3 to 4 hr, if needed. Sometimes larger doses are needed for adults.

DOSAGE ADJUSTMENT Initial dose reduced to 2 to 5 mg and increased gradually as needed and tolerated for debilitated patients.

Children ages 1 month to 5 years. 1 to 2 mg repeated q 3 to 4 hr, as needed.

Mechanism of Action

May potentiate the effects of gamma-aminobutyric acid (GABA) and other inhibitory neurotransmitters by binding to specific benzodiazepine receptors in the limbic and cortical areas of the CNS. GABA inhibits excitatory stimulation, which helps control emotional behavior. The limbic system contains a highly dense area of benzodiazepine receptors, which may explain the drug's antianxiety effects. Diazepam suppresses the spread of seizure activity caused by seizure-producing foci in the cortex, thalamus, and limbic structures.

Incompatibilities

Don't mix diazepam injection with aqueous solutions. Don't mix diazepam emulsion for I.M. injection with morphine or glycopyrrolate or administer it through an infusion set that contains polyvinyl chloride.

Contraindications

Acute angle-closure glaucoma, hypersensitivity to diazepam or its components, untreated open-angle glaucoma

Interactions

DRUGS

antacids: Altered rate of diazepam absorption
cimetidine, disulfiram, fluoxetine, isoniazid, itraconazole, ketoconazole, metoprolol, oral contraceptives, propoxyphene, propranolol, valproic acid: Decreased diazepam metabolism, increased blood level and risk of adverse effects of diazepam
CNS depressants: Increased CNS depression
digoxin: Increased serum digoxin level and risk of digitalis toxicity
levodopa: Decreased antidyskinetic effect of levodopa
probenecid: Faster onset or more prolonged effects of diazepam
ranitidine: Delayed elimination and increased blood level of diazepam
rifampin: Decreased blood diazepam level
theophyllines: Antagonized sedative effect of diazepam

ACTIVITIES

alcohol use: Increased CNS depression

Adverse Reactions

CNS: Anterograde amnesia, anxiety, ataxia, confusion, depression, dizziness, drowsiness, fatigue, headache, insomnia, lethargy, lightheadedness, sedation, sleepiness, slurred speech, tremor, vertigo
CV: Hypotension, palpitations, tachycardia
EENT: Blurred vision, diplopia, increased salivation
GI: Anorexia, constipation, diarrhea, nausea, vomiting
GU: Libido changes, urinary incontinence, urine retention
RESP: Respiratory depression
SKIN: Dermatitis
Other: Physical and psychological dependence

Nursing Considerations

•Use diazepam cautiously in patients with hepatic or renal impairment.

•Mix concentrated oral solution (Intensol) with liquid or semisolid food for administration. Use supplied calibrated dropper for accurate dosing.

•Protect diazepam injection from light. Don't use solution that's more than slightly yellow or that contains precipitate.

•Administer I.M. injection into deltoid muscle for rapid and complete absorption. Administration into other sites may cause slow, erratic absorption.

•Before administering emulsion form, ask if patient is allergic to soybeans because this form contains soybean oil.

•For an infant or a child, administer I.V. injection slowly over 3 minutes in a dose not to exceed 0.25 mg/kg.

•Administer emulsion form within 6 hours of opening ampule because this form contains no preservatives and allows rapid microbial growth. Use polyethylene-lined or glass infusion sets and polyethylene or polypropylene plastic syringes for administration. Don't use a filter with a pore size of less than 5 microns because it may break down the emulsion.

•Don't mix emulsion form with anything other than its emulsion base. Otherwise, it may become unstable and increase the risk of serious adverse reactions.

•Monitor patient for adverse reactions, especially if she has hypoalbuminemia, which increases the risk of sedation.

•**WARNING** Observe for signs of physical and psychological dependence: a strong desire or need to continue taking diazepam, a need to increase the dose to maintain drug effects, and posttherapy withdrawal symptoms, such as abdominal cramps, insomnia, irritability, nervousness, and tremor.

PATIENT TEACHING

•Instruct patient not to take more drug than prescribed, more often, or for a longer time. Warn her that physical and psychological dependence can occur, and teach her to recognize signs of dependence.

•Advise patient not to take drug to relieve everyday stress.

•Advise patient to avoid potentially hazardous activities until drug's CNS effects are known.

•Advise patient to avoid CNS depressants and alcohol during therapy.

•Instruct patient not to abruptly stop taking drug without prescriber supervision. If patient has a history of seizures, warn her that abrupt drug withdrawal may trigger them.

•Instruct patient to mix Diazepam Intensol with water, soda, or a similar beverage; applesauce; or pudding just before taking it. Caution her not to save the mixture for later. Also tell patient to use calibrated dropper that's provided to measure each dose.

•Teach patient how to self-administer a rectal form, if prescribed.

diazoxide

Hyperstat, Proglycem

Class and Category

Chemical: Benzothiadiazine derivative
Therapeutic: Antihypertensive, antihypoglycemic
Pregnancy category: C

Indications and Dosages

➤ *To manage hypoglycemia caused by hyperinsulinism*

CAPSULES, ORAL SUSPENSION

Adults and children. *Initial:* 1 mg/kg q 8 hr. *Maintenance:* 3 to 8 mg/kg/day in 2 or 3 equal doses given q 8 or 12 hr. *Maximum:* 15 mg/kg/day.

Infants and neonates. *Initial:* 3.3 mg/kg q 8 hr. *Maintenance:* 8 to 15 mg/kg/day in 2 or 3 equal doses given q 8 or 12 hr.

➤ *To treat severe hypertension in hospitalized patients*

I.V. INJECTION

Adults and children. *Initial:* 1 to 3 mg/kg by rapid bolus, repeated q 5 to 15 min until diastolic pressure falls below 100 mm Hg. Repeated in 4 hr and again in 24 hr, if needed, until oral antihypertensive therapy begins. *Maximum:* 150 mg/dose, 1.2 g/day.

Route	Onset	Peak	Duration
P.O.	In 1 hr	Unknown	8 hr
I.V.	1 min	2 to 5 min	2 to 12 hr

Mechanism of Action

Directly affects smooth muscle cells of peripheral arteries and arterioles, causing them to dilate. This action decreases peripheral resistance, which helps reduce blood pressure. Diazoxide also inhibits insulin release from the pancreas, stimulates catecholamine release, and increases hepatic glucose release.

Contraindications
Acute aortic dissection; hypersensitivity to diazoxide, thiazides, other sulfonamide derivatives, or their components; treatment of compensatory hypertension, as occurs with aortic coarctation

Interactions
DRUGS
allopurinol, colchicine, probenecid, sulfinpyrazone: Increased serum uric acid level
antihypertensives: Additive hypotensive effects
beta blockers: Increased hypotensive effects of diazoxide
diuretics, especially thiazides: Potentiated hyperglycemic, hyperuricemic, and antihypertensive effects of diazoxide
estrogens, NSAIDs, sympathomimetics: Antagonized hypotensive effects of diazoxide
insulin, oral antidiabetic drugs: Possibly decreased effectiveness of these drugs
oral anticoagulants: Increased anticoagulant effects
peripheral vasodilators, ritodrine (I.V.): Additive, possibly severe, hypotensive effects

Adverse Reactions
CNS: Anxiety, apprehension, cerebral ischemia, dizziness, euphoria, headache, insomnia, light-headedness, malaise, somnolence, weakness
CV: Bradycardia, chest pain, hypotension, palpitations, tachycardia, transient hypertension
EENT: Blurred vision, dry mouth, increased salivation, taste perversion, tinnitus, transient hearing loss
ENDO: Transient hyperglycemia
GI: Abdominal pain, anorexia, constipation, diarrhea, ileus, nausea, vomiting
MS: Gout
SKIN: Diaphoresis, flushing, pruritus, rash, sensation of warmth
Other: Extravasation with injection site cellulitis and pain; fluid and sodium retention

Nursing Considerations
• Use diazoxide cautiously in patients with uncompensated heart failure (because it can cause fluid retention and heart failure) and in patients with impaired cardiac or cerebral circulation in whom abrupt blood pressure reduction, mild tachycardia, and decreased blood perfusion may be harmful.

• Administer I.V. drug undiluted over 10 to 30 seconds. Don't give drug by I.M. or S.C. route.
• Keep patient supine during I.V. injection and for 1 hour afterward.
• Monitor blood pressure throughout treatment to check for hypertension. Before ending surveillance, measure patient's standing blood pressure if she's ambulatory.
• Frequently assess I.V. site for extravasation because the alkaline drug can irritate tissue.
• Expect to adjust dosage as prescribed if patient switches from oral suspension to capsules; suspension produces a higher blood diazoxide level.
• If diabetic patient receives I.V. diazoxide to treat hypertension, monitor for signs and symptoms of hyperglycemia because parenteral form commonly causes transient hyperglycemia.
• Monitor the blood glucose level of all patients who receive oral diazoxide to determine if drug has raised the blood glucose level to normal.
PATIENT TEACHING
• For patient receiving I.V. diazoxide, explain that she'll be on bed rest until oral therapy starts.
• Advise patient to protect oral suspension from light.
• Instruct patient to take oral drug on a regular schedule and not to skip or double doses.
• Instruct patient to check her blood glucose level regularly if she takes oral diazoxide to treat hypoglycemia.
• Caution patient not to take antidiabetic drugs unless prescribed.
• Advise patient to notify prescriber if she experiences signs of hyperglycemia, such as increased urinary frequency, increased thirst, and fruity breath.

dichloralphenazone
(all contain 325 mg of acetaminophen, 100 mg of dichloralphenazone, and 65 mg of isometheptene mucate)

Amidrine, I.D.A., Iso-Acetozone, Isocom, Midchlor, Midrin, Migquin, Migragap, Migratine, Migrazone, Migrend, Migrex, Mitride

Class and Category
Chemical: Sympathomimetic amine
Therapeutic: Analgesic
Pregnancy category: Not rated

Indications and Dosages

➤ *To relieve tension headache*

CAPSULES

Adults. 1 to 2 caps q 4 hr. *Maximum:* 8 caps/day.

➤ *To relieve migraine headache*

CAPSULES

Adults. 2 caps followed by 1 cap q hr until relief occurs. *Maximum:* 5 caps/12 hr.

Route	Onset	Peak	Duration
P.O.	30 to 60 min	1 to 3 hr	3 to 4 hr

Mechanism of Action

Acetaminophen raises the pain threshold by acting on the hypothalamus. Dichloralphenazone reduces the patient's emotional reaction to pain through its mild sedative effect. Isometheptene constricts dilated cranial and cerebral arterioles through sympathomimetic action, which reduces stimuli that lead to vascular headaches.

Contraindications

Heart disease, hepatic disease, hypersensitivity to acetaminophen or isometheptene, MAO inhibitor therapy within 14 days, severe renal disease, uncontrolled glaucoma, uncontrolled hypertension

Interactions

DRUGS

CNS depressants: Additive sedative effects
hepatic enzyme inducers, other hepatotoxic drugs: Increased risk of hepatotoxicity
MAO inhibitors: Increased risk of severe hypertension and hyperpyrexia

ACTIVITIES

alcohol use: Additive sedative effects, increased risk of hepatotoxicity

Adverse Reactions

CNS: Dizziness, drowsiness
SKIN: Rash

Nursing Considerations

•Because dichloralphenazone has vasoconstrictive and sympathomimetic actions, assess patients with peripheral vascular disease or recent angina pectoris or MI for signs and symptoms indicating aggravation or deterioration of these conditions.
•Institute safety precautions to prevent injury from falls.

PATIENT TEACHING

•**WARNING** Caution patient not to take dichloralphenazone if she has taken an MAO inhibitor within the past 14 days; doing so can cause severe hypertension or hyperpyrexia.
•Advise patient to take drug only after a headache or migraine warning sign occurs. Too-frequent use may make drug less effective and may worsen headaches.
•Instruct patient to lie down in a quiet, dark room after taking drug.
•Because of possible dizziness or drowsiness, advise patient to avoid potentially hazardous activities until drug's CNS effects are known.
•Caution patient to avoid alcohol and CNS depressants during therapy because they increase dizziness, drowsiness, and the risk of hepatotoxicity.
•Advise patient to notify prescriber if drug becomes less effective or if headaches occur more frequently.
•Teach patient how to read drug labels to avoid taking too much acetaminophen, which can cause hepatic or renal damage.
•Inform patient that decreasing the dose may prevent transient dizziness or rash.
•Instruct patient to store drug away from heat, moisture, and direct light.

dichlorphenamide

Daranide

Class and Category

Chemical: Sulfonamide derivative
Therapeutic: Antiglaucoma
Pregnancy category: C

Indications and Dosages

➤ *To manage chronic open-angle glaucoma, secondary glaucoma, and acute angle-closure glaucoma (preoperatively)*

TABLETS

Adults. *Initial:* 100 to 200 mg followed by 100 mg q 12 hr. *Maintenance:* 25 to 50 mg q.d. to t.i.d.

Route	Onset	Peak	Duration
P.O.	30 to 60 min	2 to 4 hr	6 to 12 hr

Contraindications

Adrenocortical insufficiency, hepatic insufficiency, hyperchloremic acidosis, hypersensitivity to dichlorphenamide or sulfa drugs, hypokalemia, hyponatremia, renal failure, severe obstructive pulmonary disease

Mechanism of Action

Inhibits the enzyme carbonic anhydrase, which normally exists in renal proximal tubule cells, choroid plexes of the brain, and ciliary processes of the eyes. In the eyes, enzyme inhibition decreases aqueous humor secretion, which reduces intraocular pressure.

Interactions

DRUGS

diflunisal: Increased adverse effects of dichlorphenamide, significantly decreased intraocular pressure

salicylates: Increased risk of dichlorphenamide toxicity, including CNS depression and metabolic acidosis

Adverse Reactions

CNS: Depression, disorientation, dizziness, drowsiness, lassitude, paresthesia
CV: Arrhythmias
EENT: Metallic taste, pharyngitis
ENDO: Hyperglycemia
GI: Anorexia, diarrhea, hepatic dysfunction, nausea, vomiting
GU: Phosphaturia, renal calculi, renal colic, urinary frequency
HEME: Hemolytic anemia, leukopenia, pancytopenia, thrombocytopenia
SKIN: Photosensitivity
Other: Hyperchloremia, hyperuricemia, weight loss

Nursing Considerations

•Use dichlorphenamide cautiously in patients with severe respiratory acidosis, pulmonary obstruction, or emphysema.
•Frequently monitor serum potassium level (especially in elderly patients and those taking digoxin) because diuresis may cause hypokalemia.

PATIENT TEACHING

•Instruct patient to take dichlorphenamide with food or full glass of water to decrease GI distress.
•Advise patient to avoid potentially hazardous activities until drug's CNS effects are known.
•**WARNING** Urge patient to immediately report signs of blood dyscrasias, such as sore throat, fever, unusual bleeding or bruising, numbness or tingling, and rash.
•Advise patient to avoid prolonged exposure to sunlight, to apply sunscreen, and to wear protective clothing outdoors.
•Instruct patient to take a missed dose as soon as she remembers it, unless it's almost time for the next dose.
•Advise patient to store drug at room temperature, away from moisture and heat.

diclofenac potassium

Cataflam, Voltaren Rapide (CAN)

diclofenac sodium

Apo-Diclo (CAN), Novo-Difenac (CAN), Nu-Diclo (CAN), Voltaren, Voltaren SR (CAN)

Class and Category

Chemical: Phenylacetic acid derivative
Therapeutic: Analgesic, anti-inflammatory
Pregnancy category: B

Indications and Dosages

➤ *To relieve pain and inflammation in rheumatoid arthritis*
DELAYED-RELEASE TABLETS, TABLETS
Adults. *Initial:* 150 to 200 mg/day in divided doses t.i.d. or q.i.d. *Maintenance:* 75 to 100 mg/day in divided doses t.i.d. *Maximum:* 225 mg/day.
E.R. TABLETS
Adults. *Initial:* 75 or 100 mg q.d. in the morning or evening, or 75 mg b.i.d. in the morning and evening.
RECTAL SUPPOSITORIES
Adults. 50 or 100 mg as substitute for last P.O. dose of day.

➤ *To relieve pain and inflammation in osteoarthritis*
DELAYED-RELEASE TABLETS, TABLETS
Adults. 100 to 150 mg/day in divided doses b.i.d. or t.i.d. *Maximum:* 150 mg/day.

➤ *To relieve pain in ankylosing spondylitis*
DELAYED-RELEASE TABLETS, TABLETS
Adults. 100 to 125 mg/day in 4 or 5 divided doses.

➤ *To relieve pain and dysmenorrhea*
TABLETS
Adults. 50 mg t.i.d., p.r.n.; if needed, 100 mg for first dose only.

DOSAGE ADJUSTMENT Dosage reduced, if needed, for elderly patients and those with serious renal dysfunction.

Route	Onset	Peak	Duration
P.O.*	30 min	Unknown	8 hr

Mechanism of Action
Blocks the activity of cyclooxygenase, the enzyme needed to synthesize prostaglandins, which mediate the inflammatory response and cause local vasodilation, swelling, and pain. By blocking cyclooxygenase and inhibiting prostaglandins, diclofenac reduces inflammatory symptoms. This mechanism also relieves pain because prostaglandins promote pain transmission from the periphery to the spinal cord.

Contraindications
Active GI bleeding or ulcers; asthma attacks, rhinitis, or urticaria precipitated by aspirin or other NSAIDs; hypersensitivity to diclofenac or NSAIDs

Interactions
DRUGS
acetaminophen: Increased risk of adverse renal effects with long-term concurrent use
anticoagulants, thrombolytics: Prolonged PT, increased risk of bleeding
antihypertensives: Decreased antihypertensive effectiveness
aspirin, other NSAIDs, salicylates: Increased GI irritability and bleeding, decreased diclofenac effectiveness
beta blockers: Impaired antihypertensive effects
cefamandole, cefoperazone, cefotetan, plicamycin, valproic acid: Increased risk of hypoprothrombinemia
cimetidine: Altered blood diclofenac level
colchicine, corticotropin (long-term use), glucocorticoids, potassium supplements: Increased GI irritability and bleeding
cyclosporine, gold compounds, nephrotoxic drugs: Increased risk of nephrotoxicity
digoxin: Increased serum digoxin level
insulin, oral antidiabetic drugs: Decreased effects of these drugs

lithium: Increased risk of lithium toxicity
loop diuretics: Decreased loop diuretic effectiveness
methotrexate: Increased risk of methotrexate toxicity
phenytoin: Increased blood phenytoin level
potassium-sparing diuretics: Increased risk of hyperkalemia
probenecid: Increased diclofenac toxicity
FOODS
food: Delayed absorption of delayed-release tablets
ACTIVITIES
alcohol use: Increased risk of GI irritability and bleeding

Adverse Reactions
CNS: Dizziness, drowsiness, headache
CV: Bradycardia and other arrhythmias, hypotension, vasculitis
EENT: Glaucoma, hearing loss, tinnitus
GI: Abdominal pain, constipation, diarrhea, dysphagia, elevated liver function test results, esophageal ulceration, flatulence, GI ulceration, indigestion, nausea
HEME: Eosinophilia, leukocytosis, pancytopenia, porphyria
SKIN: Pruritus, rash
Other: Fluid retention, hyperkalemia, hyperuricemia, hyponatremia, lymphadenopathy

Nursing Considerations
• Monitor liver function test results and serum uric acid level. Liver enzyme elevations usually occur within 2 months of starting diclofenac therapy.
• Report weight gain of more than 1 kg (2 lb) in 24 hours, which suggests fluid retention.
• Report signs of bleeding, such as petechiae, ecchymoses, bleeding gums, melena, and cloudy or bloody urine. Monitor patient for signs of GI irritation and ulceration, especially if patient has predisposing conditions, such as a history of GI bleeding; takes an oral corticosteroid, anticoagulant, or NSAID (long-term); smokes; is an alcoholic; is over age 60; has poor general health; or tests positive for *Helicobacter pylori.*
• Assess for hypotension. If patient takes a potassium-sparing diuretic, check for elevated serum potassium level.
PATIENT TEACHING
• Advise patient not to chew, crush, or dissolve diclofenac tablet, but to swallow it whole.

* For tablets; unknown for delayed-release and E.R. tablets.

•Instruct patient to take drug with food to minimize GI distress.

•To decrease risk of esophageal ulceration, instruct patient not to lie down for 15 to 30 minutes after taking drug.

•Warn patient to avoid potentially hazardous activities until drug's CNS effects are known.

•Instruct patient to notify prescriber if she experiences ringing or buzzing in the ears, impaired hearing, dizziness, or GI distress or bleeding.

•Advise patient to consult prescriber before taking aspirin or other OTC analgesics or using alcohol.

•Inform patient that drug increases the risk of inflammation, bleeding, ulceration, and perforation of the stomach and intestines, possibly without warning.

dicloxacillin sodium

Dycill, Dynapen, Pathocil

Class and Category

Chemical: Isoxazolyl penicillin derivative
Therapeutic: Antibiotic
Pregnancy category: B

Indications and Dosages

➤ *To treat mild to moderate upper respiratory tract and localized skin and soft-tissue infections caused by penicillinase-producing staphylococci*

CAPSULES, ORAL SOLUTION
Adults and children who weigh 40 kg (88 lb) or more. 125 mg q 6 hr.
Children who weigh less than 40 kg. 12.5 mg/kg/day divided into 4 equal doses and given q 6 hr.

➤ *To treat severe infections, such as lower respiratory tract or disseminated infections, caused by penicillinase-producing staphylococci*

CAPSULES, ORAL SOLUTION
Adults and children who weigh 40 kg or more. 250 mg q 6 hr, or higher doses, if needed. *Maximum:* 6 g/day.
Children over age 1 month who weigh less than 40 kg. 25 mg/kg/day divided into 4 equal doses and given q 6 hr, or higher doses if needed.

Mechanism of Action

Inhibits cell wall synthesis in susceptible bacteria. These bacteria assemble rigid, cross-linked cell walls in several steps. Dicloxacillin affects the final stage of cross-linking by binding with and inactivating penicillin-binding protein (the enzyme responsible for linking cell wall strands). This action inhibits cell wall synthesis and causes cell lysis and death.

Contraindications

Hypersensitivity to dicloxacillin, other penicillins, beta-lactamase inhibitors (such as piperacillin and tazobactam), cephalosporins, imipenem, or their components

Interactions

DRUGS
hepatotoxic drugs: Increased risk of hepatotoxicity
methotrexate: Decreased methotrexate clearance, increased risk of methotrexate toxicity
oral contraceptives: Decreased contraceptive action
probenecid: Increased and prolonged serum dicloxacillin concentration
tetracyclines: Decreased dicloxacillin effectiveness

FOODS
all foods: Possibly delayed absorption

Adverse Reactions

CNS: Dizziness, fatigue, fever, insomnia
EENT: Black "hairy" tongue, dry mouth, glossitis, laryngeal edema, laryngospasm, stomatitis, taste perversion
GI: Abdominal pain, anorexia, diarrhea, flatulence, nausea, pseudomembranous colitis, transient hepatitis, vomiting
GU: Nephropathy, vaginitis
MS: Prolonged muscle relaxation
SKIN: Dermatitis, erythema multiforme, pruritus, rash, urticaria, vesicular eruptions
Other: Anaphylaxis, serum sickness, superinfection

Nursing Considerations

•Before dicloxacillin therapy begins, expect to obtain body fluid and tissue samples for culture and sensitivity tests, as ordered, and review the results, if possible. Also check for history of sensitivity to penicillins, cephalosporins, and other substances.

•If diarrhea develops, notify prescriber because of possibility of pseudomembranous colitis.

PATIENT TEACHING

•Instruct patient to take dicloxacillin 1 hour before or 2 hours after meals.
•Instruct patient to take drug around the clock, not to miss a dose, and to complete the entire prescription unless directed otherwise by prescriber.
•Advise patient to take oral solution with a cold beverage but not acidic juice, such as orange juice. Explain that solution is effective for 7 days at room temperature and for 14 days if refrigerated.
•Caution patient not to open capsules and mix contents with food or liquids because an unpleasant taste and decreased drug absorption will result.
•Instruct parent to shake oral solution thoroughly and measure doses with a calibrated device for accuracy.
•Advise patient to notify prescriber if she experiences adverse GI reactions or signs of hypersensitivity or superinfection.
•If patient takes an oral contraceptive, advise her to use an additional form of contraception during therapy.
•Instruct patient to store drug away from heat, moisture, and direct light and to refrigerate—but not freeze—oral solution.

dicumarol

Class and Category

Chemical: Coumarin derivative
Therapeutic: Anticoagulant
Pregnancy category: X

Indications and Dosages

➤ *To prevent and treat pulmonary embolus, thromboembolus, and venous thrombus; to prevent thromboembolism related to atrial fibrillation and mechanical heart valves*

TABLETS

Adults. *Initial:* 200 to 300 mg on the first day. *Maintenance:* 25 to 200 mg q.d.

DOSAGE ADJUSTMENT Dosage reduced for elderly patients and those with hepatic or renal impairment.

Route	Onset	Peak	Duration
P.O.	1 to 5 days	Unknown	5 to 6 days

Mechanism of Action

Prevents coagulation by interfering with the liver's ability to synthesize vitamin K–dependent clotting factors. This in turn depletes clotting factors II (prothrombin), VII, IX, and X. Normally, clots result from a cascade of proteolytic reactions that involve several clotting factors, including vitamin K–dependent factors. These clotting factors must be converted to an activated form before the clotting cascade can continue. By depleting vitamin K–dependent clotting factors, dicumarol interferes with the clotting cascade and prevents coagulation.

Contraindications

Active bleeding; aneurysm; ascorbic acid deficiency; bacterial endocarditis; blood dyscrasia; continuous tube drainage of small intestine; CVA; diverticulitis; eclampsia or preclampsia; emaciation; hemophilia; hemorrhagic tendency; history of bleeding diathesis or warfarin-induced necrosis; leukemia; major regional lumbar block anesthesia; malnutrition; pericardial effusion; pericarditis; polyarthritis; pregnancy; prostatectomy; recent surgery on brain, eye, GI tract, or prostate; recovery from spinal puncture; severe hepatic or renal impairment; surgery resulting in large, open surfaces; threatened abortion; thrombocytopenic purpura; uncontrolled or malignant hypertension; visceral cancer; vitamin K deficiency

Interactions

DRUGS

acetaminophen, androgens, beta blockers, chlorpropamide, clofibrate, corticosteroids, cyclophosphamide, dextrothyroxine, disulfiram, erythromycin, fluconazole, gemfibrozil, glucagon, hydantoins, influenza virus vaccine, isoniazid, ketoconazole, miconazole, moricizine, propoxyphene, quinolones, streptokinase, sulfonamides, tamoxifen, thioamines, thyroid drugs, urokinase: Increased effects of dicumarol and risk of bleeding

Adverse Reactions

CNS: Fever, malaise
ENDO: Adrenal hemorrhage

GI: Abdominal cramps and distention, anorexia, diarrhea, flatulence, nausea, vomiting
GU: Menorrhagia, priapism
HEME: Hemorrhage, leukopenia
SKIN: Alopecia, pruritus, rash, urticaria
Other: Allergic reaction, purple toes syndrome

Nursing Considerations
• Use dicumarol cautiously in elderly patients and in those with hepatic or renal impairment.
• Monitor results of serial tests for PT and INR and expect to adjust dosage accordingly.
• If patient also receives heparin, expect heparin therapy to continue until INR reaches desired level: 2 to 3 times the control value for pulmonary embolus, thromboembolus, or venous thrombus; or 3 to 4.5 times the control value for thromboembolism related to atrial fibrillation or mechanical valves.
• If PT or INR are prolonged, withhold one dose of dicumarol, as prescribed. To reverse anticoagulation immediately, give vitamin K, as prescribed. If patient has severe bleeding, expect to administer blood to offset vitamin K's delayed onset.
• Assess for signs of hemorrhage, such as gingival bleeding, ecchymosis, epistaxis, hematuria, and melena.
• To avoid excessive bleeding, apply pressure to I.M. or venipuncture sites for up to 5 minutes.

PATIENT TEACHING
• Instruct patient to take dicumarol at the same time every day.
• Inform patient that drug's full effects may not occur for 2 to 7 days.
• Instruct patient to have frequent coagulation tests, as prescribed.
• Advise patient to stabilize her intake of foods high in vitamin K. Urge her to consult prescriber before starting a reducing diet, altering eating habits, or taking new vitamins or other nutritional supplements; these activities may alter her vitamin K intake.
• Caution patient to avoid activities that may cause bleeding. Advise the use of a soft toothbrush and an electric razor.
• Encourage patient to consult prescriber before taking OTC drugs, including herbs, which may affect dicumarol's anticoagulant effect.
• Instruct patient to take a missed dose as soon as she remembers unless it's nearly time

for the next dose. Urge her to report missed doses to prescriber.
• Caution patient to immediately notify prescriber if signs of bleeding occur, such as abdominal pain or swelling; back pain; bloody or black stools; bloody urine; coughing up blood; joint pain, swelling, or stiffness; severe or continuing headache; and vomiting blood or material that looks like coffee grounds.
• Urge patient to carry medical identification and tell all health care providers that she takes dicumarol.
• Explain that coagulation will gradually return to normal after therapy stops. Remind her to continue watching for signs of bleeding.

dicyclomine hydrochloride

Bentyl, Bentylol (CAN), Formulex (CAN), Spasmoban (CAN)

Class and Category
Chemical: Tertiary amine
Therapeutic: Anticholinergic, antispasmodic
Pregnancy category: Not rated

Indications and Dosages
➤ *To control diarrhea and GI tract spasms*
CAPSULES, TABLETS
Adults and adolescents. 10 to 20 mg t.i.d. or q.i.d., increased as needed and tolerated. *Maximum:* 160 mg/day.
Children ages 6 to 12. 10 mg t.i.d. or q.i.d.
E.R. TABLETS
Adults and adolescents. 30 mg b.i.d.
SYRUP
Adults and adolescents. 10 to 20 mg t.i.d. or q.i.d., increased as needed and tolerated. *Maximum:* 60 mg/day.
Children ages 2 to 13. 10 mg t.i.d. or q.i.d.
Children ages 6 months to 2 years. 5 to 10 mg t.i.d. or q.i.d.
I.M. INJECTION
Adults. 20 mg q 4 to 6 hr. Dosage adjusted as needed and tolerated.

Contraindications
Adhesions between iris and lens, GI obstruction, hemorrhagic shock, hepatic disease, hiatal hernia, hypersensitivity to any anticholinergic, ileus, intestinal atony in elderly or debilitated patients, myasthenia gravis, myocar-

dial ischemia, narrow-angle glaucoma, obstructive uropathy, renal disease, severe ulcerative colitis, tachycardia, toxic megacolon

Mechanism of Action
Inhibits acetylcholine's muscarinic actions at postganglionic parasympathetic receptors in smooth muscles, secretory glands, and the CNS. These actions relax smooth muscles and diminish GI, GU, and biliary tract secretions.

Interactions
DRUGS
adsorbent antidiarrheals, antacids: Decreased dicyclomine absorption
amantadine, anticholinergics, phenothiazines, tricyclic antidepressants: Increased dicyclomine effects
antimyasthenics: Reduced intestinal motility
atenolol: Increased atenolol effects
cyclopropane: Risk of ventricular arrhythmias
haloperidol: Decreased antipsychotic effect of haloperidol
ketoconazole: Decreased ketoconazole absorption
metoclopramide: Decreased effect of metoclopramide on GI motility
opioid analgesics: Increased risk of ileus, severe constipation, and urine retention
potassium chloride, especially wax-matrix preparations: Possibly GI ulcers
urinary alkalizers (calcium or magnesium antacids, carbonic anhydrase inhibitors, citrates, sodium bicarbonate): Delayed excretion and increased risk of adverse effects of dicyclomine

Adverse Reactions
CNS: Agitation, dizziness, drowsiness, dyskinesia, excitement, fever, insomnia, lethargy, light-headedness (with I.M. use), nervousness, paresthesia, syncope
CV: Palpitations, tachycardia
EENT: Blurred vision, cycloplegia, dry mouth, loss of taste, mydriasis, nasal congestion, photophobia
GI: Constipation, dysphagia, heartburn, ileus, vomiting
GU: Impotence, urine retention
SKIN: Decreased sweating, flushing, pruritus
Other: Heatstroke; injection site pain, redness, and swelling

Nursing Considerations
•Assess for tachycardia before giving dicyclomine because it may increase heart rate.
•Don't give drug by I.V. route.
•Monitor for symptoms of hypersensitivity, such as agitation and pruritus. They usually resolve within 48 hours after stopping drug.
•During long-term use, assess for chronic constipation and fecal impaction and take apropriate measures, as prescribed.
PATIENT TEACHING
•Instruct patient to store dicyclomine in a tightly sealed container at room temperature, protected from moisture and direct light. Advise her not to refrigerate syrup.
•Inform patient that drug relieves symptoms but doesn't cure underlying disorder.
•For best results, instruct patient to take drug 30 to 60 minutes before eating.
•Advise patient not to take an antacid or antidiarrheal within 2 hours of taking dicyclomine.
•Inform patient that blurred vision, dizziness, or drowsiness may occur.
•To prevent constipation, advise patient to eat high-fiber foods and drink at least 8 glasses of water daily.
•**WARNING** Urge patient to avoid getting overheated during exercise or in hot weather because heatstroke may result. Inform patient that hot baths or saunas may cause dizziness or fainting.
•Instruct patient to change position slowly to avoid light-headedness.
•Inform patient that stopping drug abruptly may cause vomiting and dizziness.
•Advise patient to take a missed dose as soon as she remembers unless it's nearly time for the next dose. Caution her not to double-dose.

difenoxin hydrochloride and atropine sulfate

Motofen

Class, Category, and Schedule
Chemical: Meperidine analogue (difenoxin), tertiary amine belladonna alkaloid (atropine)
Therapeutic: Antidiarrheal
Pregnancy category: C
Controlled substance: Schedule IV

Indications and Dosages
➤ *To treat acute and chronic diarrhea*
TABLETS
Adults and adolescents. 2 mg (difenoxin) immediately and then 1 mg (difenoxin) after each loose stool or q 3 to 4 hr, p.r.n. *Maximum:* 8 mg (difenoxin)/day.
DOSAGE ADJUSTMENT Dosage reduced for patients with hepatic or renal dysfunction.

Mechanism of Action
Directly affects circular smooth muscles of the GI tract, reducing intestinal motility. Subtherapeutic doses of atropine help prevent drug abuse.

Contraindications
Diarrhea caused by pseudomembranous enterocolitis or enterotoxin-producing bacteria, such as *Escherichia coli, Salmonella* sp., or *Shigella* sp.; hypersensitivity to atropine, difenoxin, diphenoxylate, or their components; narrow-angle glaucoma; obstructive jaundice

Interactions
DRUGS
barbiturates, narcotics, tranquilizers: Possibly potentiated effects of these drugs
MAO inhibitors: Possibly hypertensive crisis
naltrexone: Possibly precipitated withdrawal symptoms (in patient physically dependent on difenoxin) and intereference with difenoxin's therapeutic effects
ACTIVITIES
alcohol use: Possibly potentiated effects of difenoxin

Adverse Reactions
CNS: Confusion, dizziness, drowsiness, euphoria, fatigue, headache, insomnia, lethargy, light-headedness, nervousness, sedation
EENT: Dry mouth
GI: Abdominal distention and pain, anorexia, constipation, nausea, pancreatitis, vomiting
SKIN: Pruritus, urticaria
Other: Physical and psychological dependence

Nursing Considerations
•Closely monitor patients who are elderly or very ill or who have respiratory problems; they're more sensitive to drug's effects and may require a lower dosage.

PATIENT TEACHING
•Inform patient that diarrhea may not be controlled for 12 to 24 hours but that abdominal cramps usually subside in 30 to 90 minutes. Advise patient to consult prescriber if diarrhea doesn't improve within 2 days.
•Instruct patient to continue taking drug until diarrhea has stopped for 24 to 36 hours.
•Urge patient to consult prescriber before consuming alcohol or CNS depressants.
•Advise patient to avoid potentially hazardous activities until drug's CNS effects are known.
•Instruct patient to protect drug from heat, moisture, and direct light.

diflunisal
Apo-Diflunisal (CAN), Dolobid, Novo-Diflunisal (CAN)

Class and Category
Chemical: Difluorophenyl, salicylic acid derivative
Therapeutic: Analgesic, anti-inflammatory
Pregnancy category: C (first trimester), Not rated (later trimesters)

Indications and Dosages
➤ *To relieve mild to moderate pain*
TABLETS
Adults. 1 g followed by 0.5 g q 8 to 12 hr. *Maximum:* 1.5 g/day.
➤ *To reduce inflammation in osteoarthritis or rheumatoid arthritis*
TABLETS
Adults. 0.5 to 1 g/day in divided doses b.i.d. *Maximum:* 1.5 g/day.
DOSAGE ADJUSTMENT Dosage reduced for elderly patients and those who use diuretics; who could be harmed by prolonged bleeding time; or who have compromised cardiac function, conditions that cause fluid retention, hepatic or renal impairment, hypertension, or upper GI disease.

Route	Onset	Peak	Duration
P.O.*	1 hr	2 to 3 hr	8 to 12 hr

* For analgesia; unknown for anti-inflammatory effects.

Mechanism of Action

Blocks the activity of cyclooxygenase, the enzyme needed to synthesize prostaglandins, which mediate the inflammatory response and cause local vasodilation, swelling, and pain. By blocking cyclooxygenase and inhibiting prostaglandins, this NSAID reduces inflammatory symptoms. This mechanism also relieves pain because prostaglandins promote pain transmission from the periphery to the spinal cord.

Contraindications

Asthma attacks, rhinitis, or urticaria precipitated by aspirin or other NSAIDs; hypersensitivity to diflunisal

Interactions

Drugs

acetaminophen: Increased risk of adverse renal effects with long-term use of both drugs
antacids: Decreased blood diflunisal level
antihypertensives: Decreased antihypertensive effects
aspirin, other NSAIDs, salicylates: Increased GI irritability and bleeding, decreased diflunisal effectiveness
beta blockers: Impaired antihypertensive effects of beta blocker
cefamandole, cefoperazone, cefotetan, plicamycin, valproic acid: Increased risk of hypoprothrombinemia
colchicine, corticotropin (long-term use), glucocorticoids, potassium supplements: Increased GI irritability and bleeding
cyclosporine, gold compounds, nephrotoxic drugs: Increased risk of nephrotoxicity
digoxin: Increased serum digoxin level
heparin, oral anticoagulants, thrombolytics: Prolonged PT, increased risk of bleeding
hydrochlorothiazide: Increased blood hydrochlorothiazide level
insulin, oral antidiabetic drugs: Increased hypoglycemic effects
loop diuretics: Decreased loop diuretic effectiveness
methotrexate: Increased risk of methotrexate toxicity
phenytoin: Increased blood phenytoin level
probenecid: Increased diflunisal toxicity

Activities

alcohol use: Increased GI irritability and bleeding

Adverse Reactions

CNS: Dizziness, drowsiness, headache, insomnia
EENT: Tinnitus
GI: Abdominal pain, constipation, diarrhea, esophageal irritation, GI bleeding, indigestion, nausea, vomiting
SKIN: Rash

Nursing Considerations

• Use diflunisal cautiously in elderly patients, those who have renal dysfunction or history of upper GI disease, and those who should avoid prolonged bleeding time.
• Assess the pain's type, location, and intensity before and 1 to 2 hours after giving drug.
• Assess patient carefully because long-term or high-dose therapy may mask fever.

Patient Teaching

• Teach patient not to crush or chew diflunisal tablets.
• Instruct patient to take tablet with a full glass of water and not to lie down for 30 minutes afterward to avoid esophageal irritation.
• Inform patient that drug will start working in about 1 week but that full effects may not occur for several weeks.
• Caution patient to avoid acetaminophen, alcohol, aspirin, and other salicylates during diflunisal therapy, unless directed otherwise by prescriber.
• Instruct patient to promptly notify prescriber about black stools, bloody vomitus, ringing in ears, and severe stomach pain.
• Advise patient to avoid potentially hazardous activities until drug's CNS effects are known.
• Advise patient to tell health care providers about diflunisal therapy before surgery, including dental surgery. Therapy should stop for 1 week before procedure.

digoxin

Lanoxicaps, Lanoxin, Lanoxin Elixir Pediatric, Lanoxin Injection, Lanoxin Injection Pediatric, Novo-Digoxin (CAN)

Class and Category

Chemical: Digitalis glycoside
Therapeutic: Antiarrhythmic, cardiotonic
Pregnancy category: C

Indications and Dosages

➤ *To treat heart failure, atrial flutter, atrial fibrillation, and paroxysmal atrial tachycardia with rapid digitalization*

CAPSULES, I.V. INJECTION

Adults. *Loading:* 10 to 15 mcg/kg in 3 divided doses q 6 to 8 hr, with first dose equal to 50% of total dose. *Maintenance:* 125 to 350 mcg/day q.d. or b.i.d.

Children over age 10. *Loading:* 8 to 12 mcg/kg in 3 or more divided doses, with first dose equal to 50% of total dose. Subsequent doses given q 6 to 8 hr. *Maintenance:* 2 to 3 mcg/kg/day q.d.

Children ages 6 to 10. *Loading:* 15 to 30 mcg/kg in 3 or more divided doses, with first dose equal to 50% of total dose. Subsequent doses given q 6 to 8 hr. *Maintenance:* 4 to 8 mcg/kg/day in 2 divided doses.

Children ages 2 to 5. *Loading:* 25 to 35 mcg/kg in 3 or more divided doses, with first dose equal to 50% of total dose. Subsequent doses given q 6 to 8 hr. *Maintenance:* 6 to 9 mcg/kg/day in 2 divided doses.

Infants ages 1 to 24 months. *Loading:* 30 to 50 mcg/kg in 3 or more divided doses, with first dose equal to 50% of total dose. Subsequent doses given q 6 to 8 hr. *Maintenance:* 7.5 to 12 mcg/kg/day in 2 divided doses.

Full-term neonates. *Loading:* 20 to 30 mcg/kg in 3 or more divided doses, with first dose equal to 50% of total dose. Subsequent doses given q 6 to 8 hr. *Maintenance:* 5 to 8 mcg/kg/day in 2 divided doses.

Premature neonates. *Loading:* 15 to 25 mcg/kg in 3 or more divided doses, with first dose equal to 50% of total dose. Subsequent doses given q 6 to 8 hr. *Maintenance:* 4 to 6 mcg/kg/day in 2 divided doses.

ELIXIR, TABLETS

Adults. *Loading:* 10 to 15 mcg/kg total dose given in 3 divided doses q 6 to 8 hr, with first dose equal to 50% of total dose. *Maintenance:* 125 to 500 mcg/day.

Children over age 10. *Loading:* 10 to 15 mcg/kg total dose given in 3 divided doses q 6 to 8 hr, with first dose equal to 50% of total dose. *Maintenance:* 2.5 to 5 mcg/kg/day.

Children ages 5 to 10. *Loading:* 20 to 35 mcg/kg in 3 divided doses q 6 to 8 hr. *Maintenance:* 5 to 10 mcg/kg/day in 2 divided doses.

Children ages 2 to 5. *Loading:* 30 to 40 mcg/kg in 3 divided doses q 6 to 8 hr. *Maintenance:* 7.5 to 10 mcg/kg/day in 2 divided doses.

Infants ages 1 to 24 months. *Loading:* 35 to 60 mcg/kg in 3 divided doses q 6 to 8 hr. *Maintenance:* 10 to 15 mcg/kg/day in 2 divided doses.

Full-term neonates. *Loading:* 25 to 35 mcg/kg in 3 divided doses q 6 to 8 hr. *Maintenance:* 6 to 10 mcg/kg/day in 2 divided doses.

Premature neonates. *Loading:* 20 to 30 mcg/kg in 3 divided doses q 6 to 8 hr. *Maintenance:* 5 to 7.5 mcg/kg/day in 2 divided doses.

DOSAGE ADJUSTMENT Dosage carefully adjusted for patients who are elderly or debilitated or have implanted pacemakers because toxicity may develop at doses tolerated by most patients.

Route	Onset	Peak	Duration
P.O.	30 to 120 min	6 to 8 hr	3 to 4 days
I.V.	5 to 30 min	1 to 5 hr	3 to 4 days

Mechanism of Action

Increases the force and velocity of myocardial contraction, resulting in positive inotropic effects. Digoxin produces antiarrhythmic effects by decreasing the conduction rate and increasing the effective refractory period of the AV node.

Contraindications

Hypersensitive carotid sinus syndrome, hypersensitivity to digoxin, presence or history of digitalis toxicity or idiosyncratic reaction to digoxin, ventricular fibrillation, ventricular tachycardia unless heart failure occurs unrelated to digoxin therapy

Interactions

DRUGS

adsorbent antidiarrheals, such as kaolin and pectin; bulk laxatives; cholestyramine; colestipol; oral neomycin; sulfasalazine: Inhibited digoxin absorption

amiodarone, propafenone: Elevated blood digoxin level, possibly to toxic level

antacids: Inhibited digoxin absorption

antiarrhythmics, pancuronium, parenteral calcium salts, rauwolfia alkaloids, sympathomimetics: Possibly increased risk of arrhythmias

diltiazem, verapamil: Increased blood digoxin level, possibly excessive bradycardia

edrophonium: Excessive slowing of heart rate

erythromycin, neomycin, tetracycline: Possibly increased blood digoxin level

hypokalemia-causing drugs, potassium-wasting diuretics: Increased risk of digitalis toxicity from hypokalemia

indomethacin: Decreased renal clearance and increased blood level of digoxin

magnesium sulfate (parenteral): Possibly cardiac conduction changes and heart block
quinidine, quinine: Increased blood digoxin level
spironolactone: Increased half-life and risk of adverse effects of digoxin
succinylcholine: Increased risk of digoxin-induced arrhythmias
sucralfate: Decreased digoxin absorption

FOODS
high-fiber food: Inhibited digoxin absorption

Adverse Reactions

CNS: Confusion, depression, drowsiness, extreme weakness, headache, syncope
CV: Arrhythmias, heart block
EENT: Blurred vision, colored halos around objects
GI: Abdominal discomfort or pain, anorexia, diarrhea, nausea, vomiting
Other: Electrolyte imbalances

Nursing Considerations

•Administer parenteral digoxin undiluted, or dilute with a fourfold or greater volume of sterile water for injection, NS, or D_5W for I.V. administration. Once diluted, administer immediately. Discard if solution is markedly discolored or contains precipitate.
•Before giving each dose, take patient's apical pulse and notify prescriber if pulse is below 60 beats/minute (or other specified level).
•Monitor closely for signs of digitalis toxicity: altered mental status, arrhythmias, heart block, nausea, vision disturbances, and vomiting. If they appear, notify prescriber, check serum digoxin level as ordered, and expect to withhold drug until level is known. Monitor ECG tracing continuously.
•If patient has acute or unstable chronic atrial fibrillation, assess for drug effectiveness. Ventricular rate may not normalize even when serum drug level falls within therapeutic range; raising the dosage probably won't produce a therapeutic effect and may lead to toxicity.
•Frequently obtain ECG tracings as ordered in elderly patients because of their smaller body mass and reduced renal clearance. Elderly patients, especially those with coronary insufficiency, are more susceptible to arrhythmias—particularly ventricular fibrillation—if digitalis toxicity occurs.
•Monitor serum potassium level regularly because hypokalemia predisposes to digitalis

toxicity and serious arrhythmias. Also monitor potassium level frequently when giving potassium salts because hyperkalemia in patients receiving digoxin can be fatal.

PATIENT TEACHING
•Stress the importance of taking digoxin exactly as prescribed. Warn patient about possible toxicity from taking too much and decreased effectiveness from taking too little.
•Instruct patient to take drug at the same time each day to help increase compliance.
•Teach patient how to take her pulse, and instruct her to do so before each dose. Urge her to notify prescriber if pulse falls below 60 beats/minute or suddenly increases.
•Inform patient that small, white 0.25-mg tablets can easily be confused with other drugs. Caution against carrying drug in anything other than original labeled container.
•Emphasize the need to use the special dropper supplied with elixir to ensure accurate dose measurement.
•Instruct patient to take a missed dose as soon as she remembers if within 12 hours of scheduled dose. If not, urge her to notify prescriber immediately.
•Urge patient to notify prescriber if she experiences adverse reactions, such as GI distress or pulse changes.
•Instruct patient to carry medical identification that indicates her need for digoxin.
•Advise patient to consult prescriber before using other drugs, including OTC preparations.

digoxin immune Fab (ovine)

Digibind

Class and Category

Chemical: Digoxin-specific antigen-binding fragments
Therapeutic: Digitalis glycoside antidote
Pregnancy category: C

Indications and Dosages

➤ *To treat acute toxicity from a known amount of digoxin elixir or tablets*

I.V. INJECTION
Adults and children. Individualized dosage based on amount ingested. Dose (mg) = dose ingested (mg) multiplied by 0.8 and then di-

vided by 0.5, multiplied by 38, and rounded up to next whole vial.

➤ *To treat acute toxicity from a known amount of digoxin capsules, digitoxin tablets, or I.V. injection of digoxin or digitoxin*

I.V. INJECTION
Adults and children. Individualized dosage based on amount ingested. Dose (mg) = dose ingested (mg) divided by 0.5, then multiplied by 38 and rounded up to next whole vial.

➤ *To treat acute toxicity from an unknown amount of digoxin or digitoxin during long-term therapy*

I.V. INJECTION
Adults and children. Individualized dosage for digoxin toxicity: dose (mg) = serum digoxin level (ng/ml) multiplied by body weight (kg), then divided by 100, and then multiplied by 38. Individualized dosage for digitoxin toxicity: dose (mg) = serum digitoxin level (ng/ml) multiplied by body weight (kg) and then divided by 1,000, multiplied by 38, and rounded up to next whole vial.

DOSAGE ADJUSTMENT Higher dose delivered, as prescribed, if the dose based on ingested amount differs substantially from the dose based on serum digoxin or digitoxin level. Dose repeated after several hours, if needed.

Route	Onset	Peak	Duration
I.V.	15 to 30 min	Unknown	8 to 12 hr

Mechanism of Action
Binds with digoxin or digitoxin molecules. The resulting complex is excreted through the kidneys. As the free serum digoxin level declines, tissue-bound digoxin enters the serum and also is bound and excreted.

Contraindications
Hypersensitivity to digoxin immune Fab

Adverse Reactions
CV: Increased ventricular rate (in atrial fibrillation), worsening of heart failure or low cardiac output
Other: Allergic reaction (difficulty breathing, urticaria), febrile reaction, hypokalemia

Nursing Consideratiosns
• Expect each 38-mg vial of purified digoxin immune Fab to bind about 0.5 mg of digoxin or digitoxin.
• Reconstitute for I.V. use by dissolving 38 mg in 4 ml of sterile water for injection to yield 9.5 mg/ml. Mix gently. Further dilute with NS to a convenient volume for I.V. infusion. For very small doses, reconstituted 38-mg vial may be diluted with 34 ml of NS to yield 1 mg/ml.
• WARNING Before administering digoxin immune Fab to high-risk patient, test for allergic reaction as prescribed by diluting 0.1 ml of reconstituted drug in 9.9 ml of sodium chloride for injection and then injecting 0.1 ml (9.5 mcg/0.1 ml) intradermally. After 20 minutes, observe for an urticarial wheal surrounded by erythema. Alternatively, perform a scratch test by placing one drop of 9.5 mcg/0.1 ml dilution on patient's skin and making a ¼" scratch through the drop with a sterile needle. Inspect site in 20 minutes. Test is considered positive if it produces a wheal surrounded by erythema. If test causes a systemic reaction, apply tourniquet above test site, notify prescriber, and prepare to respond to anaphylaxis. Be aware that if a skin or systemic reaction occurs, additional drug shouldn't be given unless essential; if more of the drug must be given, expect prescriber to pretreat patient with corticosteroids and diphenhydramine. Prescriber should be on standby to treat anaphylaxis.
• For an infant, reconstitute digoxin immune Fab as ordered and administer with a tuberculin syringe.
• When administering to a child, monitor for fluid volume overload.
• When giving a large dose, expect a faster onset but watch closely for febrile reaction.
• Administer I.V. infusion through a 0.22-micron membrane filter over 30 minutes. Keep in mind that drug may be given by rapid I.V. injection if cardiac arrest is imminent.
• Monitor serum potassium level frequently, especially during first few hours of therapy. The potassium level may drop rapidly.
PATIENT TEACHING
• Inform patient of the purpose of digoxin immune Fab and how it will be administered.
• Advise patient to notify you immediately if she experiences adverse reactions, especially difficulty breathing and urticaria.

dihydroergotamine mesylate

D.H.E. 45, Dihydroergotamine-Sandoz (CAN), Migranal

Class and Category
Chemical: Semisynthetic ergot alkaloid
Therapeutic: Antimigraine
Pregnancy category: X

Indications and Dosages
➤ *To treat acute migraine with or without aura*
I.V. INJECTION
Adults. 1 mg, repeated in 1 hr, if needed. *Maximum:* 6 mg/wk.
I.M. INJECTION
Adults. 1 mg at first sign of headache, repeated q hr up to 3 mg, if needed. *Maximum:* 3 mg/24 hr, 6 mg/wk.
NASAL SPRAY
Adults. 1 spray (0.5 mg) in each nostril, repeated in 15 min for a total dose of 2 sprays in each nostril or 2 mg. *Maximum:* 3 mg/24 hr, 4 mg/wk.

Route	Onset	Peak	Duration
I.V.	In 5 min	15 min to 2 hr	About 8 hr
I.M.	15 to 30 min	15 min to 2 hr	3 to 4 hr
Nasal	In 30 min	30 to 60 min	Unknown

Contraindications
Coronary artery disease, hemiplegic or basilar migraine, hepatic or renal impairment, hypersensitivity to dihydroergotamine or other ergot alkaloids, malnutrition, peripheral vascular disease or after vascular surgery, sepsis, severe pruritus, uncontrolled hypertension

Interactions
DRUGS
beta blockers: Possibly peripheral vasoconstriction and peripheral ischemia, increased risk of gangrene
macrolides: Possibly increased risk of vasospasm, acute ergotism with peripheral ischemia
nitrates: Decreased antianginal effects of nitrates

other ergot drugs, including ergoloid mesylates, ergonovine, methylergonovine, methysergide, and sumatriptan: Increased risk of serious adverse effects from nasal dihydroergotamine
systemic vasoconstrictors: Risk of severe hypertension

Mechanism of Action
Produces intracranial and peripheral vasoconstriction by binding to all known 5-hydroxytryptamine$_1$ (5-HT$_1$) receptors, alpha$_1$- and alpha$_2$-adrenergic receptors, and dopaminergic receptors. Activation of 5-HT$_1$ receptors on intracranial blood vessels probably constricts large intracranial arteries and closes arteriovenous anastomoses to relieve migraine headache. Activation of 5-HT$_1$ receptors on sensory nerves in the trigeminal system also may inhibit the release of pro-inflammatory neuropeptides.

Peripherally, dihydroergotamine causes vasoconstriction by stimulating alpha-adrenergic receptors. At therapeutic doses, it inhibits norepinephrine reuptake, increasing vasoconstriction. The drug constricts veins more than arteries, increasing venous return while decreasing venous stasis and pooling.

Adverse Reactions
CNS: Anxiety, confusion, dizziness, fatigue, headache, paresthesia, somnolence, weakness
CV: Bradycardia, chest pain, peripheral vasospasm (calf or heel pain with exertion, cool and cyanotic hands and feet, leg weakness, weak or absent pulses), tachycardia
EENT: Abnormal vision; dry mouth; epistaxis, nasal congestion or rhinitis, and sore nose (nasal spray); miosis; pharyngitis; sinusitis; taste perversion
GI: Diarrhea, nausea, vomiting
MS: Muscle stiffness
SKIN: Localized edema of face, feet, fingers, and lower legs; sensation of heat or warmth; sudden diaphoresis

Nursing Considerations
•**WARNING** Monitor for signs of dihydroergotamine overdose, such as abdominal pain, confusion, delirium, dizziness, dyspnea, head-

ache, nausea, pain in legs or arms, paresthesia, seizures, and vomiting.
• Assess peripheral pulses, skin sensation, warmth, and capillary refill. After giving nasal dihydroergotamine, monitor for signs of widespread blood vessel constriction and adverse reactions caused by decreased circulation to many body areas.

PATIENT TEACHING
• Instruct patient to use nasal spray when headache pain—not aura—begins.
• Teach her to prime spray pump by squeezing it four times.
• Advise patient to wait 15 minutes between each set of nasal sprays.
• Encourage patient to lie down in a quiet, dark room after using drug.
• Instruct patient to use more drug if headache returns or worsens but not to exceed maximum prescribed amount or dosing schedule.
• Instruct patient to discard residual nasal spray in an open ampule after 8 hours.
• If patient experiences a headache different from her usual migraines, caution her not to use dihydroergotamine and to notify prescriber.
• Inform patient that nasal form of drug won't relieve pain other than throbbing headaches.
• Advise patient to avoid alcohol, which can exacerbate or cause headaches.
• Warn patient about possible dizziness during or after a migraine for which she took dihydroergotamine.

dihydrotachysterol

DHT, DHT Intensol, Hytakerol

Class and Category

Chemical: Sterol derivative, vitamin D analogue
Therapeutic: Antihypocalcemic, antihypoparathyroid
Pregnancy category: C

Indications and Dosages

➤ *To treat hypocalcemic and idiopathic tetany*

CAPSULES, ORAL SOLUTION, TABLETS
Adults and adolescents. *Initial:* 0.75 to 2.5 mg q.d. for 3 days for acute cases; 0.25 to 0.5 mg q.d. for 3 days for less acute cases. *Maintenance:* 0.25 mg/wk to 1 mg q.d., as needed to maintain normal serum calcium level.

➤ *To treat hypoparathyroidism*

CAPSULES, ORAL SOLUTION, TABLETS
Adults and adolescents. *Initial:* 0.75 to 2.5 mg q.d. for several days. *Maintenance:* 0.2 to 1 mg q.d.
Children. *Initial:* 1 to 5 mg q.d. for 4 days and then continued or decreased to one-quarter the dose. *Maintenance:* 0.5 to 1.5 mg q.d.

Route	Onset	Peak	Duration
P.O.	Several hr	Unknown	Up to 9 wk

Mechanism of Action
Stimulates intestinal calcium absorption and mobilizes bone calcium when parathyroid hormone and renal tissue fail to raise the serum calcium level.

Contraindications
Hypercalcemia, hypersensitivity to vitamin D, hypervitaminosis D, malabsorption syndrome, renal dysfunction

Interactions
DRUGS
aluminum-containing antacids: Possibly increased serum aluminum level, leading to toxicity
barbiturates, phenytoin: Decreased half-life and therapeutic effects of vitamin D
calcium-containing drugs, thiazide diuretics: Risk of hypercalcemia in patients with hypoparathyroidism
cholestyramine, colestipol, mineral oil: Decreased vitamin D absorption
digitalis glycosides: Possibly hypercalcemia; possibly potentiated effects of digitalis glycosides, resulting in arrhythmias
magnesium-containing antacids: Risk of hypermagnesemia, especially in patients with chronic renal failure
phosphorus-containing drugs: Increased risk of hyperphosphatemia
vitamin D analogues: Increased risk of vitamin D toxicity

Adverse Reactions
Other: Vitamin D toxicity (long-term, high-dose therapy)

Nursing Considerations
• After thyroid surgery, expect to give 0.25 mg once daily with 6 g of oral calcium lactate until danger of tetany has passed.

•Monitor serum calcium level regularly to determine dosage schedule and to detect or prevent hypercalcemia. Be aware that the difference between therapeutic and toxic doses may be small.

•Monitor closely for signs of vitamin D toxicity: abdominal cramps, amnesia, anorexia, ataxia, coma, constipation, depression, diarrhea, disorientation, hallucinations, headache, hypotonia, lethargy, nausea, syncope, tinnitus, vertigo, vomiting, and weakness. Renal impairment may cause albuminuria, polydipsia, and polyuria. Delayed treatment can result in death from cardiac and renal failure caused by widespread calcification of soft tissues, including the heart, blood vessels, kidneys, and lungs.

•If toxicity occurs, notify prescriber and expect to stop dihydrotachysterol immediately. Place patient on bed rest, administer fluids and a laxative, and place her on a low-calcium diet as ordered. For hypercalcemic crisis with dehydration, prepare to give I.V. NS and a loop diuretic (such as furosemide or ethacrynic acid) to increase urinary calcium excretion.

PATIENT TEACHING

•Stress the importance of not exceeding prescribed dihydrotachysterol dosage because of the risk of vitamin D toxicity.

•If patient detects signs of toxicity, caution her not to take the next dose and to notify prescriber immediately.

•Advise patient to drop solution directly into her mouth or to mix it with fruit juice, cereal, or other food.

•Instruct patient to take a missed dose as soon as she remembers unless it's nearly time for the next dose. Warn her not to double the dose.

•Advise patient to avoid OTC drugs and dietary supplements that contain aluminum, calcium, phosphorus, or vitamin D, unless directed by prescriber. Also advise her to avoid antacids that contain magnesium.

•Urge patient to keep follow-up appointments and to have her serum calcium level measured periodically.

diltiazem hydrochloride

Apo-Diltiaz (CAN), Cardizem, Cardizem CD, Cardizem SR, Dilacor XR, Novo-Diltiazem (CAN), Nu-Diltiaz (CAN)

Class and Category

Chemical: Benzothiazepine derivative
Therapeutic: Antianginal, antiarrhythmic, antihypertensive
Pregnancy category: C

Indications and Dosages

➤ *To treat Prinzmetal's (variant) angina and chronic stable angina*

TABLETS

Adults and adolescents. *Initial:* 30 mg t.i.d. or q.i.d. a.c. and h.s., increased q 1 or 2 days as appropriate. *Maximum:* 360 mg/day in divided doses t.i.d. or q.i.d.

➤ *To control hypertension*

E.R. CAPSULES

Adults and adolescents. *Initial:* 180 to 240 mg q.d., adjusted after 14 days as appropriate. *Maximum:* 360 mg/day.

S.R. CAPSULES

Adults and adolescents. *Initial:* 60 to 120 mg b.i.d., adjusted after 14 days as appropriate. *Maximum:* 360 mg/day.

TABLETS

Adults and adolescents. *Initial:* 30 mg t.i.d. or q.i.d. a.c. and h.s., increased q 1 or 2 days as appropriate. *Maximum:* 360 mg/day in divided doses t.i.d. or q.i.d.

➤ *To treat atrial fibrillation, atrial flutter, and paroxysmal supraventricular tachycardia*

I.V. INFUSION OR INJECTION

Adults and adolescents. 0.25 mg/kg given by bolus over 2 min. If response is inadequate after 15 min, 0.35 mg/kg given by bolus over 2 min. Then 10 mg/hr for continued reduction of heart rate after bolus dose, increased by 5 mg/hr, as needed. *Maximum:* 15 mg/hr for up to 24 hr.

Route	Onset	Peak	Duration
P.O.	30 to 60 min	In 2 wk	Unknown
P.O. (E.R.)	2 to 3 hr	In 2 wk	Unknown
P.O. (S.R.)	Unknown	In 2 wk	Unknown
I.V.	In 3 min	2 to 7 min	30 min to 10 hr*

* For infusion; 1 to 3 hr for injection.

Mechanism of Action

Diltiazem inhibits calcium movement into coronary and vascular smooth-muscle cells by blocking slow calcium channels in cell membranes, as shown. This action decreases intracellular calcium, which:
• inhibits smooth-muscle cell contractions
• decreases myocardial oxygen demand by relaxing coronary and vascular smooth muscle, reducing peripheral vascular resistance and systolic and diastolic blood pressures
• slows AV conduction time and prolongs AV nodal refractoriness
• interrupts the reentry circuit in AV nodal reentrant tachycardias.

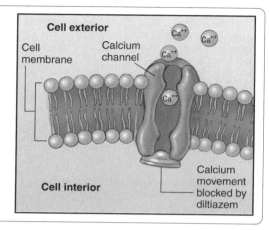

Cell exterior
Cell membrane
Calcium channel
Cell interior
Calcium movement blocked by diltiazem

Incompatibilities

Don't give diltiazem through same I.V. line as acetazolamide, acyclovir, aminophylline, ampicillin sodium/sulbactam sodium, cefamandole, cefoperazone, diazepam, furosemide, heparin, hydrocortisone sodium succinate, methylprednisolone sodium succinate, mezlocillin, nafcillin, phenytoin, rifampin, or sodium bicarbonate.

Contraindications

Acute MI; cardiogenic shock; Lown-Ganong-Levine or Wolff-Parkinson-White syndrome, second- or third-degree AV block, and sick sinus syndrome, unless artificial pacemaker is in place; pulmonary edema; systolic blood pressure below 90 mm Hg; ventricular tachycardia (wide complex)

Interactions

DRUGS

anesthetics (hydrocarbon inhalation): Additive hypotension
beta blockers: Possibly increased risk of adverse cardiovascular effects
carbamazepine, cyclosporine, quinidine, theophyllines: Decreased hepatic clearance and increased serum levels of these drugs, leading to toxicity
cimetidine: Decreased diltiazem metabolism, increased blood diltiazem level
digoxin: Increased blood digoxin level
lithium: Possibly neurotoxicity
NSAIDs: Possibly antagonized antihypertensive effect of diltiazem

prazocin: Possibly increased risk of hypotension
procainamide: Possibly increased risk of prolonged QT interval

Adverse Reactions

CNS: Abnormal gait, amnesia, depression, dizziness, dream disturbances, extrapyramidal reactions, hallucinations, headache, insomnia, nervousness, paresthesia, personality change, somnolence, syncope, tremor, weakness
CV: Angina, atrial flutter, AV block (first-, second-, and third-degree), bradycardia, bundle-branch block, heart failure, hypotension, palpitations, peripheral edema, PVCs, sinus arrest, sinus tachycardia, 12-lead ECG abnormalities, ventricular fibrillation, ventricular tachycardia
EENT: Amblyopia, dry mouth, epistaxis, eye irritation, gingival bleeding and hyperplasia, gingivitis, nasal congestion, retinopathy, taste perversion, tinnitus
ENDO: Hyperglycemia
GI: Anorexia, constipation, diarrhea, elevated liver function test results, indigestion, nausea, thirst, vomiting
GU: Acute renal failure, impotence, nocturia, polyuria, sexual dysfunction
HEME: Hemolytic anemia, leukopenia, prolonged bleeding time, thrombocytopenia
MS: Arthralgia, muscle spasms, myalgia
RESP: Dyspnea
SKIN: Alopecia, diaphoresis, erythema multiforme, exfoliative dermatitis, flushing, leukocytoclastic vasculitis, petechiae, photo-

sensitivity, pruritus, purpura, Stevens-Johnson syndrome, toxic epidermal necrolysis, urticaria
Other: Angioedema, hyperuricemia, weight gain

Nursing Considerations

• Use diltiazem cautiously in patients with impaired hepatic or renal function, and monitor liver and renal function test results, as appropriate; drug is metabolized mainly in liver and excreted by kidneys.
• **WARNING** Monitor blood pressure, pulse rate, and heart rate and rhythm by continuous ECG as appropriate during diltiazem therapy. Keep emergency equipment and drugs readily available.
• Assess for signs of heart failure, such as sudden and unexplained weight gain, dyspnea, and peripheral edema.
• If patient also receives digoxin, monitor for signs of digitalis toxicity, such as nausea, vomiting, halo vision, and elevated serum digoxin level.
• Administer sublingual nitroglycerin, as prescribed, during diltiazem therapy.
• Expect to discontinue drug if adverse skin reactions, which are usually transient, persist.

PATIENT TEACHING
• Explain that tablets can be crushed, but capsules must be swallowed whole.
• Advise patient to take a missed dose as soon as she remembers, unless it's almost time for the next dose. Caution her against doubling the dose. Urge her to contact prescriber if more than one dose is missed.
• **WARNING** Instruct patient not to stop taking drug suddenly because life-threatening problems may result.
• Instruct patient to store diltiazem at room temperature in a dry place.
• Advise patient to monitor blood pressure and pulse rate regularly and to report significant changes to prescriber.
• Urge patient to notify prescriber if she experiences chest pain, difficulty breathing, dizziness, fainting, irregular heartbeat, rash, or swollen ankles.
• Instruct patient to maintain good oral hygiene, perform gum massage, and see a dentist every 6 months to prevent gingival bleeding and hyperplasia and gingivitis.
• Urge patient to wear sunscreen and protective clothing when outdoors.

dimenhydrinate

Dinate, Dramanate, Gravol (CAN), Hydrate

Class and Category

Chemical: Ethanolamine derivative
Therapeutic: Antiemetic, antivertigo
Pregnancy category: B

Indications and Dosages

➤ *To treat nausea, vomiting, dizziness, or vertigo associated with motion sickness*

CHEWABLE TABLETS, ORAL SOLUTION, SYRUP, TABLETS
Adults and adolescents. 50 to 100 mg q 4 to 6 hr, p.r.n. *Maximum:* 400 mg/24 hr.
Children ages 6 to 12. 25 to 50 mg q 6 to 8 hr, p.r.n. *Maximum:* 150 mg/24 hr.
Children ages 2 to 6. 12.5 to 25 mg q 6 to 8 hr, p.r.n. *Maximum:* 75 mg/24 hr.

I.M. INJECTION
Adults and adolescents. 50 mg q 4 hr, p.r.n.
Children. 1.25 mg/kg or 37.5 mg/m^2 q 6 hr, p.r.n. *Maximum:* 300 mg/day.

I.V. INFUSION OR INJECTION
Adults and adolescents. 50 mg in 10 ml of NS administered slowly, over at least 2 min, q 4 hr, p.r.n.
Children. 1.25 mg/kg or 37.5 mg/m^2 in 10 ml of NS administered slowly, over at least 2 min, q 6 hr, p.r.n. *Maximum:* 300 mg/day.

Route	Onset	Peak	Duration
P.O.	Unknown	Unknown	3 to 6 hr
I.M.	20 to 30 min	Unknown	3 to 6 hr
I.V.	Immediate	Unknown	3 to 6 hr

Mechanism of Action

May inhibit vestibular stimulation and labyrinthine stimulation and function by acting on the otolith system and, with larger doses, on the semicircular canals.

Contraindications

Age less than 1 month, hypersensitivity to dimenhydrinate or its components

Interactions

DRUGS
aminoglycosides, other ototoxic drugs: Masked symptoms of ototoxicity
anticholinergics, drugs with anticholinergic activity: Potentiated anticholinergic effects of dimenhydrinate

apomorphine: Possibly decreased emetic response to apomorphine in treatment of poisoning
barbiturates, other CNS depressants: Possibly increased CNS depression
MAO inhibitors: Increased anticholinergic and CNS depressant effects of dimenhydrinate
ACTIVITIES
alcohol use: Possibly increased CNS depression

Adverse Reactions

CNS: Confusion, drowsiness, hallucinations, nervousness, paradoxical stimulation
CV: Hypotension, palpitations, tachycardia
EENT: Blurred vision, diplopia, dry eyes, dry mouth, nasal congestion
GI: Anorexia, constipation, diarrhea, epigastric discomfort, nausea, vomiting
GU: Dysuria
HEME: Hemolytic anemia
RESP: Thickening of bronchial secretions, wheezing
SKIN: Photosensitivity, rash, urticaria
Other: Anaphylaxis

Nursing Considerations

•**WARNING** Be aware that I.V. dimenhydrinate shouldn't be administered to premature or full-term neonates. Some I.V. preparations may contain benzyl alcohol, which can cause a fatal toxic syndrome characterized by CNS, respiratory, circulatory, and renal impairment and metabolic acidosis.
•**WARNING** Be aware that 50-mg/ml concentration of dimenhydrinate is intended for I.M. use. For I.V. use, the solution must be diluted further with at least 10 ml of diluent, such as D$_5$W or NS, for each milliliter of dimenhydrinate.
•Monitor patients with prostatic hyperplasia, stenosing peptic ulcer, pyloroduodenal obstruction, bladder neck obstruction, angle-closure glaucoma, bronchial asthma, or cardiac arrhythmias for worsening of these conditions caused by anticholinergic effects.
•Monitor elderly patients for signs of increased sensitivity to dimenhydrinate, such as excessive drowsiness, confusion, and restlessness.
•Assess patients, especially children and elderly patients, for evidence of paradoxical stimulation, such as nightmares, unusual excitement, nervousness, restlessness, or irritability.
•Store parenteral drug at 15° to 30° C (59° to 86° F); don't freeze.

PATIENT TEACHING

•Because dimenhydrinate may cause drowsiness, instruct patient to avoid potentially hazardous activities until drug's CNS effects are known.
•Advise patient to inform health care providers about dimenhydrinate therapy, especially if she's being evaluated for medical conditions that are affected by this drug, such as appendicitis.
•Instruct patient to avoid alcohol, sedatives, and tranquilizers while receiving this drug.
•Encourage patient to use sunscreen to prevent photosensitivity reactions.

diphenhydramine hydrochloride

Allerdryl (CAN), Banophen, Benadryl, Benadryl Allergy, Diphenhist CapTabs, Genahist, Hyrexin, Nytol QuickCaps, Siladryl, Sleep-Eze D Extra Strength, Unisom SleepGels Maximum Strength

Class and Category

Chemical: Ethanolamine derivative
Therapeutic: Antianaphylactic adjunct, antidyskinetic, antiemetic, antihistamine, antitussive (syrup), antivertigo, sedative-hypnotic
Pregnancy category: B

Indications and Dosages

➤ *To treat hypersensitivity reactions, such as perennial and seasonal allergic rhinitis, vasomotor rhinitis, allergic conjunctivitis, uncomplicated allergic skin eruptions, and transfusion reactions*
CAPSULES, TABLETS
Adults and adolescents. 25 to 50 mg q 4 to 6 hr, p.r.n. *Maximum:* 300 mg/day.
Children ages 6 to 12. 12.5 to 25 mg q 4 to 6 hr. *Maximum:* 150 mg/day.
Children up to age 6. 6.25 to 12.5 mg q 4 to 6 hr.
ELIXIR
Adults and adolescents. 25 to 50 mg q 4 to 6 hr, p.r.n. *Maximum:* 300 mg/day.
Children. 1.25 mg/kg q 4 to 6 hr. *Maximum:* 300 mg/day.
I.V. OR I.M. INJECTION
Adults and adolescents. 10 to 50 mg q 4 to 6 hr up to 100 mg/dose, if needed. *Maximum:* 400 mg/day.

Children. 1.25 mg/kg q 4 to 6 hr. *Maximum:* 300 mg/day.

➤ *To treat sleep disorders*

CAPSULES, TABLETS

Adults and adolescents. 50 mg 20 to 30 min before bedtime.

➤ *To provide antitussive effects*

ELIXIR

Adults and adolescents. 25 mg q 4 hr. *Maximum:* 100 mg/24 hr.

Children ages 6 to 12. 12.5 mg q 4 to 6 hr. *Maximum:* 75 mg/day.

Children ages 2 to 6. 6.25 mg q 4 to 6 hr. *Maximum:* 25 mg/day.

➤ *To prevent motion sickness or treat vertigo*

CAPSULES, ELIXIR, TABLETS

Adults and adolescents. 25 to 50 mg q 4 to 6 hr, p.r.n. *Maximum:* 300 mg/day.

Children. 1 to 1.5 mg/kg q 4 to 6 hr, p.r.n. *Maximum:* 300 mg/day.

I.V. OR I.M. INJECTION

Adults and adolescents. *Initial:* 10 mg. Increased to 20 to 50 mg q 2 to 3 hr, if needed. *Maximum:* 100 mg/dose, 400 mg/day.

Children. 1 to 1.5 mg/kg I.M. q 4 to 6 hr, p.r.n. *Maximum:* 300 mg/day.

➤ *To treat symptoms of Parkinson's disease and drug-induced extrapyramidal reactions in elderly patients who can't tolerate more potent antidyskinetic drugs*

CAPSULES, ELIXIR, TABLETS

Adults. 25 mg t.i.d. increased gradually to 50 mg q.i.d., if needed. *Maximum:* 300 mg/day.

I.V. OR I.M. INJECTION

Adults and adolescents. 10 to 50 mg q.i.d., as needed. *Maximum:* 100 mg/dose, 400 mg/day.

Route	Onset	Peak	Duration
P.O.	15 to 60 min	1 to 3 hr	6 to 8 hr
I.V.	Immediate	1 to 3 hr	6 to 8 hr
I.M.	30 min	1 to 3 hr	6 to 8 hr

Contraindications

Angle-closure glaucoma, bladder neck obstruction, concurrent use of MAO inhibitors, hypersensitivity to diphenhydramine or its components, lower respiratory tract symptoms (including asthma), pyloroduodenal obstruction, stenosing peptic ulcer, symptomatic benign prostatic hyperplasia

Mechanism of Action

Binds to central and peripheral H_1 receptors, competing with histamine for these sites and preventing it from reaching its site of action. By blocking histamine, diphenhydramine produces antihistamine effects, inhibiting respiratory, vascular, and GI smooth-muscle contraction; decreasing capillary permeability, which reduces wheals, flares, and itching; and decreasing salivary and lacrimal gland secretions.

Diphenhydramine produces antidyskinetic effects, possibly by inhibiting acetylcholine in the CNS. It also produces antitussive effects by directly suppressing the cough center in the medulla oblongata. Diphenhydramine's antiemetic and antivertigo effects may be related to its ability to bind to CNS muscarinic receptors and depress vestibular stimulation and labyrinthine function. Its sedative effects are related to its CNS depressant action.

Interactions

DRUGS

apomorphine: Possibly decreased emetic response to apomorphine in treatment of poisoning

barbiturates, other CNS depressants: Possibly increased CNS depression

MAO inhibitors: Increased anticholinergic and CNS depressant effects of diphenhydramine

ACTIVITIES

alcohol use: Possibly increased CNS depression

Adverse Reactions

CNS: Confusion, dizziness, drowsiness
CV: Arrhythmias, palpitations, tachycardia
EENT: Blurred vision, diplopia
GI: Epigastric distress, nausea
HEME: Agranulocytosis, hemolytic anemia, thrombocytopenia
RESP: Thickened bronchial secretions
SKIN: Photosensitivity

Nursing Considerations

•Expect to give parenteral form of diphenhydramine only when oral ingestion isn't possible.
•Keep elixir container tightly closed. Protect elixir and parenteral forms from light.

•Expect to discontinue drug at least 72 hours before skin tests for allergies because drug may inhibit cutaneous histamine response, thus producing false-negative results.

PATIENT TEACHING

•Instruct patient to take diphenhydramine at least 30 minutes before exposure to situations that may cause motion sickness.

•Advise her to take drug with food to minimize GI distress.

•Because drug may cause drowsiness, advise patient to avoid potentially hazardous activities until its CNS effects are known.

•Urge patient to avoid alcohol while taking diphenhydramine.

•Instruct her to use sunscreen to prevent photosensitivity reactions.

diphenoxylate hydrochloride and atropine sulfate

Lofene, Logen, Lomocot, Lomotil, Lonox, Vi-Atro

Class, Category, and Schedule

Chemical: Belladonna alkaloid, tertiary amine (atropine), phenylpiperidine derivative opioid (diphenoxylate)
Therapeutic: Antidiarrheal
Pregnancy category: C
Controlled substance: Schedule V

Indications and Dosages

➤ *To treat acute and chronic diarrhea*

ORAL SOLUTION, TABLETS

Adults and adolescents. *Initial:* 5 mg of diphenoxylate and 0.05 mg of atropine t.i.d. or q.i.d. *Maintenance:* 5 mg of diphenoxylate and 0.05 mg of atropine q.d., p.r.n. *Maximum:* 20 mg of diphenoxylate daily.

DOSAGE ADJUSTMENT Dosage reduced as soon as symptoms are controlled. Expect prescriber to consider alternative treatment if no improvement occurs after 10 days at maximum dosage. Dosage also reduced in elderly or very ill patients and in those with respiratory problems.

Route	Onset	Peak	Duration
P.O.	45 to 60 min	Unknown	3 to 4 hr

Mechanism of Action

Directly affects circular smooth muscles of the GI tract, reducing intestinal motility. Subtherapeutic doses of atropine are added to diphenoxylate to reduce its potential for abuse.

Contraindications

Diarrhea caused by pseudomembranous enterocolitis or enterotoxin-producing bacteria; hypersensitivity to atropine, diphenoxylate, or their components; obstructive jaundice; ulcerative colitis

Interactions

DRUGS

anticholinergics: Possibly enhanced effects of atropine
barbiturates, tranquilizers, and other habit-forming CNS depressants: Potentiated CNS depression, possibly increased risk of drug dependence
MAO inhibitors: Possibly hypertensive crisis
naltrexone: Withdrawal symptoms if patient is physically dependent on diphenoxylate
opioid analgesics: Increased risk of severe constipation, additive CNS depression

ACTIVITIES

alcohol use: Possibly potentiated CNS depression

Adverse Reactions

CNS: Confusion, depression, dizziness, drowsiness, euphoria, fever, headache, hyperthermia, lethargy, malaise, paresthesia, restlessness, sedation
CV: Tachycardia
EENT: Gingival hyperplasia
GI: Abdominal cramps or pain, anorexia, ileus, nausea, pancreatitis, toxic megacolon, vomiting
GU: Urine retention
RESP: Respiratory depression
SKIN: Dry skin and mucous membranes, flushing, pruritus, urticaria
Other: Anaphylaxis, physical and psychological dependence

Nursing Considerations

•**WARNING** Use diphenoxylate-atropine combination with extreme caution in patients with abnormal hepatic or renal function because drug can cause hepatic coma. Monitor liver function test results as appropriate during long-term therapy.

•**WARNING** Monitor for respiratory depression, especially in elderly or very ill patients and in those with respiratory problems; expect to give lower doses as prescribed.

•If severe fluid or electrolyte imbalance develops, expect to withhold drug as ordered until imbalance is corrected. Drug-induced ileus or toxic megacolon may cause fluid retention in the intestine, aggravating dehydration and electrolyte imbalance.

•Closely monitor patient with ulcerative colitis because drug has caused toxic megacolon. Notify prescriber immediately about unexpected adverse reactions, especially abdominal distention and hypoactive or absent bowel sounds.

•During long-term therapy, assess for tolerance to drug's antidiarrheal effects.

PATIENT TEACHING

•Caution patient not to exceed the prescribed dosage because of the risk of adverse reactions, including drug dependence.

•Stress the importance of keeping drug away from children because overdose can cause permanent brain damage in them.

•Instruct patient to take drug with food if GI distress occurs.

•Advise patient to avoid potentially hazardous activities until drug's CNS effects are known.

•Urge patient to avoid alcohol and CNS depressants because of additive effects.

•Instruct patient to notify prescriber if diarrhea isn't improved or controlled within 48 hours or if a fever develops.

dipyridamole

Apo-Dipyridamole FC (CAN), Apo-Dipyridamole SC (CAN), Novo-Dipiradol (CAN), Persantine

Class and Category

Chemical: Pyrimidine
Therapeutic: Coronary vasodilator, diagnostic aid, platelet aggregation inhibitor
Pregnancy category: B

Indications and Dosages

➤ *To prevent thromboembolic complications of cardiac valve replacement*

TABLETS

Adults. 75 to 100 mg q.i.d. with coumarin or indanedione derivative anticoagulant.

➤ *To aid diagnosis during thallium perfusion imaging of myocardium*

I.V. INFUSION

Adults. 0.57 mg/kg in 50 ml of D_5W infused over 4 min. *Maximum:* 60 mg.

Route	Onset	Peak	Duration
I.V.	Unknown	3.8 to 8.7 min*	Unknown

Mechanism of Action

May increase the intraplatelet level of adenosine, which causes coronary vasodilation and inhibits platelet aggregation. Dipyridamole also may increase the intraplatelet level of cAMP and may inhibit formation of the potent platelet activator stimulant thromboxane A_2, which decreases platelet activation. Vasodilation and increased blood flow occur preferentially in nondiseased coronary vessels, which results in redistribution of blood away from significantly diseased vessels. These changes in perfusion are observed during thallium imaging studies.

Contraindications

Asthma (I.V.), hypersensitivity to dipyridamole or its components, hypotension, unstable angina pectoris

Interactions

DRUGS

adenosine: Potentiated effects of adenosine
cefamandole, cefoperazone, cefotetan, plicamycin, valproic acid: Possibly hypoprothrombinemia and increased risk of bleeding
heparin, NSAIDs, thrombolytics: Possibly increased risk of bleeding
theophylline: Reversal of coronary vasodilation caused by dipyridamole, possibly false-negative thallium imaging result

Adverse Reactions

CNS: Dizziness, headache

---

* After start of infusion, for increased velocity of coronary artery blood flow.

CV: Angina, arrhythmias, ECG changes (specifically ST-segment and T-wave changes)
GI: Abdominal pain, diarrhea, nausea, vomiting
RESP: Dyspnea
SKIN: Flushing, pruritus, rash

Nursing Considerations
•Protect I.V. form of dipyridamole from direct light and freezing.
•Monitor blood pressure, pulse rate and rhythm, and breath sounds every 10 to 15 minutes during I.V. infusion.
•Keep parenteral aminophylline available to relieve adverse reactions to dipyridamole infusion.
•At therapeutic doses, expect adverse reactions to be minimal and transient. They typically resolve with long-term use.
PATIENT TEACHING
•Urge patient to take drug at least 1 hour before or 2 hours after meals for faster absorption. If she experiences GI distress, advise her to take drug with meals or milk.
•Advise patient to take drug at evenly spaced intervals.
•Inform patient that drug commonly is taken with other anticoagulants.
•Urge her to keep appointments for coagulation tests.
•Instruct patient to seek immediate emergency treatment if chest pain occurs.
•Caution patient to consult prescriber before taking aspirin and other OTC NSAIDs because of increased risk of bleeding.
•Advise patient to notify all health care providers about dipyridamole use.

dirithromycin

Dynabac

Class and Category
Chemical: Semisynthetic macrolide
Therapeutic: Antibiotic
Pregnancy category: C

Indications and Dosages
➤ *To treat acute bacterial exacerbations and secondary bacterial infections in patients with bronchitis caused by* Moraxella catarrhalis *or* Streptococcus pneumoniae, *and uncomplicated skin and soft-tissue infections caused by methicillin-susceptible* Staphylococcus aureus

TABLETS
Adults and adolescents. 500 mg q.d. for 7 days.
➤ *To treat streptococcal pharyngitis*
TABLETS
Adults and adolescents. 500 mg q.d. for 10 days.
➤ *To treat community-acquired pneumonia caused by* Legionella pneumophila, Mycoplasma pneumoniae, *or* S. pneumoniae
TABLETS
Adults and adolescents. 500 mg q.d. for 14 days.

Mechanism of Action
Binds with the 50S ribosomal subunit of the 70S ribosome in susceptible bacteria. This action inhibits RNA-dependent protein synthesis in bacterial cells, causing them to die.

Contraindications
Concurrent use of astemizole, cisapride, or pimozide; hypersensitivity to dirithromycin, erythromycin, other macrolide antibiotics, or their components; known, potential, or suspected bacteremia

Interactions
DRUGS
antacids, H₂-receptor antagonists: Increased dirithromycin absorption
astemizol, terfenadine: Possibly life-threatening arrhythmias
theophylline: Possibly increased serum theophylline level

Adverse Reactions
CNS: Dizziness, headache, weakness
GI: Abdominal pain, diarrhea, nausea, pseudomembranous colitis, vomiting
SKIN: Pruritus, rash, urticaria

Nursing Considerations
•Use dirithromycin cautiously in patients with impaired hepatic function. Monitor liver function test results as indicated because drug is metabolized in liver.
PATIENT TEACHING
•Instruct patient to take dirithromycin at the same time each day with food or within 1 hour of eating.
•Caution patient not to cut, chew, or crush tablets.
•Advise patient to store drug at room temperature in a dry place.

•Instruct patient to complete the full course of therapy, even if she feels better before it's finished.
•Advise patient to notify prescriber immediately if GI problems persist.

disopyramide

Rythmodan (CAN)

disopyramide phosphate

Norpace, Norpace CR, Rythmodan-LA (CAN)

Class and Category
Chemical: Substituted pyramide derivative
Therapeutic: Class IA antiarrhythmic
Pregnancy category: C

Indications and Dosages
➤ *To rapidly control ventricular arrhythmias*
CAPSULES
Adults. *Loading:* 300 mg (200 mg if patient weighs less than 50 kg [110 lb]). If no response to loading dose within 6 hr, 200 mg given q 6 hr. If no response within 48 hr, drug discontinued or dosage carefully increased to 250 to 300 mg q 6 hr.
➤ *To treat ventricular arrhythmias*
CAPSULES
Adults. 400 to 800 mg/day in divided doses q 6 hr, limited to 400 mg/day if patient weighs less than 50 kg. *Maximum:* 800 mg/day.
Children ages 12 to 18. 6 to 15 mg/kg/day in divided doses q 6 hr.
Children ages 4 to 12. 10 to 15 mg/kg/day in divided doses q 6 hr.
Children ages 1 to 4. 10 to 20 mg/kg/day in divided doses q 6 hr.
Children younger than age 1. 10 to 30 mg/kg/day in divided doses q 6 hr.
DOSAGE ADJUSTMENT Initial dosage reduced to 100 mg q 6 to 8 hr for adults with cardiomyopathy or possible cardiac decompensation. In patients with renal insufficiency, dosage reduced to 100 mg q 6 hr if creatinine clearance exceeds 40 ml/min/1.73 m^2 or hepatic function is impaired; 100 mg q 8 hr if creatinine clearance is 30 to 40 ml/min/1.73 m^2; 100 mg q 12 hr if creatinine clearance is 15 to 29 ml/min/1.73 m^2; and 100 mg q 24 hr if creatinine clearance is less than 15 ml/min/1.73 m^2.
E.R. CAPSULES, E.R. TABLETS
Adults. 400 to 800 mg/day in divided doses q 12 hr, limited to 200 mg q 12 hr if patient weighs less than 50 kg. *Maximum:* 800 mg/day.

Mechanism of Action
Inhibits sodium influx through fast channels of myocardial cell membranes, thus increasing the recovery period after repolarization. Disopyramide decreases automaticity in the His-Purkinje system and conduction velocity in the atria, ventricles, and accessory pathways. It prolongs the QRS and QT intervals in normal sinus rhythm and atrial arrhythmias. The drug has a potent negative inotropic effect. It also acts as an anticholinergic and increases peripheral vascular resistance.

Contraindications
Cardiogenic shock, congenital QT-interval prolongation, hypersensitivity to disopyramide or its components, second- or third-degree AV block (without pacemaker), sick sinus syndrome

Interactions
DRUGS
antiarrhythmics: Widened QRS complex, prolonged QT interval, risk of arrhythmias, serious negative inotropic effects
anticholinergics: Possibly additive anticholinergic effects
cisapride: Possibly increased risk of prolonged QT interval
clarithromycin, erythromycin: Increased blood disopyramide level
digoxin: Increased serum digoxin level
hydantoins, rifampin: Decreased blood disopyramide level
insulin, oral antidiabetic drugs: Possibly intensified antidiabetic effects
quinidine: Increased blood disopyramide level, decreased blood quinidine level, or both
verapamil: Widened QRS complex, prolonged QT interval, possibly death

Adverse Reactions
CNS: Depression, dizziness, fatigue, fever, headache, insomnia, nervousness, syncope
CV: Chest pain; conduction disturbances; edema; heart failure (new or worsened); hypercholesterolemia; hypertriglyceridemia; hypotension; palpitations; proarrhythmias, including torsades de pointes; ventricular fibrillation; ventricular tachycardia
EENT: Blurred vision; dry eyes, mouth, nose, and throat

ENDO: Gynecomastia, hypoglycemia
GI: Abdominal distention, anorexia, constipation, diarrhea, vomiting
GU: Impotence, urinary frequency and urgency, urine retention
HEME: Reversible agranulocytosis (rare), thrombocytopenia
MS: Muscle weakness
RESP: Dyspnea
SKIN: Decreased sweating, pruritus, rash, reversible cholestatic jaundice
Other: Hypokalemia, lupus erythematosus–like symptoms

Nursing Considerations

• **WARNING** Because of disopyramide's anticholinergic activity, avoid using drug in patients with glaucoma, myasthenia gravis, or urine retention.
• Use disopyramide cautiously and expect to reduce dosage in patients with impaired hepatic or renal function. Monitor hepatic and renal function, as ordered. Be aware that E.R. form shouldn't be given to patients with severe renal insufficiency.
• When changing from immediate-release to E.R. form, expect to start maintenance schedule 6 hours after last immediate-release dose.
• At therapeutic doses in hemodynamically uncompromised patients, expect drug to reduce cardiac output without decreasing resting sinus rate or affecting blood pressure. Keep in mind, however, that 2 mg/kg given I.V. over 3 minutes can increase heart rate and total peripheral resistance.
• Monitor heart rate and rhythm by continuous ECG.
• Assess serum electrolyte levels, especially the potassium level, because drug may be ineffective in hypokalemia and its toxic effects enhanced in hyperkalemia.
• If patient takes quinidine, expect to start disopyramide 6 to 12 hours after the last dose of quinidine. If patient takes procainamide, expect to start disopyramide 3 to 6 hours after the last dose of procainamide. A loading dose may not be required in either case.

PATIENT TEACHING
• Warn patient not to stop taking disopyramide abruptly; doing so may cause life-threatening cardiac problems.
• Advise patient to take a missed dose as soon as possible after she remembers, unless it's nearly time for the next dose. Caution her

against doubling the dose. Urge her to notify prescriber if she misses more than one dose.
• Instruct patient to store drug at room temperature in a dry place.
• Instruct patient to check her pulse rate regularly and report significant changes to prescriber.
• Urge patient to notify prescriber about blurred vision, constipation, difficulty urinating, dizziness, dry mouth, and trouble breathing.
• Advise patient to avoid potentially hazardous activities until drug's CNS effects are known.
• Instruct patient to rise slowly from a lying or sitting position to reduce dizziness.
• Urge patient to avoid becoming overheated during hot weather or exercise because of risk of heatstroke.

disulfiram

Antabuse

Class and Category

Chemical: Thiuram derivative
Therapeutic: Alcohol abuse deterrent
Pregnancy category: Not rated

Indications and Dosages

➤ *As adjunct to maintain sobriety in treatment of chronic alcoholism*

TABLETS
Adults. *Initial:* Up to 500 mg q.d. for 1 to 2 wk. *Maintenance:* 125 to 500 mg q.d. *Maximum:* 500 mg q.d.

Route	Onset	Peak	Duration
P.O.	In 1 to 2 hr	Unknown	Up to 14 days

Mechanism of Action

Interferes with the enzyme responsible for hepatic oxidation of acetaldehyde to acetate, which occurs during alcohol catabolism. Ingestion of even a small amount of alcohol after taking disulfiram raises the blood acetaldehyde level to 5 to 10 times normal. Disulfiram doesn't alter the rate at which alcohol is eliminated. Its major metabolite, diethyldithiocarbamate, inhibits norepinephrine synthesis and may be responsible for the drug's hypotensive effect.

Contraindications

Alcohol intoxication; coronary artery occlusion; hypersensitivity to disulfiram, its components, rubber, pesticides, or fungicides; psychosis; recent use of alcohol, alcohol-containing preparations, metronidazole, or paraldehyde; severe myocardial disease

Interactions

Drugs

alfentanil: Decreased plasma clearance and prolonged duration of action of alfentanil
amoxicillin-clavulanate, bacampicillin: Possibly disulfiram-alcohol reaction
ascorbic acid: Possibly interference with disulfiram-alcohol reaction
CNS depressants: Possibly increased CNS depressant effects of either drug
isoniazid: Increased risk of additive neurotoxic effect of disulfiram; possibly increased adverse CNS effects
metronidazole: Risk of CNS toxicity, resulting in confusion and psychosis
oral anticoagulants: Possibly increased anticoagulant effects
paraldehyde: Decreased paraldehyde metabolism, increased blood paraldehyde level
phenytoin: Possibly increased blood phenytoin level and risk of phenytoin toxicity
tricyclic antidepressants: Possibly temporary delirium

Foods

caffeine: Possibly increased cardiovascular and CNS effects of caffeine

Activities

alcohol use: Disulfiram-alcohol reaction (if used within 14 days of disulfiram therapy)

Adverse Reactions

CNS: Drowsiness, headache, peripheral neuropathy, psychotic reaction, tiredness
EENT: Blurred vision, garlic or metallic taste, optic atrophy, optic neuritis
GU: Impotence
SKIN: Rash

Nursing Considerations

• Know that disulfiram is given only to patients who are highly motivated to stop drinking and who are receiving psychotherapy or substance abuse counseling.
• Be aware that alcohol content of patient's other drugs should be checked before starting therapy.

•**WARNING** Never give drug to patient without her knowledge or who is intoxicated.
• If needed, crush tablet and mix with fluids before administration.
• Don't give drug within 14 days of patient's ingestion of a substance that contains alcohol.
• Expect alcohol ingestion during disulfiram therapy to produce a severe reaction that lasts from 30 minutes to several hours. Symptoms may include angina, anxiety, blurred vision, confusion, diaphoresis, dyspnea, heart failure, hypotension, nausea, palpitations, sinus tachycardia, syncope, thirst, throbbing headache, throbbing in neck, vertigo, vomiting, and weakness. A deep sleep usually follows.
•**WARNING** Be aware that ingestion of three or more alcoholic beverages with a disulfiram dose greater than 500 mg/day may cause respiratory depression, arrhythmias, and cardiac arrest.
• If patient takes phenytoin, monitor blood phenytoin level before and during disulfiram therapy, and adjust dosage of either drug as prescribed. Drug interactions may not occur if disulfiram therapy starts before phenytoin therapy. Be aware that a subtherapeutic phenytoin level may result if disulfiram therapy stops.
• If patient takes an oral anticoagulant, monitor PT before and during disulfiram therapy, and adjust anticoagulant dosage as prescribed. Drug interactions may not occur if disulfiram therapy starts before warfarin therapy. If disulfiram therapy stops, be prepared to adjust warfarin dosage to avoid loss of hypoprothrombinemic effects.
• Expect some adverse reactions, such as drowsiness, headache, and impotence, to subside over time or with a brief dosage reduction.
• Because one-fifth of a disulfiram dose may stay in the body for 1 week or longer, know that alcohol ingestion may continue to produce unpleasant symptoms for up to 2 weeks after therapy stops.
• Expect therapy to last months to years, depending on patient's ability to abstain from alcohol.

Patient Teaching

• Teach patient's household and family members about precautions needed and risks associated with disulfiram therapy.
• Inform patient that drug doesn't cure alcoholism but does help deter alcohol consumption.

•If patient reports daytime drowsiness, advise her to take drug in the evening.
•Warn patient to avoid alcohol-containing substances, such as vinegar, cough syrup, and sauces, during therapy because a disulfiram-alcohol reaction may occur after ingesting as little as 15 ml of 100-proof alcohol. Encourage patient to avoid alcohol-containing liniments and lotions as well.
•Teach patient what to expect if a disulfiram-alcohol reaction occurs. Inform her that a deep sleep usually follows the reaction.
•Advise patient that a reaction can occur up to 14 days after therapy stops and that a severe reaction may cause respiratory depression, arrhythmias, and cardiac arrest.
•Instruct patient to carry medical identification that indicates drug, describes possible reactions, and lists someone to notify in case of emergency.

dobutamine hydrochloride

Dobutrex

Class and Category
Chemical: Synthetic catecholamine
Therapeutic: Cardiac stimulant
Pregnancy category: Not rated

Indications and Dosages
➤ *To treat low cardiac output and heart failure*
I.V. INFUSION
Adults. 2.5 to 10 mcg/kg/min as continuous infusion adjusted according to hemodynamic response.
Children. 5 to 20 mcg/kg/min as continuous infusion adjusted according to hemodynamic response.

Route	Onset	Peak	Duration
I.V.	1 to 2 min	Unknown	Under 5 min

Incompatibilities
Don't combine dobutamine with cefamandole, cefazolin, hydrocortisone sodium succinate, cephalothin, penicillin, sodium ethycrynate, and sodium heparin because of incompatibility. Don't mix dobutamine with alkaline solutions, such as sodium bicarbonate, because of possible physical incompatibility. Don't use diluents that contain sodium bisulfite or ethanol.

Mechanism of Action
Primarily stimulates beta$_1$-adrenergic receptors, and mildly stimulates beta$_2$- and alpha$_1$-adrenergic receptors. Beta$_1$-receptor stimulation produces a positive inotropic effect on the myocardium. This increases cardiac output by boosting myocardial contractility and stroke volume. Increased myocardial contractility raises coronary blood flow and myocardial oxygen consumption. Systolic blood pressure typically rises as a result of increased stroke volume. Other hemodynamic effects include decreased systemic vascular resistance, which reduces afterload, and decreased ventricular filling pressure, which reduces preload.

Contraindications
Hypersensitivity to dobutamine or its components, idiopathic hypertrophic subaortic stenosis

Interactions
DRUGS
beta blockers: Possibly increased alpha-adrenergic activity and peripheral resistance
bretylium: Potentiated vasopressor activity, possibly arrhythmias
cyclopropane, halothane: Possibly serious arrhythmias
guanethidine: Decreased hypotensive effect of guanethidine, possibly resulting in severe hypertension
thyroid hormones: Increased cardiovascular effects of thyroid hormones or dobutamine
tricyclic antidepressants: Possibly potentiated cardiovascular and vasopressor effects of dobutamine, resulting in arrhythmias, hyperpyrexia, or severe hypertension

Adverse Reactions
CNS: Fever, headache, nervousness, restlessness
CV: Angina, bradycardia, hypertension, hypotension, palpitations, PVCs, tachycardia
GI: Nausea, vomiting
RESP: Dyspnea
SKIN: Extravasation with tissue necrosis and sloughing, rash
Other: Hypokalemia

Nursing Considerations
•Avoid giving dobutamine to patients with uncorrected hypovolemia. Expect prescriber

To order whole blood or plasma volume ex-

to order whole blood or plasma volume expanders to correct hypovolemia. Also avoid giving dobutamine to patients with acute MI because it can intensify or extend myocardial ischemia.
•Use drug cautiously in patients who are allergic to sulfites because drug may cause anaphylactic-like signs and symptoms; commercially available dobutamine injections contain sodium bisulfite. Also use drug cautiously in patients with atrial fibrillation because drug increases AV conduction. Keep in mind that patient should be adequately digitalized before administration.
•Dilute concentrate with at least 50 ml of compatible I.V. solution. A common dilution is 500 mg (40 ml from 250-ml bag) in 210 ml of D_5W or NS to yield 2,000 mcg/ml. Or dilute 1,000 mg (80 ml from 250-ml bag) in 170 ml of D_5W or NS to yield 4,000 mcg/ml. Adjust maximum concentration according to patient's fluid requirements as prescribed. Don't exceed a concentration of 5,000 mcg/ml. Discard solution after 24 hours.
•Inspect parenteral solution for particles and discoloration before administering it.
•Administer I.V. drug using an infusion pump.
•Monitor blood pressure frequently during therapy, preferably by continuous intra-arterial monitoring; a systolic pressure increase of 10 to 20 mm Hg may indicate a dobutamine-induced increase in cardiac output.
•If hypotension develops, expect to reduce dosage or discontinue drug.
•Monitor heart rate and rhythm continuously for PVCs, which may result from drug's stimulatory effect on the heart's conduction system, and sinus tachycardia, which results from positive chronotropic effect of beta stimulation and may increase the heart rate by 5 to 15 beats/minute.
•Monitor hemodynamic parameters, such as central venous pressure, pulmonary artery wedge pressure, and cardiac output, as indicated, to assess drug's effectiveness.
•WARNING Monitor serum potassium level to check for hypokalemia, a rare result of $beta_2$ stimulation that causes electrolyte imbalance.
•Monitor urine output hourly, as appropriate, to assess for improved renal blood flow.
•Be aware that dobutamine isn't indicated for long-term treatment of heart failure because it may not be effective and may increase the risk of hospitalization and death.

PATIENT TEACHING
•Explain the need for frequent hemodynamic monitoring.

docusate calcium
(dioctyl calcium sulfosuccinate)
Albert Docusate (CAN), DC Softgels, Docucal-P, Doxidan (CAN), Pro-Cal-Sof, Sulfolax, Surfak

docusate potassium
(dioctyl potassium sulfo-succinate)
Diocto-K, Kasof

docusate sodium
(dioctyl sodium sulfosuccinate)
Afko-Lube, Afko-Lube Lax, Bilax, Colace, Colax, Correctol Stool Softener Soft Gels, Dialose, Diocto, Dioeze, DOK, D.O.S. Softgels, Ex-Lax Light Formula (CAN), Modane Soft, Regulax SS, Silace

Class and Category
Chemical: Anionic surfactant
Therapeutic: Laxative, stool softener
Pregnancy category: C

Indications and Dosages
➤ *To treat constipation*
CAPSULES (DOCUSATE CALCIUM)
Adults and adolescents. 240 mg h.s. until bowel movements are normal.
Children age 6 and older. 50 to 150 mg h.s.
CAPSULES, LIQUID, SYRUP, TABLETS (DOCUSATE SODIUM)
Adults and adolescents. 50 to 500 mg h.s.
Children ages 6 to 12. 40 to 120 mg h.s.
Children ages 3 to 6. 20 to 60 mg h.s.
Children under age 3. 10 to 40 mg h.s.
CAPSULES, TABLETS (DOCUSATE POTASSIUM)
Adults and adolescents. 100 mg t.i.d. until bowel movements are normal.
Children age 6 and older. 100 mg h.s.

Route	Onset	Peak	Duration
P.O.	24 to 72 hr	Unknown	Unknown

Mechanism of Action
Acts as a surfactant that softens stool by decreasing the surface tension between the oil and water in fecal matter. This action lets more fluid penetrate the stool, thus forming a softer fecal mass.

Contraindications

Fecal impaction; hypersensitivity to docusate salts or their components; intestinal obstruction; nausea, vomiting, or other symptoms of appendicitis; undiagnosed abdominal pain

Interactions
DRUGS

mineral oil: Increased mineral oil absorption, increased risk of toxicity
tetracycline: Decreased tetracycline absorption

Adverse Reactions

CNS: Dizziness, syncope
CV: Palpitations
GI: Abdominal cramps and distention, diarrhea, nausea, perianal irritation, vomiting
MS: Muscle weakness

Nursing Considerations

•WARNING Expect long-term or excessive use of docusate to cause dependence on laxatives for bowel movements, electrolyte imbalances, osteomalacia, steatorrhea, and vitamin and mineral deficiencies.
•Assess for laxative abuse syndrome, especially in women with depression, personality disorders, or anorexia nervosa.

PATIENT TEACHING

•Instruct patient not to use docusate when she's experiencing abdominal pain, nausea, or vomiting.
•Advise patient to take docusate with a full glass of water or milk.
•To help prevent constipation, encourage patient to increase her fiber intake, exercise regularly, and drink 6 to 8 glasses (240 ml/glass) of water daily.
•Instruct patient to notify prescriber about rectal bleeding; symptoms of electrolyte imbalances, such as dizziness, light-headedness, muscle cramping, and weakness; and unrelieved constipation.

dofetilide

Tikosyn

Class and Category

Chemical: Methanesulfonanilide derivative
Therapeutic: Class III antiarrhythmic
Pregnancy category: C

Indications and Dosages

➤ *To convert symptomatic atrial fibrillation or flutter to normal sinus rhythm or to maintain normal sinus rhythm in patients converted from symptomatic atrial fibrillation or flutter*

CAPSULES

Adults. *Initial:* 500 mcg b.i.d. for patients with creatinine clearance greater than 60 ml/min/1.73 m². *Maintenance:* Dosage based on QTc interval. If, 2 to 3 hr after initial dose, QTc interval increase is 15% of baseline or less, initial dose given b.i.d. *Maximum:* 500 mcg b.i.d.
DOSAGE ADJUSTMENT Initial dose reduced to 250 mcg b.i.d. for patients with creatinine clearance of 40 to 60 ml/min/1.73 m² and to 125 mcg b.i.d. for creatinine clearance of 20 to 39 ml/min/1.73 m², as prescribed. If, 2 to 3 hr after initial dose, QTc interval has increased by at least 15% or is more than 500 msec (more than 550 msec in patients with ventricular conduction abnormalities), dosage is decreased by 50%, as prescribed; however, for patients receiving lowest initial dose of 125 mcg b.i.d., dosage is reduced to 125 mcg q.d., as prescribed. During next four doses (given q 2 to 3 hr, as prescribed), if QTc interval increases to more than 500 msec (more than 550 msec in patients with ventricular conduction abnormalities), expect to discontinue therapy, as prescribed.

Route	Onset	Peak	Duration
P.O.	Unknown	2 hr	4 hr

Mechanism of Action

Selectively blocks potassium channels in myocardial cell membranes involved in cardiac repolarization. By blocking potassium channels, dofetilide prolongs ventricular refractoriness (widens QT interval), effective refractory period, and action potential duration. These actions terminate or prevent reentrant tachyarrhythmias, such as atrial fibrillation, atrial flutter, and ventricular tachycardia.

Contraindications

Cardiac conduction disturbances without an artificial pacemaker, congenital or acquired QT prolongation syndrome, hypersensitivity to dofetilide or its components, severe renal impairment (creatinine clearance less than 20 ml/min/1.73 m²)

Interactions
DRUGS

amiloride, cimetidine, co-trimoxazole, ketoconazole, megestrol, metformin, triamterene, trimethoprim: Possibly increased blood dofetilide level

azole antifungals, diltiazem, nefazodone, norfloxacin, protease inhibitors, quinine, selective serotonin reuptake inhibitors, zafirlukast: Possibly increased blood dofetilide level and risk of dofetilide toxicity

bepridil, cisapride, macrolide antibiotics, phenothiazines, tricyclic antidepressants: Possibly prolonged QT interval

class I and III antiarrhythmics, especially amiodarone: Possibly prolonged QT interval and increased risk of dofetilide-induced proarrhythmias

diuretics (potassium-depleting): Increased risk of torsades de pointes in patients with hypokalemia or hypomagnesemia

verapamil: Possibly increased blood dofetilide level and increased risk of torsades de pointes

FOODS

grapefruit juice: Increased blood dofetilide level

ACTIVITIES

marijuana use: Increased blood dofetilide level

Adverse Reactions

CNS: Cerebral ischemia, CVA, dizziness, facial or flaccid paralysis, headache, insomnia, paresthesia, slurred speech, syncope
CV: AV block, bradycardia, cardiac arrest, chest pain, edema, MI, tachycardia, ventricular arrhythmias (including torsades de pointes and ventricular tachycardia)
GI: Abdominal pain, diarrhea, hepatic dysfunction, nausea
MS: Back pain, muscle weakness
RESP: Cough, dyspnea, respiratory tract infection
SKIN: Jaundice, rash
Other: Angioedema, flulike symptoms, weight gain

Nursing Considerations

•**WARNING** If patient has previously received amiodarone drug therapy, be aware that dofetilide therapy should not be initiated until blood amiodarone level is less than 0.3 mcg/ml or until amiodarone has been withdrawn for at least 3 months.
•Evaluate and document QTc interval before and during dofetilide therapy.

•Place patient on continuous ECG monitoring for at least 3 days, as ordered, during dofetilide therapy.
•**WARNING** If patient does not convert to normal sinus rhythm within 24 hours of starting dofetilide, expect to prepare her for possible synchronized electrical cardioversion.
•Be prepared to reevaluate renal function and QTc every 3 months, as ordered, during dofetilide therapy.
•When switching to dofetilide therapy from class I or other class III antiarrhythmics, or after withdrawing previous antiarrhythmic treatment, monitor patient's continuous ECG for at least 30 hours, as ordered.
•If patient requires a drug that may interact with dofetilide, expect to discontinue dofetilide, as prescribed, for 2 or more days before starting the other drug.
•**WARNING** Monitor laboratory test results for hypokalemia or hypomagnesemia, especially in patients who are taking diuretics, because of the increased risk of dofetilide-induced torsades de pointes.
•Frequently monitor female patients for adverse reactions, including prolonged QTc interval and torsades de pointes, because women have approximately 12% to 18% lower renal clearance of drug than men and therefore a greater risk of experiencing adverse drug reactions.

PATIENT TEACHING

•Advise patient to swallow dofetilide capsules with water.
•Instruct patient to avoid drinking grapefruit juice while taking this drug.
•Inform patient that she may be hospitalized for at least 3 days if dofetilide dosage is increased.
•Teach patient how to measure pulse rate and blood pressure during dofetilide therapy.
•Advise patient to report any chest discomfort immediately, including a fluttering sensation or palpitations.
•Advise patient to consult prescriber before using any over-the-counter drugs, nutritional supplements, or herbal products.
•Instruct patient to keep follow-up appointments to monitor heart rhythm.

dolasetron mesylate

Anzemet

Class and Category
Chemical: Carboxylate monomethanesulfonate
Therapeutic: Antiemetic
Pregnancy category: B

Indications and Dosages
➤ *To prevent nausea and vomiting due to chemotherapy*
ORAL SOLUTION, TABLETS
Adults and children over age 16. 100 mg within 1 hr before chemotherapy.
Children ages 2 to 16. 1.8 mg/kg within 1 hr before chemotherapy. *Maximum:* 100 mg.
I.V. INJECTION
Adults and children over age 16. 1.8 mg/kg or 100 mg as a single dose within 30 min before chemotherapy.
Children ages 2 to 16. 1.8 mg/kg as a single dose within 30 min before chemotherapy. *Maximum:* 100 mg.
➤ *To prevent postoperative nausea and vomiting*
ORAL SOLUTION, TABLETS
Adults and children over age 16. 100 mg within 2 hr before surgery.
Children ages 2 to 16. 1.2 mg/kg within 2 hr before surgery. *Maximum:* 100 mg.
I.V. INJECTION
Adults and children over age 16. 12.5 mg 15 min before end of anesthesia.
Children ages 2 to 16. 0.35 mg/kg 15 min before end of anesthesia. *Maximum:* 12.5 mg/dose.
➤ *To treat postoperative nausea and vomiting*
I.V. INJECTION
Adults and children over age 16. 12.5 mg as a single dose as soon as symptoms develop.
Children ages 2 to 16. 0.35 mg/kg as a single dose as soon as symptoms develop. *Maximum:* 12.5 mg/dose.

Mechanism of Action
With its active metabolite hydrodolasetron, prevents activation of the serotonin 5-HT$_3$ receptors located peripherally on the vagal nerve terminals and centrally in the chemoreceptor trigger zone, thereby decreasing the vomiting reflex.

Contraindications
Hypersensitivity to dolasetron or its components

Interactions
DRUGS
atenolol: Possibly decreased clearance of dolasetron
cimetidine: Possibly increased blood dolasetron level
rifampin: Possibly decreased blood dolasetron level

Adverse Reactions
CNS: Headache
CV: Hypertension, hypotension
GI: Diarrhea
SKIN: Rash
Other: Injection site pain

Nursing Considerations
•Expect to administer up to 100 mg of dolasetron I.V. in 30 seconds or to dilute drug in NS, D$_5$W, D$_5$.45NS, or lactated Ringer's solution and infuse for up to 15 minutes, as prescribed.
•Flush I.V. line with compatible solution before and after drug administration.
•Expect to prepare an oral solution of dolasetron for patients unable to swallow tablets by diluting injection solution with apple or apple-grape juice.
•**WARNING** Monitor patients receiving dolasetron for ECG changes, including prolonged PR, QTc, and JT intervals and widened QRS complex.
PATIENT TEACHING
•Advise parents of pediatric patients and patients who have difficulty swallowing that oral solution can be prepared by diluting injection form of drug with apple or apple-grape juice.
•Inform patient that oral solution may be refrigerated for up to 48 hours but should be discarded after 2 hours at room temperature.

donepezil hydrochloride
Aricept

Class and Category
Chemical: Piperidine derivative
Therapeutic: Antidementia
Pregnancy category: C

Indications and Dosages
➤ *To treat mild to moderate dementia of the Alzheimer type*
TABLETS
Adults. *Initial:* 5 mg h.s. After 4 to 6 wk, dosage increased to 10 mg h.s., as indicated. *Maximum:* 10 mg/day.

Mechanism of Action

Reversibly inhibits acetylcholinesterase and improves acetylcholine's concentration at cholinergic synapses. Raising the acetylcholine level in the cerebral cortex may improve cognition. Donepezil becomes less effective as Alzheimer's disease progresses and the number of intact cholinergic neurons declines.

Contraindications

Hypersensitivity to donepezil, piperidine derivatives, or their components

Interactions
DRUGS

anticholinergics: Possibly interference with activity of these drugs
carbamazepine, dexamethasone, phenobarbital, phenytoin, rifampin: Increased donepezil elimination rate
cholinergic agonists, neuromuscular blockers: Possibly synergistic effects of these drugs
ketoconazole, quinidine: Inhibited donepezil metabolism
NSAIDs: Possibly increased gastric acid secretion and increased risk of GI bleeding

Adverse Reactions

CNS: Depression, dizziness, dream disturbances, fatigue, headache, insomnia, somnolence, syncope
GI: Anorexia, constipation, diarrhea, nausea, vomiting
GU: Urinary frequency
MS: Arthralgia, muscle spasms
SKIN: Ecchymosis

Nursing Considerations

• Use donepezil cautiously in patients with bladder obstruction because drug's weak peripheral cholinergic effect could obstruct outflow.
• Use drug cautiously in patients with asthma, COPD, or other pulmonary disorders because drug has a weak affinity for peripheral cholinesterase, which may increase bronchoconstriction and bronchial secretions.
• If patient has cardiac disease, monitor heart rate and rhythm for bradycardia, which may result from increased vagal tone caused by drug's inhibition of peripheral cholinesterase. Reduced heart rate may be especially significant if patient has sick sinus syndrome,

bradycardia, or other supraventricular arrhythmia.
• Take safety precautions if patient experiences dizziness or other adverse CNS reactions.
PATIENT TEACHING
• Advise patient to take donepezil just before going to bed.
• Inform her that drug may be taken with or without food.
• Instruct patient to avoid potentially hazardous activities, such as driving, until drug's CNS effects are known. Encourage her to take safety precautions to prevent falling if she experiences adverse reactions, such as dizziness.
• Inform patient with history of peptic ulcer disease or gastric irritation that drug may aggravate these conditions by increasing gastric acid secretion.
• Caution patient to avoid NSAIDs during therapy because of risk of GI bleeding. Urge her to notify prescriber immediately if she notices black, tarry stools.

dopamine hydrochloride

Intropin, Revimine (CAN)

Class and Category

Chemical: Catecholamine
Therapeutic: Cardiac stimulant, vasopressor
Pregnancy category: C

Indications and Dosages

➤ *To correct hypotension that is unresponsive to adequate fluid volume replacement or occurs as part of shock syndrome caused by bacteremia, chronic cardiac decompensation, drug overdose, MI, open-heart surgery, renal failure, trauma, or other major systemic illnesses; to improve low cardiac output*

I.V. INFUSION
Adults. 0.5 to 3 mcg/kg/min for vasodilation of renal arteries; 2 to 10 mcg/kg/min for positive inotropic effects and increased cardiac output; 10 mcg/kg/min, increased gradually according to patient's response, for increased systolic and diastolic blood pressures.
DOSAGE ADJUSTMENT Initial dosage reduced to 10% of usual amount if patient has received MAO inhibitor in previous 2 to 3 wk.

Children. 1 to 5 mcg/kg/min increased gradually in increments of 2.5 to 5 mcg/kg/min to achieve desired results. *Maximum:* 20 mcg/kg/min.

Route	Onset	Peak	Duration
I.V.	In 5 min	Unknown	Up to 10 min

Mechanism of Action

Stimulates dopamine$_1$ (D$_1$) and dopamine$_2$ (D$_2$) postsynaptic receptors. D$_1$ receptors mediate vasodilation in renal, mesenteric, coronary, and cerebral blood vessels. D$_2$ receptors, when stimulated, inhibit norepinephrine release. In higher doses, dopamine also stimulates alpha$_1$ and alpha$_2$ receptors, causing vascular smooth-muscle contraction.

At doses of 0.5 to 3 mcg/kg/min, this naturally occurring catecholamine mainly affects dopaminergic receptors in renal, mesenteric, coronary, and cerebral vessels, resulting in vasodilation, increased renal blood flow, improved GFR, and increased urine output. At doses of 2 to 10 mcg/min, dopamine stimulates beta$_1$-adrenergic receptors, increasing cardiac output while maintaining dopaminergic-induced vasodilation. At doses of 10 mcg/kg/min or more, alpha-adrenergic agonism takes over, causing increased peripheral vascular resistance and renal vasoconstriction.

Incompatibilities

Don't add dopamine to 5% sodium bicarbonate, alkaline I.V. solutions, oxidizing agents, or iron salts.

Contraindications

Pheochromocytoma, uncorrected ventricular fibrillation, ventricular tachycardia, and other tachyarrhythmias

Interactions

DRUGS

alpha blockers, haloperidol, loxapine, phenothiazines, thioxanthenes: Antagonized peripheral vasoconstriction with high doses of dopamine
anesthetics, such as chloroform, enflurane, halothane, isoflurane, and methoxyflurane: Increased risk of severe atrial and ventricular arrhythmias
antihypertensives, diuretics used as antihypertensives: Possibly decreased antihypertensive effects of these drugs
beta blockers: Antagonized beta receptor-mediated inotropic effects of dopamine
digitalis glycosides: Possibly increased risk of arrhythmias and additive inotropic effects
diuretics: Possibly increased diuretic effects of dopamine or diuretic
doxapram: Possibly increased vasopressor effects of dopamine or doxapram
ergot alkaloids: Enhanced peripheral vasoconstriction
guanadrel, guanethidine: Possibly decreased hypotensive effects of these drugs and potentiated vasopressor response to dopamine, resulting in hypertension and arrhythmias
levodopa: Possibly increased risk of arrhythmias
MAO inhibitors: Prolonged and intensified cardiac stimulation and vasopressor effect of dopamine
maprotiline, tricyclic antidepressants: Possibly potentiated cardiovascular and vasopressor effects of dopamine, resulting in arrhythmias, hyperpyrexia, or severe hypertension
mecamylamine, methyldopa: Possibly decreased hypotensive effects of these drugs and enhanced vasopressor effect of dopamine
methylphenidate: Possibly potentiated vasopressor effect of dopamine
nitrates: Possibly decreased antianginal effects of nitrates; possibly decreased vasopressor effect of dopamine, resulting in hypotension
oxytocic drugs: Possibly severe hypertension
phenoxybenzamine: Possibly antagonized peripheral vasoconstriction of dopamine, causing hypotension and tachycardia
phenytoin: Possibly sudden bradycardia and hypotension
rauwolfia alkaloids: Possibly decreased hypotensive effects of these drugs
sympathomimetics: Possibly increased adverse cardiovascular and other effects
thyroid hormones: Increased risk of coronary insufficiency

Adverse Reactions

CNS: Headache
CV: Angina, bradycardia, hypertension, hypotension, palpitations, peripheral vasoconstriction, sinus tachycardia, ventricular arrhythmias
GI: Nausea, vomiting

RESP: Dyspnea
SKIN: Extravasation with tissue necrosis

Nursing Considerations

•If possible, avoid giving dopamine to patients with occlusive vascular disease, such as atherosclerosis, Buerger's disease, diabetic endarteritis, or Raynaud's disease, because of the risk of decreased peripheral circulation.
•Use drug cautiously in patients with cardiac disease, particularly coronary artery disease, because dopamine increases myocardial oxygen demand. Also use drug cautiously in patients who are allergic to sulfites, which are contained in some forms of dopamine.
•Inspect parenteral solution for particles and discoloration before administration.
•Dilute dopamine concentrate with a compatible I.V. solution before administering. Typical dilution is 400 mg in 250 ml to yield 1.6 mg/ml. Don't exceed 3.2 mg/ml.
•If patient has hypovolemia, ensure adequate fluid resuscitation before giving drug.
•Give drug by I.V. infusion using an infusion pump.
•WARNING When the infusion rate exceeds 20 mcg/kg/min, monitor patient for excessive vasoconstriction and loss of renal vasodilating effects. Avoid using an infusion rate above 50 mcg/kg/min.
•If you must infuse more than 20 mcg/kg/min of dopamine to maintain blood pressure, expect to infuse norepinephrine as prescribed.
•To avoid extravasation and tissue necrosis, administer infusion through a central catheter. If you must administer drug through a peripheral line, inspect site frequently for signs of extravasation and necrosis. If you detect such signs, start a new I.V. line for dopamine infusion, discontinue previous I.V. line, and notify prescriber immediately.
•If drug extravasates, expect prescriber to give 5 to 10 mg of phentolamine diluted in 10 to 15 ml of NS, as prescribed. Phentolamine infiltrates directly into area to antagonize vasoconstriction and minimize sloughing and tissue necrosis.
•Titrate dopamine gradually to minimize hypotension, especially after a high infusion rate.
•Monitor blood pressure continuously with an intra-arterial line, as indicated.
•Place patient on continuous ECG monitor-

ing, and assess heart rate and rhythm for arrhythmias.
•Monitor hemodynamic parameters, such as central venous pressure, pulmonary artery wedge pressure, and cardiac output, as indicated, to assess drug's effectiveness.
•Monitor urine output hourly as appropriate to assess patient for improved renal blood flow.

PATIENT TEACHING

•Explain the need for frequent hemodynamic monitoring.

doxapram hydrochloride

Dopram

Class and Category

Chemical: Pyrrolidinone derivative
Therapeutic: Respiratory stimulant
Pregnancy category: B

Indications and Dosages

➤ *To stimulate respiration in COPD-related acute respiratory insufficiency*
I.V. INFUSION
Adults and adolescents. 1 to 2 mg/min titrated according to respiratory response. *Maximum:* 3 mg/min for up to 2 hr.

➤ *To treat respiratory depression after anesthesia*
I.V. INFUSION
Adults and adolescents. 5 mg/min until desired response occurs and then reduced to 1 to 3 mg/min. *Maximum:* Cumulative dose of 4 mg/kg or 300 mg.
I.V. INJECTION
Adults and adolescents. 0.5 to 1 mg/kg, repeated q 5 min, if needed. *Maximum:* 1.5 mg/kg as a single dose or 2 mg/kg q 5 min.

Route	Onset	Peak	Duration
I.V.	20 to 40 sec	1 to 2 min	5 to 12 min

Mechanism of Action

Activates peripheral carotid, aortic, and other chemoreceptors to stimulate respiration, resulting in increased tidal volume and respiratory rate. Doxapram also may increase respiratory rate and tidal volume by directly stimulating the respiratory center in the medulla oblongata.

Incompatibilities
To avoid precipitation and gas formation, don't mix doxapram with alkaline solutions, such as aminophylline, sodium bicarbonate, or 2.5% thiopental.

Contraindications
Age less than 1 month; CVA; head injury; hypersensitivity to doxapram or its components; mechanical disorders of ventilation, including acute asthma, flail chest, muscle paresis, pneumothorax, and pulmonary fibrosis; seizure disorder; severe cardiovascular disorder; severe hypertension

Interactions
DRUGS
chloroform, cyclopropane, enflurane, halothane, isoflurane, methoxyflurane, trichloroethylene: Possibly adverse myocardial effects if doxapram given within 10 minutes of these drugs
CNS stimulants: Possibly excessive CNS stimulation, resulting in arrhythmias, insomnia, irritability, nervousness, or seizures
MAO inhibitors, sympathomimetics: Additive vasopressor effects
skeletal muscle relaxants: Masked residual effects of muscle relaxants

Adverse Reactions
CNS: Disorientation, dizziness, headache
CV: Arrhythmias, including sinus tachycardia; hypertension
GI: Diarrhea, hiccups, nausea, vomiting
GU: Urine retention
RESP: Bronchospasm, cough, dyspnea
SKIN: Diaphoresis
Other: Injection site pain, redness, swelling, and thrombophlebitis

Nursing Considerations
•Avoid giving doxapram to patients receiving mechanical ventilation.
•Maintain a patent airway, and assess for optimal oxygenation before administering drug.
•Monitor I.V. insertion site for extravasation and signs of thrombophlebitis or local skin irritation.
•If hypertension or dyspnea develops suddenly, stop infusion as directed.
•Assess for early signs of overdose, including enhanced deep tendon reflexes, skeletal muscle hyperactivity, and tachycardia.
PATIENT TEACHING
•Explain the need for frequent pulse and blood pressure monitoring.

doxazosin mesylate
Cardura, Cardura-1 (CAN), Cardura-2 (CAN), Cardura-4 (CAN)

Class and Category
Chemical: Quinazoline derivative
Therapeutic: Antihypertensive, benign prostatic hyperplasia therapeutic agent
Pregnancy category: C

Indications and Dosages
➤ *To manage hypertension*
TABLETS
Adults. *Initial:* 1 mg q.d. Doubled q 1 to 2 wk, if needed to achieve desired blood pressure. *Maximum:* 16 mg/day.

➤ *To treat benign prostatic hyperplasia (BPH)*
TABLETS
Adults. *Initial:* 1 mg q.d. Doubled q 1 to 2 wk, if needed, based on signs and symptoms. *Maximum:* 8 mg/day.

Route	Onset	Peak	Duration
P.O.	1 to 2 hr*	2 to 6 hr†	24 hr†

Mechanism of Action
Competitively inhibits alpha$_1$-adrenergic receptors in the sympathetic nervous system, causing peripheral vasodilation and reduced peripheral vascular resistance. This action increases heart rate and decreases blood pressure, especially in a standing position. Doxazosin also relaxes smooth muscle of the bladder neck, prostate, and prostate capsule, which reduces urethral resistance and pressure and urinary outflow resistance, which helps treat BPH.

Contraindications
Hypersensitivity to doxazosin, prazosin, terazosin, or their components

Interactions
DRUGS
antihypertensives, diuretics: Enhanced hypotensive effects
cimetidine: Possibly increased serum doxazosin level

---

* For hypertension; in 2 wk for BPH.
† For hypertension; unknown for BPH.

dopamine: Antagonized vasopressor effect of high-dose dopamine
ephedrine, metaraminol, methoxamine, phenylephrine: Possibly decreased vasopressor effects of these drugs
epinephrine: Possibly severe hypotension and tachycardia
NSAIDs: Possibly loss of hypotensive activity from sodium or fluid accumulation

Adverse Reactions
CNS: Dizziness, drowsiness, headache, nervousness, restlessness, vertigo
CV: Arrhythmias, including sinus tachycardia; first-dose orthostatic hypotension; palpitations; peripheral edema
EENT: Rhinitis
GI: Nausea
RESP: Dyspnea

Nursing Considerations
• Don't give doxazosin to hypotensive patients.
• Use drug cautiously in patients with hepatic disease (because normal dosage may cause exaggerated effects) and in elderly patients (because hypotensive response may be more pronounced).
• **WARNING** Monitor for orthostatic hypotension (which may cause syncope) early in therapy, especially after exercise and in patients with hypovolemia.
• Monitor blood pressure for 2 to 6 hours after first dose and with each dose increase because orthostatic hypotension commonly occurs during this time. Adjust dose as prescribed, based on standing blood pressure.
• Carefully monitor patients with renal disease for exaggerated effects, such as first-dose orthostatic hypotension.
• Monitor urination, checking for difficulty urinating and urine retention, to assess drug's effects on BPH.
PATIENT TEACHING
• Inform patient that she may take doxazosin in the morning or evening and with food, if desired.
• Instruct patient to change position slowly to minimize effects of orthostatic hypotension.
• Advise patient to avoid standing for long periods, exercising, using alcohol, and going outside in hot weather; these activities may exacerbate orthostatic hypotension.
• Advise patient to avoid potentially hazardous activities until drug's CNS effects are known.

doxepin hydrochloride
Novo-Doxepin (CAN), Sinequan, Triadapin (CAN)

Class and Category
Chemical: Dibenzoxepin derivative
Therapeutic: Antidepressant
Pregnancy category: Not rated

Indications and Dosages
➤ *To treat mild to moderate depression or anxiety*
CAPSULES, ORAL SOLUTION
Adults and adolescents. 75 to 150 mg q.d. h.s. *Maximum:* 150 mg q.d.
➤ *To treat mild to moderate depression or anxiety with organic disease*
CAPSULES, ORAL SOLUTION
Adults and adolescents. 25 to 50 mg q.d.
➤ *To treat severe depression or anxiety*
CAPSULES, ORAL SOLUTION
Adults and adolescents. 50 mg t.i.d., gradually increased to 300 mg q.d., as indicated.

Route	Onset	Peak	Duration
P.O.	2 to 3 wk	Unknown	Unknown

Mechanism of Action
May block serotonin and norepinephrine reuptake by adrenergic nerves. In this way, the tricyclic antidepressant raises serotonin and norepinephrine levels at nerve synapses, which may elevate mood and reduce depression.

Incompatibilities
Don't mix doxepin solution with carbonated beverages or grape juice.

Contraindications
Acute recovery phase of MI; concurrent use of MAO inhibitor; glaucoma; hypersensitivity to doxepin, other tricyclic antidepressants, or their components; urine retention

Interactions
DRUGS
amantadine, anticholinergics, antidyskinetics, antihistamines: Possibly intensified anticholinergic effects, causing confusion, hallucinations, and nightmares
anticonvulsants: Possibly lowered seizure threshold and decreased effects of these drugs

antithyroid drugs: Possibly increased risk of agranulocytosis

barbiturates, carbamazepine: Increased doxepin metabolism, decreased blood doxepin level, possibly lowered seizure threshold

bupropion, clozapine, cyclobenzaprine, haloperidol, loxapine, maprotiline, molindone, phenothiazines, thioxanthenes: Possibly prolonged and intensified sedative and anticholinergic effects of either drug, possibly increased risk of seizures

cimetidine: Increased blood doxepin level from inhibited systemic clearance, resulting in increased risk of toxicity

clonidine, guanadrel, guanethidine: Increased risk of hypertension, especially during second week of doxepin therapy

CNS depressants: Possibly potentiated CNS depression, hypotension, and respiratory depression

corticosteroids: Possibly exacerbated depression

direct-acting sympathomimetics, such as epinephrine and norepinephrine: Potentiated effects of these drugs

disulfiram: Possibly transient delirium

fluoxetine: Possibly increased blood doxepin level

MAO inhibitors: Possibly hyperpyrexia, hypertension, seizures, and death

oral anticoagulants: Possibly increased anticoagulant effects of these drugs

pimozide: Increased risk of arrhythmias

probucol: Possibly prolonged QT interval and increased risk of ventricular tachycardia

thyroid hormones: Possibly increased therapeutic and toxic effects of both drugs

ACTIVITIES

alcohol use: Possibly enhanced CNS depression, hypotension, and respiratory depression

Adverse Reactions

CNS: Confusion, delirium, dream disturbances, drowsiness, fatigue, hallucinations, headache, nervousness, parkinsonism, restlessness, sedation, seizures, tremor

CV: ECG changes, orthostatic hypotension, palpitations

EENT: Blurred vision, dry mouth, taste perversion

GI: Constipation, diarrhea, heartburn, ileus, increased appetite, nausea, vomiting,

GU: Decreased libido, ejaculation disorders

SKIN: Diaphoresis, jaundice

Other: Weight gain

Nursing Considerations

•If desired, mix oral solution in 120 ml of water; milk; or orange, grapefruit, tomato, or pineapple juice.

•Expect to observe adverse reactions within a few hours after giving drug.

•Evaluate patient for therapeutic response: decreased anxiety, apprehension, depression, fear, guilt, somatic symptoms, and worry; increased energy; and more restful sleep.

•Keep in mind that abrupt withdrawal of doxepin after prolonged therapy can cause cholinergic rebound effects, including diarrhea, nausea, and vomiting.

•Plan to discontinue drug, as prescribed, several days before elective surgery to avoid hypertension.

•Monitor elderly patients for signs of parkinsonism, especially with high-dose therapy.

•Be alert for seizures. Patients with a seizure disorder may need an increased anticonvulsant dosage to maintain seizure control.

•For patients with asthma or sulfite sensitivity, know that doxepin tablets may aggravate asthma or cause allergic reactions because they contain sulfites.

•Monitor diabetic patient's blood glucose level closely; drug may alter glucose metabolism.

•If patient takes a thyroid hormone, be alert for increased responses to both drugs and, possibly, exaggerated drug-induced effects, such as arrhythmias and CNS stimulation. Untreated hypothyroidism prevents adequate response to therapy.

PATIENT TEACHING

•Instruct patient to avoid alcohol during doxepin therapy because mental alertness may decrease.

•Advise diabetic patient to measure her blood glucose level more often than usual.

doxercalciferol

Hectorol

Class and Category

Chemical: Fat-soluble vitamin D analogue
Therapeutic: Antihyperparathyroid
Pregnancy category: B

Indications and Dosages

➤ *To reduce elevated intact parathyroid hormone (iPTH) blood level in managing of secondary hyperparathyroidism in patients undergoing chronic hemodialysis*

CAPSULES

Adults. *Initial:* 10 mcg 3 times/wk (about every other day) before, during, or after dialysis. *Maintenance:* If iPTH level is decreased by 50% and above 300 picograms (pg)/ml, dosage increased by 2.5 mcg at 8-wk intervals, as needed. If iPTH level is between 150 and 300 pg/ml, initial dosage maintained. If iPTH level is less than 100 pg/ml, drug stopped for 1 wk and then restarted at a dose that's at least 2.5 mcg less than previous dose. *Maximum:* 20 mcg 3 times/wk for a total of 60 mcg/wk.

Mechanism of Action

Undergoes hepatic conversion to an active metabolite (1,25-dihydroxyvitamin D_2 [1,25-dihydroxyergocalciferol]), which increases intestinal absorption of dietary calcium and renal tubular reabsorption of urinary calcium. Together with parathyroid hormone, doxercalciferol also mobilizes calcium from bone. These effects serve to maintain the blood calcium levels in patients with chronic renal failure, which in turn prevents hyperparathyroidism.

In patients with renal failure, decreased metabolic activation of vitamin D in the kidneys leads to chronic hypocalcemia. The parathyroid gland compensates by increasing PTH secretion, but renal failure prevents it from achieving a normal blood calcium level. Thus, secondary hyperparathyroidism develops. Because doxercalciferol doesn't require renal conversion to form its active metabolite, it can regulate the blood calcium level and thus suppress PTH secretion and reduce its blood level in patients with chronic renal failure. An elevated PTH level in these patients lead to metabolic bone disease, such as renal osteodystrophy.

Contraindications

Evidence of vitamin D toxicity, hypersensitivity to doxercalciferol or its components, risk or history of hypercalcemia or hyperphosphatemia

Interactions

DRUGS

cholestyramine, mineral oil, orlistat, and other drugs that affect lipid absorption: Possibly decreased doxercalciferol absorption

magnesium-containing antacids: Possibly additive drug effects and increased risk of hypermagnesemia

vitamin D and its analogues: Possibly additive effects, resulting in increased adverse effects, such as hypercalcemia

Adverse Reactions

CNS: Dizziness, headache, malaise
CV: Peripheral edema
GI: Nausea, vomiting
RESP: Dyspnea

Nursing Considerations

•**WARNING** Be aware that patients who take vitamin D also should not take doxercalciferol because they may develop severe vitamin D toxicity and hypercalcemia.

•Be alert for signs and symptoms of vitamin D toxicity and hypercalcemia in patients receiving high-dose or long-term doxercalciferol therapy. Early signs and symptoms include bone pain, constipation, dry mouth, headache, metallic taste, myalgia, nausea, somnolence, vomiting, and weakness. Late signs and symptoms include albuminuria, anorexia, arrhythmias, azotemia, conjunctivitis (calcific), decreased libido, elevated AST and ALT levels, elevated BUN level, generalized vascular calcification, hypercholesterolemia, hypertension, hyperthermia, irritability, mild metabolic acidosis, nephrocalcinosis, nocturia, pancreatitis, photophobia, polydipsia, polyuria, pruritus, rhinorrhea, and weight loss.

•Keep emergency equipment readily available in case patient develops toxicity.

•Expect to monitor blood iPTH, calcium, and phosphorus levels before starting drug therapy and weekly during early treatment.

•For patients with renal failure who are undergoing hemodialysis, be aware that oral calcium-based or other non–aluminum-containing phosphate binders and a low phosphate diet typically are used to control the serum phosphorus level. An elevated serum phosphorus level worsens secondary hyperparathyroidism and may decrease doxercalciferol's effectiveness in reducing the blood iPTH level.

•After doxercalciferol therapy starts, expect to decrease dosage of phosphate binders to correct persistent mild hypercalcemia. Expect to increase dosage to correct persistent mild hyperphosphatemia.

• Avoid giving magnesium-containing antacids with doxercalciferol if patient receives long-term hemodialysis because doing so may lead to hypermagnesemia.

PATIENT TEACHING

• Urge patient who takes doxercalciferol to strictly follow a low-phosphorus diet and to take calcium supplements, as prescribed, to maintain blood calcium level.

• Explain the importance of periodic follow-up blood work to measure drug effectiveness. Mention that it may take several months to achieve optimal PTH suppression.

• Warn patient not to take other forms of vitamin D while taking doxercalciferol and to consult prescriber before taking any OTC drugs.

• Advise patient to contact prescriber immediately if early signs or symptoms of toxicity, such as headache or nausea, develop.

doxycycline calcium

(contains 50 mg of base per 5 ml of oral suspension)

Vibramycin

doxycycline hyclate

(contains 50 or 100 mg of base per capsule, 100 mg of base per delayed-release capsule, 100 mg of base per tablet, and 100 or 200 mg of base per injection vial)

Alti-Doxycycline (CAN), Apo-Doxy (CAN), Doryx, Doxycin (CAN), Vibramycin, Vibra-Tabs

doxycycline monohydrate

(contains 50 or 100 mg of base per capsule and 25 mg of base per 5 ml of oral suspension)

Monodox, Vibramycin

Class and Category

Chemical: Oxytetracycline derivative
Therapeutic: Antibiotic
Pregnancy category: D

Indications and Dosages

➤ *To treat cutaneous, GI, or inhalation anthrax*

CAPSULES, DELAYED-RELEASE CAPSULES, ORAL SUSPENSION, TABLETS, I.V. INFUSION

Adults, adolescents, and children who weigh more than 45 kg (99 lb). 100 mg (base) q 12 hr for 60 days.

Children who weigh less than 45 kg. 2.2 mg/kg (base) q 12 hr for 60 days.

➤ *To treat endocervical, rectal, and urethral infections caused by* Chlamydia trachomatis

CAPSULES, DELAYED-RELEASE CAPSULES, ORAL SUSPENSION, TABLETS

Adults and children over age 8 who weigh more than 45 kg. 100 mg (base) b.i.d. for 7 days. *Maximum:* 300 mg (base)/day.

Children who weigh 45 kg or less. 2.2 mg (base)/kg b.i.d. on day 1 and then 2.2 to 4.4 mg (base)/kg q.d. or 1.1 to 2.2 mg (base)/kg b.i.d.

I.V. INFUSION

Adults and children over age 8 who weigh more than 45 kg. 200 mg (base) q.d. or 100 mg (base) q 12 hr on day 1 and then 100 to 200 mg (base) q.d. or 50 to 100 mg (base) q 12 hr. *Maximum:* 300 mg (base)/day.

Children who weigh 45 kg or less. 4.4 mg (base)/kg q.d. or 2.2 mg (base)/kg q 12 hr on day 1 and then 2.2 to 4.4 mg (base)/kg q.d. or 1.1 to 2.2 mg (base)/kg q 12 hr.

➤ *To treat epididymo-orchitis caused by* C. trachomatis *or* Neisseria gonorrhoeae *or nongonococcal urethritis caused by* C. trachomatis *or* Ureaplasma urealyticum

CAPSULES, DELAYED-RELEASE CAPSULES, ORAL SUSPENSION, TABLETS

Adults and children over age 8 who weigh more than 45 kg. 100 mg (base) b.i.d. for at least 10 days. *Maximum:* 300 mg (base)/day.

Children who weigh 45 kg or less. 2.2 mg (base)/kg b.i.d. on day 1 and then 2.2 to 4.4 mg (base)/kg q.d. or 1.1 to 2.2 mg (base)/kg b.i.d.

I.V. INFUSION

Adults and children over age 8 who weigh more than 45 kg. 200 mg (base) q.d. or 100 mg (base) q 12 hr on day 1 and then 100 to 200 mg (base) q.d. or 50 to 100 mg (base) q 12 hr. *Maximum:* 300 mg (base)/day.

Children who weigh 45 kg or less. 4.4 mg (base)/kg q.d. or 2.2 mg (base)/kg q 12 hr on day 1 and then 2.2 to 4.4 mg (base)/kg q.d. or 1.1 to 2.2 mg (base)/kg q 12 hr.

➤ *To prevent malaria*

CAPSULES, DELAYED-RELEASE CAPSULES, ORAL SUSPENSION, TABLETS

Adults and children over age 8 who weigh more than 45 kg. 100 mg (base) q.d. beginning 1 to 2 wk before travel, continued daily during travel, and then daily for 4 wk after travel ends. *Maximum:* 300 mg (base)/day.

Children over age 8. 2 mg (base)/kg q.d. beginning 1 to 2 days before travel, continued daily during travel, and then daily for 4 wk after travel ends. *Maximum:* 100 mg (base) q.d.

➤ *To treat early syphilis in penicillin-allergic patients*

CAPSULES, DELAYED-RELEASE CAPSULES, ORAL SUSPENSION, TABLETS

Adults and children over age 8 who weigh more than 45 kg. 100 mg (base) b.i.d. for 2 wk. *Maximum:* 600 mg (base)/day.

Children who weigh 45 kg or less. 2.2 mg (base)/kg b.i.d. on day 1 and then 2.2 to 4.4 mg (base)/kg q.d. or 1.1 to 2.2 mg (base)/kg b.i.d.

I.V. INFUSION

Adults and children over age 8 who weigh more than 45 kg. 150 mg (base) q 12 hr for at least 10 days. *Maximum:* 300 mg (base)/day.

Children who weigh 45 kg or less. 4.4 mg (base)/kg q.d. or 2.2 mg (base)/kg q 12 hr on day 1 and then 2.2 to 4.4 mg (base)/kg q.d. or 1.1 to 2.2 mg (base)/kg q 12 hr.

➤ *To treat syphilis of more than 1 year's duration in penicillin-allergic patients*

CAPSULES, DELAYED-RELEASE CAPSULES, ORAL SUSPENSION, TABLETS

Adults and children over age 8 who weigh more than 45 kg. 100 mg (base) b.i.d. for 4 wk. *Maximum:* 300 mg (base)/day.

I.V. INFUSION

Adults and children over age 8 who weigh more than 45 kg. 150 mg (base) q 12 hr for at least 10 days. *Maximum:* 300 mg (base)/day.

Children who weigh 45 kg or less. 4.4 mg (base)/kg q.d. or 2.2 mg (base)/kg q 12 hr on day 1 and then 2.2 to 4.4 mg (base)/kg q.d. or 1.1 to 2.2 mg (base)/kg q 12 hr.

➤ *To treat all other infections caused by susceptible organisms*

CAPSULES, DELAYED-RELEASE CAPSULES, ORAL SUSPENSION, TABLETS

Adults and children over age 8 who weigh more than 45 kg. 100 mg (base) q 12 hr on day 1 and then 100 mg (base) q.d. or 50 mg (base) b.i.d. For severe infections, 100 mg (base) continued q 12 hr. *Maximum:* 300 mg (base)/day.

Children who weigh 45 kg or less. 2.2 mg (base)/kg b.i.d. on day 1 and then 2.2 to 4.4 mg (base)/kg q.d. or 1.1 to 2.2 mg (base)/kg b.i.d.

I.V. INFUSION

Adults and children over age 8 who weigh more than 45 kg. 200 mg (base) q.d. or 100 mg (base) q 12 hr on day 1 and then 100 to 200 mg (base) q.d. or 50 to 100 mg (base) q 12 hr. *Maximum:* 300 mg (base)/day.

Children who weigh 45 kg or less. 4.4 mg (base)/kg q.d. or 2.2 mg (base)/kg q 12 hr on day 1 and then 2.2 to 4.4 mg (base)/kg q.d. or 1.1 to 2.2 mg (base)/kg q 12 hr.

Mechanism of Action

Exerts a bacteriostatic effect against a wide variety of gram-positive and gram-negative organisms. Doxycycline is more lipophilic than other tetracyclines, which allows it to pass more easily through the bacterial lipid bilayer, where it binds reversibly to 30S ribosomal subunits. Bound doxycycline blocks the binding of aminoacyl transfer RNA to messenger RNA, thus inhibiting bacterial protein synthesis.

Contraindications

Hypersensitivity to any tetracycline

Interactions

DRUGS

aluminum-, calcium-, magnesium-, or zinc-containing antacids; calcium supplements; choline and magnesium salicylates; iron salts; magnesium-containing laxatives: Decreased doxycycline absorption and therapeutic effects

barbiturates, carbamazepine, phenytoin: Increased clearance and decreased effects of doxycycline

cholestyramine, colestipol: Decreased doxycycline absorption

digoxin: Increased bioavailability of digoxin, possibly leading to digitalis toxicity

oral anticoagulants: Possibly increased hypoprothrombinemic effects of these drugs

oral contraceptives: Decreased effectiveness of estrogen-containing oral contraceptives, increased risk of breakthrough bleeding

penicillins: Inhibited bactericidal action

sodium bicarbonate: Altered doxycycline absorption from increased gastric pH

FOODS

dairy products, other foods high in calcium or iron: Decreased doxycycline absorption

Adverse Reactions

CNS: Paresthesia

CV: Phlebitis

EENT: Black "hairy" tongue, glossitis, hoarseness, oral candidiasis, pharyngitis, stomatitis, tooth discoloration
GI: Anorexia; bulky, loose stools; diarrhea; dysphagia; enterocolitis; epigastric distress; esophageal ulcers; hepatotoxicity; nausea; rectal candidiasis; vomiting
GU: Anogenital lesions, dark yellow or brown urine, elevated BUN level, vaginal candidiasis
HEME: Eosinophilia, hemolytic anemia, neutropenia, thrombocytopenia, thrombocytopenic purpura
SKIN: Dermatitis, photosensitivity, rash, urticaria
Other: Anaphylaxis, injection site phlebitis

Nursing Considerations

• Avoid giving doxycycline to breast-feeding women because of the risk of enamel hypoplasia, inhibited linear skeletal growth, oral and vaginal candidiasis, photosensitivity reactions, and tooth discoloration in breast-feeding infant.
• Avoid giving drug to children younger than age 8; it may cause permanent discoloration and enamel hypoplasia of developing teeth.
• Use oral suspension cautiously in patients who are allergic to sulfites because it contains sodium metabisulfite.
• Expect to adjust dosage for patients with hepatic disease to avoid drug accumulation.
• **WARNING** Don't give doxycycline by I.M. or S.C. route.
• Give doxycycline without regard to meals. Although food and milk may delay absorption, they don't significantly reduce it.
• Observe patient frequently for injection site phlebitis, a common adverse reaction to I.V. administration.
• Monitor liver enzyme levels as appropriate to detect hepatotoxicity.
• Expect oral or parenteral doxycycline to increase risk of oral, rectal, or vaginal candidiasis—especially in elderly or debilitated patients and those on prolonged therapy—by changing the normal balance of microbial flora.
• Monitor patient closely for diarrhea, which may indicate pseudomembranous colitis. If diarrhea occurs, notify prescriber and expect to withhold doxycycline. Expect to treat pseudomembranous colitis with fluids, electrolytes, protein, and an antibiotic effective against *Clostridium difficile*.

PATIENT TEACHING

• Instruct patient to avoid taking doxycycline just before bedtime because drug may not dissolve properly when she's recumbent and may cause esophageal burning and ulceration.
• Advise patient to avoid dairy products and other foods high in calcium or iron during therapy.
• Inform patient that her urine may become dark yellow or brown during therapy.
• Instruct patient to avoid sun exposure and ultraviolet light during therapy.
• Advise patients who take an oral contraceptive to use an additional contraceptive method during therapy.
• If patient is being treated for a sexually transmitted disease, explain that her partner may need treatment as well.
• Instruct patient to notify prescriber immediately if she experiences anorexia, diarrhea, epigastric distress, nausea, and vomiting.

dronabinol

(delta-9-tetrahydrocannabinol, THC)

Marinol

Class, Category, and Schedule

Chemical: Synthetic tetrahydrocannabinol
Therapeutic: Antiemetic, appetite stimulant
Pregnancy category: C
Controlled substance: Schedule II

Indications and Dosages

➤ *To prevent nausea and vomiting caused by chemotherapy in patients unresponsive to other antiemetics*
CAPSULES
Adults. 5 mg/m^2 1 to 3 hr before and 2 to 4 hr after chemotherapy, increased by 2.5 mg/m^2, as needed. *Maximum:* 15 mg/m^2/dose or a total of 4 to 6 doses/day.
➤ *To stimulate appetite in cancer and AIDS patients*
CAPSULES
Adults. *Initial:* 2.5 mg b.i.d. before lunch and supper, increased as needed. *Maximum:* 20 mg/day in divided doses.
DOSAGE ADJUSTMENT Dosage reduced to 2.5 mg before supper or h.s. for patients who can't tolerate 5 mg/day.

Route	Onset	Peak	Duration
P.O.	Unknown	Unknown	24 hr or longer*

Mechanism of Action

May exert antiemetic effect by inhibiting the vomiting control mechanism in the medulla oblongata. As the main psychoactive substance in marijuana (*Cannabis sativa* L.), dronabinol's effects may be mediated by cannabinoid receptors in neural tissues.

Contraindications

Hypersensitivity to dronabinol, its components, sesame oil, or marijuana

Interactions

DRUGS

anticholinergics, antihistamines: Possibly increased risk of tachycardia
apomorphine: Possibly potentiated CNS depression, possibly decreased emetic response with prior use of dronabinol
CNS stimulants, such as amphetamines, and CNS depressants, such as benzodiazepines: Additive CNS effects
sympathomimetics: Possibly enhanced hypertension, tachycardia, and other adverse cardiovascular effects

ACTIVITIES

alcohol use: Additive CNS depressant effects

Adverse Reactions

CNS: Amnesia, anxiety, ataxia, confusion, delusions, depression, dizziness, drowsiness, euphoria, hallucinations, irritability, mood changes, nervousness, sleep disturbance
CV: Orthostatic hypotension, palpitations, sinus tachycardia
GI: Nausea, vomiting
Other: Physical and psychological dependence

Nursing Considerations

•WARNING Be aware that drug shouldn't be discontinued abruptly; otherwise, withdrawal syndrome may occur.
•Know that patients under age 45 may tolerate drug better than those over age 45.

---

* For appetite stimulant effects; unknown for antiemetic effects.

•Monitor for adverse reactions that mimic psychosis, such as hallucinations and, possibly, acute anxiety, especially with high doses.
•Anticipate higher risk of cardiovascular reactions, such as increased heart rate and blood pressure changes (especially orthostatic hypotension), at higher doses.
•WARNING Expect tolerance to drug to develop over time, especially if patient has smoked marijuana.
•Be aware that short-term, low-dose therapy doesn't typically lead to physical and psychological dependence, which may occur with long-term, high-dose therapy.
•Expect drug to alter REM sleep pattern, even after therapy stops.

PATIENT TEACHING

•Caution patient not to stop taking dronabinol abruptly because withdrawal symptoms may occur.
•Urge patient not to use alcohol while taking dronabinol because it may enhance CNS depression.
•Instruct patient to rise slowly to sitting or standing position to minimize effects of orthostatic hypotension.
•Advise patient to avoid potentially hazardous activities until drug's CNS effects are known.
•Inform patient that sleep pattern may be adversely affected during therapy and for sometime afterward.

droperidol

Inapsine

Class and Category

Chemical: Butyrophenone derivative
Therapeutic: Antiemetic
Pregnancy category: C

Indications and Dosages

➤ *To reduce nausea and vomiting after surgery or diagnostic procedures when other treatments are ineffective*

I.V. OR I.M. INJECTION

Adults and adolescents. Dosage individualized up to a maximum initial dose of 2.5 mg I.M. or slow I.V. Additional 1.25 mg may be administered to achieve desired effect if potential benefit outweighs potential risk.
Children ages 2 to 12. Dosage individualized up to a maximum initial dose of 0.1 mg/kg.

Additional dose may be administered to achieve desired effect if potential benefit outweighs potential risk.

DOSAGE ADJUSTMENT Initial dosage reduced for elderly, debilitated, or critically ill patients because of the increased risk of hypotension and excessive sedation.

Route	Onset	Peak	Duration
I.V., I.M.	3 to 10 min	In 30 min	2 to 4 hr

Mechanism of Action

Produces sedation by blocking postsynaptic dopamine receptors in the limbic system. Droperidol may reduce nausea by blocking dopamine receptors in the chemoreceptor trigger zone in the reticular formation of the medulla oblongata. It also may produce antiemetic effects by attaching to postsynaptic gamma-aminobutyric acid receptors in the chemoreceptor trigger zone.

Contraindications

Hypersensitivity to droperidol or its components, known or suspected prolonged QT interval (including congenital long QT syndrome)

Interactions

DRUGS

amoxapine, haloperidol, loxapine, metoclopramide, metyrosine, molindone, olanzapine, phenothiazines, pimozide, rauwolfia alkaloids, risperidone, tacrine, thioxanthenes: Possibly increased risk of severe extrapyramidal reactions

anesthetics: Possibly hypotension and peripheral vasodilation

antiarrhythmics (class I or III), antidepressants, antimalarials, benzodiazepines, diuretics, I.V. opiates, laxatives, MAO inhibitors, volatile anesthetics, and other drugs that prolong QT interval (such as some antihistamines): Increased risk of serious adverse effects of droperidol, such as prolonged QT interval and arrhythmias

antihypertensives: Possibly orthostatic hypotension

bromocriptine, levodopa: Possibly inhibited actions of these drugs

CNS depressants: Additive CNS depression

epinephrine: Possibly paradoxical reduction of blood pressure

propofol: Possibly decreased antiemetic effect of both drugs

ACTIVITIES

alcohol use: Additive CNS depression

Adverse Reactions

CNS: Anxiety, drowsiness, dystonia, restlessness
CV: Cardiac arrest, hypertension, hypotension, potentially fatal arrhythmias (such as torsades de pointes and ventricular tachycardia), prolonged QT interval, sinus tachycardia
EENT: Fixed upward position of eyeballs, laryngospasm
MS: Spasms of tongue, face, neck, and back muscles
RESP: Bronchospasm

Nursing Considerations

•WARNING Use droperidol cautiously in patients over age 65 and in patients with alcoholism, bradycardia, heart failure, hypokalemia, hypomagnesemia, parkinsonism, or pre-existing QT-interval prolongation because they're at increased risk for prolonged QT interval and potentially fatal adverse reactions. Patients who take drugs that prolong QT interval, such as some antiarrhythmics and benzodiazepines, and patients who take drugs that may cause an electrolyte imbalance, such as diuretics and laxatives, are also at increased risk.

•Expect a 12-lead ECG to be performed on all patients before droperidol administration to verify the absence of prolonged QT interval. Monitor ECG continuously for 2 to 3 hours after administering drug. Also monitor serum electrolyte levels to detect electrolyte imbalances.

•Use droperidol cautiously in patients with cardiac disease, who may not be able to compensate for drug's hypotensive effect. Monitor vital signs, including blood pressure, frequently. Be aware that hypertension and tachycardia may occur in patients with a history of pheochromocytoma.

•Expect altered level of consciousness to last up to 12 hours after drug is given. Expect dosage to be reduced if patient is taking an opioid analgesic.

•If drug causes extrapyramidal reactions, such as restlessness, dystonia, and oculogyric crisis, expect to administer an anticholinergic, such as benztropine or diphenhydramine. Be sure to maintain a patent airway and oxygenation.

•If severe hypotension develops, expect to administer phenylephrine. If hypotension is related to hypovolemia, expect to administer fluids.

PATIENT TEACHING
• Advise patient to immediately report palpitations or faintness, which may indicate an abnormal cardiac rhythm.
• Instruct patient to ask for help with ambulation on first postoperative day because altered consciousness may last up to 12 hours.
• Caution patient to avoid drinking alcohol, taking CNS depressants, driving, and operating machinery for 24 hours after receiving droperidol.

drotrecogin alfa (activated)

(recombinant human activated protein C)

Xigris

Class and Category

Chemical: Serine protease glycoprotein
Therapeutic: Anti-inflammatory, antithrombolytic
Pregnancy category: C

Indications and Dosages

➤ *To reduce high risk of death in patients with severe sepsis (associated with acute organ dysfunction)*

I.V. INFUSION
Adults. 24 mcg/kg/hr for 96 hr.

Mechanism of Action

Interferes with a number of the body's responses to severe sepsis, including increased thrombin generation and fibrin formation, impaired fibrinolysis, and systemic inflammation. Drotrecogin alfa produces its antithrombotic effect by inhibiting Factors Va and VIIIa and exhibits indirect profibrinolytic activity by inhibiting plasminogen activator inhibitor-1 and limiting the generation of activated thrombin-activatable-fibrinolysis-inhibitor.

Drotrecogin may produce its anti-inflammatory effect by inhibiting production of human tumor necrosis factor and other cytokines, preventing leukocyte adhesion to selectins, and limiting thrombin-induced inflammatory responses in the microvascular endothelium.

Incompatibilities

Don't infuse any other drugs or solutions, except D_5W, NS, LR, or dextrose and saline mixtures, through the same I.V. line as drotrecogin alfa.

Contraindications

Active internal bleeding; evidence of cerebral herniation; hemorrhagic stroke within the past 3 months; hypersensitivity to drotrecogin alfa or its components; intracranial or intraspinal surgery or severe head trauma within the past 2 months; intracranial neoplasm or lesion; presence of epidural catheter; trauma with an increased risk of life-threatening bleeding

Interactions

DRUGS
abciximab, eptifibatide, and other glycoprotein IIb/IIIa inhibitors; aspirin and other platelet inhibitors; heparin; oral anticoagulants; thrombolytics: Increased risk of bleeding

Adverse Reactions

CNS: Intracranial hemorrhage
CV: Intrathoracic bleeding
GI: GI, intra-abdominal, or retroperitoneal bleeding
GU: Genitourinary bleeding
HEME: Prolonged APTT
SKIN: Ecchymosis

Nursing Considerations

• Be aware that drotrecogin alfa is used only for patients with severe sepsis who are at high risk for death, as determined by an APACHE II score, which is a method of assessing the risk of mortality.
• Reconstitute 5-mg and 20-mg vials of drotrecogin alfa by slowly adding 2.5 ml or 10 ml of sterile water for injection, respectively, to yield a concentration of 2 mg/ml. Gently swirl—don't shake—vial until powder is completely dissolved. Use immediately or store for up to 3 hours at 15° to 30° C (59° to 86° F).
• Add reconstituted drug to NS by directing stream to side of bag to minimize agitation. Gently invert the bag to mix; don't shake. Dilute drug to a concentration of 100 to 200 mg/ml if it will be administered by I.V. infusion pump and to a final concentration of 100 to 1,000 mg/ml if it will be administered by syringe pump. Be aware that infusion bag should not be transported by a me-

chanical delivery system, such as a tube delivery system between the pharmacy and nursing unit.

•Prime infusion set for 15 minutes at a flow rate of 5 ml/hour when infusing a concentration of less than 200 mg/ml at a rate of less than 5 ml/hour. Use prepared I.V. solution within 12 hours.

•Administer drotrecogin alfa through a dedicated I.V. line or a dedicated lumen of a multilumen central venous catheter. Don't infuse any other drugs or solutions—other than D₅W, NS, LR, or dextrose and saline mixtures—through the same line.

•Be aware that the total duration of the infusion must equal 96 hours, even if you need to interrupt it for a period. For example, if you calculate that the infusion should end on 5 p.m. Friday, but then have to discontinue it to give the patient blood for 2 hours on Thursday, add those 2 hours to your estimated completion time, which would then be 7 p.m. Friday.

•WARNING Monitor patient closely for signs of bleeding; stop drotrecogin alfa infusion immediately and notify prescriber if bleeding occurs. Patients at increased risk for bleeding include those with chronic severe hepatic disease, intracranial arteriovenous malformation or aneurysm, known bleeding diathesis, recent (in the past 6 weeks) GI bleeding, or recent (in the past 3 months) ischemic stroke; those receiving concurrent therapeutic heparin (15 U/kg/hour or more); those who have recently received thrombolytic therapy (in the past 3 days), aspirin (at dosage greater than 650 mg/day) or other platelet inhibitors (in the past 7 days), or oral anticoagulants or glycoprotein IIb/IIIa inhibitors (in the past 7 days); those with any other condition in which bleeding would constitute a significant hazard or be difficult to manage because of its location; and those with a platelet count less than 30,000 × 10⁶/L or PT (as INR) greater than 3.0.

•Expect to discontinue drotrecogin alfa 2 hours before an invasive surgical or other procedure that poses a risk of bleeding and to resume administration immediately after uncomplicated, less-invasive procedures or 12 hours after major invasive procedures or surgery at the same rate of 24 mg/kg/hour, as prescribed.

•Be aware that drotrecogin alfa may prolong APTT during administration; PT may need to

be used to monitor coagulopathy status during treatment.

•Before using drotrecogin alfa, refrigerate it at 2° to 8° C (36° to 46 °F); don't freeze. Protect drug from heat and direct sunlight.

PATIENT TEACHING

•Teach patient about adverse reactions associated with drotrecogin alfa, including bleeding from gums or nose or increased bruising. Instruct her to immediately report any signs of bleeding.

•Reassure patient that she'll be monitored closely throughout therapy.

dutasteride

Class and Category
Chemical: Synthetic 4-azasteroid compound
Therapeutic: Benign prostatic hyperplasia agent
Pregnancy category: X

Indications and Dosages
➤ *To treat symptomatic benign prostatic hyperplasia*
CAPSULES
Adult males. 0.5 mg q.d.

Contraindications
Children; females; hypersensitivity to dutasteride, its components, or other 5-alpha reductase inhibitors

Interactions
DRUGS
cimetidine, ciprofloxacin, diltiazem, ketoconazole, ritonavir, verapamil, and other CYP3A4 inhibitors: Risk of decreased metabolism and enhanced effects of dutasteride

Adverse Reactions
ENDO: Gynecomastia, increased serum testosterone and thyroid-stimulating hormone levels
GU: Decreased ejaculatory volume, decreased libido, impotence

Nursing Considerations
•WARNING Be aware that dutasteride is absorbed through the skin. If you are female and pregnant or of childbearing age, do *not* handle the dutasteride capsule when administering it to a patient.

Mechanism of Action

Dutasteride reduces prostate gland enlargement by inhibiting the conversion of the male hormone testosterone to its active metabolite, 5-alpha dihydrotestosterone (DHT). DHT is the principal hormone that stimulates prostate cells to grow. As men age, they may become more sensitive to the effects of DHT, resulting in an excessive growth of prostatic cells and enlargement of the prostate. This condition, known as benign prostatic hyperplasia, may cause such signs and symptoms as urinary hesitancy, urinary urgency, and nocturia.

The intracellular enzyme 5-alpha-reductase (5α-R), which is present in the liver, prostate, and skin, converts testosterone to DHT, as shown below left. The two forms of 5α-R are type 1 and type 2. Dutasteride, a dual 5α-R inhibitor, deactivates both forms. When 5α-R is inhibited by dutasteride, the production of DHT is suppressed, as shown below right. With less circulating DHT, the prostate gland becomes smaller and the patient experiences an improvement in his symptoms.

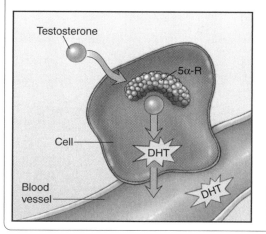
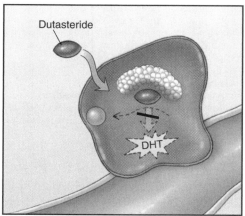

•Expect patient to undergo a digital rectal examination of the prostate before and periodically during dutasteride therapy.
•Anticipate the need to obtain a new baseline prostate-specific antigen (PSA) value after 3 to 6 months of treatment because dutasteride can decrease PSA concentration by 40% to 50%.

PATIENT TEACHING

•**WARNING** Urge patient and female partners to use reliable contraceptive method during dutasteride therapy because semen of men who take drug can harm male fetuses. Caution women and children against handling capsules.
•Advise patient to inform prescriber if he has liver disease.
•Explain how to take drug properly, and advise patient to follow instructions that accompany drug. Instruct him to swallow cap-sule whole and to notify pharmacist if capsules are cracked or leaking.
•Inform patient that drug may cause decreased ejaculatory volume, decreased libido, and impotence.
•Instruct patient to postpone blood donations for 6 months after final dose to avoid transmitting dutasteride to a pregnant female during a blood transfusion.
•Urge patient to have periodic follow-up evaluations.

dyphylline

Dilor, Lufyllin

Class and Category

Chemical: Xanthine derivative
Therapeutic: Bronchodilator
Pregnancy category: C

Indications and Dosages

➤ *To prevent or relieve bronchospasm from acute and chronic bronchial asthma, chronic bronchitis, and emphysema*

ELIXIR, TABLETS

Adults. Up to 15 mg/kg q 6 hr.

I.M. INJECTION

Adults. *Initial:* 500 mg. *Maintenance:* 250 to 500 mg q 2 to 6 hr, as needed.

Mechanism of Action

May cause bronchodilation by inhibiting phosphodiesterase enzymes. These enzymes normally inactivate cAMP and cGMP, which are responsible for bronchial smooth-muscle relaxation. Other possible mechanisms of action include calcium translocation, prostaglandin antagonism, catecholamine stimulation, and adenosine-receptor antagonism.

Contraindications

Hypersensitivity to dyphylline, xanthines, or their components; peptic ulcer disease; seizure disorder (unless controlled by anticonvulsants)

Interactions

DRUGS

beta blockers: Possibly inhibited bronchodilation by dyphylline

ephedrine: Possibly increased frequency of insomnia, nausea, and nervousness

hydrocarbon inhalation anesthetics: Possibly increased risk of ventricular arrhythmias

probenecid: Possibly decreased renal excretion of dyphylline

sucralfate: Possibly adsorption of dyphylline if drugs given within 2 hours of each other

Adverse Reactions

CNS: Headache, insomnia, irritability, nervousness, seizures, tremor

CV: Arrhythmias, hypotension, tachycardia

GI: Diarrhea, gastroesophageal reflux, nausea, vomiting

GU: Increased diuresis

Nursing Considerations

•Inspect I.M. form of dyphylline for precipitate. If precipitate is present, discard drug and obtain a new ampule.

•Give oral drug at least 1 hour after meals for best absorption. However, if drug causes GI distress, give it with food if prescribed.

•Don't give parenteral drug by I.V. route.

•Evaluate for therapeutic response: decreased respiratory rate and effort.

•Assess for signs of dyphylline toxicity, including seizures and ventricular tachycardia.

PATIENT TEACHING

•Instruct patient to take oral dyphylline with a full glass of water and on an empty stomach to promote absorption.

•Advise patient to consult prescriber about taking drug with food if she experiences GI distress.

➤━━━━━━━━━━━━━━━━━━◄

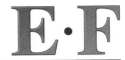

E·F

eflornithine hydrochloride

(alpha-difluoromethyl-ornithine, DFMO)

Ornidyl

Class and Category
Chemical: Difluoromethylornithine
Therapeutic: Antiprotozoal
Pregnancy category: C

Indications and Dosages

➤ *To treat the meningoencephalitic stage of* Trypanosoma brucei gambiense *infection (sleeping sickness)*

I.V. INFUSION
Adults. 100 mg/kg given over at least 45 min q 6 hr for 14 days.

Route	Onset	Peak	Duration
I.V.	Unknown	4 to 6 hr	Unknown

Mechanism of Action
Inhibits the enzyme ornithine decarboxylase, which is needed for decarboxylation of ornithine. This process is the first step in polyamine synthesis, which is needed for protozoal cell division and differentiation.

Incompatibilities
Don't administer eflornithine with any other drug.

Contraindications
Hypersensitivity to eflornithine or its components

Adverse Reactions
CNS: Asthenia, dizziness, headache, seizures
EENT: Hearing loss
GI: Abdominal pain, anorexia, diarrhea, vomiting
HEME: Anemia, eosinophilia, leukopenia, myelosuppression, thrombocytopenia
Other: Alopecia, facial edema

Nursing Considerations
•Plan to reduce eflornithine dosage as prescribed, based on renal function. Monitor creatinine clearance in patients with renal function impairment.
•Before infusion, dilute eflornithine concentrate with sterile water for injection. Using strict aseptic technique, withdraw the contents of a 100-ml vial and inject 25 ml into each of four I.V. diluent bags that contain 100 ml of sterile water. The resulting solution contains 40 mg/ml of eflornithine (5,000 mg of eflornithine in 125 ml total volume).
•Store bags of diluted eflornithine at 4° C (39° F) to reduce the risk of contamination. Use diluted drug within 24 hours.
•Expect to monitor CBC, including platelet count, before treatment, twice weekly during treatment, and weekly after therapy stops until hematologic values return to baseline.
•Take infection-control and bleeding precautions because drug may cause myelosuppression. Adjust dosage or stop therapy as prescribed, based on severity.
•Take seizure precautions during therapy.
•Consult prescriber about the need for serial audiography, if appropriate.
•Store undiluted vials at room temperature and protect from freezing and light.

PATIENT TEACHING
•Stress the importance of follow-up visits because the risk of relapse lasts for 24 months after treatment.
•Teach patient how to follow infection-control and bleeding precautions if myelosuppression occurs.
•Warn patient about risk of seizures; advise against performing potentially hazardous activities during therapy.

enalapril maleate

Vasotec

enalaprilat

Vasotec I.V.

Class and Category
Chemical: Dicarbocyl-containing ACE inhibitor
Therapeutic: Antihypertensive
Pregnancy category: C (first trimester), D (later trimesters)

Indications and Dosages

➤ *To control hypertension*

TABLETS

Adults. *Initial:* 5 mg q.d., increased after 1 to 2 wk, as needed. *Maintenance:* 10 to 40 mg q.d. or in divided doses b.i.d.

Children. 0.08 mg/kg q.d., titrated according to blood pressure response up to 5 mg q.d. *Maximum:* 0.58 mg/kg/dose or 40 mg/dose.

I.V. INJECTION

Adults. 1.25 mg q 6 hr.

DOSAGE ADJUSTMENT Initial dose reduced to 2.5 mg P.O. or 0.625 mg I.V. for patients who have sodium and water depletion from diuretic therapy, are receiving diuretics, or have a creatinine clearance below 30 ml/min/1.73 m². If response to I.V. dose is inadequate after 1 hr, I.V. dose of 0.625 mg is repeated and therapy continued at 1.25 mg q 6 hr.

➤ *To treat heart failure*

TABLETS

Adults. *Initial:* 2.5 mg q.d. or b.i.d., increased after 1 to 2 wk, as needed. *Maintenance:* 5 to 40 mg q.d. or in divided doses b.i.d.

➤ *To treat asymptomatic left ventricular dysfunction*

TABLETS

Adults. *Initial:* 2.5 mg b.i.d., increased to 20 mg/day in divided doses.

DOSAGE ADJUSTMENT Initial dosage reduced to 2.5 mg q.d. and, if possible, diuretic dosage reduced in patients who have a serum sodium level below 130 mEq/L or a serum creatinine level above 1.6 mg/dl.

Route	Onset	Peak	Duration
P.O.	1 hr	4 to 6 hr	About 24 hr
I.V.	15 min	1 to 4 hr	About 6 hr

Contraindications

History of angioedema from previous ACE inhibitor; hypersensitivity to enalapril, enalaprilat, or their components

Interactions

DRUGS

allopurinol, bone marrow depressants (such as amphotericin B and methotrexate), procainamide, systemic corticosteroids: Possibly increased risk of fatal neutropenia or agranulocytosis

cyclosporine, potassium-sparing diuretics, potassium supplements: Increased risk of hyperkalemia

diuretics, other antihypertensives: Additive hypotensive effects

lithium: Increased blood lithium level and lithium toxicity

NSAIDs: Possibly reduced antihypertensive effects of enalapril and enalaprilat

sympathomimetics: Possibly reduced therapeutic effects of enalapril and enalaprilat

FOODS

potassium-containing salt substitutes: Increased risk of hyperkalemia

ACTIVITIES

alcohol use: Possibly additive hypotensive effect

Mechanism of Action

May reduce blood pressure by affecting the renin-angiotensin-aldosterone system. By inhibiting ACE, enalapril:

• prevents conversion of angiotensin I to angiotensin II, a potent vasoconstrictor that also stimulates the adrenal cortex to secrete aldosterone

• may inhibit renal and vascular production of angiotensin II

• decreases the serum angiotensin II level and increases serum renin activity, which decreases aldosterone secretion and slightly increases serum potassium level and fluid loss

• decreases vascular tone and blood pressure

• inhibits aldosterone release, which reduces sodium and water reabsorption and increases their excretion, further reducing blood pressure.

Adverse Reactions

CNS: Ataxia, confusion, CVA, depression, dizziness, dream disturbances, fatigue, headache, insomnia, nervousness, peripheral neuropathy, somnolence, syncope, vertigo, weakness

CV: Angina, arrhythmias, cardiac arrest, hypotension, MI, orthostatic hypotension, palpitations, pulmonary embolism and infarction, Raynaud's phenomenon

EENT: Blurred vision, conjunctivitis, dry eyes and mouth, glossitis, hoarseness, lacrimation, loss of smell, pharyngitis, rhinorrhea, stomatitis, taste perversion, tinnitus

ENDO: Gynecomastia

GI: Abdominal pain, anorexia, constipation,

diarrhea, hepatic failure, hepatitis, ileus, indigestion, melena, nausea, pancreatitis, vomiting
GU: Flank pain, impotence, oliguria, renal failure, UTI
MS: Muscle spasms
RESP: Asthma, bronchitis, bronchospasm, cough, dyspnea, pneumonia, pulmonary edema, pulmonary infiltrates, upper respiratory tract infection
SKIN: Alopecia, diaphoresis, erythema multiforme, exfoliative dermatitis, flushing, pemphigus, photosensitivity, pruritus, rash, Stevens-Johnson syndrome, toxic epidermal necrolysis, urticaria
Other: Anaphylaxis, angioedema, herpes zoster, hyperkalemia

Nursing Considerations
• Use enalapril and enalaprilat cautiously in patients with impaired renal function. Be aware that drug shouldn't be given to children with a GFR of less than 30 ml/min/1.73 m^2.
• For children who can't swallow tablets, consult with prescriber and pharmacist about preparation of an oral suspension from tablets as directed by manufacturer.
• Give each I.V. dose over at least 5 minutes.
• Measure blood pressure immediately after first dose and frequently for at least 2 hours thereafter. If hypotension requires a dosage reduction, monitor blood pressure frequently for 2 hours after reduced dosage is administered and for another hour after blood pressure has stabilized.
• Monitor blood pressure regularly during therapy. If hypotension develops, place patient in a supine position and expect to give I.V. NS or other volume expander as prescribed.
• Monitor heart rate and rhythm. Expect to obtain repeated 12-lead ECG tracings.
• Monitor laboratory test results to check hepatic and renal function, leukocyte count, and serum potassium level.
• Monitor patient closely for angioedema of the face, lips, tongue, glottis, larynx, and limbs. For angioedema of the face and lips, stop drug and give an antihistamine, as prescribed. If tongue, glottis, or larynx is involved, assess patient for airway obstruction and prepare to give epinephrine 1:1,000 (0.3 to 0.5 ml) S.C. and maintain a patent airway.

PATIENT TEACHING
• Advise patient to take enalapril or enalaprilat at the same time each day.
• Instruct patient not to split, crush, or chew tablets.
• Inform patient that light-headedness and fainting may occur, especially during first few days of therapy. Advise him to change position slowly and avoid potentially hazardous activities until drug's CNS effects are known.
• Inform patient that diarrhea, excessive sweating, vomiting, and other conditions may cause dehydration, which can lead to dizziness, fainting, and very low blood pressure during therapy. Urge sufficient fluid intake to prevent dehydration and related adverse reactions. If diarrhea or vomiting is severe or prolonged, instruct patient to notify prescriber.
• Urge patient to immediately notify prescriber if angioedema and other adverse reactions, including persistent dry cough, occur.
• Advise patient to consult prescriber before using salt substitutes, potassium supplements, or other drugs (including OTC drugs) while taking drug.

enoxacin

Penetrex

Class and Category
Chemical: Fluoroquinolone
Therapeutic: Antibiotic
Pregnancy category: C

Indications and Dosages
➤ *To treat gonorrhea*
TABLETS
Adults. 400 mg as a single dose.
➤ *To treat uncomplicated UTIs*
TABLETS
Adults. 200 mg q 12 hr for 7 days.
➤ *To treat complicated UTIs*
TABLETS
Adults. 400 mg q 12 hr for 14 days.
DOSAGE ADJUSTMENT Dosage reduced to one-half in patients with creatinine clearance of 30 ml/min/1.73 m^2 or less.

Contraindications
History of tendinitis or tendon rupture, hypersensitivity to enoxacin or any quinolone antibiotic

Mechanism of Action

Normally, the enzyme DNA gyrase is responsible for unwinding and supercoiling bacterial DNA before it replicates, as shown below left. Enoxacin inhibits this enzyme, as shown below right, interfering with bacterial cell replication and causing cell death.

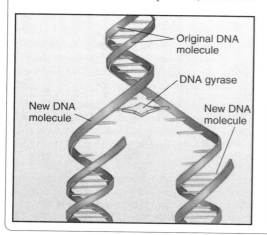

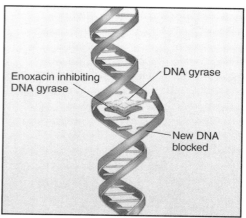

Interactions

DRUGS

aluminum-, calcium-, or magnesium-containing antacids; ferrous sulfate; magnesium-containing laxatives; sucralfate; zinc: Interference with enoxacin absorption, decreased blood enoxacin level

bismuth: Decreased enoxacin bioavailability (by about 25% if given with or up to 60 minutes after enoxacin)

cyclosporine: Possibly increased blood cyclosporine level

digoxin: Increased serum digoxin level and risk of digitalis toxicity

NSAIDs: Possibly increased risk of CNS stimulation and seizures

theophylline: Interference with theophylline metabolism, increased risk of theophylline toxicity

warfarin: Possibly increased anticoagulant effect of warfarin and increased risk of bleeding

FOODS

caffeine: Decreased caffeine clearance, increased adverse effects of caffeine, increased blood enoxacin level

Adverse Reactions

CNS: Dizziness, drowsiness, hallucinations, headache, insomnia, nervousness, seizures, vertigo
EENT: Taste perversion
GI: Abdominal pain, diarrhea, indigestion, nausea, pseudomembranous colitis, vomiting
GU: Vaginitis
MS: Tendinitis, tendon rupture
SKIN: Photosensitivity, pruritus, rash
Other: Anaphylaxis

Nursing Considerations

•Be aware that enoxacin shouldn't be given to a patient under age 18 because it may cause arthropathy.
•Use drug cautiously in patients with a history of or susceptibility to seizures.
•Obtain a specimen for culture and sensitivity tests, as ordered, but expect to begin therapy before results are available.
•Monitor closely for signs and symptoms of anaphylaxis after first dose: shock, dyspnea, facial or laryngeal edema, loss of consciousness, paresthesia, pruritus, and urticaria. If they occur, stop enoxacin immediately, notify prescriber, and prepare to treat symptoms.

•Ask if patient has a history of seizures. Take seizure and safety precautions because drug may induce seizures and other adverse CNS reactions after a single dose.
•Notify prescriber if severe or prolonged diarrhea develops; it may indicate pseudomembranous colitis.
•Monitor for pain, inflammation, and tendon rupture, especially in shoulders, hands, and ankles.
•If patient has gonorrhea, expect to obtain a serologic test for syphilis at the time of diagnosis and to repeat it 3 months after enoxacin therapy ends.

PATIENT TEACHING
•Stress the importance of taking enoxacin exactly as prescribed for the full course, even if patient feels better before it's finished.
•Instruct patient to take drug at the same times each day—1 hour before or 2 hours after meals—with 8 oz of water.
•Advise patient to avoid potentially hazardous activities until drug's CNS effects are known.
•Advise patient to notify prescriber if symptoms don't improve within a few days after therapy starts.
•Urge patient to drink plenty of fluids but to avoid caffeine during therapy.
•Caution patient not to take aluminum-, calcium-, or magnesium-containing antacids; bismuth; or products that contain iron or zinc for 8 hours before or 2 hours after taking enoxacin.
•Advise patient to avoid direct sunlight and to use sunscreen and wear protective clothing while outdoors. Urge him to notify prescriber about photosensitivity reactions.
•Instruct patient to stop taking enoxacin and notify prescriber immediately if a rash or other allergic reaction develops.
•Instruct patient to take a missed dose as soon as he remembers, unless it's nearly time for the next dose. Warn against doubling the dose.
•Instruct patient to stop taking enoxacin and notify prescriber about tendon pain or inflammation and to rest until tendinitis or tendon rupture is ruled out.

enoxaparin sodium

Lovenox

Class and Category
Chemical: Low-molecular-weight heparin
Therapeutic: Antithrombotic
Pregnancy category: B

Indications and Dosages
➤ *To prevent deep vein thrombosis after hip or knee replacement and for continued prophylaxis after hospitalization for hip replacement*
S.C. INJECTION
Adults. 30 mg q 12 hr, starting 12 to 24 hr after surgery and lasting up to 14 days. Alternatively, 40 mg q.d., starting 9 to 15 hr after hip replacement surgery. *Prophylaxis:* 40 mg q.d. for 3 wk.

➤ *To prevent deep vein thrombosis after abdominal surgery for patients with thromboembolic risk factors (age over 40, obesity, general anesthesia lasting longer than 30 minutes, cancer, or a history of deep vein thrombosis or pulmonary embolism)*
S.C. INJECTION
Adults. 40 mg q.d., starting 2 hr before surgery and lasting 7 to 10 days.

➤ *To prevent ischemic complications of unstable angina and non-Q-wave MI*
S.C. INJECTION
Adults. 1 mg/kg q 12 hr with 100 to 325 mg of aspirin q.d. for 2 to 8 days or until condition is stable.

Route	Onset	Peak	Duration
S.C.	Unknown	3 to 5 hr	Up to 24 hr

Mechanism of Action
Potentiates the action of antithrombin III, a coagulation inhibitor. By binding with antithrombin III, enoxaparin rapidly binds with and inactivates clotting factors (primarily thrombin and factor Xa). Without thrombin, fibrinogen can't convert to fibrin and clots can't form.

Incompatibilities
Don't mix enoxaparin with other I.V. fluids or drugs.

Contraindications
Active major bleeding; hypersensitivity to enoxaparin, heparin, low-molecular-weight

heparins, or pork products; thrombocytopenia and positive antiplatelet antibody test while taking low-molecular-weight heparins

Interactions
DRUGS
cefamandole, cefoperazone, cefotetan, plicamycin, valproic acid: Possibly increased risk of hemorrhage
NSAIDs; oral anticoagulants; platelet aggregation inhibitors, such as aspirin, dipyridamole, sulfinpyrazone, and ticlopidine; thrombolytics, such as alteplase, anistreplase, streptokinase, and urokinase: Possibly increased risk of bleeding

Adverse Reactions
CNS: Confusion, CVA, fever
CV: Peripheral edema, pulmonary embolism
EENT: Epistaxis
GI: Bloody stools, hematemesis, melena, nausea, vomiting
GU: Hematuria, menstrual irregularities
HEME: Anemia, hemorrhage, thrombocytopenia
RESP: Dyspnea
SKIN: Ecchymosis, persistent bleeding or oozing from mucous membranes or surgical wounds
Other: Injection site erythema, hematoma, irritation, and pain

Nursing Considerations
•Use enoxaparin with extreme caution in patients with a history of heparin-induced thrombocytopenia or an increased risk of hemorrhage. Use it cautiously in patients with bleeding diathesis, recent GI ulceration or hemorrhage, or uncontrolled hypertension. Also expect possible delayed drug elimination in elderly patients and those with renal insufficiency.
•Be aware that enoxaparin is not recommended for patients with prosthetic heart valves, especially pregnant women, because of the risk of prosthetic valve thrombosis.
•Don't give drug by I.M. injection.
•Expect to give drug with aspirin to patient with unstable angina and non-Q wave MI.
•Closely monitor for bleeding and decreased platelet count during therapy. Notify prescriber immediately if platelet count falls below 100,000/mm^3. Also expect to discontinue drug and start appropriate prescribed

therapy if patient has a thromboembolic event, such as a CVA, despite enoxaparin therapy.
•Test stool for occult blood, as ordered.
•Keep protamine sulfate nearby in case of accidental overdose.
PATIENT TEACHING
•Advise patient to notify prescriber about adverse reactions, especially bleeding.
•Instruct patient to seek immediate help if he experiences signs of thromboembolism, such as neurologic changes and severe shortness of breath.
•Stress the importance of complying with follow-up visits with prescriber.
•Teach patient or family member how to administer enoxaparin at home, if needed. Show patient how to administer by deep S.C. injection while lying down. Instruct him not to expel the air bubble from a prefilled syringe to avoid losing some of the drug. Tell him to insert the entire needle into a skin fold held between the thumb and forefinger. Remind him to alternate administration sites between the left and right anterolateral abdominal wall.
•To minimize bruising, caution patient not to rub the injection site after giving the injection.
•Review safe handling and disposal of syringes and needles.

entacapone

Comtan

Class and Category
Chemical: COMT inhibitor
Therapeutic: Antidyskinetic
Pregnancy category: C

Indications and Dosages
➤ *As adjunct to manage symptoms of Parkinson's disease*
TABLETS
Adults. 200 mg with each dose of carbidopa-levodopa. *Maximum:* 1,600 mg/day.

Contraindications
Hypersensitivity to entacapone or its components, use within 14 days of nonselective MAO inhibitor therapy

Mechanism of Action

Inhibits peripheral catechol-*O*-methyl-transferase (COMT), the major metabolizing enzyme for levodopa. During levodopa metabolism, COMT causes the formation of a levodopa metabolite that reduces the effectiveness of levodopa. By inhibiting COMT, entacapone leads to higher sustained blood levels of levodopa and its increased availability for diffusion into the CNS, where it is converted to dopamine. Depleted dopamine stores are thought to cause Parkinson's disease. By replenishing dopamine stores, entacapone increases dopaminergic stimulation in the brain and reduces the symptoms of Parkinson's disease. Carbidopa is given with levodopa because it inhibits the peripheral distribution of levodopa, making more levodopa available for transport to the brain.

Interactions

DRUGS

ampicillin, chloramphenicol, cholestyramine, erythromycin, probenecid, rifampin: Decreased biliary excretion of entacapone
apomorphine, bitolterol, dobutamine, dopamine, epinephrine, isoetharine, isoproterenol, methyldopa, norepinephrine: Possibly increased heart rate, arrhythmias, and excessive changes in blood pressure
MAO inhibitors (nonselective): Possibly inhibited entacapone metabolism

Adverse Reactions

CNS: Agitation, anxiety, asthenia, dizziness, dyskinesia, fatigue, hallucinations, hyperkinesia, hypokinesia, somnolence
EENT: Dry mouth
GI: Abdominal pain, constipation, diarrhea, indigestion, gastritis, nausea
GU: Brown-orange urine
MS: Back pain
RESP: Dyspnea
SKIN: Diaphoresis, purpura

Nursing Considerations

•**WARNING** Be aware that entacapone should not be discontinued abruptly because doing so may precipitate signs and symptoms resembling those of neuroleptic malignant syndrome, such as fever, muscle rigidity, altered level of consciousness, confusion, and elevated creatine kinase level. Patients may also experience a rapid reemergence of parkinsonian symptoms.
•Monitor for drug-induced diarrhea during first 4 to 12 weeks of entacapone therapy.
•Assist patient with activities as necessary because drug may increase occurrence of orthostatic hypotension or syncope in susceptible patients.
•Monitor for worsening dyskinesia because entacapone potentiates dopaminergic adverse effects of levodopa and may exacerbate pre-existing dyskinesia.
•Be aware that drug may be taken with selective MAO inhibitors, such as selegiline.

PATIENT TEACHING

•Instruct patient to always take entacapone with carbidopa-levodopa because drug has no antidyskinetic effect of its own.
•Inform patient that dizziness and sleepiness are more common at beginning of treatment, especially in those with hypotension.
•Advise patient not to participate in potentially hazardous activities until drug's CNS effects are known, especially if he's also taking CNS depressants.
•If patient is scheduled for surgery, instruct him to inform surgeon and anesthesiologist of entacapone use beforehand because COMT inhibitors may interact with some drugs used in surgical procedures.
•Caution patient that entacapone may increase adverse effects of carbidopa-levodopa, such as nausea and uncontrolled movements. If these adverse effects do increase, advise him to contact prescriber immediately because carbidopa-levodopa dosage may need to be lowered.
•Inform patient that urine may turn brown-orange while he's taking entacapone but that this is a harmless effect.

epinephrine

(adrenaline)

Adrenalin, Adrenalin Chloride Solution, Ana-Guard, Bronkaid Mist, Bronkaid Mistometer (CAN), EpiPen (CAN), EpiPen Auto-Injector, EpiPen Jr. (CAN), EpiPen Jr. Auto-Injector, Primatene Mist

E
F

epinephrine bitartrate

Asthmahaler Mist, Bronkaid Suspension Mist

racepinephrine

AsthmaNefrin, MicroNefrin, Nephron, Vaponefrin

Class and Category

Chemical: Catecholamine
Therapeutic: Antianaphylactic, bronchodilator, cardiac stimulant, vasopressor
Pregnancy category: C

Indications and Dosages

➤ *To treat bronchospasm*

INHALED SOLUTION (EPINEPRHINE)

Adults and children age 4 and older. 1 to 3 inhalations (10 drops) by hand-bulb nebulizer no more than q 3 hr.

INHALED SOLUTION (RACEPINEPHRINE)

Adults and children age 4 and older. 3 inhalations of 0.5 ml (10 drops) by hand-bulb nebulizer, or 0.2 to 0.5 ml (4 to 10 drops) of diluted solution given over 15 min by jet nebulizer; repeated after 3 to 4 hr, if needed.

ORAL INHALED AEROSOL (EPINEPHRINE BITARTRATE)

Adults and children age 4 and older. 1 inhalation (160 mcg) repeated after 1 min, if needed; then repeated after at least 3 hr.

ORAL INHALER (EPINEPHRINE)

Adults and children age 4 and older. 1 inhalation (200 to 275 mcg) repeated after at least 1 min, if needed; then repeated after at least 3 hr.

➤ *To treat croup*

INHALED SOLUTION (RACEPINEPHRINE)

Children. 0.05 ml/kg diluted to 3 ml in NS and given over 15 min q 2 hr, as needed. *Maximum:* 0.5 ml/dose.

➤ *To treat anaphylaxis*

I.V. INFUSION

Adults and adolescents. 100 to 250 mcg given slowly.

I.M. OR S.C. INJECTION

Adults and adolescents. 100 to 500 mcg repeated q 10 to 15 min, as needed. *Maximum:* 1 mg/dose; three doses.

Children. 10 mcg/kg repeated q 15 min for three doses. *Maximum:* 300 mcg/dose.

➤ *To treat severe anaphylactic shock*

I.V. INFUSION

Adults. 1 mcg/min titrated to 2 to 10 mcg/min for desired hemodynamic response.

➤ *To treat cardiac arrest*

I.V. INJECTION

Adults. 0.5 to 1 mg q 3 to 5 min during resuscitation.

Children. 10 mcg/kg followed by 100 mcg/kg q 3 to 5 min, if needed. If two doses produce no response, subsequent doses are increased to 200 mcg/kg q 5 min.

Neonates. 10 to 30 mcg/kg q 3 to 5 min.

Route	Onset	Peak	Duration
I.V., I.M.	Rapid	Unknown	1 to 2 min
S.C.	5 to 10 min	In 20 min	Short
Oral inhalation	1 to 5 min	In 5 to 15 min	Up to 3 hr

Mechanism of Action

Acts on alpha and beta receptors. This nonselective adrenergic agonist stimulates:
• alpha$_1$ receptors, which constricts arteries and may decrease bronchial secretions
• presynaptic alpha$_2$ receptors, which inhibits norepinephrine release by way of negative feedback
• postsynaptic alpha$_2$ receptors, which constricts arteries
• beta$_1$ receptors, which induces positive chronotropic and inotropic responses
• beta$_2$ receptors, which dilates arteries, relaxes bronchial smooth muscles, increases glycogenolysis, and prevents mast cells from secreting histamine and other substances, thus reversing bronchoconstriction and edema.

Incompatibilities

Don't mix epinephrine with alkalies or oxidizing agents, including bromine, chlorine, chromates, iodine, metal salts (as from iron), nitrites, oxygen, and permanganates, because these substances can destroy epinephrine.

Contraindications

Cerebral arteriosclerosis, coronary insufficiency, counteraction of phenothiazine-induced hypotension, dilated cardiomyopathy, general anesthesia with halogenated hydrocarbons or cyclopropane, hypersensitivity to epinephrine or its components, labor, angle-closure glaucoma, organic brain damage, shock (nonanaphylactic)

Interactions
DRUGS
alpha-adrenergic blockers, drugs with alpha-adrenergic action, rapid-acting vasodilators: Blockage of epinephrine's alpha-adrenergic effect, possibly causing severe hypotension and tachycardia

amyl nitrite, nitrates: Decreased antianginal effects

antihypertensives, diuretics used to treat hypertension: Decreased antihypertensive effects

beta blockers: Mutual inhibition of therapeutic effects, possibly severe hypertension and cerebral hemorrhage

digoxin, quinidine: Increased risk of arrhythmias

dihydroergotamine, ergoloid mesylates, ergonovine, ergotamine, methylergonovine, methysergide, oxytocin: Increased risk of vasoconstriction, causing gangrene, peripheral vascular ischemia, or severe hypertension

hydrocarbon inhalation anesthetics: Increased risk of severe atrial and ventricular arrhythmias

insulin, oral antidiabetic drugs: Decreased effects of these drugs

MAO inhibitors: Possibly increased vasopressor effect of epinephrine and hypertensive crisis

maprotiline, tricyclic antidepressants: Potentiated cardiovascular effects of epinephrine, possibly causing arrhythmias, hyperpyrexia, severe hypertension, or tachycardia

sympathomimetics: Additive CNS stimulation, increased cardiovascular effects of either drug

thyroid hormones: Increased effects of either drug

xanthines: Increased CNS stimulation, additive toxic effects

Adverse Reactions
CNS: Anxiety, chills, fever, dizziness, drowsiness, hallucinations, headache, insomnia, light-headedness, nervousness, restlessness, seizures, tremor, weakness

CV: Chest discomfort or pain; fast, irregular, or slow heartbeat; palpitations; severe hypertension

EENT: Blurred vision, dry mouth or throat, miosis

GI: Anorexia, heartburn, nausea, vomiting

GU: Dysuria

MS: Muscle twitching, severe muscle spasms

RESP: Dyspnea

SKIN: Cold skin, diaphoresis, ecchymosis, flushed or red face or skin, pallor, tissue necrosis

Other: Hyperkalemia, hypokalemia, injection site pain and stinging

Nursing Considerations
• Use epinephrine with extreme caution in patients with angina, arrhythmias, asthma, degenerative heart disease, or emphysema. Epinephrine's inotropic effect equals that of dopamine and dobutamine; its chronotropic effect exceeds that of both.

• Use drug cautiously in elderly patients and those with cardiovascular disease (other than listed above), diabetes mellitus, hypertension, hyperthyroidism, prostatic hypertrophy, and psychoneurologic disorders.

• Dilute the 1:1,000 (1-mg/ml) solution of parenteral epinephrine before I.V. administration. Be aware that some preparations contain sulfites.

• Shake suspension thoroughly before withdrawing dose; refrigerate it between uses.

• Inspect epinephrine solution or suspension before use. If it's pink or brown, air has entered a multidose vial. If it's discolored or contains particles, discard it. Also discard unused portions of parenteral epinephrine.

• When injecting drug, rotate sites because repeated injections in the same site may cause vasoconstriction and localized necrosis.

• Be aware that drug shouldn't be given by intra-arterial injection because marked vasoconstriction may cause gangrene.

• Avoid I.M. injection into buttocks. Vasoconstriction reduces oxygen tension in tissues, which may allow anaerobic Clostridium welchii to multiply and cause gas gangrene.

• Monitor for potassium imbalances. Initially, hyperkalemia occurs when hepatocytes release potassium. Hypokalemia may quickly follow as skeletal muscles take up potassium.

• To minimize insomnia, give the last dose a few hours before bedtime.

• WARNING To treat cardiac arrest, at least twice the peripheral I.V. dose of epinephrine may be given by endotracheal instillation. Two dilutions are needed for this regimen; use great caution to avoid medication errors.

PATIENT TEACHING
• Warn patient not to exceed recommended dose or shorten dosing interval because of the risk of adverse reactions and tolerance.

• Advise patient to notify prescriber if symptoms don't improve or if they improve but then worsen.
• Instruct patient to take the day's last dose a few hours before bedtime to avoid insomnia.
• Caution patient not to use inhalation solution that is pink or brown or contains particles.
• Teach patient how to use oral inhaler or inhalation solution, as needed.
• If patient also uses an oral corticosteroid inhaler, instruct him to use epinephrine inhaler first, wait 5 minutes, and then use corticosteroid inhaler to increase its effectiveness.
• Advise patient to notify prescriber immediately if he experiences blurred vision, chest pain, difficulty breathing, a fast or irregular heartbeat, or increased sweating.

epoetin alfa

(EPO, erythropoietin alfa, recombinant erythropoietin, r-HuEPO)

Epogen, Eprex (CAN), Procrit

Class and Category
Chemical: 165–amino acid glycoprotein identical to human erythropoietin
Therapeutic: Antianemic
Pregnancy category: C

Indications and Dosages
➤ *To treat anemia from renal failure*
I.V. OR S.C. INJECTION
Adults and adolescents. *Initial:* 50 to 100 U/kg 3 times/wk, increased by 25 U/kg after 8 wk if hematocrit hasn't risen by 5 or 6 points or is below desired range (30% to 36%). *Maintenance:* Dosage gradually decreased by 25 U/kg q 4 wk or more to lowest dose that keeps hematocrit at 30% to 36%. *Maximum:* 300 U/kg 3 times/wk.
Children on dialysis. 50 U/kg 3 times/wk; increased after 8 wk if hematocrit hasn't risen by 5 or 6 points and is still below desired range of 30% to 36%. *Maintenance:* Dosage gradually decreased to lowest dose that keeps hematocrit at 30% to 36%.
➤ *To treat anemia in HIV-infected patients who take zidovudine*
I.V. OR S.C. INJECTION
Adults with serum erythropoietin level of 500 mU/ml or less who receive 4,200 mg or less of zidovudine/wk. *Initial:* 100 U/kg 3 times/wk, increased by 50 to 100 U/kg q 4 to 8 wk after 8 wk of therapy. *Maintenance:* Dosage gradually titrated to maintain desired response, based on such factors as variations in zidovudine dosage and occurrence of infection or inflammation. *Maximum:* 300 U/kg 3 times/wk.
➤ *To treat anemia from chemotherapy*
S.C. INJECTION
Adults. *Initial:* 150 U/kg 3 times/wk. Dosage decreased if initial dose causes hematocrit to rapidly rise more than 4 points in 2 wk. Dosage increased after 8 wk if response is inadequate. *Maximum:* 300 U/kg 3 times/wk.
➤ *To reduce the need for blood transfusion in anemic patients who must undergo surgery*
S.C. INJECTION
Adults. 300 U/kg q.d. for 10 days before surgery, on day of surgery, and 4 days after surgery; or 600 U/kg/wk starting 3 wk before surgery for a total of 3 doses. Dose of 300 U/kg repeated on day of surgery.
DOSAGE ADJUSTMENT For patients with anemia from renal failure, dosage temporarily reduced or drug discontinued if hematocrit reaches or exceeds 36%; drug is resumed at a lower dose when hematocrit returns to desired range. For patients with anemia from zidovudine use, therapy temporarily discontinued if hematocrit reaches or exceeds 40% and is resumed at a 25% lower dose when hematocrit returns to desired range.

Route	Onset	Peak	Duration
I.V., S.C.	In 2 to 6 wk	In 2 mo	About 2 wk

Mechanism of Action
Stimulates the release of reticulocytes from the bone marrow into the bloodstream, where they develop into mature RBCs.

Incompatibilities
Don't mix epoetin alfa with any other drug.

Contraindications
Hypersensitivity to human albumin or products made from mammal cells, uncontrolled hypertension

Interactions
DRUGS
antihypertensives: Increased blood pressure (to hypertensive level), especially when hematocrit rises rapidly
heparin: Increased heparin requirement in hemodialysis patients
iron supplements: Increased iron requirement and need for increased dose

Adverse Reactions
CNS: Fatigue, headache, seizures
CV: Chest pain, deep vein thrombosis, edema, hypertension, tachycardia
GI: Diarrhea, nausea, vomiting
HEME: Polycythemia
MS: Bone pain, muscle weakness
RESP: Dyspnea
SKIN: Rash, urticaria
Other: Flulike symptoms, hyperkalemia, injection site reaction

Nursing Considerations
•Use epoetin alfa cautiously in patients who have conditions that could decrease or delay response to drug, such as aluminum intoxication, folic acid deficiency, hemolysis, infection, inflammation, iron deficiency, malignant neoplasm, osteitis (fibrosa cystica), or vitamin B_{12} deficiency.
•Also use drug cautiously in patients with cardiovascular disorders caused by hypertension, a history of seizures, vascular disease, or a hematologic disorder, such as hypercoagulation, myelodysplastic syndrome, or sickle cell disease.
•WARNING Be aware that the multidose vial of epoetin contains benzyl alcohol, which can cause a fatal toxic syndrome in neonates and immature infants characterized by CNS, respiratory, circulatory, and renal impairment and metabolic acidosis.
•Don't shake vial during preparation to avoid denaturing glycoprotein and inactivating epoetin alfa.
•Discard unused portion of single-dose vial because it contains no preservatives. Discard unused portion of multidose vial after 21 days.
•Be aware that baseline hemoglobin level should be above 10 but below 13 g/dl if drug is given to patient scheduled for surgery.
•Expect to increase heparin dose if patient receives hemodialysis because epoetin alfa can increase the RBC volume, which could cause clots to form in the dialyzer, hemodialysis vascular access, or both.

•Expect to give an iron supplement (I.V. iron dextran, if needed) because iron requirements rise when erythropoiesis consumes existing iron stores.
•Monitor drug effectiveness by checking hematocrit, typically twice weekly until it stabilizes at 30% to 36%. After that, monitoring can be less frequent.
•Take seizure precautions.
•Be aware that the risk of hypertensive or thrombotic complications increases if the hematocrit rises more than 4 points in 2 weeks.
PATIENT TEACHING
•Teach patient how to dispose of needles properly, and caution him against reusing needles.
•Advise patient that the risk of seizures is highest during the first 90 days of epoetin alfa therapy. Urge him not to engage in hazardous activities during this time.
•Stress the importance of complying with the dosage regimen and keeping follow-up medical appointments and appointments for laboratory tests.
•Encourage patient to eat iron-rich foods.
•Review possible adverse reactions, and urge patient to notify prescriber if he experiences chest pain, headache, hives, rapid heartbeat, rash, seizures, shortness of breath, or swelling.

epoprostenol sodium
(PGI_2, PGX, prostacyclin)
Flolan

Class and Category
Chemical: Natural prostaglandin
Therapeutic: Antihypertensive, vasodilator
Pregnancy category: B

Indications and Dosages
➤ *To provide long-term treatment of primary pulmonary hypertension*
I.V. INFUSION
Adults. *Initial:* 2 ng/kg/min, increased by 2 ng/kg/min q 15 min or longer until dose-limiting effects occur (abdominal, chest, or musculoskeletal pain; anxiety; bradycardia; dizziness; dyspnea; flushing; headache; hypotension; nausea; tachycardia; vomiting; or other adverse reactions). *Maintenance:* Dosage reduced by at least 4 ng/kg/min by continuous infusion.
DOSAGE ADJUSTMENT Continuous infusion rate adjusted, based on persistence, recur-

E
F

rence, or worsening of primary pulmonary hypertension and dose-related adverse reactions.

Mechanism of Action
Directly relaxes vascular smooth muscles through its action as a natural prostaglandin. This results in arterial dilation and inhibition of platelet aggregation. These actions decrease pulmonary vascular resistance, increase cardiac index and oxygen delivery, and limit thrombus formation.

Incompatibilities
Don't mix epoprostenol with other parenteral solutions or drugs.

Contraindications
Hypersensitivity to epoprostenol or its components; long-term use in patients with heart failure caused by severe left ventricular systolic dysfunction; pulmonary edema that developed while establishing epoprostenol dosage

Interactions
DRUGS
anticoagulants, antiplatelet drugs, NSAIDs: Increased risk of bleeding
antihypertensives, diuretics, vasodilators: Decreased blood pressure

Adverse Reactions
CNS: Anxiety, chills, confusion, dizziness, fever, headache, nervousness, paresthesia, syncope, weakness
CV: Bradycardia, chest pain, hypotension, tachycardia
GI: Abdominal pain, diarrhea, nausea, vomiting
HEME: Thrombocytopenia
MS: Arthralgia, jaw pain, myalgia
RESP: Dyspnea, hypoxia
SKIN: Flushing
Other: Flulike symptoms, injection site infection and pain, sepsis, weight loss or gain

Nursing Considerations
•Use epoprostenol cautiously in elderly patients because they may have decreased hepatic, renal, or cardiac function, or other diseases or may receive other drugs that can interact with epoprostenol.
•Reconstitute drug only with sterile diluent that comes with package. Don't dilute reconstituted epoprostenol.
•To make 100 ml of reconstituted solution at 3,000 ng/ml, dissolve contents of 0.5-mg vial

with 5 ml of diluent; withdraw 3 ml and add enough diluent to make 100 ml. To make 100 ml of solution at 5,000 ng/ml, dissolve contents of 0.5-mg vial with 5 ml of diluent; withdraw contents and add enough diluent to make 100 ml. To make 100 ml of solution at 10,000 ng/ml, dissolve contents of two 0.5-mg vials each with 5 ml of diluent; withdraw contents and add enough diluent to make 100 ml. To make 100 ml of solution at 15,000 ng/ml, dissolve contents of 1.5-mg vial with 5 ml of diluent; withdraw contents and add enough diluent to make 100 ml.
•Give continuous infusion through a central venous catheter. Use peripheral I.V. infusion only until central access is established.
•Use an ambulatory infusion pump that's small, lightweight, and able to deliver 2 ng/kg/min. It should have alarms for occlusion, end of infusion, and low battery. Use a polyvinyl chloride, polypropylene, or glass reservoir. Keep a backup pump and infusion set nearby to minimize disruptions in delivery.
•At room temperature, administer a single container of reconstituted solution over 8 hours. For extended use at temperatures above 77° F (25° C), use a cold pouch with frozen gel packs to keep drug at 36° to 46° F (2° to 8° C) for 12 hours.
•After a new infusion rate has been established, monitor closely for adverse reactions. Measure each blood pressure with patient standing and supine. Also, monitor heart rate for several hours after dosage adjustment.
•During prolonged infusion, monitor for dose-related adverse reactions. If they arise, expect to decrease infusion rate by 2 ng/kg/min every 15 minutes, as prescribed, until dose-limiting reactions resolve.
•Avoid abrupt withdrawal or a sudden large reduction in infusion rate, which could cause rebound pulmonary hypertension (asthenia, dizziness, and dyspnea) or death.
•Protect reconstituted drug from light and refrigerate for no more than 48 hours. Discard solution that has been frozen or that has been refrigerated for more than 48 hours.
PATIENT TEACHING
•Inform patient that epoprostenol is infused continuously through a permanent indwelling central venous catheter by a small infusion pump.
•Stress that patient must commit to long-term therapy, possibly for years.

•Teach patient or caregiver how to reconstitute drug, administer it, and care for the permanent central venous catheter.
•Urge patient to maintain prescribed infusion rate and consult prescriber before altering it.
•Caution patient that even brief interruptions in drug delivery may cause rapid worsening of symptoms.
•Instruct patient to notify prescriber if adverse reactions occur.
•Make sure patient or caregiver has ready access to emergency phone numbers.

eprosartan mesylate

Teveten

Class and Category
Chemical: Monomethanesulfonate, non-biphenyl nontetrazole angiotensin II receptor antagonist
Therapeutic: Antihypertensive
Pregnancy category: Not rated

Indications and Dosages
➤ To *control blood pressure in patients with essential hypertension*
TABLETS
Adults. *Initial:* 600 mg q.d. *Maximum:* 800 mg q.d. or in divided doses b.i.d.

Mechanism of Action
Blocks the effects of angiotensin II (a potent vasoconstrictor that's part of the renin-angiotensin-aldosterone system) by blocking its binding to angiotensin I receptors in vascular smooth muscles, adrenal glands, and other tissues. This action halts angiotensin II's negative feedback on renin secretion. Thus, circulating renin and angiotensin II levels rise and vascular resistance declines.

Contraindications
Hypersensitivity to eprosartan or its components

Adverse Reactions
CNS: Depression, dizziness, drowsiness, fatigue
CV: Hypertriglyceridemia, hypotension
EENT: Pharyngitis, rhinitis
GI: Abdominal pain
GU: Oliguria, UTI
MS: Myalgia
RESP: Cough, upper respiratory tract infection

Nursing Considerations
•Monitor for excessive hypotension if patient receives other cardiac drugs.
•Expect maximum blood pressure response after about 3 weeks.
•Be aware that, unlike ACE inhibitors, eprosartan doesn't affect bradykinin breakdown and cause the characteristic ACE cough.
PATIENT TEACHING
•Inform patient that maximum blood pressure response may not occur for 3 to 4 weeks.
•Advise patient that drug may cause dizziness, drowsiness, or very low blood pressure. Instruct him to rise slowly to sitting and standing positions.

eptifibatide

Integrilin

Class and Category
Chemical: Cyclic heptapeptide
Therapeutic: Platelet aggregation inhibitor
Pregnancy category: B

Indications and Dosages
➤ To *treat unstable angina and non–Q wave MI*
I.V. INFUSION
Adults. *Initial:* 180 mcg/kg over 1 to 2 min as soon as possible after diagnosis. *Maintenance:* 2 mcg/kg/min by continuous infusion beginning immediately after initial dose and continuing until discharge or coronary artery bypass grafting, up to 72 hr.
DOSAGE ADJUSTMENT For patients with serum creatinine levels of 2 to 4 mg/dl, initial dosage reduced to 135 mcg/kg over 1 to 2 min and maintenance dosage to 0.5 mcg/kg/min by continuous infusion. Dosage discontinued before coronary artery bypass graft surgery or if platelet count is less than 100,000/mm³.

➤ To *prevent thrombosis related to percutaneous transluminal coronary angioplasty (PTCA)*
I.V. INFUSION
Adults. *Initial:* 135 mcg/kg over 1 to 2 min immediately before procedure. *Maintenance:* 0.5 mcg/kg/min by continuous infusion beginning immediately after initial dose and continuing for 20 to 24 hr. *Maximum:* 96 hr of therapy.

Route	Onset	Peak	Duration
I.V.	Immediate	In 15 min	4 to 8 hr

Mechanism of Action
Reversibly inhibits platelet aggregation by preventing the binding of fibrinogen, von Willebrand factor, and other adhesive ligands to glycoprotein IIb/IIIa receptors on activated platelets. As a result, eptifibatide disrupts the final cross-linking stage of platelet aggregation—and thrombus formation.

Incompatibilities
Don't administer eptifibatide through the same I.V. line as furosemide.

Contraindications
Active bleeding or CVA during previous 30 days, bleeding diathesis, dependency on dialysis, history of hemorrhagic CVA, hypersensitivity to eptifibatide, major surgery during previous 4 weeks, serum creatinine level of 2 mg/dl or higher for 180 mcg/kg dose or 2 mcg/kg/min infusion, serum creatinine level of 4 mg/dl or higher for 135 mcg/kg dose or 0.5 mcg/kg/min infusion, severe uncontrolled hypertension (systolic pressure above 200 mm Hg, diastolic pressure above 110 mm Hg), thrombocytopenia (platelet count below 100,000/mm³)

Interactions
DRUGS
anticoagulants, clopidogrel, dipyridamole, NSAIDs, thrombolytics, ticlopidine: Additive pharmacologic effects, increased risk of bleeding

Adverse Reactions
CNS: Intracranial hemorrhage
CV: Hypotension
GI: Hematemesis
GU: Hematuria
HEME: Bleeding, decreased hemoglobin level, thrombocytopenia
Other: Anaphylaxis

Nursing Considerations
• Expect to obtain hematocrit, platelet count, and hemoglobin and serum creatinine levels before eptifibatide therapy to detect abnormalities. Also expect to obtain APTT and PT as a baseline.
• Withdraw bolus dose of eptifibatide from a 10-ml (2 mg/ml) vial into a syringe.
• Using a vented I.V. infusion set, administer a continuous infusion directly from the 100-ml (0.75 mg/ml) vial. Be sure to center the spike in the circle on top of the vial stopper.

• Expect to maintain APTT between 50 and 70 seconds or according to facility protocol during therapy unless patient undergoes PTCA.
• If patient undergoes PTCA, expect to maintain his activated clotting time between 200 and 250 seconds during the procedure.
• During therapy, avoid arterial and venous punctures, I.M. injections, urinary catheter use, nasotracheal or nasogastric intubation, and use of noncompressible I.V. sites, such as subclavian and jugular veins.
• Expect to discontinue eptifibatide and heparin and monitor patient closely if platelet count falls below 100,000/mm³.
• Plan to discontinue drug, as prescribed, if patient undergoes coronary artery bypass surgery.
PATIENT TEACHING
• Instruct patient to immediately report bleeding.
• Reassure patient that he'll be monitored closely throughout therapy.
• Advise patient to avoid activities that may lead to bruising and bleeding.

ergoloid mesylates
(dihydrogenated ergot alkaloids)
Gerimal, Hydergine, Hydergine LC

Class and Category
Chemical: Dihydrogenated ergot alkaloid derivative
Therapeutic: Antidementia adjunct, cerebral metabolic enhancer
Pregnancy category: Not rated

Indications and Dosages
➤ *To treat age-related decline in mental capacity*
CAPSULES, ORAL SOLUTION, S.L. TABLETS, TABLETS
Adults. 1 to 2 mg t.i.d.

Route	Onset	Peak	Duration
P.O.	3 wk or more	Unknown	Unknown

Mechanism of Action
May increase cerebral metabolism, blood flow, and oxygen uptake. These actions may increase neurotransmitter levels.

Contraindications
Acute or chronic psychosis, hypersensitivity to ergoloid mesylates or their components

Interactions
DRUGS
delavirdine, efavirenz, indinavir, nelfinavir, saquinavir: Increased risk of ergotism (blurred vision, dizziness, and headache)
dopamine: Increased risk of gangrene

Adverse Reactions
CNS: Dizziness, headache, light-headedness, syncope
CV: Bradycardia, orthostatic hypotension
EENT: Blurred vision, nasal congestion, tongue soreness (with S.L. tablets)
GI: Abdominal cramps, anorexia, nausea, vomiting
SKIN: Flushing, rash

Nursing Considerations
•Expect ergoloid mesylates to be prescribed only after a pathophysiologic cause for mental decline has been ruled out.
•Measure blood pressure and pulse rate and rhythm before therapy begins and monitor them frequently during therapy.
•If bradycardia or hypotension develops, expect to discontinue drug permanently.
PATIENT TEACHING
•Stress the importance of adhering to prescribed dosage and schedule.
•Teach caregiver to place S.L. tablet under patient's tongue and withhold food, fluids, and cigarettes until tablet dissolves.
•Instruct patient not to swallow S.L. tablets.
•Advise caregiver to skip a missed dose and resume the regular dosing schedule. Warn against doubling the dose, and urge caregiver to notify prescriber if patient misses two or more doses in a row.
•Instruct caregiver to store drug in a tightly closed, light-resistant container.
•Inform caregiver and family that drug may take 3 to 4 weeks to produce its effects.
•Stress the importance of follow-up care.

ergotamine tartrate

Ergomar (CAN), Ergostat, Gynergen (CAN), Medihaler Ergotamine (CAN)

Class and Category
Chemical: Ergot alkaloid
Therapeutic: Vascular headache suppressant
Pregnancy category: X

Indications and Dosages
➤ *To relieve vascular headaches, such as migraine, migraine variants, and cluster headaches*
S.L. TABLETS
Adults. *Initial:* 2 mg at first sign of attack and repeated q 30 min, p.r.n. *Maximum:* 6 mg/day and no more than two times/wk at least 5 days apart.
TABLETS
Adults. *Initial:* 1 to 2 mg at first sign of attack and repeated q 30 min, p.r.n. Dosage increased to 3 mg for subsequent attacks if needed and if lower dose was well tolerated. *Maximum:* 6 mg/day.
ORAL INHALATION AEROSOL
Adults: 1 (360-mcg) inhalation at first sign of attack and repeated q 5 min, p.r.n. *Maximum:* 2.16 mg/day and no more than two times/wk at least 5 days apart.

Route	Onset	Peak	Duration
P.O., S.L.	Unknown	1 to 5 hr	Unknown

Mechanism of Action
Directly stimulates vascular smooth muscles, constricting arteries and veins and depressing vasomotor centers in the brain.

Contraindications
Coronary artery disease, hypersensitivity to ergot alkaloids, hypertension, impaired hepatic or renal function, malnutrition, peripheral vascular disease (Raynaud's disease, severe arteriosclerosis, syphilitic arteritis, thromboangiitis obliterans, thrombophlebitis), pregnancy or risk of pregnancy, sepsis, severe pruritus

Interactions
DRUGS
beta blockers: Increased risk of vasoconstriction and, possibly, peripheral gangrene
erythromycin, troleandomycin: Increased risk of peripheral vasospasm and ischemia
nitrates: Increased ergotamine effects, decreased antianginal effects of nitrates, increased risk of hypertension
sumatriptan: Possibly additive vasoconstriction
vasoconstrictors: Increased risk of dangerous hypertension
ACTIVITIES
smoking: Possibly increased risk of peripheral vasoconstriction and ischemia

Adverse Reactions

CNS: Anxiety, confusion, dizziness, drowsiness, paresthesia, severe headache
CV: Chest pain, fast or slow heart rate, heart valve fibrosis, increased or decreased blood pressure, MI, weak pulse
EENT: Dry mouth, miosis, vision changes
GI: Nausea, vomiting
MS: Arm, back, or leg pain; muscle weakness in legs
SKIN: Cold, cyanotic, or pale feet or hands; pruritus
Other: Edema of face, feet, fingers, or lower legs; physical dependence

Nursing Considerations

• Use ergotamine cautiously in elderly patients.
• If patient receives long-term therapy, monitor pain control; he may need increasingly higher doses to obtain relief.
• Notify prescriber at the first sign of vasospasm and expect to discontinue drug.

PATIENT TEACHING

• Teach patient to take a tablet at the first sign of headache and to lie down in a quiet, dark room.
• Instruct patient not to swallow S.L. tablet but to let it dissolve under his tongue. Advise him not to drink, eat, or smoke until tablet has dissolved.
• Stress the importance of adhering to prescribed dosage and schedule because of drug's potential for dependence.
• Warn patient not to smoke while taking ergotamine (especially heavy smokers) because the combination of drug and nicotine, which also constricts vessels, may increase the risk of peripheral vascular ischemia.
• Advise patient to notify prescriber if usual doses fail to relieve headaches or if headache frequency or severity increases.
• Urge patient to avoid alcohol because it worsens headaches. Also suggest that patient avoid excessive cold, which may increase peripheral vasoconstriction.
• Instruct patient to notify prescriber if an infection develops because severe infection may increase sensitivity to drug.
• Advise patient to notify prescriber if he experiences chest pain; numbness, pain, or tingling in fingers or toes; pulse rate changes; swelling of face, feet, fingers, or lower legs; or vision changes.

ertapenem sodium

Invanz

Class and Category

Chemical: Synthetic 1-β methyl-carbapenem
Therapeutic: Antibiotic
Pregnancy category: B

Indications and Dosages

➤ *To treat moderate to severe infections, such as complicated intra-abdominal infections due to* Escherichia coli, Clostridium clostridioforme, Eubacterium lentum, Peptostreptococcus *species,* Bacteroides fragilis, B. distasonis, B. ovatus, B. thetaiotaomicron, *or* B. uniformis; *complicated skin and skin-structure infections due to* Staphylococcus aureus *(methicillin-susceptible strains only),* Streptococcus pyogenes, E. coli, *or* Peptostreptococcus *species; community-acquired pneumonia due to* Streptococcus pneumoniae *(penicillin-susceptible strains only, including cases with concurrent bacteremia),* Haemophilus influenzae *(beta-lactamase–negative strains only), or* Moraxella catarrhalis; *complicated UTIs (including pyelonephritis) due to* E. coli *(including cases with concurrent bacteremia) or* Klebsiella pneumoniae; *and acute pelvic infections (including postpartum endomyometritis, septic abortion, and postsurgical gynecologic infections) due to* Streptococcus agalactiae, E. coli, B. fragilis, Porphyromonas asaccharolytica, Peptostreptococcus *species, or* Prevotella bivia

I.V. INFUSION

Adults. 1 g q.d., infused over 30 min, for up to 14 days.

I.M. INJECTION

Adults. 1 g q.d. for up to 7 days.

DOSAGE ADJUSTMENT Dosage decreased to 500 mg q.d. for patients with advanced renal insufficiency (creatinine clearance less than or equal to 30 ml/min/1.73 m^2) or end-stage renal insufficiency (creatinine clearance less than or equal to 10 ml/min/1.73 m^2). For patients on hemodialysis who have received 500 mg of ertapenem within 6 hr of hemodialysis, supplemental dose of 150 mg given after hemodialysis.

Mechanism of Action

Inhibits bacterial cell wall synthesis by binding to specific penicillin-binding proteins inside the cell wall. Penicillin-binding proteins are responsible for various steps in bacterial cell wall synthesis. By binding to these proteins, ertapenem leads to bacterial cell wall lysis.

Incompatibilities

Don't mix ertapenem with other drugs. Don't dilute it with solutions containing dextrose.

Contraindications

Hypersensitivity to ertapenem, its components, or other drugs in the same class; hypersensitivity to local anesthetics (I.M. form only, because lidocaine hydrochloride 1% is used as a diluent); patients who have experienced anaphylactic reactions to beta-lactam drugs

Interactions
DRUGS

probenecid: Increased ertapenem half-life, increased and prolonged blood ertapenem level

Adverse Reactions

CNS: Agitation, anxiety, asthenia, confusion, disorientation, dizziness, fatigue, fever, headache, insomnia, mental changes, seizures, somnolence, stupor
CV: Chest pain, edema, hypertension, hypotension, tachycardia, thrombophlebitis
EENT: Oral candidiasis, pharyngitis
ENDO: Hyperglycemia
GI: Abdominal pain, acid regurgitation, constipation, diarrhea, elevated liver function test results, indigestion, nausea, vomiting
GU: Elevated serum creatinine level, RBCs and WBCs in urine, vaginitis
HEME: Anemia, decreased hematocrit, decreased WBC count, eosinophilia, neutropenia, prolonged PT, thrombocytopenia, thrombocytosis
MS: Leg pain
RESP: Cough, crackles, dyspnea, respiratory distress, wheezing
SKIN: Erythema, extravasation, pruritus, rash
Other: Anaphylaxis, death, hyperkalemia, hypokalemia, infusion site pain or redness

Nursing Considerations

• Obtain sputum, urine, or other specimens for culture and sensitivity testing, as ordered, before giving ertapenem. Expect to begin therapy before results are available.
• When preparing drug for I.V. use, reconstitute 1 g of drug with 10 ml of sterile water for injection, 0.9% sodium chloride injection, or bacteriostatic water for injection. Don't use solutions that contain dextrose. Shake well to dissolve. Immediately transfer reconstituted drug to 50 ml of NS. Use within 6 hours if stored at room temperature or within 24 hours if refrigerated at 5° C (41° F). Don't freeze. Administer I.V. infusion over 30 minutes.
• Inspect drug for particles and discoloration after reconstitution.
• For I.M. injection, reconstitute 1 g of drug with 3.2 ml of 1% lidocaine hydrochloride injection (*without* epinephrine). Shake thoroughly to form solution. Use within 1 hour after preparation. Withdraw contents of vial and inject deep into a large muscle mass such as the gluteal muscles.
• **WARNING** Don't administer reconstituted I.M. solution by I.V. route because of the potential for adverse reactions from the lidocaine hydrochloride injection used to reconstitute drug.
• Monitor patient closely for a life-threatening anaphylactic reaction. Patients with a history of hypersensitivity to penicillin, cephalosporins, other beta-lactams, or other allergens are at increased risk.
• **WARNING** If ertapenem triggers an anaphylactic reaction, discontinue drug, notify prescriber immediately, and provide appropriate therapy. Anaphylaxis requires immediate treatment with epinephrine as well as airway management and administration of oxygen and I.V. corticosteroids, as needed.
• Be aware that patients with a history of seizures, other CNS disorders that predispose them to seizures (such as brain lesions), or compromised renal function may be at increased risk for seizures. Administer anticonvulsants, as ordered.
• Monitor patient for diarrhea during or shortly after drug therapy; diarrhea may signal pseudomembranous colitis.
• Be aware that because ertapenem is excreted in breast milk, its use by nursing mothers is carefully evaluated.
PATIENT TEACHING
• Instruct patient receiving ertapenem to immediately report signs of an anaphylactic reaction, such as rash, itching, or shortness of breath, or signs of superinfection, such as

severe diarrhea or white patches on tongue or in mouth.

erythromycin

(contains 250, 333, or 500 mg of base per delayed-release capsule, delayed-release tablet, or tablet)

Apo-Erythro (CAN), E-Mycin, Erybid (CAN), ERYC, Ery-Tab, Ilotycin, Novo-Rythro Encap (CAN), PCE

erythromycin estolate

(contains 250 mg of base per capsule or tablet, or 125 or 250 mg of base per 5 ml of oral suspension)

Ilosone, Novo-Rythro (CAN)

erythromycin ethylsuccinate

(contains 1 g of base per 1.6 g of oral suspension or tablet)

Apo-Erythro-ES (CAN), E.E.S., EryPed, Erythro, Novo-Rythro (CAN)

erythromycin gluceptate

(contains 500 or 1,000 mg of base per vial)

Ilotycin

erythromycin lactobionate

(contains 500 or 1,000 mg of base per vial)

Erythrocin

erythromycin stearate

(contains 125 or 250 mg of base per 5 ml of oral suspension, or 250 or 500 mg of base per tablet)

Apo-Erythro-S (CAN), Erythrocin, Erythrocot, My-E, Novo-Rythro (CAN), Wintrocin

Class and Category
Chemical: Macrolide
Therapeutic: Antiacne, antibiotic
Pregnancy category: B

Indications and Dosages
➤ *To treat mild to moderate upper respiratory tract infections caused by* Haemophilus influenzae, Streptococcus pneumoniae, *or* Streptococcus pyogenes *(group A beta-hemolytic streptococcus)*
CAPSULES, CHEWABLE TABLETS, DELAYED-RELEASE CAPSULES, DELAYED-RELEASE TABLETS, ORAL SUSPENSION, TABLETS, I.V. INFUSION
Adults. 250 to 500 mg (base) q 6 hr for 10 days.

Children. 250 to 500 mg (base) q.i.d. or 20 to 50 mg (base)/kg/day in divided doses for 10 days. For *H. influenzae* infections, erythromycin ethylsuccinate is administered with 150 mg/kg/day of sulfisoxazole. *Maximum:* Adult dosage, or 6 g/day for erythromycin ethylsuccinate.
➤ *To treat lower respiratory tract infections caused by* S. pneumoniae *or* S. pyogenes *(group A beta-hemolytic streptococcus)*
CAPSULES, CHEWABLE TABLETS, DELAYED-RELEASE CAPSULES, DELAYED-RELEASE TABLETS, ORAL SUSPENSION, TABLETS, I.V. INFUSION
Adults. 250 to 500 mg (base) q 6 hr for 10 days.
Children. 250 to 500 mg (base) q.i.d. or 20 to 50 mg (base)/kg/day in divided doses for 10 days. *Maximum:* Adult dosage.
➤ *To treat respiratory tract infections caused by* Mycoplasma pneumoniae
CAPSULES, CHEWABLE TABLETS, DELAYED-RELEASE CAPSULES, DELAYED-RELEASE TABLETS, ORAL SUSPENSION, TABLETS, I.V. INFUSION
Adults. 500 mg (base) q 6 hr for 5 to 10 days or up to 3 wk for severe infections.
➤ *To treat mild to moderate skin and soft-tissue infections caused by* S. pyogenes *or* Staphylococcus aureus
CAPSULES, CHEWABLE TABLETS, DELAYED-RELEASE CAPSULES, DELAYED-RELEASE TABLETS, ORAL SUSPENSION, TABLETS, I.V. INFUSION
Adults. 250 mg (base) q 6 hr or 500 mg (base) q 12 hr for 10 days. *Maximum:* 4 g (base)/day.
Children. 250 to 500 mg (base) q.i.d. or 20 to 50 mg (base)/kg/day in divided doses for 10 days. *Maximum:* Adult dosage.
➤ *To treat acne vulgaris*
DELAYED-RELEASE CAPSULES, DELAYED-RELEASE TABLETS, TABLETS
Adults and adolescents. *Initial:* 250 mg (base) q 6 hr, 333 mg (base) q 8 hr, or 500 mg (base) q 12 hr for 4 wk. *Maintenance:* 333 to 500 mg (base) q.d.
➤ *To treat pertussis (whooping cough) caused by* Bordetella pertussis
CAPSULES, CHEWABLE TABLETS, DELAYED-RELEASE CAPSULES, DELAYED-RELEASE TABLETS, ORAL SUSPENSION, TABLETS, I.V. INFUSION
Children. 500 mg (base) q.i.d. or 40 to 50 mg (base)/kg/day in divided doses for 5 to 14 days.

➤ *To treat diphtheria*
CAPSULES, CHEWABLE TABLETS, DELAYED-RELEASE CAPSULES, DELAYED-RELEASE TABLETS, ORAL SUSPENSION, TABLETS, I.V. INFUSION
Adults and children. 500 mg (base) q 6 hr for 10 days.

➤ *To treat erythrasma*
CAPSULES, CHEWABLE TABLETS, DELAYED-RELEASE CAPSULES, DELAYED-RELEASE TABLETS, ORAL SUSPENSION, TABLETS, I.V. INFUSION
Adults and children. 250 mg (base) t.i.d. for 21 days.

➤ *To treat intestinal amebiasis*
CAPSULES, CHEWABLE TABLETS, DELAYED-RELEASE CAPSULES, DELAYED-RELEASE TABLETS, ORAL SUSPENSION, TABLETS, I.V. INFUSION
Adults. 250 mg (base) q 6 hr for 10 to 14 days.
Children. 30 to 50 mg (base)/kg/day in divided doses for 10 to 14 days

➤ *To treat pelvic inflammatory disease caused by* Neisseria gonorrhoeae
CAPSULES, CHEWABLE TABLETS, DELAYED-RELEASE CAPSULES, DELAYED-RELEASE TABLETS, ORAL SUSPENSION, TABLETS, I.V. INFUSION
Adults. 500 mg (base) I.V. q 6 hr for 3 days and then 250 mg (base) P.O. or I.V. q 6 hr for 7 days.

➤ *To treat newborn conjunctivitis*
I.V. INFUSION
Neonates. 50 mg (base)/kg/day in four divided doses for 14 days.

➤ *To treat pneumonia in neonates*
I.V. INFUSION
Neonates. 50 mg (base)/kg/day in divided doses for 21 days.

➤ *To treat urogenital infections caused by* Chlamydia trachomatis *during pregnancy*
CAPSULES, CHEWABLE TABLETS, DELAYED-RELEASE CAPSULES, DELAYED-RELEASE TABLETS, ORAL SUSPENSION, TABLETS
Adults. 500 mg (base) on an empty stomach q 6 hr for 7 days; or 250 mg (base) on an empty stomach q 6 hr for at least 14 days.

➤ *To treat nongonococcal urethritis or uncomplicated urethral, endocervical, or rectal infections caused by* C. trachomatis
CAPSULES, CHEWABLE TABLETS, DELAYED-RELEASE CAPSULES, DELAYED-RELEASE TABLETS, ORAL SUSPENSION, TABLETS
Adults. 500 mg (base) q 6 hr for 7 days. If patient can't tolerate high doses, 250 mg (base) q 6 hr for 14 days.

➤ *To treat primary syphilis*
CAPSULES, CHEWABLE TABLETS, DELAYED-RELEASE CAPSULES, DELAYED-RELEASE TABLETS, ORAL SUSPENSION, TABLETS
Adults. 20 to 40 g (base) in divided doses over 10 to 15 days.

➤ *To treat Legionnaire's disease*
CAPSULES, CHEWABLE TABLETS, DELAYED-RELEASE CAPSULES, DELAYED-RELEASE TABLETS, ORAL SUSPENSION, TABLETS, I.V. INFUSION
Adults. 1 to 4 g (base)/day in divided doses for 10 to 14 days.

➤ *To treat rheumatic fever*
CAPSULES, CHEWABLE TABLETS, DELAYED-RELEASE CAPSULES, DELAYED-RELEASE TABLETS, ORAL SUSPENSION, TABLETS, I.V. INFUSION
Adults. 250 mg (base) q 12 hr.

➤ *To prevent bacterial endocarditis in patients with penicillin allergy who plan dental or upper respiratory tract surgery*
CAPSULES, CHEWABLE TABLETS, DELAYED-RELEASE CAPSULES, DELAYED-RELEASE TABLETS, ORAL SUSPENSION, TABLETS, I.V. INFUSION
Adults. 1 g (base) given 1 to 2 hr before procedure and then 500 mg (base) 6 hr after initial dose.
Children. 20 mg (base)/kg given 2 hr before procedure and then 10 mg (base)/kg 6 hr after initial dose.

➤ *To treat listeriosis*
CAPSULES, CHEWABLE TABLETS, DELAYED-RELEASE CAPSULES, DELAYED-RELEASE TABLETS, ORAL SUSPENSION, TABLETS, I.V. INFUSION
Adults. 250 mg (base) q 6 hr or 500 mg (base) q 12 hr. *Maximum:* 4 g (base)/day.

Mechanism of Action
Binds with the 50S ribosomal subunit of the 70S ribosome in many types of aerobic, anaerobic, gram-positive, and gram-negative bacteria. This action inhibits RNA-dependent protein synthesis in bacterial cells, causing them to die.

Contraindications
Astemizole, cisapride, pimozide, or terfenadine therapy; hypersensitivity to erythromycin, macrolide antibiotics, or their components; hepatic disease (erythromycin estolate)

Interactions
DRUGS
alfentanil: Decreased alfentanil clearance, prolonged alfentanil action

astemizole, cisapride, terfenadine: Increased risk of cardiotoxicity, torsades de pointes, ventricular tachycardia, and death
atorvastatin, lovastatin, pravastatin, simvastatin: Increased risk of rhabdomyolysis
carbamazepine, valproic acid: Possibly inhibited metabolism of these drugs, increasing their blood levels and risk of toxicity
chloramphenicol, lincomycins: Antagonized effects of these drugs
cyclosporine: Increased risk of nephrotoxicity
digoxin: Increased serum digoxin level and risk of digitalis toxicity
ergotamine: Decreased ergotamine metabolism, increased risk of vasospasm from ergotamine use
hepatotoxic drugs: Increased risk of hepatotoxicity
midazolam, triazolam: Increased pharmacologic effects of these drugs
oral contraceptives: Failed contraception, hepatotoxicity
ototoxic drugs: Increased risk of ototoxicity if patient with impaired renal function receives high doses of erythromycin
penicillins: Interference with bactericidal effects of penicillins
sildenafil: Increased effects of sildenafil
warfarin: Prolonged PT and risk of hemorrhage, especially in elderly patients
xanthines (except dyphylline): Increased serum theophylline level and risk of theophylline toxicity

ACTIVITIES
alcohol use: Increased alcohol level (by 40%) with I.V. erythromycin

Adverse Reactions

CNS: Fatigue, fever, malaise, weakness
CV: Prolonged QT interval, torsades de pointes, ventricular arrhythmias
EENT: Hearing loss, oral candidiasis
GI: Abdominal cramps and pain, diarrhea, hepatotoxicity, nausea, vomiting
GU: Vaginal candidiasis
SKIN: Erythema, jaundice, pruritus, rash
Other: Fluid overload (from I.V. infusion), injection site inflammation and phlebitis

Nursing Considerations

•Before administering the first erythromycin dose, expect to obtain body fluid or tissue sample for culture and sensitivity testing.
•Reconstitute parenteral form before administration. Add at least 10 ml of preservative-free sterile water for injection to each 500-mg vial or at least 20 ml of diluent to each 1-g vial.
•For prolonged infusion, expect to infuse a buffered solution up to 24 hours after dilution.
•For intermittent infusion, dilute the dose if needed in 100 to 250 ml of NS or D₅W and administer slowly over 20 to 60 minutes.
•When giving I.V. erythromycin gluceptate, dilute the solution if needed to 1 g/L in NS or D₅W injection for slow, continuous infusion. Diluted solution remains potent for 7 days if refrigerated.
•When giving I.V. erythromycin lactobionate, dilute the solution if needed to 1 to 5 mg/ml in NS, LR, or other electrolyte solution for slow, continuous infusion. Diluted solution remains potent for 14 days if refrigerated and for 24 hours at room temperature.
•Be aware that infusions prepared in piggyback infusion bottles remain potent for 30 days if frozen, 24 hours if refrigerated, or 8 hours at room temperature. Don't store infusions prepared in the ADD-vantage system.
•Don't use diluent that contains benzyl alcohol if parenteral erythromycin is intended for a neonate. It may cause a fatal toxic syndrome of CNS depression, hypotension, metabolic acidosis, renal failure, respiratory problems, and, possibly, seizures and intracranial hemorrhage.
•Periodically monitor liver function test results to detect signs of hepatotoxicity, which is most common with erythromycin estolate use. Signs typically appear within 2 weeks after continuous therapy starts and resolve when therapy stops.
•Assess hearing regularly, especially in elderly patients and those who receive 4 g or more/day or have hepatic or renal disease. Hearing impairment begins 36 hours to 8 days after treatment starts and usually begins to improve 1 to 14 days after therapy stops.
•During I.V. therapy, assess patient for signs of fluid overload, such as acute dyspnea and crackles.
•Monitor infants for vomiting or irritability with feeding because infantile hypertrophic pyloric stenosis has been reported following erythromycin therapy.

PATIENT TEACHING
•Stress the importance of completing the prescribed therapy, even if patient feels better before it's finished.

•Advise patient to notify prescriber if symptoms worsen or don't improve after a few days of therapy.
•Teach patient how to administer prescribed drug form. Instruct him to swallow capsules or tablets whole. For an oral suspension, teach him to use the measuring device provided to ensure accurate doses. Remind him to shake the suspension before measuring a dose.
•Advise patient to take any oral form with a full glass of water on an empty stomach (except erythromycin ethylsuccinate, which is better absorbed with food).
•If GI distress occurs, instruct patient to take oral form with food.
•Instruct patient to promptly notify prescriber about allergic reactions, hearing changes, or signs of hepatic dysfunction.

escitalopram oxalate

Lexapro

Class and Category
Chemical: Pure S+ enantiomer of racemic bicyclic phthalane derivative citalopram
Therapeutic: Antidepressant
Pregnancy category: C

Indications and Dosages
➤ *To treat major depression*
TABLETS
Adults. *Initial:* 10 mg q.d. in morning or evening, increased to 20 mg q.d. after one or more wk, as needed.
DOSAGE ADJUSTMENT Dosage shouldn't exceed 10 mg q.d. for elderly patients and those with hepatic impairment.

Mechanism of Action
Inhibits reuptake of the neurotransmitter serotonin by CNS neurons, thereby increasing the amount of serotonin available in nerve synapses. An elevated serotonin level may result in elevated mood and reduced depression.

Contraindications
Hypersensitivity to escitalopram, citalopram or its components; use within 14 days of MAO inhibitor therapy

Interactions
DRUGS
carbamazepine: Possibly increased clearance of escitalopram
CNS drugs: Additive CNS effects
lithium: Possible enhancement of the serotonergic effects of escitalopram
MAO inhibitors: Possibly hyperpyretic episodes, hypertensive crisis, serotonin syndrome, and severe seizures
metoprolol: Increased metoprolol plasma levels with decreased cardioselectivity of metoprolol
naratriptan, sumatriptan, zolmitriptan: Possibly weakness, hyperreflexia, and incoordination
St. John's wort: Increased risk of serotonin syndrome
sibutramine: Increased risk of serotonin syndrome
ACTIVITIES
alcohol use: Possibly increased cognitive and motor effects of alcohol

Adverse Reactions
CNS: Dizziness, fatigue, insomnia, somnolence
EENT: Dry mouth, rhinitis, sinusitis
ENDO: Syndrome of inappropriate ADH secretion
GI: Abdominal pain, constipation, decreased appetite, diarrhea, indigestion, nausea
GU: Anorgasmia, decreased libido, ejaculation disorders, impotence
SKIN: Increased sweating

Nursing Considerations
•Use escitalopram cautiously in patients with history of mania or seizures, patients with severe renal impairment, or those with diseases or conditions that produce altered metabolism or hemodynamic responses.
•Monitor patient for hypo-osmolarity of serum and urine and for hyponatremia, which may indicate escitalopram-induced syndrome of inappropriate ADH secretion.
•Observe patient for signs of misuse or abuse, such as development of tolerance; increasing dosage of drug without approval; and drug-seeking behavior because escitalopram's potential for physical and psychological dependence is unknown.
•Be aware that prescriber should reassess patient periodically to determine continued need for therapy and appropriate dosage.

•Inform patient that alcohol use isn't recommended during escitalopram therapy because it may decrease his ability to think clearly and perform motor skills.
•Advise patient to avoid potentially hazardous activities until drug's CNS effects are known.
•Instruct patient that drug shouldn't be taken with citalopram hydrobromide because of potentially additive effects.
•Tell patient that improvement may not be noticed for 1 to 4 weeks after therapy begins. Emphasize the importance of continuing therapy as prescribed.
•Warn patient not to stop taking drug abruptly. Explain that gradual tapering helps to avoid withdrawal symptoms.
•Urge patient to inform prescriber of any over-the-counter drugs he takes because of potential for interactions.

esmolol hydrochloride

Brevibloc

Class and Category
Chemical: Beta blocker
Therapeutic: Antiarrhythmic, antihypertensive
Pregnancy category: C

Indications and Dosages
➤ *To treat supraventricular tachycardia*
I.V. INFUSION
Adults. *Loading:* 500 mcg/kg over 1 min. *Maintenance:* If response to loading dose is adequate after 5 min, 50 mcg/kg/min infused for 4 min. If response is inadequate after 5 min, another 500 mcg/kg may be given over 1 min followed by 100 mcg/kg/min for 4 min. Sequence repeated, as needed, until adequate response occurs, increasing maintenance dosage by 50 mcg/kg/min at each step. *Maximum:* 200 mcg/kg/min for 48 hr.
Children. 50 mcg/kg/min titrated q 10 min up to 300 mcg/kg/min.
➤ *To treat intraoperative and postoperative tachycardia and hypertension*
I.V. INFUSION
Adults. *Initial:* 250 to 500 mcg/kg over 1 min. *Maintenance:* 50 mcg/kg/min infused over 4 min. If response is inadequate after 5 min, another 250 to 500 mcg/kg may be given over 1 min followed by 100 mcg/kg/min for

4 min. Sequence repeated, as needed, up to 4 times, increasing by 50 mcg/kg/min each time. *Maximum:* 200 mcg/kg/min for 48 hr.
DOSAGE ADJUSTMENT Subsequent loading doses omitted, increments decreased to 25 mcg/kg/min, and titration intervals increased to 10 min as heart rate approaches desired level or if blood pressure decreases too much.

Route	Onset	Peak	Duration
I.V.	Immediate	Unknown	10 to 20 min

Mechanism of Action
Inhibits stimulation of beta$_1$ receptors primarily in the heart, which decreases cardiac excitability, cardiac output, and myocardial oxygen demand. Esmolol also decreases renin release from the kidneys, which helps reduce blood pressure.

Incompatibilities
Don't mix esmolol with 5% sodium bicarbonate injection.

Contraindications
Cardiogenic shock, hypersensitivity to beta blockers, overt heart failure, second- or third-degree heart block, sinus bradycardia

Interactions
DRUGS
antihypertensives: Possibly hypotension
insulin, oral antidiabetic drugs: Possibly masking of signs and symptoms of hypoglycemia caused by these drugs
MAO inhibitors: Possibly severe hypertension if esmolol is administered within 14 days of discontinuing MAO inhibitor therapy
neuromuscular blockers: Possibly potentiated and prolonged action of these drugs
phenytoin: Possibly increased cardiac depression
reserpine: Possibly bradycardia and hypotension
sympathomimetics, xanthine derivatives: Possibly inhibited therapeutic effects of both drugs

Adverse Reactions
CNS: Anxiety, confusion, depression, dizziness, fatigue, fever, headache, syncope
CV: Bradycardia, chest pain, decreased peripheral circulation, heart block, hypotension
GI: Nausea, vomiting
RESP: Dyspnea, wheezing
SKIN: Diaphoresis, flushing, pallor
Other: Infusion site pain, redness, and swelling

Nursing Considerations

• Use esmolol cautiously if patient has supraventricular arrhythmias with decreased cardiac output, hypotension, or other hemodynamic compromise or is taking drugs that decrease peripheral resistance or myocardial filling, contractility, or impulse generation.

• Also use drug cautiously in patients with impaired renal function because drug is excreted by the kidneys. Patients with end-stage renal disease have an increased risk of adverse reactions.

• Avoid giving esmolol for intraoperative or postoperative hypertension that results mainly from vasoconstriction caused by hypothermia.

• Expect to give lowest possible dose to patients with allergies, asthma, bronchitis, or emphysema. If bronchospasm develops, expect to discontinue infusion immediately and give a beta$_2$ stimulating drug, as ordered.

• Don't give 250 mg/ml (2,500 mg/10 ml) dosage strength by direct I.V. push. Dilute it to a 10-mg/ml infusion by first removing 20 ml from 500 ml of a compatible I.V. solution, such as D$_5$W or D$_5$NS, and then adding 5 g of esmolol to the solution.

• Use diluted solution within 24 hours if stored at room temperature.

• Use a 100-mg vial (prediluted to 10 mg/ml) to give loading dose. For a 70-kg (154-lb) patient, loading dose for 500 mcg/kg/min would be 3.5 ml.

• Monitor blood pressure and heart rate frequently during therapy. Keep in mind that hypotension can occur at any dose but usually is dose-related. Hypotension typically reverses within 30 minutes after dose is decreased or infusion is stopped.

• Inspect infusion site regularly for evidence of thrombophlebitis (pain, redness, or swelling at site). Infusions of 20 mg/ml are more likely to cause serious vein irritation than those of 10 mg/ml. Extravasation of 20 mg/ml may cause a serious local reaction and, possibly, skin necrosis. Don't infuse more than 10 mg/ml into a small vein or through a butterfly catheter.

PATIENT TEACHING

• Urge patient to report adverse reactions immediately.

• Reassure patient that his blood pressure, heart rate, and response to therapy will be monitored throughout esmolol therapy.

esomeprazole magnesium

Nexium

Class and Category

Chemical: Substituted benzimidazole
Therapeutic: Antiulcer agent
Pregnancy category: B

Indications and Dosages

➤ *To treat gastroesophageal reflux disease (GERD)*

DELAYED-RELEASE CAPSULES

Adults. 20 to 40 mg q.d. for 4 to 8 wk; may be repeated for another 4 to 8 wk if ulcer hasn't healed. *Maintenance:* 20 mg q.d. for up to 6 mo.

➤ *As adjunct to treat duodenal or gastric ulcer associated with* Helicobacter pylori

DELAYED-RELEASE CAPSULES

Adults. 40 mg q.d. in combination with amoxicillin 1,000 mg b.i.d. and clarithromycin 500 mg b.i.d. for 10 days.

DOSAGE ADJUSTMENT Maximum dosage 20 mg q.d. for patients with severe hepatic insufficiency.

Mechanism of Action

Interferes with gastric acid secretion by inhibiting the hydrogen-potassium-adenosine triphosphatase (H$^+$, K$^+$-ATPase) enzyme system, or proton pump, in gastric parietal cells. Normally, the proton pump uses energy from the hydrolysis of ATPase to drive H$^+$ and chloride (Cl$^-$) out of parietal cells and into the stomach lumen in exchange for potassium (K$^+$), which leaves the stomach lumen and enters parietal cells. After this exchange, H$^+$ and Cl$^-$ combine in the stomach to form hydrochloric acid (HCl). Esomeprazole irreversibly inhibits the final step in gastric acid production by blocking the exchange of intracellular H$^+$ and extracellular K$^+$, thus preventing H$^+$ from entering the stomach and additional HCl from forming.

Contraindications

Hypersensitivity to esomeprazole or its components

Interactions

DRUGS

diazepam: Possibly increased blood diazepam level

digoxin, iron salts, ketoconazole: Possibly decreased absorption of these drugs
FOODS
all foods: Decreased bioavailability of esomeprazole

Adverse Reactions
CNS: Headache
EENT: Dry mouth
GI: Abdominal pain, constipation, diarrhea, flatulence, nausea

Nursing Considerations
•Administer esomeprazole at least 1 hour before meals because food decreases drug's bioavailability.
•**WARNING** Monitor patients taking drug with amoxicillin and clarithromycin to treat *H. pylori*–associated ulcer for severe diarrhea. Severe diarrhea may be a sign of pseudomembranous colitis, a serious adverse reaction to antibiotics. Be prepared to obtain stool cultures, as ordered, if diarrhea occurs.
PATIENT TEACHING
•If patient has difficulty swallowing esomeprazole capsules, advise him to open capsule and sprinkle pellets into a tablespoon of cool applesauce. Tell patient not to chew pellets and to discard any unused pellets once capsule has been opened.
•Inform patient that he may take antacids while using esomeprazole but that he should notify prescriber if he feels the need to take them.

estazolam
ProSom

Class, Category, and Schedule
Chemical: Benzodiazepine
Therapeutic: Sedative-hypnotic
Pregnancy category: X
Controlled substance: Schedule IV

Indications and Dosages
➤ *To treat insomnia*
TABLETS
Adults. 1 to 2 mg h.s.
DOSAGE ADJUSTMENT Starting dose reduced to 0.5 mg for small or debilitated elderly patients.

Route	Onset	Peak	Duration
P.O.	Unknown	Unknown	6 to 8 hr

Mechanism of Action
May potentiate the effects of gamma-aminobutyric acid (GABA) and other inhibitory neurotransmitters by binding to specific benzodiazepine receptors in the limbic and cortical areas of the CNS. By binding to these receptors, estazolam increases GABA's inhibitory effects and blocks cortical and limbic arousal.

Contraindications
Acute angle-closure glaucoma; hypersensitivity to estazolam, other benzodiazepines, or their components; pregnancy; psychosis

Interactions
DRUGS
carbamazepine: Possibly increased blood carbamazepine level
cimetidine, diltiazem, disulfiram, erythromycin, fluoxetine, fluvoxamine, itraconazole, nefazodone, oral contraceptives, propoxyphene, ranitidine, verapamil: Possibly increased blood level and impaired hepatic metabolism of estazolam
clozapine: Possibly cardiac arrest or respiratory depression
CNS depressants: Possibly potentiated CNS depression
levodopa: Possibly decreased therapeutic effects of levodopa
FOODS
grapefruit juice: Possibly increased blood level and impaired hepatic metabolism of estazolam
ACTIVITIES
alcohol use: Possibly potentiated CNS depression

Adverse Reactions
CNS: Amnesia, anxiety, ataxia, confusion, delusions, depression, dizziness, drowsiness, euphoria, headache, hypokinesia, irritability, malaise, nervousness, slurred speech, tremor
CV: Chest pain, palpitations, tachycardia
EENT: Blurred vision, dry mouth, increased salivation, photophobia
GI: Abdominal pain, constipation, diarrhea, nausea, thirst, vomiting
GU: Libido changes
SKIN: Diaphoresis
Other: Physical or psychological dependence

Nursing Considerations
•Use estazolam with extreme caution in patients with a history of drug or alcohol abuse

because of the risk of addiction. Expect to give drug for no more than 12 weeks for the same reason.
•Use drug cautiously in elderly or debilitated patients and those with depression or impaired hepatic, renal, or respiratory function.
•Expect to discontinue estazolam gradually to prevent withdrawal symptoms. Avoid stopping it abruptly if patient has a history of seizures.

PATIENT TEACHING
•Warn patient not to exceed prescribed dosage or to take estazolam longer than prescribed because of the risk of addiction.
•Because estazolam can reduce alertness, advise patient to avoid potentially hazardous activities until drug's CNS effects are known.
•Advise patient not to drink alcohol or take other CNS depressants during estazolam therapy because of the risk of additive effects.
•Warn elderly or debilitated patients and those with impaired renal or hepatic function about the risk of excessive sedation or mental impairment. Urge patient to notify prescriber if these problems occur.
•Caution patient who takes 2-mg dosage for a long time against stopping drug abruptly; withdrawal symptoms may develop.

estradiol

Estrace, Estring

estradiol cypionate

depGynogen, Depo-Estradiol, Depogen, Dura-Estrin, E-Cypionate, Estragyn LA 5, Estro-Cyp, Estrofem, Estro-L.A.

estradiol transdermal system

Alora, Climara, Esclim, Estraderm, Fem-Patch, Vivelle, Vivelle-Dot

estradiol valerate

Clinagen LA 40, Delestrogen, Dioval 40, Dioval XX, Duragen-20, Estra-L 40, Estro-Span, Femogex (CAN), Gynogen L.A. 20, Gynogen L.A. 40, Menaval-20, Valergen 10, Valergen 20, Valergen 40

ethinyl estradiol

Estinyl

Class and Category

Chemical: Estrogenic derivative, steroid hormone

Therapeutic: Antineoplastic, antiosteoporotic, ovarian hormone replacement
Pregnancy category: X

Indications and Dosages

➤ *To treat menopausal symptoms*

TABLETS (ESTRADIOL)

Adult menopausal and postmenopausal females. Starting on day 5 of a cycle, 0.5 to 2 mg q.d. in cycles of 3 wk on, 1 wk off.

Adult postmenopausal females with an intact uterus who are receiving concomitant progestin therapy. 0.5 to 2 mg q.d. with a daily progestin; or 0.5 to 2 mg q.d. on days 1 through 25 of a 28-day cycle, with a progestin beginning on day 12 or 16 and continuing through day 25 of the cycle, then no drugs on days 26 through 28, as prescribed.

TABLETS (ETHINYL ESTRADIOL)

Adult menopausal and postmenopausal females. 0.02 to 0.05 mg q.d. in cycles of 3 wk on, 1 wk off.

Adult postmenopausal females with an intact uterus who are receiving concomitant progestin therapy. 0.02 to 0.05 mg q.d. with a daily progestin; or 0.02 to 0.05 mg q.d. on days 1 through 25 of a 28-day cycle, with a progestin beginning on day 12 or 16 and continuing through day 25 of the cycle, then no drugs on days 26 through 28, as prescribed.

DOSAGE ADJUSTMENT Dosage may be reduced to less than 1 mg/day (estradiol) or 0.05 mg/day (ethinyl estradiol) for patients with vaginal or vulvar symptoms only.

I.M. INJECTION (ESTRADIOL CYPIONATE IN OIL)

Adult females. 1 to 5 mg as a single dose q 3 to 4 wk as needed.

I.M. INJECTION (ESTRADIOL VALERATE IN OIL)

Adult females. 10 to 20 mg q 4 wk as needed.

TRANSDERMAL (ALORA, ESTRADERM, VIVELLE, VIVELLE-DOT)

Adult menopausal and postmenopausal females. *Initial:* 0.025 to 0.05 mg/day in cycles of 3 wk on, 1 wk off. One patch applied to trunk or buttocks and replaced twice/wk (q 3 to 4 days). Titrate dosage to control symptoms, as prescribed.

TRANSDERMAL (CLIMARA)

Adult females. *Initial:* 0.05 mg/day. One patch applied to trunk or buttocks and replaced q wk. Titrate dosage to control symptoms, as prescribed. Follow a cyclic schedule, as prescribed, unless patient has had a hysterectomy.

E
F

TRANSDERMAL (ESCLIM)

Adult females. *Initial:* 0.025 mg/day. One patch applied to upper arm, upper thigh, or buttocks and replaced twice/wk (q 3 to 4 days). Titrate dosage to control symptoms, as prescribed. Follow a cyclic schedule, as prescribed, unless patient has had a hysterectomy.

TRANSDERMAL (FEMPATCH)

Adult females. *Initial:* 0.025 mg/day. One patch applied to buttocks and replaced q wk. If symptoms are not relieved after 4 to 6 wk, increased to two patches q wk, as prescribed. Follow a cyclic schedule, as prescribed, unless patient has had a hysterectomy.

➤ *To treat menopausal symptoms as combination therapy in patients with an intact uterus*

TRANSDERMAL estradiol (ALORA, ESTRADERM, VIVELLE, VIVELLE-DOT) IN COMBINATION WITH ESTRADIOL AND NORETHINDRONE ACETATE (COMBIPATCH)

Adult females. 0.05 mg/day estradiol-only transdermal system applied for first 14 days of a 28-day cycle and replaced twice/wk, according to product directions. Estradiol and norethindrone acetate transdermal system applied for remaining 14 days of 28-day cycle and replaced twice/wk during this period.

➤ *To treat postmenopausal vaginal and urogenital symptoms*

VAGINAL CREAM (ESTRACE)

Adult females. *Initial:* 2 to 4 g (200 to 400 mcg) q.d. for 1 to 2 wk. Then, dosage gradually reduced to one-half of initial dose, as prescribed, for 1 to 2 wk. *Maintenance:* 1 g (100 mcg) q.d. 1 to 3 times/wk for 3 wk, followed by 1 wk of no drugs. Repeat cyclically as needed.

VAGINAL RING (ESTRING)

Adult females. One ring (7.5 mcg of estradiol/ 24 hrs) inserted into upper third of vaginal vault and replaced q 3 mo.

➤ *To prevent osteoporosis secondary to estrogen deficiency due to either natural or surgical menopause*

TABLETS (ESTRADIOL)

Adult females. At least 0.5 mg q.d. cyclically or continuously, titrated as needed to control concurrent menopausal symptoms, as prescribed.

TABLETS (ETHINYL ESTRADIOL)

Adult females. At least 0.02 mg q.d. cyclically or continuously, as prescribed.

TRANSDERMAL (ALORA, VIVELLE-DOT)

Adult females. *Initial:* 0.025 mg/day continuously. One patch applied to lower abdomen or buttocks and replaced twice/wk. Titrate dosage to control symptoms and maintain bone density, as prescribed.

TRANSDERMAL (CLIMARA)

Adult females. *Initial:* 0.025 or 0.05 mg/day. One patch applied to trunk or buttocks and replaced q wk. Titrate dosage to control symptoms, as prescribed. Follow a cyclic schedule, as prescribed, unless patient has had a hysterectomy.

TRANSDERMAL (ESTRADERM)

Adult females. *Initial:* 0.05 mg/day. One patch applied to trunk or buttocks and replaced twice/wk. Titrate dosage to control symptoms, as prescribed. Follow a cyclic schedule, as prescribed, unless patient has had a hysterectomy.

➤ *To treat estrogen deficiency due to oophorectomy, primary ovarian failure, or female hypogonadism*

TABLETS (ESTRADIOL)

Adult females. 0.5 to 2 mg q.d. continuously or in cycles of 3 wk on, 1 wk off.

TABLETS (ETHINYL ESTRADIOL)

Adult females. For primary ovarian failure or oophorectomy, 0.05 mg t.i.d. initially, then 0.05 mg q.d. after a few weeks, cyclically or continuously. For female hypogonadism, 0.05 mg q.d. to t.i.d. for first 2 wk of a theoretical menstrual cycle. A progestin may be added, as prescribed, during last half of cycle to help induce menses.

I.M. INJECTION (ESTRADIOL CYPIONATE IN OIL)

Adult females. 1.5 to 2 mg q mo (for female hypogonadism only).

I.M. INJECTION (ESTRADIOL VALERATE IN OIL)

Adult females. 10 to 20 mg q mo as needed.

TRANSDERMAL (ALORA, ESTRADERM, VIVELLE)

Adult females. *Initial:* 0.05 mg/day. One patch applied to trunk or buttocks and replaced twice/wk. Titrate dosage to control symptoms, as prescribed. Follow a cyclic schedule, as prescribed, unless patient has had a hysterectomy.

TRANSDERMAL (CLIMARA)

Adult females. *Initial:* 0.05 mg/day. One patch applied to trunk or buttocks and replaced q wk. Titrate dosage to control symptoms, as prescribed. Follow a cyclic schedule, as prescribed, unless patient has had a hysterectomy.

TRANSDERMAL (ESCLIM)
Adult females. *Initial:* 0.025 mg/day. One patch applied to upper arm, upper thigh, or buttocks and replaced twice/wk (q 3 to 4 days). Titrate dosage to control symptoms, as prescribed. Follow a cyclic schedule, as prescribed, unless patient has had a hysterectomy.

TRANSDERMAL (FEMPATCH)
Adult females. *Initial:* 0.025 mg. One patch applied to buttocks and replaced q wk. If symptoms are not relieved after 4 to 6 wk, increased to two patches q wk, as prescribed. Follow a cyclic schedule, as prescribed, unless patient has had a hysterectomy.

➤ *To treat dysfunctional uterine bleeding caused by hormonal imbalance in patients with a hypoplastic or atrophic endometrium and without uterine disease*

TRANSDERMAL (CLIMARA)
Adult females. *Initial:* 0.05 mg/day. One patch applied to trunk or buttocks and replaced q wk. Titrate dosage to control symptoms, as prescribed. Follow a cyclic schedule, as prescribed.

TRANSDERMAL (FEMPATCH)
Adult females. *Initial:* 0.025 mg/day. One patch applied to buttocks and replaced q wk. If symptoms are not relieved after 4 to 6 wk, increased to two patches q wk, as prescribed. Follow a cyclic schedule, as prescribed.

➤ *To provide palliative treatment for inoperable, progressive breast cancer in selected men and postmenopausal women*

TABLETS (ESTRADIOL)
Adults. 10 mg t.i.d. for at least 3 mo.

TABLETS (ETHINYL ESTRADIOL)
Adults. 1 mg t.i.d. for at least 3 mo.

➤ *To treat advancing inoperable prostate cancer*

TABLETS (ESTRADIOL)
Adult males. 1 to 2 mg b.i.d. or t.i.d., adjusted or continued, as prescribed, according to patient response.

TABLET (ETHINYL ESTRADIOL)
Adult males. 0.15 to 3 mg q.d., adjusted or continued, as prescribed, according to patient response.

I.M. INJECTION (ESTRADIOL VALERATE)
Adult males. 30 mg q 1 to 2 wk, adjusted or continued, as prescribed, according to patient response.

Mechanism of Action
Increases the rate of DNA and RNA synthesis in the cells of female reproductive organs, pituitary gland, hypothalamus, and other target organs. In the hypothalamus, estrogens reduce the release of gonadotropin-releasing hormone, which decreases pituitary release of follicle-stimulating hormone and luteinizing hormone. In women, these hormones are required for normal genitourinary and other essential body functions. At the cellular level, estrogens increase cervical secretions, cause endometrial cell proliferation, and improve uterine tone. Estrogen replacement helps maintain genitourinary function and reduces vasomotor symptoms when estrogen production declines as a result of menopause, surgical removal of ovaries, or other estrogen deficiency states. Estrogen replacement also helps prevent osteoporosis by inhibiting bone resorption.

In men, estrogens inhibit pituitary secretion of luteinizing hormone and decrease testicular secretion of testosterone. These actions may decrease prostate tumor growth and lower the level of prostate-specific antigen (PSA).

Contraindications
Active thrombophlebitis or thromboembolic disorders; hypersensitivity to estradiol, ethinyl estradiol, or their components; hypersensitivity to tartrazine dye (contained in 0.02-mg estradiol and ethinyl estradiol tablets); known or suspected breast cancer or estrogen-dependent cancer; pregnancy; undiagnosed abnormal genital bleeding

Interactions
DRUGS
aminocaproic acid: Possibly increased hypercoagulability caused by aminocaproic acid
barbiturates, carbamazepine, hydantoins, rifabutin, rifampin: Possibly reduced activity of estradiol
bromocriptine: Possibly decreased therapeutic effects of bromocriptine
calcium: Possibly increased calcium absorption
corticosteroids: Increased therapeutic and toxic effects of corticosteroids

cyclosporine: Increased risk of hepatotoxicity and nephrotoxicity

didanosine, lamivudine, zalcitabine: Possibly pancreatitis

hepatotoxic drugs, such as isoniazid: Increased risk of hepatitis and hepatotoxicity

oral antidiabetic drugs: Decreased therapeutic effects of these drugs

somatrem, somatropin: Possibly accelerated epiphyseal maturation

tamoxifen: Possibly decreased therapeutic effects of tamoxifen

vitamin C: Decreased metabolism and possibly increased adverse effects of estradiol

warfarin: Decreased anticoagulant effect

FOODS

grapefruit juice: Decreased metabolism and possibly increased adverse effects of estradiol

ACTIVITIES

smoking: Increased risk of CVA, pulmonary embolism, thrombophlebitis, and transient ischemic attack

Adverse Reactions

CNS: CVA, depression, dizziness, headache, migraine headache

CV: MI, peripheral edema, pulmonary embolism, thromboembolism, thrombophlebitis

EENT: Intolerance of contact lenses, vision changes

ENDO: Breast enlargement, pain, tenderness, or tumors; gynecomastia; hyperglycemia

GI: Abdominal cramps or pain, anorexia, constipation, diarrhea, elevated liver function test results, gallbladder obstruction, hepatitis, increased appetite, nausea, pancreatitis, vomiting

GU: Amenorrhea, breakthrough bleeding, cervical erosion, clear vaginal discharge, decreased libido (males), dysmenorrhea, impotence, increased libido (females), prolonged or heavy menstrual bleeding, testicular atrophy, vaginal candidiasis

SKIN: Acne, alopecia, hirsutism, jaundice, melasma, oily skin, purpura, rash, seborrhea, urticaria

Other: Folic acid deficiency, hypercalcemia (in metastatic bone disease), weight gain

Nursing Considerations

•**WARNING** Be aware that estradiol (Estrace) and ethinyl estradiol (Estinyl) are distinct and separate products and that their dosing is not equivalent.

•Administer oral preparations with or immediately after food to decrease nausea.

•For I.M. injection of estradiol cypionate or estradiol valerate, roll vial and syringe between palms to evenly disperse drug. Use at least a 21-gauge needle because of viscosity of oil-based solution. Use a dry, sterile syringe. Inject deep into upper outer quadrant of gluteal muscle. Aspirate before injection to avoid injection into a blood vessel.

•Be aware that, in patients who are converting from oral estrogen to transdermal system, oral estrogen should be discontinued 1 week before skin patches are applied.

•Expect to begin prophylaxis treatment against osteoporosis as soon as possible after menopause.

•Be aware that estrogen therapy should be given cyclically or combined with a progestin for 10 to 14 days per month in women with an intact uterus to minimize the risk of endometrial hyperplasia.

•**WARNING** Be aware that severe hypercalcemia may occur in patients with bone metastasis due to breast cancer because estrogens influence the metabolism of calcium and phosphorus. Monitor for toxic effects of increased calcium absorption in patients who are predisposed to hypercalcemia or nephrolithiasis.

•**WARNING** Assess patient for possible contact lens intolerance or changes in vision or visual acuity because estrogens can cause keratoconus, leading to increased curvature of the cornea. Be prepared to discontinue drug immediately, as prescribed, if patient experiences sudden partial or complete loss of vision or sudden onset of proptosis, diplopia, or migraine.

•Monitor PT test results of patients receiving warfarin for loss of anticoagulant effect because estrogens increase production of clotting factors VII, VIII, IX, and X and promote platelet aggregation.

•Monitor for elevated liver function test results because estrogens and progestins may exacerbate such conditions as acute intermittent or variegate hepatic porphyria.

•Closely monitor patients with hypertension for increases in blood pressure because estrogens may cause fluid retention. Also monitor patients with asthma, heart disease, migraines, renal disease, or seizure disorder for exacerbation of these conditions.

•Monitor for peripheral edema or mild

weight gain because estrogens can cause sodium and fluid retention.

•Frequently monitor blood glucose levels in patients with diabetes mellitus because estrogens may cause decreased insulin sensitivity and alterations in glucose tolerance.

•Expect to discontinue estrogen combination therapy in any woman who develops signs or symptoms of thromboembolic or cerebrovascular disease.

•Be aware that exogenous estradiol and progestins may exacerbate mood disorders, including depression. Monitor for depression, mood changes, anxiety, fatigue, dizziness, or insomnia. If significant depression occurs, expect to discontinue hormone replacement therapy.

•Assess skin for melasma (tan or brown patches), which may develop on forehead, cheeks, temples, and upper lip. These patches may persist after drug is discontinued.

•Monitor blood PSA level in patients with inoperable prostate cancer to determine if patient is responding to hormone therapy. If patient responds (usually within 3 months), expect therapy to continue until disease is significantly advanced.

•Monitor thyroid function test results in patients with hypothyroidism because long-term use of ethinyl estradiol may result in decreased effectiveness of thyroid replacement therapy.

•Expect to discontinue estrogen therapy several weeks before major surgery, as prescribed, because certain procedures are associated with prolonged immobilization and therefore pose an increased risk of thromboembolism.

PATIENT TEACHING

•Advise patient to remain recumbent for at least 30 minutes after applying estradiol vaginal cream. Inform her that she may use a sanitary napkin (but not a tampon) to protect clothing after application.

•Teach patient proper application and use of transdermal patch. Instruct her not to apply patch to breasts, waistline, or other areas where it may not adhere properly. Advise her to rotate application sites at least weekly and to remove old patch before applying new one. If patch falls off, instruct her to reapply it to another area or to apply a new patch and continue the original treatment schedule. Caution her not to expose patch to sun for

prolonged periods. Inform her that she may bathe while wearing the patch.

•Teach patient proper use of estradiol vaginal ring. Instruct her to insert ring in upper third of vagina, to keep it there for 90 days, and then to remove it and insert a new ring. Alternatively, patient may remove ring within 90-day dosage period, rinse it with lukewarm (not hot or boiling) water, and reinsert it as needed for personal hygiene.

•Inform patient receiving estradiol treatment that she should have an annual pelvic examination, including a Papanicolaou test, to screen for cervical dysplasia.

•Inform patient that a cyclic combination regimen of estradiol and a progestin may cause monthly withdrawal bleeding.

estradiol and norethindrone acetate

Activella, CombiPatch

Class and Category

Chemical: Estrogen derivative, steroid hormone
Therapeutic: Antiosteoporotic, ovarian hormone replacement
Pregnancy category: X

Indications and Dosages

➤ *To treat estrogen deficiency due to hypogonadism, oophorectomy, or primary ovarian failure in patients with an intact uterus*

TRANSDERMAL (COMBIPATCH)

Adult females. Continuous combined regimen for women who don't want to resume menses: 0.05-mg estradiol/0.14-mg norethindrone acetate/day transdermal system (9-cm^2 CombiPatch) is worn continuously on lower abdomen; may be increased to 0.05-mg estradiol/0.25-mg norethindrone acetate/day system (16-cm^2 CombiPatch), as prescribed, if a greater progestin dose is desired. New system is applied twice/wk (q 3 to 4 days) during a 28-day cycle.

Adult females. Continuous sequential regimen in combination with an estradiol-only transdermal delivery system: 0.05-mg/day estradiol transdermal system (Vivelle) is worn for first 14 days of a 28-day cycle and is replaced twice/wk according to product directions. For remaining 14 days of 28-day cycle, 0.05-mg estradiol/0.14-mg norethindrone acetate/day transdermal system (9-cm² CombiPatch) is worn on lower abdomen; may be increased to 0.05-mg estradiol/ 0.25-mg norethindrone acetate/day system (16-cm² CombiPatch), as prescribed, if a greater progestin dose is desired. Combi-Patch system is replaced twice/wk (q 3 to 4 days) during this period in the cycle.

➤ *To treat menopausal symptoms and to prevent osteoporosis due to estrogen deficiency in postmenopausal women with an intact uterus*

TABLETS (ACTIVELLA)

Adult females. 1 tablet (1 mg estradiol and 0.5 mg norethindrone acetate) q.d.

TRANSDERMAL (COMBIPATCH)

Adult females. Continuous combined regimen for women who don't want to resume menses: 0.05-mg estradiol/0.14-mg norethindrone acetate/day transdermal system (9-cm² CombiPatch) is worn continuously on lower abdomen; may be increased to 0.05-mg estradiol/0.25-mg norethindrone acetate/day system (16-cm² CombiPatch), as prescribed, if a greater progestin dose is desired. New system is applied twice/wk (q 3 to 4 days) during a 28-day cycle.

Adult females. Continuous sequential regimen in combination with an estradiol-only transdermal delivery system: 0.05-mg/day estradiol transdermal system (Vivelle) is worn for first 14 days of a 28-day cycle and is replaced twice/wk according to product directions. For remaining 14 days of 28-day cycle, 0.05-mg estradiol/0.14-mg norethindrone acetate/day transdermal system (9-cm² CombiPatch) is worn on lower abdomen; may be increased to 0.05-mg estradiol/ 0.25-mg norethindrone acetate/day system (16-cm² CombiPatch), as prescribed, if a greater progestin dose is desired. Combi-Patch system is replaced twice/wk (q 3 to 4 days) during this period in the cycle.

Route	Onset	Peak	Duration
Transdermal	Unknown	In 24 hr	Unknown

Contraindications

Active thrombophlebitis or thromboembolic disorders; endometrial hyperplasia; hepatic disorders; hypersensitivity to estradiol, norethindrone, or their components; jaundice; known or suspected breast cancer or history of breast cancer from estrogen use;

known or suspected estrogen-dependent cancer; pregnancy; undiagnosed abnormal genital bleeding; vaginal disorders

Mechanism of Action

Estradiol increases the rate of DNA and RNA synthesis in the cells of female reproductive organs, pituitary gland, hypothalamus, and other target organs. In the hypothalamus, estrogens decrease the release of gonadotropin-releasing hormone, which reduces pituitary release of follicle-stimulating hormone and luteinizing hormone. In women, these hormones are required for normal genitourinary and other essential body functions. At the cellular level, estrogens increase cervical secretions, cause endometrial cell proliferation, and improve uterine tone. Estrogen replacement helps maintain genitourinary function and reduces vasomotor symptoms when estrogen production declines as a result of menopause, surgical removal of ovaries, or other estrogen deficiency states. Estrogen replacement also helps prevent osteoporosis by inhibiting bone resorption.

Norethindrone is a progestin. Progestins prolong some of the positive effects of estrogens on HDL cholesterol. Norethindrone diffuses freely into target cells of the female reproductive tract, mammary glands, hypothalamus, and pituitary gland and binds to the progesterone cell receptor. It converts a proliferative endometrium into a secretory one in women with adequate estrogen replacement, reducing endometrial growth and the risk of endometrial cancer compared with women who have an intact uterus and take unopposed estrogens. Norethindrone also decreases nuclear estradiol receptors and suppresses epithelial DNA synthesis in endometrial tissues.

Interactions

DRUGS

aminocaproic acid: Possibly increased hypercoagulability caused by aminocaproic acid
barbiturates, carbamazepine, hydantoins, rifabutin, rifampin: Possibly reduced activity of estradiol and norethindrone
bromocriptine: Possibly decreased therapeutic effects of bromocriptine

calcium: Possibly increased calcium absorption

corticosteroids: Increased therapeutic and toxic effects of corticosteroids

cyclosporine: Increased risk of hepatotoxicity and nephrotoxicity

didanosine, lamivudine, zalcitabine: Possibly pancreatitis

hepatotoxic drugs, such as isoniazid: Increased risk of hepatitis and hepatotoxicity

oral antidiabetic drugs: Decreased therapeutic effects of these drugs

somatrem, somatropin: Possibly accelerated epiphyseal maturation

tamoxifen: Possibly decreased therapeutic effects of tamoxifen

vitamin C: Decreased metabolism and possibly increased adverse effects of estradiol and norethindrone

warfarin: Decreased anticoagulant effect

FOODS

grapefruit juice: Decreased metabolism and possibly increased adverse effects of estradiol and norethindrone

ACTIVITIES

smoking: Increased risk of CVA, pulmonary embolism, thrombophlebitis, and transient ischemic attack

Adverse Reactions

CNS: CVA, depression, dizziness, headache, migraine headache

CV: MI, peripheral edema, pulmonary embolism, thromboembolism, thrombophlebitis

EENT: Intolerance of contact lenses, vision changes

ENDO: Breast enlargement, pain, tenderness, or tumors; gynecomastia; hyperglycemia

GI: Abdominal cramps or pain, anorexia, constipation, diarrhea, elevated liver function test results, gallbladder obstruction, hepatitis, increased appetite, nausea, pancreatitis, vomiting

GU: Amenorrhea, breakthrough bleeding, cervical erosion, clear vaginal discharge, decreased libido (males), dysmenorrhea, impotence, increased libido (females), prolonged or heavy menstrual bleeding, testicular atrophy, vaginal candidiasis

SKIN: Acne, alopecia, hirsutism, jaundice, melasma, oily skin, purpura, rash, seborrhea, urticaria

Other: Folic acid deficiency, hypercalcemia (in metastatic bone disease), weight gain

Nursing Considerations

•**WARNING** Be aware that severe hypercalcemia may occur in patients with bone metastasis due to breast cancer because estrogens influence the metabolism of calcium and phosphorus. Monitor for toxic effects of increased calcium absorption in patients who are predisposed to hypercalcemia or nephrolithiasis.

•**WARNING** Assess patient for possible contact lens intolerance or changes in vision or visual acuity because estrogens can cause keratoconus, leading to increased curvature of the cornea. Be prepared to discontinue drug immediately, as prescribed, if patient experiences sudden partial or complete loss of vision or sudden onset of proptosis, diplopia, or migraine.

•Monitor PT test results of patients receiving warfarin for loss of anticoagulant effect because estrogens increase production of clotting factors VII, VIII, IX, and X and promote platelet aggregation.

•Monitor for elevated liver function test results because estrogen and progestins may exacerbate such conditions as acute intermittent or variegate hepatic porphyria.

•Closely monitor patients with hypertension for increases in blood pressure because estrogens may cause fluid retention. Also monitor patients with asthma, heart disease, renal disease, migraines, or seizure disorder for exacerbation of these conditions.

•Monitor for peripheral edema or mild weight gain because estrogens can cause sodium and fluid retention.

•Observe patients, especially those with diabetes mellitus, for changes in glucose tolerance when estrogen therapy is initiated or discontinued. Patients with diabetes mellitus may develop altered glucose tolerance secondary to decreased insulin sensitivity.

•Be aware that exogenous estradiol and norethindrone may exacerbate mood disorders, including depression. Monitor for depression, mood changes, anxiety, fatigue, dizziness, or insomnia. If significant depression occurs, expect to discontinue hormone replacement therapy.

•Assess skin for melasma (tan or brown patches), which may develop on forehead, cheeks, temples, and upper lip. These patches may persist after drug is discontinued.

•Expect to discontinue estrogen combination

therapy in any woman who develops signs or symptoms of thromboembolic or cerebrovascular disease.

•Expect to discontinue estrogen therapy several weeks before major surgery, as prescribed, because certain procedures are associated with prolonged immobilization and therefore pose an increased risk of thromboembolism.

PATIENT TEACHING

•Teach patient proper application and use of CombiPatch transdermal system. Instruct her to tear pouch open, rather than using scissors, and to remove stiff protective liner covering adhesive without touching adhesive. Tell her not to cut or trim the patch. Advise her to apply patch to a clean, dry, and hairless part of lower abdomen, with sticky side to skin. Caution her not to apply patch to breasts; to injured, irritated, callused, or scarred areas; or to areas where it may not adhere properly, such as waistline.

•Advise patient to rotate application sites at least weekly and to remove old patch before applying new one. If patch falls off, instruct her to reapply it to another area, or to apply a new patch and continue the original treatment schedule. Caution her not to expose patch to sun for prolonged periods. Inform her that she may bathe while wearing the patch.

•Advise patient taking estradiol and norethindrone not to smoke because smoking increases the risk of deep vein thrombosis, MI, and other thromboembolic disorders.

•Inform patient that estradiol and norethindrone regimen may cause monthly withdrawal bleeding.

•Advise patient receiving estradiol treatment to have an annual pelvic examination, including a Papanicolaou (Pap) smear, to screen for cervical dysplasia.

estrogens (conjugated)

C.E.S. (CAN), Congest (CAN), Premarin

estrogens (conjugated) and medroxyprogesterone

Prempro

synthetic estrogens, A (conjugated)

Cenestin

Class and Category

Chemical: Estrogen derivative, steroid hormone

Therapeutic: Antiosteoporotic, ovarian hormone replacement

Pregnancy category: X

Indications and Dosages

➤ *To treat atrophic vaginitis, vasomotor menopausal symptoms, and vulvar atrophy*

TABLETS

Adults. 0.3 to 1.25 mg q.d. in cycles of 3 wk on, 1 wk off. Or combination product (0.625 mg of conjugated estrogens and 2.5 mg of medroxyprogesterone) q.d.

➤ *To treat atrophic vaginitis and vulvar atrophy*

VAGINAL CREAM

Adults. 0.5 to 2 g q.d. in cycles of 3 wk on, 1 wk off.

➤ *To prevent osteoporosis*

TABLETS

Adults. 0.625 mg q.d. continuously or in cycles of 3 wk on, 1 wk off. Or combination product (0.625 mg of conjugated estrogens and 2.5 mg of medroxyprogesterone) q.d.

➤ *To provide palliative treatment for advanced androgen-dependent prostate cancer*

TABLETS

Adults. 1.25 to 2.5 mg t.i.d.

➤ *To provide palliative treatment for metastatic breast cancer*

TABLETS

Adults. 10 mg t.i.d. for 3 mo or longer.

➤ *To treat dysfunctional uterine bleeding*

I.V. INFUSION, I.M. INJECTION

Adults. 25 mg, repeated in 6 to 12 hr if needed.

➤ *To treat estrogen deficiency from oophorectomy or primary ovarian failure*

TABLETS

Adults. 1.25 mg q.d. continuously or in cycles of 3 wk on, 1 wk off.

➤ *To treat female hypogonadism*

TABLETS

Adults. 2.5 to 7.5 mg/day in divided doses t.i.d. for 20 days followed by 10 days off. Cycle repeated until breakthrough bleeding occurs. If bleeding begins during 10-day rest period, 20-day course of 2.5 to 7.5 mg/day in divided doses t.i.d. should begin during last 5 days of rest period and should be given with oral progestin. If bleeding begins during 20-day course, therapy is discontinued and then resumed on day 5 of bleeding.

Mechanism of Action
Increase the rate of DNA and RNA synthesis in the cells of female reproductive organs, hypothalamus, pituitary glands, and other target organs. In the hypothalamus, estrogens reduce the release of gonadotropin-releasing hormone, which decreases pituitary release of follicle-stimulating hormone and luteinizing hormone. In women, these hormones are required for normal genitourinary and other essential body functions. At the cellular level, estrogens increase cervical secretions, cause endometrial cell proliferation, and increase uterine tone. Estrogen replacement helps maintain genitourinary function and reduce vasomotor symptoms when estrogen production declines as a result of menopause, surgical removal of ovaries, or other estrogen deficiency states. Estrogen replacement also helps prevent osteoporosis by inhibiting bone resorption so that resorption doesn't exceed bone formation.

In men, estrogens inhibit pituitary secretion of luteinizing hormone and decrease testicular secretion of testosterone. These actions may decrease prostate tumor growth and lower the level of prostate-specific antigen.

Incompatibilities
Don't combine I.V. estrogens with acid solutions, ascorbic acid, and protein hydrolysate because they're incompatible.

Contraindications
Abnormal or undiagnosed vaginal bleeding; breast, endometrial, or estrogen-dependent cancer; hypersensitivity to conjugated estrogens or their components; pregnancy; thromboembolic disorders

Interactions
DRUGS
aminocaproic acid: Possibly increased hypercoagulability caused by aminocaproic acid
barbiturates, carbamazepine, hydantoins, rifabutin, rifampin: Possibly reduced activity of estrogen and medroxyprogesterone

bromocriptine: Possibly interference with bromocriptine's therapeutic effects
calcium: Possibly increased calcium absorption
corticosteroids: Increased therapeutic and toxic effects of corticosteroids
cyclosporine: Increased risk of hepatotoxicity and nephrotoxicity
didanosine, lamivudine, zalcitabine: Possibly pancreatitis
hepatotoxic drugs, such as isoniazid: Increased risk of hepatitis and hepatotoxicity
oral antidiabetic drugs: Decreased therapeutic effects of these drugs
somatrem, somatropin: Possibly accelerated epiphyseal maturation
tamoxifen: Possibly interference with tamoxifen's therapeutic effects
warfarin: Decreased anticoagulant effect
ACTIVITIES
smoking: Increased risk of CVA, pulmonary embolism, thrombophlebitis, and transient ischemic attack

Adverse Reactions
CNS: CVA, depression, dizziness, headache, migraine headache
CV: MI, peripheral edema, pulmonary embolism, thromboembolism, thrombophlebitis
EENT: Intolerance of contact lenses
ENDO: Breast enlargement, pain, tenderness, or tumors; gynecomastia; hyperglycemia
GI: Abdominal cramps or pain, anorexia, constipation, diarrhea, gallbladder obstruction, hepatitis, increased appetite, nausea, pancreatitis, vomiting
GU: Amenorrhea, breakthrough bleeding, cervical erosion, clear vaginal discharge, decreased libido (males), dysmenorrhea, impotence, increased libido (females), prolonged or heavy menstrual bleeding, testicular atrophy, vaginal candidiasis
SKIN: Acne, alopecia, hirsutism, jaundice, melasma, oily skin, purpura, rash, seborrhea, urticaria
Other: Folic acid deficiency, hypercalcemia (in metastatic bone disease), weight gain

Nursing Considerations
• Reconstitute conjugated estrogens with NS, dextrose, or invert sugar solution and use within a few hours. Discard solution that contains precipitate.
• Assess for peripheral edema, a sign of fluid retention.

•Evaluate patient's fluid intake and output, watching for positive fluid balance.
•Assess for signs of depression, such as changes in mental status, affect, and mood.
•Monitor serum calcium level to detect severe hypercalcemia in patients with bone metastasis from breast cancer.
•Expect to discontinue drug during periods of immobilization, 4 weeks before elective surgery, and if jaundice develops.

PATIENT TEACHING
•Urge patient to immediately report breakthrough bleeding to prescriber.
•Instruct patient to perform a monthly breast self-examination and comply with all prescribed follow-up examinations, especially endometrial tests, because natural and synthetic estrogens increase the risk of breast and endometrial cancer.
•Encourage patient to stay active to reduce the risk of thrombophlebitis.
•Inform male patient that prolonged use of estrogens may cause gynecomastia and female patient that long-term use may increase risk of heart disease, stroke and breast cancer.

etanercept

Enbrel

Class and Category

Chemical: Dimeric recombinant human p75 tumor necrosis factor receptor (TNFR)
Therapeutic: Disease-modifying antirheumatoid drug
Pregnancy category: B

Indications and Dosages

➤ *To reduce signs and symptoms of active rheumatoid or psoriatic arthritis alone or in combination with methotrexate*

Mechanism of Action

Etanercept reduces joint inflammation associated with rheumatoid arthritis by binding with tumor necrosis factor (TNF), a cytokine, or protein, that plays an important role in normal inflammatory and immune responses.

In rheumatoid arthritis, the immune and inflammatory disease process triggers the release of TNF, primarily from macrophages. TNF then binds to TNF receptors on cell membranes, as shown below left. This action renders TNF biologically active and triggers a cascade of inflammatory events that results in increased inflammation of the synovial membrane, the release of destructive lysosomal enzymes, and further joint destruction.

Etanercept binds specifically to TNF and prevents it from binding with TNF receptors on the cell membranes, as shown below right. This action renders the bound TNF biologically inactive, prevents TNF-mediated cellular responses, and results in significant reduction in inflammatory activity.

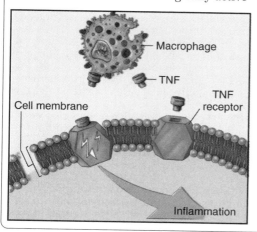

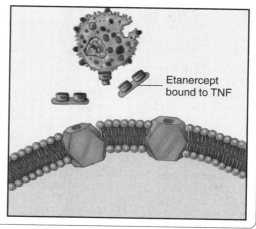

S.C. INJECTION
Adults. 25 mg twice/wk for up to 2 yr.
➤ *To reduce signs and symptoms of juve-*
nile rheumatoid arthritis
S.C. INJECTION
Children ages 4 to 17. 0.4 mg/kg twice/wk,
3 to 4 days apart, for 3 to 7 mo. *Maximum:*
25 mg twice/wk.

Incompatibilities
Don't combine etanercept with other drugs.

Contraindications
Hypersensitivity to etanercept, hamster protein,
or their components, sepsis or risk of sepsis

Adverse Reactions
CNS: Asthenia, chills, fever, headache
CV: Hypertension, hypotension
EENT: Pharyngitis, rhinitis, sinusitis
GI: Abdominal abscess, abdominal pain,
cholecystitis, diarrhea, indigestion, nausea,
vomiting
GU: Pyelonephritis
MS: Septic arthritis
RESP: Bronchitis, cough, pneumonia, upper
respiratory tract infection
SKIN: Cellulitis, foot abscess, leg ulcer, pru-
ritus, rash
Other: Injection site edema, erythema, and
pain; sepsis; varicella infection

Nursing Considerations
•WARNING Don't use the diluent provided
with etanercept (bacteriostatic water for injection, USP, with 0.9% benzyl alcohol) for
patients with benzyl alcohol hypersensitivity.
Use sterile water for injection instead.
•WARNING If you have a latex allergy, don't
handle needle cover of diluent syringe because it contains dry natural rubber (latex).
•WARNING Expect to discontinue etanercept
if patient develops sepsis because of increased risk of death.
•Be aware that live virus vaccines should
not be given to patients taking etanercept
because drug decreases patient's immune
response and places him at increased risk for
secondary transmission of vaccine virus.
•Monitor patients with immunosuppression
for active signs and symptoms of acute or
chronic infection, including chills, fever, and
tachycardia, because etanercept decreases

patient's defenses against infection. Be aware
that drug also increases patient's risk of developing malignant tumors.
•Continue to administer corticosteroids,
NSAIDs, and other analgesics, as prescribed,
during etanercept therapy.
PATIENT TEACHING
•Inform patient that etanercept is given by a
small injection under the skin, and teach him
proper injection technique if prescriber has
recommended self-administration.
•Help patient prepare and inject first few
doses.
•Advise patient to use dissolved powder as
soon as possible. Explain that dissolved
powder may be kept in refrigerator for up to
6 hours after mixing and then should be discarded.
•Instruct patient to rotate injection sites among
the thigh, stomach, and upper arms and to
avoid areas that are tender, red, bruised, or
hard. Advise him to make sure that each site is
at least 1″ away from a previous site.
•Urge patient to discard used needles and
syringes in a puncture-resistant container
and not to reuse them. Instruct him to return
container to prescriber for proper disposal.
•Advise patient to consult prescriber immediately if he develops a cold or other infection while taking etanercept because drug
may decrease his ability to fight infection.
•Caution patient who has never had chickenpox to contact prescriber right away if he
is exposed because he may develop a more
serious infection.

ethacrynic acid
Edecrin

ethacrynate sodium
Edecrin

Class and Category
Chemical: Ketone derivative of anyloxyacetic
acid
Therapeutic: Diuretic
Pregnancy category: B

Indications and Dosages
➤ *To promote diuresis in heart failure; he-*
patic cirrhosis; renal disease; ascites of
short duration caused by cancer, idio-

pathic edema, or lymphedema; and
edema in children (excluding infants
with congenital heart disease or nephrotic syndrome)

ORAL SOLUTION, TABLETS
Adults. *Initial:* 50 to 100 mg/day as a single
dose or in divided doses. Dosage increased
by 25 to 50 mg/day, if needed. *Maintenance:*
50 to 200 mg/day. *Maximum:* 400 mg/day.
Children (except infants). *Initial:* 25 mg q.d.
Dosage increased in 25-mg increments daily,
if needed.

I.V. INFUSION
Adults. *Initial:* 50 mg or 0.5 to 1 mg/kg. Dose
repeated in 2 to 4 hr, if needed, then q 4 to 6
hr based on patient response. In an emergency, dose repeated q 1 hr, if needed. *Maximum:* 100 mg as a single dose.

Route	Onset	Peak	Duration
P.O.	30 min	2 hr	6 to 8 hr
I.V.	5 min	15 to 30 min	2 hr

Mechanism of Action
Probably inhibits the sulfhydryl-catalyzed
enzyme systems that cause sodium and
chloride resorption in the proximal and
distal tubules and the ascending limb of
the loop of Henle. These inhibitory effects
increase urinary excretion of sodium,
chloride, and water, causing profound diuresis. The drug also increases the excretion of potassium, hydrogen, calcium,
magnesium, bicarbonate, ammonium, and
phosphate.

Contraindications
Anuria; hypersensitivity to ethacrynic acid,
ethacrynate sodium, sulfonylureas, or their
components; infancy; severe diarrhea

Interactions
DRUGS
ACE inhibitors, antihypertensives: Possibly
hypotension
aminoglycosides: Increased risk of ototoxicity
amiodarone: Increased risk of arrhythmias
amphotericin B: Increased risk of electrolyte
imbalances, nephrotoxicity, and ototoxicity
anticoagulants, thrombolytics: Possibly potentiated anticoagulation and risk of hemorrhage

corticosteroids: Increased risk of gastric
hemorrhage
digoxin: Increased risk of digitalis toxicity
insulin, oral antidiabetic drugs: Possibly increased blood glucose level and decreased
therapeutic effects of these drugs
lithium: Increased risk of lithium toxicity
neuromuscular blockers: Possibly increased
neuromuscular blockade
NSAIDs: Possibly decreased effects of ethacrynic acid
sympathomimetics: Possibly interference
with hypotensive effects of ethacrynic acid
and ethacrynate sodium
ACTIVITIES
alcohol use: Possibly potentiated hypotensive
and diuretic effects of ethacrynic acid and
ethacrynate sodium

Adverse Reactions
CNS: Confusion, fatigue, headache, malaise,
nervousness
CV: Orthostatic hypotension
EENT: Blurred vision, hearing loss, ototoxicity (ringing or buzzing in ears), sensation of
fullness in ears, yellow vision
ENDO: Hyperglycemia, hypoglycemia
GI: Abdominal pain, anorexia, diarrhea, dysphagia, GI bleeding (I.V. form), nausea, vomiting
GU: Hematuria (I.V. form), interstitial nephritis, polyuria
HEME: Agranulocytosis, severe neutropenia,
thrombocytopenia
SKIN: Rash
Other: Hyperuricemia, hypochloremic alkalosis, hypokalemia, hypomagnesemia, hyponatremia, hypovolemia, infusion site irritation
and pain

Nursing Considerations
•**WARNING** Use ethacrynic acid and ethacrynate sodium cautiously in patients with advanced hepatic cirrhosis, especially those
who also have a history of electrolyte imbalance or hepatic encephalopathy; both forms
of drug may lead to lethal hepatic coma.
•Dilute ethacrynate sodium with D_5W or NS
for I.V. infusion. Discard unused portion after
24 hours.
•Don't use diluted ethacrynate sodium that's
cloudy or opalescent.
•Infuse I.V. ethacrynate sodium slowly over
30 minutes.
•Weigh patient daily and assess for signs of
electrolyte imbalances and dehydration.

Monitor blood pressure and fluid intake and output, and check laboratory test results. Notify prescriber about significant changes. Prescriber may reduce dosage or temporarily discontinue drug.
•If hypokalemia develops, administer replacement potassium, as ordered.
•Monitor blood glucose level frequently, especially if patient has diabetes mellitus; both forms of drug may cause hyperglycemia or hypoglycemia.
•Notify prescriber if patient experiences hearing loss, vertigo, or ringing, buzzing, or sense of fullness in his ears. Drug may need to be discontinued.

PATIENT TEACHING
•Instruct patient to take the last dose of ethacrynic acid several hours before bedtime to avoid sleep interruption from diuresis. If patient receives once-daily dosing, advise him to take the dose in the morning to avoid sleep disturbance caused by nocturia.
•Suggest that patient take drug with food or milk to reduce GI distress.
•Advise patient to change position slowly to minimize effects of orthostatic hypotension, especially if he also takes an antihypertensive.
•Unless contraindicated, urge patient to eat more high-potassium foods and to take a potassium supplement, if prescribed, to prevent hypokalemia.
•Caution patient not to drink alcohol, stand for prolonged periods, or exercise during hot weather because these activities may exacerbate orthostatic hypotension.
•Instruct patient to notify prescriber if he experiences diarrhea; buzzing, fullness, or ringing in his ears; hearing loss; severe nausea; vertigo; or vomiting. Drug may need to be discontinued.
•Remind diabetic patient to check his blood glucose level frequently to detect alterations.

ethambutol hydrochloride

Etibi (CAN), Myambutol

Class and Category
Chemical: Diisopropylethylene diamide derivative
Therapeutic: Antitubercular
Pregnancy category: Not rated

Indications and Dosages
➤ *As adjunct to treat tuberculosis and atypical mycobacterial infections caused by* Mycobacterium tuberculosis
TABLETS
Adults and adolescents who haven't received previous antitubercular therapy. 15 mg/kg q.d.
Adults and adolescents who have received previous antitubercular therapy. 25 mg/kg q.d.; after 60 days, decreased to 15 mg/kg q.d.

Mechanism of Action
May suppress bacterial multiplication by interfering with RNA synthesis in susceptible bacteria that are actively dividing.

Contraindications
Hypersensitivity to ethambutol or its components, optic neuritis

Interactions
DRUGS
other neurotoxic drugs: Increased risk of neurotoxicity, such as optic and peripheral neuritis

Adverse Reactions
CNS: Burning sensation or weakness in arms and legs, confusion, disorientation, fever, headache, paresthesia
EENT: Blurred vision, decreased visual acuity, eye pain, optic neuritis, red-green color blindness
GI: Abdominal pain, anorexia, nausea, vomiting
MS: Arthralgia, gouty arthritis
SKIN: Rash

Nursing Considerations
•Expect prescriber to refer patient for an ophthalmologic examination that includes tests for visual fields, acuity, and red-green color blindness before taking ethambutol and monthly thereafter, especially if therapy is prolonged or dosage exceeds 15 mg/kg/day.
•Expect to give at least one other antitubercular drug with ethambutol, as prescribed, because bacterial resistance to a single drug may develop quickly.
•Monitor laboratory test results for increased serum uric acid level if patient has gouty arthritis or impaired renal function.

•Obtain a monthly sputum specimen, as ordered, to check bacteriologic response in sputum-positive patient.
•Keep in mind that successful drug therapy typically takes 6 to 12 months but may take years.

PATIENT TEACHING
•Teach patient to recognize ethambutol's possible adverse reactions.
•Advise patient to take drug with food if he experiences adverse GI reactions.
•Instruct patient to take a missed dose as soon as he remembers, unless it's nearly time for the next dose. Caution him not to double-dose.
•Inform patient that therapy may last months or years and that compliance is essential.
•Advise patient to notify prescriber if no improvement occurs within 3 weeks; if bothersome or severe adverse reactions occur; if his vision changes; or if a rash, fever, or joint pain (signs of hypersensitivity) develops.

ethchlorvynol

Placidyl

Class, Category, and Schedule
Chemical: Chlorinated tertiary acetylenic carbinol
Therapeutic: Sedative-hypnotic
Pregnancy category: C
Controlled substance: Schedule IV

Indications and Dosages
➤ *To provide short-term relief from insomnia*
CAPSULES
Adults. 0.5 to 1 g h.s. for no longer than 1 wk.

Route	Onset	Peak	Duration
P.O.	15 to 60 min	Unknown	5 hr

Mechanism of Action
Exerts sedative-hypnotic, muscle relaxant, and anticonvulsant effects possibly by depressing the reticular activating system.

Contraindications
Hypersensitivity to ethchlorvynol or its components, porphyria

Interactions
DRUGS
CNS depressants, tricyclic antidepressants: Increased CNS depression
oral anticoagulants: Decreased anticoagulant effects
ACTIVITIES
alcohol use: Increased CNS depression

Adverse Reactions
CNS: Ataxia, dizziness, facial numbness, fatigue, light-headedness, syncope, unsteadiness, weakness
CV: Hypotension
EENT: Blurred vision, unpleasant aftertaste
GI: Epigastric pain, indigestion, nausea, vomiting
HEME: Thrombocytopenia
SKIN: Jaundice, rash, urticaria
Other: Physical and psychological dependence

Nursing Considerations
•If patient awakens too early after taking 0.5 or 0.75 g of ethchlorvynol at bedtime, ask prescriber if he may take a single supplemental dose of 200 mg.
•Assess for signs of addiction if patient has taken drug for 2 weeks or longer.
•Be aware that ethchlorvynol shouldn't be given for longer than 1 week. If patient has received prolonged therapy, expect to discontinue drug gradually to prevent withdrawal symptoms. Notify prescriber if you detect withdrawal symptoms: diaphoresis, hallucinations, irritability, muscle twitching, nausea, nervousness, restlessness, seizures, sleep disturbance, tremor, vomiting, and weakness.
PATIENT TEACHING
•Caution patient not to exceed prescribed dosage or dosing frequency because of ethchlorvynol's habit-forming potential. Instruct him not to use drug for more than 1 week.
•Advise patient to take drug with food or milk to minimize adverse GI reactions.
•If patient has taken long-term ethchlorvynol therapy, warn against stopping drug abruptly; advise him to contact prescriber for guidelines to reduce dosage.
•Direct patient to avoid alcohol and other CNS depressants during therapy because they increase the risk of adverse reactions.
•Advise patient to avoid potentially hazardous activities until drug's CNS effects are known.

ethionamide

Trecator-SC

Class and Category

Chemical: Thiamide analogue of isonicotinic acid
Therapeutic: Antitubercular
Pregnancy category: Not rated

Indications and Dosages

➤ *As adjunct to treat tuberculosis*

TABLETS

Adults. 0.5 to 1 g/day in divided doses q 8 to 12 hr, together with other antituberculars. *Maximum:* 1 g/day.
Children. 15 to 20 mg/kg/day in divided doses q 8 to 12 hr, together with other antituberculars. *Maximum:* 750 mg/day.

Mechanism of Action

May inhibit peptide synthesis, resulting in bacteriostatic action against *Mycobacterium tuberculosis.*

Contraindications

Hypersensitivity to ethionamide or its components, severe hepatic damage

Interactions

DRUGS

cycloserine: Increased risk of adverse CNS effects, especially seizures
other neurotoxic drugs: Increased risk of neurotoxicity, such as optic and peripheral neuritis

Adverse Reactions

CNS: Burning or pain in arms and legs, clumsiness, confusion, depression, mental or mood changes, paresthesia, unsteadiness
CV: Orthostatic hypotension
EENT: Blurred vision, eye pain, increased salivation, metallic taste, optic neuritis, stomatitis, vision loss
ENDO: Goiter, hypoglycemia, hypothyroidism
GI: Anorexia, hepatitis, nausea, vomiting
SKIN: Jaundice, rash

Nursing Considerations

•Use ethionamide cautiously in patients with a history of hypersensitivity to isoniazid, niacin, pyrazinamide, or chemically related drugs; they also may be hypersensitive to ethionamide.
•Expect to give another antitubercular with ethionamide to decrease the risk of development of bacterial resistance.
•Also plan to give pyridoxine to prevent or minimize peripheral neuritis (numbness, tingling, burning, or pain in hands and feet), especially if patient has already had isoniazid-induced peripheral neuritis.
•Monitor liver function test results, and assess for signs of impaired function, such as hepatitis and jaundice.
•Question patient regularly about vision changes. Notify prescriber if patient reports blurred vision, eye pain, or loss of vision or visual acuity.
•Monitor compliance with therapy; treatment may need to continue for 1 to 2 years or indefinitely.

PATIENT TEACHING

•Advise patient to take ethionamide with food if adverse GI reactions occur.
•Instruct patient to take a missed dose as soon as he remembers unless it's nearly time for the next dose. Caution him not to double-dose.
•Advise patient to notify prescriber if no improvement occurs within 3 weeks; if bothersome or severe adverse reactions occur; if his vision changes; or if he experiences numbness, tingling, burning, or pain in his hands and feet.
•Inform patient that therapy may have to continue for months or years and that compliance is essential.

ethosuximide

Zarontin

Class and Category

Chemical: Succinimide derivative
Therapeutic: Anticonvulsant
Pregnancy category: Not rated

Indications and Dosages

➤ *To manage absence seizures in a patient who also has generalized tonic-clonic seizures*

CAPSULES, SYRUP

Adults and children age 6 and older. *Initial:* 500 mg q.d. *Maintenance:* Increased by 250 mg q 4 to 7 days until control is achieved with minimal adverse reactions.

E
F

Children ages 3 to 6. *Initial:* 250 mg q.d. *Maintenance:* Increased by 250 mg q 4 to 7 days until control is achieved with minimal adverse reactions.

Mechanism of Action
Elevates the seizure threshold and reduces the frequency of attacks by depressing the motor cortex and elevating the threshold of CNS response to convulsive stimuli.

Contraindications
Hypersensitivity to ethosuximide, succinimides, or their components

Interactions
DRUGS
carbamazepine, phenobarbital, phenytoin, primidone: Possibly decreased blood ethosuximide level
CNS depressants: Possibly increased CNS depression
haloperidol: Possibly decreased blood haloperidol level
loxapine, MAO inhibitors, maprotiline, molindone, phenothiazines, pimozide, tricyclic antidepressants: Possibly lowered seizure threshold and reduced therapeutic effect of ethosuximide
valproic acid: Increased or decreased blood ethosuximide level
ACTIVITIES
alcohol use: Possibly increased CNS depression

Adverse Reactions
CNS: Aggressiveness, ataxia, decreased concentration, dizziness, drowsiness, euphoria, fatigue, headache, hyperactivity, irritability, lethargy, nightmares, sleep disturbance
EENT: Gingival hypertrophy, myopia, tongue swelling
GI: Abdominal and epigastric pain, abdominal cramps, anorexia, diarrhea, hiccups, indigestion, nausea, vomiting
GU: Increased libido, microscopic hematuria, vaginal bleeding
HEME: Agranulocytosis, aplastic anemia, eosinophilia, leukopenia, pancytopenia
SKIN: Erythematous and pruritic rash, hirsutism, Stevens-Johnson syndrome, systemic lupus erythematosus, urticaria
Other: Weight loss

Nursing Considerations
• Use ethosuximide with extreme caution in patients with hepatic or renal disease.
• Give other anticonvulsants concurrently, as prescribed, to control generalized tonic-clonic seizures.
• Monitor CBC and platelet count and assess for signs of infection, such as cough, fever, and pharyngitis. Also routinely evaluate liver and renal function test results.
• Take safety precautions because drug may cause adverse CNS reactions, such as dizziness and drowsiness.
PATIENT TEACHING
• Stress the importance of complying with ethosuximide regimen.
• Advise patient to take a missed dose as soon as he remembers unless it's nearly time for the next dose. Warn him not to double-dose.
• Instruct patient not to engage in potentially hazardous activities until drug's CNS effects are known.
• Caution patient not to stop taking drug abruptly; doing so increases the risk of absence seizures.

ethotoin
Peganone

Class and Category
Chemical: Hydantoin derivative
Therapeutic: Anticonvulsant
Pregnancy category: C

Indications and Dosages
➤ *To treat tonic-clonic and simple or complex partial seizures as initial or adjunct therapy, or when other drugs are ineffective*
TABLETS
Adults and adolescents. *Initial:* 0.5 to 1 g on the first day in four to six divided doses, increased over several days until desired response is reached. *Maintenance:* 2 to 3 g/day in four to six divided doses. *Maximum:* 3 g/day.
Children. *Initial:* Up to 750 mg/day, based on weight and age, in four to six divided doses, adjusted as needed and tolerated. *Maintenance:* 0.5 to 1 g/day in four to six divided doses. *Maximum:* 3 g/day.
DOSAGE ADJUSTMENT For debilitated patients, initial dosage lowered to reduce the risk of adverse reactions.

Mechanism of Action

Limits the spread of seizure activity and the start of new seizures by:
• regulating voltage-dependent sodium and calcium channels in neurons
• inhibiting calcium movement across neuronal membranes
• enhancing sodium-potassium adenosine triphosphatase activity in neurons and glial cells.

These actions may result from ethotoin's ability to slow the recovery rate of inactivated sodium channels.

Contraindications

Hematologic disorders; hepatic dysfunction; hypersensitivity to ethotoin, phenytoin, other hydantoins, or their components

Interactions
DRUGS

acetaminophen: Increased risk of hepatotoxicity with long-term acetaminophen use
amiodarone: Possibly increased blood ethotoin level and risk of toxicity
antacids: Possibly decreased ethotoin effectiveness
bupropion, clozapine, loxapine, MAO inhibitors, maprotiline, phenothiazines, pimozide, thioxanthenes: Possibly lowered seizure threshold and decreased therapeutic effects of ethotoin; possibly intensified CNS depressant effects of these drugs
chloramphenicol, cimetidine, disulfiram, fluconazole, isoniazid, methylphenidate, metronidazole, omeprazole, phenylbutazone, ranitidine, salicylates, sulfonamides, trimethoprim: Possibly impaired metabolism of these drugs and increased risk of ethotoin toxicity
corticosteroids, cyclosporine, digoxin, disopyramide, doxycycline, furosemide, levodopa, mexiletine, quinidine: Decreased therapeutic effects of these drugs
diazoxide: Possibly decreased therapeutic effects of both drugs
estrogens, progestins: Decreased therapeutic effects of these drugs, increased blood ethotoin level
folic acid, leucovorin: Increased ethotoin metabolism, decreased seizure control
haloperidol: Possibly lowered seizure threshold and decreased therapeutic effects of ethotoin; possibly decreased blood haloperidol level

insulin, oral antidiabetic drugs: Possibly increased blood glucose level and decreased therapeutic effects of these drugs
lidocaine: Increased lidocaine metabolism, leading to reduced concentration
methadone: Possibly increased methadone metabolism, leading to withdrawal symptoms
molindone: Possibly lowered seizure threshold and impaired absorption and decreased therapeutic effects of ethotoin
oral anticoagulants: Possibly impaired metabolism of these drugs and increased risk of ethotoin toxicity; possibly increased anticoagulant effect initially, but decreased effect with prolonged therapy
oral contraceptives containing estrogen and progestin: Possibly breakthrough bleeding and decreased contraceptive effectiveness
rifampin: Possibly decreased therapeutic effects of ethotoin
streptozocin: Possibly decreased therapeutic effects of streptozocin
sucralfate: Possibly decreased ethotoin absorption
tricyclic antidepressants: Possibly lowered seizure threshold and decreased therapeutic effects of ethotoin; possibly decreased blood level of tricyclic antidepressants
valproic acid: Possibly decreased blood ethotoin level, increased blood valproic acid level
vitamin D analogues: Decreased vitamin D analogue activity; risk of anticonvulsant-induced rickets and osteomalacia
xanthines: Possibly inhibited ethotoin absorption and increased clearance of xanthines
ACTIVITIES
alcohol use: Possibly decreased ethotoin effectiveness, enhanced CNS depressant effects

Adverse Reactions

CNS: Clumsiness, confusion, drowsiness, excitement, peripheral neuropathy, sedation, slurred speech, stuttering, tremor
EENT: Nystagmus
GI: Constipation, diarrhea, nausea, vomiting
HEME: Agranulocytosis, leukopenia, thrombocytopenia
SKIN: Rash, Stevens-Johnson syndrome, toxic epidermal necrolysis
Other: Lymphadenopathy, systemic lupus erythematosus

Nursing Considerations

• Obtain CBC and differential before treatment and at monthly intervals for the first few months of ethotoin therapy, as ordered.

E
F

•**WARNING** Be aware that ethotoin shouldn't be discontinued abruptly because of a risk of causing status epilepticus. Plan to reduce dosage gradually or substitute another drug, as prescribed.

•Monitor patient for signs and symptoms of infection or unusual bleeding because ethotoin may cause hematologic toxicity.

•Because of ethotoin's potential for hepatotoxicity, monitor liver function test results and expect drug to be discontinued if test results are abnormal.

•Notify prescriber immediately and expect ethotoin to be discontinued and substituted with another drug if patient develops depressed blood counts, enlarged lymph nodes, or rash.

•Be aware that ethotoin may be substituted for phenytoin without loss of seizure control if patient develops severe gingival hyperplasia or other adverse reactions. Expect ethotoin dosage to be four to six times greater than phenytoin dosage.

•Institute and maintain seizure precautions according to facility protocol.

PATIENT TEACHING

•Instruct patient to take ethotoin exactly as prescribed and not to discontinue drug abruptly.

•Advise patient to take drug with food to enhance absorption and reduce adverse GI effects.

•Advise patient to report easy bruising, epistaxis, fever, malaise, petechiae, or sore throat to prescriber immediately.

•Instruct patient to keep medical appointments to monitor drug effectiveness and check for adverse reactions. Explain the need for periodic laboratory tests.

•Urge patient to avoid alcohol during therapy.

•Caution patient to avoid hazardous activities until drug's adverse effects are known.

•Encourage patient to wear or carry medical identification indicating his diagnosis and drug therapy.

etidronate disodium

Didronel

Class and Category

Chemical: Bisphosphonate
Therapeutic: Antihypercalcemic, bone resorption inhibitor
Pregnancy category: B (oral), C (parenteral)

Indications and Dosages

➤ *To treat Paget's disease of bone (osteitis deformans)*

TABLETS

Adults. 5 to 10 mg/kg/day for up to 6 mo, or 11 to 20 mg/kg/day for up to 3 mo.

➤ *To prevent and treat heterotopic ossification after total hip replacement*

TABLETS

Adults. 20 mg/kg/day for 1 mo before surgery and then 20 mg/kg/day for 3 mo after surgery for a total of 4 mo of treatment.

➤ *To prevent and treat heterotopic ossification after spinal cord injury*

TABLETS

Adults. 20 mg/kg/day for 2 wk and then 10 mg/kg/day for 10 wk for a total of 12 wk of treatment.

➤ *To treat moderate to severe hypercalcemia caused by cancer*

I.V. INFUSION

Adults. *Initial:* 7.5 mg/kg/day infused over at least 2 hr for 3 to 7 successive days. Oral etidronate therapy may begin at 20 mg/kg/day for 30 days on the day after last infusion.

DOSAGE ADJUSTMENT Dosage reduced if patient has renal impairment. Drug not administered if serum creatinine level exceeds 5 mg/dl.

Mechanism of Action

Inhibits normal and abnormal bone resorption by reducing bone turnover and slowing the remodeling of pagetic or heterotopic bone. Etidronate also decreases the elevated cardiac output that's seen in Paget's disease of bone and reduces local increases in skin temperature. It also inhibits the abnormal bone resorption that may occur with cancer and reduces the amount of calcium that enters the blood from resorbed bone.

Contraindications

Hypersensitivity to etidronate, bisphosphonates, or their components; severe renal impairment

Interactions

DRUGS

aluminum-, calcium-, or magnesium-containing antacids; aluminum-, calcium-, iron-, or

magnesium-containing vitamin and mineral supplements: Decreased etidronate absorption
FOODS
high-calcium food, such as milk and other dairy products: Decreased etidronate absorption

Adverse Reactions
EENT: Altered taste, metallic taste
GI: Diarrhea, elevated liver function test results, nausea
GU: Nephrotoxicity
MS: Bone fractures, bone pain
Other: Hypocalcemia

Nursing Considerations
•Anticipate beginning etidronate therapy as soon as possible after spinal cord injury, preferably before evidence of heterotopic ossification exists.
•Expect etidronate not to inhibit healing of spinal fractures, affect prosthesis, or disrupt trochanter attachment when used after total hip replacement.
•Give oral form 2 hours before meals to prevent decreased absorption.
•Dilute parenteral form in at least 250 ml of NS.
•Give parenteral form slowly over at least 2 hours.
•Store diluted parenteral solution at room temperature for up to 48 hours.
•**WARNING** Monitor for hypocalcemia if patient receives parenteral form for more than 3 days.
•When treating hypercalcemia, expect to continue drug for up to 90 days if serum calcium level remains within acceptable range.
PATIENT TEACHING
•Instruct patient to take etidronate tablets on an empty stomach—2 hours before meals, antacids, or calcium supplements. Urge him to drink a full glass of water with tablets and to avoid taking drug with milk or other high-calcium foods.
•Advise patient to take a missed dose as soon as he remembers and as long as 2 hours have elapsed since his last meal. Instruct him not to eat for another 2 hours. Warn against double-dosing.
•Inform patient with Paget's disease that his response to etidronate may be slow and may continue for months after treatment.

etodolac
Lodine, Lodine XL

Class and Category
Chemical: Pyranoindoleacetic acid derivative
Therapeutic: Analgesic, anti-inflammatory
Pregnancy category: C (first trimester), Not rated (later trimesters)

Indications and Dosages
➤ *To manage osteoarthritis*
CAPSULES, TABLETS
Adults. *Initial:* 800 to 1,200 mg/day in divided doses. *Maintenance:* 600 to 1,200 mg/day in divided doses. *Maximum:* 1,200 mg/day for patients who weigh 60 kg (132 lb) or more; 20 mg/kg/day for patients who weigh less than 60 kg.
E.R. TABLETS
Adults. 400 to 1,000 mg/day.
➤ *To relieve mild to moderate pain*
CAPSULES, TABLETS
Adults. *Initial:* 400 mg and then 200 to 400 mg q 6 to 8 hr. *Maximum:* 1,200 mg/day for patients who weigh 60 kg or more; 20 mg/kg/day for patients who weigh less than 60 kg.

Route	Onset	Peak	Duration
P.O.	30 min	1 to 2 hr	4 to 12 hr

Mechanism of Action
Blocks the activity of cyclooxygenase, the enzyme needed for prostaglandin synthesis. Prostaglandins, important mediators of the inflammatory response, cause local vasodilation with swelling and pain. By inhibiting cyclooxygenase and prostaglandins, this NSAID causes inflammatory symptoms and pain to subside.

Contraindications
Angioedema, asthma, bronchospasm, nasal polyps, rhinitis, or urticaria induced by aspirin, iodides, or NSAIDs; hypersensitivity to etodolac or its components

Interactions
DRUGS
ACE inhibitors: Possibly decreased hypotensive effects of these drugs
acetaminophen (long-term use): Increased risk of adverse renal effects
antacids: Decreased blood etodolac level
antiplatelets, oral anticoagulants, thrombolytics: Prolonged PT (with warfarin), increased risk of bleeding

cidofovir: Possibly nephrotoxicity
corticosteroids: Increased risk of adverse GI effects
cyclosporine: Increased nephrotoxic effects
digoxin: Increased blood digoxin level and risk of digitalis toxicity
insulin, oral antidiabetic drugs: Increased risk of hypoglycemia
lithium: Increased blood lithium level and, possibly, toxicity
loop diuretics: Possibly decreased effects of loop diuretics
methotrexate: Increased risk of methotrexate toxicity
salicylates: Decreased blood etodolac level, increased risk of adverse GI effects

ACTIVITIES
alcohol use, smoking: Increased risk of adverse GI effects

Adverse Reactions

CNS: Chills, dizziness, drowsiness, fever, malaise
CV: Edema, heart failure
EENT: Tinnitus
GI: Abdominal pain, constipation, diarrhea, elevated liver function test results, flatulence, gastritis, GI bleeding, GI perforation, hepatitis, indigestion, nausea, vomiting
GU: Dysuria, elevated serum creatinine level, hematuria, renal failure or insufficiency
HEME: Anemia, easy bruising, thrombocytopenia
SKIN: Pruritus, urticaria, vesiculobullous or other rash

Nursing Considerations

• Administer etodolac with food to minimize adverse GI reactions.
• If patient also takes acetaminophen, monitor fluid intake and output and BUN and serum creatinine levels for signs of adverse renal reactions.

PATIENT TEACHING
• Instruct patient to take etodolac with food or after meals if adverse GI reactions occur.
• Caution him to avoid aspirin or aspirin-containing products while taking drug.
• Advise patient not to smoke or drink alcoholic beverages during therapy because these activities increase the risk of adverse GI reactions.
• Inform patient that he may experience dizziness or drowsiness.

• Instruct him to notify prescriber immediately if he experiences blood in urine, easy bruising, itching, rash, signs of GI bleeding, swelling, or yellow eyes or skin.

famotidine

Act (CAN), Apo-Famotidine (CAN), Dyspep HB (CAN), Gen-Famotidine (CAN), Mylanta-AR, Novo-Famotidine (CAN), Nu-Famotidine (CAN), Pepcid, Pepcid AC, Pepcid RPD

Class and Category

Chemical: Thiazole derivative
Therapeutic: Antiulcer agent, gastric acid secretion inhibitor
Pregnancy category: B

Indications and Dosages

➤ *To provide short-term treatment of active duodenal ulcer*

ORAL SUSPENSION, TABLETS (CHEWABLE, ORAL DISINTEGRATING, AND REGULAR)
Adults and adolescents. 40 mg q.d. h.s. or 20 mg b.i.d.
Children. 0.5 mg/kg/day as a single dose h.s. or in divided doses b.i.d.

I.V. INFUSION OR INJECTION
Adults and adolescents over age 16. 20 mg q 12 hr, infused over 15 to 30 min or injected over at least 2 min.
Children ages 1 to 16. *Initial:* 0.25 mg/kg q 12 hr, infused over 15 to 30 min or injected over at least 2 min. *Maximum:* 40 mg/day.

➤ *To prevent recurrence of duodenal ulcer*

ORAL SUSPENSION, TABLETS (CHEWABLE, ORAL DISINTEGRATING, AND REGULAR)
Adults and adolescents. 20 mg q.d. h.s.

➤ *To provide short-term treatment for active, benign gastric ulcer*

ORAL SUSPENSION, TABLETS (CHEWABLE, ORAL DISINTEGRATING, AND REGULAR)
Adults and adolescents. 40 mg q.d. h.s.
Children. 0.5 mg/kg/day as a single dose h.s. or in divided doses b.i.d.

I.V. INFUSION OR INJECTION
Adults and adolescents over age 16. 20 mg q 12 hr.
Children ages 1 to 16. *Initial:* 0.25 mg/kg q 12 hr. *Maximum:* 40 mg/day.

➤ *To treat gastroesophageal reflux disease*
ORAL SUSPENSION, TABLETS (CHEWABLE, ORAL DISINTE-
GRATING, AND REGULAR)
Adults and adolescents. 20 mg b.i.d. for up
to 6 wk.
Children who weigh more than 10 kg (22 lb).
1 to 2 mg/kg/day in divided doses b.i.d.
Children who weigh less than 10 kg. 1 to
2 mg/kg/day in divided doses t.i.d.
I.V. INFUSION OR INJECTION
Children ages 1 to 16. *Initial:* 0.25 mg/kg q
12 hr. *Maximum:* 40 mg/day.
➤ *To treat esophagitis caused by gastro-
esophageal reflux*
ORAL SUSPENSION, TABLETS (CHEWABLE, ORAL DISINTE-
GRATING, AND REGULAR)
Adults and adolescents. 20 to 40 mg b.i.d. for
up to 12 wk.
➤ *To treat gastric hypersecretory condi-
tions, such as Zollinger-Ellison syn-
drome*
ORAL SUSPENSION, TABLETS (CHEWABLE, ORAL DISINTE-
GRATING, AND REGULAR)
Adults and adolescents. *Initial:* 20 mg q 6 hr.

Dosage adjusted, if needed, based on patient
response.
I.V. INFUSION OR INJECTION
Adults and adolescents. 20 mg q 12 hr.
➤ *To prevent heartburn and indigestion*
TABLETS (CHEWABLE, ORAL DISINTEGRATING, AND
REGULAR)
Adults and adolescents. 10 mg 1 hr before
eating. *Maximum:* 20 mg q 24 hr.
➤ *To treat heartburn and indigestion*
TABLETS (CHEWABLE, ORAL DISINTEGRATING, AND
REGULAR)
Adults and adolescents. 10 mg at onset of
symptoms. *Maximum:* 20 mg q 24 hr for up to
2 wk unless advised otherwise by prescriber.
DOSAGE ADJUSTMENT Oral or parenteral
dosage reduced or dosing interval increased
(to 36 to 48 hr), if needed, in patients with
renal insufficiency and creatinine clearance
of 49 ml/min/1.73 m^2 or less.

Route	Onset	Peak	Duration
P.O.	1 hr	1 to 4 hr	10 to 12 hr
I.V.	In 30 min	0.5 to 3 hr	10 to 12 hr

Mechanism of Action
In normal digestion, parietal cells in the
gastric epithelium secrete hydrogen (H$^+$)
ions, which combine with chloride ions
(Cl$^-$) to form hydrochloric acid (HCl), as
shown below left. However, HCl can in-
flame, ulcerate, and perforate the gastric
and intestinal mucosa that's normally protected by mucus. Famotidine, an H$_2$-recep-
tor antagonist, reduces HCl formation by
preventing histamine from binding with
H$_2$ receptors on the surface of parietal
cells, as shown below right. By doing so,
the drug helps prevent peptic ulcers from
forming and helps heal existing ones.

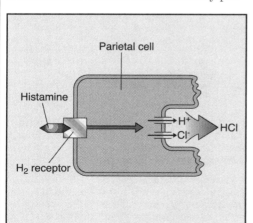

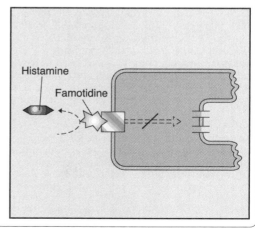

Contraindications

Hypersensitivity to famotidine, other H_2-receptor antagonists, or their components

Interactions

DRUGS

antacids, sucralfate: Possibly decreased absorption of famotidine
bone marrow depressants: Increased risk of blood dyscrasias
itraconazole, ketoconazole: Possibly decreased absorption of these drugs

ACTIVITIES

alcohol use: Possibly increased blood alcohol level

Adverse Reactions

CNS: Dizziness, fever, headache, insomnia, mental or mood changes
CV: Arrhythmias, palpitations
EENT: Dry mouth, laryngeal edema, tinnitus
GI: Abdominal pain, anorexia, constipation, diarrhea, hepatitis, nausea, vomiting
HEME: Aplastic anemia, leukopenia, neutropenia, pancytopenia, thrombocytopenia
RESP: Bronchospasm, dyspnea, wheezing
SKIN: Alopecia, dry skin, erythema multiforme, exfoliative dermatitis, jaundice, pruritus, rash, Stevens-Johnson syndrome, toxic epidermal necrolysis, urticaria
Other: Anaphylaxis, angioedema, facial edema, hyperuricemia

Nursing Considerations

•Shake famotidine oral suspension vigorously for 5 to 10 seconds before administration.
•Dilute injection form (2 ml) with NS or other solution to 5 to 10 ml; give I.V. injection over at least 2 minutes. Or dilute in 100 ml of D_5W and infuse over 15 to 30 minutes. Or infuse premixed injection (20 mg/50 ml NS) over 15 to 30 minutes.
•WARNING Be aware that Pepcid AC chewable tablets contain aspartame, which can be dangerous for patients with phenylketonuria.

PATIENT TEACHING

•Instruct patient to store famotidine oral suspension at room temperature (below 86° F [30° C]) and protect it from freezing. Teach her to shake the bottle vigorously for 5 to 10 seconds after adding water and right before use.
•Advise patient who uses Pepcid RPD to store drug in unopened package. For each dose, instruct her to open blister pack with dry hands, place a tablet on her tongue, let it dissolve, and swallow it with saliva.
•If patient uses chewable tablets, instruct her to chew them thoroughly before swallowing.
•If patient also takes antacids, instruct her to wait 30 to 60 minutes after taking famotidine, if possible, before taking antacid.
•Caution patient to avoid alcohol and smoking during famotidine therapy because they irritate the stomach and can delay ulcer healing.

felbamate

Felbatol

Class and Category

Chemical: Dicarbamate
Therapeutic: Anticonvulsant
Pregnancy category: C

Indications and Dosages

➤ *To treat partial seizures in patients who don't respond to other drugs*

ORAL SUSPENSION, TABLETS

Adults and adolescents over age 14. *Initial:* 1,200 mg/day in divided doses t.i.d. or q.i.d. Dosage increased over several weeks based on patient response. *Maximum:* 3,600 mg/day.
Children ages 2 to 14. *Initial:* 15 mg/kg/day in divided doses t.i.d. or q.i.d. Dosage increased over several weeks based on patient response. *Maximum:* 3,600 mg/day or 45 mg/kg/day.

➤ *As adjunct to treat generalized or partial seizures associated with Lennox-Gastaut syndrome in children*

ORAL SUSPENSION, TABLETS

Children ages 2 to 14. *Initial:* 15 mg/kg/day in divided doses t.i.d. or q.i.d. while decreasing other anticonvulsant drugs by 20% to control their blood levels. Felbamate dosage increased by 15 mg/kg/day q wk. *Maximum:* 3,600 mg/day or 45 mg/kg/day.

Contraindications

Hepatic dysfunction; history of blood dyscrasias; hypersensitivity to felbamate, other carbamates, or their components

Mechanism of Action
May exert its anticonvulsant effects by antagonizing the effects of the amino acid glycine. When glycine binds to *N*-methyl-D-aspartate (NMDA) receptors in the CNS, the frequency at which receptor-gated calcium ion channels open is increased—an important factor in initiating seizures. Felbamate may raise the seizure threshold by blocking NMDA receptors so that glycine can't bind to them.

Interactions
DRUGS
carbamazepine: Decreased blood carbamazepine level and increased felbamate clearance, resulting in decreased blood felbamate level
fosphenytoin, phenytoin: Increased blood phenytoin level and increased felbamate clearance, resulting in decreased blood felbamate level
methsuximide: Increased adverse effects of methsuximide
oral contraceptives: Possibly decreased effectiveness of oral contraceptives
phenobarbital: Decreased blood felbamate level, increased blood phenobarbital level and risk of adverse effects
valproic acid: Increased blood valproic acid level and increased risk of adverse effects

Adverse Reactions
CNS: Abnormal gait, aggressiveness, agitation, anxiety, dizziness, drowsiness, fever, headache, insomnia, mood changes, tremor
EENT: Altered taste, diplopia, rhinitis
GI: Abdominal pain, anorexia, constipation, diarrhea, elevated liver function test results, hepatic failure, indigestion, nausea, vomiting
HEME: Aplastic anemia, leukopenia, pancytopenia, thrombocytopenia
RESP: Upper respiratory tract infection
SKIN: Photosensitivity, purpura, rash
Other: Anaphylaxis, lymphadenopathy, weight loss

Nursing Considerations
•Check liver function test results before starting felbamate therapy, and expect to monitor test results every 1 to 2 weeks during treatment. Notify prescriber immediately and expect to discontinue drug if test results become abnormal.

•Plan to taper dosage by one-third every 4 to 5 days as prescribed. If patient receives adequate amounts of other anticonvulsant drugs, felbamate may be discontinued without tapering, if needed.
•**WARNING** Assess for signs of aplastic anemia and bone marrow depression, which may occur with felbamate use. Signs may not appear until several months after therapy begins. Expect to stop felbamate therapy if bone marrow depression develops.
•If patient receives adjunctive therapy, expect adverse reactions to resolve as other anticonvulsant dosages decrease.

PATIENT TEACHING
•Direct patient to shake suspension before using and to use a calibrated spoon or container to measure each dose.
•Instruct patient to store felbamate oral suspension and tablets at room temperature.
•Because drug may cause photosensitivity, urge patient to protect her skin from sun and to avoid sunlamps and tanning booths.
•Inform patient that dizziness and drowsiness may occur. Advise her to avoid potentially hazardous activities until drug's CNS effects are known.
•Warn patient not to stop taking felbamate abruptly.
•Advise patient to return for ordered liver function tests and to report yellow skin or eyes and dark urine to prescriber.
•Instruct patient to tell prescriber if she experiences bleeding, infection, or fatigue.
•Advise patient to carry medical identification that indicates her condition and drug therapy.
•Because felbamate decreases oral contraceptive effectiveness, discuss alternate contraceptive methods.

felodipine
Plendil, Renedil (CAN)

Class and Category
Chemical: Dihydropyridine derivative
Therapeutic: Antihypertensive
Pregnancy category: C

Indications and Dosages
➤ *To manage essential hypertension alone or with other antihypertensives*
E.R. TABLETS
Adults. *Initial:* 5 mg q.d. Dosage adjusted q

2 wk to 2.5 to 10 mg q.d. based on patient response.
DOSAGE ADJUSTMENT Initial or maintenance dosage reduced, if needed, in patients who are over age 65 or have impaired hepatic function.

Route	Onset	Peak	Duration
P.O.	2 to 5 hr	Unknown	16 to 24 hr

Mechanism of Action
May slow the movement of extracellular calcium into myocardial and vascular smooth-muscle cells by deforming calcium channels in cell membranes, inhibiting ion-controlled gating mechanisms, and interfering with calcium release from the sarcoplasmic reticulum. The effect of all these actions is a decrease in intracellular calcium ions, which inhibits contraction of smooth-muscle cells and dilates coronary and systemic arteries. As with other calcium channel blockers, felodipine's actions result in increased oxygen to the myocardium and reduced peripheral resistance, blood pressure, and afterload.

Contraindications
Hypersensitivity to felodipine or its components

Interactions
DRUGS
anesthetics (hydrocarbon inhalation): Possibly hypotension
antihypertensives, prazocin: Increased risk of hypotension
beta blockers: Increased adverse effects of beta blockers
cimetidine: Increased felodipine bioavailability
digoxin: Transiently increased blood digoxin level and risk of digitalis toxicity
estrogens: Possibly increased fluid retention and decreased therapeutic effect of felodipine
lithium: Increased risk of neurotoxicity
NSAIDs, sympathomimetics: Possibly decreased therapeutic effect of felodipine
procainamide, quinidine: Increased risk of prolonged Q-T interval
FOODS
grapefruit juice: Doubled felodipine bioavailability

Adverse Reactions
CNS: Asthenia, dizziness, drowsiness, fatigue, headache, paresthesia, syncope, weakness
CV: Chest pain, hypotension, palpitations, peripheral edema, tachycardia
EENT: Gingival hyperplasia, pharyngitis, rhinitis
GI: Abdominal cramps, constipation, diarrhea, indigestion, nausea
HEME: Agranulocytosis
MS: Back pain
RESP: Cough
SKIN: Flushing, rash

Nursing Considerations
• Use felodipine cautiously in patients with heart failure or reduced ventricular function.
• Monitor blood pressure during dosage titration and throughout felodipine therapy, especially in elderly patients.
• Expect drug bioavailability to increase by up to twofold when felodipine is taken with grapefruit juice.
• WARNING Be aware that felodipine may cause severe hypotension with syncope, which may lead to reflex tachycardia. This can precipitate angina in patients with coronary artery disease or a history of angina.
• Monitor for signs of overdose, such as excessive peripheral vasodilation, marked hypotension and, possibly, bradycardia. If you detect such signs, place patient in supine position with legs elevated and give I.V. fluids, as prescribed. Expect to give I.V. atropine for bradycardia.
PATIENT TEACHING
• Instruct patient to swallow tablets whole and not to crush or chew them.
• Caution patient not to alter her intake of grapefruit juice during therapy.
• Advise patient to store felodipine at room temperature and to protect it from light.
• Instruct patient to monitor her pulse rate and blood pressure.
• Teach patient how to minimize gingival hyperplasia.
• Advise patient to notify prescriber immediately if she experiences palpitations, pronounced dizziness, or swelling of hands or feet.

fenofibrate
Tricor

Class and Category
Chemical: Aryloxisobutyric acid derivative
Therapeutic: Antihyperlipidemic
Pregnancy category: C

Indications and Dosages
➤ *To decrease serum triglyceride and VLDL levels in patients at risk for pancreatitis*
CAPSULES
Adults. *Initial:* 67 mg/day with food. *Maximum:* 201 mg/day in divided doses with meals.
DOSAGE ADJUSTMENT For patients with creatinine clearance of less than 50 ml/min/1.73 m^2, dosage increased only after drug's therapeutic and renal effects are known.

Route	Onset	Peak	Duration
P.O.	6 to 8 wk	2 wk	Unknown

Mechanism of Action
May increase the lipolysis of triglyceride-rich lipoproteins and decrease the synthesis of fatty acids and triglycerides by enhancing the activation of lipoprotein lipase and acyl-coenzyme A synthetase. Fenofibrate also may:
• increase hepatic elimination of cholesterol as bile salts
• promote the catabolism of larger, less dense LDLs with a high-binding affinity for cellular LDL receptors.

Contraindications
Gallbladder disease, hypersensitivity to fenofibrate or its components, severe hepatic or renal impairment

Interactions
DRUGS
bile acid sequestrants: Decreased fenofibrate absorption
cyclosporine: Increased risk of nephrotoxicity
HMG-CoA reductase inhibitors (atorvastatin, cerivastatin, fluvastatin, lovastatin, pravastatin, simvastatin): Increased risk of myopathy, rhabdomyolysis, and acute renal failure
oral anticoagulants: Increased risk of bleeding
FOODS
all foods: Increased fenofibrate bioavailability

Adverse Reactions
CNS: Dizziness
EENT: Eye irritation, rhinitis, vitreous floaters
GI: Cholecystitis, cholelithiasis, constipation, eructation, flatulence, hepatotoxicity, pancreatitis, vomiting
GU: Decreased libido
HEME: Agranulocytosis, thrombocytopenia
MS: Myalgia, myositis, rhabdomyolysis
RESP: Allergic alveolitis
SKIN: Photosensitivity, pruritus, rash, urticaria
Other: Flulike symptoms

Nursing Considerations
• As prescribed, discontinue drugs known to increase the serum triglyceride level, such as beta blockers, estrogens, and thiazides, before starting fenofibrate.
• Give drug with a full glass of water with meals.
• Administer 1 hour before or 4 hours after bile acid sequestrants.
• Monitor results of liver and renal function and glucose tolerance tests.
• Monitor serum triglyceride level at 4- to 8-week intervals. If level doesn't decrease after 2 months at maximum dosage, expect to discontinue therapy.
PATIENT TEACHING
• Stress that fenofibrate will be effective only if patient carefully follows prescriber's instructions about diet and exercise.
• Instruct patient to protect drug from heat, moisture, and direct light.
• Advise patient to undergo laboratory tests, as directed, to determine drug's effectiveness. They include liver function tests after 3 to 6 months and hematocrit, hemoglobin, and WBC count periodically during first year.
• Instruct patient to notify prescriber immediately if she experiences chills, fever, or sore throat. Also urge her to tell prescriber about unexplained muscle pain, tenderness, or weakness, especially if accompanied by fatigue or fever.

fenoldopam mesylate
Corlopam

Class and Category
Chemical: Dopamine agonist
Therapeutic: Antihypertensive
Pregnancy category: B

Indications and Dosages

➤ *To treat severe hypertension when rapid, but quickly reversible, emergency reduction of blood pressure is clinically indicated, including malignant hypertension with deteriorating end-organ function*

I.V. INFUSION

Adults. *Initial:* 0.025 to 0.3 mcg/kg/min, individualized according to patient weight and desired effect. *Usual:* 0.01 to 1.6 mcg/kg/min. *Maximum:* 1.6 mcg/kg/min for up to 48 hr.

Route	Onset	Peak	Duration
I.V.	Rapid	Unknown	Unknown

Mechanism of Action

Stimulates dopamine-1 postsynaptic receptors, which mediate renal and mesenteric vasodilation. This vasodilating activity lowers blood pressure and total peripheral resistance while increasing renal blood flow.

Contraindications

Hypersensitivity to fenoldopam or its components

Interactions

DRUGS

antihypertensives: Additive hypotensive effect
dopamine antagonists, metoclopramide: Possibly decreased effects of fenoldopam

Adverse Reactions

CNS: Anxiety, headache, light-headedness
CV: Hypotension, ST- and T-wave changes, tachycardia
EENT: Increased intraocular pressure
GI: Abdominal pain, nausea
SKIN: Diaphoresis, flushing
Other: Hypokalemia, injection site pain

Nursing Considerations

• Reconstitute by adding 40 mg of fenoldopam (4 ml of concentrate) to 1,000 ml of NS or D₅W, or 20 mg of fenoldopam (2 ml of concentrate) to 500 ml of NS or D₅W, or 10 mg of fenoldopam (1 ml of concentrate) to 250 ml of NS or D₅W to produce a final fenoldopam concentration of 40 mcg/ml.
• Infuse through a mechanical infusion pump for proper control of infusion rate.

• Expect to titrate dosage in increments of 0.05 to 0.1 mcg/kg/min, as prescribed.
• Expect to monitor heart rate and blood pressure every 15 minutes during fenoldopam therapy because most of drug's effect on blood pressure occurs within 15 minutes of any dosage change.
• Be aware that patient may be started on oral antihypertensive therapy, as prescribed, any time after blood pressure is stable during fenoldopam infusion.
• Discard any reconstituted solution not used within 24 hours.
• **WARNING** Assess for signs of increased myocardial oxygen demand, especially in patients with heart failure or a history of angina, because fenoldopam may produce a rapid decline in blood pressure, resulting in symptomatic hypotension and a dose-dependent increase in heart rate.
• Monitor serum potassium level because fenoldopam decreases serum potassium concentrations, which may result in hypokalemia, exacerbate arrhythmias, or precipitate conduction abnormalities, especially in patients with cardiac disease.
• Monitor patients with glaucoma or increased intraocular pressure for changes in vision because fenoldopam causes a dose-dependent increase in intraocular pressure.
• Be alert for possible allergic- or anaphylactic-type reaction to sodium metabisulfite, a component of fenoldopam injection, especially in patients with asthma.

PATIENT TEACHING

• Inform patient that she'll be switched to an oral antihypertensive once her blood pressure is controlled.
• Instruct patient to expect frequent monitoring of vital signs.

fenoprofen calcium

Nalfon

Class and Category

Chemical: Propionic acid derivative
Therapeutic: Analgesic, anti-inflammatory, antirheumatic
Pregnancy category: Not rated

Indications and Dosages

➤ *To manage mild to moderate pain*

CAPSULES, TABLETS

Adults. 200 mg q 4 to 6 hr, as needed.

➤ *To relieve pain, stiffness, and swelling from rheumatoid arthritis or osteoarthritis*
CAPSULES, TABLETS
Adults. 300 to 600 mg t.i.d. or q.i.d. *Maximum:* 3,200 mg/day.

Route	Onset	Peak	Duration
P.O.	15 to 30 min*	Unknown†	4 to 6 hr‡

Mechanism of Action
Blocks the activity of cyclooxygenase, the enzyme necessary for prostaglandin synthesis. Prostaglandins, important mediators in the inflammatory response, cause local vasodilation with swelling and pain. With the blocking of cyclooxygenase and the inhibition of prostaglandins, inflammatory symptoms subside. Pain relief also is achieved by inhibiting prostaglandins because they play a role in pain transmission from the periphery to the spinal cord.

Contraindications
Angioedema, asthma, bronchospasm, nasal polyps, rhinitis, or urticaria induced by aspirin, iodides, or NSAIDs; hypersensitivity to fenoprofen or its components; renal impairment; severe hepatic impairment

Interactions
DRUGS
acetaminophen: Increased risk of renal impairment with concurrent long-term use
antacids: Decreased fenoprofen effectiveness
anticoagulants, cefamandole, cefoperazone, cefotetan, heparin, plicamycin, thrombolytics, valproic acid: Increased risk of bleeding
antineoplastics: Increased adverse hematologic effects
cyclosporine: Increased risk of nephrotoxicity
diuretics, triamterene: Decreased effectiveness of these drugs
glucocorticoids, NSAIDs, potassium supplements: Increased adverse GI effects

---
* For analgesia; 2 days for antirheumatic effects.
† For analgesia; 2 to 3 wk for antirheumatic effects.
‡ For analgesia; unknown for antirheumatic effects.

insulin, oral antidiabetic drugs: Increased risk of hypoglycemia
lithium: Increased risk of lithium toxicity
methotrexate: Increased risk of methotrexate toxicity
phenobarbital: Possibly decreased elimination half-life of fenoprofen
salicylates: Increased risk of GI bleeding
ACTIVITIES
alcohol use, smoking: Increased risk of GI bleeding

Adverse Reactions
CNS: Agitation, confusion, dizziness, drowsiness, headache, sleep disturbance, tremor, weakness
CV: Palpitations, peripheral edema, tachycardia, vasodilation
EENT: Blurred vision, dry or sore mouth, hearing loss, tinnitus
GI: Abdominal cramps, distention, and pain; anorexia; constipation; diarrhea; flatulence; GI ulceration; indigestion; nausea; vomiting
GU: Dysuria
MS: Muscle spasms and twitching, myalgia
RESP: Dyspnea
SKIN: Diaphoresis, erythema, pruritus, urticaria

Nursing Considerations
• Monitor renal function, blood pressure, PT, and CBC before and periodically during fenoprofen therapy.
• Give drug with food, milk, or antacids to decrease adverse GI reactions.
• **WARNING** In patient who receives long-term therapy, assess for signs of toxicity, such as agitation; blurred vision; coma; confusion; drowsiness; elevated BUN and serum creatinine levels; indigestion; nausea; rash; seizures; severe headache; slow, labored breathing; tinnitus; and vomiting.
PATIENT TEACHING
• Advise patient to take fenoprofen with food, milk, or antacids to minimize GI distress. Also direct her to take drug with a full glass of water and to remain upright for 30 minutes after taking drug to decrease the risk of drug lodging in the esophagus and causing irritation.
• Instruct patient to swallow drug whole and not to crush, break, chew, or open capsules.
• Caution patient to avoid alcohol, aspirin, and other NSAIDs, unless prescribed, while taking fenoprofen.

•If patient also takes an anticoagulant, advise her to watch for and immediately report bleeding problems, such as bloody or tarry stools and bloody vomitus.
•Caution patient to avoid potentially hazardous activities until drug's CNS effects are known.

fentanyl citrate

Actiq, Sublimaze

fentanyl transdermal system

Duragesic

Class, Category, and Schedule
Chemical: Opioid, phenylpiperidine derivative
Therapeutic: Analgesic, anesthesia adjunct
Pregnancy category: C
Controlled substance: Schedule II

Indications and Dosages
➤ *To provide surgical premedication*
I.M. INJECTION
Adults. 0.05 to 0.1 mg 30 to 60 min before surgery.
➤ *As adjunct to regional anesthesia*
I.V. OR I.M. INJECTION
Adults. 0.05 to 0.1 mg I.M. or slow I.V. over 1 to 2 min.
➤ *To manage postoperative pain in post-anesthesia care unit*
I.M. INJECTION
Adults. 0.05 to 0.1 mg. Repeated in 1 to 2 hr, if needed.
➤ *To treat breakthrough pain in cancer patients who have developed a tolerance to opioid therapy*
TRANSMUCOSAL LOZENGE
Adults. *Initial:* 200 mcg placed between cheek and gum for up to 15 min followed by second dose 15 min after first dose ends, if needed. Dosage increased according to patient's needs.
➤ *To relieve severe chronic pain that doesn't respond to less potent drugs*
TRANSDERMAL SYSTEM
Adults. *Initial:* 1 25-mcg/hr patch, replaced q 72 hr (or 48 hr, if needed). Dosage increased after first 72 hr and then q 6 days. For dosage above 100 mcg/hr, more than 1 patch is used.
DOSAGE ADJUSTMENT For patients with long-term opioid use, dosage adjusted based on previous day's requirement. For cancer patients who need more than 800 mcg/day for breakthrough pain, dosage altered or another long-acting opioid given, as prescribed.

Route	Onset	Peak	Duration
I.V.	1 to 2 min	3 to 5 min	30 to 60 min
I.M.	7 to 15 min	20 to 30 min	1 to 2 hr
Trans-dermal	12 to 24 hr	Unknown	Over 72 hr

Mechanism of Action
Binds to opioid receptor sites in the CNS, altering the perception of and emotional response to pain by inhibiting the ascending pain pathways. Fentanyl also may alter neurotransmitter release from afferent nerves that are responsive to painful stimuli. The drug also produces respiratory depression by acting directly on respiratory centers in the brain stem.

Contraindications
Asthma, hypersensitivity to narcotics, myasthenia gravis, significant respiratory depression, upper airway obstruction (for I.V. or I.M. form); acute or chronic pain, body weight less than 10 kg (22 lb), doses that exceed 5 mcg/kg in adults or 15 mcg/kg in children (for transmucosal form); acute or postoperative pain, age less than 12 (or less than 18 if weight is less than 50 kg [110 lb]), dosage that exceeds 25 mcg/hr at the start of therapy, hypersensitivity to fentanyl (or alfentanil, sufentanil, or adhesives), treatment of mild to moderate pain that's responsive to nonopioid drugs (for transdermal form)

Interactions
DRUGS
anticholinergics, antidiarrheals (such as loperamide and paregoric): Increased risk of severe constipation
antihypertensives, diuretics: Possibly potentiated hypotension
benzodiazepines: Possibly reduced fentanyl dose required for anesthesia induction
buprenorphine: Possibly decreased therapeutic effects of buprenorphine
CNS depressants: Possibly increased CNS and respiratory depression and hypotension
cytochrome P-450 inducers (such as rifampin, carbamazepine, and phenytoin): Possibly

induced metabolism and increased clearance of fentanyl

erythromycin, itraconazole, ketoconazole, ritonavir: Possibly increased opioid effect of transdermal fentanyl

hydroxyzine: Possibly increased analgesic effect of fentanyl and increased CNS depression and hypotension

MAO inhibitors: Possibly unpredictable, even fatal, effects if taken within 14 days of fentanyl

metoclopramide: Possibly antagonized effect of metoclopramide on gastric motility

nalbuphine, pentazocine: Possibly antagonized analgesic, respiratory depressant, and CNS depressant effects of fentanyl; possibly additive hypotensive and CNS and respiratory depressant effects of both drugs

naloxone: Antagonized analgesic, hypotensive, CNS, and respiratory depressant effects of fentanyl

naltrexone: Possibly blocked therapeutic effects of fentanyl

neuromuscular blockers: Possibly prevention or reversal of muscle rigidity induced by fentanyl

ACTIVITIES

alcohol use: Increased CNS and respiratory depression and hypotension

Adverse Reactions

CNS: Agitation, amnesia, anxiety, asthenia, ataxia, confusion, delusions, depression, dizziness, drowsiness, euphoria, fever, hallucinations, headache, lack of coordination, light-headedness, nervousness, paranoia, sedation, seizures, sleep disturbance, slurred speech, syncope, tremor, weakness, yawning

CV: Asystole, bradycardia, chest pain, edema, hypotension, orthostatic hypotension, tachycardia

EENT: Blurred vision, dry mouth, laryngospasm, rhinitis, sneezing

GI: Anorexia, constipation, ileus, indigestion, nausea, vomiting

GU: Urinary hesitancy, urine retention

RESP: Apnea, depressed cough reflex, dyspnea, hypoventilation

SKIN: Diaphoresis, exfoliative dermatitis, localized skin redness and swelling (with transdermal form), pruritus, rash

Other: Drug tolerance, physical or psychological dependence with long-term use, weight loss

Nursing Considerations

• To reduce skin irritation, spray allergy inhaler triamcinolone on patient's skin, as prescribed, before applying fentanyl patch.
• Expect blood fentanyl level to be prolonged if patient chews or swallows transmucosal form because drug is absorbed slowly from GI tract.
• Be aware that 100 mcg of fentanyl is equivalent in potency to 10 mg of morphine.
• To achieve optimum pain control with the lowest possible fentanyl dose, also plan to give a nonopioid analgesic, such as acetaminophen, as prescribed.
• To prevent withdrawal symptoms after long-term use, expect to taper drug dosage gradually, as prescribed.
• Assess patient for withdrawal symptoms after dosage reduction or conversion to another opioid analgesic.
• For patient with bradycardia, implement cardiac monitoring, as ordered, and assess heart rate and rhythm frequently during fentanyl therapy because drug may further slow heart rate.
• **WARNING** Expect respiratory depressant effects to last longer than analgesic effects. Also be prepared for residual drug to potentiate the effects of subsequent doses. Residual drug can be detected for at least 6 hours after I.V. dose and 17 hours after dose of other forms.
• **WARNING** Assess for signs of overdose, such as cardiopulmonary arrest, hypoventilation, pupil constriction, respiratory and CNS depression, seizures, and shock. Give naloxone (possibly in repeated doses), as prescribed. Be prepared to assist with endotracheal intubation and mechanical ventilation and to provide fluids.
• Monitor the blood glucose level of diabetic patients who are receiving transdermal fentanyl because each unit contains about 2 g of sugar.

PATIENT TEACHING

• Instruct patient to avoid alcohol and other CNS depressants during fentanyl therapy unless prescribed.
• Advise patient not to stop taking drug unless directed by prescriber because withdrawal symptoms may occur. Ease the patient's fears about drug dependence.
• For transdermal form, instruct patient to choose a site with intact (not irritated or irradiated) skin on a flat surface, such as the chest, back, flank, or upper arm, and, if appropriate, to clip, not shave, hair from the site and clean it with water (no soaps, lotions, oils, or alcohol). After site preparation, instruct pa-

tient to press patch firmly in place with palm for 30 seconds, making sure edges are sealed. If patch loosens, tell her to tape edges down but not cover the entire patch. If more than one patch is needed, the edges shouldn't touch or overlap. Instruct patient to remove patch after 72 hours, fold it in half with adhesive sides together, and flush it down the toilet. Remind her not to reuse a site for at least 3 days.
•Inform patient that fever, saunas, hot tubs, heating pads, and electric blankets may increase transdermal absorption and adverse reactions.
•For transmucosal form, instruct patient to open package just before use and to save plastic cap for disposal of unused portion of lozenge. Tell her to place lozenge between her cheek and gum and to suck, not chew, it for 15 minutes. Show her how to move lozenge from one side of her mouth to the other, using the handle provided separately.
•For transmucosal form, tell patient to see dentist regularly and to brush teeth and floss after each meal because of increased risk of dental caries.
•For transmucosal form, inform diabetic patient that each unit contains 2 g of sugar. Instruct him to monitor his blood glucose levels closely.

ferrous fumarate

(contains 100 mg of elemental iron per capsule or per 5 ml of oral suspension, 33 mg of elemental iron per chewable tablet or per 5 ml of oral suspension, 106 mg of elemental iron per E.R. capsule, 15 mg of elemental iron per 0.6 ml of oral solution, and 20 to 115 mg of elemental iron per tablet)

Femiron, Feostat, Feostat Drops, Ferretts, Fumasorb, Fumerin, Hemocyte, Ircon, Neo-Fer (CAN), Nephro-Fer, Novofumar (CAN), Palafer (CAN), Span-FF

ferrous gluconate

(contains 10 mg of elemental iron per capsule, 34 mg of elemental iron per 5 ml of elixir, 37 mg of elemental iron per E.R. tablet, 35 mg of elemental iron per 5 ml of syrup, and 34 to 38 mg of elemental iron per tablet)

Apo-Ferrous Gluconate (CAN), Fergon, Ferralet, Ferralet Slow Release, Fertinic (CAN), Novoferrogluc (CAN), Simron

ferrous sulfate

(contains 50 mg of elemental iron per capsule, 60 mg of elemental iron per dried capsule, 30 to 50 mg of elemental iron per dried E.R. capsule, 50 mg of elemental iron per dried E.R. tablet, 65 mg of elemental iron per dried tablet, 44 mg of elemental iron per 5 ml of elixir, 60 to 65 mg of elemental iron per enteric-coated tablet, 65 to 105 mg of elemental iron per E.R. tablet, 15 mg of elemental iron per 0.6 ml of oral solution, 18 mg of elemental iron per 0.5 ml of oral solution, 25 mg of elemental iron per ml of oral solution, 30 or 60 mg of elemental iron per 5 ml of oral solution, and 39 to 65 mg of elemental iron per tablet)

Apo-Ferrous Sulfate (CAN), Feosol, Feratab, Fer-gen-sol, Fer-In-Sol Capsules, Fer-In-Sol Drops, Fer-In-Sol Syrup, Fer-Iron Drops, Fero-Grad (CAN), Fero-Gradumet, Ferospace, Ferralyn Lanacaps, Ferra-TD, Mol-Iron, Novoferrosulfa (CAN), PMS-Ferrous Sulfate (CAN), Slow-Fe

iron, carbonyl

(contains 50 mg of elemental iron per caplet)

Feosol

Class and Category

Chemical: Trace element, mineral
Therapeutic: Antianemic, nutritional supplement
Pregnancy category: Not rated

Indications and Dosages

➤ *To prevent iron deficiency based on U.S. and Canadian recommended daily allowances*

CAPLETS, CAPSULES, CHEWABLE TABLETS, DRIED CAPSULES, DRIED E.R. CAPSULES, DRIED E.R.. TABLETS, DRIED TABLETS, ELIXIR, ENTERIC-COATED TABLETS, E.R. CAPSULES, E.R. TABLETS, ORAL SOLUTION, ORAL SUSPENSION, SYRUP, TABLETS

Male adults and children age 11 and older. 10 mg (8 to 10 mg Canadian) of elemental iron daily.
Female adults and children age 11 and older. 10 to 15 mg (8 to 13 mg Canadian) of elemental iron daily.
Pregnant females. 30 mg (17 to 22 mg Canadian) of elemental iron daily.
Breast-feeding females. 15 mg (8 to 13 mg Canadian) of elemental iron daily.

Children ages 7 to 10. 10 mg (8 to 10 mg Canadian) of elemental iron daily.
Children ages 4 to 6. 10 mg (8 mg Canadian) of elemental iron daily.
Children from birth to age 3. 6 to 10 mg (0.3 to 6 mg Canadian) of elemental iron daily.

➤ *To replace iron in deficiency states*
CAPLETS, CAPSULES, CHEWABLE TABLETS, DRIED CAPSULES, DRIED E.R. CAPSULES, DRIED E.R. TABLETS, DRIED TABLETS, ELIXIR, ENTERIC-COATED TABLETS, E.R. CAPSULES, E.R. TABLETS, ORAL SOLUTION, ORAL SUSPENSION, SYRUP, TABLETS
Adults and adolescents. 100 to 200 mg of elemental iron t.i.d. for 4 to 6 mo.
Children ages 2 to 12 who weigh 30 to 50 kg (66 to 110 lb). 50 to 100 mg/day of elemental iron in divided doses t.i.d. or q.i.d. for 4 to 6 mo.
Children ages 6 months to 2 years. Up to 6 mg/kg/day of elemental iron in divided doses t.i.d. or q.i.d. for 4 to 6 mo.
Infants under age 6 months. 10 to 25 mg/day of elemental iron in divided doses t.i.d. or q.i.d. for 4 to 6 mo.

➤ *To provide iron supplementation during pregnancy*
CAPLETS, CAPSULES, CHEWABLE TABLETS, DRIED CAPSULES, DRIED E.R. CAPSULES, DRIED E.R. TABLETS, DRIED TABLETS, ELIXIR, ENTERIC-COATED TABLETS, E.R. CAPSULES, E.R. TABLETS, ORAL SOLUTION, ORAL SUSPENSION, SYRUP, TABLETS
Pregnant females. 15 to 30 mg of elemental iron q.d. during second and third trimesters.
DOSAGE ADJUSTMENT Dosage increased if needed for elderly patients, who sometimes don't absorb iron as easily as younger adults.

Mechanism of Action
Acts to normalize RBC production by binding with hemoglobin or by being oxidized and stored as hemosiderin or aggregated ferritin in reticuloendothelial cells of the liver, spleen, and bone marrow. Iron is an essential component of hemoglobin, myoglobin, and several enzymes, including cytochromes, catalase, and peroxidase. Iron is needed for catecholamine metabolism and normal neutrophil function.

Contraindications
Hemochromatosis, hemolytic anemias, hemosiderosis, hypersensitivity to iron salts or their components, other anemic conditions unless accompanied by iron deficiency

Interactions
DRUGS
acetohydroxamic acid: Reduced absorption of both drugs
antacids, calcium supplements: Decreased absorption and effectiveness of iron supplement
ascorbic acid (with doses of 200 mg or more): Increased iron absorption
cholestyramine, cimetidine: Decreased iron absorption
ciprofloxacin, enoxacin, etidronate, lomefloxacin, norfloxacin, ofloxacin, oral tetracyclines: Decreased effectiveness of these drugs
dimercaprol: Possibly combination with iron in body to form a harmful chemical
levodopa: Possibly chelation with iron, decreasing levodopa absorption and blood level
levothyroxine: Decreased levothyroxine effectiveness and, possibly, hypothyroidism
methyldopa: Decreased methyldopa absorption and efficacy
penicillamine: Decreased penicillamine absorption because penicillamine chelates heavy metals
vitamin E: Decreased vitamin E absorption
FOODS
coffee; eggs; foods that contain bicarbonates, carbonates, oxalates, or phosphates; milk and milk products; tea that contains tannic acid; whole-grain breads and cereals and other high-fiber foods: Decreased iron absorption and effectiveness
ACTIVITIES
alcohol abuse (acute or chronic): Increased serum iron level

Adverse Reactions
CNS: Dizziness, fever, headache, paresthesia, syncope
CV: Chest pain, tachycardia
EENT: Metallic taste, tooth discoloration
GI: Abdominal cramps, constipation, epigastric pain, nausea, stool discoloration, vomiting
HEME: Hemochromatosis, hemolysis, hemosiderosis
RESP: Dyspnea
SKIN: Diaphoresis, flushing, rash, urticaria

Nursing Considerations
•Give iron tablets and capsules with a full glass of water or juice. Don't crush enteric-coated tablets or open capsules.
•Because iron solutions may stain teeth, dilute and administer with a straw or place drops in back of patient's throat. Mix the

elixir form in water. Fer-In-Sol Drops or Syrup may be mixed with water or juice.
•To maximize absorption, give iron salts 1 hour before or 2 hours after meals. If GI irritation occurs, give with or just after meals.
•Protect liquid form from freezing.
•Be aware that at usual dosages, serum hemoglobin level usually normalizes in about 2 months unless blood loss continues. Treatment lasts for 3 to 6 months to help replenish iron stores.
•**WARNING** Monitor for signs of iron overdose, which may include abdominal pain, diarrhea (possibly bloody), nausea, severe vomiting, and sharp abdominal cramps. In case of iron toxicity or accidental iron overdose (a leading cause of fatal poisoning in children under age 6), give deferoxamine, as prescribed. As few as 3 adult iron tablets can cause serious poisoning in young children.
•Don't give antacids, coffee, tea, dairy products, eggs, or whole-grain cereals or breads within 1 hour before or 2 hours after giving iron salts.
•Remember that unabsorbed iron turns stool green or black and can mask blood in stool. Check stool for occult blood, as ordered.

PATIENT TEACHING
•Instruct patient not to chew any solid dosage form of iron except for chewable tablets.
•Inform patient that symptoms of iron deficiency may include decreased stamina, learning problems, shortness of breath, and tiredness.
•To improve iron absorption, encourage patient to eat lean red meat, chicken, turkey, and fish as well as foods rich in vitamin C (such as citrus fruits and fresh vegetables).
•Urge patient to avoid foods that impair iron absorption, including dairy products, eggs, spinach, and high-fiber foods, such as whole-grain breads and cereals and bran. Also advise her to avoid drinking coffee or tea within 1 hour of iron intake.
•Caution patient not to take antacids or calcium supplements within 1 hour before and 2 hours after taking iron supplement.
•Inform patient that her stool should become dark green or black during therapy. Advise her to notify prescriber if it doesn't.
•To minimize tooth stains from liquid iron, instruct patient to mix each dose with water, fruit juice, or tomato juice and to drink it with a straw. When patient must take liquid

iron by dropper, direct her to place drops well back on the tongue and to follow with water or juice. Inform patient that iron stains can be removed by brushing with baking soda (sodium bicarbonate) or medicinal peroxide (hydrogen peroxide 3%).
•Advise patient to consult prescriber before taking large amounts of iron for longer than 6 months.
•Warn patient about the high risk of accidental poisoning, and urge her to keep iron preparations out of the reach of children.

filgrastim
(granulocyte colony-stimulating factor, rG-CSF)
Neupogen

Class and Category
Chemical: Granulocyte colony-stimulating factor
Therapeutic: Antineutropenic, hematopoietic stimulator
Pregnancy category: C

Indications and Dosages
➤ *To prevent infection after myelosuppressive chemotherapy*
I.V. INFUSION
Adults. 5 mcg/kg q.d. over 15 to 30 min. Increased, if needed, by 5 mcg/kg with each chemotherapy cycle.
S.C. INJECTION
Adults. 5 mcg/kg q.d. for up to 2 wk. Increased, if needed, by 5 mcg/kg with each chemotherapy cycle.
➤ *To reduce the duration of neutropenia after bone marrow transplantation*
I.V. INFUSION
Adults. 10 mcg/kg q.d. over 4 hr or as a continuous infusion over 24 hr.
S.C. INFUSION
Adults. 10 mcg/kg as a continuous infusion over 24 hr.
➤ *To enhance peripheral blood progenitor cell collection in autologous hematopoietic stem cell transplantation*
S.C. INFUSION OR INJECTION
Adults. 10 mcg/kg as continuous infusion over 24 hr or a single injection, beginning 4 days before first leukapheresis and continuing until last day of leukapheresis.

> *To reduce the occurrence and duration of neutropenia in congenital neutropenia*

S.C. INJECTION

Adults. 6 mcg/kg b.i.d.

> *To reduce the occurrence and duration of neutropenia in idiopathic or cyclic neutropenia*

S.C. INJECTION

Adults. 5 mcg/kg q.d.

DOSAGE ADJUSTMENT Dosage reduced for patients whose absolute neutrophil count remains above 10,000/mm^3.

Route	Onset	Peak	Duration
I.V.	In 5 min	Unknown	Unknown

Mechanism of Action

Is pharmacologically identical to human granulocyte colony-stimulating factor, an endogenous hormone synthesized by monocytes, endothelial cells, and fibroblasts. Filgrastim induces the formation of neutrophil progenitor cells by binding directly to receptors on the surface of granulocytes, which then divide and differentiate. It also potentiates the effects of mature neutrophils, which reduces fever and the risk of infection raised by severe neutropenia.

Incompatibilities

Don't mix filgrastim in vial or syringe with NS because precipitate will form.

Contraindications

Hypersensitivity to filgrastim, its components, or proteins derived from *Escherichia coli*

Interactions

DRUGS

lithium: Increased neutrophil production

Adverse Reactions

CNS: Fever, headache
CV: Transient supraventricular tachycardia
GI: Splenomegaly
HEME: Leukocytosis
MS: Arthralgia; myalgia; pain in arms, legs, lower back, or pelvis
SKIN: Pruritus, rash
Other: Anaphylaxis, injection site pain and redness

Nursing Considerations

• Warm filgrastim to room temperature before injection. Discard drug if stored longer than 6 hours at room temperature or 24 hours in refrigerator.
• Withdraw only one dose from a vial; don't repuncture the vial.
• Don't shake the solution.
• For continuous infusion, dilute in D$_5$W (not NS) to produce less than 15 mcg/ml.
• For S.C. dose larger than 1 ml, give by divided doses in more than one injection site.
• After chemotherapy, administer filgrastim over 15 to 30 minutes. Don't administer within 24 hours before or after cytotoxic chemotherapy.
• Monitor CBC, hematocrit, and platelet count two or three times weekly, as appropriate.
• Inform prescriber and expect to discontinue drug if leukocytosis develops or absolute neutrophil count consistently exceeds 10,000/mm^3.
• Anticipate decreased response to drug if patient has received extensive radiation therapy or long-term chemotherapy.

PATIENT TEACHING

• Teach patient how to prepare, administer, and store filgrastim. Caution her not to reuse needle, syringe, or vial.
• Provide patient with puncture-resistant container for needle and syringe disposal.
• Stress the importance of returning for follow-up laboratory tests.

finasteride

Propecia, Proscar

Class and Category

Chemical: 4-Azasteroid compound
Therapeutic: Benign prostatic hyperplasia agent, hair growth stimulant
Pregnancy category: X

Indications and Dosages

> *To treat symptomatic benign prostatic hyperplasia*

TABLETS

Adults. 5 mg q.d.

> *To treat male-pattern baldness*

TABLETS

Adults. 1 mg q.d.

Route	Onset	Peak	Duration
P.O.*	Unknown	8 hr	24 hr†
P.O.‡	In 3 mo	Unknown	Unknown

Mechanism of Action
Inhibits 5-alpha reductase, an intracellular enzyme that converts testosterone to its metabolite (5-alpha dihydrotestosterone) in the liver, prostate, and skin. This metabolite is a potent androgen that's partially responsible for benign prostatic hyperplasia and hair loss.

Contraindications
Age (childhood), hypersensitivity to finasteride, sex (female)

Interactions
DRUGS
theophylline: Decreased blood theophylline level

Adverse Reactions
CNS: Dizziness, headache
EENT: Lip swelling
ENDO: Gynecomastia
GI: Abdominal pain, diarrhea
GU: Decreased ejaculatory volume, decreased libido, impotence
MS: Back pain
SKIN: Rash

Nursing Considerations
•Expect patient to have a digital rectal examination of the prostate before and periodically during finasteride therapy.
PATIENT TEACHING
•**WARNING** Urge patient and female partners to use reliable contraception during finasteride therapy because semen of men who take drug can harm male fetuses. Caution women and children against handling broken tablets.
•Explain how to take drug properly, and advise patient to follow instructions that accompany drug.
•Inform patient that drug may cause decreased ejaculatory volume, decreased libido, and impotence.

---

* For benign prostatic hyperplasia.
† With single-dose therapy; 2 wk with multiple-dose therapy.
‡ For male-pattern baldness.

•Urge patient to have periodic follow-up tests and checkups to determine drug effectiveness.

flavoxate hydrochloride
Urispas

Class and Category
Chemical: Flavone derivative
Therapeutic: Urinary tract antispasmodic
Pregnancy category: B

Indications and Dosages
➤ *To relieve dysuria, nocturia, suprapubic pain, urinary frequency and urgency, and urinary incontinence caused by cystitis, prostatitis, urethrocystitis, or urethrotrigonitis*
TABLETS
Adults and adolescents. 100 to 200 mg t.i.d. or q.i.d.

Route	Onset	Peak	Duration
P.O.	55 min	112 min	Unknown

Mechanism of Action
Relaxes muscles by cholinergic blockade and counteracts smooth-muscle spasms in the urinary tract.

Contraindications
Achalasia; GI hemorrhage; hypersensitivity to flavoxate or its components; obstruction of the duodenum, ileum, or pylorus; obstructive uropathies of the lower urinary tract

Interactions
DRUGS
bethanechol, metoclopramide: Possibly antagonized GI motility effects of these drugs

Adverse Reactions
CNS: Confusion, decreased concentration, dizziness, drowsiness, fever, headache, nervousness, vertigo
CV: Palpitations, tachycardia
EENT: Accommodation disturbances, blurred vision, dry mouth, eye pain, photophobia, worsening of glaucoma
GI: Constipation, nausea, vomiting
GU: Dysuria
HEME: Eosinophilia, leukopenia
SKIN: Decreased sweating, dermatoses, urticaria

Nursing Considerations
•Monitor for eye pain if patient has glaucoma because flavoxate's anticholinergic effects may worsen glaucoma.

PATIENT TEACHING
•Caution patient about possible dry mouth and photophobia. Advise her to wear sunglasses outdoors, and suggest sugarless candy or gum, ice chips, sips of water, or saliva substitute for dry mouth.
•Advise patient to avoid potentially hazardous activities until drug's CNS effects are known.
•Caution patient not to become overheated or to take hot baths or saunas because drug reduces sweating, which can lead to dizziness, fainting, or heatstroke.
•Instruct patient to notify prescriber immediately if she experiences confusion, drowsiness, dysuria, headache, high fever, hives, nausea, nervousness, palpitations, rash, tachycardia, vertigo, vision problems, vomiting, or worsening dry mouth.

flecainide acetate
Tambocor

Class and Category
Chemical: Benzamide derivative
Therapeutic: Class IC antiarrhythmic
Pregnancy category: C

Indications and Dosages
➤ *To prevent and suppress recurrent life-threatening ventricular tachycardia*

TABLETS
Adults. *Initial:* 100 mg q 12 hr (q 8 hr for some patients). Increased by 50 mg b.i.d. q 4 days, if needed, until response occurs. *Maintenance:* Up to 150 mg q 12 hr. *Maximum:* 400 mg/day.
DOSAGE ADJUSTMENT Initial dose reduced to 100 mg/day or 50 mg q 12 hr for patients with creatinine clearance of less than 35 ml/min/1.73 m².
➤ *To prevent paroxysmal atrial fibrillation or flutter or paroxysmal supraventricular tachycardia*

TABLETS
Adults. *Initial:* 50 mg q 12 hr (q 8 hr for some patients). Increased by 50 mg b.i.d. q 4 days, if needed, until response occurs. *Maintenance:* Up to 150 mg q 12 hr. *Maximum:* 300 mg/day.

Mechanism of Action
Achieves antiarrhythmic effect by inhibiting fast sodium channels of myocardial cell membranes, which increase myocardial recovery after repolarization, and by depressing the upstroke of the action potential. Flecainide also produces its antiarrhythmic effect by:
•slowing intracardiac conduction, which slightly increases the duration of the action potential in atrial and ventricular muscle, thus prolonging the PR interval, QRS complex, and QT interval
•shortening the action potential of Purkinje fibers without affecting surrounding myocardial tissue
•inhibiting extracellular calcium influx (at high doses)
•stopping paroxysmal reentrant supraventricular tachycardias by acting on antegrade pathways of dysfunctional AV conduction
•decreasing conduction in the accessory pathways in patients with Wolff-Parkinson-White syndrome.

Contraindications
Cardiogenic shock, hypersensitivity to flecainide or its components, recent MI, right bundle-branch block associated with left hemiblock or second- or third-degree AV block unless pacemaker is present

Interactions
DRUGS
amiodarone: Increased blood flecainide level
beta blockers, disopyramide, verapamil: Possibly myocardial depression and increased blood levels of both drugs
calcium channel blockers: Increased risk of arrhythmias
digoxin: Possibly increased blood digoxin level
urinary acidifiers: Possibly increased flecainide elimination and decreased therapeutic effects
urinary alkalizers: Possibly decreased elimination and increased therapeutic effects of flecainide
FOODS
acidic juices, foods that decrease urine pH below 5.0: Increased flecainide elimination and decreased therapeutic effects

foods that increase urine pH above 7.0, strict vegetarian diet: Decreased flecainide elimination and increased therapeutic effects

ACTIVITIES

smoking: Increased flecainide clearance

Adverse Reactions

CNS: Anxiety, depression, dizziness, drowsiness, fatigue, headache, light-headedness, tremor, weakness
CV: Arrhythmias, chest pain, heart failure, hypotension
EENT: Blurred vision
GI: Abdominal pain, anorexia, constipation, hepatic dysfunction, nausea, vomiting
RESP: Dyspnea
SKIN: Rash

Nursing Considerations

• Monitor urine pH at the start of flecainide therapy.
• Check blood pressure, fluid intake and output, and weight regularly during therapy.
• Monitor blood trough level of flecainide, as appropriate; therapeutic level is 0.2 to 1 mcg/ml.
• Expect drug to cause mild to moderate negative inotropic effects, minimal cardiovascular effects, and no effect on blood pressure, heart rate, and left ventricular function.
• **WARNING** Because hypokalemia or hyperkalemia may interfere with flecainide's therapeutic effects, monitor serum potassium level before and during therapy and notify prescriber immediately if potassium imbalance develops. Also monitor for and notify prescriber about prolonged PR interval, QRS complex, or QT interval; chest pain; hypotension; and signs of heart failure. Keep in mind that drug can cause fatal proarrhythmias, which is why it isn't considered a first-line antiarrhythmic.
• Expect prolonged flecainide therapy to raise blood alkaline phosphatase level.

PATIENT TEACHING

• Instruct patient to take flecainide at regular intervals to maintain a constant blood level.
• Advise patient to take a missed dose as soon as she remembers if it's within 6 hours of the scheduled time.
• Teach patient how to take her pulse, and instruct her to record it daily, along with her weight. Advise her to bring record to follow-up visits.

• Encourage family members to obtain instruction in basic cardiac life support.
• Advise patient to notify prescriber immediately about chest pain, difficulty breathing, and dizziness.
• Caution patient not to stop taking drug suddenly but to taper dosage gradually according to prescriber's instructions.

fluconazole

Diflucan

Class and Category

Chemical: Triazole derivative
Therapeutic: Antifungal
Pregnancy category: C

Indications and Dosages

➤ *To treat oral and esophageal candidiasis*

ORAL SUSPENSION, TABLETS, I.V. INJECTION

Adults and adolescents. 200 mg on day 1 followed by 100 mg q.d. for at least 2 (oral) or 3 (esophageal) wk after symptoms resolve.
Children. 3 mg/kg q.d. for at least 2 (oral) or 3 (esophageal) wk and then for 2 wk after esophageal symptoms resolve.

➤ *To treat systemic candidiasis*

ORAL SUSPENSION, TABLETS, I.V. INJECTION

Adults and adolescents. 400 mg on day 1, followed by 200 mg q.d. for at least 4 wk and then for 2 wk after symptoms resolve.

➤ *To treat cryptococcal meningitis*

ORAL SUSPENSION, TABLETS, I.V. INJECTION

Adults and adolescents. 400 mg q.d. until patient responds to treatment, then 200 to 400 mg q.d. for 10 to 12 wk after CSF culture is negative. *Maintenance:* 200 mg q.d. to suppress relapse.
Children. 6 to 12 mg/kg/day for 10 to 12 wk after CSF culture is negative.

➤ *To prevent candidiasis after bone marrow transplantation*

ORAL SUSPENSION, TABLETS, I.V. INJECTION

Adults and adolescents. 400 mg q.d. starting several days before procedure if severe neutropenia is expected and continued for 7 days after absolute neutrophil count exceeds 1,000/mm^3.

➤ *To treat vaginal candidiasis*

CAPSULES, ORAL SUSPENSION, TABLETS

Adults. 150 mg as a single dose.

DOSAGE ADJUSTMENT Dosage reduced for patients with hepatic or renal impairment. Dosage reduced by 50% for patients with creatinine clearance of 11 to 50 ml/min/1.73 m^2.

Mechanism of Action
Damages fungal cells by interfering with a cytochrome P-450 enzyme needed to convert lanosterol to ergosterol, an essential part of the fungal cell membrane. Decreased ergosterol synthesis causes increased cell permeability, which allows cell contents to leak. Fluconazole also may inhibit endogenous respiration, interact with membrane phospholipids, inhibit transformation of yeasts to mycelial forms, inhibit purine uptake, and impair triglyceride and phospholipid biosynthesis.

Incompatibilities
Don't add fluconazole to I.V. bag that contains any other drug.

Contraindications
Hypersensitivity to fluconazole or its components

Interactions
DRUGS
astemizole, terfenadine: Increased blood levels of these drugs
cimetidine: Decreased blood fluconazole level
cyclosporine: Increased blood cyclosporine level
glipizide, glyburide, tolbutamide: Increased risk of hypoglycemia
hydrochlorothiazide: Increased blood fluconazole level from decreased excretion
isoniazid, rifampin: Decreased fluconazole effects
nonsedating antihistamines: Increased blood antihistamine level, increased risk of cardiotoxicity
oral anticoagulants: Increased anticoagulant effects
phenytoin: Increased blood phenytoin level
rifabutin: Increased blood rifabutin level
theophylline: Increased blood theophylline level
zidovudine: Increased blood zidovudine level

Adverse Reactions
CNS: Chills, dizziness, drowsiness, fever, headache, seizures

GI: Abdominal pain, anorexia, constipation, diarrhea, hepatic failure, nausea, vomiting
HEME: Agranulocytosis, leukopenia, thrombocytopenia
SKIN: Exfoliative dermatitis, photosensitivity, rash

Nursing Considerations
• Expect to obtain BUN and serum creatinine levels and culture and sensitivity and liver function test results before therapy starts.
• Refrigerate, but don't freeze, fluconazole oral suspension. Shake well before administering.
• Discard I.V. solution that's cloudy or contains precipitate. Don't infuse more than 200 mg/hr or add supplemental drugs to infusion.
• Monitor hepatic and renal function periodically during therapy, and notify prescriber if you detect signs of dysfunction.
• Assess for rash every 8 hours during therapy, and notify prescriber if rash occurs.
• If patient receives an oral anticoagulant, monitor coagulation test results and assess for bleeding.
• Monitor for symptoms of overdose, such as hallucinations and paranoia. If they occur, provide supportive treatment, gastric lavage, and, possibly, hemodialysis, which can reduce blood fluconazole level by half after about 3 hours.
PATIENT TEACHING
• Instruct patient to take fluconazole tablets or oral suspension 30 minutes before or 2 hours after meals. Inform her that tablets may be crushed for easier swallowing.
• Advise patient to complete entire course of therapy, even if she feels better.
• If patient takes an oral antidiabetic drug, caution her to monitor blood glucose level frequently because of increased risk of hypoglycemia.
• Instruct patient to take a missed dose as soon as she remembers, unless it's within 4 hours of next dose. Warn against double-dosing.
• Advise patient to notify prescriber immediately about diarrhea, headache, nausea, rash, right upper quadrant abdominal pain, or vomiting.
• Suggest that breast-feeding patient consult prescriber about possible breast-feeding discontinuation during therapy.

fluconazole acetate
Florinef

Class and Category
Chemical: Glucocorticoid
Therapeutic: Mineralocorticoid replacement
Pregnancy category: C

Indications and Dosages
➤ *To treat primary and secondary chronic adrenocortical insufficiency*
TABLETS
Adults and adolescents. *Usual:* 100 mcg q.d. Dosage may range from 100 mcg 3 times/wk to 200 mcg q.d.
Children. 50 to 100 mcg q.d.
➤ *To treat salt-losing adrenogenital syndrome*
TABLETS
Adults. 100 to 200 mcg q.d.
Children. 50 to 100 mcg q.d.
DOSAGE ADJUSTMENT Dosage reduced to 50 mcg q.d. if transient hypertension develops during therapy.

Route	Onset	Peak	Duration
P.O.	Unknown	Unknown	1 to 2 days

Mechanism of Action
Enhances sodium reabsorption, hydrogen and potassium excretion, and water retention by the distal renal tubules, much like aldosterone, an endogenous mineralocorticoid. In large doses, fludrocortisone can inhibit endogenous adrenocortical secretion, thymic activity, and pituitary corticotropin excretion. It also can promote glycogen deposits in the liver and induce a negative nitrogen balance when protein intake is deficient.

Contraindications
Hypersensitivity to fludrocortisone, adrenocorticoids, or their components; systemic fungal infections

Interactions
DRUGS
digoxin: Increased risk of digitalis toxicity and arrhythmias from hypokalemia
phenytoin, rifampin: Decreased fludrocortisone effects
potassium-wasting drugs, such as loop diuretics and amphotericin B: Increased risk of severe hypokalemia

Adverse Reactions
CNS: Dizziness, headache, mental changes, seizures
CV: Arrhythmias, heart failure, hypertension, peripheral edema
EENT: Cataracts (with long-term use), increased intraocular pressure
ENDO: Adrenal insufficiency, growth suppression in children, hyperglycemia
GI: Anorexia, nausea, vomiting
GU: Menstrual irregularities
HEME: Easy bruising
MS: Arthralgia, muscle weakness, myalgia, osteoporosis (with long-term use), tendon contractures
SKIN: Acne, diaphoresis, rash, urticaria
Other: Hypokalemia, hypokalemic alkalosis, impaired wound healing, weight gain

Nursing Considerations
•Monitor blood pressure, fluid status, and serum electrolyte levels periodically during fludrocortisone therapy. Assess for signs of heart failure, including adventitious breath sounds, peripheral edema, and weight gain.
•Monitor for signs and symptoms of overdose, such as cardiomegaly, edema, excessive weight gain, hypertension, and hypokalemia. These effects usually subside a few days after therapy stops. Potassium supplementation may be needed.
•Notify prescriber if patient experiences dizziness, headache, hypertension, hypokalemia, signs of infection, or weight gain.
PATIENT TEACHING
•Instruct patient to take a missed dose of fludrocortisone as soon as she remembers if it's within 12 hours of scheduled time. Warn against double-dosing. Advise her to notify prescriber if she misses more than one dose or if nausea or vomiting prevents her from taking drug.
•Instruct patient to reduce dietary sodium and to eat more potassium-rich foods during therapy.
•Direct patient to weigh herself each morning before breakfast and to notify prescriber if she gains more than 2 lb (0.9 kg) per day or 5 lb (2.3 kg) per week. Instruct her to monitor how tightly her rings and shoes fit.
•Advise patient to notify prescriber about stressful events—such as dental extractions, emotional upset, illness, surgery, and trauma—because a dosage increase may be required.

•Instruct patient to notify prescriber about dizziness, fever, fluid retention, headache, joint pain, irregular heart rate, muscle weakness, or palpitations.
•Inform patient that drug may delay wound healing.
•Caution patient not to stop taking drug abruptly but to taper dosage gradually, as prescribed.
•Urge patient to carry medical identification that documents her corticosteroid use.

flumazenil

Anexate (CAN), Romazicon

Class and Category

Chemical: Imidazobenzodiazepine derivative
Therapeutic: Benzodiazepine antidote
Pregnancy category: C

Indications and Dosages

➤ *To reverse sedation from benzodiazepine therapy*

I.V. INJECTION
Adults. 0.2 mg, repeated after 45 to 60 sec if response is inadequate and then repeated q 1 min, if needed. If sedation recurs, regimen is repeated q 20 min or more. *Maximum:* 1 mg over 5 min or 3 mg in 1-hr period.

➤ *To reverse benzodiazepine toxicity or suspected overdose*

I.V. INJECTION
Adults. 0.2 mg followed by 0.3 mg 30 to 60 sec later if response is inadequate and then 0.5 mg repeated q 1 min. If sedation recurs, regimen is repeated q 20 min. *Maximum:* 3 mg in 1-hr period.

Route	Onset	Peak	Duration
I.V.	1 to 2 min	6 to 10 min	Variable

Mechanism of Action

Antagonizes the CNS effects of benzodiazepines by competing for their binding sites.

Contraindications

Evidence of tricyclic antidepressant overdose; hypersensitivity to flumazenil, benzodiazepines, or their components; use of benzodiazepine to control intracranial pressure, status epilepticus, or a potentially life-threatening condition

Interactions
DRUGS
benzodiazepines: Benzodiazepine withdrawal symptoms, including seizures
tetracyclic or tricyclic antidepressant overdose: High risk of seizures
FOODS
all foods: Increased flumazenil clearance (by half) with food ingestion during I.V. injection

Adverse Reactions
CNS: Agitation, anxiety, ataxia, confusion, dizziness, drowsiness, emotional lability, fatigue, headache, hypoesthesia, insomnia, paresthesia, resedation, seizures, tremor, vertigo
CV: Hot flashes, hypertension, palpitations
EENT: Blurred vision, diplopia, dry mouth
GI: Nausea, vomiting
RESP: Dyspnea, hyperventilation, hypoventilation
SKIN: Diaphoresis, flushing, rash
Other: Injection site pain and thrombophlebitis

Nursing Considerations
•Use flumazenil cautiously in patients with cardiac disease. Assess for increased stress or anxiety from benzodiazepine withdrawal because cardiac patient's blood pressure may rise.
•Give flumazenil undiluted or diluted in a syringe with D$_5$W, NS, or LR solution. Administer over 15 to 30 seconds directly into tubing of a free-flowing compatible I.V. solution. Use a large vein, if possible, to minimize pain at site. Avoid extravasation because drug may irritate tissue.
•Be aware that drug may cause signs of benzodiazepine withdrawal in drug-dependent patient. Also, abrupt awakening from benzodiazepine overdose can cause agitation, dysphoria, and increased adverse reactions.
•Be aware that benzodiazepine reversal may cause an anxiety or a panic attack for patient with a history of these episodes. Expect to adjust dosage carefully.
•Monitor for signs of resedation and hypoventilation for at least 2 hours after giving flumazenil because drug has a short half-life. Be aware that patient shouldn't be discharged until the risk of resedation has resolved.

PATIENT TEACHING
•Caution patient to avoid alcohol and OTC drugs for 10 to 24 hours after flumazenil administration.
•Advise patient to avoid potentially hazardous activities for 18 to 24 hours after discharge.
•Inform patient and family that agitation, emotional lability, and panic attack (if patient has a history of such episodes) can follow flumazenil administration. Instruct them to watch for depression, difficulty breathing, flushing, hyperventilation, insomnia, palpitations, and tremor.

flunisolide

AeroBid, AeroBid-M, Bronalide (CAN), Nasalide, Nasarel, Rhinalar (CAN)

Class and Category

Chemical: Corticosteroid
Therapeutic: Antiasthmatic, anti-inflammatory
Pregnancy category: C

Indications and Dosages

➤ *To provide maintenance treatment of asthma, alone or with oral corticosteroids*
INHALATION AEROSOL
Adults and adolescents age 15 and older. 500 mcg (2 inhalations) b.i.d., in the morning and evening. *Maximum:* 2,000 mcg/day (4 inhalations b.i.d.).
Children ages 6 to 15. 500 mcg (2 inhalations) b.i.d. *Maximum:* 1,000 mcg/day.
➤ *To relieve symptoms of seasonal or perennial rhinitis*
NASAL SOLUTION
Adults. 50 mcg (2 sprays) b.i.d. in each nostril. *Maximum:* 400 mcg/day (16 sprays).
Children. 25 mcg (1 spray) t.i.d. in each nostril. *Maximum:* 200 mcg/day (8 sprays).

Route	Onset	Peak	Duration
Inhalation	In 4 wk	Unknown	Unknown
Nasal	3 to 7 days	Unknown	4 to 6 hr

Contraindications

Hypersensitivity to flunisolide or its components, primary treatment of status asthmaticus or other acute asthma episodes that require emergency treatment, recent nasal surgery (nasal form), untreated localized infection of nasal mucosa (nasal form)

Mechanism of Action

Inhibits cells involved in the inflammatory response of asthma, such as mast cells, eosinophils, basophils, lymphocytes, macrophages, and neutrophils. Also inhibits production or secretion of chemical mediators, such as histamine, eicosanoids, leukotrienes, and cytokines.

Adverse Reactions

CNS: Anxiety, chills, depression, dizziness, headache, hyperactivity, insomnia, irritability, lethargy, mood changes, nervousness, tremor, vertigo
CV: Hypertension
EENT: Candidiasis (oral and throat), dry mouth and throat, earache, eye infection, hoarseness, loss of smell or taste, mouth irritation, pharyngitis, rhinitis, sinusitis, sneezing
GI: Abdominal pain, anorexia, constipation, diarrhea, flatulence, heartburn, increased appetite, indigestion, nausea, vomiting
GU: Menstrual irregularities
HEME: Eosinophilia
RESP: Bronchitis, dyspnea, pleurisy, pneumonia
SKIN: Acne, eczema, pruritus, rash, urticaria
Other: Growth suppression (children), lymphadenopathy

Nursing Considerations

•Use flunisolide cautiously in patients with ocular herpes simplex; pulmonary tuberculosis; or untreated systemic bacterial, fungal, parasitic, or viral infection.
•If patient receives an oral corticosteroid, expect to taper corticosteroid dosage slowly 1 week after changing to flunisolide. For patient who receives prednisone, plan to reduce its dosage by no more than 2.5 mg/day at weekly intervals, beginning at least 1 week after flunisolide therapy starts.
•WARNING Assess patient who switches from systemic corticosteroid to flunisolide for signs of adrenal insufficiency (fatigue, hypotension, lassitude, nausea, vomiting, weakness) during initial treatment and during stress, trauma, surgery, infection, or other electrolyte-depleting conditions. Notify prescriber immediately if you suspect adrenal insufficiency.
•Monitor growth in children because of increased risk of growth suppression associated with intranasal corticosteroid drugs such as flunisolide.
PATIENT TEACHING
•Teach patient how to use flunisolide inhaler properly. When starting a new canister, advise

her to spray it once into the air (avoiding her eyes) to check for mist.
•Instruct patient to gargle or rinse after each use to help prevent mouth and throat dryness, relieve throat irritation, and prevent oropharyngeal infection.
•Urge patient to contact prescriber if symptoms haven't improved after 3 weeks.
•**WARNING** Caution patient not to use flunisolide to relieve acute bronchospasm.
•If patient switches from an oral corticosteroid to flunisolide, advise her to carry medical identification indicating the need for supplemental systemic corticosteroids during stress or severe asthma attack. Advise her to ask prescriber how to respond to these problems.
•Caution patient to avoid exposure to chickenpox and measles and to contact prescriber immediately if exposure occurs.

fluoxetine hydrochloride

Prozac, Prozac Weekly, Sarafem

Class and Category
Chemical: Phenylpropylamine derivative
Therapeutic: Antibulimic, antidepressant, antiobsessive-compulsive
Pregnancy category: C

Indications and Dosages
➤ *To treat depression*
CAPSULES, ORAL SOLUTION, TABLETS (PROZAC, PROZAC WEEKLY)
Adults. *Initial:* 20 mg q.d. in the morning. Dosage increased q 4 to 8 wk as needed. Dosage greater than 20 mg/day given b.i.d. morning and noon. *Maximum:* 80 mg/day.
DELAYED-RELEASE CAPSULES
Adults. 90 mg/wk, beginning 7 days after last 20-mg q.d. dose.
➤ *To treat obsessive-compulsive disorder*
CAPSULES, ORAL SOLUTION, TABLETS (PROZAC, PROZAC WEEKLY)
Adults. *Initial:* 20 mg q.d. in the morning. Dosage increased q 4 to 8 wk as needed. Dosage greater than 20 mg/day given b.i.d. morning and noon. *Maximum:* 80 mg/day.
➤ *To treat moderate to severe bulimia nervosa*
CAPSULES, ORAL SOLUTION, TABLETS (PROZAC, PROZAC WEEKLY)
Adults. 60 mg q.d. in the morning. Some patients may be prescribed a lower dose, which is titrated to 60 mg/day as tolerated.

➤ *To treat panic disorder with or without agoraphobia*
CAPSULES, ORAL SOLUTION, TABLETS (PROZAC, PROZAC WEEKLY)
Adults. *Initial:* 10 mg q.d. Dosage increased in 1 wk to 20 mg/day, as needed. *Maximum:* 60 mg/day.
➤ *To treat premenstrual dysmorphic disorder*
CAPSULES (SARAFEM)
Adults. 20 mg q.d. Dosage increased as needed. *Maximum:* 80 mg/day.
DOSAGE ADJUSTMENT Dose or frequency reduced for patients with hepatic impairment or concurrent illness, those who take multiple medications, and for elderly patients.

Route	Onset	Peak	Duration
P.O.*	1 to 6 wk†	Unknown	Unknown

Mechanism of Action
Selectively inhibits reuptake of the neurotransmitter serotonin by CNS neurons and increases the amount of serotonin that's available in nerve synapses. An elevated serotonin level may result in elevated mood and, consequently, reduced depression.

Contraindications
Hypersensitivity to selective serotonin reuptake inhibitors or their components, use within 14 days of MAO inhibitor therapy

Interactions
DRUGS
alprazolam, diazepam: Possibly prolonged half-life of these drugs
astemizole: Increased risk of serious arrhythmias
buspirone: Decreased buspirone effects
clozapine, fluphenazine, haloperidol, maprotiline, trazodone: Increased risk of adverse effects
lithium: Increased or decreased blood lithium level
MAO inhibitors: Possibly severe and life-threatening adverse effects
phenytoin: Increased blood phenytoin level and risk of toxicity
pimozide: Possibly bradycardia
serotonergics (such as amphetamines and other psychostimulants, antidepressants, and dopamine agonists): Serotonin syndrome

* Capsules, oral solution, and tablets.
† For depression and bulimia; 5 wk for obsessive-compulsive disorder.

tricyclic antidepressants: Increased risk of adverse effects, including seizures
tryptophan: Increased risk of central and peripheral toxicity
warfarin: Increased risk of bleeding

Adverse Reactions
CNS: Anxiety, chills, dream disturbances, drowsiness, fatigue, fever, headache, hypomania, insomnia, mania, nervousness, restlessness, seizures, somnolence, tremor, vertigo, weakness, yawning
CV: Hypotension, palpitations
EENT: Abnormal vision, dry mouth, pharyngitis, sinusitis
ENDO: Galactorrhea, gynecomastia, hypoglycemia
GI: Anorexia, diarrhea, indigestion, nausea
GU: Decreased libido, ejaculation disorders, impotence
HEME: Altered platelet function, unusual bleeding
MS: Arthralgia, myalgia
RESP: Dyspnea
SKIN: Diaphoresis, pruritus, rash, urticaria
Other: Flulike symptoms, hyponatremia, weight loss

Nursing Considerations
•Use fluoxetine cautiously in patients with a history of seizures.
•**WARNING** Avoid giving fluoxetine within 14 days of an MAO inhibitor or starting MAO inhibitor therapy within 5 weeks of discontinuing fluoxetine.
•**WARNING** If patient receives another drug that raises serotonin level (such as dopamine agonists, MAO inhibitors and other antidepressants, tryptophan, and amphetamines and other psychostimulants), assess for serotonin syndrome, a rare but serious adverse effect of selective serotonin reuptake inhibitors. Signs and symptoms include agitation, confusion, diaphoresis, diarrhea, fever, hyperactive reflexes, poor coordination, restlessness, shaking, talking or acting with uncontrolled excitement, tremor, and twitching.
•Monitor patients with diabetes mellitus for altered blood glucose levels because drug may cause hypoglycemia during therapy and hyperglycemia when therapy stops. Expect to adjust dosage of antidiabetic drug, as prescribed.
•Expect patient to be reevaluated periodically to determine whether therapy should be continued.

PATIENT TEACHING
•**WARNING** Inform patient that fluoxetine increases the risk of serotonin syndrome, a rare but serious complication. Teach patient to recognize its signs and symptoms, including diarrhea, fever, hyperactive reflexes, increased sweating, mood changes, rapid heart rate, restlessness, and shivering or shaking, and advise her to notify prescriber immediately if they occur.
•Caution patient to avoid potentially hazardous activities until drug's CNS effects are known.
•Advise patient to consult prescriber before taking OTC or prescription drugs, if a rash or hives develop, or if she becomes or intends to become pregnant during therapy.
•Inform patient that drug may take several weeks to achieve full effects.
•Instruct patient to schedule and maintain follow-up appointments for reevaluation of symptoms.

fluphenazine decanoate
Modecate (CAN), Modecate Concentrate (CAN), Prolixin Decanoate

fluphenazine enanthate
Moditen Enanthate (CAN), Prolixin Enanthate

fluphenazine hydrochloride
Apo-Fluphenazine (CAN), Moditen HCl (CAN), Permitil, Permitil Concentrate, PMS Fluphenazine (CAN), Prolixin, Prolixin Concentrate

Class and Category
Chemical: Phenothiazine, propylpiperazine derivative
Therapeutic: Antipsychotic
Pregnancy category: Not rated

Indications and Dosages
➤ *To control psychotic disorders*
ELIXIR, ORAL SOLUTION, TABLETS (FLUPHENAZINE HYDROCHLORIDE)
Adults and adolescents. *Initial:* 2.5 to 10 mg/day in divided doses q 6 to 8 hr. When symptoms are controlled, dosage reduced to 1 to 5 mg q.d. *Maximum:* 20 mg/dose with caution.
Children. 250 to 750 mcg q.d. to q.i.d.
I.M. INJECTION (FLUPHENAZINE HYDROCHLORIDE)
Adults and adolescents. *Initial:* 1.25 mg, increased as clinical condition tolerates up to 2.5 to 10 mg/day in divided doses q 6 to 8 hr. *Maximum:* 10 mg/day.

DOSAGE ADJUSTMENT For elderly or debilitated patients, dosage reduced to 1 to 2.5 mg/day in divided doses q 6 to 8 hr.

I.M. OR S.C. INJECTION (FLUPHENAZINE DECANOATE OR ENANTHATE)

Adults. *Initial:* 12.5 to 25 mg q 1 to 4 wk, as needed (decanoate). For doses over 50 mg, next dose increased cautiously by 12.5 mg. Or 25 mg q 2 wk, with dose and dosing interval adjusted based on patient response (enanthate). *Maximum:* 100 mg/dose.

Adolescents and children age 12. *Initial:* 6.25 to 18.75 mg/wk (decanoate), increased to 12.5 to 25 mg q 1 to 3 wk, according to clinical condition.

Children ages 5 to 12. 3.125 to 12.5 mg q 1 to 3 wk (decanoate), according to clinical condition.

Route	Onset	Peak	Duration
P.O.	In 1 hr	Variable	6 to 8 hr
I.M.*	In 1 hr	Variable	6 to 8 hr
I.M., S.C.†	In 24 to 72 hr	Variable	1 to 6 wk‡

Mechanism of Action
May block postsynaptic dopamine receptor sites in the CNS. This action may depress areas of the brain that control activity and aggression, including the cerebral cortex, hypothalamus, and limbic system.

Incompatibilities
Don't mix fluphenazine hydrochloride oral solution with beverages that contain caffeine, such as coffee and cola; tannins, such as tea; or pectins, such as apple juice. They're physically incompatible.

Contraindications
Blood dyscrasias, bone marrow depression, cerebral arteriosclerosis, coma, concomitant use of large amounts of another CNS depressant, coronary artery disease, hepatic dysfunction, hypersensitivity to phenothiazines, myeloproliferative disorders, severe CNS depression, severe hypertension or hypotension, subcortical brain damage

---

* For hydrochloride.
† For decanoate and enanthate.
‡ For decanoate; 2 wk for enanthate.

Interactions
DRUGS
adsorbent antidiarrheals, aluminum- or magnesium-containing antacids: Possibly inhibited absorption of fluphenazine
amantadine, anticholinergics: Possibly intensified adverse effects of both drugs
amphetamines: Possibly decreased therapeutic effects of both drugs
antihypertensives: Possibly severe hypotension
antithyroid drugs: Increased risk of agranulocytosis
beta blockers: Possibly increased blood levels and risk of adverse effects of both drugs
bromocriptine: Decreased bromocriptine effects
CNS depressants: Possibly prolonged and intensified CNS depression
erythromycin: Possibly inhibited fluphenazine metabolism
guanethidine: Decreased hypotensive effect of guanethidine
levodopa: Possibly decreased antidyskinetic effect of levodopa
lithium: Possibly neurotoxicity (disorientation, extrapyramidal reactions, unconsciousness)
meperidine: Excessive sedation and hypotension
metrizamide: Increased risk of seizures when injected in subarachnoid area during fluphenazine therapy
oral anticoagulants: Possibly decreased anticoagulant effects
pimozide, other drugs that prolong QT interval: Prolonged QT interval and risk of arrhythmias
thiazide diuretics: Increased risk of hyponatremia, hypotension, and water intoxication
tricyclic antidepressants: Possibly prolonged and intensified sedation
ACTIVITIES
alcohol use: Possibly increased CNS depression and increased risk of heatstroke

Adverse Reactions
CNS: Ataxia, cerebral edema, dizziness, drowsiness, headache, insomnia, light-headedness, nervousness, seizures, slurred speech, syncope, worsening psychotic symptoms
CV: AV conduction disorders, bradycardia, cardiac arrest, hypercholesterolemia, hypertension, orthostatic hypotension, QT prolongation, shock, ST-segment depression, tachycardia
EENT: Blurred vision, dry mouth, glaucoma, increased salivation, laryngeal edema, laryn-

gospasm, miosis, mydriasis, nasal congestion, papillary hypertrophy of the tongue, parotid gland enlargement, photophobia, pigmentary retinopathy, ptosis
ENDO: Breast engorgement (females), galactorrhea, hyperglycemia, hypoglycemia, mastalgia, syndrome of inappropriate ADH secretion
GI: Anorexia, constipation, diarrhea, fecal impaction, ileus, increased appetite, nausea, vomiting
GU: Amenorrhea, bladder paralysis, decreased libido, enuresis, menstrual irregularities, polyuria, urinary frequency, urinary incontinence, urine retention
HEME: Anemia, aplastic anemia, eosinophilia, leukopenia, thrombocytopenia, thrombocytopenic or nonthrombocytopenic purpura
RESP: Bronchospasm, dyspnea, increased respiratory depth
SKIN: Contact dermatitis, dry skin, eczema, erythema, jaundice, photosensitivity, pruritus, seborrhea
Other: Heatstroke, hyponatremia, lupuslike symptoms, weight gain

Nursing Considerations
•Use fluphenazine cautiously in patients with a history of glaucoma or renal impairment.
•For I.M. and S.C. injection, use at least a 21G needle.
•Monitor temperature; a significant, unexplained rise can indicate intolerance and a need to discontinue drug. Notify prescriber immediately if this occurs.
•Assess for signs of hepatic failure, such as jaundice.
•Notify prescriber about worsening psychotic symptoms: agitation, catatonic state, confusion, depression, hallucinations, lethargy, paranoid reactions.

PATIENT TEACHING
•If patient takes elixir form of fluphenazine, instruct her to keep it in an amber or opaque bottle because drug is sensitive to light.
•Advise patient not to mix oral solution with beverages that contain caffeine (coffee, cola), tannins (tea), or pectins (apple juice).
•Caution patient about possible dizziness or light-headedness.
•Teach patient how to prevent heatstroke, orthostatic hypotension, and photosensitivity reactions.
•Warn patient not to stop taking fluphenazine abruptly.

flurazepam hydrochloride
Apo-Flurazepam (CAN), Dalmane, Novo-Flupam (CAN), Somnol (CAN)

Class, Category, and Schedule
Chemical: Benzodiazepine
Therapeutic: Sedative-hypnotic
Pregnancy category: Not rated
Controlled substance: Schedule IV

Indications and Dosages
➤ *To treat insomnia characterized by difficulty falling asleep, frequent nocturnal awakenings, or early-morning awakening*
CAPSULES
Adults. 15 to 30 mg h.s.
DOSAGE ADJUSTMENT Initial dose reduced to 15 mg for elderly or debilitated patients until individual response is known.

Route	Onset	Peak	Duration
P.O.	15 to 45 min	Unknown	7 to 8 hr

Mechanism of Action
May potentiate the effects of gamma-aminobutyric acid (GABA) and other inhibitory neurotransmitters by binding to specific benzodiazepine receptor sites in the limbic and cortical areas of the CNS. By binding to these receptor sites, flurazepam increases GABA's inhibitory effects and blocks cortical and limbic arousal.

Contraindications
Acute angle-closure glaucoma, breast-feeding, hypersensitivity to other benzodiazepines, itraconazole or ketoconazole therapy, psychosis

Interactions
DRUGS
cimetidine, diltiazem, disulfiram, erythromycin, fluoxetine, fluvoxamine, itraconazole, nefazodone, estrogen-containing oral contraceptives, propoxyphene, ranitidine, verapamil: Possibly increased blood level and impaired hepatic metabolism of flurazepam
clozapine: Possibly cardiac arrest or respiratory depression
CNS depressants: Possibly potentiated CNS depression
levodopa: Possibly decreased therapeutic effects of levodopa

FOODS
grapefruit juice: Possibly increased blood level and impaired hepatic metabolism of flurazepam
ACTIVITIES
alcohol use: Possibly potentiated CNS and respiratory depression

Adverse Reactions
CNS: Amnesia, anxiety, ataxia, confusion, delusions, depression, dizziness, drowsiness, euphoria, headache, hypokinesia, irritability, malaise, nervousness, slurred speech, tremor
CV: Chest pain, palpitations, tachycardia
EENT: Blurred vision, dry mouth, increased salivation, photophobia
GI: Abdominal pain, constipation, diarrhea, nausea, thirst, vomiting
GU: Libido changes
SKIN: Diaphoresis
Other: Physical or psychological dependence

Nursing Considerations
•Use flurazepam cautiously in patients with severe mental depression or reduced respiratory function; drug may intensify depression and lead to respiratory depression.
•Expect to use lowest effective dose in elderly or debilitated patients to minimize the risk of ataxia, confusion, dizziness, and oversedation.
•Monitor liver function test results, as appropriate.
PATIENT TEACHING
•Instruct patient not to exceed prescribed flurazepam dosage and not to stop drug abruptly.
•Caution patient about possible morning dizziness or drowsiness.
•Because flurazepam can reduce alertness, advise patient to avoid potentially hazardous activities until drug's CNS effects are known.
•Caution patient to avoid alcohol and CNS depressants during therapy.
•Advise patient to notify prescriber if she becomes or intends to become pregnant during therapy.
•Inform patient that her sleep may be disturbed for the first few nights after stopping drug.

flurbiprofen
Ansaid, Froben (CAN), Froben SR (CAN), Novo-Flurprofen (CAN)

Class and Category
Chemical: Propionic acid derivative
Therapeutic: Antiarthritis, anti-inflammatory
Pregnancy category: B (first trimester), Not rated (later trimesters)

Indications and Dosages
➤ *To treat acute or chronic rheumatoid arthritis and osteoarthritis*
E.R. CAPSULES
Adults. 200 mg q.d. in the evening.
TABLETS
Adults. *Initial:* 200 to 300 mg/day in divided doses b.i.d. to q.i.d. *Maximum:* 300 mg/day (100 mg/dose).

Mechanism of Action
Blocks the activity of cyclooxygenase, the enzyme necessary for prostaglandin synthesis. Prostaglandins, important mediators in the inflammatory response, cause local vasodilation with swelling and pain. They also play a role in pain transmission from the periphery to the spinal cord. By blocking cyclooxygenase and inhibiting prostaglandins, this NSAID causes inflammatory symptoms and pain to subside.

Contraindications
Angioedema, asthma, bronchospasm, nasal polyps, rhinitis, or urticaria induced by aspirin, iodides, or NSAIDs; hypersensitivity to NSAIDs

Interactions
DRUGS
acetaminophen: Increased risk of renal impairment with long-term use of both drugs
antacids: Decreased flurbiprofen effectiveness
anticoagulants, cefamandole, cefoperazone, cefotetan, heparin, plicamycin, thrombolytics, valproic acid: Increased risk of bleeding
antineoplastics: Increased adverse hematologic effects
cyclosporine: Increased risk of nephrotoxicity
diuretics, triamterene: Decreased effectiveness of these drugs
glucocorticoids, other NSAIDs, potassium supplements: Increased adverse GI effects
insulin, oral antidiabetic drugs: Increased risk of hypoglycemia
lithium: Increased risk of lithium toxicity
methotrexate: Increased risk of methotrexate toxicity
salicylates: Increased risk of GI bleeding

ACTIVITIES
alcohol use, smoking: Increased risk of GI bleeding

Adverse Reactions
CNS: Anxiety, depression, dizziness, drowsiness, forgetfulness, headache, insomnia, malaise, nervousness, tremor, weakness
CV: Arrhythmias, heart failure, hypertension, hypotension, palpitations, peripheral edema, tachycardia
EENT: Amblyopia, blurred vision, rhinitis, stomatitis, tinnitus, vision changes
GI: Abdominal cramps or distress, anorexia, constipation, diarrhea, flatulence, GI bleeding, increased appetite, indigestion, nausea, vomiting
GU: Hematuria, renal failure, UTI
HEME: Agranulocytosis, eosinophilia, leukopenia, neutropenia, pancytopenia, thrombocytopenia
SKIN: Flushing, rash

Nursing Considerations
•Use flurbiprofen cautiously in patients with renal disease.
•Expect elderly patients to receive the lowest effective dose for the shortest possible duration to reduce their risk of adverse renal and GI reactions.
•Monitor for evidence of GI bleeding, such as abdominal pain, decreased serum hemoglobin level, and tarry stools.
•Assess for signs of heart failure, such as dyspnea, peripheral edema, and sudden weight gain.
•Monitor serum creatinine level or creatinine clearance; expect to reduce dosage to avoid excessive accumulation of flurbiprofen.

PATIENT TEACHING
•Encourage patient to take flurbiprofen with food or milk to avoid GI distress.
•Caution patient about possible blurred vision, dizziness, and drowsiness.
•Advise patient to avoid aspirin, alcohol, and smoking during flurbiprofen therapy.
•Instruct patient to notify prescriber if black stools, edema, persistent headache, rash, or vision changes develop.

fluticasone propionate
Flonase, Flovent, Flovent Rotadisk

Class and Category
Chemical: Trifluorinated corticosteroid
Therapeutic: Antiasthmatic, anti-inflammatory
Pregnancy category: C

Indications and Dosages
➤ *To prevent asthma attacks, alone or with oral corticosteroids*
INHALATION AEROSOL
Adults and children age 12 and older using bronchodilator therapy. *Initial:* 88 mcg inhaled b.i.d. *Maximum:* 440 mcg inhaled b.i.d.
Adults and children age 12 and older switching from another inhaled corticosteroid. *Initial:* 88 to 220 mcg inhaled b.i.d. *Maximum:* 440 mcg inhaled b.i.d.
Adults and children age 12 and older using oral corticosteroid therapy. *Initial and maximum:* 880 mcg inhaled b.i.d.
ROTADISK INHALATION POWDER
Adults and children age 12 and older using bronchodilator therapy. *Initial:* 100 mcg inhaled b.i.d. *Maximum:* 500 mcg inhaled b.i.d.
Adults and children age 12 and older switching from another inhaled corticosteroid. *Initial:* 100 to 250 mcg inhaled b.i.d. *Maximum:* 500 mcg inhaled b.i.d.
Adults and children age 12 and older using oral corticosteroid therapy. *Initial and maximum:* 1,000 mcg inhaled b.i.d.
Children ages 4 to 11 using bronchodilator therapy. *Initial:* 50 mcg inhaled b.i.d. *Maximum:* 100 mcg inhaled b.i.d.
Children ages 4 to 11 switching from another inhaled corticosteroid. *Initial:* 50 mcg inhaled b.i.d. *Maximum:* 100 mcg inhaled b.i.d.
➤ *To prevent or treat seasonal or perennial allergic rhinitis*
NASAL SUSPENSION
Adults and children age 12 and older. *Initial:* 100 mcg (2 sprays) in each nostril q.d. or 50 mcg (1 spray) in each nostril b.i.d, as needed. *Maintenance:* 50 mcg (1 spray) in each nostril q.d., as tolerated and needed. *Maximum:* 200 mcg/day (4 sprays).
Children ages 4 to 11. 50 or 100 mcg (1 or 2 sprays) in each nostril q.d. in the morning, as needed. *Maximum:* 200 mcg/day (4 sprays).

Route	Onset	Peak	Duration
Inhalation*	In 24 hr	1 to 2 wk	Several days
Nasal	12 hr to 3 days	4 to 7 days	1 to 2 wk

* Aerosol and Rotadisk.

Mechanism of Action
Inhibits cells involved in the inflammatory response of asthma, such as mast cells, eosinophils, basophils, lymphocytes, macrophages, and neutrophils. Fluticasone also inhibits production or secretion of chemical mediators, such as histamine, eicosanoids, leukotrienes, and cytokines.

Contraindications
Hypersensitivity to fluticasone or its components, primary treatment of status asthmaticus or other acute asthma episodes that require intensive measures, untreated nasal mucosal infection (nasal suspension)

Interactions
DRUGS
ketoconazole, ritonavir and other strong cytochrome P450 3A4 inhibitors (long-term use): Possibly increased blood fluticasone level

Adverse Reactions
CNS: Aggressiveness, agitation, depression, difficulty speaking, dizziness, fatigue, fever, headache, insomnia, malaise, restlessness
EENT: Allergic rhinitis, cataracts, conjunctivitis, dry mouth and throat, eye irritation, glaucoma, laryngitis, loss of voice, nasal congestion or discharge, nasal sinus pain, oropharyngeal candidiasis, otitis media, pharyngitis, sinusitis, tonsillitis
ENDO: Adrenal insufficiency, cushingoid symptoms, growth suppression in children, hyperglycemia
GI: Abdominal pain, diarrhea, indigestion, nausea, vomiting
GU: Dysmenorrhea
HEME: Easy bruising
MS: Arthralgia, myalgia
RESP: Asthma exacerbation, bronchitis, bronchospasm, chest congestion and tightness, cough, dyspnea, upper respiratory tract infection, wheezing
SKIN: Dermatitis, ecchymosis, rash, urticaria
Other: Flulike symptoms, weight gain

Nursing Considerations
•Use fluticasone cautiously in patients with ocular herpes simplex, pulmonary tuberculosis, or untreated systemic bacterial, fungal, parasitic, or viral infection.
•If patient takes a systemic corticosteroid, expect to taper dosage by no more than 2.5 mg/day at weekly intervals, starting 1 week after fluticasone therapy begins.
•**WARNING** If prescriber switches patient from systemic corticosteroid to fluticasone, assess for signs of adrenal insufficiency (fatigue, hypotension, lassitude, nausea, vomiting, weakness) early in treatment and when patient is exposed to stress, trauma, surgery, infection, or other electrolyte-depleting conditions or procedures. Notify prescriber immediately if this condition develops.
•As prescribed, administer a fast-acting inhaled bronchodilator if bronchospasm occurs immediately after fluticasone use. Expect to stop fluticasone and start another drug therapy.
•Expect to titrate fluticasone to lowest effective dosage after asthma has stabilized.
PATIENT TEACHING
•Advise patient to use fluticasone regularly, as prescribed. Caution her not to use it to relieve acute bronchospasm.
•Instruct patient to shake canister and to use inhaler according to package insert instructions. On first use, advise her to spray once into the air (away from her eyes) and look for a fine mist.
•If 2 inhalations are prescribed, direct patient to wait at least 1 minute between them.
•Instruct patient to gargle and rinse her mouth after each dose to help prevent dry mouth and throat, relieve throat irritation, and prevent oropharyngeal yeast infection.
•If patient uses more than one inhaler, instruct her to use fluticasone last, at least 5 minutes after previous inhaler.
•Explain that symptoms may improve within 2 days but that full improvement may not occur for 1 to 2 weeks or longer.
•Caution patient not to increase dosage but to contact prescriber after 1 week if symptoms continue or worsen.
•Instruct patient to notify prescriber immediately if she has asthma attacks that don't respond to bronchodilators during fluticasone therapy.
•If patient is switching from an oral corticosteroid to fluticasone, urge her to carry medical identification indicating the need for supplemental systemic corticosteroids during stress or severe asthma attack.

fluvastatin sodium
Lescol, Lescol XL

Class and Category
Chemical: Heptenoic acid derivative
Therapeutic: Antihyperlipidemic
Pregnancy category: X

Indications and Dosages
➤ *As adjunct to lower cholesterol level in primary hypercholesterolemia, to decrease progression of coronary atherosclerosis*
CAPSULES
Adults. 20 to 40 mg h.s. *Maximum:* 40 mg b.i.d.
EXTENDED-RELEASE TABLETS
Adults. 80 mg h.s. *Maximum:* 80 mg/day.

Route	Onset	Peak	Duration
P.O.	In 1 to 2 wk	In 4 to 6 wk	Unknown
P.O. (E.R.)	In 2 wk	In 4 wk	Unknown

Mechanism of Action
Interferes with the hepatic enzyme hydroxymethylglutaryl-coenzyme A reductase. By doing so, fluvastatin reduces the formation of mevalonic acid (a cholesterol precursor), thus interrupting the pathway by which cholesterol is synthesized. When the cholesterol level declines in hepatic cells, LDLs are consumed, which also reduces the amount of circulating total cholesterol and serum triglycerides.

Contraindications
Acute hepatic disease, breast-feeding, hypersensitivity to fluvastatin or its components, pregnancy, unexplained persistently elevated liver enzyme levels

Interactions
DRUGS
bile acid sequestrants: Possibly decreased fluvastatin bioavailability
cimetidine, omeprazole, ranitidine: Significantly increased blood fluvastatin level
cyclosporine, erythromycin, gemfibrozil, niacin: Increased risk of severe myopathy, rhabdomyolysis, and acute renal failure
itraconazole, ketoconazole: Increased risk of myopathy
oral contraceptives: Increased risk of bleeding
rifampin: Significantly decreased blood fluvastatin level, increased plasma clearance

ACTIVITIES
alcohol use: Increased bioavailability and blood level of fluvastatin

Adverse Reactions
CNS: Dizziness, fatigue, headache, insomnia, weakness
EENT: Pharyngitis, rhinitis, sinusitis
GI: Abdominal cramps and pain, constipation, diarrhea, flatulence, indigestion, nausea, vomiting
GU: UTI
MS: Arthritis, back pain, myalgia, myositis, rhabdomyolysis
RESP: Bronchitis, cough, upper respiratory tract infection
SKIN: Pruritus, rash

Nursing Considerations
•**WARNING** Expect to discontinue fluvastatin therapy if serum CK level rises sharply or myopathy is suspected.
PATIENT TEACHING
•Urge patient to comply with monthly laboratory tests early in treatment.
•Instruct patient to follow low-fat diet, as prescribed.
•Advise patient to notify prescriber promptly about muscle pain or unexplained weakness.

fluvoxamine maleate

Luvox

Class and Category
Chemical: Aralkylketone derivative
Therapeutic: Antiobsessional
Pregnancy category: C

Indications and Dosages
➤ *To treat obsessive-compulsive disorder*
TABLETS
Adults. *Initial:* 50 mg h.s., increased by 50 mg q 4 to 7 days, if needed. *Maximum:* 300 mg/day.
Children ages 8 to 17. *Initial:* 25 mg h.s., increased by 25 mg q 4 to 7 days, if needed. *Maximum:* 200 mg/day.
DOSAGE ADJUSTMENT Doses divided for adults taking more than 100 mg/day and children taking more than 50 mg/day; given in 2 equal doses b.i.d. or 2 unequal doses with larger dose h.s.

Route	Onset	Peak	Duration
P.O.	3 to 10 wk	Unknown	Unknown

Mechanism of Action

May potentiate serotonin's action by blocking its reuptake at neuronal membranes. An elevated serotonin level may result in elevated mood and, consequently, reduced depression and anxiety, which often accompany obsessive-compulsive disorder.

Contraindications

Astemizole or cisapride therapy, hypersensitivity to fluvoxamine maleate or its components, use within 14 days of MAO inhibitor therapy

Interactions

DRUGS

antihistamines: Increased risk of impaired mental and motor skills
astemizole, cisapride, terfenadine: Possibly fatal QT prolongation
benzodiazepines: Decreased benzodiazepine clearance, possibly impaired memory and motor skills
buspirone: Decreased buspirone effects, increased blood fluvoxamine level, paradoxical worsening of obsessive-compulsive disorder
carbamazepine: Increased risk of carbamazepine toxicity
clozapine: Increased blood clozapine level
diltiazem: Increased risk of bradycardia
haloperidol: Increased blood haloperidol level, possibly delayed recall and reduced memory and attention span
lithium: Possibly increased serotonin reuptake action of fluvoxamine
MAO inhibitors: Possibly serious or fatal reactions (such as agitation, autonomic instability, coma, delirium, fluctuating vital signs, hyperthermia, myoclonus, and rigidity)
methadone: Possibly significantly increased blood methadone level, increased risk of methadone toxicity
metoprolol, propranolol: Increased blood levels of these drugs, possibly reduced diastolic blood pressure and heart rate induced by these drugs
serotonergics (such as amphetamines and other psychostimulants, antidepressants, and dopamine agonists): Serotonin syndrome
sympathomimetics: Possibly increased effects of sympathomimetics and increased risk of serotonin syndrome

tacrine: Increased blood level and therapeutic and adverse effects of tacrine
theophylline: Decreased theophylline clearance, increased risk of theophylline toxicity
tricyclic antidepressants: Increased blood levels of antidepressants
warfarin: Increased blood warfarin level, prolonged PT

FOODS

caffeine: Possibly decreased hepatic clearance of caffeine

ACTIVITIES

smoking: Increased fluvoxamine metabolism

Adverse Reactions

CNS: Agitation, anxiety, apathy, chills, confusion, depression, dizziness, drowsiness, fatigue, headache, hypomania, insomnia, malaise, mania, nervousness, sedation, tremor, vertigo, yawning
CV: Palpitations, tachycardia
EENT: Altered taste, blurred vision, dry mouth
GI: Anorexia, constipation, diarrhea, flatulence, indigestion, nausea, vomiting
GU: Decreased libido, ejaculation disorders, impotence, urinary frequency, urine retention
MS: Muscle twitching
RESP: Dyspnea, upper respiratory tract infection
SKIN: Diaphoresis, rash
Other: Flulike symptoms, weight gain

Nursing Considerations

• Use fluvoxamine cautiously in patients with cardiovascular disease, impaired hepatic or renal function, mania, seizures, or suicidal tendencies.
• WARNING Be aware that fluvoxamine shouldn't be given within 14 days of an MAO inhibitor.
• WARNING If patient receives another drug that raises the serotonin level by a different mechanism, assess for serotonin syndrome, a rare but serious complication of certain selective serotonin reuptake inhibitors. Signs and symptoms include agitation, confusion, diaphoresis, diarrhea, fever, hyperactive reflexes, lack of coordination, muscle twitching, restlessness, shivering, talking or acting with uncontrolled excitement, and tremor. Drugs that raise the serotonin level include MAO inhibitors, tryptophan, amphetamines and other psychostimulants,

E
F

antidepressants (buspirone, lithium), and dopamine agonists.

PATIENT TEACHING

• Caution patient not to drink alcohol during fluvoxamine therapy.

• Advise patient to avoid potentially hazardous activities until drug's CNS effects are known.

• **WARNING** Inform patient that fluvoxamine increases the risk of a rare but serious problem: serotonin syndrome. Urge her to notify prescriber immediately if symptoms develop.

• Caution patient not to stop taking drug abruptly. Explain that gradual tapering helps avoid withdrawal symptoms.

fondaparinux sodium

Arixtra

Class and Category

Chemical: Synthetic pentasaccharide Factor Xa inhibitor
Therapeutic: Antithrombolytic
Pregnancy category: B

Indications and Dosages

➤ *To provide prophylaxis against deep vein thrombosis, which may lead to pulmonary embolism in patients undergoing hip fracture surgery, hip replacement surgery, or knee replacement surgery*

S.C. INJECTION

Adults. *Initial*: After hemostasis has been established, 2.5 mg S.C. 6 to 8 hr after surgery, followed by 2.5 mg S.C. q.d. for 5 to 9 days. *Maximum*: 2.5 mg S.C. q.d. for 11 days.

Mechanism of Action

Selectively binds to antithrombin III, which enhances the inactivation of clotting Factor Xa by antithrombin III. Inactivation of Factor Xa interrupts the blood coagulation pathway, which then inhibits thrombin formation. Without thrombin, fibrinogen can't convert to fibrin and clots can't form.

Incompatibilities

Don't mix fondaparinux sodium with other injections or infusions.

Contraindications

Active major bleeding, bacterial endocarditis, body weight less than 50 kg (110 lb), fonda-parinux-induced thrombocytopenia associated with a positive in vitro test for antiplatelet antibodies, hypersensitivity to fondaparinux, severe renal impairment (creatinine clearance less than 30 ml/min/1.73 m^2)

Interactions

DRUGS

abciximab, thrombolytics, other drugs that enhance risk of bleeding: Increased risk of hemorrhage

Adverse Reactions

CNS: Confusion, dizziness, fever, headache, insomnia
CV: Edema, hypotension
GI: Constipation, diarrhea, elevated liver function test results, indigestion, nausea, vomiting
GU: Urine retention, UTI
HEME: Anemia, bleeding, hematoma, postoperative hemorrhage, thrombocytopenia
SKIN: Bullous eruption, increased wound drainage, rash, purpura
Other: Generalized pain; hypokalemia; injection site bleeding, rash, and pruritus

Nursing Considerations

• Inspect fondaparinux for particles or discoloration before administration.

• Alternate injection sites during treatment, using the left and right anterolateral or left and right posterolateral abdominal wall. Don't expel air bubble from prefilled syringe before injection to prevent expelling drug from syringe. Don't give drug by I.M. injection.

• **WARNING** Closely monitor patients who have had epidural or spinal anesthesia or a spinal puncture for signs of neurologic impairment. They're at risk for developing an epidural or spinal hematoma, which can put them at risk for paralysis.

• Closely monitor patient for bleeding (such as ecchymosis, epistaxis, hematemesis, hematuria, and melena), especially those at risk for decreased drug elimination (such as elderly patients and patients with mild to moderate renal impairment) and those at increased risk for bleeding (such as patients with congenital or acquired bleeding disorders; active ulcerative GI disease; hemorrhagic stroke; recent brain, spinal, or ophthalmologic surgery; diabetic retinopathy; or a history of heparin-induced thrombocytopenia; and those being treated concomitantly with platelet inhibitors).

•Perform periodic CBC, including platelet count, as ordered. Expect prescriber to discontinue drug if platelet count falls below 100,000/mm³. Be aware that routine coagulation tests, such as PT and INR, are not used to monitor fondaparinux therapy; an anti-Xa assay may be used instead. Also, test stools for occult blood, as ordered.

•Monitor renal function test results, as ordered. Expect to discontinue drug if severe renal impairment or labile renal function occurs during fondaparinux therapy.

•Store drug at controlled room temperature.

PATIENT TEACHING

•Inform patient that fondaparinux can't be taken orally.

•Instruct patient to seek immediate help if he experiences signs of thromboembolism, such as neurologic changes and severe shortness of breath.

•Inform patient about the increased risk of bleeding. Instruct her or family member to watch for and report abdominal or lower back pain, black stools, bleeding gums, bloody urine, or severe headaches.

•Teach patient or family member how to administer fondaparinux by S.C. injection at home, if needed. Instruct her not to expel air bubble from a prefilled syringe to avoid expelling some of the drug. Tell her to insert the entire needle into a skinfold held between thumb and forefinger, and remind her to alternate administration sites.

•Caution patient not to rub injection site after administering drug to minimize bruising.

•Review safe handling and disposal of syringes and needles.

•Advise patient to keep follow-up appointments and undergo ordered laboratory tests.

formoterol fumarate dihydrate

Foradil Aerolizer, Oxeze Turbuhaler (CAN)

Class and Category

Chemical: Racemic acid salt
Therapeutic: Bronchodilator
Pregnancy category: C

Indications and Dosages

➤ *To prevent asthma-induced bronchospasm*

POWDER FOR ORAL INHALATION
Adults and children age 5 and older. 12 mcg q 12 hr through inhaler device. *Maximum:* 24 mcg/day.

➤ *To prevent exercise-induced bronchospasm*
POWDER FOR ORAL INHALATION
Adults and adolescents age 12 and older. 12 mcg at least 15 min before exercise q 12 hr p.r.n. *Maximum:* 24 mcg/day.

➤ *To provide long-term treatment of bronchospasm in patients with chronic bronchitis and emphysema*
POWDER FOR ORAL INHALATION
Adults. 12 mcg q 12 hr through inhaler device. *Maximum:* 24 mcg/day.

Route	Onset	Peak	Duration
Oral inhalation	1 to 3 min	Unknown	12 hr

Mechanism of Action

Selectively attaches to beta$_2$ receptors on bronchial membranes, stimulating the intracellular enzyme adenyl cyclase to convert adenosine triphosphate to cAMP. The resulting increase in the intracellular cAMP level relaxes bronchial smooth-muscle cells, stabilizes mast cells, and inhibits histamine release.

Contraindications

Acute asthma, hypersensitivity to formoterol fumarate or its components

Interactions
DRUGS

adrenergics: Possibly increased sympathetic effects of formoterol
beta blockers: Decreased effects of formoterol, possibly severe bronchospasm
corticosteroids, non-potassium-sparing diuretics, xanthine derivatives: Possibly increased hypokalemic effect of formoterol
disopyramide, MAO inhibitors, phenothiazines, procainamide, quinidine, tricyclic antidepressants: Possibly prolonged QTc interval, increasing risk of ventricular arrhythmias

Adverse Reactions

CNS: Dizziness, fatigue, headache, insomnia, malaise, tremor

CV: Angina, arrhythmias, hypertension, hypotension, palpitations, tachycardia
EENT: Dry mouth; laryngeal spasm, irritation, or swelling; hoarseness; rhinitis and tonsillitis (in children)
ENDO: Hyperglycemia
GI: Abdominal pain, gastroenteritis, indigestion (in children); nausea
MS: Muscle spasms
RESP: Bronchitis, bronchospasm (paradoxical or hypersensitivity-induced), cough, upper respiratory tract infection
SKIN: Dermatitis, rash
Other: Hypokalemia, metabolic acidosis, viral infection (in children)

Nursing Considerations
•Administer formoterol capsules only by oral inhalation.
•Store capsules in original blister pack, and open immediately before use.
•To use delivery system, place capsule in well of inhaler device. Press and release buttons on side of device to pierce capsule. Have patient inhale rapidly and deeply through mouthpiece; drug is dispersed into airways as patient inhales.
•**WARNING** Monitor patient for worsening or deteriorating asthma because drug isn't rapid-acting and shouldn't be used as a substitute for corticosteroid therapy.
•Monitor patient closely for paradoxical bronchospasm; if this occurs, discontinue drug immediately and notify prescriber.
•Monitor patients with a history of cardiovascular disorders, especially coronary insufficiency, arrhythmias, or hypertension. Notify prescriber of any significant increases in pulse rate or blood pressure or exacerbation of chronic conditions because formoterol may produce cardiovascular reactions, including angina, arrhythmias, hypertension or hypotension, palpitations, and tachycardia. Drug may need to be discontinued if such reactions occur.

PATIENT TEACHING
•Advise patient, especially if she has significant cardiac history, to inform prescriber of any other drugs she takes before beginning formoterol therapy to prevent harmful drug interactions.
•Instruct patient to use manufacturer's plastic device for inhaling formoterol, to always use new inhaler that comes with each refill,

and not to use a spacer. Tell her never to swallow capsules.
•Teach patient how to properly store drug and inhaler. Instruct her to avoid exposing capsules to moisture and to always handle them with dry hands because powder inside capsules must be dry to be inhaled. Also advise her to keep inhaler in a dry place and *not* to wash it.
•Teach patient proper use of formoterol delivery system. Instruct her to remove capsule from blister pack just before use, to place capsule in well of inhaler device, to press and release buttons on side of device to pierce capsule, and then to inhale rapidly and deeply through mouthpiece. Emphasize that she should only inhale, *not exhale*, into device.
•Instruct patient who currently uses oral or inhaled corticosteroids to continue using them, as prescribed, even if she feels better after starting formoterol.
•Caution patient not to increase formoterol dosage or frequency without consulting prescriber because she may need a rapid-acting bronchodilator.
•Urge patient to notify prescriber if her symptoms worsen, if formoterol becomes less effective, or if she needs more inhalations of her short-acting beta$_2$-agonist than usual because this may indicate that her asthma is worsening.
•Instruct patient to notify prescriber immediately if she experiences palpitations, chest pain, rapid heart rate, tremor, or nervousness while taking formoterol because dosage may need to be adjusted.

fosfomycin tromethamine
Monurol

Class and Category
Chemical: Phosphonic acid derivative
Therapeutic: Antibiotic
Pregnancy category: B

Indications and Dosages
➤ *To treat uncomplicated UTIs (acute cystitis) caused by* Enterococcus faecalis *or* Escherichia coli
GRANULES FOR ORAL SOLUTION
Women age 18 and older. 3 g as a single dose mixed with water.

Route	Onset	Peak	Duration
P.O.	2 to 3 days	48 hr	Unknown

Mechanism of Action

Disrupts the formation of bacterial cell walls by blocking cell wall precursors. Specifically, fosfomycin inactivates enolpyruvyl transferase, which irreversibly blocks the condensation of uridine diphosphate-*N*-acetylglucosamine with phospho *enol*pyruvate, a preliminary step in bacterial cell wall synthesis. Fosfomycin also decreases adherence of bacteria to epithelial cells of the urinary tract.

Contraindications

Hypersensitivity to fosfomycin or its components

Interactions

DRUGS

metoclopramide: Decreased blood level and urinary excretion of fosfomycin

Adverse Reactions

CNS: Asthenia, dizziness, fever, headache, insomnia, nervousness, paresthesia, somnolence
EENT: Dry mouth, pharyngitis, rhinitis
GI: Abdominal pain, anorexia, constipation, diarrhea, flatulence, indigestion, nausea, vomiting
GU: Dysmenorrhea, dysuria, hematuria, menstrual irregularities, vaginitis
MS: Back pain
SKIN: Pruritus, rash
Other: Flulike symptoms, lymphadenopathy

Nursing Considerations

• Use fosfomycin cautiously in patients with impaired renal function because drug clearance may be decreased.
• Expect to obtain urine specimens for culture and sensitivity tests before and after therapy.
• To reconstitute granules, pour contents of single-dose packet into 90 to 120 ml (3 to 4 oz) of water (not hot water) and stir. Administer immediately after dissolving.
• WARNING Expect adverse reactions to increase if more than one dose is used to treat a single episode of acute cystitis.

PATIENT TEACHING

• Explain how to reconstitute fosfomycin, and instruct patient to take drug immediately after it dissolves. Caution her not to take dry granules or mix with hot water.
• To treat each episode of acute cystitis, advise patient to use only a single dose, as prescribed, to avoid increasing the risk of adverse reactions.
• Urge patient to notify prescriber if symptoms don't improve in 2 to 3 days.
• Instruct patient to return to prescriber for further urine testing after taking fosfomycin.

fosinopril sodium

Monopril

Class and Category

Chemical: Phosphinic acid derivative
Therapeutic: Antihypertensive, vasodilator
Pregnancy category: C (first trimester), D (later trimesters)

Indications and Dosages

➤ *To manage blood pressure, alone or with other antihypertensives*

TABLETS

Adults. *Initial:* 10 mg q.d. *Maintenance:* 20 to 40 mg q.d. *Maximum:* 80 mg/day.
➤ *To treat heart failure*

TABLETS

Adults. 10 mg q.d.
DOSAGE ADJUSTMENT Initial dosage reduced to 5 mg q.d., if needed, for patients with acute heart failure, moderate to severe renal failure, or recent aggressive diuresis. Dosage may be increased over several weeks to maximum of 40 mg q.d.

Route	Onset	Peak	Duration
P.O.	1 hr	2 to 6 hr	24 hr

Contraindications

Hypersensitivity to fosinopril, other ACE inhibitors, or their components

Interactions

DRUGS

allopurinol, bone marrow depressants, procainamide, systemic corticosteroids: Increased risk of potentially fatal neutropenia or agranulocytosis
antacids: Impaired fosinopril absorption
cyclosporine, potassium-sparing diuretics, potassium supplements: Increased risk of hyperkalemia

diuretics, other antihypertensives: Possibly additive hypotension
lithium: Increased blood lithium level and risk of lithium toxicity
NSAIDs: Possibly decreased antihypertensive effect of fosinopril

FOODS
salt substitutes: Increased risk of hyperkalemia

ACTIVITIES
alcohol use: Possibly additive hypotension

Mechanism of Action
May reduce blood pressure by affecting renin-angiotensin-aldosterone system. By inhibiting angiotensin-converting enzyme, fosinopril:
• prevents conversion of angiotensin I to angiotensin II, a potent vasoconstrictor that also stimulates the adrenal cortex to secrete aldosterone
• may inhibit renal and vascular production of angiotensin II
• decreases serum angiotensin II level and increases serum renin activity, which decreases aldosterone secretion, slightly increasing the serum potassium level and fluid loss
• decreases vascular tone and blood pressure
• inhibits aldosterone release, which reduces sodium and water reabsorption and increases their excretion, further reducing blood pressure.

Adverse Reactions
CNS: Confusion, depression, dizziness, drowsiness, fatigue, fever, headache, insomnia, mood changes, sleep disturbance, syncope, tremor, vertigo, weakness
CV: Angina, arrhythmias (including AV conduction disorders, bradycardia, and tachycardia), claudication, hypotension, MI, orthostatic hypotension, palpitations
EENT: Dry mouth, epistaxis, eye irritation, hoarseness, rhinitis, sinus problems, taste perversion, tinnitus, vision changes
GI: Abdominal distention and pain, anorexia, constipation, diarrhea, flatulence, hepatic failure, hepatitis, hepatomegaly, nausea, pancreatitis, vomiting
GU: Decreased libido, flank pain, renal insufficiency, sexual dysfunction, urinary frequency

MS: Arthralgia, gout, myalgia
RESP: Asthma; bronchitis; bronchospasm; dry, persistent, tickling cough; dyspnea; tracheobronchitis; upper respiratory tract infection
SKIN: Diaphoresis, jaundice, photosensitivity, pruritus, rash, urticaria
Other: Anaphylaxis, angioedema, hyperkalemia, weight gain

Nursing Considerations
• Monitor serum potassium level before and during fosinopril therapy, as appropriate.
• Observe patient being treated for heart failure for at least 2 hours after giving drug to detect hypotension or orthostatic hypotension. If either develops, notify prescriber and monitor patient until blood pressure stabilizes. Keep in mind that orthostatic hypotension is unlikely to develop in patients with a systolic blood pressure over 100 mm Hg who receive a 10-mg dose.
• If patient also receives an antacid, separate administration times by at least 2 hours.
• If patient also receives a diuretic or another antihypertensive, expect to reduce its dosage over 2 to 3 days before starting fosinopril. If blood pressure isn't controlled with fosinopril alone, other antihypertensive therapy may resume, as prescribed. If so, observe for excessive hypotension.
• **WARNING** If angioedema affects the face, glottis, larynx, limbs, lips, mucous membranes, or tongue, notify prescriber immediately. Expect to discontinue fosinopril and start appropriate therapy at once. If airway obstruction threatens, promptly give 0.3 to 0.5 ml of epinephrine solution 1:1,000 S.C., as prescribed.

PATIENT TEACHING
• Instruct patient to take fosinopril at the same time each day to improve compliance and maintain drug's therapeutic effect.
• Emphasize the importance of taking fosinopril as prescribed, even if patient feels well. Caution her not to stop taking drug without consulting prescriber.
• Explain that drug helps control—but doesn't cure—hypertension and that patient may need lifelong therapy.
• **WARNING** Urge patient to seek immediate medical attention for difficulty breathing or swallowing, hoarseness, or swelling of the face, lips, tongue, or throat.

•Instruct patient to notify prescriber about persistent, severe nausea, vomiting, and diarrhea; resulting dehydration may lead to hypotension.

•Advise patient not to take other drugs or use salt substitutes without consulting prescriber.

•Encourage patient to keep scheduled appointments with prescriber to monitor blood pressure, blood test results, and progress.

•Caution patient about possible dizziness.

•To minimize effects of orthostatic hypotension, advise patient to rise slowly from a lying or sitting position and to dangle legs over bed for several minutes before standing.

•Reinforce prescriber's recommendations for lifestyle changes, such as smoking cessation, stress reduction, dietary improvements, alcohol avoidance, and regular exercise.

•If patient is a woman of childbearing age, urge her to use contraception during therapy because drug may harm fetus.

•Advise patient to use caution during exercise and hot weather because of the increased risk of dehydration from excessive sweating.

fosphenytoin sodium

Cerebyx

Class and Category

Chemical: Hydantoin derivative
Therapeutic: Anticonvulsant
Pregnancy category: D

Indications and Dosages

➤ *To treat status epilepticus*

I.V. INFUSION, I.M. INJECTION

Adults and adolescents. *Initial:* 15 to 20 mg of phenytoin equivalent (PE)/kg I.V. at 100 to 150 PE/min. *Maintenance:* 4 to 6 mg PE/kg/day I.V. or I.M. in divided doses b.i.d. to q.i.d. *Maximum:* 30 mg PE/kg as total loading dose.

Children. *Initial:* 15 to 20 mg PE/kg I.V. given at up to 3 mg PE/kg/min. *Maintenance:* 4 to 6 mg PE/kg/day I.V. or I.M. in divided doses b.i.d. to q.i.d.

➤ *To prevent or treat seizures during and after neurosurgery*

I.V. INFUSION, I.M. INJECTION

Adults and adolescents. *Initial:* 10 to 20 mg PE/kg I.V., not to exceed 150 mg PE/min. *Maintenance:* 4 to 6 mg PE/kg/day I.V. or I.M. in divided doses b.i.d. to q.i.d. *Maximum:* 30 mg PE/kg as total loading dose.

Mechanism of Action

Is converted from fosphenytoin (a prodrug) to phenytoin, which limits the spread of seizure activity and the start of new seizures. Phenytoin does so by regulating voltage-dependent sodium and calcium channels in neurons, inhibiting calcium movement across neuronal membranes, and enhancing the sodium-potassium-adenosine triphosphatase activity in neurons and glial cells. These actions may stem from phenytoin's ability to slow the recovery rate of inactivated sodium channels.

Contraindications

Hypersensitivity to fosphenytoin, phenytoin, other hydantoins, or their components

Interactions

DRUGS

acetaminophen (long-term use): Increased risk of hepatotoxicity

acyclovir: Decreased blood phenytoin level, loss of seizure control

alfentanil: Increased clearance and decreased effectiveness of alfentanil

amiodarone, fluoxetine: Possibly increased blood phenytoin level and risk of toxicity

antacids: Possibly decreased phenytoin effectiveness

antineoplastics: Increased phenytoin metabolism

beta blockers: Increased myocardial depression

bupropion, clozapine, loxapine, MAO inhibitors, maprotiline, phenothiazines, pimozide, thioxanthenes: Possibly lowered seizure threshold and decreased therapeutic effects of phenytoin, possibly intensified CNS depressant effects of these drugs

calcium: Possibly impaired phenytoin absorption

calcium channel blockers: Possibly increased blood phenytoin level

carbamazepine: Decreased blood carbamazepine level, possibly increased blood phenytoin level and risk of toxicity

chloramphenicol, cimetidine, disulfiram, isoniazid, methylphenidate, metronidazole, phenylbutazone, ranitidine, salicylates, sulfonamides, trimethoprim: Possibly impaired metabolism of these drugs, increased risk of phenytoin toxicity

CNS depressants: Possibly increased CNS depression
corticosteroids, cyclosporine, digoxin, disopyramide, doxycycline, furosemide, levodopa, mexiletine, quinidine: Decreased therapeutic effects of these drugs
diazoxide: Possibly decreased therapeutic effects of both drugs
dopamine: Possibly sudden hypotension or cardiac arrest after I.V. fosphenytoin administration
estrogen- and progestin-containing contraceptives: Possibly breakthrough bleeding and decreased contraceptive effectiveness
estrogens, progestins: Decreased therapeutic effects, increased blood phenytoin level
felbamate: Possibly impaired metabolism and increased blood level of phenytoin
fluconazole, itraconazole, ketoconazole, miconazole: Increased blood phenytoin level
folic acid: Increased phenytoin metabolism, decreased seizure control
haloperidol: Possibly lowered seizure threshold and decreased therapeutic effects of phenytoin; possibly decreased blood haloperidol level
insulin, oral antidiabetic drugs: Possibly increased blood glucose level and decreased therapeutic effects of these drugs
lamotrigine: Possibly decreased therapeutic effects of lamotrigine
lidocaine: Possibly decreased blood lidocaine level, increased myocardial depression
lithium: Increased risk of lithium toxicity
methadone: Possibly increased methadone metabolism, leading to withdrawal symptoms
molindone: Possibly lowered seizure threshold, impaired absorption, and decreased therapeutic effects of phenytoin
omeprazole: Possibly increased blood phenytoin level
oral anticoagulants: Possibly impaired metabolism of these drugs and increased risk of phenytoin toxicity; possibly increased anticoagulant effects initially and then decreased effects with prolonged therapy
rifampin: Possibly decreased therapeutic effects of phenytoin
streptozocin: Possibly decreased therapeutic effects of streptozocin
sucralfate: Possibly decreased phenytoin absorption
tricyclic antidepressants: Possibly lowered seizure threshold and decreased therapeutic

effects of phenytoin; possibly decreased blood antidepressant level
valproic acid: Decreased blood phenytoin level, increased blood valproic acid level
vitamin D analogues: Decreased vitamin D analogue activity
xanthines: Possibly inhibited phenytoin absorption and increased clearance of xanthines
zaleplon: Increased clearance and decreased effectiveness of zaleplon
ACTIVITIES
alcohol use: Possibly decreased phenytoin effectiveness

Adverse Reactions
CNS: Agitation, amnesia, asthenia, ataxia, cerebral edema, chills, coma, confusion, CVA, delusions, depression, dizziness, emotional lability, encephalitis, encephalopathy, extrapyramidal reactions, fever, headache, hemiplegia, hostility, hypoesthesia, lack of coordination, malaise, meningitis, nervousness, neurosis, paralysis, personality disorder, positive Babinski's sign, seizures, somnolence, speech disorders, stupor, subdural hematoma, syncope, transient paresthesia, tremor, vertigo
CV: Atrial flutter, bradycardia, bundle-branch block, cardiac arrest, cardiomegaly, edema, heart failure, hypertension, hypotension, orthostatic hypotension, palpitations, PVCs, shock, tachycardia, thrombophlebitis
EENT: Amblyopia, conjunctivitis, diplopia, dry mouth, earache, epistaxis, eye pain, gingival hyperplasia, hearing loss, hyperacusis, increased salivation, loss of taste, mydriasis, nystagmus, pharyngitis, photophobia, rhinitis, sinusitis, taste perversion, tinnitus, tongue swelling, visual field defects
ENDO: Diabetes insipidus, hyperglycemia, ketosis
GI: Anorexia, constipation, diarrhea, dysphagia, elevated liver function test results, flatulence, gastritis, GI bleeding, hepatic necrosis, hepatitis, ileus, indigestion, nausea, vomiting
GU: Albuminuria, dysuria, incontinence, oliguria, polyuria, renal failure, urine retention, vaginal candidiasis
HEME: Anemia, easy bruising, leukopenia, thrombocytopenia
MS: Arthralgia, back pain, leg cramps, muscle twitching, myalgia, myasthenia, myoclonus, myopathy

RESP: Apnea, asthma, atelectasis, bronchitis, dyspnea, hemoptysis, hyperventilation, hypoxia, increased cough, increased sputum production, pneumonia, pneumothorax
SKIN: Contact dermatitis, diaphoresis, maculopapular or pustular rash, photosensitivity, skin discoloration, skin nodule, Stevens-Johnson syndrome, transient pruritus, urticaria
Other: Cachexia, cryptococcosis, dehydration, facial edema, flulike symptoms, hyperkalemia, hypokalemia, hypophosphatemia, infection, injection site reaction, lymphadenopathy, sepsis

Nursing Considerations
•Express the dosage, concentration, and infusion rate of fosphenytoin in PE units. Misreading an order or a label could result in massive overdose.
•Refrigerate unopened fosphenytoin at 2° to 8° C (36° to 46° F), but don't freeze.
•Dilute drug in D_5W or NS to 1.5 to 25 mg PE/ml.
•Inspect parenteral solution before administration. Discard solution that contains particles or is discolored.
•Be aware that drug shouldn't be given I.M. for status epilepticus because I.V. route allows faster onset and peak.
•Keep in mind that I.V. fosphenytoin administration doesn't require use of a filter, as with phenytoin administration.
•Don't give fosphenytoin solution faster than 150 mg PE/minute because of the risk of hypotension. For a 50-kg (110-lb) patient, infusion typically takes 5 to 7 minutes. Fosphenytoin can be given more rapidly than I.V. phenytoin.
•Follow loading dose with maintenance dosage of oral or parenteral phenytoin or parenteral fosphenytoin, as prescribed.
•As prescribed, give I.V. benzodiazepine (such as lorazepam or diazepam) with fosphenytoin; otherwise, drug's full antiepileptic effect won't be immediate.
•Monitor ECG, blood pressure, and respiratory function for 10 to 20 minutes after infusion ends.
•Expect to obtain blood fosphenytoin (phenytoin) level 2 hours after I.V. infusion or 4 hours after I.M. injection. Therapeutic level generally ranges from 10 to 20 mcg/ml; steady-state may take several days to several weeks to reach.

•Be aware that I.V. or I.M. fosphenytoin may be substituted for oral phenytoin sodium at same total daily dose and frequency. If prescribed, give daily amount in two or more divided doses to maintain seizure control.
•When switching between phenytoin and fosphenytoin, remember that small differences in phenytoin bioavailability can lead to significant changes in blood phenytoin level and an increased risk of toxicity.
•If drug causes transient, infusion-related paresthesia and pruritus, decrease or discontinue infusion, as ordered.
•Monitor CBC for thrombocytopenia or leukopenia—signs of hematologic toxicity. Also monitor serum albumin level and results of renal and liver function tests.
•Anticipate increased frequency and severity of adverse reactions after I.V. administration in patients with hepatic or renal impairment or hypoalbuminemia.
•Discontinue drug, as ordered, if signs of hypersensitivity develop: acute hepatotoxicity (hepatic necrosis and hepatitis), fever, lymphadenopathy, and skin reactions during first 2 months of therapy.
•Monitor blood phenytoin level to detect early signs of toxicity, such as diplopia, nausea, severe confusion, slurred speech, and vomiting. Expect to reduce or stop drug if such signs develop.
•**WARNING** Monitor for seizures; at toxic levels, phenytoin is excitatory.
•**WARNING** If patient has bradycardia or heart block rhythm, notify prescriber and expect to withhold drug because severe cardiovascular reactions and death have occurred.
•Expect to provide vitamin D supplement if patient has inadequate dietary intake and is receiving long-term anticonvulsant treatment.
•Document type, onset, and characteristics of seizures as well as response to treatment.
PATIENT TEACHING
•Inform patient that fosphenytoin typically is used for short-term treatment.
•Instruct patient to notify prescriber immediately about bothersome symptoms, especially rash and swollen glands.
•Because gingival hyperplasia may develop during long-term therapy, emphasize the importance of good oral hygiene and gum massage.
•Urge patient to consume adequate amounts of vitamin D.

frovatriptan succinate

Frova

Class and Category

Chemical: Selective 5-hydroxytryptamine$_1$ (5-HT$_1$) receptor agonist, triptan
Therapeutic: Antimigraine agent
Pregnancy category: C

Indications and Dosages

➤ *To treat acute migraine with or without aura*

TABLETS

Adults. 2.5 mg, repeated in 2 hr if needed. *Maximum:* 7.5 mg/day.

Mechanism of Action

Binds to selective 5-HT$_1$ receptors (5-HT$_{1B}$ and 5-HT$_{1D}$) on extracerebral and intracranial arteries to inhibit excessive dilation of these vessels. This action may decrease carotid arterial blood flow, thus relieving acute migraines. Frovatriptan may also relieve pain by inhibiting the release of proinflammatory neuropeptides and reducing transmission of trigeminal nerve impulses from sensory nerve endings during a migraine attack.

Contraindications

Basilar or hemiplegic migraines; cerebrovascular, peripheral vascular, or ischemic or vasospastic coronary artery disease (CAD); hypersensitivity to frovatriptan or its components; uncontrolled hypertension; use within 24 hours of other serotonin-receptor agonists or of ergotamine-containing or ergot-type drugs

Interactions

DRUGS

dihydroergotamine mesylate, other ergotamine-containing drugs: Possibly prolonged vasospastic reaction
fluoxetine, other selective serotonin-reuptake inhibitors: Possibly weakness, hyperreflexia, and incoordination
oral contraceptives, propranolol: Possibly increased blood frovatriptan level

Adverse Reactions

CNS: Anxiety, dizziness, dysesthesia, fatigue, headache, hypoesthesia, insomnia, paresthesia
CV: Arrhythmias (such as bradycardia and tachycardia), chest pain, coronary artery vasospasm, ECG changes, MI, myocardial ischemia (transient), palpitations, ventricular fibrillation, ventricular tachycardia
EENT: Abnormal vision, dry mouth, indigestion, rhinitis, sinusitis, tinnitus
GI: Abdominal pain, diarrhea, indigestion, vomiting
MS: Skeletal pain
SKIN: Diaphoresis, flushing
Other: Generalized pain

Nursing Considerations

•Be aware that frovatriptan is used cautiously in patients with peripheral vascular disease because drug may cause vasospastic reactions, leading to vascular and colonic ischemia with abdominal pain and bloody diarrhea. Assess patient's peripheral circulation and bowel sounds during therapy.
•Don't administer frovatriptan within 24 hours of another 5-HT$_1$ receptor agonist, such as sumatriptan or rizatriptan, or of an ergotamine-containing or ergot-type drug, such as dihydroergotamine or methysergide.
•Administer tablet with fluids.
•Assess patient for headache before administering second dose. Don't administer more than three 2.5-mg tablets a day.
•**WARNING** Be aware that some patients have experienced serious adverse cardiac reactions—including fatal ones—after using 5-HT$_1$ receptor agonists. However, these reactions are extremely rare; most were reported in patients with risk factors for CAD.
•Assess cardiovascular status and institute continuous ECG monitoring, as ordered, immediately after drug administration in patients with cardiovascular risk factors because they're at risk for asymptomatic cardiac ischemia.
•Assess for arrhythmias, chest pain, and other signs of heart disease in patients with risk factors for CAD. Expect to periodically assess cardiovascular status of patients on long-term therapy.
•Be aware that the safety of treating more than four migraine attacks in 30 days (on average) has not been established.
•Regularly monitor blood pressure of hypertensive patients during therapy because frovatriptan may produce a transient increase in blood pressure.

PATIENT TEACHING
•Instruct patient to read and follow manufacturer's instructions for using frovatriptan to ensure maximum therapeutic results.
•Remind patient not to exceed prescribed daily dosage.
•Encourage patient to lie down in a dark, quiet room after taking drug to help relieve migraine.
•Instruct patient to seek emergency care for chest, jaw, or neck tightness after drug use because drug may cause coronary artery vasospasm.
•Urge patient to report palpitations to prescriber.
•Caution patient about possible adverse CNS effects, and advise her to avoid hazardous activities until drug's CNS effects are known.

furazolidone

Furoxone

Class and Category

Chemical: MAO inhibitor, nitrofuran derivative
Therapeutic: Antibiotic, antiprotozoal
Pregnancy category: C

Indications and Dosages

➤ *To treat bacterial diarrhea and cholera*
ORAL SUSPENSION, TABLETS
Adults and adolescents. 100 mg q 6 hr for 5 to 7 days.
Infants and children age 1 month and older. 1.25 mg/kg q 6 hr for 5 to 7 days. *Maximum:* 8.8 mg/kg/day.
➤ *To treat giardiasis*
ORAL SUSPENSION, TABLETS
Adults and adolescents. 100 mg q 6 hr for 7 to 10 days.
Infants and children age 1 month and older. 1.25 to 2 mg/kg q 6 hr for 7 to 10 days. *Maximum:* 8.8 mg/kg/day.

Mechanism of Action

May interfere with several bacterial enzyme systems through DNA strand damage. Furazolidone also prevents the inactivation of tyramine by GI and hepatic MAO because it is similar in structure and actions to MAO inhibitors.

Contraindications

Age less than 1 month; hypersensitivity to furazolidone, other nitrofurans, or their components

Interactions
DRUGS
levodopa: Increased therapeutic and adverse effects (particularly hypertension) of levodopa
meperidine: Possibly agitation, apnea, coma, diaphoresis, fever, and seizures
other MAO inhibitors, sedatives, sympathomimetics, tranquilizers, tricyclic antidepressants: Possibly sudden and severe hypertensive crisis
selective serotonin reuptake inhibitors: Increased risk of serotonin syndrome
FOODS
foods and beverages with high content of tyramine or other vasopressor amines: Possibly sudden and severe hypertensive crisis
ACTIVITIES
alcohol use: Possibly disulfiram-like reaction

Adverse Reactions
CNS: Headache, malaise
ENDO: Hypoglycemia
GI: Abdominal pain, diarrhea, nausea, vomiting
GU: Darkened urine
HEME: Hemolytic anemia, leukopenia
Other: Allergic reaction (arthralgia, dyspnea, fever, hypotension, urticaria, vesicular morbilliform rash)

Nursing Considerations
•Ask patient if she has a history of blood disorders—especially glucose-6-phosphate dehydrogenase (G6PD) deficiency—before giving furazolidone.
•As ordered, check G6PD level before giving furazolidone to whites of Mediterranean and Near Eastern origin, Asians, or blacks; G6PD deficiency may worsen drug's hemolytic effect.
•If no response occurs within 7 days, expect to discontinue drug because organism is resistant. Provide therapy with other antibiotics, as prescribed.
•If giardiasis symptoms persist, expect to obtain three stool specimens for analysis several days apart, starting 3 to 4 weeks after treatment ends.

PATIENT TEACHING
•Instruct patient to take drug at evenly spaced intervals around the clock.
•Advise patient to take drug with food if GI distress occurs.
•Direct patient to take a missed dose as soon as she remembers, unless it's nearly time for the next scheduled dose. Caution against double-dosing.
•Instruct patient to take furazolidone for the full time prescribed because stopping too soon could result in reinfection.
•Advise patient to store furazolidone between 59° and 86° F (15° and 30° C), protected from moisture and light.
•Inform patient that drug may cause dizziness and usually turns urine brown.
•Instruct patient to avoid alcohol during therapy and for 4 days afterward.
•Give patient a list of products to avoid during furazolidone therapy and for at least 2 weeks afterward, such as foods and beverages that contain tyramine and other vasopressor amines (for example, ripe cheese, beer, red and white wine, and smoked or pickled meat, poultry, or fish), OTC appetite suppressants, cough and cold medicines, and other drugs, unless prescribed.
•Instruct patient to notify prescriber if she experiences difficult breathing, fever, flushing, itching, muscle aches, or rash.

furosemide

Apo-Furosemide (CAN), Furoside (CAN), Lasix, Lasix Special (CAN), Myrosemide, Novosemide (CAN), Uritol (CAN)

Class and Category
Chemical: Sulfonamide
Therapeutic: Antihypertensive, diuretic
Pregnancy category: C

Indications and Dosages
➤ *To reduce edema caused by cirrhosis, heart failure, and renal disease, including nephrotic syndrome*
ORAL SOLUTION, TABLETS
Adults. 20 to 80 mg as a single dose, increased by 20 to 40 mg q 6 to 8 hr until desired response occurs. *Maximum:* 600 mg/day.
Children. 2 mg/kg as a single dose, increased by 1 to 2 mg/kg q 6 to 8 hr until desired response occurs. *Maximum:* 6 mg/kg/dose.

I.V. INFUSION, I.V. OR I.M. INJECTION
Adults. 20 to 40 mg as a single dose, increased by 20 mg q 2 hr until desired response occurs.
Children. 1 mg/kg as a single dose, increased by 1 mg/kg q 2 hr until desired response occurs. *Maximum:* 6 mg/kg/dose.
DOSAGE ADJUSTMENT Initial single dose limited to 20 mg for elderly patients.
➤ *To manage mild to moderate hypertension, as adjunct to treat acute pulmonary edema and hypertensive crisis*
ORAL SOLUTION, TABLETS
Adults. *Initial:* 40 mg b.i.d., adjusted until desired response occurs. *Maximum:* 600 mg/day.
I.V. INFUSION OR INJECTION
Adults with normal renal function. 40 to 80 mg as a single dose over several minutes.
Adults with acute renal failure or pulmonary edema. 100 to 200 mg as a single dose over several minutes.
DOSAGE ADJUSTMENT For patients with acute pulmonary edema without hypertensive crisis, dosage reduced to 40 mg followed by 80 mg 1 hr later if therapeutic response doesn't occur.

Route	Onset	Peak	Duration
P.O.	20 to 60 min	1 to 2 hr	6 to 8 hr
I.V.	5 min	In 30 min	2 hr
I.M.	30 min	Unknown	2 hr

Mechanism of Action
Inhibits sodium and water reabsorption in the loop of Henle and increases urine formation. As the body's plasma volume decreases, aldosterone production increases, which promotes sodium reabsorption and the loss of potassium and hydrogen ions. Furosemide also increases the excretion of calcium, magnesium, bicarbonate, ammonium, and phosphate. By reducing intracellular and extracellular fluid volume, the drug reduces blood pressure and decreases cardiac output. Over time, cardiac output returns to normal.

Incompatibilities
Don't mix furosemide (a milky, buffered alkaline solution) with highly acidic solutions.

Contraindications

Anuria unresponsive to furosemide; hypersensitivity to furosemide, sulfonamides, or their components

Interactions

DRUGS

ACE inhibitors: Possibly first-dose hypotension
aminoglycosides, cisplatin: Increased risk of ototoxicity
amiodarone: Increased risk of arrhythmias from hypokalemia
chloral hydrate: Possibly diaphoresis, hot flashes, and hypertension
digoxin: Increased risk of digitalis toxicity related to hypokalemia
insulin, oral antidiabetic drugs: Increased blood glucose level
lithium: Increased risk of lithium toxicity
NSAIDs: Possibly decreased diuresis
phenytoin, probenecid: Possibly decreased therapeutic effects of furosemide
propranolol: Possibly increased blood propranolol level
thiazide diuretics: Possibly profound diuresis and electrolyte imbalances

ACTIVITIES

alcohol use: Possibly increased hypotensive and diuretic effects of furosemide

Adverse Reactions

CNS: Dizziness, fever, headache, paresthesia, restlessness, vertigo, weakness
CV: Orthostatic hypotension, shock, thromboembolism, thrombophlebitis
EENT: Blurred vision, ototoxicity, stomatitis, tinnitus, transient hearing loss (rapid I.V. injection), yellow vision
ENDO: Hyperglycemia
GI: Abdominal cramps, anorexia, constipation, diarrhea, indigestion, nausea, pancreatitis, vomiting
GU: Bladder spasms, glycosuria
HEME: Agranulocytosis (rare), anemia, aplastic anemia (rare), azotemia, hemolytic anemia, leukopenia, thrombocytopenia
MS: Muscle spasms
SKIN: Erythema multiforme, exfoliative dermatitis, jaundice, photosensitivity, pruritus, purpura, rash, urticaria
Other: Allergic reaction (interstitial nephritis, necrotizing vasculitis, systemic vasculitis), dehydration, hyperuricemia, hypochloremia, hypokalemia, hyponatremia, hypovolemia

Nursing Considerations

•**WARNING** Use furosemide cautiously in patients with advanced hepatic cirrhosis, especially those who also have a history of electrolyte imbalance or hepatic encephalopathy; drug may lead to lethal hepatic coma.
•Obtain patient's weight before and periodically during furosemide therapy to monitor fluid loss.
•For once-a-day dosing, give drug in the morning so patient's sleep won't be interrupted by increased need to urinate.
•Prepare drug for infusion with NS, LR, or D$_5$W.
•Administer drug slowly I.V. over 1 to 2 minutes to prevent ototoxicity.
•Expect patient to have periodic hearing tests during prolonged or high-dose I.V. therapy.
•Monitor blood pressure and hepatic and renal function as well as BUN, blood glucose, and serum creatinine, electrolyte, and uric acid levels, as appropriate.
•Be aware that elderly patients are more susceptible to hypotensive and electrolyte-altering effects and thus are at greater risk for shock and thromboembolism.
•If patient is at high risk for hypokalemia, give potassium supplements along with furosemide, as prescribed.
•Expect to discontinue furosemide at maximum dosage if oliguria persists for more than 24 hours.
•Be aware that furosemide may worsen left ventricular hypertrophy and adversely affect glucose tolerance and lipid metabolism.
•Notify prescriber if patient experiences hearing loss, vertigo, or ringing, buzzing, or sense of fullness in her ears. Drug may need to be discontinued.

PATIENT TEACHING

•Instruct patient to take furosemide at the same time each day to maintain therapeutic effects. Urge her to take it as prescribed, even if she feels well.
•Instruct patient to take the last dose of furosemide several hours before bedtime to avoid sleep interruption from diuresis. If patient receives once-daily dosing, advise her to take the dose in the morning to avoid sleep disturbance caused by nocturia.
•Advise patient to change position slowly to minimize effects of orthostatic hypotension and to take furosemide with food or milk to reduce GI distress.
•Caution patient about drinking alcoholic

E
F

beverages, standing for prolonged periods, and exercising in hot weather because these actions increase the hypotensive effect of furosemide.
•Emphasize the importance of weight and diet control, especially limiting sodium intake.
•Unless contraindicated, urge patient to eat more high-potassium foods and to take a potassium supplement, if prescribed, to prevent hypokalemia.
•Instruct patient to keep follow-up appointments with prescriber to monitor progress. Urge her to notify prescriber about persistent, severe nausea, vomiting, and diarrhea because they may cause dehydration.
•Inform diabetic patient that furosemide may increase blood glucose level, and advise her to check her blood glucose level frequently.

G·H·I

gabapentin
Neurontin

Class and Category
Chemical: Cyclohexane-acetic acid derivative
Therapeutic: Anticonvulsant
Pregnancy category: C

Indications and Dosages
➤ *To manage postherpetic neuralgia*
CAPSULES, ORAL SOLUTION, TABLETS
Adults. *Initial:* 300 mg on day 1, increased to 300 mg b.i.d. on day 2, increased to 300 mg t.i.d. on day 3, and increased gradually thereafter according to pain response, up to 600 mg t.i.d. *Maximum:* 1800 mg/day.
➤ *As adjunct to treat partial seizures*
CAPSULES, ORAL SOLUTION, TABLETS
Adults and adolescents. *Initial:* 300 mg t.i.d., increased gradually according to clinical response. *Maintenance:* 900 to 1,800 mg/day. *Maximum:* 3,600 mg/day.
DOSAGE ADJUSTMENT Dosage reduced to 300 mg b.i.d. if creatinine clearance is 30 to 60 ml/min/1.73 m^2; to 300 mg q.d. if creatinine clearance is 15 to 29 ml/min/1.73 m^2; and to 300 mg q.o.d. if creatinine clearance is less than 15 ml/min/1.73 m^2.

Mechanism of Action
Is structurally similar to endogenous gamma-aminobutyric acid (GABA), the most common inhibitory neurotransmitter in the brain. Although gababentin's exact mechanism of action is unknown, GABA is known to inhibit the rapid firing of neurons, which is associated with seizures.

Contraindications
Hypersensitivity to gabapentin or its components

Interactions
DRUGS
aluminum- and magnesium-containing antacids: Decreased gabapentin bioavailability

CNS depressants: Increased CNS depression
ACTIVITIES
alcohol use: Increased CNS depression

Adverse Reactions
CNS: Agitation, altered proprioception, amnesia, anxiety, apathy, aphasia, asthenia, ataxia, cerebellar dysfunction, chills, CNS tumors, decreased or absent reflexes, delusions, depersonalization, depression, dizziness, dream disturbances, dysesthesia, dystonia, emotional lability, euphoria, facial paralysis, fatigue, fever, hallucinations, headache, hemiplegia, hostility, hyperkinesia, hyperreflexia, hypoesthesia, hypotonia, intracranial hemorrhage, lack of coordination, malaise, migraine headache, nervousness, paranoia, paresis, paresthesia, positive Babinski's sign, psychosis, sedation, seizures, somnolence, stupor, subdural hematoma, suicidal tendencies, syncope, tremor, vertigo
CV: Angina, hypertension, hypotension, murmur, palpitations, peripheral edema, peripheral vascular insufficiency, tachycardia, vasodilation
EENT: Abnormal vision, amblyopia, blepharospasm, cataracts, conjunctivitis, diplopia, dry eyes and mouth, earache, epistaxis, eye hemorrhage, eye pain, gingival bleeding, gingivitis, glossitis, hearing loss, increased salivation, inner ear infection, loss of taste, nystagmus, pharyngitis, photophobia, ptosis (bilateral or unilateral), rhinitis, sensation of fullness in ears, stomatitis, taste perversion, tinnitus, tooth discoloration, visual field defects
GI: Abdominal pain, anorexia, constipation, diarrhea, fecal incontinence, flatulence, gastroenteritis, hemorrhoids, hepatomegaly, increased appetite, indigestion, melena, nausea, thirst, vomiting
GU: Decreased libido, impotence
HEME: Anemia, decreased WBC count, leukopenia, thrombocytopenia
MS: Arthralgia, arthritis, back pain, bone fractures, dysarthria, joint stiffness or swelling, muscle twitching, myalgia, positive Romberg test, tendinitis
RESP: Apnea, cough, dyspnea, pneumonia
SKIN: Abrasion, acne, alopecia, cyst, diaphoresis, dry skin, eczema, hirsutism, pruritus, purpura, rash, seborrhea, urticaria
Other: Facial edema, lymphadenopathy, viral infection, weight gain or loss

G
H
I

Nursing Considerations
•As needed, open gabapentin capsules and mix contents with water, fruit juice, applesauce, or pudding before administration.
•Administer initial dose at bedtime to minimize adverse reactions, especially ataxia, dizziness, fatigue, and somnolence.
•Give drug at least 2 hours after giving an antacid.
•Don't exceed 12 hours between doses on a 3-times-a-day schedule.
•Be aware that routine monitoring of blood gabapentin level isn't necessary.
•WARNING To discontinue drug or switch to an alternate anticonvulsant, expect to change gradually over at least 1 week, as prescribed, to avoid loss of seizure control.
•Monitor renal function test results, and expect to adjust dosage, if necessary.
PATIENT TEACHING
•If patient has trouble swallowing gabapentin capsules, advise him to open them and sprinkle contents in juice or on soft food immediately before use.
•Instruct patient not to take drug within 2 hours after taking an antacid.
•Advise patient to take a missed dose as soon as he remembers. If the next scheduled dose is less than 2 hours away, tell him to wait 1 to 2 hours before taking it and then resume his regular dosing schedule. Caution against double-dosing.
•Caution patient not to stop taking drug abruptly.
•Inform patient about possible ataxia, dizziness, drowsiness, and nystagmus. Advise him to avoid potentially hazardous activities until drug's CNS effects are known.
•To prevent complications from adverse oral reactions (such as gingivitis), encourage patient to use good oral hygiene and to seek routine dental care.
•Inform patient that drug's adverse effects usually are mild to moderate and decline with continued use.
•Urge patient to keep follow-up appointments with prescriber to check progress.

galantamine hydrobromide
Reminyl

Class and Category
Chemical: Tertiary alkaloid
Therapeutic: Antidementia agent
Pregnancy category: B

Indications and Dosages
➤ *To treat mild to moderate Alzheimer's-type dementia*
ORAL SOLUTION, TABLETS
Adults. *Initial:* 4 mg b.i.d. Dosage increased by 8 mg/day q 4 wk, if tolerated. *Maximum:* 12 mg b.i.d.
DOSAGE ADJUSTMENT For patients with moderately impaired hepatic or renal function, maximum dosage shouldn't exceed 16 mg/day.

Route	Onset	Peak	Duration
P.O.	Unknown	About 1 hr	Unknown

Mechanism of Action
Reduces acetylcholine metabolism by competitively and reversibly inhibiting the brain enzyme acetylcholinesterase. Acetylcholine-producing neurons degenerate in the brains of patients with Alzheimer's disease. Inhibition of acetylcholinesterase increases the amount of acetylcholine, which is necessary for nerve impulse transmission.

Contraindications
Hypersensitivity to galantamine hydrobromide or its components, severe hepatic or renal impairment (creatinine clearance less than 9 ml/min/1.73 m^2)

Interactions
DRUGS
amitriptyline, fluoxetine, fluvoxamine, quinidine: Possibly decreased galantamine clearance
anticholinergics: Possibly interference with cholinesterase activity
cholinergic agonists, cholinesterase inhibitors, neuromuscular blockers: Possibly exaggerated effects of these drugs and galantamine
cimetidine: Possibly increased galantamine bioavailability
ketoconazole, paroxetine: Increased galantamine bioavailability

Adverse Reactions
CNS: Depression, dizziness, fatigue, headache, insomnia, somnolence, syncope, tremor
CV: Bradycardia
EENT: Rhinitis

GI: Abdominal pain, anorexia, diarrhea, indigestion, nausea, vomiting
GU: Hematuria, UTI
HEME: Anemia
Other: Weight loss

Nursing Considerations
•Administer galantamine twice daily with morning and evening meals, and ensure adequate fluid intake to prevent GI symptoms.
•If therapy is interrupted for several days, expect to restart drug at lowest dose because drug's benefits are lost when it is discontinued.
•Monitor patient's heart rate closely because drug can have vagotonic effects on heart's sinoatrial and atrioventricular nodes, which can lead to bradycardia.
•Monitor patients, especially those at risk for ulcer disease and those using NSAIDs, for symptoms of active or occult GI bleeding because gastric acid secretion may increase as a result of increased cholinergic activity.
•Monitor patients with severe asthma or obstructive pulmonary disease for exacerbation of symptoms because galantamine has cholinergic-like effects that may precipitate bronchospasm.
•Continue to assess patient for progressive deterioration of mental status because drug becomes less effective as Alzheimer's disease progresses and the number of intact cholinergic neurons declines.

PATIENT TEACHING
•Instruct patient or caregiver to administer drug with morning and evening meals.
•Advise patient or caregiver to notify prescriber immediately if therapy is stopped for several days. Prescriber may restart drug at lowest dose.
•Advise patient not to drive or perform activities requiring high levels of alertness, especially during first weeks of treatment, because drug may cause dizziness and drowsiness.
•Inform patient and family members that drug isn't a cure for Alzheimer's disease.

gatifloxacin

Tequin

Class and Category
Chemical: Fluoroquinolone
Therapeutic: Antibiotic
Pregnancy category: C

Indications and Dosages
➤ *To treat acute bacterial exacerbations of chronic bronchitis caused by* Haemophilus influenzae, H. parainfluenzae, Moraxella catarrhalis, Staphylococcus aureus, *or* Streptococcus pneumoniae
TABLETS, I.V. INFUSION
Adults. 400 mg q.d. for 5 days.
➤ *To treat complicated UTIs caused by* Escherichia coli, Klebsiella pneumoniae, *or* Proteus mirabilis; *and acute pyelonephritis caused by* E. coli
TABLETS, I.V. INFUSION
Adults. 400 mg q.d. for 7 to 10 days.
➤ *To treat acute sinusitis due to* H. influenzae *or* S. pneumoniae
TABLETS, I.V. INFUSION
Adults. 400 mg q.d. for 10 days.
➤ *To treat community-acquired pneumonia caused by* Chlamydia pneumoniae, H. influenzae, H. parainfluenzae, Legionella pneumophila, M. catarrhalis, Mycoplasma pneumoniae, S. aureus, *or* S. pneumoniae
TABLETS, I.V. INFUSION
Adults. 400 mg q.d. for 7 to 14 days.
➤ *To treat uncomplicated cystitis caused by* E. coli, K. pneumoniae, *or* P. mirabilis
TABLETS, I.V. INFUSION
Adults. 400 mg as a single dose or 200 mg q.d. for 3 days.
➤ *To treat uncomplicated urethral gonorrhea in men, and cervical and acute rectal gonorrhea in women caused by* Neisseria gonorrhoeae
TABLETS, I.V. INFUSION
Adults. 400 mg as a single dose.
DOSAGE ADJUSTMENT For patients with creatinine clearance of less than 40 ml/min/1.73 m² and those receiving hemodialysis or continuous peritoneal dialysis, initial dose of 400 mg is followed by reduced dosage of 200 mg q.d., as prescribed. No dosage adjustment is required for single-dose treatments or for treatment of uncomplicated cystitis.

Contraindications
Hypersensitivity to gatifloxacin, other fluoroquinolones, or their components

Interactions
DRUGS
aluminum-, magnesium-, or zinc-containing antacids: Reduced GI absorption and blood level of gatifloxacin

iron: Possibly reduced effectiveness of gatifloxacin
oral antidiabetic drugs: Possibly altered glucose control
probenecid: Increased blood level and sustained half-life of gatifloxacin

Mechanism of Action

Interferes with bacterial cell replication by inhibiting the bacterial enzyme DNA gyrase, which is essential for replication, transcription, and repair of bacterial DNA. Gatifloxacin also inhibits topoisomerase IV, an enzyme involved in the partitioning of chromosomal DNA during bacterial cell division.

Adverse Reactions

CNS: Chills, dizziness, fever, headache, insomnia, nightmares, paresthesia, tremor, vertigo
CV: Chest pain, palpitations, peripheral edema, vasodilation
ENDO: Hyperglycemia, hypoglycemia
EENT: Abnormal vision, glossitis, mouth ulcers, oral candidiasis, pharyngitis, stomatitis, taste perversion, tinnitus
GI: Abdominal pain, constipation, diarrhea, indigestion, nausea, vomiting
GU: Dysuria, hematuria, vaginitis
MS: Back pain
RESP: Dyspnea
SKIN: Diaphoresis, rash
Other: Infusion site inflammation

Nursing Considerations

• Administer oral gatifloxacin at least 4 hours before or after preparations containing aluminum, magnesium, zinc, or iron.
• Reconstitute gatifloxacin concentrate for infusion with an appropriate amount of D_5W, NS, 0.45NS, D_5LR, 5% sodium bicarbonate, Plasma-Lyte 56 and D_5W, or M/6 sodium lactate to create a final concentration of 2 mg/ml. Use solutions prepared with 5% sodium bicarbonate immediately, as prescribed. Be aware that no further dilution is needed when using premixed flexible bags.
• Don't add other drugs to gatifloxacin injection or infuse gatifloxacin through same I.V. line as other drugs. Inspect I.V. solution before infusion. Use only if solution remains clear and light yellow or greenish yellow. Discard if particulate matter is present.

• Infuse I.V. solution over 60 minutes, using an infusion pump to avoid too-rapid or bolus administration.
• **WARNING** Be aware that gatifloxacin may caused prolonged QTc interval, leading to an increased risk of ventricular arrhythmia in susceptible patients, especially those with hypokalemia and those taking quinidine, procainamide, amiodarone, or sotalol.
• Monitor patient for nightmares and insomnia because gatifloxacin may cause excessive CNS stimulation. If patient develops these symptoms, notify prescriber immediately and expect to discontinue drug.
• Monitor blood glucose level in patients with diabetes to detect hypoglycemia or hyperglycemia, which may be caused by gatifloxacin.
• Be aware that use of any fluoroquinolone may increase the risk of tendon rupture.

PATIENT TEACHING
• Instruct patient to complete the full course of gatifloxacin therapy, as prescribed.
• Advise patient to take drug at least 4 hours before or after preparations containing aluminum, magnesium, iron, or zinc.
• Instruct patient to notify prescriber at first sign of allergic reaction, such as rash.
• Advise patient to notify prescriber immediately if he experiences tendon pain, inflammation, or rupture.
• Advise diabetic patient taking oral antidiabetic drugs to monitor his blood glucose level frequently and to notify prescriber of significant changes.

gemfibrozil

Apo-Gemfibrozil (CAN), Gen-Fibro (CAN), Lopid, Novo-Gemfibrozil (CAN), Nu-Gemfibrozil (CAN)

Class and Category

Chemical: Fibric acid derivative, phenoxypentanoic acid
Therapeutic: Antihyperlipidemic
Pregnancy category: C

Indications and Dosages

➤ *As adjunct (with diet) to treat hyperlipidemia types IIb, IV, and V*
CAPSULES, TABLETS
Adults. 600 mg a.c. b.i.d.

Route	Onset	Peak	Duration
P.O.	2 to 5 days	4 wk	Unknown

Mechanism of Action

May decrease hepatic triglyceride production by reducing VLDL synthesis, inhibiting peripheral lipolysis, and decreasing hepatic extraction of free fatty acids. Gemfibrozil also may inhibit the synthesis and increase the clearance of apolipoprotein B, a carrier molecule for VLDL. In addition, it may accelerate the turnover and removal of total cholesterol from the liver while increasing cholesterol excretion into the feces. As a result of these actions, triglyceride, total cholesterol, and VLDL levels decrease; the HDL level increases; and the LDL level is unaffected.

Contraindications

Gallbladder disease, hepatic or severe renal dysfunction, hypersensitivity to gemfibrozil or its components

Interactions

DRUGS

chenodiol, ursodiol: Decreased effectiveness of gemfibrozil
HMG-CoA reductase inhibitors: Increased risk of rhabdomyolysis and acute renal failure
oral anticoagulants: Increased anticoagulant effects

Adverse Reactions

CNS: Chills, fatigue, headache, hypoesthesia, paresthesia, seizures, somnolence, syncope, vertigo
CV: Vasculitis
EENT: Blurred vision, cataracts, hoarseness, retinal edema, taste perversion
GI: Abdominal or epigastric pain, cholelithiasis, colitis, diarrhea, flatulence, heartburn, hepatoma, nausea, pancreatitis, vomiting
GU: Decreased male fertility, dysuria, impotence
HEME: Anemia, bone marrow hypoplasia, eosinophilia, leukopenia, thrombocytopenia
MS: Arthralgia, back pain, myalgia, myasthenia, myopathy, myositis, rhabdomyolysis, synovitis
RESP: Cough
SKIN: Eczema, jaundice, pruritus, rash
Other: Anaphylaxis, angioedema, increased risk of bacterial and viral infections, lupus-like symptoms, weight loss

Nursing Considerations

• Monitor serum triglyceride and cholesterol levels, as appropriate.
• Periodically review CBC and liver function test results during therapy, as ordered.
• If serum triglyceride and cholesterol levels don't improve within 3 months, expect to switch to a different drug, as prescribed.

PATIENT TEACHING

• Instruct patient to take gemfibrozil 30 minutes before breakfast and 30 minutes before dinner.
• Advise patient to take a missed dose as soon as he remembers, unless it's nearly time for the next dose. Caution against double-dosing.
• Stress the importance of a low-fat diet, regular exercise, alcohol avoidance, and smoking cessation, as appropriate.
• Caution patient to avoid potentially hazardous activities until drug's CNS effects are known.
• Instruct patient to notify prescriber if he experiences chills; cough; fever; hoarseness; lower back, side, or muscle pain; painful or difficult urination; severe abdominal pain with nausea and vomiting; tiredness; or weakness.
• If patient also takes an oral anticoagulant, urge him to report unusual bleeding or bruising; anticoagulant dosage may need to be reduced.
• Advise patient to keep scheduled appointments with prescriber to check progress.

gentamicin sulfate

Cidomycin (CAN), Garamycin, G-Mycin, Jenamicin

Class and Category

Chemical: Aminoglycoside derived from *Micromonospora purpurea*
Therapeutic: Antibiotic
Pregnancy category: D

Indications and Dosages

➤ *To treat serious bacterial infections caused by aerobic gram-negative organisms and some gram-positive organisms, including Citrobacter sp., Enterobacter sp., Escherichia coli, Klebsiella sp., Proteus sp., Pseudomonas aeruginosa, Serratia sp., Staphylococcus aureus, and many strains of Streptococcus sp.*

I.V. INFUSION, I.M. INJECTION
Adults and adolescents. 1 to 1.7 mg/kg q 8 hr for 7 to 10 days.
Children. 2 to 2.5 mg/kg q 8 hr for 7 to 10 days.
Infants. 2.5 mg/kg q 8 to 16 hr for 7 to 10 days.
Premature or full-term neonates up to age 1 week. 2.5 mg/kg q 12 to 24 hr for 7 to 10 days.

INTRATHECAL (INTRALUMBAR OR INTRAVENTRICULAR) INJECTION
Adults and adolescents. 4 to 8 mg q.d.
Infants and children age 3 months and older. 1 to 2 mg q.d.

➤ *To treat uncomplicated UTIs*

I.V. INFUSION, I.M. INJECTION
Adults and adolescents who weigh more than 60 kg (132 lb). 160 mg q.d. or 80 mg q 12 hr.
Adults and adolescents who weigh less than 60 kg. 3 mg/kg q.d. or 1.5 mg/kg q 12 hr.
DOSAGE ADJUSTMENT Supplemental dose of 1 to 1.7 mg/kg (2 to 2.5 mg/kg for children) given by I.M. injection or I.V. infusion after hemodialysis, based on infection severity.

> **Mechanism of Action**
> Binds to negatively charged sites on the outer cell membrane of bacteria, thereby disrupting the membrane's integrity. Gentamicin also binds to bacterial ribosomal subunits and inhibits protein synthesis. Both actions lead to cell death.

Incompatibilities
Don't administer gentamicin through same I.V. line as other drugs, especially beta-lactam antibiotics (penicillins and cephalosporins), because substantial mutual inactivation may occur. Give drugs through separate sites.

Contraindications
Hypersensitivity or serious toxic reaction to other aminoglycosides, hypersensitivity to gentamicin or its components

Interactions
DRUGS
aminoglycosides (concurrent use of two or more): Decreased bacterial uptake of each drug, increased risk of ototoxicity and nephrotoxicity
cephalosporins, enflurane, methoxyflurane, vancomycin: Increased risk of nephrotoxicity

loop diuretics: Increased risk of ototoxicity and nephrotoxicity
neuromuscular blockers: Prolonged respiratory depression, increased neuromuscular blockade
penicillins: Inactivation of gentamicin by certain penicillins, increased risk of nephrotoxicity

Adverse Reactions
CNS: Acute organic mental syndrome, confusion, depression, fever, headache, increased protein in cerebrospinal fluid, lethargy, myasthenia gravis–like syndrome, neurotoxicity (dizziness, hearing loss, tinnitus, vertigo), peripheral neuropathy or encephalopathy (muscle twitching, numbness, seizures, skin tingling), pseudotumor cerebri
CV: Hypertension, hypotension, palpitations
EENT: Blurred vision, increased salivation, laryngeal edema, ototoxicity, stomatitis, vision changes
GI: Anorexia, nausea, splenomegaly, transient hepatomegaly, vomiting
GU: Nephrotoxicity
HEME: Anemia, eosinophilia, granulocytopenia, increased or decreased reticulocyte count, leukopenia, thrombocytopenia
MS: Arthralgia, leg cramps
RESP: Pulmonary fibrosis, respiratory depression
SKIN: Alopecia, generalized burning sensation, pruritus, purpura, rash, urticaria
Other: Anaphylaxis, injection site pain, superinfection, weight loss

Nursing Considerations
•Before gentamicin therapy begins, expect to obtain a body fluid or tissue specimen for culture and sensitivity testing, as ordered, or check test results, if available.
•Be aware that drug is best absorbed when administered by I.V. route. The blood level is unpredictable after I.M. administration.
•For I.V. use, dilute each dose with 50 to 200 ml of NS or D_5W to yield no more than 1 mg/ml. Administer slowly over 30 to 60 minutes.
•Don't administer gentamicin through same I.V. line as other drugs without first consulting pharmacist.
•Expect to adjust dosage based on peak and trough blood drug levels drawn after third maintenance dose, as prescribed.
•Don't give gentamicin by S.C. route because it may be painful.

• When assisting with intrathecal injection, use only 2 mg/ml of preservative-free preparation. Drug may be injected directly or delivered by implanted reservoir.
• Don't give gentamicin to pregnant patient because drug can cause hearing loss in fetus.
• **WARNING** When giving pediatric injectable form of drug, be alert for allergic reactions—including anaphylaxis and, possibly, life-threatening asthmatic episodes—because drug contains sodium bisulfite.
• Assess for signs of other infections because gentamicin may cause overgrowth of nonsusceptible organisms.
• Be aware that premature infants, neonates, and elderly patients have an increased risk of nephrotoxicity.

PATIENT TEACHING
• Stress the importance of completing the full course of gentamicin therapy.
• Instruct patient to immediately report adverse reactions, such as hearing loss, to avoid permanent effects.

glimepiride

Amaryl

Class and Category
Chemical: Sulfonylurea
Therapeutic: Antidiabetic
Pregnancy category: C

Indications and Dosages
➤ *To control blood glucose level in type 2 diabetes mellitus*

TABLETS
Adults. 1 to 2 mg q.d. with first meal of the day. *Maintenance:* 1 to 4 mg q.d., increased by 1 to 2 mg q 1 to 2 wk as needed for blood glucose control. *Maximum:* 8 mg/day.
DOSAGE ADJUSTMENT Initial dosage reduced to 1 mg q.d. if needed for patients with renal impairment.

➤ *As adjunct (with insulin) to control blood glucose level*

TABLETS
Adults. 8 mg q.d. with low-dose insulin.

Route	Onset	Peak	Duration
P.O.	2 to 3 hr	Unknown	Over 24 hr

Mechanism of Action
Stimulates insulin release from beta cells in the pancreas. The drug also increases peripheral tissue sensitivity to insulin, either by enhancing insulin binding to cellular receptors or by increasing the number of insulin receptors.

Contraindications
Diabetes complicated by pregnancy; diabetic coma; hypersensitivity to glimepiride, sulfonylureas, or their components; ketoacidosis; sole therapy for type 1 diabetes mellitus

Interactions
DRUGS
ACE inhibitors, anabolic steroids, androgens, azole antifungals, bromocriptine, chloramphenicol, disopyramide, fibric acid derivatives, guanethidine, H_2-receptor antagonists, insulin, magnesium salts, MAO inhibitors, methyldopa, octreotide, oral anticoagulants, oxyphenbutazone, phenylbutazone, probenecid, quinidine, salicylates, sulfonamides, tetracycline, theophylline, tricyclic antidepressants, urinary acidifiers: Increased risk of hypoglycemia
asparaginase, calcium channel blockers, cholestyramine, clonidine, corticosteroids, danazol, diazoxide, estrogen, glucagon, hydantoins, isoniazid, lithium, morphine, nicotinic acid, oral contraceptives, phenothiazines, rifabutin, rifampin, sympathomimetics, thiazide diuretics, thyroid drugs, urinary alkalinizers: Increased risk of hyperglycemia
beta blockers: Possibly hyperglycemia or masking of hypoglycemia signs
digoxin: Increased risk of digitalis toxicity
pentamidine: Initially hypoglycemia and then hyperglycemia if beta cell damage occurs
ACTIVITIES
alcohol use: Altered blood glucose control (usually hypoglycemia)

Adverse Reactions
CNS: Abnormal gait, anxiety, asthenia, chills, depression, dizziness, fatigue, headache, hypertonia, hypoesthesia, insomnia, malaise, migraine headache, nervousness, paresthesia, somnolence, syncope, tremor, vertigo
CV: Arrhythmias, edema, hypertension, vasculitis

EENT: Blurred vision, conjunctivitis, eye pain, pharyngitis, retinal hemorrhage, rhinitis, taste perversion, tinnitus
ENDO: Hypoglycemia
GI: Anorexia, constipation, diarrhea, elevated liver function test results, epigastric discomfort or fullness, flatulence, heartburn, hunger, nausea, proctocolitis, trace blood in stool, vomiting
GU: Darkened urine, decreased libido, dysuria, polyuria
HEME: Agranulocytosis, aplastic anemia, eosinophilia, hemolytic anemia, hepatic porphyria, leukopenia, pancytopenia
MS: Arthralgia, leg cramps, myalgia
RESP: Dyspnea
SKIN: Allergic skin reactions, diaphoresis, eczema, erythema multiforme, exfoliative dermatitis, flushing, jaundice, lichenoid reactions, maculopapular or morbilliform rash, photosensitivity, urticaria
Other: Disulfiram-like reaction

Nursing Considerations
•Monitor fasting blood glucose level to determine response to glimepiride. Expect to check glycosylated hemoglobin level every 3 to 6 months to evaluate long-term blood glucose control.
•Arrange for dietary consultation and diabetic teaching, if appropriate. Ask dietitian to discuss with patient the amount of alcohol he can consume without risking hypoglycemia.
•Expect to switch patient to insulin therapy, as prescribed, during physical stress, such as infection, surgery, and trauma.
•WARNING Expect a higher risk of hypoglycemia when giving glimepiride to a malnourished or debilitated patient or one with renal, hepatic, pituitary, or adrenal insufficiency.

Patient Teaching
•Instruct patient to take glimepiride just before the first meal of the day. Caution him not to skip the meal after taking drug.
•Urge patient not to skip doses or increase dosage without consulting prescriber.
•Urge patient to report signs of hypoglycemia, such as anxiety, confusion, dizziness, excessive sweating, headache, and nausea.
•Encourage patient to carry candy or other simple sugars to treat mild hypoglycemia.
•Advise patient to consult prescriber before taking any OTC drug.
•Urge patient to carry identification indicating that he has diabetes.

•Teach patient how to monitor his blood glucose level.
•Teach patient about exercise, diet, signs of hyperglycemia and hypoglycemia, hygiene, foot care, and ways to avoid infection.
•Instruct patient to notify prescriber if he experiences darkened urine, difficulty controlling his blood glucose level, easy bruising, fever, rash, sore throat, or unusual bleeding.
•If photosensitivity is a problem, instruct patient to avoid direct sunlight and to wear sunscreen.

glipizide
Glucotrol, Glucotrol XL

Class and Category
Chemical: Sulfonylurea
Therapeutic: Antidiabetic
Pregnancy category: C

Indications and Dosages
➤ *To control blood glucose level in type 2 diabetes mellitus*

E.R. TABLETS
Adults. *Initial:* 5 mg q.d. with breakfast. Dosage increased by 5 mg/day q 3 mo, if needed. *Maintenance:* 5 to 10 mg q.d. *Maximum:* 20 mg/day.

TABLETS
Adults. *Initial:* 5 mg 30 min before first meal of the day. Dosage adjusted by 2.5 to 5 mg q 2 to 3 days. For daily dose of 15 mg or less, give as a single dose. For dose above 15 mg/day, give in 2 divided doses. *Maximum:* 40 mg/day.

➤ *As adjunct to or replacement for insulin therapy in type 2 diabetes mellitus*

CAPSULES, TABLETS
Adults who need more than 20 U insulin/day. 5 mg q.d., while decreasing insulin dosage by one-half. Further insulin reductions are based on clinical response.
DOSAGE ADJUSTMENT Initial dosage reduced to 2.5 mg q.d. if needed for patients over age 65 and those with hepatic disease.

Route	Onset	Peak	Duration
P.O.	10 to 30 min	30 min to 2 hr	12 to 24 hr
P.O. (E.R.)	Unknown	Unknown	18 to 24 hr

Mechanism of Action

Stimulates insulin release from beta cells in the pancreas. Glipizide also increases peripheral tissue sensitivity to insulin, either by enhancing insulin binding to cellular receptors or by increasing the number of insulin receptors.

Contraindications

Diabetes complicated by pregnancy; diabetic coma; hypersensitivity to glipizide, sulfonylureas, or their components; ketoacidosis; sole therapy for type 1 diabetes mellitus

Interactions

DRUGS

ACE inhibitors, anabolic steroids, androgens, azole antifungals, bromocriptine, chloramphenicol, disopyramide, fibric acid derivatives, guanethidine, H$_2$-receptor antagonists, insulin, magnesium salts, MAO inhibitors, methyldopa, octreotide, oral anticoagulants, oxyphenbutazone, phenylbutazone, probenecid, quinidine, salicylates, sulfonamides, tetracycline, theophylline, tricyclic antidepressants, urinary acidifiers: Increased risk of hypoglycemia
asparaginase, calcium channel blockers, cholestyramine, clonidine, corticosteroids, danazol, diazoxide, estrogen, glucagon, hydantoins, isoniazid, lithium, morphine, nicotinic acid, oral contraceptives, phenothiazines, rifabutin, rifampin, sympathomimetics, thiazide diuretics, thyroid drugs, urinary alkalizers: Increased risk of hyperglycemia
beta blockers: Possibly hyperglycemia or masking of hypoglycemia signs
digitalis glycosides: Increased risk of digitalis toxicity
pentamidine: Initially hypoglycemia and then hyperglycemia if beta cell damage occurs

FOODS

all foods: Possibly delayed drug absorption of tablets if taken within 30 minutes of meal

ACTIVITIES

alcohol use: Altered blood glucose control (usually hypoglycemia)

Adverse Reactions

CNS: Abnormal gait, anxiety, asthenia, chills, depression, dizziness, fatigue, headache, hypertonia, hypoesthesia, insomnia, malaise, migraine headache, nervousness, paresthesia, somnolence, syncope, tremor, vertigo
CV: Arrhythmias, edema, hypertension, vasculitis
EENT: Blurred vision, conjunctivitis, eye pain, pharyngitis, retinal hemorrhage, rhinitis, taste perversion, tinnitus
ENDO: Hypoglycemia
GI: Anorexia, constipation, diarrhea, elevated liver function test results, epigastric discomfort or fullness, flatulence, heartburn, hunger, nausea, proctocolitis, trace blood in stool, vomiting
GU: Darkened urine, decreased libido, dysuria, polyuria
HEME: Agranulocytosis, aplastic anemia, eosinophilia, hemolytic anemia, hepatic porphyria, leukopenia, pancytopenia
MS: Arthralgia, leg cramps, myalgia
RESP: Dyspnea
SKIN: Allergic skin reactions, diaphoresis, eczema, erythema multiforme, exfoliative dermatitis, flushing, jaundice, lichenoid reactions, maculopapular or morbilliform rash, photosensitivity, urticaria
Other: Disulfiram-like reaction

Nursing Considerations

• To improve blood glucose control, administer glipizide in divided doses instead of once a day, as prescribed.
• Check blood glucose level at least 3 times daily for a patient switching from insulin to glipizide. Patients who take more than 40 U of insulin daily may need hospitalization during transition.
• Discontinue insulin when dosage drops below 20 U daily, as prescribed, for patient receiving combination therapy.
• If patient gradually loses responsiveness to glipizide, expect to give a second antidiabetic drug to maintain blood glucose control, as prescribed.
• Monitor fasting blood glucose level to determine response to drug. Expect to check glycosylated hemoglobin level every 3 to 6 months or as ordered to evaluate long-term blood glucose control.
• Arrange for a dietary consultation and diabetic teaching, if appropriate. Ask dietitian to discuss with patient the amount of alcohol he can consume without risking hypoglycemia.
• Expect to switch patient to insulin therapy, as prescribed, during physical stress, such as infection, surgery, or trauma.
• **WARNING** Expect a higher risk of hypoglycemia when giving glipizide to a malnour-

G
H
I

ished or debilitated patient or one with renal, hepatic, pituitary, or adrenal insufficiency.

PATIENT TEACHING

•Instruct patient to take glipizide tablets 30 minutes before the first meal of the day. Caution him not to skip the meal after taking drug.

•Advise patient not to skip doses or increase dosage without consulting prescriber.

•Urge patient to report signs of hypoglycemia, such as anxiety, confusion, dizziness, excessive sweating, headache, and nausea.

•Encourage patient to carry candy or other simple sugars to treat mild hypoglycemia.

•Caution patient to consult prescriber before taking any OTC drugs.

•Urge patient to carry identification indicating that he has diabetes.

•Teach patient how to monitor his blood glucose level.

•Teach patient about exercise, diet, signs of hyperglycemia and hypoglycemia, hygiene, foot care, and ways to avoid infection.

•Instruct patient to notify prescriber if he experiences darkened urine, easy bruising, fever, hypoglycemia or hyperglycemia, rash, sore throat, and unusual bleeding.

•If photosensitivity is a problem, instruct patient to avoid direct sunlight and to wear sunscreen.

glucagon

Glucagon Diagnostic Kit, Glucagon Emergency Kit

Class and Category

Chemical: Synthetic hormone
Therapeutic: Antihypoglycemic, diagnostic aid adjunct
Pregnancy category: B

Indications and Dosages

➤ *To provide emergency treatment of severe hypoglycemia*

I.V., I.M., OR S.C. INJECTION

Adults and children who weigh more than 20 kg (44 lb). 1 mg, repeated in 15 min, if needed.

Children who weigh 20 kg or less. 0.5 mg, or 0.02 to 0.03 mg/kg, repeated in 15 min, if needed.

➤ *To provide diagnostic assistance by inhibiting bowel peristalsis in radiologic examination of GI tract*

I.V. INJECTION

Adults. 0.25 to 2 mg before procedure. Dose, route, and timing vary with segment of GI tract examined and length of procedure.

Route	Onset	Peak	Duration
I.V.	5 to 20 min*†	Unknown	90 min*‡
I.M.	15 to 26 min*§	Unknown	90 min*‖
S.C.	30 to 45 min*	Unknown	90 min*

Mechanism of Action

Increases production of adenylate cyclase, which catalyzes the conversion of adenosine triphosphate to cAMP, a process that in turn activates phosphorylase. Phosphorylase promotes the breakdown of glycogen to glucose (glycogenolysis) in the liver. As a result, the blood glucose level increases and GI smooth muscles relax.

Incompatibilities

Don't mix glucagon with sodium chloride or solutions that have a pH of 3.0 to 9.5; use with dextrose solutions instead.

Contraindications

Hypersensitivity to glucagon or its components, pheochromocytoma

Interactions

DRUGS

oral anticoagulants: Possibly interference with anticoagulant metabolism, increasing anticoagulant effects

Adverse Reactions

CV: Hypotension (with hypersensitivity reaction), tachycardia
GI: Nausea, vomiting
RESP: Bronchospasm, respiratory distress
SKIN: Urticaria

---

* For antihypoglycemic action.
† 45 sec to 1 min for smooth-muscle relaxation action.
‡ 9 to 25 min for smooth-muscle relaxation action.
§ 4 to 10 min for smooth-muscle relaxation action.
‖ 12 to 32 min for smooth-muscle relaxation action.

Nursing Considerations

•Rouse patient as quickly as possible because prolonged hypoglycemia can cause cerebral damage.

•For I.V. use, reconstitute a 1-mg vial of glucagon with 1 ml of diluent or a 10-mg vial with 10 ml of diluent. Don't give more than 1 mg/ml. For large doses, dilute with sterile water for injection.

•Before injecting glucagon, place unconscious patient on his side to prevent aspiration of vomitus when he regains consciousness.

•Administer by slow I.V. injection to decrease the risk of adverse reactions, such as tachycardia and vomiting.

•If patient doesn't respond to glucagon, expect to administer I.V. dextrose.

•When patient has regained consciousness, give him oral carbohydrates to restore hepatic glycogen stores and prevent secondary hypoglycemia.

•Keep in mind that glucagon isn't effective in patients with depleted hepatic glycogen stores caused by such conditions as adrenal insufficiency, chronic hypoglycemia, and starvation.

PATIENT TEACHING

•Instruct patient to monitor his blood glucose level, especially when signs of hypoglycemia occur.

•Teach patient and family members how to recognize signs of hypoglycemia and when to notify prescriber.

•Advise patient to carry candy or other simple sugars with him to treat early hypoglycemia.

•Emphasize the importance of a consistent diet, regular exercise, and proper use of insulin or an oral antidiabetic drug.

•Make sure unstable diabetic patients and family members know how to give glucagon subcutaneously in case of hypoglycemia. Instruct family members to keep patient on his side and give him a carbohydrate when he awakens. Advise against giving fluids by mouth until patient is fully conscious.

•Instruct patient and family members to call for emergency medical assistance after glucagon treatment, especially if patient can't ingest oral glucose or if he's taking the sulfonylurea chlorpropamide, in case secondary hypoglycemia occurs.

glyburide
(glibenclamide)

Albert Glyburide (CAN), Apo-Glyburide (CAN), DiaBeta, Euglucon (CAN), Gen-Glybe (CAN), Glynase PresTab, Medi-Glybe (CAN), Micronase, Novo-Glyburide (CAN), Nu-Glyburide (CAN)

Class and Category

Chemical: Sulfonylurea
Therapeutic: Antidiabetic
Pregnancy category: C (B for Glynase PresTab and Micronase)

Indications and Dosages

➤ *To control blood glucose level in type 2 diabetes mellitus*

MICRONIZED TABLETS

Adults. *Initial:* 1.5 to 3 mg q.d. with first meal of the day, increased by up to 1.5 mg at weekly intervals, if needed. *Maintenance:* 0.75 to 12 mg as a single dose or in divided doses with meals.

NONMICRONIZED TABLETS

Adults. *Initial:* 2.5 to 5 mg q.d. with first meal of the day, increased by up to 2.5 mg at weekly intervals, if needed. *Maintenance:* 1.25 to 20 mg/day as a single dose or in divided doses with meals.

DOSAGE ADJUSTMENT During conversion from insulin to glyburide for adults who use more than 40 U insulin/day, initial dosage adjusted to 5-mg nonmicronized tablet or 3-mg micronized tablet as a single dose with 50% of usual insulin dose; glyburide dosage increased gradually, as needed. For adults who use less than 40 U insulin/day, usual glyburide dosage is used when insulin is discontinued.

For elderly patients, initial dosage possibly reduced to 1.25-mg nonmicronized tablet q.d. and gradually increased by 2.5 mg/wk, as needed; or 0.75- to 3-mg micronized tablet q.d. and gradually increased by 1.5 mg/wk, as needed.

Route	Onset	Peak	Duration
P.O.*	1 hr	2.3 to 3.5 hr	12 to 24 hr
P.O.†	15 to 60 min	1 to 3 hr	24 hr

* Micronized.
† Nonmicronized.

Mechanism of Action
Stimulates insulin release from beta cells in the pancreas. Glyburide also increases peripheral tissue sensitivity to insulin either by enhancing insulin binding to cellular receptors or by increasing the number of insulin receptors.

Contraindications
Diabetes complicated by pregnancy; diabetic coma; hypersensitivity to glyburide, sulfonylureas, or their components; ketoacidosis; sole therapy for type 1 diabetes mellitus

Interactions
DRUGS
ACE inhibitors, anabolic steroids, androgens, azole antifungals, bromocriptine, chloramphenicol, disopyramide, fibric acid derivatives, guanethidine, H_2-receptor antagonists, insulin, magnesium salts, MAO inhibitors, methyldopa, octreotide, oral anticoagulants, oxyphenbutazone, phenylbutazone, probenecid, quinidine, salicylates, sulfonamides, tetracycline, theophylline, tricyclic antidepressants, urinary acidifiers: Increased risk of hypoglycemia
asparaginase, calcium channel blockers, cholestyramine, clonidine, corticosteroids, danazol, diazoxide, estrogen, glucagon, hydantoins, isoniazid, lithium, morphine, nicotinic acid, oral contraceptives, phenothiazines, rifabutin, rifampin, sympathomimetics, thiazide diuretics, thyroid drugs, urinary alkalinizers: Increased risk of hyperglycemia
beta blockers: Possibly hyperglycemia or masking of hypoglycemia signs
digitalis glycosides: Increased risk of digitalis toxicity
pentamidine: Initial hypoglycemia and then hyperglycemia if beta cell damage occurs
FOODS
high-fat foods: Reduced bioavailability of nonmicronized glyburide
ACTIVITIES
alcohol use: Altered blood glucose control (usually hypoglycemia)

Adverse Reactions
CNS: Abnormal gait, anxiety, asthenia, chills, depression, dizziness, fatigue, headache, hypertonia, hypoesthesia, insomnia, malaise, migraine headache, nervousness, paresthesia, somnolence, syncope, tremor, vertigo
CV: Arrhythmias, edema, hypertension, vasculitis
EENT: Blurred vision, conjunctivitis, eye pain, pharyngitis, retinal hemorrhage, rhinitis, taste perversion, tinnitus
ENDO: Hypoglycemia
GI: Anorexia, constipation, diarrhea, elevated liver function test results, epigastric discomfort or fullness, flatulence, heartburn, hunger, nausea, proctocolitis, trace blood in stool, vomiting
GU: Decreased libido, dysuria, polyuria
HEME: Agranulocytosis, aplastic anemia, eosinophilia, hemolytic anemia, hepatic porphyria, leukopenia, pancytopenia
MS: Arthralgia, leg cramps, myalgia
RESP: Dyspnea
SKIN: Allergic skin reactions, diaphoresis, eczema, erythema multiforme, exfoliative dermatitis, flushing, jaundice, lichenoid reactions, maculopapular or morbilliform rash, photosensitivity, urticaria
Other: Disulfiram-like reaction

Nursing Considerations
• Give glyburide as a single dose before the first meal of the day. If patient takes more than 10 mg daily or if severe GI distress occurs, give in 2 divided doses before meals.
• Monitor fasting blood glucose level to determine patient's response to glyburide. Expect to check glycosylated hemoglobin level every 3 to 6 months or as ordered to evaluate long-term blood glucose control.
• When patient switches from insulin to glyburide, check blood glucose level 3 times daily before meals.
• Be aware that micronized tablets aren't equal to nonmicronized tablets; they contain smaller particles, which affects drug bioavailability.
• **WARNING** Expect a higher risk of hypoglycemia when giving drug to a malnourished or debilitated patient or one with renal, hepatic, pituitary, or adrenal insufficiency.
• Administer insulin as needed and prescribed during periods of increased stress, such as infection, surgery, and trauma.
• Arrange for diabetic teaching and consultation between patient and dietitian, if appropriate.

PATIENT TEACHING

• Instruct patient to take glyburide just before the day's first meal. Caution him not to skip the meal after taking drug.
• Advise patient not to take nonmicronized glyburide with a high-fat meal because doing so can reduce drug bioavailability.
• Caution patient to avoid skipping doses, discontinuing glyburide, or taking OTC drugs without first consulting prescriber.
• Teach patient how to monitor his blood glucose level and when to notify prescriber.
• Urge patient to report signs of hypoglycemia, such as anxiety, confusion, dizziness, excessive sweating, headache, and nausea.
• Suggest that patient carry candy or other simple sugars to treat mild hypoglycemia.
• Urge patient to avoid alcohol because it increases the risk of hypoglycemia.
• Advise patient to carry identification indicating that he has diabetes.
• Teach patient about exercise, diet, signs of hyperglycemia and hypoglycemia, hygiene, foot care, and ways to avoid infection.
• Instruct patient to notify prescriber if he experiences easy bruising, fever, hypoglycemia or hyperglycemia, rash, sore throat, and unusual bleeding.
• If photosensitivity is a problem, instruct patient to avoid direct sunlight and to wear sunscreen.

glyburide and metformin hydrochloride

Glucovance

Class and Category

Chemical: Sulfonylurea (glyburide), dimethylbiguanide (metformin)
Therapeutic: Antidiabetic
Pregnancy category: B

Indications and Dosages

➤ *To reduce blood glucose level as initial therapy in patients with type 2 diabetes mellitus*

TABLETS

Adults. *Initial:* 1.25 mg/250 mg q.d. or b.i.d. Dosage increased by 1.25 mg/250 mg/day q 2 wk as needed.

➤ *To reduce blood glucose level in patients with type 2 diabetes mellitus who are not adequately controlled on either a sulfonylurea or metformin alone*

TABLETS

Adults. *Initial:* 2.5 mg/500 mg or 5 mg/500 mg b.i.d. Dosage increased, as prescribed, by 5 mg/500 mg/day. *Maximum:* 20 mg/2,000 mg/day.

DOSAGE ADJUSTMENT For patients currently receiving glyburide or another sulfonylurea, metformin, or a combination of these drugs, expect initial dosage prescribed to be equal to or less than that currently being taken.

Route	Onset	Peak	Duration
P.O. (glyburide)	45 to 60 min	1.5 to 3 hr	24 hr
P.O. (metformin)	Days to 1 wk	2 wk	2 wk after drug is discontinued

G
H
I

Mechanism of Action

Glyburide and metformin work in complementary ways to improve glucose control. Glyburide stimulates insulin release from beta cells in the pancreas. It also increases peripheral tissue sensitivity to insulin either by enhancing insulin binding to cellular receptors or by increasing the number of insulin receptors.

Metformin hydrochloride may promote the storage of excess glucose as glycogen in the liver, thus reducing glucose production. Metformin also may improve glucose use by skeletal muscle and adipose tissue by facilitating glucose transport across cell membranes. It also may increase the number of insulin receptors on cell membranes and make them more sensitive to insulin.

Contraindications

Acute or chronic metabolic acidosis; diabetes complicated by pregnancy; diabetic coma; heart failure requiring drug treatment; hypersensitivity to glyburide, metformin, biguanides, sulfonylureas, or their components; ketoacidosis; renal disease or dysfunction (serum creatinine level of 1.5 mg/dl or more in males or 1.4 mg/dl or more in females); type 1 diabetes

Interactions

DRUGS

glyburide and metformin hydrochloride

calcium channel blockers, corticosteroids, diuretics, estrogens, isoniazid, nicotinic acid, oral contraceptives, phenothiazine, phenytoin, sympathomimetics, thiazide diuretics, thyroid hormones: Possibly hyperglycemia, possibly hypoglycemia when these drugs are withdrawn

vitamin B$_{12}$: Probably decreased vitamin B$_{12}$ absorption

glyburide component only

beta-adrenergic blockers, chloramphenicol, highly protein-bound drugs, MAO inhibitors NSAIDs, oral anticoagulants, probenecid, salicylates, sulfonamides: Potentiated hypoglycemic action of glyburide, possibly hyperglycemia when these drugs are withdrawn

ciprofloxacin: Potentiated hypoglycemic action of glyburide

miconazole (oral): Possibly severe hypoglycemia

metformin hydrochloride component only

cimetidine: Increased blood metformin level, possibly increased risk of hypoglycemia

furosemide: Increased blood metformin level, decreased blood furosemide level

nifedipine: Enhanced absorption of metformin

FOODS

all foods: Delayed and reduced absorption of metformin

ACTIVITIES

alcohol use: Altered blood glucose control (usually hyperglycemia), possibly potentiated effect of metformin on lactate metabolism

Adverse Reactions

CNS: Headache
ENDO: Hypoglycemia
GI: Abdominal pain, diarrhea, indigestion, nausea, vomiting
HEME: Megaloblastic anemia, thrombocytopenia
RESP: Upper respiratory tract infection
Other: Lactic acidosis

Nursing Considerations

•Administer glyburide and metformin as a single dose before first meal of the day. If patient takes more than 10 mg of the glyburide component daily or if severe GI distress occurs, expect to divide dose and give b.i.d. before morning and evening meals.

•**WARNING** Monitor renal function, as ordered, before beginning therapy and at least annually thereafter because significant renal impairment can result in tissue hypoperfusion and hypoxemia, leading to lactic acidosis.

•**WARNING** Expect to discontinue glyburide and metformin for 48 hours before and after radiographic tests involving I.V. administration of iodinated contrast materials because iodinated media increase the risk of renal failure and lactic acidosis during drug therapy.

•**WARNING** Monitor malnourished or debilitated patients and those with renal, hepatic, pituitary, or adrenal insufficiency because they're at increased risk for hypoglycemia. Expect to monitor vitamin B$_{12}$ blood levels at least every 2 to 3 years in patients with inadequate vitamin B$_{12}$ or calcium intake or absorption because prolonged drug use may result in decreased vitamin B$_{12}$ absorption.

•Monitor fasting blood glucose level to determine patient's response to drug. Expect to monitor glycosylated hemoglobin (HbA$_{1c}$) level every 3 to 6 months, as ordered, to evaluate long-term blood glucose control.

•Frequently monitor blood glucose level to detect hyperglycemia and to assess the need for supplemental insulin during periods of increased stress, such as infection, surgery, and trauma.

•When patient switches from insulin to glyburide and metformin, expect to increase frequency of blood glucose monitoring to t.i.d. before meals.

•In pregnant females, expect to discontinue drug at least 2 weeks before expected delivery date, as prescribed, to avoid profound hypoglycemia in neonate.

•Arrange for diabetes teaching and consultation with a dietitian or certified diabetes educator, if possible.

PATIENT TEACHING

•Instruct patient to take glyburide and metformin with morning meal if taking once a day, or with morning and evening meals if taking twice a day. Caution him not to skip meal after taking drug.

•Advise patient not to skip doses, discontinue drug, or take OTC drugs without first consulting prescriber because hyperglycemia may result.

•Inform patient that most common adverse

effects are minor, including diarrhea, nausea, and upset stomach, and typically occur during first few weeks of therapy; advise him that taking drug with meals reduces these effects.

•Teach patient how to monitor his blood glucose level and when to notify prescriber.
•Advise patient to expect laboratory monitoring of HbA_{1c} level every 3 months until blood glucose level is controlled.
•Instruct patient to report signs of hypoglycemia, such as anxiety, confusion, dizziness, excessive sweating, headache, and nausea.
•Advise patient to carry identification indicating that he has diabetes, and suggest that he carry candy to treat mild hypoglycemia.
•Teach patient about exercise, diet, signs of hyperglycemia and hypoglycemia, hygiene, foot care, and ways to avoid infection.
•Instruct patient to notify prescriber if he experiences easy bruising, unusual bleeding, fever, hypoglycemia or hyperglycemia, rash, or sore throat because drug may need to be discontinued.
•Advise patient to avoid alcohol because it increases the risk of hypoglycemia.
•Inform pregnant patient that she may be taken off glyburide and metformin and switched to insulin therapy, as prescribed, at least 2 weeks before expected delivery date.

glycopyrrolate

Robinul, Robinul Forte

Class and Category

Chemical: Quaternary ammonium compound
Therapeutic: Antiarrhythmic, anticholinergic, cholinergic adjunct
Pregnancy category: B

Indications and Dosages

➤ *To treat peptic ulcer disease*
TABLETS
Adults and adolescents. 1 to 2 mg b.i.d. or t.i.d. *Maximum:* 8 mg/day.
I.V. OR I.M. INJECTION
Adults and adolescents. 0.1 to 0.2 mg q 4 hr, p.r.n. *Maximum:* 4 doses/day.

➤ *To reduce gastric acid and respiratory secretions before anesthesia*

I.M. INJECTION
Adults and adolescents. 0.0044 mg/kg 30 to 60 min before anesthesia or when preanesthesia sedative or narcotic is given.
Children over age 2. 0.0044 to 0.0088 mg/kg 30 to 60 min before anesthesia or when preanesthesia sedative or narcotic is given.

➤ *To counteract intraoperative and anesthesia-induced arrhythmias*
I.V. INJECTION
Adults and adolescents. 0.1 mg, repeated q 2 to 3 min, if needed.
Children over age 2. 0.0044 mg/kg. Dose repeated q 2 to 3 min, if needed. *Maximum:* 0.1 mg as a single dose.

➤ *As cholinergic adjunct in curariform block*
I.V. INJECTION
Adults and children over age 2. 0.2 mg glycopyrrolate for each 1 mg of neostigmine or each 5 mg of pyridostigmine when given together.

Route	Onset	Peak	Duration
P.O.	60 min	Unknown	8 to 12 hr
I.V.	1 min	Unknown	2 to 3 hr*
I.M., S.C.	15 to 30 min	30 to 45 min	2 to 3 hr*

Mechanism of Action

Inhibits acetylcholine's action on postganglionic muscarinic receptors throughout the body. Depending on the receptors' location, glycopyrrolate produces various effects, such as:
•reducing the volume and acidity of gastric secretions
•controlling excessive bronchial, pharyngeal, and tracheal secretions and dilating the bronchi
•inhibiting vagal stimulation of the heart
•relaxing smooth muscle in the GI and GU tracts.

Incompatibilities

Don't mix glycopyrrolate with alkaline drugs or solutions that have a pH over 6.0 because

---

* For vagal blocking effect; up to 7 hr for reduction of saliva.

drug stability may be affected. A pH over 6.0 may occur if glycopyrrolate is mixed with dexamethasone sodium phosphate or LR solution. Gas or precipitate may form if glycopyrrolate is mixed in same syringe as chloramphenicol, diazepam, dimenhydrinate, methohexital sodium, pentobarbital sodium, secobarbital sodium, sodium bicarbonate, or thiopental sodium.

Contraindications

Angle-closure glaucoma, asthma, hemorrhage with unstable cardiovascular status, hepatic disease, hypersensitivity to anticholinergics, ileus, intestinal atony, myasthenia gravis, obstructive GI or urinary disorders, toxic megacolon, ulcerative colitis

Interactions
DRUGS

anticholinergics, tricyclic antidepressants: Possibly increased anticholinergic effects
antidiarrheals (adsorbent): Decreased glycopyrrolate absorption, leading to decreased therapeutic effectiveness
antimyasthenics: Possibly reduced intestinal motility
atenolol: Possibly potentiated effects of atenolol
calcium- or magnesium-containing antacids, carbonic anhydrase inhibitors, citrates, sodium bicarbonate: Possibly reduced excretion of glycopyrrolate and increased therapeutic and adverse effects
cyclopropane: Possibly ventricular arrhythmias
digoxin: Possibly potentiated digoxin effects
haloperidol, phenothiazines: Possibly decreased effectiveness of these drugs
ketoconazole: Possibly decreased ketoconazole absorption
metoclopramide: Possibly antagonized effects of metoclopramide
opioids: Possibly severe constipation and urine retention, risk of ileus
potassium chloride: Possibly increased severity of potassium chloride–induced gastric lesions

Adverse Reactions

CNS: Confusion, dizziness, drowsiness, headache, insomnia, nervousness, weakness
CV: Bradycardia (with low doses), palpitations, tachycardia (with high doses)
EENT: Blurred vision, cycloplegia, dry mouth, increased intraocular pressure, loss of taste,

mydriasis, nasal congestion, photophobia, taste perversion
GI: Abdominal distention, constipation, dysphagia, nausea, vomiting
GU: Impotence, urinary hesitancy, urine retention
RESP: Dyspnea
SKIN: Decreased sweating (may lead to heat exhaustion), flushing, urticaria

Nursing Considerations

• Use glycopyrrolate cautiously in patients with arrhythmias, bradycardia, heart failure, hypertension, hyperthyroidism, or tachycardia because drug's anticholinergic effect can worsen these conditions.
• Give tablet form 30 to 60 minutes before meals.
• As needed and prescribed, give 2-mg dose at bedtime to ensure overnight control of symptoms.
• For I.V. use, administer by direct injection without diluting. Or inject into tubing of a flowing I.V. solution unless it contains an alkaline drug or sodium bicarbonate.
• Use continuous cardiac monitoring, as ordered, to assess for arrhythmias during drug administration.
• **WARNING** Check all doses carefully because even a slight overdose can lead to toxicity.
• To prevent overheating caused by decreased sweating, adjust the room temperature and make sure patient is well hydrated.
PATIENT TEACHING
• Advise patient to take glycopyrrolate tablets 30 to 60 minutes before meals.
• Instruct patient to consult prescriber before taking any OTC drugs.
• Caution patient about possible drowsiness and dizziness.
• Suggest that he use sugarless hard candy, ice, or saliva substitute to relieve dry mouth.
• Instruct patient to avoid exertion and hot environments because he's prone to heat exhaustion while taking glycopyrrolate.
• Urge patient to maintain hydration by drinking at least 8 glasses of water daily, unless contraindicated.
• Instruct patient to notify prescriber if he experiences abdominal distention, difficulty breathing, difficulty urinating, eye pain, irregular heartbeat or palpitations, sensitivity to light, or severe constipation.
• Advise patient to wear sunglasses in bright light.
• Inform male patient that reversible impotence may occur during therapy.

•If urinary hesitancy occurs, advise patient to void before taking each dose.

granisetron hydrochloride

Kytril

Class and Category
Chemical: Carbazole
Therapeutic: Antiemetic
Pregnancy category: B

Indications and Dosages
➤ *To prevent nausea and vomiting caused by chemotherapy*
ORAL SOLUTION, TABLETS
Adults and adolescents. 1 mg up to 1 hr before chemotherapy and repeated 12 hr later; or 2 mg up to 1 hr before chemotherapy.
I.V. INFUSION
Adults and adolescents. 10 mcg/kg diluted and infused over 5 min, starting 30 min before chemotherapy; or 10 mcg/kg undiluted and infused over 30 sec, starting 30 min before chemotherapy.
➤ *To prevent nausea and vomiting caused by radiation therapy*
ORAL SOLUTION, TABLETS
Adults and adolescents. 2 mg q.d. given 1 hr before radiation therapy.
➤ *To prevent or treat postoperative nausea and vomiting*
I.V. INJECTION
Adults and adolescents. 1 mg administered over 30 sec before induction of anesthesia or immediately before reversal anesthesia for prevention. 1 mg administered over 30 sec after surgery for treatment.

Mechanism of Action
Has a high affinity for serotonin receptors along vagal nerve endings in the intestines. Because of this affinity, granisetron prevents the nausea and vomiting that usually result when serotonin is released by damaged enterochromaffin cells.

Incompatibilities
Don't mix granisetron in same solution as other drugs.

Contraindications
Hypersensitivity to granisetron or its components

Adverse Reactions
CNS: Asthenia, chills, CNS stimulation, drowsiness, fever, headache, insomnia, somnolence
CV: Hypertension
EENT: Taste perversion
GI: Abdominal pain, anorexia, constipation, diarrhea, elevated liver function test results, nausea, vomiting
HEME: Anemia, leukopenia, thrombocytopenia
SKIN: Alopecia

Nursing Considerations
•For use with chemotherapy, dilute I.V. preparation of granisetron with NS or D_5W to a total volume of 20 to 50 ml. Mixture may be stored for up to 24 hours. Use only on days when chemotherapy is given.
•For use with surgery, administer I.V. injection undiluted over 30 seconds.
PATIENT TEACHING
•Inform patient that granisetron is given orally or I.V. before chemotherapy to help prevent nausea.
•Instruct patient to take tablet without food to avoid reducing drug bioavailability.
•Advise patient to report constipation, fever, severe diarrhea, or severe headache to prescriber. Also caution him about possible drowsiness.
•Suggest that patient use sugarless hard candy to help alleviate nausea.

guaifenesin

Anti-Tuss, Balminil Expectorant (CAN), Benylin-E (CAN), Breonesin, Calmylin Expectorant (CAN), Diabetic Tussin EX, Fenesin, Gee-Gee, Genatuss, GG-CEN, Glycotuss, Glytuss, Guiatuss, Halotussin, Humibid L.A., Humibid Sprinkle, Hytuss, Hytuss 2X, Naldecon Senior EX, Organidin NR, Pneumomist, Resyl (CAN), Robitussin, Scot-tussin Expectorant, Sinumist-SR, Touro EX, Uni-tussin

Class and Category
Chemical: Glyceryl guaiacolate
Therapeutic: Expectorant
Pregnancy category: C

Indications and Dosages
➤ *To relieve cough, especially when secretions are thick*
CAPSULES, ORAL SOLUTION, SYRUP, TABLETS
Adults and adolescents. 200 to 400 mg q 4 hr. *Maximum:* 2,400 mg/day.

CAPSULES, ORAL SOLUTION, SYRUP
Children ages 6 to 12. 100 to 200 mg q 4 hr. *Maximum:* 1,200 mg/day.

E.R. CAPSULES OR TABLETS
Adults and adolescents. 600 to 1,200 mg q 12 hr. *Maximum:* 2,400 mg/day.
Children ages 6 to 12. 600 mg q 12 hr. *Maximum:* 1,200 mg/day.
Children ages 2 to 6. 300 mg q 12 hr. *Maximum:* 600 mg/day.

ORAL SOLUTION, SYRUP
Children ages 2 to 6. 50 to 100 mg q 4 hr. *Maximum:* 600 mg/day.
Children ages 6 months to 2 years. 25 to 50 mg q 4 hr (individualized). *Maximum:* 300 mg/day.

Route	Onset	Peak	Duration
P.O.	30 min	Unknown	4 to 6 hr

Mechanism of Action
Increases fluid and mucus removal from the upper respiratory tract by increasing the volume of secretions and reducing their adhesiveness and surface tension.

Contraindications
Hypersensitivity to guaifenesin

Adverse Reactions
CNS: Dizziness, headache
GI: Nausea and vomiting (with large doses)
SKIN: Rash, urticaria

Nursing Considerations
• As prescribed and as appropriate, give liquid forms of guaifenesin to children.
• Don't expect guaifenesin alone to suppress cough. As prescribed, administer with other drugs, such as codeine.
• Watch for signs of more serious condition, such as cough that lasts longer than 1 week, fever, persistent headache, and rash.
PATIENT TEACHING
• Instruct patient to take each dose with a full glass of water.
• Instruct patient to increase fluid intake (unless contraindicated) to help thin secretions.
• Advise patient not to take drug longer than 1 week and to notify prescriber about fever, persistent headache, or rash.

guanadrel sulfate
Hylorel

Class and Category
Chemical: Guanidine derivative
Therapeutic: Antihypertensive
Pregnancy category: B

Indications and Dosages
➤ *To manage hypertension*
TABLETS
Adults. 5 mg b.i.d., increased to 20 to 75 mg/day in divided doses t.i.d. or q.i.d., if needed.
DOSAGE ADJUSTMENT Initial dosage reduced to 5 mg q.d. if needed for patients with renal impairment or creatinine clearance of 30 to 60 ml/min/1.73 m². Then dosage adjusted after at least 7 days. Initial dosage reduced to 5 mg q.o.d. if needed for patients with creatinine clearance of less than 30 ml/min/1.73 m². Then dosage adjusted after at least 2 wk.

Route	Onset	Peak	Duration
P.O.	30 min to 2 hr	4 to 6 hr	4 to 14 hr

Mechanism of Action
Exerts its antihypertensive effect at peripheral sympathetic nerve endings. Through an uptake mechanism, guanadrel is stored in adrenergic neurons, where it displaces norepinephrine from its storage sites. This action blocks the normal release of norepinephrine in response to nerve impulses, which depletes norepinephrine stores in the synapses and relaxes vessel walls, thus reducing peripheral resistance and blood pressure.

Contraindications
Heart failure not caused by hypertension, hypersensitivity to guanadrel or its components, MAO inhibitor use within 1 week of guanadrel use, pheochromocytoma

Interactions
DRUGS
alpha blockers, beta blockers, rauwolfia alkaloids: Possibly orthostatic hypotension or bradycardia
amphetamines, appetite suppressants, cyclobenzaprine, haloperidol, loxapine, maprotiline, methylphenidate, phenothiazines, thioxanthenes, tricyclic antidepressants: Decreased antihypertensive effect of guanadrel
anticholinergics: Possibly decreased inhibition of gastric acid secretion
barbiturates, opioids: Increased hypotensive effect
MAO inhibitors: Possibly severe blood pressure increase

NSAIDs: Possibly sodium and water retention and decreased antihypertensive effect of guanadrel

sympathomimetics: Possibly reduced antihypertensive effect of guanadrel, leading to hypertension; possibly potentiated effects of sympathomimetics

vasodilators: Increased orthostatic hypotension

ACTIVITIES

alcohol use: Increased hypotensive effect

Adverse Reactions

CNS: Confusion, drowsiness, fatigue, headache, light-headedness, paresthesia, sleep disturbance
CV: Chest pain, orthostatic hypotension, palpitations, peripheral edema
EENT: Blurred vision, dry mouth and throat, glossitis
GI: Abdominal cramps or pain, anorexia, constipation, diarrhea, indigestion, nausea, vomiting
GU: Difficult ejaculation, hematuria, impotence, nocturia, urinary frequency or urgency
MS: Arthralgia, back or neck pain, joint inflammation, leg cramps, muscle weakness, myalgia
RESP: Cough, dyspnea
Other: Excessive weight gain or loss

Nursing Considerations

•Use guanadrel cautiously in patients with asthma because drug may aggravate this condition. Monitor patient for acute dyspnea, wheezing, and other signs of asthma attack. Notify prescriber immediately if they develop.
•WARNING Assess for signs of overdose, such as blurred vision, dizziness, and syncope.
•Be aware that elderly patients have a greater risk of experiencing dizziness and syncope.
•Assess for signs of fluid retention and heart failure, including crackles, a new S_3 heart sound, and sudden weight gain.

PATIENT TEACHING

•Inform patient that guanadrel doesn't cure high blood pressure but does help control it.
•Instruct patient to take drug at the same time each day to improve compliance and blood pressure control.
•Caution patient about possible dizziness, light-headedness, and fainting, especially when getting up from a lying or sitting position. Advise him to rise slowly, especially in the morning, and to sit with his feet dangling for 1 to 2 minutes before standing up.
•Instruct patient to sit or lie down immediately if he feels dizzy.

•To prevent fainting, advise patient to avoid alcohol, standing for long periods, excessive exercise, and exposure to hot weather.
•Instruct patient to check with prescriber before taking OTC drugs during guanadrel therapy.
•Advise patient to follow a low-sodium diet to help reduce blood pressure and prevent fluid retention.

guanethidine monosulfate

Apo-Guanethidine (CAN), Ismelin

Class and Category

Chemical: Guanidine derivative
Therapeutic: Antihypertensive
Pregnancy category: C

Indications and Dosages

➤ *To manage moderate to severe hypertension and renal hypertension*

TABLETS

Adults. *Initial:* 10 to 12.5 mg q.d., increased as needed by 10 to 12.5 mg q wk. *Maintenance:* 25 to 50 mg q.d. Some patients may need up to 300 mg q.d.
Children. 0.2 mg/kg q.d., increased p.r.n. by 0.2 mg/kg q 7 to 10 days. *Maximum:* 3 mg/kg q 24 hr.

DOSAGE ADJUSTMENT Initial dosage increased to 25 to 50 mg q.d. for adult hospitalized patients because they can be monitored more closely. Then dosage increased by 25 to 50 mg q.o.d., p.r.n.

Route	Onset	Peak	Duration
P.O.	Unknown	8 hr*	Unknown*

Mechanism of Action

Exerts its antihypertensive effect at peripheral sympathetic nerve endings. Through an uptake mechanism, guanethidine is stored in adrenergic neurons, where it displaces norepinephrine from its storage sites. This action blocks the normal release of norepinephrine in response to nerve impulses, which depletes norepinephrine stores in the synapses and relaxes vessel walls, thus reducing peripheral resistance and blood pressure.

* For single dose; 1 to 3 wk for multiple doses.

Contraindications

Heart failure not caused by hypertension, hypersensitivity to guanethidine or its components, MAO inhibitor use within 1 week of guanethidine use, pheochromocytoma

Interactions

DRUGS

alpha blockers, beta blockers, rauwolfia alkaloids: Possibly orthostatic hypotension or bradycardia

amphetamines, appetite suppressants, cyclobenzaprine, haloperidol, loxapine, maprotiline, methylphenidate, phenothiazines, thioxanthenes, tricyclic antidepressants: Decreased antihypertensive effect of guanethidine

anticholinergics: Possibly decreased inhibition of gastric acid secretion

barbiturates, opioids: Increased hypotensive effect

insulin, oral antidiabetic drugs: Possibly increased antidiabetic effect of these drugs

MAO inhibitors: Possibly severe blood pressure increase

NSAIDs: Possibly sodium and water retention and decreased antihypertensive effect of guanethidine

sympathomimetics: Possibly reduced antihypertensive effect of guanethidine, leading to hypertension; possibly potentiated effects of sympathomimetics

vasodilators: Increased orthostatic hypotension

ACTIVITIES

alcohol use: Increased hypotensive effect

Adverse Reactions

CNS: Depression, dizziness, fatigue, headache, lassitude, paresthesia, syncope
CV: Angina, bradycardia, orthostatic hypotension, palpitations, peripheral edema
EENT: Blurred vision, dry mouth, glossitis, nasal congestion, parotid gland tenderness, ptosis
GI: Anorexia, constipation, diarrhea (severe), indigestion, nausea, vomiting
GU: Ejaculation disorders, elevated BUN level, impotence, nocturia, priapism, urinary frequency
HEME: Anemia, leukopenia, thrombocytopenia
MS: Leg cramps, muscle twitching, myalgia
RESP: Asthma exacerbation, dyspnea
SKIN: Alopecia, dermatitis
Other: Weight gain

Nursing Considerations

• As prescribed, discontinue MAO inhibitor therapy at least 1 week before starting guanethidine.
• Because guanethidine has cumulative effects, give a small initial dose and increase gradually, as prescribed. When blood pressure is controlled, expect to reduce dosage to lowest effective level.
• Monitor for orthostatic hypotension, which occurs most often when arising in the morning and is exacerbated by hot weather, exercise, and alcohol. Assess supine and standing blood pressures, especially after dosage adjustments.
• Measure daily weight to help detect fluid retention. Also observe for edema and other signs of heart failure. A thiazide diuretic may be prescribed to decrease sodium and fluid retention.
• Notify prescriber if severe diarrhea occurs. Drug may need to be discontinued.
• Monitor febrile patient for increased hypotension and adverse reactions because fever decreases drug requirements.
• As ordered, stop giving guanethidine 2 weeks before surgery to reduce the risk of cardiac arrest during anesthesia.

PATIENT TEACHING

• Teach patient how to recognize signs of orthostatic hypotension, and advise changing position slowly. Inform patient that symptoms are worse in the morning and exacerbated by exercise, hot weather, alcohol, and hot showers.
• Instruct patient to report fainting, frequent dizziness, and severe diarrhea.
• Caution patient to avoid alcohol because it may increase the risk of orthostatic hypotension.
• Instruct patient to weigh himself daily at the same time, on the same scale, and wearing the same amount of clothing. Advise him to report signs of fluid retention, such as reduced urine volume, sudden weight increase, and limb swelling.
• Urge patient to consult prescriber before taking OTC drugs during guanethidine therapy.
• If a diabetic patient takes insulin or a sulfonylurea, instruct him to monitor his blood glucose level more frequently to check for hypoglycemia.
• Advise patient to follow a low-sodium diet

to help reduce blood pressure and prevent fluid retention.

guanfacine hydrochloride

Tenex

Class and Category
Chemical: Dichlorobenzine derivative
Therapeutic: Antihypertensive
Pregnancy category: B

Indications and Dosages
➤ *To manage hypertension, alone or with other antihypertensives*
TABLETS
Adults. 1 mg q.d. h.s., increased if needed to 2 mg after 3 to 4 wk. Then increased to 3 mg if needed after another 3 to 4 wk. *Maintenance:* 2 or 3 mg q.d.
DOSAGE ADJUSTMENT Twice-daily dosing used if blood pressure tends to rise at the end of 24-hr period.

Route	Onset	Peak	Duration
P.O.	Unknown*	8 to 12 hr†	24 hr

Mechanism of Action
Decreases sympathetic nerve impulse outflow from the brain's vasomotor center to the heart and blood vessels by stimulating central alpha$_2$-adrenergic receptors. This action reduces peripheral vascular resistance, renovascular resistance, heart rate, and blood pressure. Prolonged use of guanfacine may reduce total peripheral vascular resistance, slightly reducing the heart rate. Guanfacine also stimulates growth hormone secretion, reduces circulating levels of plasma catecholamines, and reduces left ventricular hypertrophy.

Contraindications
Hypersensitivity to guanfacine

---

* For single dose; in 1 wk for multiple doses.
† For single dose; 1 to 3 mo for multiple doses.

Interactions
DRUGS
CNS depressants: Possibly increased CNS depression
NSAIDs, sympathomimetics, tricyclic antidepressants: Possibly decreased antihypertensive effect of guanfacine
other antihypertensives: Possibly increased antihypertensive effect, resulting in hypotension
ACTIVITIES
alcohol use: Possibly increased CNS depression

Adverse Reactions
CNS: Anxiety, confusion, depression, dizziness, drowsiness, headache, nervousness, weakness
CV: Bradycardia, orthostatic hypotension
EENT: Conjunctivitis, dry mouth
GI: Constipation, nausea
GU: Decreased libido, impotence
SKIN: Dermatitis, diaphoresis, pruritus, purpura, rash

Nursing Considerations
• Use guanfacine cautiously in patients with cerebrovascular disease, chronic renal or hepatic failure, recent MI, or severe coronary insufficiency.
• Give drug at bedtime to minimize daytime sedation.
• WARNING Expect to discontinue drug by decreasing dosage gradually over 2 to 4 days. Typically, if patient hasn't had drug for 2 or more days, he may experience withdrawal symptoms, including abdominal cramps, anxiety, chest pain, diaphoresis, headache, increased salivation, insomnia, irregular heart rate and rhythm, nausea, nervousness, restlessness, tremor, and vomiting.
• If you suspect that patient has drug-related depression, notify prescriber immediately and expect to discontinue drug.
PATIENT TEACHING
• Instruct patient to take guanfacine at bedtime to reduce daytime drowsiness.
• Caution patient about possible drowsiness, and advise him to avoid potentially hazardous activities until drug's CNS effects are known.
• Urge patient to avoid alcohol and other CNS depressants while taking guanfacine.
• Advise patient to report rash.
• Inform male patient that drug may cause impotence. Suggest that he discuss impotence with prescriber, if it occurs.

G H I

•Caution patient not to stop taking drug abruptly because doing so can cause a dangerous rise in blood pressure along with anxiety and nervousness.

halazepam

Paxipam

Class, Category, and Schedule
Chemical: Benzodiazepine
Therapeutic: Antianxiety
Pregnancy category: D
Controlled substance: Schedule IV

Indications and Dosages
➤ *To manage anxiety*
TABLETS
Adults. 20 to 40 mg t.i.d. or q.i.d. *Optimal:* 80 to 160 mg/day.
DOSAGE ADJUSTMENT Dosage reduced to 20 mg q.d. or b.i.d. if needed for debilitated patients.

Route	Onset	Peak	Duration
P.O.	Slow	Unknown	6 to 8 hr

Mechanism of Action
May potentiate the effects of gamma-aminobutyric acid (GABA) and other inhibitory neurotransmitters by binding to specific benzodiazepine receptor sites in the limbic and cortical areas of the CNS. By binding to these receptor sites, halazepam increases the inhibitory effects of GABA and blocks cortical and limbic arousal.

Contraindications
Acute angle-closure glaucoma, hypersensitivity to halazepam or its components, itraconazole or ketoconazole therapy, psychosis

Interactions
DRUGS
antacids: Possibly altered rate of halazepam absorption
barbiturates, CNS depressants, narcotics: Increased CNS depression, possibly sedation and impaired motor function
cimetidine, diltiazem, disulfiram, erythromycin, fluoxetine, fluvoxamine, isoniazid, itraconazole, ketoconazole, metoprolol, nefazodone, oral contraceptives, propoxyphene,
propranolol, ranitidine, valproic acid, verapamil: Decreased clearance, increased blood level, and increased risk of adverse effects of halazepam
clozapine: Possibly respiratory depression
digoxin: Increased blood digoxin level and risk of digitalis toxicity
levodopa: Decreased antidyskinetic effect
neuromuscular blockers: Increased or blocked neuromuscular blockade
theophyllines: Decreased sedative effect of halazepam
ACTIVITIES
alcohol use: Increased CNS depression, possibly sedation and impaired motor function
smoking: Decreased halazepam effectiveness

Adverse Reactions
CNS: Agitation, anxiety, ataxia, confusion, depression, dizziness, drowsiness, euphoria, headache, irritability, nervousness, slurred speech, tremor, weakness
CV: Angina, palpitations, sinus tachycardia
EENT: Diplopia, dry mouth, tinnitus
GI: Abdominal cramps or pain, constipation, diarrhea, increased salivation, nausea, vomiting
GU: Decreased libido, dysuria
MS: Arthralgia
SKIN: Pruritus, rash

Nursing Considerations
•Use halazepam cautiously in patients with impaired hepatic or renal function, seizure disorders, or suicidal tendencies.
•Be aware that risk of halazepam addiction and abuse is relatively high.
•Monitor renal and liver function test results, as appropriate, during long-term treatment.
•Expect to withdraw drug gradually over 2 weeks to avoid withdrawal symptoms, which include anxiety, confusion, insomnia, psychosis, and seizures.
PATIENT TEACHING
•Instruct patient to take halazepam exactly as prescribed and not to stop taking it abruptly because withdrawal symptoms may occur.
•Caution patient to avoid alcohol and other CNS depressants during therapy. Advise patient to avoid OTC drugs, such as cough and cold remedies, because they may contain CNS depressants.
•Advise patient to avoid potentially hazardous activities until drug's CNS effects are known.

•Instruct patient to report depression, difficulty voiding, double vision, persistent drowsiness, and rash.
•Explain that drug's full effects may not occur for 6 weeks.

haloperidol

Apo-Haloperidol (CAN), Haldol, Novo-Peridol (CAN), Peridol (CAN)

haloperidol decanoate

Haldol Decanoate, Haldol LA (CAN)

haloperidol lactate

Haldol Concentrate

Class and Category
Chemical: Butyrophenone derivative
Therapeutic: Antidyskinetic, antipsychotic
Pregnancy category: C (haloperidol decanoate), Not rated (haloperidol, haloperidol lactate)

Indications and Dosages
➤ *To treat psychotic disorders*
ORAL SOLUTION, TABLETS
Adults and adolescents. 0.5 to 5 mg b.i.d. or t.i.d. *Maximum:* Usually 100 mg/day.
Children ages 3 to 12. 0.05 mg/kg/day in divided doses b.i.d. or t.i.d. Increased by 0.5 mg q 5 to 7 days, if needed. *Maximum:* 0.15 mg/kg/day.
➤ *To treat nonpsychotic behavior disorders and Tourette's syndrome*
ORAL SOLUTION, TABLETS
Adults and adolescents. 0.5 to 5 mg b.i.d. or t.i.d. *Maximum:* Usually 100 mg/day.
Children ages 3 to 12. 0.05 to 0.075 mg/kg/day in divided doses b.i.d. or t.i.d. Increased by 0.5 mg q 5 to 7 days, if needed. *Maximum:* 0.075 mg/kg/day.
DOSAGE ADJUSTMENT Initial dosage reduced to 0.5 to 2 mg b.i.d. or t.i.d. if needed for elderly or debilitated patients.
➤ *To treat acute psychotic episodes*
I.M. INJECTION
Adults and adolescents. *Initial:* 2 to 5 mg followed by subsequent doses as frequently as q 60 min. Alternatively, if symptoms are controlled, dose may be repeated q 4 to 8 hr. *Maximum:* Usually 100 mg/day. First oral dose may be given 12 to 24 hr after last parenteral dose.

➤ *To provide long-term antipsychotic therapy for patients who require parenteral therapy*
LONG-ACTING I.M. (DECANOATE) INJECTION
Adults. *Initial:* 10 to 15 times the daily oral dose up to 100 mg. Repeated q 4 wk, if needed. *Maximum:* 300 mg/mo.

Route	Onset	Peak	Duration
I.M.*	Unknown	3 to 4 days†	Unknown

Mechanism of Action
May block postsynaptic dopamine receptors in the limbic system and increase brain turnover of dopamine, producing an antipsychotic effect.

Contraindications
Blood dyscrasias, bone marrow depression, cerebral arteriosclerosis, coma, concomitant use of large amounts of other CNS depressants, coronary artery disease, epilepsy, hepatic dysfunction, hypersensitivity to haloperidol or its components, Parkinson's disease, severe hypertension or hypotension, severe CNS depression, subcortical brain damage

Interactions
DRUGS
amphetamines: Possibly decreased stimulant effects of amphetamines and decreased antipsychotic effect of haloperidol
anticholinergics, antidyskinetics, antihistamines: Increased anticholinergic effect and risk of decreased antipsychotic effect of haloperidol
anticonvulsants: Possibly decreased effectiveness of anticonvulsants and decreased blood haloperidol level
bromocriptine: Possibly decreased effectiveness of bromocriptine
bupropion: Lowered seizure threshold, increased risk of major motor seizure
CNS depressants: Increased CNS depression and risk of respiratory depression and hypotension
diazoxide: Possibly hypoglycemia
dopamine (high-dose therapy): Possibly decreased vasoconstriction

---

* For haloperidol decanoate and lactate.
† For haloperidol decanoate only; 30 to 45 min for haloperidol lactate.

ephedrine: Possibly decreased vasopressor effect of ephedrine
epinephrine: Possibly severe hypotension and tachycardia
fluoxetine: Increased risk of severe and frequent extrapyramidal effects
guanadrel, guanethidine: Decreased hypotensive effects of these drugs
levodopa, pergolide: Possibly decreased therapeutic effects of these drugs
lithium: Increased risk of neurotoxicity
MAO inhibitors, maprotiline, tricyclic antidepressants: Increased sedative and anticholinergic effects of these drugs
metaraminol: Possibly decreased vasopressor effect of metaraminol
methoxamine: Decreased vasopressor effect, shortened duration of action of methoxamine
methyldopa: Possibly disorientation, slowed or difficult thought processes
phenylephrine: Decreased vasopressor response to phenylephrine
ACTIVITIES
alcohol use: Increased CNS depression and risk of respiratory depression and hypotension

Adverse Reactions

CNS: Agitation, anxiety, confusion, drowsiness, euphoria, extrapyramidal reactions that may be irreversible (akathisia, pseudoparkinsonism, tardive dyskinesia), hallucinations, headache, insomnia, neuroleptic malignant syndrome, restlessness, slurred speech, tremor, vertigo
CV: Cardiac arrest, hypertension, orthostatic hypotension, QT prolongation, ventricular tachycardia
EENT: Blurred vision, dry mouth, increased salivation (all drug forms); stomatitis (oral solution)
ENDO: Breast engorgement, galactorrhea
GI: Constipation, nausea, vomiting
GU: Decreased libido, difficult ejaculation, impotence, menstrual irregularities, urine retention
HEME: Anemia, leukocytosis, leukopenia
SKIN: Diaphoresis, photosensitivity, rash
Other: Heatstroke, weight gain

Nursing Considerations
•Before giving oral solution, dilute it with a beverage, such as cola or orange, apple, or tomato juice.
•Administer haloperidol decanoate (long-acting form prepared in sesame oil to pro-duce slow, sustained release) by deep I.M. injection into gluteal muscle using Z-track technique and 21G needle. Don't give more than 3 ml at one site. Expect to reach a stable plasma level after third or fourth dose.
•If injection solution has a slight yellow discoloration, be aware that this change doesn't affect potency.
•Monitor for tardive dyskinesia (potentially irreversible involuntary movements) in patients receiving long-term therapy, especially elderly women who take large doses.
•If extrapyramidal reactions occur during the first few days of treatment, reduce dosage, as prescribed.
•Avoid stopping haloperidol abruptly unless severe adverse reactions occur.
•Monitor for signs of neuroleptic malignant syndrome, a rare but possibly fatal disorder linked to antipsychotic drugs. Signs include altered mental status, arrhythmias, fever, and muscle rigidity.

PATIENT TEACHING
•Advise patient to take haloperidol exactly as prescribed and not to stop taking it abruptly because withdrawal symptoms may occur.
•To prevent oral mucosal irritation, instruct patient to dilute liquid form with juice or cola before taking it.
•Caution patient to avoid skin contact with oral solution because it may cause a rash.
•Advise patient to take tablets with food or a full glass of milk or water to reduce GI distress.
•Instruct patient to maintain adequate fluid intake and to take precautions against heatstroke.
•Urge patient not to drink alcohol during therapy.
•If sedation occurs, caution patient to avoid driving and other potentially hazardous activities.
•Instruct patient to report repetitive movements, tremor, and vision changes to prescriber.

heparin calcium
Calcilean (CAN), Calciparine
heparin sodium
Hepalean (CAN), Heparin Leo (CAN), Heparin Lock Flush, Liquaemin

Class and Category
Chemical: Glycosaminoglycan
Therapeutic: Anticoagulant
Pregnancy category: C

Indications and Dosages
➤ *To prevent and treat deep vein thrombosis and pulmonary embolism, to treat peripheral arterial embolism, and to prevent thromboembolism before and after cardioversion of chronic atrial fibrillation*
I.V. INFUSION OR INJECTION
Adults. *Loading:* 35 to 70 U/kg or 5,000 U by injection. Then 20,000 to 40,000 U infused over 24 hr.
Children. *Loading:* 50 U/kg by injection. Then 100 U/kg infused q 4 hr or 20,000 U/m² infused over 24 hr.
I.V. INJECTION
Adults. *Initial:* 10,000 U. *Maintenance:* 5,000 to 10,000 U q 4 to 6 hr.
Children. *Initial:* 50 U/kg. *Maintenance:* 100 U/kg/dose q 4 hr.
I.V. OR S.C. INJECTION
Adults. *Loading:* 5,000 U I.V., then 10,000 to 20,000 U S.C. *Maintenance:* 8,000 to 10,000 U S.C. q 8 hr or 15,000 to 20,000 U S.C. q 12 hr.
➤ *To diagnose and treat disseminated intravascular coagulation (DIC)*
I.V. INFUSION OR INJECTION
Adults. 50 to 100 U/kg q 4 hr. Drug may be discontinued if no improvement occurs in 4 to 8 hr.
Children. 25 to 50 U/kg q 4 hr. Drug may be discontinued if no improvement occurs in 4 to 8 hr.
➤ *To prevent postoperative thromboembolism*
S.C. INJECTION
Adults. 5,000 U 2 hr before surgery and then 5,000 U q 8 to 12 hr for 7 days or until patient is fully ambulatory.
➤ *To prevent clots in patients undergoing open-heart and vascular surgery*
I.V. INFUSION OR INJECTION
Adults. 300 U/kg for procedures that last less than 60 min; 400 U/kg for procedures that last longer than 60 min. *Minimum:* 150 U/kg.
Children. 300 U/kg for procedures that last less than 60 min. Then dosage is based on coagulation test results. *Minimum:* 150 U/kg.
➤ *To maintain heparin lock patency*

I.V. INJECTION
Adults. 10 to 100 U/ml heparin flush solution (enough to fill device) after each use of device.

Route	Onset	Peak	Duration
I.V.	Immediate	Minutes	Unknown
S.C.	In 20 to 60 min	Unknown	Unknown

Mechanism of Action
Binds with antithrombin III, enhancing antithrombin III's inactivation of the coagulation enzymes thrombin (factor IIa) and factors Xa and XIa. At low doses, heparin inhibits factor Xa and prevents the conversion of prothrombin to thrombin. Thrombin is necessary for the conversion of fibrinogen to fibrin; without fibrin, clots can't form. At high doses, heparin inactivates thrombin, preventing fibrin formation and existing clot extension.

Incompatibilities
Don't mix heparin with any other drug unless you have an order to do so and have checked with pharmacist. Heparin is incompatible with many drugs and solutions, especially ones that contain a phosphate buffer, sodium bicarbonate, or sodium oxalate.

Contraindications
Hypersensitivity to heparin or its components; severe thrombocytopenia; uncontrolled bleeding, except in DIC

Interactions
DRUGS
antihistamines, digoxin, nicotine, tetracyclines: Decreased anticoagulant effect of heparin
aspirin, NSAIDs, platelet aggregation inhibitors, sulfinpyrazone: Increased platelet inhibition and risk of bleeding
cefamandole, cefoperazone, cefotetan, methimazole, plicamycin, propylthiouracil, valproic acid: Possibly hypoprothrombinemia and increased risk of bleeding
chloroquine, hydroxychloroquine: Possibly thrombocytopenia and increased risk of hemorrhage
ethacrynic acid, glucocorticoids, salicylates: Increased risk of bleeding and GI ulceration and hemorrhage

nitroglycerin (I.V.): Possibly decreased anticoagulant effect of heparin
probenecid: Possibly increased anticoagulant effect of heparin
thrombolytics: Increased risk of hemorrhage
ACTIVITIES
smoking: Decreased anticoagulant effect of heparin

Adverse Reactions

CNS: Chills, dizziness, fever, headache, peripheral neuropathy
CV: Chest pain
EENT: Epistaxis, gingival bleeding, rhinitis
GI: Abdominal distention and pain, hematemesis, melena, nausea, vomiting
GU: Hematuria, hypermenorrhea
HEME: Easy bruising, excessive bleeding from wounds, thrombocytopenia
MS: Back pain, myalgia, osteoporosis
RESP: Dyspnea, wheezing
SKIN: Alopecia, cyanosis, petechiae, pruritus, urticaria
Other: Anaphylaxis; injection site hematoma, irritation, pain, redness, and ulceration

Nursing Considerations

• Use heparin cautiously in alcoholics; menstruating women; and patients with mild hepatic or renal disease or a history of allergies, asthma, or GI ulcer.
•WARNING Administer heparin only by S.C. or I.V. route; I.M. injection causes hematoma, irritation, and pain.
• Avoid injecting any drugs by I.M. route during heparin therapy to decrease the risk of bleeding and hematoma.
• Administer S.C. heparin into the anterior abdominal wall, above the iliac crest, and 5 cm (2″) or more away from the umbilicus. To minimize subcutaneous tissue trauma, lift adipose tissue away from deep tissues; don't aspirate for blood before injecting drug; don't move needle while injecting drug; and don't massage the injection site before or after injection. Keep in mind that you can apply gentle pressure to the site after you withdraw the needle.
• Alternate injection sites, and observe for signs of bleeding and hematoma formation.
• To prepare heparin for continuous infusion, invert container at least six times to prevent drug from pooling. Anticipate slight discoloration of prepared solution; this doesn't indicate a change in potency.

• During continuous I.V. therapy, expect to obtain APTT after 8 hours of therapy. Use the arm opposite the infusion site.
• For intermittent I.V. therapy, expect to adjust dose based on coagulation test results performed 30 minutes earlier. Therapeutic range is typically 1.5 to 2.5 times the control.
• Take safety precautions to prevent bleeding, such as having patient use a soft-bristled toothbrush and an electric razor.
• Monitor blood test results and observe for signs of bleeding, such as ecchymosis, epistaxis, hematemesis, hematuria, melena, and petechiae.
• Make sure all health care providers know that patient is receiving heparin.
• Keep protamine sulfate on hand to use as an antidote for heparin. Be aware that each milligram of protamine sulfate neutralizes 100 U of heparin.
• Be aware that prescriber may order oral anticoagulants before discontinuing heparin to avoid increased coagulation caused by heparin withdrawal. Heparin may be discontinued when full therapeutic effect of oral anticoagulant is achieved.
• Know that women over age 60 have the highest risk of hemorrhage during therapy.
PATIENT TEACHING
• Explain that heparin can't be taken orally.
• Inform patient about the increased risk of bleeding; urge her to avoid injuries and to use a soft-bristled toothbrush and an electric razor.
• Advise patient to avoid drugs that interact with heparin, such as aspirin and ibuprofen.
• Instruct patient and family to watch for and report abdominal or lower back pain, black stools, bleeding gums, bloody urine, excessive menstrual bleeding, nosebleeds, and severe headaches.
• Inform patient that temporary hair loss may occur.
• Advise patient to wear or carry appropriate medical identification.

hydralazine hydrochloride

Apo-Hydralazine (CAN), Apresoline (CAN), Novo-Hylazin (CAN)

Class and Category

Chemical: Phthalazine derivative

Therapeutic: Antihypertensive, vasodilator
Pregnancy category: C

Indications and Dosages
➤ *To manage essential hypertension, alone or with other antihypertensives*

TABLETS

Adults. *Initial:* 40 mg/day in divided doses b.i.d. or q.i.d. for first 2 to 4 days and then increased to 100 mg/day in divided doses b.i.d. or q.i.d. for remainder of first wk. *Maximum:* Usually 200 mg/day, but sometimes 300 to 400 mg/day.

Children. 0.75 mg/kg/day in divided doses b.i.d. or q.i.d., increased gradually over 3 to 4 wk. *Maximum:* 7.5 mg/kg or 200 mg/day.

➤ *To manage severe essential hypertension when drug can't be taken orally or when need to reduce blood pressure is urgent*

I.V. OR I.M. INJECTION

Adults. 5 to 40 mg, repeated as needed.
Children. 1.7 to 3.5 mg/kg/day in divided doses q 4 to 6 hr, as needed.

Incompatibilities
Don't mix hydralazine in I.V. infusion solutions.

Route	Onset	Peak	Duration
P.O.	20 to 30 min	1 to 2 hr	2 to 4 hr
I.V.	5 to 20 min	10 to 80 min	2 to 6 hr
I.M.	10 to 30 min	1 hr	2 to 6 hr

Contraindications
Coronary artery disease, hypersensitivity to hydralazine or its components, mitral valve disease

Interactions
DRUGS

beta blockers: Increased effects of both drugs
diazoxide, MAO inhibitors, other antihypertensives: Risk of severe hypotension
epinephrine: Possibly decreased vasopressor effect of epinephrine
NSAIDs: Decreased hydralazine effects
sympathomimetics: Possibly decreased antihypertensive effect of hydralazine

FOODS

all foods: Possibly increased bioavailability of hydralazine

Mechanism of Action
May act in a manner that resembles organic nitrates and sodium nitroprusside, except that hydralazine is selective for arteries. It:
• exerts a direct vasodilating effect on vascular smooth muscle
• interferes with calcium movement in vascular smooth muscle by altering cellular calcium metabolism
• dilates arteries rather than veins, which minimizes orthostatic hypotension and increases cardiac output and cerebral blood flow
• causes a reflex autonomic response that increases the heart rate, cardiac output, and left ventricular ejection fraction
• has a positive inotropic effect on the heart.

Adverse Reactions
CNS: Chills, fever, headache, peripheral neuritis
CV: Angina, edema, orthostatic hypotension, palpitations, tachycardia
EENT: Lacrimation, nasal congestion
GI: Anorexia, constipation, diarrhea, nausea, vomiting
RESP: Dyspnea
SKIN: Blisters, flushing, pruritus, rash, urticaria
Other: Lupus-like symptoms, especially with high doses; lymphadenopathy

Nursing Considerations
• Monitor CBC, lupus erythematosus cell preparation, and ANA titer before therapy and periodically as appropriate during long-term treatment.
• Anticipate that drug may change color in solution. Consult pharmacist if color change occurs.
• Be aware that hydralazine may undergo color changes when exposed to a metal filter.
• Give tablets with food to increase bioavailability.
• Monitor blood pressure and pulse rate regularly and weigh patient daily during therapy.
• Check blood pressure with patient in lying, sitting, and standing positions, and watch for signs of orthostatic hypotension. Expect orthostatic hypotension to be most common in

G
H
I

the morning, during hot weather, and with exercise.

•**WARNING** Expect to discontinue drug immediately if patient experiences lupus-like symptoms, such as arthralgia, fever, myalgia, pharyngitis, and splenomegaly.

•Expect prescriber to withdraw drug gradually to avoid a rapid increase in blood pressure.

•Expect to treat peripheral neuritis with pyridoxine.

PATIENT TEACHING

•Instruct patient to take hydralazine tablets with food.

•Advise patient to change position slowly, especially in the morning. Caution her that hot showers may increase hypotension.

•Instruct patient to immediately notify prescriber about fever, muscle and joint aches, and sore throat.

•Urge patient to report numbness and tingling in her limbs, which may require treatment with another drug.

•Caution patient against stopping drug abruptly because doing so may cause severe hypertension.

hydrochlorothiazide

Esidrix, Hydro-chlor, Hydro-D, Hydro-DIURIL, Microzide, Neo-Codema (CAN), Novo-Hydrazide (CAN), Oretic, Urozide (CAN)

Class and Category

Chemical: Benzothiadiazide
Therapeutic: Antihypertensive, diuretic
Pregnancy category: B

Indications and Dosages

➤ *To manage hypertension*

CAPSULES

Adults. 12.5 mg/day.

ORAL SOLUTION, TABLETS

Adults. 25 to 100 mg/day as a single dose or in divided doses b.i.d.

Children age 6 months and older. 1 to 2 mg/kg/day as a single dose or in divided doses b.i.d.

Infants under age 6 months. Up to 3 mg/kg/day.

➤ *As adjunct to treat edema caused by cirrhosis, corticosteroids, estrogen, heart failure, or renal disorders*

ORAL SOLUTION, TABLETS

Adults. 25 to 100 mg b.i.d., q.d., or q.o.d for 3 to 5 days/wk.

Children age 6 months and older. 1 to 2 mg/kg/day as a single dose or in divided doses b.i.d.

Infants under age 6 months. Up to 3 mg/kg/day.

Route	Onset	Peak	Duration
P.O.	2 hr	4 hr	6 to 12 hr

Contraindications

Anuria; hypersensitivity to hydrochlorothiazide, other thiazides, sulfonamide derivatives, or their components; renal failure

Interactions

DRUGS

amantadine: Possibly increased blood level and risk of toxicity of amantadine

amiodarone: Increased risk of arrhythmias from hypokalemia

amphotericin B, corticosteroids: Increased electrolyte depletion, especially potassium

antihypertensives: Increased antihypertensive effects

calcium: Possibly increased serum calcium level

cholestyramine, colestipol: Reduced GI absorption of hydrochlorothiazide

diazoxide: Increased antihypertensive and hyperglycemic effects of hydrochlorothiazide

diflunisal: Possibly increased blood hydrochlorothiazide level

digoxin: Increased risk of digitalis toxicity from hypokalemia

dopamine: Possibly increased diuretic effects of both drugs

insulin, oral antidiabetic drugs: Possibly increased blood glucose level

lithium: Decreased lithium clearance, increased risk of lithium toxicity

neuromuscular blockers: Possibly enhanced neuromuscular blockade from hypokalemia

NSAIDs: Decreased diuretic effect of hydrochlorothiazide, increased risk of renal failure

oral anticoagulants: Possibly decreased anticoagulant effects

sympathomimetics: Possibly decreased antihypertensive effect of hydrochlorothiazide

vitamin D: Increased risk of hypercalcemia

Adverse Reactions

CNS: Dizziness, headache, insomnia, paresthesia, vertigo, weakness

Mechanism of Action

A thiazide diuretic, hydrochlorothiazide promotes the movement of sodium (Na^+), chloride (Cl^-), and water (H_2O) from blood in the peritubular capillaries into the nephron's distal convoluted tubule, as shown at right. Initially, hydrochlorothiazide may decrease extracellular fluid volume, plasma volume, and cardiac output, which helps explain blood pressure reduction. It also may reduce blood pressure by causing direct dilation of arteries. After several weeks, extracellular fluid volume, plasma volume, and cardiac output return to normal, and peripheral vascular resistance remains decreased.

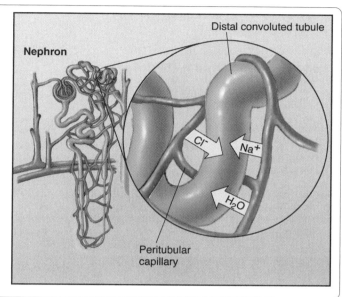

CV: Hypotension, orthostatic hypotension, vasculitis
EENT: Blurred vision, dry mouth
ENDO: Hyperglycemia
GI: Abdominal cramps, anorexia, constipation, diarrhea, indigestion, jaundice, nausea, vomiting
GU: Decreased libido, impotence, interstitial nephritis, nocturia, polyuria, renal failure
HEME: Agranulocytosis, aplastic anemia, hemolytic anemia, leukopenia, neutropenia, thrombocytopenia
MS: Muscle spasms and weakness
SKIN: Alopecia, exfoliative dermatitis, photosensitivity, purpura, rash, urticaria
Other: Anaphylaxis, dehydration, hypercalcemia, hyperuricemia, hypochloremia, hypokalemia, hyponatremia, hypovolemia, metabolic alkalosis, weight loss

Nursing Considerations

•Give hydrochlorothiazide in the morning and early in the evening to avoid nocturia.
•Monitor fluid intake and output, daily weight, blood pressure, and serum levels of electrolytes, especially potassium.
•Assess for signs of hypokalemia, such as muscle spasms and weakness.

•Monitor BUN and serum creatinine levels regularly.
•Frequently monitor blood glucose level as ordered in diabetic patients, and expect to increase antidiabetic drug dosage, as needed.
•If patient has a history of gouty arthritis, expect an increased risk of gout attacks during therapy.

PATIENT TEACHING

•Advise patient to take hydrochlorothiazide in the morning and early in the evening to avoid awakening during the night to urinate.
•Instruct patient to take drug with food or milk if adverse GI reactions occur.
•Direct patient to weigh herself at the same time each day wearing the same amount of clothing and to notify prescriber if she gains more than 2 lb (0.9 kg) per day or 5 lb (2.3 kg) per week.
•Instruct patient to eat a diet high in potassium-rich food, including citrus fruits, bananas, tomatoes, and dates.
•Advise patient to change position slowly to minimize effects of orthostatic hypotension.
•Urge patient to notify prescriber about decreased urination, muscle cramps and weakness, and unusual bleeding or bruising.

hydrocodone and ibuprofen

Vicoprofen

Class, Category, and Schedule

Chemical: Opioid and phenanthrene derivative (hydrocodone), propionic acid derivative (ibuprofen)
Therapeutic: Analgesic
Pregnancy category: C
Controlled substance: Schedule III

Indications and Dosages

➤ *To relieve acute pain*

TABLETS

Adults. 1 tablet (7.5 mg of hydrocodone, 200 mg of ibuprofen) q 4 to 6 hr, p.r.n., for up to 5 days. *Maximum:* 5 tablets (37.5 mg of hydrocodone, 1,000 mg of ibuprofen)/day.

Route	Onset	Peak	Duration
P.O.	10 to 30 min	30 to 60 min	4 to 6 hr

Mechanism of Action

Exerts a synergistic analgesic effect through two mechanisms of action. Hydrocodone, a mu opiate-receptor agonist, alters the perception of pain at the spinal cord and higher CNS levels by blocking the release of inhibitory neurotransmitters, such as gamma-aminobutyric acid and acetylcholine. It also alters the emotional response to pain.

Ibuprofen blocks the activity of cyclooxygenase, the enzyme necessary for prostaglandin synthesis. Prostaglandins, important mediators in the inflammatory response, cause local vasodilation with swelling and pain. They also play a role in pain transmission from the periphery to the spinal cord. With the inhibition of cyclooxygenase and prostaglandin synthesis, inflammatory symptoms subside.

Contraindications

Hypersensitivity to aspirin, hydrocodone, ibuprofen, narcotics, other NSAIDs, or their components; respiratory depression; severe asthma; upper airway obstruction

Interactions

DRUGS

ACE inhibitors (such as benazepril, captopril, and enalapril): Possibly decreased therapeutic effects of ACE inhibitors

anticholinergics: Increased risk of ileus
aspirin, corticosteroids, NSAIDs: Possibly increased risk of GI ulceration and hemorrhage
CNS depressants: Increased CNS depression
diuretics: Possibly decreased diuresis, increased risk of renal failure
lithium: Increased blood lithium level, increased risk of lithium toxicity
methotrexate: Increased blood methotrexate level, increased risk of methotrexate toxicity
MAO inhibitors (such as furazolidone, phenelzine, procarbazine, selegiline, tranylcypromine): Increased risk of adverse CNS effects
naloxone: Possibly withdrawal symptoms in physically dependent patients
naltrexone: Possibly prolonged respiratory depression and cardiac arrest
oral anticoagulants: Increased risk of GI bleeding
tricyclic antidepressants: Possibly increased adverse effects of hydrocodone or potentiated antidepressant effects

ACTIVITIES

alcohol use: Possibly increased CNS depression

Adverse Reactions

CNS: Anxiety, confusion, depression, dizziness, euphoria, fatigue, fever, headache, insomnia, irritability, lethargy, nervousness, paresthesia, sedation, slurred speech, somnolence, tremor, weakness
CV: Arrhythmias, peripheral edema, hypotension, orthostatic hypotension, palpitations
EENT: Dry mouth, mouth ulcers, pharyngitis, rhinitis, sinusitis, tinnitus, vision changes
GI: Anorexia, constipation, dysphagia, esophagitis, flatulence, gastritis, gastroenteritis, indigestion, nausea, vomiting
GU: Impotence, urinary frequency, urine retention
RESP: Bronchitis, dyspnea, respiratory depression
SKIN: Diaphoresis, flushing, pruritus, rash, urticaria
Other: Physical and psychological dependence

Nursing Considerations

•Expect to give hydrocodone and ibuprofen for short-term pain relief only (no more than 10 days).
•Expect prolonged use of drug to produce physical and psychological dependence; physical dependence may cause withdrawal symptoms when drug is discontinued.

•Assess carefully for adverse reactions when giving drug to elderly patients; they are especially sensitive to drug and are at increased risk for constipation.

•**WARNING** Monitor for signs of overdose, such as blurred vision; cold, clammy skin; confusion; dizziness; dyspnea; headache; hearing loss; malaise; mental or mood changes; nausea; respiratory depression; sinus bradycardia; tinnitus; and vomiting. Notify prescriber immediately if they develop.

PATIENT TEACHING

•Inform patient that hydrocodone and ibuprofen may cause drowsiness and dizziness.

•Advise patient to avoid potentially hazardous activities until drug's CNS effects are known.

•Caution patient not to take more than prescribed dosage because of the risk of dependence.

•Urge patient to avoid using alcohol during drug therapy.

•Advise patient to change position slowly to minimize effects of orthostatic hypotension.

•If patient reports dry mouth, suggest that she use sugarless candy or gum or ice chips.

hydrocodone bitartrate and acetaminophen

Allay, Anexsia, Anolor DH 5, Bancap-HC, Co-Gesic, Dolacet, Dolagesic, Duocet, Hycomed, Hyco-Pap, Hydrocet, Hydrogesic, Lorcet-HD, Lorcet Plus, Lortab, Margesic-H, Oncet, Panacet, Panlor, Polygesic, Stagesic, T-Gesic, Ugesic, Vanacet, Vendone, Vicodin, Vicodin ES, Zydone

Class, Category, and Schedule

Chemical: Opioid and phenanthrene derivative (hydrocodone), para-aminophenol derivative (acetaminophen)
Therapeutic: Analgesic
Pregnancy category: C
Controlled substance: Schedule III

Indications and Dosages

➤ *To treat moderate to severe back pain and pain from arthralgia, cancer, dental procedures, headache, and myalgia*

CAPSULES

Adults. 1 capsule (5 mg of hydrocodone, 500 mg of acetaminophen) q 4 to 6 hr, p.r.n.; or 2 capsules (10 mg of hydrocodone, 1,000 mg of acetaminophen) q 6 hr, p.r.n. *Maximum:* 8 capsules (40 mg of hydrocodone, 4,000 mg of acetaminophen)/24 hr.

ORAL SOLUTION

Adults. 5 to 15 ml (2.5 mg of hydrocodone, 167 mg of acetaminophen/5 ml) q 4 to 6 hr, p.r.n., for up to 6 days.

TABLETS

Adults. 1 or 2 tablets (2.5 mg of hydrocodone, 500 mg of acetaminophen/tablet) q 4 to 6 hr, p.r.n.; or 1 tablet (5 mg of hydrocodone, 500 mg of acetaminophen) q 4 to 6 hr, p.r.n., up to 2 tablets q 6 hr, p.r.n.; or 1 tablet (7.5 mg hydrocodone, 650 mg acetaminophen) q 4 to 6 hr, p.r.n., up to 2 tablets q 6 hr, p.r.n.; or 1 tablet (7.5 mg of hydrocodone, 750 mg of acetaminophen) q 4 to 6 hr, p.r.n.; or 1 tablet (10 mg of hydrocodone, 650 mg of acetaminophen) q 4 to 6 hr, p.r.n. *Maximum:* 40 mg of hydrocodone, 4,000 mg of acetaminophen/day.

Route	Onset	Peak	Duration
P.O.	10 to 30 min	30 to 60 min	4 to 6 hr

Mechanism of Action

Exerts a synergistic analgesic effect through two mechanisms of action. Hydrocodone, a mu opiate-receptor agonist, alters the perception of pain at the spinal cord and higher CNS levels by blocking the release of inhibitory neurotransmitters, such as gamma-aminobutyric acid and acetylcholine. It also alters the emotional response to pain.

Acetaminophen increases the pain threshold at the CNS level by inhibiting cyclooxygenase, an enzyme involved in prostaglandin synthesis. Prostaglandins, important mediators in the inflammatory response, cause local vasodilation with swelling and pain. They also play a role in pain transmission from the periphery to the spinal cord. With the inhibition of cyclooxygenase and prostaglandin synthesis, inflammatory symptoms subside.

Contraindications

Acute asthma; hypersensitivity to acetaminophen, aspirin, hydrocodone, narcotics, NSAIDs, or their components; respiratory depression; upper airway obstruction

Interactions

DRUGS

anticholinergics: Increased risk of ileus, severe constipation, and urine retention

antidiarrheals (antiperistaltic): Increased risk of CNS depression and severe constipation

barbiturate anesthetics: Possibly increased respiratory and CNS depression

chlorpromazine, thioridazine: Increased risk of adverse and toxic effects of hydrocodone

CNS depressants: Increased risk of CNS and respiratory depression and hypotension

diuretics, other antihypertensives: Increased risk of hypotension

MAO inhibitors (such as furazolidone, phenelzine, procarbazine, selegiline, tranylcypromine) within 14 days of receiving hydrocodone and acetaminophen: Increased risk of adverse CNS effects

metoclopramide: Possibly antagonized effect of metoclopramide on GI motility

naloxone: Possibly withdrawal symptoms in physically dependent patients

naltrexone: Possibly prolonged respiratory depression or cardiac arrest

other opioid analgesics: Risk of increased CNS and respiratory depression and hypotension

ACTIVITIES

alcohol use: Increased risk of CNS depression

Adverse Reactions

CNS: Confusion, dizziness, drowsiness, euphoria, headache, lethargy, restlessness, sedation, syncope
CV: Hypotension, orthostatic hypotension, tachycardia
EENT: Dry mouth, laryngeal edema, laryngospasm, vision changes
GI: Anorexia, constipation, nausea, vomiting
GU: Dysuria, urine retention
RESP: Atelectasis, bronchospasm, respiratory depression, wheezing
SKIN: Diaphoresis, flushing, pruritus, rash, urticaria
Other: Physical and psychological dependence

Nursing Considerations

•Expect prolonged use of hydrocodone and acetaminophen to produce physical and psychological dependence; physical dependence may cause withdrawal symptoms when drug is discontinued.
•Assess carefully for adverse reactions when giving drug to elderly patients; they're especially sensitive to drug and are at increased risk for constipation.
•**WARNING** Monitor for signs of overdose, such as blurred vision; cold, clammy skin; confusion; dizziness; dyspnea; headache; hearing loss; malaise; mental or mood changes; nausea; respiratory depression; sinus bradycardia; tinnitus; and vomiting. Notify prescriber immediately if they develop.

PATIENT TEACHING

•Inform patient that hydrocodone and acetaminophen may cause dizziness and drowsiness.
•Advise patient to avoid potentially hazardous activities until drug's CNS effects are known.
•Caution patient not to take more than prescribed dosage because of risk of dependence.
•Urge patient to avoid using alcohol during drug therapy.
•Advise patient to change position slowly to minimize effects of orthostatic hypotension.
•If patient reports dry mouth, suggest that she use sugarless candy or gum or ice chips.

hydrocortisone

(cortisol)

Cortef, Hydrocortone

hydrocortisone acetate

Hydrocortone Acetate

hydrocortisone cypionate

Cortef

hydrocortisone sodium phosphate

Hydrocortone Phosphate

hydrocortisone sodium succinate

A-hydroCort, Solu-Cortef

Class and Category

Chemical: Glucocorticoid
Therapeutic: Adrenocorticoid replacement, anti-inflammatory
Pregnancy category: Not rated

Indications and Dosages

➤ *To treat severe inflammation or acute adrenal insufficiency*

ORAL SUSPENSION, TABLETS (HYDROCORTISONE, HYDRO-
CORTISONE CYPIONATE)

Adults. 20 to 240 mg/day as a single dose or
in divided doses.

I.V. INFUSION OR I.V., I.M., OR S.C. INJECTION (HYDRO-
CORTISONE SODIUM PHOSPHATE); I.M. INJECTION (HYDRO-
CORTISONE)

Adults. 15 to 240 mg/day as a single dose or
in divided doses. *Usual:* ½ to ⅓ the oral dose.

DOSAGE ADJUSTMENT Dosage increased above
240 mg/day if needed to treat acute disease.

I.V. INFUSION; I.V. OR I.M. INJECTION (HYDROCORTISONE
SODIUM SUCCINATE)

Adults. 100 to 500 mg q 2, 4, or 6 hr.

➤ *To treat joint and tissue inflammation*

INTRA-ARTICULAR INJECTION (HYDROCORTISONE ACETATE)

Adults. 25 to 37.5 mg injected into large joints
or bursae as a single dose, or 10 to 25 mg
injected into small joints as a single dose.

INTRALESIONAL INJECTION (HYDROCORTISONE ACETATE)

Adults. 5 to 12.5 mg injected into tendon
sheaths as a single dose, or 12.5 to 25 mg injected into ganglia as a single dose.

SOFT-TISSUE INJECTION (HYDROCORTISONE ACETATE)

Adults. 25 to 50 mg as a single dose. Sometimes a dose of up to 75 mg is needed.

Route	Onset	Peak	Duration
P.O. (hydro-cortisone)	Unknown	1 hr	1.25 to 1.5 days
P.O. (cypi-onate)	Unknown	1 to 2 hr	Unknown
I.V. (phos-phate, suc-cinate)	Rapid	Unknown	Unknown
I.M. (hydro-cortisone)	Unknown	4 to 8 hr	Unknown
I.M. (phos-phate)	Rapid	1 hr	Unknown
I.M. (succi-nate)	Rapid	1 hr	Variable
Other* (acetate)	Unknown	24 to 48 hr	3 days to 4 wk

Contraindications

Hypersensitivity to hydrocortisone or its
components, idiopathic thrombocytopenic
purpura (I.M.), recent vaccination with live-
virus vaccine, systemic fungal infection

---

* Intra-articular, intralesional, and soft-tissue
  injection.

Mechanism of Action

Binds to intracellular glucocorticoid receptors and suppresses the inflammatory
and immune responses by:
•inhibiting neutrophil and monocyte accumulation at the inflammation site and
suppressing their phagocytic and bactericidal activity
•stabilizing lysosomal membranes
•suppressing the antigen response of macrophages and helper T cells
•inhibiting the synthesis of cellular mediators of the inflammatory response, such as
cytokines, interleukins, and prostaglandins.

Interactions

DRUGS

acetaminophen: Increased risk of hepatotoxicity
*amphotericin B, carbonic anhydrase inhibi-
tors:* Possibly severe hypokalemia
anabolic steroids, androgens: Increased risk
of edema and severe acne
anticholinergics: Possibly increased intraocular pressure
anticoagulants, thrombolytics: Increased risk
of GI ulceration and hemorrhage, possibly
decreased therapeutic effects of these drugs
asparaginase: Increased risk of hyperglycemia and toxicity
aspirin, NSAIDs: Increased risk of GI distress and bleeding
digoxin: Possibly hypokalemia-induced arrhythmias and digitalis toxicity
*ephedrine, phenobarbital, phenytoin, rifam-
pin:* Decreased blood hydrocortisone level
estrogens, oral contraceptives: Possibly increased therapeutic and toxic effects of hydrocortisone
insulin, oral antidiabetic drugs: Possibly increased blood glucose level
isoniazid: Possibly decreased therapeutic effects of isoniazid
mexiletine: Possibly decreased blood mexiletine level
neuromuscular blockers: Possibly increased
neuromuscular blockade, causing respiratory
depression or apnea
*potassium-depleting drugs, such as thiazide
diuretics:* Possibly severe hypokalemia
potassium supplements: Possibly decreased
effects of these supplements
somatrem, somatropin: Possibly decreased
therapeutic effects of these drugs
streptozocin: Increased risk of hyperglycemia

G
H
I

vaccines: Decreased antibody response and increased risk of neurologic complications

ACTIVITIES

alcohol use: Increased risk of GI distress and bleeding

Adverse Reactions

CNS: Ataxia, behavioral changes, depression, dizziness, euphoria, fatigue, headache, increased intracranial pressure with papilledema, insomnia, malaise, mood changes, paresthesia, seizures, steroid psychosis, syncope, vertigo
CV: Arrhythmias (from hypokalemia), fat embolism, heart failure, hypertension, hypotension, thromboembolism, thrombophlebitis
EENT: Exophthalmos, glaucoma, increased intraocular pressure, nystagmus, posterior subcapsular cataracts
ENDO: Adrenal insufficiency during stress, cushingoid symptoms (buffalo hump, central obesity, moon face, supraclavicular fat pad enlargement), diabetes mellitus, growth suppression in children, hyperglycemia, negative nitrogen balance from protein catabolism
GI: Abdominal distention, hiccups, increased appetite, nausea, pancreatitis, peptic ulcer, ulcerative esophagitis, vomiting
GU: Amenorrhea, glycosuria, menstrual irregularities, perineal burning or tingling
HEME: Easy bruising, leukocytosis
MS: Arthralgia; aseptic necrosis of femoral and humeral heads; compression fractures; muscle atrophy, twitching, or weakness; myalgia; osteoporosis; spontaneous fractures; steroid myopathy; tendon rupture
SKIN: Acne; altered skin pigmentation; diaphoresis; erythema; hirsutism; necrotizing vasculitis; petechiae; purpura; rash; scarring; sterile abscess; striae; subcutaneous fat atrophy; thin, fragile skin; urticaria
Other: Anaphylaxis, hypocalcemia, hypokalemia, hypokalemic alkalosis, impaired wound healing, masking of signs of infection, metabolic alkalosis, suppressed skin test reaction, weight gain

Nursing Considerations

• Be aware that systemic hydrocortisone shouldn't be given to immunocompromised patients, such as those with fungal and other infections, including amebiasis, hepatitis B, tuberculosis, vaccinia, and varicella.
• Give daily dose of hydrocortisone in the morning to mimic the normal peak in adrenocortical secretion of corticosteroids.
• When possible, give oral dose with food or milk to avoid GI distress.

• Don't give acetate injectable suspension by I.V. route.
• Give hydrocortisone sodium succinate as a direct I.V. injection over 30 seconds to several minutes, or as an intermittent or a continuous infusion. For infusion, dilute to 1 mg/ml or less with D_5W, NS, or D_5NS.
• Inject I.M. form deep into gluteal muscle, and rotate injection sites to prevent muscle atrophy. S.C. injection may cause atrophy and sterile abscess.
• Be aware that high-dose therapy shouldn't be given for longer than 48 hours. Be alert for depression or psychotic episodes during high-dose therapy.
• Regularly monitor weight, blood pressure, and serum electrolyte levels during therapy.
• Expect hydrocortisone to exacerbate infections or mask their signs and symptoms.
• Monitor blood glucose level in diabetic patients, and increase insulin or oral antidiabetic drug dosage, as prescribed.
• Know that elderly patients are at high risk for osteoporosis during long-term therapy.
• Anticipate the possibility of acute adrenal insufficiency with stress, such as emotional upset, fever, surgery, and trauma. Increase hydrocortisone dosage, as prescribed.
• **WARNING** Avoid withdrawing drug suddenly after long-term therapy because adrenal crisis can result. Expect to reduce dosage gradually as prescribed and monitor response.

PATIENT TEACHING

• Advise patient to take daily dose of hydrocortisone at 9 a.m.
• Instruct patient to take tablets or oral suspension with milk or food.
• Caution patient not to stop taking drug abruptly without first consulting prescriber.
• Instruct patient to report early signs of adrenal insufficiency: anorexia, difficulty breathing, dizziness, fainting, fatigue, joint pain, muscle weakness, and nausea.
• Inform patient that easy bruising may occur.
• Advise patient on long-term therapy to have periodic eye examinations.
• If patient receives long-term therapy, urge her to carry or wear medical identification.

hydromorphone hydrochloride

(dihydromorphinone)

Dilaudid, Dilaudid-5, Dilaudid-HP, Hydrostat IR, PMS-Hydromorphone (CAN), PMS-Hydromorphone Syrup (CAN)

Class, Category, and Schedule

Chemical: Phenanthrene derivative, semisynthetic opioid derivative
Therapeutic: Analgesic
Pregnancy category: C
Controlled substance: Schedule II

Indications and Dosages

➤ *To relieve moderate to severe pain*

ORAL SOLUTION

Adults. 2.5 to 10 mg q 3 to 6 hr, p.r.n.

TABLETS

Adults. 2 mg q 3 to 6 hr, p.r.n. Increased to 4 mg or more q 4 to 6 hr, if indicated.

I.V. INJECTION

Adults. 1 mg q 3 hr, p.r.n.

I.M. OR S.C. INJECTION

Adults. 1 or 2 mg q 3 to 6 hr, p.r.n. Increased to 3 or 4 mg q 4 to 6 hr, if needed for severe pain.

SUPPOSITORIES

Adults. 3 mg q 4 to 8 hr, p.r.n.

Route	Onset	Peak	Duration
P.O.	30 min	1.5 to 2 hr	4 hr
I.V.	10 to 15 min	15 to 30 min	2 to 3 hr
I.M.	15 min	30 to 60 min	4 to 5 hr
S.C.	15 min	30 to 90 min	4 hr
P.R.	30 min	Unknown	4 hr

Mechanism of Action

May bind with opioid receptors in the spinal cord and higher levels in the CNS. In this way, hydromorphone is believed to stimulate mu and kappa receptors, thus altering the perception of and emotional response to pain.

Contraindications

Acute asthma; hypersensitivity to hydromorphone, other narcotics, or their components; increased intracranial pressure; severe respiratory depression; upper respiratory tract obstruction

Interactions

DRUGS

anticholinergics: Increased risk of ileus, severe constipation, or urine retention
antihypertensives, diuretics, guanadrel, guanethidine, mecamylamine: Increased risk of orthostatic hypotension
barbiturate anesthetics: Increased sedative effect of hydromorphone
belladonna alkaloids, difenoxin and atropine, diphenoxylate and atropine, kaolin pectin, loperamide, paregoric: Increased risk of CNS depression and severe constipation
buprenorphine, butorphanol, dezocine, nalbuphine, pentazocine: Possibly potentiated or suppressed symptoms of spontaneous narcotic withdrawal
CNS depressants, other opioid analgesics: Additive CNS depression and hypotension
hydroxyzine: Increased analgesia, CNS depression, and hypotension
metoclopramide: Decreased effect of metoclopramide on GI motility
naloxone: Possibly withdrawal symptoms in physically dependent patients
naltrexone: Possibly prolonged respiratory depression or cardiac arrest
neuromuscular blockers: Additive CNS depression

ACTIVITIES

alcohol use: Increased CNS depression

Adverse Reactions

CNS: Anxiety, confusion, dizziness, drowsiness, euphoria, hallucinations, headache, nervousness, restlessness, sedation, somnolence, tremor, weakness
CV: Hypertension, orthostatic hypotension, palpitations, tachycardia
EENT: Blurred vision, diplopia, dry mouth, laryngeal edema, laryngospasm, nystagmus, tinnitus
GI: Abdominal cramps, anorexia, biliary tract spasm, constipation, hepatotoxicity, nausea, vomiting
GU: Dysuria, urine retention
RESP: Dyspnea, respiratory depression, wheezing
SKIN: Diaphoresis, flushing
Other: Injection site pain, redness, and swelling; physical and psychological dependence

Nursing Considerations

•To improve analgesic action, give hydromorphone before pain becomes intense.
•Give I.V. form by direct injection over at least 2 minutes. For infusion, mix drug with D_5W, NS, or Ringer's solution.
•Monitor for respiratory depression when using I.V. route. Keep resuscitation equipment and naloxone nearby.
•Rotate I.M. and S.C. injection sites.
•Assess for constipation.

G
H
I

•Monitor for signs of physical dependence or abuse.
•Anticipate that drug may mask or worsen gallbladder pain.

PATIENT TEACHING
•Instruct patient to take hydromorphone exactly as prescribed and before pain becomes severe.
•Advise patient to take drug with food to avoid GI distress.
•Instruct patient to refrigerate suppositories before use.
•Caution patient to avoid alcohol and OTC drugs during therapy, unless prescriber approves.
•Instruct patient to report constipation, difficulty breathing, severe nausea, or vomiting.
•Inform patient that drug may cause drowsiness and sedation. Advise her to avoid potentially hazardous activities until drug's CNS effects are known.
•Advise patient to change position slowly to minimize effects of orthostatic hypotension.

hydroxyzine hydrochloride

Apo-Hydroxyzine (CAN), Atarax, Multipax (CAN), Novo-Hydroxyzin (CAN)

hydroxyzine pamoate
Vistaril

Class and Category
Chemical: Piperazine derivative
Therapeutic: Antianxiety, antiemetic, antihistamine, sedative-hypnotic
Pregnancy category: C

Indications and Dosages
➤ *To relieve anxiety and induce sedation and hypnosis*
CAPSULES, ORAL SUSPENSION, SYRUP, TABLETS
Adults and adolescents. 50 to 100 mg as a single dose.
Children. 600 mcg/kg as a single dose.
I.M. INJECTION
Adults and adolescents. 50 to 100 mg q 4 to 6 hr, p.r.n. (antianxiety); 50 mg as a single dose (sedative-hypnotic).
➤ *To treat pruritus*
CAPSULES, ORAL SUSPENSION, SYRUP, TABLETS
Adults and adolescents. 25 to 100 mg t.i.d. or q.i.d., p.r.n.
Children. 500 mcg/kg q 6 hr, p.r.n.

➤ *To provide antiemetic effects*
CAPSULES, ORAL SUSPENSION, SYRUP, TABLETS
Adults and adolescents. 25 to 100 mg t.i.d. or q.i.d., p.r.n.
Children. 500 mcg/kg q 6 hr, p.r.n.
I.M. INJECTION
Adults and adolescents. 25 to 100 mg, p.r.n.
Children. 1.1 mg/kg as a single dose.
➤ *As adjunct to permit reduction in preoperative and postoperative narcotic dosage*
I.M. INJECTION
Adults and adolescents. 25 to 100 mg given with prescribed narcotic.
Children. 1.1 mg/kg given with prescribed narcotic.
DOSAGE ADJUSTMENT For elderly patients, treatment is started at lowest possible dosage.

Route	Onset	Peak	Duration
P.O.	15 to 60 min	Unknown	4 to 6 hr
I.M.	20 to 30 min	Unknown	4 to 6 hr

Mechanism of Action
Competes with histamine for histamine$_1$ receptor sites on the surfaces of effector cells. This suppresses the results of histaminic activity: edema, flare, and pruritus. Hydroxyzine's antiemetic effect may stem from its central anticholinergic actions. Its sedative actions occur at the subcortical level of the CNS and are dose-related.

Contraindications
Breast-feeding; hypersensitivity to cetirizine, hydroxyzine, or their components

Interactions
DRUGS
CNS depressants: Increased CNS depression
ACTIVITIES
alcohol use: Increased CNS depression

Adverse Reactions
CNS: Drowsiness, involuntary motor activity, seizures, tremor
EENT: Dry mouth
Other: Injection site pain

Nursing Considerations
•Don't give hydroxyzine by S.C. or I.V. route because tissue necrosis may occur.

•Inject I.M. form deep into a large muscle, using the Z-track method.
•Observe for oversedation if patient takes another CNS depressant.

PATIENT TEACHING
•Urge patient to avoid alcohol.
•Caution patient about drowsiness; tell her to avoid potentially hazardous activities until drug's CNS effects are known.

hyoscyamine sulfate

Anaspaz, A-Spas S/L, Cystospaz, Cystospaz-M, Donnamar, ED-SPAZ, Gastrosed, Levbid, Levsin, Levsinex Timecaps, Levsin/SL, Symax SL, Symax SR

Class and Category

Chemical: Belladonna alkaloid, tertiary amine
Therapeutic: Antimuscarinic, antispasmodic
Pregnancy category: C

Indications and Dosages

➤ *To treat peptic ulcers and GI tract disorders caused by spasm*

ELIXIR, ORAL SOLUTION
Adults and adolescents. 0.125 to 0.25 mg q 4 to 6 hr.
Children. Dosage individualized by weight.
E.R. CAPSULES
Adults and adolescents. 0.375 mg q 12 hr.
E.R. TABLETS
Adults and adolescents. 0.375 to 0.75 mg q 12 hr. *Maximum:* 1.5 mg/day.
TABLETS
Adults and adolescents. 0.125 to 0.5 mg t.i.d. or q.i.d.
Children. Dosage individualized by weight.
I.V., I.M., OR S.C. INJECTION
Adults and adolescents. 0.25 to 0.5 mg q 4 to 6 hr.
Children. Dosage individualized by weight.

➤ *To control salivation and excessive secretions during surgical procedures*

I.V. INJECTION
Adults and adolescents. 0.5 mg 30 to 60 min before procedure.

Contraindications

Acute hemorrhage and hemodynamic instability; angle-closure glaucoma; hepatic disease; hypersensitivity to hyoscyamine, other anticholinergics, or their components; ileus; intestinal atony; myasthenia gravis; myocardial ischemia; obstructive GI disease; obstructive uropathy; renal disease; severe ulcerative colitis; tachycardia; toxic megacolon

Route	Onset	Peak	Duration
P.O.*	20 to 30 min	30 to 60 min	4 hr
P.O. (E.R.)†	20 to 30 min	40 to 90 min	12 hr
I.V., I.M., S.C.	2 to 3 min	15 to 30 min	4 hr

Mechanism of Action

Competitively inhibits acetylcholine at autonomic postganglionic cholinergic receptors. Because the most sensitive receptors are in the salivary, bronchial, and sweat glands, hyoscyamine acts mainly to reduce salivary, bronchial, and sweat gland secretions. It also causes GI smooth muscle to contract and decreases gastric secretion and GI motility. In addition, hyoscyamine causes the bladder detrusor muscle to contract; reduces nasal and oropharyngeal secretions; and decreases airway resistance from relaxation of smooth muscle in the bronchi and bronchioles.

Interactions

DRUGS
anticholinergics: Possibly increased anticholingeric effects
antidiarrheals (adsorbent): Possibly decreased therapeutic effects of hyoscyamine
calcium- and magnesium-containing antacids, carbonic anhydrase inhibitors, citrates, sodium bicarbonate, urinary alkalinizers: Possibly potentiated therapeutic and adverse effects of hyoscyamine
haloperidol: Possibly decreased therapeutic effects of haloperidol
ketoconazole: Possibly reduced ketoconazole absorption

---

* For tablets only; for elixir and oral solution, onset is 5 to 20 min, and peak and duration are unknown.
† For E.R. tablets only; for E.R. capsules, onset and peak are unknown, and duration is 12 hr.

metoclopramide: Possibly antagonized therapeutic effects of metoclopramide
opioid analgesics: Increased risk of severe constipation and ileus

Adverse Reactions
CNS: Drowsiness, insomnia
EENT: Blurred vision; dry mouth, nose, and throat; photophobia
ENDO: Decreased lactation
GI: Constipation
GU: Impotence, urine retention
SKIN: Decreased sweating
Other: Heatstroke, injection site redness and urticaria

Nursing Considerations
•Use hyoscyamine cautiously in patients with arrhythmias, autonomic neuropathy, coronary artery disease, heart failure, hiatal hernia with reflux esophagitis, hypertension, hyperthyroidism, renal failure, or tachycardia.
•Give drug 30 to 60 minutes before meals and at bedtime. Give bedtime dose at least 2 hours after the day's last meal.
•Anticipate that tablets may not disintegrate and may appear in stool.
•WARNING Expect an increased risk of drug-induced heatstroke in hot or humid weather because hyoscyamine decreases sweating.
•WARNING Be aware that lower doses may paradoxically decrease the heart rate and that higher doses affect nicotinic receptors in autonomic ganglia, causing delirium, disorientation, hallucinations, and restlessness.
•Monitor urine output, and be alert for urine retention.

PATIENT TEACHING
•Instruct patient to void before taking each dose and to notify prescriber if she has trouble urinating during hyoscyamine therapy.
•Advise patient to take drug 30 to 60 minutes before meals and at bedtime. Bedtime dose should be taken at least 2 hours after the day's last meal.
•Inform patient that drug may cause drowsiness. Advise her to avoid potentially hazardous activities until drug's CNS effects are known.
•If patient reports dry mouth, suggest using sugarless hard candy or gum.
•Inform male patient that drug may cause impotence. If it occurs, suggest that he discuss it with prescriber.
•Advise patient to avoid exposure to high temperatures and to increase fluid intake, unless contraindicated.

ibuprofen

Actiprofen Caplets (CAN), Advil, Apo-Ibuprofen (CAN), Bayer Select Ibuprofen Pain Relief Formula Caplets, Children's Advil, Children's Motrin, Dolgesic, Excedrin IB, Genpril, Haltran, Ibifon 600 Caplets, Ibuprin, Ibuprohm Caplets, Ibu-Tab, Medipren, Midol IB, Motrin, Motrin-IB, Novo-Profen (CAN), Nu-Ibuprofen (CAN), Nuprin, Pamprin-IB, Q-Profen, Rufen, Trendar

Class and Category
Chemical: Propionic acid derivative
Therapeutic: Analgesic, anti-inflammatory, antipyretic
Pregnancy category: Not rated

Indications and Dosages
➤ *To relieve pain in rheumatoid arthritis and osteoarthritis*
CAPSULES, CHEWABLE TABLETS, ORAL SUSPENSION, TABLETS
Adults. 300 mg q.i.d., or 400, 600, or 800 mg t.i.d. or q.i.d. *Range:* 1.2 to 3.2 g/day.

➤ *To relieve mild to moderate pain*
CAPSULES, CHEWABLE TABLETS, ORAL SUSPENSION, TABLETS
Adults. 400 mg q 4 to 6 hr, p.r.n.

➤ *To relieve acute migraine pain*
CAPSULES, CHEWABLE TABLETS, ORAL SUSPENSION, TABLETS
Adults. 200 to 400 mg at onset of migraine pain. *Maximum:* 400 mg/day.

➤ *To relieve pain in primary dysmenorrhea*
CAPSULES, CHEWABLE TABLETS, ORAL SUSPENSION, TABLETS
Adults. 400 mg q 4 hr, p.r.n.

➤ *To relieve pain in juvenile arthritis*
CAPSULES, CHEWABLE TABLETS, ORAL SUSPENSION, TABLETS
Children. 30 to 70 mg/kg/day in divided doses t.i.d. or q.i.d.; 20 mg/kg/day for mild disease.

➤ *To relieve minor aches, pains, and dysmenorrhea and to reduce fever*
CAPSULES, CHEWABLE TABLETS, ORAL SUSPENSION, TABLETS
Adults. 200 to 400 mg q 4 to 6 hr. *Maximum:* 1.2 g/day.

➤ *To reduce fever*
CAPSULES, CHEWABLE TABLETS, ORAL SUSPENSION, TABLETS
Children ages 6 months to 12 years. 5 to 10 mg/kg q 4 to 6 hr. *Maximum:* 40 mg/kg/day.

Contraindications
Angioedema, asthma, bronchospasm, nasal polyps, rhinitis, or urticaria caused by hypersensitivity to aspirin, ibuprofen, iodides, or other NSAIDs

Route	Onset	Peak	Duration
P.O.*	30 min	Unknown	4 to 6 hr
P.O.†	Up to 7 days	1 to 2 wk	Unknown
P.O.‡	In 1 hr	2 to 4 hr	6 to 8 hr

Mechanism of Action

Blocks the activity of cyclooxygenase, the enzyme needed to synthesize prostaglandins, which mediate the inflammatory response and cause local vasodilation, swelling, and pain. By blocking cyclooxygenase and inhibiting prostaglandins, this NSAID reduces inflammatory symptoms and relieves pain. Ibuprofen's antipyretic action probably stems from its effect on the hypothalamus, which increases peripheral blood flow, causing vasodilation and heat dissipation.

Interactions

DRUGS

acetaminophen: Possibly increased renal effects with long-term use of both drugs
antihypertensives: Decreased effectiveness of these drugs
aspirin, other NSAIDs: Increased risk of bleeding and adverse GI effects
bone marrow depressants: Possibly increased leukopenic and thrombocytopenic effects of bone marrow depressants
cefamandole, cefoperazone, cefotetan: Increased risk of hypoprothrombinemia and bleeding
colchicine, platelet aggregation inhibitors: Increased risk of GI bleeding, hemorrhage, and ulcers
corticosteroids, potassium supplements: Increased risk of adverse GI effects
cyclosporine: Increased risk of nephrotoxicity from both drugs, increased blood cyclosporine level
digoxin: Increased blood digoxin level and risk of digitalis toxicity
diuretics (loop, potassium-sparing, and thiazide): Decreased diuretic and antihypertensive effects
gold compounds, nephrotoxic drugs: Increased risk of adverse renal effects

heparin, oral anticoagulants, thrombolytics: Increased anticoagulant effects, increased risk of hemorrhage
insulin, oral antidiabetic drugs: Possibly increased hypoglycemic effects of these drugs
lithium: Increased blood lithium level
methotrexate: Decreased methotrexate clearance, increased risk of methotrexate toxicity
plicamycin, valproic acid: Increased risk of hypoprothrombinemia and GI bleeding, hemorrhage, and ulcers
probenecid: Possibly increased blood level, effectiveness, and risk of toxicity of ibuprofen

ACTIVITIES

alcohol use: Increased risk of adverse GI effects

Adverse Reactions

CNS: Aseptic meningitis, dizziness, headache, nervousness
CV: Fluid retention, heart failure, peripheral edema
EENT: Amblyopia, epistaxis, stomatitis, tinnitus
GI: Abdominal cramps, distention, or pain; anorexia; constipation; diarrhea; elevated liver function test results; epigastric discomfort; flatulence; gastritis; GI bleeding, hemorrhage, perforation, or ulceration; heartburn; hepatitis; indigestion; nausea; vomiting
GU: Cystitis, hematuria, renal failure (acute)
HEME: Agranulocytosis, anemia, aplastic anemia, eosinophilia, hemolytic anemia, neutropenia, prolonged bleeding time, thrombocytopenia
RESP: Bronchospasm, dyspnea, wheezing
SKIN: Blisters, erythema multiforme, photosensitivity, pruritus, rash, Stevens-Johnson syndrome, urticaria
Other: Anaphylaxis, angioedema, flulike symptoms, weight gain

Nursing Considerations

•Give ibuprofen with food or after meals to reduce GI distress.
•Although drug's analgesic effect occurs at low doses, expect to give at least 400 mg four times a day for anti-inflammatory effect.
•Be aware that higher doses may be prescribed for rheumatoid arthritis than for osteoarthritis.
•Assess for signs of GI bleeding and ulceration, which can occur without warning during long-term therapy.
•Monitor hepatic and renal function periodically during long-term therapy.

---

* For analgesic effects.
† For anti-inflammatory effects.
‡ For antipyretic effects.

•Be aware that ibuprofen oral suspension may contain sucrose, which may affect blood glucose level in patients with diabetes.
•Anticipate that ibuprofen's anti-inflammatory and antipyretic actions may mask signs and symptoms of infection.
PATIENT TEACHING
•Instruct patient to take ibuprofen tablets with a full glass of water and to avoid lying down for 15 to 30 minutes afterward to prevent esophageal irritation.
•Advise patient to take drug with food or after meals to reduce GI distress.
•Instruct patient to consult prescriber before taking drug for more than 3 days for fever or 10 days for pain.
•Inform patient with phenylketonuria that Motrin chewable tablets contain aspartame.
•Inform patient that full therapeutic effect for arthritis may take 2 weeks or longer.
•Advise patient to avoid taking two different NSAIDs at the same time, unless directed by prescriber.
•Urge patient to avoid alcohol, aspirin, and corticosteroids while taking ibuprofen.
•Suggest that patient wear sunscreen and protective clothing when outdoors to minimize photosensitivity.
•Advise patient to report flulike symptoms, rash, signs of GI bleeding, swelling, vision changes, and weight gain.

ibutilide fumarate

Corvert

Class and Category
Chemical: Methanesulfonanilide derivative
Therapeutic: Class III antiarrhythmic
Pregnancy category: C

Indications and Dosages
➤ *To rapidly convert recent-onset atrial flutter or fibrillation to sinus rhythm*
I.V. INFUSION
Adults who weigh 60 kg (132 lb) or more. 1 mg over 10 min. Repeated 10 min after first dose is finished if arrhythmia persists.
Adults who weigh less than 60 kg. 0.01 mg/kg over 10 min. Repeated 10 min after first dose is finished if arrhythmia persists.
DOSAGE ADJUSTMENT Infusion discontinued if arrhythmia is terminated or if sustained or nonsustained ventricular tachycardia or prolonged QT or QTc interval develops.

Mechanism of Action
May promote sodium movement through slow inward sodium channels in myocardial cell membranes. Ibutilide also may inhibit a component of potassium channels in myocardial cell membranes involved in cardiac repolarization. These actions prolong the cardiac action potential by delaying repolarization and increasing atrial and ventricular refractoriness. As a result, the sinus rate slows and AV conduction is delayed.

Contraindications
Hypersensitivity to ibutilide or its components

Interactions
DRUGS
amiodarone, astemizole, disopyramide, maprotiline, phenothiazines, procainamide, quinidine, sotalol, tricyclic antidepressants: Possibly prolonged QT interval, leading to increased risk of proarrhythmias

Adverse Reactions
CNS: Headache, syncope
CV: AV block, bradycardia, bundle-branch block, heart failure, hypertension, hypotension, idioventricular rhythm, orthostatic hypotension, palpitations, prolonged QT interval, sinus and supraventricular tachycardia, supraventricular arrhythmias, ventricular arrhythmias, ventricular tachycardia (sustained and nonsustained)
GI: Nausea
GU: Renal failure

Nursing Considerations
•Before giving ibutilide, check serum electrolyte levels and expect to correct abnormalities, as prescribed. Be especially alert for hypokalemia and hypomagnesemia, which can lead to arrhythmias.
•Give drug undiluted, or dilute it in 50 ml of NS or D_5W. Add contents of 10-ml vial (0.1 mg/ml) to 50 ml of solution to obtain 0.017 mg/ml. Use polyvinyl chloride plastic bags or polyolefin bags for ibutilide admixtures. Administer within 24 hours (48 hours if refrigerated).
•Infuse drug slowly over 10 minutes.
•As ordered, monitor cardiac rhythm continuously during drug infusion and for at least

4 hours afterward—longer if arrhythmias appear or if patient has abnormal hepatic function. Observe for ventricular ectopy.
•Make sure that a defibrillator and drugs to treat sustained ventricular tachycardia are available during therapy and when monitoring patient after therapy.

PATIENT TEACHING
•Inform patient that ibutilide will be administered by I.V. infusion and that his heart rhythm will be monitored continuously during the infusion.
•Ask patient to report chest pain, faintness, numbness, tingling, palpitations, and shortness of breath.
•Advise patient to keep follow-up appointments to monitor heart rhythm.

imipenem and cilastatin sodium

Primaxin (CAN), Primaxin ADD-Vantage, Primaxin IM, Primaxin IV

Class and Category

Chemical: Thienamycin derivative (imipenem), heptenoic acid derivative (cilastatin sodium)
Therapeutic: Antibiotic
Pregnancy category: C

Indications and Dosages

➤ *To treat severe or life-threatening bacterial infections (including endocarditis, pneumonia, and septicemia as well as bone, joint, intra-abdominal, skin, and soft-tissue infections) caused by gram-positive anaerobic organisms, such as most staphylococci and streptococci and some enterococci (including* Enterococcus faecalis); *most strains of* Enterobacteriaceae *(including* Citrobacter *sp.,* Enterobacter *sp.,* Escherichia coli, Klebsiella *sp.,* Morganella morganii, Proteus mirabilis, Providencia stuartii, *and* Serratia marcescens); *and many gram-negative aerobic and anaerobic species (including* Bacteroides *sp.,* Campylobacter *sp.,* Clostridium *sp.,* Haemophilus influenzae, Legionella *sp.,* Neisseria gonorrhoeae, *and* Pseudomonas aeruginosa)

I.V. INFUSION (DOSAGES BASED ON IMIPENEM CONTENT)
Adults and adolescents. 500 mg q 6 hr to 1,000 mg q 6 to 8 hr. *Maximum:* 50 mg/kg or 4 g/day, whichever is lower.
Children age 3 months and older. 15 to 25 mg/kg q 6 hr. *Maximum:* 2,000 to 4,000 mg/day.
Infants ages 4 weeks to 3 months who weigh 1,500 g (3 lb, 3 oz) or more. 25 mg/kg q 6 hr. *Maximum:* 2,000 to 4,000 mg/day.
Neonates ages 1 to 4 weeks who weigh 1,500 g or more. 25 mg/kg q 8 hr. *Maximum:* 2,000 to 4,000 mg/day.
Neonates under age 1 week who weigh 1,500 g or more. 25 mg/kg q 12 hr. *Maximum:* 2,000 to 4,000 mg/day.

➤ *To treat moderate infections caused by the organisms listed above*

I.V. INFUSION (DOSAGES BASED ON IMIPENEM CONTENT)
Adults and adolescents. 500 mg q 6 to 8 hr up to 1,000 mg q 8 hr. *Maximum:* 50 mg/kg or 4 g/day, whichever is lower.
Children age 3 months and older. 15 to 25 mg/kg q 6 hr. *Maximum:* 2,000 to 4,000 mg/day.
Infants ages 4 weeks to 3 months who weigh 1,500 g or more. 25 mg/kg q 6 hr. *Maximum:* 2,000 to 4,000 mg/day.
Neonates ages 1 to 4 weeks who weigh 1,500 g or more. 25 mg/kg q 8 hr. *Maximum:* 2,000 to 4,000 mg/day.
Neonates under age 1 week who weigh 1,500 g or more. 25 mg/kg q 12 hr. *Maximum:* 2,000 to 4,000 mg/day.

I.M. INJECTION (DOSAGES BASED ON IMIPENEM CONTENT)
Adults and adolescents. 500 to 750 mg q 12 hr. *Maximum:* 1,500 mg/day.
Children. 10 to 15 mg/kg q 6 hr.

➤ *To treat mild infections caused by the organisms listed above*

I.V. INFUSION (DOSAGES BASED ON IMIPENEM CONTENT)
Adults and adolescents. 250 to 500 mg q 6 hr. *Maximum:* 50 mg/kg or 4 g/day, whichever is lower.
Children age 3 months and older. 15 to 25 mg/kg q 6 hr. *Maximum:* 2,000 (for fully susceptible organisms) to 4,000 (for moderately susceptible organisms) mg/day.
Infants ages 4 weeks to 3 months who weigh 1,500 g or more. 25 mg/kg q 6 hr. *Maximum:* 2,000 to 4,000 mg/day.
Neonates ages 1 to 4 weeks who weigh 1,500 g or more. 25 mg/kg q 8 hr. *Maximum:* 2,000 to 4,000 mg/day.

G
H
I

Neonates under age 1 week who weigh 1,500 g or more. 25 mg/kg q 12 hr. *Maximum:* 2,000 to 4,000 mg/day.

I.M. INJECTION (DOSAGES BASED ON IMIPENEM CONTENT)
Adults and adolescents. 500 to 750 mg q 12 hr. *Maximum:* 1,500 mg/day.
Children. 10 to 15 mg/kg q 6 hr.
➤ *To treat uncomplicated UTIs caused by the organisms listed above*

I.V. INFUSION (DOSAGES BASED ON IMIPENEM CONTENT)
Adults and adolescents. 250 mg q 6 hr. *Maximum:* 50 mg/kg or 4 g/day, whichever is lower.
➤ *To treat complicated UTIs caused by the organisms listed above*

I.V. INFUSION (DOSAGES BASED ON IMIPENEM CONTENT)
Adults and adolescents. 500 mg q 6 hr. *Maximum:* 50 mg/kg or 4 g/day, whichever is lower.
DOSAGE ADJUSTMENT Dosage reduced based on creatinine clearance for patients with impaired renal function.

Mechanism of Action

Produces two related actions. During bacterial cell wall synthesis, imipenem selectively binds to penicillin-binding proteins that are responsible for cell wall formation. This action causes bacterial cells to rapidly lyse and die. Cilastatin sodium inhibits imipenem's breakdown in the kidneys, thus maintaining a high imipenem level in the urinary tract.

Incompatibilities

Don't administer imipenem and cilastatin through same I.V. line as beta-lactam antibiotics or aminoglycosides.

Contraindications

Hypersensitivity to imipenem, its components, other beta–lactam antibiotics, or amide-type local anesthetics (I.M.); meningitis (I.V.); severe heart block or shock (I.M.)

Interactions

DRUGS
cyclosporine: Increased adverse CNS effects of both drugs
ganciclovir: Increased risk of seizures
probenecid: Slightly increased blood level and half-life of imipenem

Adverse Reactions

CNS: Confusion, dizziness, fever, seizures, somnolence, tremor, weakness

CV: Hypotension
EENT: Oral candidiasis
GI: Diarrhea, nausea, pseudomembranous colitis, vomiting
RESP: Wheezing
SKIN: Diaphoresis, pruritus, rash, urticaria
Other: Anaphylaxis, injection site thrombophlebitis

Nursing Considerations

•Obtain body fluid and tissue specimens for culture and sensitivity testing, as ordered, before giving first dose of imipenem and cilastatin. Expect to start therapy before test results are available.
•For I.V. administration, add about 10 ml of diluent to each 250- or 500-mg vial and shake well. Transfer this reconstituted drug to at least 100 ml of prescribed I.V. solution. After the transfer, add another 10 ml of diluent to each vial, shake, and then transfer to infusion container. Shake infusion container until clear. To reconstitute piggyback bottles, add 100 ml of diluent to each 250- or 500-mg infusion bottle, and shake well.
•Administer reconstituted drug within 4 to 10 hours, depending on diluent used (24 to 48 hours if refrigerated). Color may range from clear to yellow; don't administer solution that contains particles.
•Infuse 500-mg or smaller dose over 20 to 30 minutes and 750- to 1,000-mg dose over 40 to 60 minutes.
•Inject I.M. form into a large muscle mass.
•Expect increased risk of imipenem-induced seizures in patients with brain lesions, head trauma, or history of CNS disorders and in those receiving more than 2 g of drug daily.
•Assess for signs and symptoms of allergic reaction and bacterial or fungal superinfection.
PATIENT TEACHING
•Inform patient that imipenem and cilastatin must be given by infusion or injection.
•Instruct patient to report discomfort at I.V. insertion site.
•Advise patient to report itching, signs of superinfection (such as diarrhea and sore mouth), and hives.

imipramine hydrochloride

Apo-Imipramine (CAN), Impril (CAN), Norfranil, Novopramine (CAN), Tipramine, Tofranil

imipramine pamoate

Tofranil-PM

Class and Category

Chemical: Dibenzazepine derivative
Therapeutic: Antidepressant
Pregnancy category: Not rated

Indications and Dosages

➤ *To treat depression*

CAPSULES

Adults. *Initial:* 75 mg/day h.s., gradually increased as needed and tolerated. *Maximum:* 300 mg/day (hospitalized patients), 200 mg/day (outpatients).

TABLETS

Adults. *Initial:* 25 to 50 mg t.i.d. or q.i.d., gradually increased as needed and tolerated. *Maximum:* 300 mg/day (hospitalized patients), 200 mg/day (outpatients).

DOSAGE ADJUSTMENT Initial dosage reduced to 25 mg h.s. for depressed elderly patients and then adjusted as needed and tolerated up to 100 mg/day in divided doses.

Adolescents. *Initial:* 25 to 50 mg/day in divided doses, adjusted as needed and tolerated. *Maximum:* 100 mg/day.

Children ages 6 to 12. 10 to 30 mg/day in divided doses b.i.d.

➤ *As adjunct to treat childhood enuresis*

TABLETS

Children age 6 and older. 25 mg 1 hr before h.s. Increased to 50 mg if no response occurs within 1 wk and child is under age 12; increased to 75 mg if child is age 12 or older. *Maximum:* 2.5 mg/kg/day.

Route	Onset	Peak	Duration
P.O.	2 to 3 wk*	Unknown	Unknown

Contraindications

Acute recovery period after MI; hypersensitivity to imipramine, other tricyclic antidepressants, or their components; use within 2 weeks of MAO inhibitor therapy

Interactions

DRUGS

amantadine, anticholinergics, antidyskinetics, antihistamines: Risk of increased anticholin-

---

* For antidepressant effect.

Mechanism of Action

May interfere with reuptake of serotonin (and possibly other neurotransmitters) at presynaptic neurons, thus enhancing serotonin's effects at postsynaptic receptors. Mood elevation may result from restoration of normal levels of neurotransmitters at nerve synapses. This tricyclic antidepressant also blocks acetylcholine receptors, which may explain how it relieves enuresis.

ergic effects, including confusion, hallucinations, and nightmares
anticonvulsants: Increased risk of CNS depression, increased risk of seizures, decreased effectiveness of imipramine
antithyroid drugs: Possibly agranulocytosis
barbiturates, carbamazepine: Possibly decreased blood level and effectiveness of imipramine
cimetidine, fluoxetine: Possibly increased blood imipramine level
clonidine, guanadrel, guanethidine: Possibly decreased antihypertensive effects of these drugs, increased CNS depression (clonidine)
CNS depressants: Increased CNS depression, respiratory depression, and hypotension
disulfiram, ethchlorvynol: Risk of delirium, increased CNS depression (ethchlorvynol)
estramustine, estrogen-containing oral contraceptives, estrogens: Risk of increased bioavailability of imipramine, increased depression
MAO inhibitors: Increased risk of hypertensive crisis, severe seizures, and death
oral anticoagulants: Possibly increased anticoagulant activity
pimozide, probucol: Risk of arrhythmias
sympathomimetics (including ophthalmic epinephrine and vasoconstrictive local anesthetics): Increased risk of arrhythmias, hyperpyrexia, hypertension, tachycardia
thyroid hormones: Risk of increased therapeutic and adverse effects of both drugs

ACTIVITIES

alcohol use: Increased CNS depression, increased alcohol effects
sun exposure: Increased risk of photosensitivity

Adverse Reactions

CNS: Anxiety, ataxia, chills, confusion, CVA, delirium, dizziness, drowsiness, excitation,

extrapyramidal reactions, fever, hallucinations, headache, insomnia, nervousness, nightmares, parkinsonism, seizures, tremor
CV: Arrhythmias, orthostatic hypotension, palpitations
EENT: Blurred vision, dry mouth, increased intraocular pressure, pharyngitis, taste perversion, tinnitus, tongue swelling
ENDO: Gynecomastia, syndrome of inappropriate ADH secretion
GI: Constipation, diarrhea, heartburn, ileus, increased appetite, nausea, vomiting
GU: Impotence, libido changes, testicular swelling, urine retention
HEME: Agranulocytosis, bone marrow depression
RESP: Wheezing
SKIN: Alopecia, diaphoresis, jaundice, photosensitivity, pruritus, rash, urticaria
Other: Allergic reaction, facial edema, weight gain

Nursing Considerations
• Use imipramine cautiously in patients with a history of urine retention or angle-closure glaucoma because drug's anticholinergic effects may cause urine retention and increased intraocular pressure.
• **WARNING** Don't administer MAO inhibitors within 2 weeks of imipramine therapy. Otherwise, patient may experience hypertensive crisis, seizures, and death.
• Frequently assess for adverse reactions during first 2 hours of therapy.
• Monitor supine and standing blood pressure for orthostatic hypotension before and during imipramine therapy and before dosage increases.
• Anticipate increased risk of arrhythmias in patients with a history of cardiac disease.
• When drug is used for depression, expect mood elevation to take 2 to 3 weeks.
• Avoid abrupt withdrawal of drug in patients who receive long-term therapy. Such withdrawal may cause headache, malaise, nausea, sleep disturbance, and vomiting.
• Taper drug gradually, as ordered, a few days before surgery to avoid the risk of hypertension during surgery.
• Obtain CBC, as ordered, if patient experiences signs and symptoms of infection, such as fever or pharyngitis.
• Limit drug access for potentially suicidal patient.

PATIENT TEACHING
• Advise patient to take imipramine exactly as prescribed. Warn him that stopping drug abruptly may cause headache, malaise, nausea, trouble sleeping, and vomiting.
• Advise patient to report chills, difficulty urinating, dizziness, excessive sedation, fever, palpitations, signs of an allergic reaction, and sore throat.
• Caution patient to avoid potentially hazardous activities until drug's CNS effects are known.
• Urge patient to avoid alcohol during imipramine therapy because of the risk of increased CNS depression and alcohol effects.
• Suggest that patient eat small, frequent meals to help relieve nausea.
• Instruct patient to avoid prolonged exposure to sunlight because of the risk of photosensitivity.
• Inform male patient about possible impotence and increased or decreased libido.
• If patient reports dry mouth, suggest sugarless candy or gum to relieve it. Tell him to check with prescriber if dry mouth persists after 2 weeks.

immune globulin intravenous (human)
(IGIV, immune serum globulin, ISG, IVIG)
Gamimune N 5% S/D, Gamimune N 10% S/D, Gammagard S/D, Gammagard S/D 0.5 g, Gammar-P IV, Iveegam EN, Polygam S/D, Sandoglobulin, Venoglobulin-I, Venoglobulin-S 5%, Venoglobulin-S 10%

immune globulin intramuscular (human)
(gamma globulin, IG)
BayGam

Class and Category
Chemical: Polyvalent antibody
Therapeutic: Antibacterial, anti–Kawasaki disease agent, antipolyneuropathy agent, antiviral, immunizing agent, platelet count stimulator
Pregnancy category: C

Indications and Dosages

➤ *To treat primary immunodeficiency*

I.V. INFUSION (GAMMAR-P IV)

Adults. 200 to 400 mg/kg q 3 to 4 wk.

Adolescents and children. 200 mg/kg q 3 to 4 wk.

I.V. INFUSION (IVEEGAM EN)

Adults. 200 mg/kg q mo.

I.V. INFUSION (SANDOGLOBULIN)

Adults and children. 200 mg/kg q mo. If response is inadequate, dose may be increased to 300 mg/kg or dosing frequency may be increased.

I.V. INFUSION (GAMIMUNE N 5% S/D OR 10% S/D)

Adults. 100 to 200 mg/kg q mo. If response is inadequate, dose may be increased to as high as 400 mg/kg or dosing frequency may be increased.

I.V. INFUSION (GAMMAGARD S/D, POLYGAM S/D)

Adults. 200 to 400 mg/kg initially, then at least 100 mg/kg q mo thereafter. If response is inadequate, dose or frequency may be adjusted.

I.V. INFUSION (VENOGLOBULIN-I)

Adults and children. 200 mg/kg q mo. If response is inadequate, dose may be increased to 300 to 400 mg/kg q mo or dosing frequency may be increased.

I.V. INFUSION (VENOGLOBULIN-S 5% OR 10%)

Adults and children. 200 mg/kg q mo. If response is inadequate, dose may be increased to as high as 400 mg/kg or dosing frequency may be increased.

I.M. INJECTION (BAYGAM)

Adults. 0.66 ml/kg (at least 200 mg/kg) q 3 to 4 wk; initial dose may be doubled.

➤ *To treat idiopathic thrombocytopenic purpura (ITP)*

I.V. INFUSION (GAMIMUNE N 5% S/D)

Adults and children. 400 mg/kg/day for 5 days. Alternatively, 1,000 mg/kg for 1 or 2 days for patients not at risk for increased fluid volume.

I.V. INFUSION (GAMIMUNE N 10% S/D)

Adults and children. 1,000 mg/kg for 1 or 2 days for patients at risk for increased fluid volume.

DOSAGE ADJUSTMENT In acute ITP of childhood, I.V. Sandoglobulin therapy may be discontinued after 2nd day of 5-day course if initial platelet count response is adequate (30,000 to 50,000/mm^3). In chronic ITP, an additional I.V. infusion of 400 mg/kg (of either Sandoglobulin or Gamimune) may be prescribed if platelet count falls below 30,000/mm^3 or if patient develops significant bleeding. If response remains inadequate, an additional I.V. infusion of 800 to 1,000 mg/kg may be given.

I.V. INFUSION (GAMMAGARD S/D)

Adults. 1 g/kg. If response is inadequate, up to three separate doses may be administered on alternate days.

I.V. INFUSION (SANDOGLOBULIN)

Adults and adolescents. 400 mg/kg/day for 2 to 5 consecutive days.

I.V. INFUSION (VENOGLOBULIN-I)

Adults and children. *Induction:* Cumulative dose up to 2 g/kg over 2 to 7 consecutive days. *Maintenance (adults):* 2 g/kg as a single dose q 2 wk as needed to maintain platelet count above 30,000/mm^3 or prevent bleeding episodes. *Maintenance (children):* 1 g/kg as a single dose q 2 wk as needed to maintain platelet count above 30,000/mm^3 or prevent bleeding episodes.

I.V. INFUSION (VENOGLOBULIN-S 5% OR 10%)

Adults and children. Cumulative dose up to 2,000 mg/kg over 5 consecutive days.

DOSAGE ADJUSTMENT An additional I.V. infusion of 1,000 mg/kg may be administered to maintain a platelet count of 30,000/mm^3 in children or 20,000/mm^3 in adults or to prevent bleeding episodes.

➤ *As adjunct to treat Kawasaki disease*

I.V. INFUSION (GAMMAGARD S/D)

Adults and adolescents. 1 g/kg as a single dose; alternatively, 400 mg/kg/day for 4 consecutive days.

I.V. INFUSION (IVEEGAM EN, VENOGLOBULIN-S 5% OR 10%)

Adults and adolescents. 2 g/kg as a single dose; alternatively, Iveegam EN may be given at 400 mg/kg q.d. for 4 days.

➤ *To decrease the risk of graft-versus-host disease, interstitial pneumonia, septicemia, and other infections during first 100 days after bone marrow transplantation*

I.V. INFUSION (GAMIMUNE N 5% S/D OR 10% S/D)

Adults over age 20. 500 mg/kg on 7th and 2nd days before transplant (or at time conditioning therapy for transplantation begins), and then weekly through 90th day after transplant.

➤ *As adjunct to treat bacterial infections secondary to B-cell chronic lymphocytic leukemia*

G
H
I

I.V. INFUSION (GAMMAGARD S/D, POLYGAM S/D)
Adults and adolescents. 400 mg/kg q 3 to 4 wk.
➤ *To prevent bacterial infection in children with HIV who are immunosuppressed*
I.V. INFUSION (GAMIMUNE N 5% S/D OR 10% S/D)
Children. 400 mg/kg q.d. every 28 days.
➤ *To prevent hepatitis A*
I.M. INJECTION (BAYGAM)
Adults with household or institutional contacts. 0.01 ml/lb (0.02 ml/kg).
Adults traveling to areas where hepatitis A is common. 0.02 ml/kg if staying less than 3 mo, 0.06 ml/kg (repeated q 4 to 6 mo) if staying 3 mo or longer.
➤ *To prevent or lessen severity of measles (rubeola) in susceptible persons*
I.M. INJECTION (BAYGAM)
Adults. 0.11 ml/lb (0.2 ml/kg) for persons exposed fewer than 6 days previously.
➤ *To provide passive immunization against varicella in immunosuppressed patients*
I.M. INJECTION (BAYGAM)
Adults. 0.6 to 1.2 ml/kg if varicella-zoster immune globulin (human) is unavailable.
➤ *To reduce the risk of infection and fetal damage in women who have been exposed to rubella in early pregnancy*
I.M. INJECTION (BAYGAM)
Adults. 0.55 ml/kg.

Route	Onset	Peak	Duration
I.V.	Unknown	Unknown	21 to 28 days

Mechanism of Action

Releases antibody-specific globulins to produce an antibody-antigen reaction that results in bacterial lysis and facilitates bacterial phagocytosis. In treatment of ITP, immune globulin blocks iron receptors on macrophages to increase immunoglobulin action. Immune globulin also increases cytokine production and improves B-cell immune function by regulating T-cell and macrophage activity. Newly formed antigen-antibody complexes produce split complement components that cause bacterial lysis.

In Kawasaki disease and bacterial infections secondary to B-cell chronic lymphocytic leukemia, immune globulin neutralizes bacterial and viral toxins that harm the immune and inflammatory responses.

Incompatibilities

Don't mix immune globulin with any other drugs, including other immune globulins, or with any I.V. solutions other than D_5W or manufacturer's supplied diluent because effects of doing so are unknown.

Contraindications

Hypersensitivity to immune globulin (human) or its components, IgA deficiency in patients with known antibody to IgA

Interactions
DRUGS
vaccines, live virus: Possibly decreased response to vaccine

Adverse Reactions
CNS: Headache, malaise
CV: Tachycardia
GI: Nausea, vomiting
MS: Arthralgia, back pain, myalgia
RESP: Dyspnea

Nursing Considerations

• Before administering immune globulin, monitor patient's fluid volume and BUN and serum creatinine levels, as ordered, to determine if he's at risk for acute renal failure. Those at increased risk include patients with existing renal insufficiency, diabetes mellitus, volume depletion, sepsis, or paraproteinemia; those taking concomitant nephrotoxic drugs; and those over age 65. Expect drug to be discontinued if renal function deteriorates.
• When preparing drug for administration, verify that the appropriate form of immune globulin is being used—either immune globulin intramuscular for I.M. injection or immune globulin intravenous for I.V. infusion.
• To reconstitute drug for infusion, follow manufacturer's guidelines and use only diluent recommended by manufacturer. Don't shake solution; excessive shaking causes foaming. If drug or diluent is cold, drug may take up to 20 minutes to dissolve.
• If drug is reconstituted outside of sterile laminar airflow conditions, administer it immediately and discard unused portions.
• Consult manufacturer's guidelines to determine appropriate flow rate for initiating infusion. Expect to increase flow rate after 15 to 30 minutes, according to guidelines.

•**WARNING** Monitor for an acute inflammatory reaction in patients who have never received immune globulin therapy before, in those whose last treatment was more than 8 weeks before, and in those whose initial infusion rate exceeded 1 ml/minute. Within 30 minutes to 1 hour after beginning of infusion, assess for chills, fever, facial flushing, feeling of tightness in chest, dizziness, nausea and vomiting, diaphoresis, and hypotension. Notify prescriber immediately if such symptoms occur, and be prepared to stop infusion until symptoms have subsided.

•**WARNING** After immune globulin administration, monitor patient closely for aseptic meningitis. Notify prescriber if patient develops drowsiness, fever, nausea and vomiting, nuchal rigidity, photophobia, painful eye movements, or severe headache.

•Be aware that immune globulin intravenous is made from human plasma and therefore may contain infectious agents, such as viruses. However, the risk of transmitting a virus by infusion has been reduced by screening blood donors, testing donated blood, and inactivating or removing certain viruses from the product.

PATIENT TEACHING

•Instruct patient to immediately report any symptoms he experiences after receiving immune globulin.

•Inform patient that he'll need to postpone live virus vaccines for up to 11 months after receiving immune globulin because drug may delay or inhibit his response to vaccine.

inamrinone

(amrinone)

Inocor

Class and Category

Chemical: Bipyridine derivative
Therapeutic: Cardiac inotrope
Pregnancy category: C

Indications and Dosages

➤ *To treat heart failure in patients who haven't responded sufficiently to digoxin, diuretics, or vasodilators*

I.V. INFUSION

Adults. *Initial:* 0.75 mg/kg by bolus administered over 2 to 3 min and repeated after 30 min, if needed. *Maintenance:* 5 to 10 mcg/kg/min by infusion. *Maximum:* 10 mg/kg/day.

Route	Onset	Peak	Duration
I.V.	2 to 5 min	In 10 min	30 min to 2 hr

Mechanism of Action

Inhibits phosphodiesterase enzymes that normally degrade myocardial cAMP. This action increases intracellular levels of cAMP, which regulates intracellular and extracellular calcium balance. An increased intracellular cAMP level enhances the influx of calcium into the cell, thereby increasing the force of myocardial contractions. Inamrinone also acts directly on peripheral vascular smooth-muscle cells, causing relaxation and dilation. This action reduces preload and afterload.

Incompatibilities

Don't administer inamrinone through same I.V. line as furosemide to prevent precipitate formation. Don't dilute inamrinone in solution that contains dextrose because a chemical interaction occurs over 24 hours.

Contraindications

Hypersensitivity to inamrinone, bisulfites, or their components; severe aortic or pulmonary valvular disease

Interactions

DRUGS

disopyramide: Possibly severe hypotension

Adverse Reactions

CNS: Fever
CV: Chest pain, hypotension, pericarditis, supraventricular tachycardia, ventricular arrhythmias
GI: Abdominal pain, anorexia, elevated liver function test results, hepatotoxicity, nausea, vomiting
HEME: Elevated erythrocyte sedimentation rate, thrombocytopenia (especially with high-dose or prolonged treatment)
MS: Myositis
RESP: Hypoxemia, pleuritis
SKIN: Jaundice
Other: Infusion site burning

Nursing Considerations

•**WARNING** Be aware that inamrinone may increase the risk of ventricular arrhythmias in patients with atrial flutter or fibrillation. To minimize this risk, expect to pretreat such patients with digoxin.

•Administer inamrinone undiluted or diluted in NS or 0.45NS to a concentration of 1 to 3 mg/ml, as prescribed. Use diluted solution within 24 hours.

•**WARNING** Monitor vital signs regularly. If blood pressure falls significantly, slow or stop inamrinone infusion and notify prescriber.

•Monitor weight, cardiac index, central venous pressure, pulmonary artery wedge pressure, and fluid intake and output as appropriate to assess effectiveness of therapy.

•**WARNING** Assess frequently for signs of thrombocytopenia, such as bruising or bleeding and altered platelet count. If signs appear, expect to decrease inamrinone dose or discontinue drug.

PATIENT TEACHING

•Instruct patient to notify you or another nurse if he becomes dizzy, which may indicate hypotension.

indapamide

Apo-Indapamide (CAN), Gen-Indapamide (CAN), Lozide (CAN), Lozol, Novo-Indapamide (CAN), Nu-Indapamide (CAN)

Class and Category

Chemical: Sulfonamide
Therapeutic: Antihypertensive, diuretic
Pregnancy category: B

Indications and Dosages

➤ *To treat edema caused by heart failure*

TABLETS

Adults. 2.5 mg q.d. in the morning, increased to 5 mg/day after 1 wk, if indicated.

➤ *To manage hypertension*

TABLETS

Adults. 2.5 mg q.d., increased to 5 mg after 4 wk, if needed.

Route	Onset	Peak	Duration
P.O.*	1 to 2 hr	Unknown	36 hr
P.O.†	1 to 2 wk	8 to 12 wk	Up to 8 wk

Contraindications

Anuria; hypersensitivity to thiazide diuretics, related diuretics, or sulfonamide-derived drugs

---

* For edema.
† For hypertension (with multiple doses).

Mechanism of Action

Acts mainly on the distal convoluted tubules, where it enhances excretion of sodium, chloride, and water by inhibiting sodium ion movement across renal tubules. The resulting decrease in plasma and extracellular fluid volume decreases peripheral vascular resistance and reduces blood pressure. This thiazide diuretic also may cause arterial vasodilation by blocking calcium channels in smooth-muscle cells.

Interactions

DRUGS

amiodarone: Increased risk of arrhythmias if hypokalemia develops
cholestyramine, colestipol: Decreased indapamide absorption
diazoxide: Increased risk of hyperglycemia
digoxin: Increased risk of digitalis toxicity if hypokalemia develops
hypotension-producing drugs: Increased antihypertensive or diuretic effects
lithium: Increased risk of lithium toxicity
neuromuscular blockers: Possibly increased neuromuscular blockade, risk of respiratory depression
oral anticoagulants: Possibly decreased anticoagulant effects

Adverse Reactions

CNS: Anxiety, dizziness, drowsiness, fatigue, fever, headache, mood changes, nervousness, sleep disturbance, vertigo, weakness
CV: Arrhythmias, hypercholesterolemia, orthostatic hypotension, palpitations
EENT: Dry mouth
ENDO: Hyperglycemia, hypoglycemia
GI: Anorexia, constipation, diarrhea, hepatitis, nausea, pancreatitis, thirst, vomiting
GU: Impotence, nocturia
MS: Gout, muscle spasms
SKIN: Jaundice, necrotizing vasculitis, photosensitivity, pruritus, rash, urticaria
Other: Dilutional hypochloremia and hyponatremia, hypokalemia, metabolic alkalosis, weight loss

Nursing Considerations

•Administer indapamide with food or milk to reduce adverse GI reactions.

- Give drug early in the day to avoid nocturia.
- Weigh patient daily, and monitor fluid intake and output, blood pressure, and serum electrolyte levels.
- Monitor BUN and serum creatinine levels regularly, as appropriate.
- If muscle cramps and weakness develop from hypokalemia, expect prescriber to order a potassium supplement or potassium-sparing diuretic.
- When managing hypertension, expect therapeutic response to take several weeks.

PATIENT TEACHING
- Advise patient to take indapamide early in the day to avoid nighttime urination and with food or milk to minimize GI distress.
- Encourage patient to eat high-potassium foods, such as oranges and bananas.
- Direct patient to change position slowly to minimize effects of orthostatic hypotension.
- Instruct patient to weigh himself daily at the same time and wearing similar clothing. Direct him to report a weight gain of more than 2 lb (0.9 kg) per day or 5 lb (2.3 kg) per week.
- Inform patient about possible photosensitivity.
- If patient reports dry mouth, suggest sugarless gum or hard candy to relieve it.

indomethacin

Apo-Indomethacin (CAN), Indocid (CAN), Indocin, Indocin SR, Novo-Methacin (CAN), Nu-Indo (CAN)

indomethacin sodium trihydrate

Apo-Indomethacin (CAN), Indameth, Indocid (CAN), Indocid PDA (CAN), Indocin, Indocin I.V., Novomethacin (CAN)

Class and Category

Chemical: Indoleacetic acid derivative
Therapeutic: Antigout, anti-inflammatory, antirheumatic
Pregnancy category: Not rated

Indications and Dosages

➤ *To relieve symptoms of ankylosing spondylitis, osteoarthritis, and rheumatoid arthritis*

CAPSULES, ORAL SUSPENSION
Adults. 25 to 50 mg b.i.d. to q.i.d., increased by 25 or 50 mg/day q wk, if needed. *Maxi-*

mum: 200 mg/day. After adequate response, dosage reduced as low as possible.

E.R. CAPSULES (ANTIRHEUMATIC)
Adults. 75 mg q.d., increased to 75 mg b.i.d, if needed.

SUPPOSITORIES
Adults. 50 mg up to q.i.d.

➤ *To relieve symptoms of juvenile arthritis*
CAPSULES, ORAL SUSPENSION, SUPPOSITORIES
Children. 1.5 to 2.5 mg/kg/day in divided doses t.i.d. or q.i.d. *Maximum:* 4 mg/kg/day or 150 to 200 mg/day, whichever is less. After adequate response, oral dosage reduced as low as possible.

➤ *To relieve symptoms of acute gouty arthritis*

CAPSULES, ORAL SUSPENSION
Adults. *Initial:* 100 mg. Increased up to 50 mg t.i.d. *Maximum:* 200 mg/day. After pain relief achieved, dosage tapered until drug is discontinued altogether.

SUPPOSITORIES
Adults. 50 mg up to q.i.d. *Maximum:* 200 mg/day.

➤ *To treat inflammation and relieve acute shoulder pain from bursitis or tendinitis*
CAPSULES, ORAL SUSPENSION
Adults. 75 to 150 mg/day in divided doses t.i.d. or q.i.d. for 7 to 14 days.

SUPPOSITORIES
Adults. 50 mg up to q.i.d. *Maximum:* 200 mg/day.

DOSAGE ADJUSTMENT Dosage reduced for elderly patients.

➤ *To treat hemodynamically significant patent ductus arteriosus in premature infants who weigh 500 to 1,750 g (1 to 3.9 lb)*
I.V. INJECTION
Infants over age 7 days. *Initial:* 200 mcg/kg (0.2 mg/kg) over 5 to 10 sec; 1 or 2 additional doses of 250 mcg/kg (0.25 mg/kg) given at 12- to 24-hr intervals, if needed.
Neonates ages 2 to 7 days. *Initial:* 200 mcg/kg (0.2 mg/kg) over 5 to 10 sec; 1 or 2 additional doses of 200 mcg/kg (0.2 mg/kg) given at 12- to 24-hr intervals, if needed.
Neonates under age 48 hours. *Initial:* 200 mcg/kg (0.2 mg/kg) over 5 to 10 sec; 1 or 2 additional doses of 100 mcg/kg (0.1 mg/kg) given at 12- to 24-hr intervals, if needed.

G
H
I

Route	Onset	Peak	Duration
P.O.*	2 to 4 hr	2 to 5 days	Unknown
P.O.†	30 min	Unknown	4 to 6 hr
P.O.‡	In 7 days	1 to 2 wk	Unknown

Mechanism of Action

Blocks the activity of cyclooxygenase, the enzyme needed to synthesize prostaglandins, which mediate the inflammatory response and cause local vasodilation, swelling, and pain. By blocking cyclooxygenase and inhibiting prostaglandins, this NSAID reduces inflammatory symptoms and helps relieve pain.

Incompatibilities

Don't give indomethacin suspension with alkaline antacids or liquids. Don't mix reconstituted indomethacin sodium with I.V. infusion solutions.

Contraindications

Allergy or hypersensitivity to aspirin, indomethacin, iodides, other NSAIDs, or their components; history of proctitis or recent rectal bleeding (suppositories)

Interactions
DRUGS

Note: All effects listed are for oral forms and suppositories unless indicated.
acetaminophen: Increased risk of adverse renal effects (with long-term use of both drugs)
aluminum- and magnesium-containing antacids: Possibly decreased blood indomethacin level
aminoglycosides: Increased risk of aminoglycoside toxicity
antihypertensives: Decreased effectiveness of these drugs
aspirin, other NSAIDs: Increased risk of adverse GI effects and non-GI bleeding
bone marrow depressants: Possibly increased leukopenic or thrombocytopenic effects of these drugs
cefamandole, cefoperazone, cefotetan: Increased risk of hypoprothrombinemia and bleeding

colchicine, platelet aggregation inhibitors: Increased risk of GI bleeding, hemorrhage, and ulcers
corticosteroids, potassium supplements: Increased risk of adverse GI effects
cyclosporine: Increased risk of nephrotoxicity from both drugs, increased blood cyclosporine level
diflunisal: Increased blood indomethacin level and risk of GI bleeding
digoxin: Increased blood digoxin level and risk of digitalis toxicity (all forms)
diuretics (thiazide, loop, and potassium-sparing): Decreased diuretic and antihypertensive effects
gold compounds, nephrotoxic drugs: Increased risk of adverse renal effects
heparin, oral anticoagulants, thrombolytics: Increased anticoagulant effects and risk of hemorrhage
lithium: Increased blood lithium level and risk of toxicity
methotrexate: Increased risk of methotrexate toxicity
plicamycin, valproic acid: Increased risk of hypoprothrombinemia and GI bleeding, hemorrhage, and ulcers
probenecid: Increased blood level and effectiveness of indomethacin, increased risk of indomethacin toxicity
zidovudine: Increased blood zidovudine level and risk of toxicity, increased risk of indomethacin toxicity
ACTIVITIES

alcohol use: Increased risk of adverse GI effects

Adverse Reactions

Note: All reactions are for oral forms and suppositories unless indicated.
CNS: Confusion, depression, dizziness, drowsiness, fatigue, hallucinations, headache, intraventricular hemorrhage (I.V.), peripheral neuropathy, seizures, syncope, vertigo
CV: Arrhythmias, chest pain, edema, fluid retention (all forms), heart failure, hypertension, pulmonary hypertension (I.V.)
EENT: Blurred vision, corneal and retinal damage, epistaxis, hearing loss, tinnitus
ENDO: Hypoglycemia (I.V.)
GI: Abdominal cramps or pain, abdominal distention (I.V.), anorexia, constipation, diarrhea, epigastric discomfort, GI bleeding (all

---

* For antigout effects.
† For anti-inflammatory effects.
‡ For antirheumatic effects.

forms), hepatic dysfunction (I.V.), ileus (I.V.), indigestion, intestinal perforation (I.V.), nausea, pancreatitis, peptic ulcer, vomiting (all forms)
GU: Hematuria, interstitial nephritis, nephrotic syndrome, oliguria (I.V.), proteinuria, renal dysfunction (I.V.), vaginal bleeding
HEME: Agranulocytosis, aplastic anemia, bone marrow depression, disseminated intravascular coagulation, hemolytic anemia, iron deficiency anemia, leukopenia, thrombocytopenia, unusual bleeding or bruising (all forms)
SKIN: Ecchymosis, erythema multiforme, erythema nodosum, photosensitivity, pruritus, rash, Stevens-Johnson syndrome, toxic epidermal necrolysis, urticaria
Other: Anaphylaxis, angioedema, hyperkalemia (I.V.), hyponatremia (I.V.), injection site irritation

Nursing Considerations
• Give oral indomethacin with food, a full glass of water (not suspension), or an antacid to reduce GI distress.
• Shake suspension well before administering.
• Give up to 100 mg of daily dose (not E.R. capsules) at bedtime to reduce nighttime pain and morning stiffness in arthritis patients.
• Make sure suppository stays in rectum at least 1 hour to improve absorption.
• To reconstitute I.V. form, add 1 to 2 ml of preservative-free sodium chloride for injection or preservative-free sterile water to vial. A solution made with 1 ml of diluent contains 100 mcg (0.1 mg) of indomethacin/0.1 ml. A solution made with 2 ml of diluent contains 50 mcg (0.05 mg) of indomethacin/0.1 ml. Use solution immediately because it contains no preservatives. Discard unused portion.
• Be aware that scheduled I.V. doses may be withheld if infant or neonate has anuria or a significant decrease in urine output (less than 0.6 ml/kg/hr).
• When using I.V. form, avoid extravasation to protect surrounding tissue.
• Anticipate a second course (another 3 doses) of I.V. indomethacin if patent ductus arteriosus fails to close or reopens. After two courses, surgery may be performed.
• Because indomethacin causes sodium retention, monitor weight and blood pressure, especially if patient has hypertension.

• When drug is used to treat gouty arthritis, expect its action to peak in 24 to 36 hours and significant swelling to gradually disappear over 3 to 5 days.
• Be aware that E.R. form shouldn't be used to treat gouty arthritis.
• Expect to use suppositories for patients who can't swallow oral form.
• To evaluate drug effectiveness, assess for reduced pain and inflammation and improved joint mobility.
• Be alert for signs of GI bleeding and ulceration, which can occur without warning.
• Be aware that drug shouldn't be used for long-term therapy because of increased risk of adverse reactions.
• Be aware that drug's anti-inflammatory action may mask signs of infection.
• Expect patient to have intermittent checkups during long-term therapy and an ophthalmologic examination if vision changes develop.

PATIENT TEACHING
• Advise patient to take indomethacin capsules with a full glass of water and to avoid lying down for 15 to 30 minutes after taking drug. This helps prevent drug from lodging in esophagus and causing irritation. Caution him not to open or crush capsules.
• Instruct patient to take drug with food or an antacid to reduce GI distress.
• Instruct patient to make sure suppository stays in rectum at least 1 hour.
• Urge patient to avoid alcohol during therapy.
• Remind patient that improvement may not occur for 2 to 4 weeks after starting indomethacin and that he should continue taking drug, as prescribed.
• Inform breast-feeding patient that drug appears in breast milk and may cause seizures in infants. Urge her to use another feeding method during indomethacin therapy.
• Caution against prolonged sun exposure during therapy.
• Urge patient to notify prescriber immediately about bloody or black, tarry stools; changes in vision or hearing; fever; itching; rash; sore throat; swelling in arms or legs; and weight gain.
• Stress the importance of undergoing ordered laboratory tests and eye examinations during long-term therapy.

infliximab

Remicade

Class and Category

Chemical: Monoclonal antibody
Therapeutic: Anti-inflammatory
Pregnancy category: C

Indications and Dosages

➤ *To control moderate to severe Crohn's disease long term*

I.V. INFUSION

Adults. *Induction:* 5 mg/kg over 2 hr, repeated 2 and 6 wk after first infusion. *Maintenance:* 5 mg/kg over 2 hr q 8 wk.

DOSAGE ADJUSTMENT For patients who respond then lose response, dosage may be increased up to 10 mg/kg or frequency increased to q 4 wk. For patients with fistulizing Crohn's disease, 5-mg/kg infusion repeated 2 and 6 wk after first infusion.

➤ *As adjunct to reduce signs and symptoms, inhibit progression of structural damage, and improve physical function in patients with moderate to severe active rheumatoid arthritis who haven't adequately responded to methotrexate alone*

I.V. INFUSION

Adults. 3 mg/kg, with methotrexate, repeated 2 and 6 wk after first infusion and then q 8 wk thereafter.

DOSAGE ADJUSTMENT For patients who have an inadequate response to combination treatment, infliximab dosage increased up to 10 mg/kg or dosing frequency increased to q 4 wk.

Mechanism of Action

Binds with cytokine tumor necrosis factor-alpha (TNF-alpha), thus preventing it from binding with its receptors. As a result, TNF-alpha can't induce proinflammatory cytokines (such as interleukins) and increase endothelial permeability (a change that normally enhances leukocyte migration). These actions lead to reduced infiltration of inflammatory cells into inflamed areas of the intestine and joints.

Incompatibilities

Don't infuse infliximab in same I.V. line with other drugs or through plasticized polyvinyl chloride infusion equipment or devices.

Contraindications

Hypersensitivity to infliximab, murine proteins, or their components; moderate or severe (NYHA Class III or IV) heart failure

Adverse Reactions

CNS: Chills, dizziness, fatigue, fever, headache, syncope
CV: Chest pain, hypertension, hypotension
EENT: Oral candidiasis, pharyngitis, rhinitis, sinusitis
GI: Abdominal hernia; abdominal pain; cholecystitis; diarrhea; intestinal obstruction, perforation, or stenosis; nausea; splenic infarction; splenomegaly; vomiting
GU: Kidney infection, ureteral obstruction, UTI, vaginal candidiasis, vaginitis
HEME: Thrombocytopenia
MS: Back pain, myalgia
RESP: Bronchitis, cough, dyspnea, pneumonia, tuberculosis, upper respiratory tract infection, wheezing
SKIN: Facial flushing, pruritus, rash, urticaria
Other: Lupuslike symptoms, lymphoma

Nursing Considerations

• WARNING Because infliximab increases the risk of developing tuberculosis and reactivating latent tuberculosis, expect prescriber to evaluate patient's risk and to start tuberculosis treatment, as appropriate, before starting infliximab.

• WARNING Be aware that infliximab increases the risk of serious or fatal opportunistic infections, including histoplasmosis, listeriosis, and pneumocystosis. Expect prescriber to carefully evaluate patient's risk before starting drug.

• To reconstitute infliximab, use a 21G (or smaller) needle to add 10 ml of sterile water for injection to each vial of drug. Swirl to mix; don't shake. Be aware that solution may foam and be clear or light yellow.

• Withdraw a volume equal to amount of reconstituted drug from a 250-ml glass bottle or polypropylene or polyolefin infusion bag of NS. Then add the reconstituted infliximab to the bottle to dilute it to 250 ml. Use within 3 hours.

• Administer I.V. infusion over at least 2 hours, using a polyethylene-lined infusion set with an in-line, sterile, nonpyrogenic, low-protein-binding filter that is 1.2 microns or less in pore size. Don't reuse infusion set.

• Be prepared to stop infusion if a hypersensitivity reaction occurs. Keep acetaminophen, antihistamines, corticosteroids, and epineph-

rine on hand for immediate use. A reaction may occur 2 hours to 12 days after infusion.
•WARNING Assess patient for signs and symptoms of infection, especially if patient receives immunosuppressant therapy or has a chronic infection. Upper respiratory tract infections and UTIs are most common, but sepsis and fatal opportunistic infections have occurred.
•WARNING Be aware that infliximab shouldn't be given to patients with NYHA Class III or IV congestive heart failure because it may worsen the condition or cause death. If such a patient does receive infliximab, expect to discontinue drug if congestive heart failure worsens.

PATIENT TEACHING
•Inform patient that infliximab should take effect within 1 to 2 weeks.
•Urge patient to report signs of infection, such as burning with urination, cough, and sore throat, as well as signs of infusion reaction, such as chest pain, chills, dyspnea, facial flushing, fever, itching, headache, and rash. Infusion reaction may occur up to 12 days after receiving drug.

ipecac syrup

Ipecac Syrup

Class and Category

Chemical: Cephaelis acuminata or *Cephaelis ipecacuanha* derivative
Therapeutic: Emetic
Pregnancy category: C

Indications and Dosages

➤ *To induce vomiting after drug overdose and certain types of poisoning*

SYRUP
Adults and children over age 12. 15 to 30 ml followed by 240 ml of water. Dose repeated if vomiting doesn't begin within 20 to 30 min.
Children ages 1 to 12. 15 ml preceded or followed by 120 to 240 ml of water. Dose repeated if vomiting doesn't begin within 20 to 30 min.
Infants ages 6 months to 1 year. 5 to 10 ml preceded or followed by 120 to 240 ml of water.

Route	Onset	Peak	Duration
P.O.	20 to 30 min	Unknown	20 to 25 min

Contraindications

Loss of gag reflex, poisoning with strychnine or corrosives (such as alkaloid substances, petroleum distillates, and strong acids), seizures, semiconsciousness or unconsciousness, severe inebriation, shock

Mechanism of Action

Induces vomiting by irritating the gastric mucosa and stimulating the medullary chemoreceptor trigger zone in the CNS.

Interactions

DRUGS
activated charcoal: Neutralization of emetic effect

Adverse Reactions

CNS: Depression, drowsiness
EENT: Aspiration of vomitus, coughing
GI: Diarrhea, indigestion

Nursing Considerations

•Give ipecac syrup only to conscious patients, and follow with adequate water. Give young or frightened children water before or after ipecac.
•Expect vomiting to begin 20 to 30 minutes after patient takes drug.
•If vomiting doesn't occur within 30 minutes of second dose, prepare for gastric lavage.
•Don't give ipecac after ingestion of petroleum distillates, such as gasoline, or caustic substances (to avoid further injury to esophagus).
•If activated charcoal also will be given to treat overdose or poisoning, expect to give it after patient vomits or 30 minutes after second dose if no vomiting occurs because activated charcoal will adsorb ipecac and inhibit its action.
•Know that arrhythmias, atrial fibrillation, bradycardia, fatal myocarditis, hypotension, myalgia, or muscle stiffness or weakness may develop if patient takes excessive dose or fails to vomit after taking drug.

PATIENT TEACHING
•Inform patient of ipecac's effects.
•Instruct adult patient to drink 8 oz (240 ml) of water after taking drug. Instruct a child to drink 4 to 8 oz (120 to 240 ml) of water before or after taking drug.
•Inform patient or parents of child that diarrhea may occur after taking drug.
•Urge parents to keep ipecac syrup at home (along with the telephone number of a poison control center), and teach them how to administer it in case of poisoning.
•WARNING Advise parents that ipecac syrup has replaced ipecac fluid extract and ipecac

G
H
I

tincture and that they should check their home supply and update it, if needed. Inform them that ipecac fluid extract is 14 times more concentrated than ipecac syrup and can cause serious, possibly toxic effects if administered incorrectly.

ipratropium bromide

Apo-Ipravent (CAN), Atrovent, Kendral-Ipratropium (CAN)

Class and Category
Chemical: Quaternary *N*-methyl isopropyl derivative of noratropine
Therapeutic: Anticholinergic, bronchodilator
Pregnancy category: B

Indications and Dosages
➤ *To treat bronchitis and COPD*
INHALATION AEROSOL
Adults and adolescents. 2 to 4 inhalations (36 to 72 mcg) t.i.d. or q.i.d. *Maximum:* Up to 12 inhalations (216 mcg)/24 hr.
INHALATION SOLUTION FOR NEBULIZER
Adults and adolescents. 250 to 500 mcg dissolved in preservative-free sterile NS q 6 to 8 hr. For severe COPD exacerbations, 500 mcg q 4 to 8 hr.

➤ *To treat perennial and allergic rhinitis*
NASAL SPRAY
Adults and children age 6 and older. 2 sprays of 0.03% (21 mcg/spray) per nostril b.i.d. or t.i.d. *Maximum:* 12 sprays (252 mcg)/24 hr.
➤ *To treat rhinorrhea from common cold*
NASAL SPRAY
Adults and children age 5 and older. 2 sprays of 0.06% (42 mcg/spray) per nostril t.i.d. or q.i.d. for up to 4 days. *Maximum:* 16 sprays (672 mcg)/24 hr.

Route	Onset	Peak	Duration
Inhalation	5 to 15 min	1 to 2 hr	3 to 8 hr
Nasal	5 min	1 to 4 hr	4 to 8 hr

Contraindications
Hypersensitivity to atropine, ipratropium bromide, or their components; hypersensitivity to peanuts, soya lecithin, soybeans, or related products (with aerosol inhaler)

Interactions
DRUGS
anticholinergics: Increased anticholinergic effects
tacrine: Decreased effects of both drugs

Adverse Reactions
CNS: Dizziness, insomnia

Mechanism of Action
After acetylcholine is released from cholinergic fibers, ipratropium prevents it from attaching to muscarinic receptors on membranes of smooth-muscle cells, as shown at right. By blocking acetycholine's effects in the bronchi and bronchioles, ipratropium relaxes smooth muscles and causes bronchodilation.

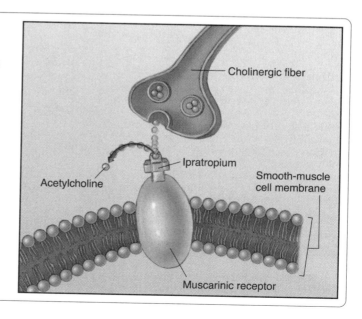

CV: Bradycardia (nasal spray), hypertension, palpitations
EENT: Dry mouth, laryngospasm, taste perversion (all drug forms); blurred vision, eye irritation and pain, glaucoma or worsening of existing glaucoma (if nasal spray comes in contact with eyes); epistaxis, nasal dryness and irritation, pharyngitis, rhinitis, sinusitis, tinnitus (with nasal spray)
GI: Constipation, ileus, nausea
GU: Prostatitis, urine retention
MS: Arthritis
RESP: Bronchitis, bronchospasm, cough, dyspnea, increased sputum production
SKIN: Dermatitis, rash, urticaria
Other: Angioedema, flulike symptoms

Nursing Considerations
• Use ipratropium cautiously in patients with angle-closure glaucoma, benign prostatic hyperplasia, or bladder neck obstruction.
• As prescribed, mix ipratropium inhalation solution with preservative-free albuterol, and preservative-free ipratropium inhalation solution with cromolyn inhalation solution. Use within 1 hour.
• When using a nebulizer, apply a mouthpiece to prevent drug from leaking out around mask and causing blurred vision or eye pain.

PATIENT TEACHING
• Caution patient not to use ipratropium to treat acute bronchospasm.
• Teach patient proper use of inhaler or nasal spray. Instruct him to shake inhaler well with each use.
• Advise patient to keep spray out of his eyes because it may irritate them or blur his vision. If spray comes in contact with his eyes, instruct patient to flush them with cool tap water and to contact prescriber.
• Instruct patient to rinse mouth after each nebulizer or inhaler treatment to help minimize throat dryness and irritation.
• If patient is using 0.06% nasal spray for a common cold, advise him to use it no longer than 4 days.
• Teach patient how to determine whether canister is empty by counting and recording number of doses.
• Advise patient to report decreased response to ipratropium as well as difficulty voiding, eye pain, palpitations, and vision changes.

ipratropium bromide and albuterol sulfate
Combivent, DuoNeb

Class and Category
Chemical: Quarternary *N*-methyl isopropyl derivative of noratropine (ipratropium); selective beta$_2$-adrenergic agonist, sympathomimetic (albuterol)
Therapeutic: Bronchodilator
Pregnancy category: C

Indications and Dosages
➤ *To treat bronchospasm in patients with COPD who require more than one bronchodilator*
INHALATION AEROSOL (COMBIVENT)
Adults. 2 inhalations (36 mcg ipratropium, 180 mcg albuterol base) q.i.d. and as needed. *Maximum:* 12 inhalations (216 mcg ipratropium, 1.08 g albuterol base)/24 hr.
INHALATION SOLUTION FOR NEBULIZER (DUONEB)
Adults. 3 ml (0.5 mg ipratropium, 2.5 mg albuterol base) q.i.d. *Maximum:* 2 additional 3-ml doses/24 hr, p.r.n.

Route	Onset	Peak	Duration
Inhalation aerosol	In 15 min	1 hr	4 to 5 hr
Inhalation solution	5 to 15 min	1 to 2 hr	Up to 5 hr

Mechanism of Action
Prevents acetylcholine (after its release from cholinergic fibers) from attaching to muscarinic receptors on membranes of smooth-muscle cells. By blocking acetylcholine's effects in the bronchi and bronchioles, ipratropium relaxes smooth muscles and causes bronchodilation. Albuterol attaches to beta$_2$ receptors on bronchial cell membranes, which stimulates the intracellular enzyme adenylate cyclase to convert adenosine triphosphate to cyclic adenosine monophosphate (cAMP). This reaction decreases intracellular calcium level and increases intracellular cAMP. Together, these effects relax bronchial smooth-muscle cells and inhibit histamine release.

Contraindications

Hypersensitivity to albuterol, ipratropium, or their components; hypersensitivity to atropine or its derivatives; hypersensitivity to peanuts, soya lecithin, soybeans, or related products (with aerosol inhaler)

Interactions

DRUGS

anticholinergics, such as atropine: Possibly additive effects of ipratropium
beta blockers: Possibly mutual inhibition of therapeutic effects
MAO inhibitors, tricyclic antidepressants: Possibly potentiation of albuterol's adverse cardiovascular effects
non-potassium-sparing diuretics, such as loop and thiazide diuretics: Increased risk of hypokalemia
sympathomimetic bronchodilators, such as theophylline: Increased risk of adverse cardiovascular effects

Adverse Reactions

CNS: Drowsiness, headache, nervousness, tremor
CV: Chest pain, increased heart rate, palpitations
EENT: Acute eye pain, altered taste, blurred vision, dry mouth, pharyngitis, sinusitis, sore throat, voice alterations, worsened angle-closure glaucoma
GI: Constipation, diarrhea, indigestion, nausea
GU: UTI
MS: Back pain, leg cramps, muscle aches
RESP: Bronchitis, cough, exacerbation of COPD, paradoxical bronchospasm, pneumonia, upper respiratory tract infection, wheezing
SKIN: Flushing
Other: Hypokalemia

Nursing Considerations

• Prime the aerosol inhaler with three priming sprays if giving it for the first time or if it hasn't been used for more than 24 hours.
• As prescribed, administer nebulized dose using a mouthpiece or properly fitting face mask attached to a jet nebulizer connected to an air compressor with adequate airflow.
• **WARNING** Avoid spraying drug directly into patient's eyes because it may cause vision disturbances. In a patient with angle-closure glaucoma, be aware that spraying drug directly into his eyes may precipitate an acute attack or exacerbate the condition.

• Monitor urine output if patient has a history of prostatic hyperplasia or bladder-neck obstruction because drug may aggravate these conditions and cause urine retention.
• Frequently monitor heart rate and rhythm and blood pressure in patients with a history of arrhythmias, coronary artery insufficiency, or hypertension because the drug may cause adverse cardiovascular effects in these patients. If adverse cardiovascular effects occur, expect to discontinue drug.
• Monitor serum potassium level because drug may cause transient hypokalemia.
• Although immediate hypersensitivity reactions are rare, monitor patient for angioedema, bronchospasm, oropharyngeal edema, pruritus, rash, urticaria, and anaphylaxis.

PATIENT TEACHING

• Teach patient how to use inhaler or nebulizer properly. Instruct him to shake aerosol inhaler well before use and to wait 1 minute between inhalations.
• Instruct patient to rinse mouth after each nebulizer or inhaler treatment to help minimize throat dryness and irritation.
• Advise patient to keep drug out of his eyes because it may irritate them or blur his vision. If drug comes in contact with his eyes, instruct patient to flush them with cool tap water and to contact prescriber immediately.
• Caution patient not to use more than the prescribed dose because of the risk of serious adverse reactions and possibly death. Advise patient to contact prescriber immediately if doses become less effective.
• Advise patient to contact prescriber before using other inhaled drugs.

irbesartan

Avapro

Class and Category

Chemical: Nonpeptide angiotensin II antagonist
Therapeutic: Antihypertensive
Pregnancy category: C (first trimester), D (later trimesters)

Indications and Dosages

➤ *To manage hypertension, alone or with other antihypertensives*

TABLETS

Adults and adolescents. *Initial:* 150 mg q.d. *Maximum:* 300 mg q.d.

DOSAGE ADJUSTMENT Initial dosage reduced to 75 mg q.d. for patients with hypovolemia or hyponatremia from such causes as hemodialysis or vigorous diuretic therapy.
Children ages 6 to 12. *Initial:* 75 mg q.d. *Maximum:* 150 mg q.d.

Route	Onset	Peak	Duration
P.O.	Unknown	In 4 to 6 wk	Unknown

Mechanism of Action
Selectively blocks binding of the potent vasoconstrictor angiotensin (AT) II to AT_1 receptor sites in many tissues, including vascular smooth muscle and adrenal glands. This inhibits the vasoconstrictive and aldosterone-secreting effects of AT II, which reduces blood pressure.

Contraindications
Hypersensitivity to irbesartan or its components

Interactions
DRUGS
diuretics: Possibly additive hypotensive effects

Adverse Reactions
CNS: Anxiety, dizziness, fatigue, headache, nervousness
CV: Chest pain, hypotension, peripheral edema, tachycardia
EENT: Pharyngitis, rhinitis
GI: Abdominal pain, diarrhea, heartburn, indigestion, nausea, vomiting
GU: UTI
MS: Musculoskeletal pain
RESP: Upper respiratory tract infection
SKIN: Rash

Nursing Considerations
•If patient has known or suspected hypovolemia, provide treatment, such as I.V. NS, as prescribed, to correct this condition before beginning irbesartan therapy. Or expect to begin therapy with a lower dosage.
•Frequently monitor blood pressure to evaluate drug's effectiveness.
•If blood pressure isn't controlled with irbesartan alone, expect to also give a diuretic, such as hydrochlorothiazide, as prescribed.
•WARNING If patient receives a diuretic or another antihypertensive during irbesartan therapy, frequently monitor his blood pressure because he's at risk for developing hypotension.

•If patient experiences symptomatic hypotension, expect to discontinue drug temporarily. Immediately place patient in supine position and prepare to administer I.V. NS, as prescribed. Expect to resume drug therapy after blood pressure stabilizes.
•If patient receives a diuretic, provide adequate hydration, as appropriate, to help prevent hypovolemia. Also monitor patient for signs and symptoms of hypovolemia, such as hypotension, dizziness, and fainting.
•WARNING Monitor patient for increased BUN and serum creatinine levels if he has heart failure or impaired renal function because drug may cause acute renal failure. If increases are significant or persistent, notify prescriber immediately.

PATIENT TEACHING
•Advise patient to take drug at the same time each day to maintain its therapeutic effect.
•Explain the importance of regular exercise, proper diet, and other lifestyle changes in controlling hypertension.
•Caution patient to avoid hazardous activities until drug's CNS effects are known.
•Instruct patient to consult prescriber before taking any new drug.
•To reduce the risk of dehydration and hypotension, advise patient to drink adequate fluids during hot weather and exercise.
•Instruct patient to contact prescriber if severe nausea, vomiting, or diarrhea occurs and continues because of the risk of dehydration and hypotension.
•Advise female patient to notify prescriber immediately about known or suspected pregnancy. Explain that if she becomes pregnant, prescriber may replace irbesartan with another antihypertensive that's safe to use during pregnancy.
•Urge patient to keep follow-up appointments with prescriber to monitor progress.

iron dextran

(contains 50 mg of elemental iron per milliliter)
DexFerrum, DexIron (CAN), InFeD

Class and Category
Chemical: Iron salt, mineral
Therapeutic: Antianemic agent
Pregnancy category: C

Indications and Dosages

➤ *To treat iron deficiency anemia*
I.V. INFUSION
Adults and children who weigh over 15 kg (33 lb). Dose (ml) = 0.0442 (desired hemoglobin − observed hemoglobin) × lean body weight (in kg) + (0.26 × lean body weight). Alternatively, consult dosage table in package insert. *Maximum:* 2 ml (100 mg)/day.
Children over age 4 months who weigh 5 to 15 kg (11 to 33 lb). Dose (ml) = 0.0442 (desired hemoglobin − observed hemoglobin) × weight (kg) + (0.26 × weight). Alternatively, consult dosage table in package insert. *Maximum:* 1 ml (50 mg)/day.
➤ *To replace iron lost in blood loss*
I.V. INFUSION
Adults. Replacement iron (mg) = ml of blood loss × hematocrit.

Mechanism of Action

Restores hemoglobin and replenishes iron stores. Iron, an essential component of hemoglobin, myoglobin, and several enzymes (including cytochromes, catalase, and peroxidase), is needed for catecholamine metabolism and normal neutrophil function.

In iron dextran therapy, iron binds to available protein parts after the drug has been split into iron and dextran by cells of the reticuloendothelial system. The bound iron forms hemosiderin or ferritin, physiologic forms of iron, and transferrin, which replenish hemoglobin and depleted iron stores. Dextran is metabolized or excreted.

Incompatibilities

Don't mix iron dextran with blood for transfusion, other drugs, or parenteral nutrition solutions for I.V. infusion.

Contraindications

Anemia other than iron deficiency, hypersensitivity to iron dextran or its components

Interactions

None known.

Adverse Reactions

CNS: Chills, disorientation, dizziness, fever, headache, malaise, paresthesia, seizures, syncope, unconsciousness, weakness
CV: Arrhythmias, bradycardia, chest pain, shock, hypertension, hypotension, tachycardia
EENT: Altered taste
GI: Abdominal pain, diarrhea, nausea, vomiting
GU: Hematuria
HEME: Leukocytosis
MS: Arthralgia, arthritis, backache, myalgia, rhabdomyolysis
RESP: Bronchospasm, dyspnea, respiratory arrest, wheezing
SKIN: Cyanosis, diaphoresis, rash, pruritus, purpura, urticaria
Other: Anaphylaxis, infusion site phlebitis

Nursing Considerations

•Expect oral iron therapy to be discontinued before iron dextran therapy is initiated. Iron dextran is administered only when oral therapy is not feasible; it also may be administered by I.M. injection.
•Expect to monitor hemoglobin level, hematocrit, serum ferritin level, and transferrin saturation, as ordered, before, during, and after iron dextran therapy.
•**WARNING** Before initiating therapy, administer a test dose of 0.5 ml of iron dextran gradually over 30 seconds, as prescribed, and monitor patient closely for an anaphylactic reaction.
•Wait 1 to 2 hours before administering the remainder of the dose. Infuse undiluted iron dextran slowly, at a rate not to exceed 1 ml/minute (50 mg/minute).
•**WARNING** Monitor patient closely for signs and symptoms of anaphylaxis, such as severe hypotension, loss of consciousness, collapse, dyspnea, and seizures, during and after infusion. Patients with a history of asthma or known allergies are at increased risk for anaphylaxis and, possibly, death. Institute emergency resuscitation measures as needed, including epinephrine administration, as prescribed.
•**WARNING** Assess blood pressure frequently after drug administration because hypotension is a common adverse effect that may be related to infusion rate; avoid rapid infusion.
•Be aware that patient may exhibit adverse reactions, including arthralgia, backache, chills, and vomiting, 1 to 2 days after drug therapy. Symptoms should resolve within 3 to 4 days.
•Assess patients with a history of rheumatoid arthritis for exacerbation of joint pain and swelling.

• Monitor patients with preexisting cardiovascular disease for an exacerbation due to drug's adverse effects.
• Assess patient for iron overload, characterized by sedation, decreased activity, pale eyes, and bleeding in GI tract and lungs.
• Store iron dextran at 15° to 30° C (59° to 86° F).

PATIENT TEACHING
• Instruct patient to immediately report signs of an adverse reaction, such as shortness of breath, wheezing, or rash, during iron dextran therapy.
• Advise patient not to take any oral iron preparations without first consulting prescriber.
• Inform patient that symptoms of iron deficiency may include decreased stamina, learning problems, shortness of breath, and fatigue. Encourage patient to plan periods of activity and rest in order to avoid excessive fatigue.
• Stress the importance of following dosage regimen and of keeping follow-up medical appointments and appointments for laboratory tests.

iron sucrose

(contains 100 mg of elemental iron per 5 ml)
Venofer

Class and Category
Chemical: Iron salt, mineral
Therapeutic: Antianemic
Pregnancy category: B

Indications and Dosages
➤ *To treat iron deficiency anemia in hemodialysis patients receiving erythropoietin*

I.V. INJECTION OR INFUSION
Adults. *Initial:* 100 mg of elemental iron during dialysis. *Usual:* 100 mg of elemental iron q wk to 3 times/wk to a total dose of 1,000 mg. Dosage repeated as needed to maintain target levels of hemoglobin and hematocrit and acceptable blood iron level. *Maximum:* 100 mg/dose.

Incompatibilities
Don't mix with other drugs or parenteral nutrition solutions for I.V. infusion.

Contraindications
Anemia other than iron deficiency, hypersensitivity to iron salts or their components, iron overload

Mechanism of Action
Acts to replenish iron stores lost during dialysis because of increased erythropoiesis and insufficient absorption of iron from the GI tract. Iron is an essential component of hemoglobin, myoglobin, and several enzymes, including cytochromes, catalase, and peroxidase, and is needed for catecholamine metabolism and normal neutrophil function. Iron sucrose injection also normalizes RBC production by binding with hemoglobin or being stored as ferritin in reticuloendothelial cells of the liver, spleen, and bone marrow.

Interactions
DRUGS
chloramphenicol: Possibly decreased effectiveness of iron sucrose
oral iron preparations: Possibly reduced absorption of oral iron supplements

Adverse Reactions
CNS: Dizziness, fever, headache, malaise
CV: Chest pain, hypertension, hypotension
GI: Abdominal pain, diarrhea, elevated liver function test results, nausea, vomiting
MS: Leg cramps, muscle weakness, myalgia
RESP: Cough, dyspnea, pneumonia
SKIN: Pruritus
Other: Anaphylaxis, fluid overload, infusion or injection site redness

Nursing Considerations
• To reconstitute iron sucrose injection for infusion, dilute 100 mg of elemental iron in a maximum of 100 ml of NS immediately before infusion. Infuse over at least 15 minutes. Discard any unused diluted solution.
• Administer drug directly into a dialysis line by slow I.V. injection or by infusion at a rate of 20 mg/minute, not to exceed 100 mg per injection.
• **WARNING** Monitor closely for signs and symptoms of anaphylaxis, such as severe hypotension, loss of consciousness, collapse, dyspnea, or seizures, during and after drug administration. Institute emergency resuscitation measures as needed.
• **WARNING** Assess blood pressure frequently after drug administration because hypotension is a common adverse reaction that may be related to infusion rate (avoid rapid infusion) or total cumulative dose.

G
H
I

•Expect to monitor hemoglobin, hematocrit, serum ferritin, and transferrin saturation, as ordered, before, during, and after iron sucrose therapy. Make sure that serum iron levels are tested 48 hours after last dose. Notify prescriber and expect to discontinue therapy if blood iron levels are normal or elevated, to prevent iron toxicity.
•Assess patient for possible iron overload, characterized by sedation, decreased activity, pale eyes, and bleeding in GI tract and lungs.

PATIENT TEACHING
•Advise patient not to take any oral iron preparations during iron sucrose therapy without first consulting prescriber.
•Inform patient that symptoms of iron deficiency may include decreased stamina, learning problems, shortness of breath, and fatigue.

isocarboxazid

Marplan

Class and Category
Chemical: Hydrazine derivative
Therapeutic: Antidepressant
Pregnancy category: C

Indications and Dosages
➤ *To treat major depression*
TABLETS
Adults and adolescents over age 16. *Initial:* 10 mg b.i.d., increased by 10 mg/day every 2 to 4 days, as needed and tolerated. *Maximum:* 60 mg/day.

Route	Onset	Peak	Duration
P.O.	7 to 10 days	Unknown	10 days

Mechanism of Action
Irreversibly binds to MAO, reducing its activity and increasing levels of neurotransmitters, including serotonin and the catecholamine neurotransmitters dopamine, epinephrine, and norepinephrine. This regulation of CNS neurotransmitters helps to ease depression. With long-term use, isocarboxazid results in down-regulation (desensitization) of alpha$_2$- or beta-adrenergic and serotonin receptors after 2 to 4 weeks, which also produces an antidepressant effect.

Contraindications
Cardiovascular disease; cerebrovascular disease; heart failure; hepatic disease; history of headaches; hypersensitivity to isocarboxazid or its components; hypertension; pheochromocytoma; severe renal impairment; use of anesthetics, antihypertensives, bupropion, buspirone, carbamazepine, CNS depressants, cyclobenzaprine, dextromethorphan, meperidine, selective serotonin reuptake inhibitors, sympathomimetics, or tricyclic antidepressants; use within 14 days of another MAO inhibitor

Interactions
DRUGS
anticholinergics, antidyskinetics, antihistamines: Increased anticholinergic effect, prolonged CNS depression (with antihistamines)
anticonvulsants: Increased CNS depression, possibly altered seizure pattern
antihypertensives, diuretics: Increased hypotensive effect
bromocriptine: Possibly interference with bromocriptine effects
bupropion: Increased risk of bupropion toxicity
buspirone, guanadrel, guanethidine: Increased risk of hypertension
caffeine-containing drugs: Increased risk of dangerous arrhythmias and severe hypertension
carbamazepine, cyclobenzaprine, maprotiline, other MAO inhibitors: Increased risk of hyperpyretic crisis, hypertensive crisis, severe seizures, and death; altered pattern of seizures (with carbamazepine)
CNS depressants: Increased CNS depression
dextromethorphan: Increased risk of excitation, hypertension, and hyperpyrexia
doxapram: Increased vasopressor effects of either drug
fluoxetine, paroxetine, sertraline, trazodone, tricyclic antidepressants: Increased risk of life-threatening serotonin syndrome
haloperidol, loxapine, molindone, phenothiazines, pimozide, thioxanthenes: Prolonged and intensified anticholinergic, hypotensive, and sedative effects of these drugs or isocarboxazid
insulin, oral antidiabetic drugs: Increased hypoglycemic effects
levodopa: Increased risk of sudden, moderate to severe hypertension
local anesthetics (with epinephrine or levonordefrin): Possibly severe hypertension

meperidine, other opioid analgesics: Increased risk of coma, hyperpyrexia, hypotension, immediate excitation, rigidity, seizures, severe hypertension, severe respiratory depression, shock, sweating, and death
methyldopa: Increased risk of hallucinations, headache, hyperexcitability, and severe hypertension
methylphenidate: Increased CNS stimulant effects
metrizamide: Decreased seizure threshold and increased risk of seizures
oral anticoagulants: Increased anticoagulant activity
phenylephrine (nasal or ophthalmic): Potentiated vasopressor effect of phenylephrine
rauwolfia alkaloids: Increased risk of moderate to severe hypertension, CNS depression (when isocarboxazid is added to rauwolfia alkaloid therapy), CNS excitation and hypertension (when rauwolfia alkaloid is added to isocarboxazid therapy)
spinal anesthetics: Increased risk of hypotension
sympathomimetics: Prolonged and intensified cardiac stimulant and vasopressor effects
tryptophan: Increased risk of confusion, disorientation, hyperreflexia, hyperthermia, hyperventilation, mania or hypomania, and shivering

FOODS
aged cheese; avocados; bananas; fava or broad beans; cured meat or sausage; overripe fruit; pickled or smoked fish, meats or poultry; protein extract; soy sauce; yeast extract; and other foods high in tyramine or other pressor amines: Increased risk of dangerous arrhythmias and severe hypertensive crisis

ACTIVITIES
alcohol-containing products that also may contain tyramine, such as beer (including reduced-alcohol and alcohol-free beer), hard liquor, liqueurs, sherry, and wines (red and white): Increased risk of hypertensive crisis

Adverse Reactions
CNS: Agitation, dizziness, drowsiness, fever, headache, insomnia, intracranial bleeding, overstimulation, restlessness, sedation, tremor, weakness
CV: Bradycardia, chest pain, edema, hypertensive crisis, orthostatic hypotension, palpitations, tachycardia

EENT: Blurred vision, dry mouth, mydriasis, photophobia, yellowing of sclera
GI: Abdominal pain, anorexia, constipation, diarrhea, elevated liver function test results, increased appetite, nausea
GU: Darkened urine, oliguria, sexual dysfunction
HEME: Leukopenia
MS: Muscle spasms, myoclonus, neck stiffness
SKIN: Clammy skin, diaphoresis, jaundice, rash
Other: Unusual weight gain

Nursing Considerations
•Monitor patient's blood pressure during isocarboxazid therapy to detect hypertensive crisis and decrease the risk of orthostatic hypotension.
•**WARNING** Notify prescriber immediately if patient has signs and symptoms of hypertensive crisis (drug's most serious adverse effect), such as chest pain, headache, neck stiffness, and palpitations. Expect to stop drug immediately if these occur.
•Keep phentolamine readily available to treat hypertensive crisis. Give 5 mg by slow I.V. infusion, as prescribed, to reduce blood pressure without causing excessive hypotension. Use external cooling measures, as prescribed, to manage fever.
•To avoid hypertensive crisis, expect to wait 10 to 14 days, as prescribed, when switching patient from one MAO inhibitor to another or when switching from a dibenzazepine-related drug, such as amitriptyline or perphenazine.
•Monitor patient with a history of epilepsy for seizures because isocarboxazid may alter seizure threshold. Institute seizure precautions according to facility protocol.
•Monitor liver function test results and assess patient for abdominal pain, darkened urine, and jaundice because isocarboxazid may cause hepatic dysfunction.
•Expect to observe some therapeutic effect in 7 to 10 days, but keep in mind that full effect may not occur for 4 to 8 weeks.
•Be aware that, for maintenance therapy, the smallest dose possible should be used. Once clinical effect has been achieved, expect to decrease the dosage slowly over several weeks.
•Keep dietary restrictions in place for at least 2 weeks after stopping isocarboxazid

because of the slow recovery from drug's enzyme-inhibiting effects.
•Ideally, expect to stop drug 10 days before elective surgery, as prescribed, to avoid hypotension.
•Anticipate that coadministration with a selective serotonin reuptake inhibitor may cause confusion, diaphoresis, diarrhea, seizures, and other less severe symptoms.
•Monitor severely depressed patient for suicidal tendencies. If they arise, institute suicide precautions, as appropriate and according to facility policy, and notify prescriber immediately.
•Monitor patient for sudden insomnia. If it develops, notify prescriber and be prepared to give drug early in the day.

PATIENT TEACHING
•Inform patient and family members that therapeutic effects of isocarboxazid may take several weeks to appear and that he should continue taking drug as prescribed.
•Caution patient to rise slowly from a lying or sitting position to minimize effects of orthostatic hypotension.
•**WARNING** Instruct patient to avoid the following foods, beverages, and drugs during isocarboxazid therapy and for 2 weeks afterward: alcohol-free and reduced-alcohol beer and wine; appetite suppressants; beer; broad beans; cheese (except cottage and cream cheese); chocolate and caffeine in large quantities; dry sausage (including Genoa salami, hard salami, Lebanon bologna, and pepperoni); hay fever drugs; inhaled asthma drugs; liver; meat extract; OTC cold and cough medicines (including those containing dextromethorphan); nasal decongestants (tablets, drops, or spray); pickled herring; products that contain tyramine; protein-rich foods that may have undergone protein changes by aging, fermenting, pickling, or smoking; sauerkraut; sinus drugs; weight-loss preparations; yeast extracts (including brewer's yeast in large quantities); yogurt; and wine.
•Advise patient to notify prescriber immediately about chest pain, dizziness, headache, nausea, neck stiffness, palpitations, rapid heart rate, sweating, and vomiting.
•Advise patient to inform all health care providers (including dentists) that he takes an MAO inhibitor because certain drugs are contraindicated within 2 weeks of therapy.

•Urge patient to avoid potentially hazardous activities until drug's adverse effects are known.
•Urge patient with diabetes mellitus who's taking insulin or an oral antidiabetic drug to monitor blood glucose level frequently during therapy because isocarboxazid may affect glucose control.
•Caution patient not to stop taking drug abruptly to avoid recurrence of original symptoms.

isoetharine hydrochloride

Arm-a-Med Isoetharine (0.062%, 0.125%, 0.167%, 0.2%, 0.25%), Beta-2 (1%), Bronkosol (1%), Dey-Lute Isoetharine (0.08%, 0.1%, 0.17%, 0.25%)

isoetharine mesylate

Bronkometer (0.61%)

Class and Category

Chemical: Catecholamine
Therapeutic: Bronchodilator
Pregnancy category: Not rated

Indications and Dosages

➤ *To prevent and treat reversible bronchospasm from chronic bronchitis or emphysema*

INHALATION AEROSOL
Adults and adolescents. 1 or 2 inhalations (340 or 680 mcg) q 4 hr.
INHALATION SOLUTION FOR HAND-BULB NEBULIZER
Adults. 3 to 7 inhalations of undiluted 0.5% or 1% solution q 4 hr.
INHALATION SOLUTION FOR NEBULIZER
Adults. 2.5 to 10 mg over 15 to 20 min. Repeated q 4 hr, p.r.n.

Route	Onset	Peak	Duration
Inhalation	5 min	5 to 15 min	2 to 3 hr

Mechanism of Action

Attaches to beta$_2$ receptors on bronchial cell membranes, which stimulates the intracellular enzyme adenylate cyclase to convert adenosine triphosphate to cAMP. Increased intracellular levels of cAMP help relax bronchial smooth-muscle cells, stabilize mast cells, and inhibit histamine release.

Contraindications

Hypersensitivity to isoetharine, sympatho-mimetic amines, or their components

Interactions

DRUGS

beta blockers: Decreased effects of both drugs
cyclopropane, halothane: Increased risk of arrhythmias
ephedrine: Increased cardiac stimulation
epinephrine: Increased effects of epinephrine
guanethidine: Decreased hypotensive effects
isoproterenol: Excessive cardiac stimulation
MAO inhibitors: Increased risk of hypertensive crisis, increased vascular effects of isoetharine
methyldopa: Increased vasopressor response
nitrates: Possibly decreased effects of both drugs
oxytocic drugs: Increased risk of hypotension
rauwolfia alkaloids: Increased risk of hypertension
tricyclic antidepressants: Increased risk of arrhythmias

Adverse Reactions

CNS: Anxiety, dizziness, headache, insomnia, tremor, vertigo, weakness
CV: Angina, arrhythmias, hypertension, palpitations, tachycardia
EENT: Choking sensation, eyelid or lip swelling, laryngospasm, taste perversion
GI: Nausea, vomiting
RESP: Bronchospasm, cough, paradoxical increased airway resistance (with excessive use), wheezing
SKIN: Dermatitis, flushing, pruritus, urticaria
Other: Angioedema, facial edema

Nursing Considerations

• Dilute 1% isoetharine inhalation solution with 1 to 4 ml of sterile NS; 0.062% to 0.25% solutions don't need to be diluted before use.
• Don't use a solution that's pink or darker than light yellow or one that contains precipitate.
• Wait 1 minute after initial inhaler dose to assess whether patient needs a second dose.
• Monitor blood pressure and pulse rate, and observe for arrhythmias during therapy.

PATIENT TEACHING

• Teach patient how to use isoetharine inhaler or nebulizer.
• Instruct patient to take drug exactly as directed and not to exceed dosage.
• Instruct patient not to take other drugs, even OTC drugs, unless prescribed.

• Teach patient how to determine when canister needs to be replaced by counting and recording number of doses.
• Instruct patient to report chest pain, difficulty breathing, failure to respond to usual isoetharine dose, irregular heartbeat, productive cough, or tremor.

isoniazid

(isonicotinic acid hydrazide, INH)

Isotamine (CAN), Laniazid, Nydrazid, PMS-Isoniazid (CAN)

Class and Category

Chemical: Isonicotinic acid derivative
Therapeutic: Antibiotic, antitubercular
Pregnancy category: C

Indications and Dosages

➤ *To prevent tuberculosis*

SYRUP, TABLETS, I.M. INJECTION

Adults and adolescents. 300 mg q.d.
Children. 10 mg/kg q.d. (up to 300 mg).

➤ *As adjunct to treat active tuberculosis*

SYRUP, TABLETS

Adults and adolescents. 300 mg q.d. or 15 mg/kg (up to 900 mg) 2 or 3 times/wk, based on treatment regimen.
Children. 10 to 20 mg/kg (up to 300 mg) q.d. or 20 to 40 mg/kg (up to 900 mg) 2 or 3 times/wk, based on treatment regimen.

I.M. INJECTION

Adults and adolescents. 5 mg/kg (up to 300 mg) q.d. or 15 mg/kg (up to 900 mg) 2 or 3 times/wk, based on treatment regimen.
Children. 10 to 20 mg/kg (up to 300 mg) q.d. or 20 to 40 mg/kg (up to 900 mg) 2 or 3 times/wk, based on treatment regimen.

Mechanism of Action

Interferes with lipid and nucleic acid synthesis in actively growing tubercule bacilli cells. Isoniazid also disrupts bacterial cell wall synthesis and may interfere with mycolic acid synthesis in mycobacterial cells.

Contraindications

History of serious adverse reactions (such as hepatic injury) from isoniazid, hypersensitivity to isoniazid or its components

G
H
I

Interactions

DRUGS

acetaminophen: Increased risk of hepatotoxicity and, possibly, nephrotoxicity

alfentanil: Decreased alfentanil clearance and increased duration of alfentanil's effects

aluminum-containing antacids: Decreased isoniazid absorption

benzodiazepines: Decreased benzodiazepine clearance

carbamazepine: Increased blood carbamazepine level and toxicity, increased risk of isoniazid toxicity

corticosteroids: Decreased isoniazid effects

cycloserine: Increased risk of adverse CNS effects and CNS toxicity

disulfiram: Changes in behavior and coordination

enflurane: Increased risk of high-output renal failure

halothane: Increased risk of hepatotoxicity and hepatic encephalopathy

hepatotoxic drugs, rifampin: Increased risk of hepatotoxicity

ketoconazole: Possibly decreased blood ketoconazole level and resistance to antifungal treatment

meperidine: Risk of hypotensive episodes or CNS depression

nephrotoxic drugs: Increased risk of nephrotoxicity

oral anticoagulants: Increased anticoagulant effects

phenytoin: Increased blood phenytoin level, increased risk of phenytoin toxicity

theophylline: Increased blood theophylline level

FOODS

tyramine-containing foods, such as cheese and fish: Increased responses to tyramine contained in foods, possibly resulting in chills; diaphoresis; headache; light-headedness; and red, itchy, clammy skin

ACTIVITIES

alcohol use: Increased risk of hepatotoxicity and increased isoniazid metabolism

Adverse Reactions

CNS: Clumsiness, confusion, dizziness, encephalopathy, fatigue, fever, hallucinations, neurotoxicity, paresthesia, peripheral neuritis, psychosis, seizures, weakness

CV: Vasculitis

EENT: Optic neuritis

ENDO: Gynecomastia, hyperglycemia

GI: Abdominal pain, anorexia, elevated liver function test results, epigastric distress, hepatitis, nausea, vomiting

GU: Glycosuria

HEME: Agranulocytosis, aplastic anemia, eosinophilia, hemolytic anemia, sideroblastic anemia, thrombocytopenia

MS: Arthralgia, joint stiffness

SKIN: Jaundice, pruritus, rash

Other: Hypocalcemia, hypophosphatemia, injection site irritation, lupuslike symptoms, lymphadenopathy

Nursing Considerations

• Administer isoniazid cautiously to diabetic, alcoholic, or malnourished patients and those at risk for developing peripheral neuritis.

• Give drug 1 hour before or 2 hours after meals to promote absorption. If GI distress occurs, give drug with a small amount of food or an antacid that doesn't contain aluminum 1 hour before or 2 hours after meal.

• Monitor results of liver enzyme studies, which may be ordered monthly, because isoniazid can cause severe (and possibly fatal) hepatitis.

• Be aware that about 50% of patients metabolize isoniazid more slowly, which may lead to increased toxic effects. Monitor for such adverse reactions as peripheral neuritis; if they occur, expect to decrease dosage.

• Give isoniazid with other antitubercular drugs, as prescribed, to prevent development of resistant organisms.

• Be aware that patients with advanced HIV infection may experience more severe adverse reactions in greater numbers.

PATIENT TEACHING

• Instruct patient to take isoniazid exactly as prescribed and not to stop taking it without first consulting prescriber. Explain that treatment may take months or years.

• Direct patient to take drug on an empty stomach 1 hour before or 2 hours after meals. If GI distress occurs, instruct him to take drug with food or an antacid that doesn't contain aluminum.

• Advise patient to watch for and report signs of hepatic dysfunction, including darkened urine, decreased appetite, fatigue, and jaundice.

• Caution patient not to drink alcohol while taking isoniazid because alcohol increases the risk of hepatitis.

•Provide patient with a list of tyramine-containing foods to avoid when taking isoniazid, such as cheese, fish, salami, red wine, and yeast extracts. Inform him that consuming these foods during isoniazid therapy may cause unpleasant adverse reactions, such as chills, pounding heartbeat, and sweating.
•Inform patient that he'll need periodic laboratory tests and physical examinations.
•Instruct patient to report fever, nausea, numbness and tingling in arms and legs, rash, vision changes, vomiting, and yellowing of skin.

isoproterenol

(isoprenaline)

Isuprel

isoproterenol hydrochloride

Isuprel, Isuprel Mistometer

isoproterenol sulfate

Medihaler-Iso

Class and Category
Chemical: Catecholamine
Therapeutic: Antiarrhythmic, bronchodilator
Pregnancy category: B (inhalation), C (I.V. infusion)

Indications and Dosages
➤ *To treat bronchospasm in asthma and to prevent and treat bronchospasm in COPD*
INHALATION AEROSOL (ISOPROTERENOL HYDROCHLORIDE)
Adults and adolescents. 1 oral inhalation (120 to 131 mcg), repeated in 2 to 5 min. Inhalations repeated q 3 to 4 hr, p.r.n.
INHALATION AEROSOL (ISOPROTERENOL SULFATE)
Adults and adolescents. 1 oral inhalation (80 mcg), repeated in 2 to 5 min. Inhalations repeated q 4 to 6 hr, p.r.n.
INHALATION SOLUTION FOR NEBULIZER (ISOPROTERENOL)
Adults and adolescents. 2.5 mg diluted and administered over 10 to 20 min. Repeated q 4 hr, p.r.n.
Children. 0.05 to 0.1 mg/kg (up to 1.25 mg) diluted and administered over 10 to 20 min. Repeated q 4 hr, p.r.n.
➤ *To manage bronchospasm during anesthesia*
I.V. INJECTION (ISOPROTERENOL HYDROCHLORIDE)
Adults. 0.01 to 0.02 mg, repeated p.r.n.

➤ *To treat bradycardia with significant hemodynamic change, such as third-degree heart block or prolonged QT intervals*
I.V. INFUSION (ISOPROTERENOL HYDROCHLORIDE)
Adults. *Initial:* 2 mcg/min. Titrated according to heart rate, as ordered. *Maximum:* 10 mcg/min.

Route	Onset	Peak	Duration
I.V.*	Unknown	Unknown	1 to 2 hr
I.V.†	In 5 min	Unknown	10 min
Inhalation	In 5 min	5 to 15 min	In 3 hr

Mechanism of Action
Stimulates beta$_1$ receptors in the myocardium and cardiac conduction system, resulting in positive inotropic and chronotropic effects. Isoproterenol also shortens the AV conduction time and refractory period in patients with AV block. This action increases the ventricular rate and halts bradycardia and associated syncope.
  In addition, isoproterenol attaches to beta$_2$ receptors on bronchial cell membranes. This action stimulates the intracellular enzyme adenylate cyclase to convert adenosine triphosphate to cyclic adenosine monophosphate (cAMP). An increased intracellular level of cAMP relaxes bronchial smooth-muscle cells, stabilizes mast cells, and inhibits histamine release.

Contraindications
Angina pectoris, heart block or tachycardia from digitalis toxicity, ventricular arrhythmias that require inotropic therapy (I.V. form); hypersensitivity to isoproterenol or its components, such as sulfite in some preparations (inhalation form); tachyarrhythmias (I.V. and inhalation forms)

Interactions
DRUGS
Note: All interactions listed are for I.V. form unless indicated.
alpha blockers, other drugs with this action: Possibly decreased peripheral vasoconstrict-

* For treatment of bronchospasm.
† For treatment of bradycardia.

ing and hypertensive effects of isoproterenol
anesthetics (hydrocarbon inhalation): Increased risk of atrial and ventricular arrhythmias
astemizole, cisapride, drugs that prolong QTc interval, terfenadine: Possibly prolonged QTc interval
beta blockers (ophthalmic): Decreased effects of isoproterenol, increased risk of bronchospasm, wheezing, decreased pulmonary function, and respiratory failure
beta blockers (systemic): Increased risk of bronchospasm, decreased effects of both drugs (including inhalation form of isoproterenol)
digoxin: Increased risk of arrhythmias, hypokalemia, and digitalis toxicity
diuretics, other antihypertensives: Possibly decreased antihypertensive effects
ergot alkaloids: Increased vasoconstriction and vasopressor effects
MAO inhibitors: Intensified and extended cardiac stimulation and vasopressor effects
quinidine, other drugs that affect myocardial reaction to sympathomimetics: Increased risk of arrhythmias
theophylline: Increased risk of cardiotoxicity, decreased blood theophylline level
thyroid hormones: Increased effects of both drugs, increased risk of coronary insufficiency in patients with coronary artery disease
tricyclic antidepressants: Increased vasopressor response, increased risk of prolonged QTc interval and arrhythmias

Adverse Reactions

CNS: Dizziness, headache, insomnia, nervousness, syncope, tremor, weakness
CV: Angina, arrhythmias, bradycardia, hypertension, hypotension, palpitations, tachycardia, ventricular arrhythmias
EENT: Dry mouth, oropharyngeal edema, taste perversion
ENDO: Hyperglycemia
GI: Heartburn, nausea, vomiting
MS: Muscle spasms and twitching
RESP: Bronchitis, bronchospasm, cough, dyspnea, increased sputum production, pulmonary edema, wheezing
SKIN: Dermatitis, diaphoresis, erythema multiforme, flushing, pallor, pruritus, rash, Stevens-Johnson syndrome, urticaria
Other: Angioedema, hypokalemia

Nursing Considerations

• Expect to give lowest possible dose of isoproterenol for shortest possible time to minimize tolerance.
• Don't administer I.V. form if it is pink or brown or contains precipitate.
• Administer infusion through large vein, and monitor for signs of extravasation.
• Monitor blood pressure, cardiac rhythm, central venous pressure, and urine output when giving I.V. drug. Adjust infusion rate to response, as ordered.
• Notify prescriber immediately if heart rate increases significantly or exceeds 110 beats/minute during I.V. infusion.
• Know that drug may increase pulse pressure and cause hypotension. Expect to reduce I.V. infusion slowly to decrease risk of hypotension.
• **WARNING** Be aware that isoproterenol markedly increases the risk of arrhythmias. If an arrhythmia develops, expect to give a cardioselective beta blocker, such as atenolol, as prescribed.
• Be aware that isoproterenol isn't used regularly to treat asthma, decreased cardiac output, hypotension, or shock because it increases the risk of arrhythmias, hypotension, and ischemia.
• **WARNING** If isoproterenol aggravates a ventilation-perfusion problem, expect patient's blood oxygen level to fall even as his breathing seems to improve.

PATIENT TEACHING
• Instruct patient not to use isoproterenol inhaler more often than prescribed because excessive use may cause cardiac and respiratory problems.
• Teach patient how to use the inhaler, and observe his technique. Provide a spacer, as needed.
• Instruct patient to wait 2 to 5 minutes before taking second inhalation.
• Advise patient to rinse his mouth after inhalation to remove drug residue and minimize mouth dryness.
• Inform patient that saliva may appear pink after inhalation.
• If patient also uses a corticosteroid inhaler, tell him to take isoproterenol first and then wait at least 2 minutes before taking corticosteroid.
• Instruct patient to report chest pain, dizziness, hyperglycemic symptoms (such as ab-

dominal cramps, lethargy, nausea, and vomiting), insomnia, irregular heartbeat, palpitations, tremor, and weakness.
• Advise patient to also report reduced drug effectiveness, increased use of inhaler, and increased symptoms after taking drug.

isosorbide dinitrate

Apo-ISDN (CAN), Cedocard-SR (CAN), Coradur (CAN), Coronex (CAN), Dilatrate-SR, Isordil Tembids, Isordil Titradose, Sorbitrate

isosorbide mononitrate

IMDUR, ISMO, Monoket

Class and Category
Chemical: Organic nitrate
Therapeutic: Antianginal, vasodilator
Pregnancy category: C

Indications and Dosages
➤ *To treat or prevent angina*
CHEWABLE TABLETS
Adults. 5 mg q 2 to 3 hr, p.r.n. (dinitrate).
E.R. CAPSULES
Adults. 40 to 80 mg q 8 to 12 hr (dinitrate).
E.R. TABLETS
Adults. 20 to 80 mg q 8 to 12 hr (dinitrate); 30 to 60 mg q.d., increased gradually as tolerated to 120 mg q.d. (mononitrate).
S.L. TABLETS
Adults. 2.5 to 5 mg q 2 to 3 hr, p.r.n. (dinitrate).
TABLETS
Adults. 5 to 40 mg q 6 hr, adjusted as needed (dinitrate); 20 mg in 2 doses given 7 hr apart (mononitrate).

Route	Onset	Peak	Duration
P.O.*	1 hr†	Unknown	5 to 6 hr
P.O. (chewable)*	In 3 min	Unknown	30 min to 2 hr
P.O. (E.R.)*	30 min	Unknown	6 to 8 hr
P.O. (S.L.)*	In 3 min	Unknown	2 hr

* For dinitrate.
† For mononitrate, onset also is 1 hr; peak and duration are unknown.

Contraindications
Angle-closure glaucoma; cerebral hemorrhage; concurrent use of sildenafil; head trauma; hypersensitivity to isosorbide, other nitrates, or their components; orthostatic hypotension; severe anemia

Interactions
DRUGS
acetylcholine, norepinephrine: Possibly decreased effectiveness of these drugs
antihypertensives, calcium channel blockers, opioid analgesics, other vasodilators: Increased risk of orthostatic hypotension
aspirin: Increased blood level and pharmacologic action of isosorbide
sildenafil: Increased risk of hypotension and death
sympathomimetics: Increased risk of hypotension, possibly decreased therapeutic effects of isosorbide
ACTIVITIES
alcohol use: Increased risk of orthostatic hypotension

Adverse Reactions
CNS: Agitation, confusion, dizziness, headache, insomnia, restlessness, syncope, vertigo, weakness
CV: Arrhythmias, orthostatic hypotension, palpitations, peripheral edema, tachycardia
EENT: Blurred vision, diplopia (all drug forms); sublingual burning (S.L. form)
GI: Abdominal pain, diarrhea, indigestion, nausea, vomiting
GU: Dysuria, impotence, urinary frequency
HEME: Hemolytic anemia
MS: Arthralgia, muscle twitching
RESP: Bronchitis, pneumonia, upper respiratory tract infection
SKIN: Diaphoresis, flushing, rash

Nursing Considerations
• Use isosorbide cautiously in patients with hypovolemia or mild hypotension. Monitor for increased hypotension and reduced cardiac output.
• Give drug 1 hour before or 2 hours after meals. Give with meals if patient experiences severe headaches or adverse GI reactions.
• Know that patient may experience daily headaches from isosorbide's vasodilating effects. Give acetaminophen, as prescribed, to relieve pain.

G
H
I

Mechanism of Action

Isosorbide may interact with nitrate receptors in vascular smooth-muscle cell membranes. By interacting with nitrate receptors' sulfhydryl groups, the drug is reduced to nitric oxide. Nitric oxide activates the enzyme guanylate cyclase, increasing intracellular formation of cyclic guanosine monophosphate (cGMP). An increased cGMP level may relax vascular smooth muscle by forcing calcium out of muscle cells, causing vasodilation. This improves cardiac output by reducing primarily preload but also afterload.

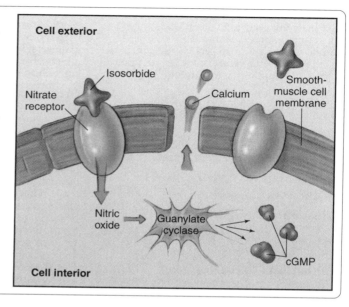

•**WARNING** Be aware that abrupt drug discontinuation may cause angina and increase the risk of MI.
•Monitor blood pressure frequently during isosorbide therapy.
•Keep drug away from heat and light.

PATIENT TEACHING
•Teach patient and family to recognize signs and symptoms of angina, including chest pain, fullness, or pressure, which commonly is accompanied by sweating and nausea. Pain may radiate down the left arm or into the neck or jaw. Inform female patients and those with diabetes mellitus or hypertension that they may experience only fatigue and shortness of breath.
•Advise patient not to crush or chew isosorbide E.R. capsules or tablets or S.L. tablets unless specifically ordered to do so.
•Instruct patient to place S.L. tablet under tongue and not to swallow it, but to let it dissolve. Explain that moisture in mouth promotes drug absorption and that tingling or burning in the mouth indicates drug effectiveness.
•Advise patient to chew chewable tablets well and to keep them in his mouth for 1 to 2 minutes before swallowing to enhance drug absorption.

•Instruct patient to take drug before any situation or activity that might precipitate angina.
•Advise patient to carry isosorbide with him at all times.
•Caution patient that abrupt drug discontinuation may cause angina and increase the risk of MI.
•Instruct patient to report blurred vision, fainting, increased angina attacks, rash, and severe or persistent headaches.
•Teach patient to reduce the effects of orthostatic hypotension by changing position slowly. Advise him to lie down if he becomes dizzy.
•Inform patient that drug commonly causes headache, which typically resolves after a few days of continuous therapy. Suggest that patient take acetaminophen as needed and as prescribed.
•Advise patient to avoid potentially hazardous activities until drug's CNS effects are known.
•Urge patient to avoid alcohol consumption during isosorbide therapy.
•Instruct patient to store drug in a tightly closed container away from light and heat.

isotretinoin

Accutane

Class and Category
Chemical: Retinoid
Therapeutic: Acne inhibitor
Pregnancy category: X

Indications and Dosages
➤ *To treat severe recalcitrant nodular acne*
CAPSULES
Adults. *Initial:* 0.5 mg to 1 mg/kg/day in two divided doses, increased as needed up to 2 mg/kg/day given in two divided doses. *Maximum:* 2 mg/kg/day. Course of therapy given for 15 to 20 wk with second course given, as needed, after a period of 2 mo or more off therapy.

Mechanism of Action
Inhibits sebaceous gland function and keratinization, which results in diminished nodular formation associated with recalcitrant nodular acne.

Contraindications
Hypersensitivity to isotretinoin or any of its components, hypersensitivity to parabens, pregnancy

Interactions
DRUGS
corticosteroids (systemic): Possibly increased risk of osteoporosis
oral contraceptives including microdosed progesterone preparations, medroxyprogesterone injection, levonorgestrel implants: Possibly decreased effectiveness of contraceptive
phenytoin: Possibly increased risk of osteomalacia
tetracyclines: Increased risk of benign intracranial hypertension
vitamin A supplements: Increased risk of additive toxic effects

Adverse Reactions
CNS: Aggressive or violent behavior, depression, dizziness, drowsiness, emotional instability, fatigue, headache, insomnia, lethargy, malaise, nervousness, paresthesias, pseudotumor cerebri, psychosis, seizures, stroke, suicidal ideation, syncope, weakness
CV: Chest pain, decreased high-density lipoprotein level, edema, elevated creatinine phosphokinase level, hypercholesteremia, hypertriglyceridemia, palpitation, stroke, tachycardia, vascular thrombotic disease, vasculitis
ENDO: Abnormal menses, alterations in blood glucose levels
EENT: Bleeding and inflammation of gums, cataracts, color vision disorder, conjunctivitis, corneal opacities, decreased night vision, dry mouth or nose, dry eyes, epistaxis, eyelid inflammation, hearing impairment, keratitis, optic neuritis, photophobia, tinnitus, visual disturbances, voice alteration
GI: Colitis, hepatitis, ileitis, inflammatory bowel disease, liver enzyme elevation, nausea, pancreatitis
GU: Glomerulonephritis, hematuria, proteinuria, WBCs in urine
HEME: Anemia, agranulocytosis, neutropenia, platelet count elevation, sedimentation rate elevation, thrombocytopenia
MS: Arthralgia, arthritis, back pain (children), bone abnormalities, calcification of tendons and ligaments, premature epiphyseal closure, tendonitis
RESP: Bronchospasms, respiratory infection
SKIN: Alopecia, bruising, disseminated herpes simplex, dry lips or skin, eruptive xanthomas, eczema, facial erythema, flushing, fulminant acne, hair abnormalities, hirsutism, hyperpigmentation, increased sunburn susceptibility, infections, nail dystrophy, paronychia, peeling of palms and soles, photoallergic or photosensitizing reactions, pruritus, pyogenic granuloma, rash, seborrhea, skin fragility, sweating, urticaria
Other: Abnormal wound healing, alkaline phosphatase increase, allergic reactions, hyperuricemia, lymphadenopathy, weight loss

Nursing Considerations
•Ensure that women of childbearing age have had two negative urine or serum pregnancy tests with a sensitivity of at least 50 mIU/ml, joined the Accutane Survey, signed the consent form, and watched the videotape provided by manufacturer prior to beginning isotretinoin therapy.
•**WARNING** Notify prescriber if elevated serum triglyceride levels can't be controlled or if symptoms of pancreatitis occur (abdominal pain, nausea, vomiting). Drug may need to be discontinued because fatal hemorrhagic pancreatitis has occurred with drug use.
•Obtain serum lipid level before therapy and periodically thereafter, as ordered, to detect elevated lipid levels that result from isotretinoin therapy.

G
H
I

•Monitor liver enzyme levels periodically, as ordered, because drug can cause hepatitis.
•Assess patient frequently for adverse reactions and report to prescriber any that occur; drug may have serious adverse effects that require discontinuation.

PATIENT TEACHING
•Instruct patient to take isotretinoin with food or milk.
•Advise women of child-bearing age that two forms of contraceptives must be used simultaneously (unless absolute abstinence is a chosen method) 1 month before therapy and for 1 month after therapy has stopped because of potential for fetal harm. Inform women who use oral contraceptives that drug may lessen effectiveness of oral contraceptives. Urge patient to notify prescriber immediately if pregnancy occurs.
•Urge patient to report headache, nausea, vomiting and visual disturbances immediately to prescriber because drug will need to be discontinued immediately and the patient referred to a neurologist.
•Caution patient and family that isotretinoin may cause aggressive or violent behavior, depression, psychosis, and suicidal ideation. Instruct patient to notify prescriber immediately if changes in mood occur.
•Tell patient to report hearing changes or tinnitus, visual difficulties, abdominal pain, rectal bleeding, or severe diarrhea to prescriber because drug may need to be discontinued.
•Advise patient to avoid potentially hazardous activities until drug's CNS effects are known. Caution her that changes in night vision may occur suddenly.
•Caution patient not to donate blood during therapy and for one month after therapy has stopped because blood might be given to a pregnant woman.
•Warn patient that transient exacerbation of acne may occur, especially during initial therapy and to notify prescriber if this occurs.
•Instruct patient to avoid wax epilation and skin resurfacing procedures during therapy and for at least 6 months thereafter because of scarring potential.
•Caution patient to avoid exposure to direct sunlight or UV light and to wear sunscreen when outdoors.
•Inform patient that decreased tolerance to contact lenses may occur during and after therapy.

•Alert patient to the potential for mild musculoskeletal adverse reactions that may occur with therapy, which usually clear rapidly after drug is discontinued. Urge patient to notify prescriber if symptoms become bothersome or serious because drug may need to be discontinued.
•Advise patient not to take vitamin A supplements while on drug therapy because of potential additive toxic effects.
•Instruct patient to notify all prescribers of isotretinoin use because of potential interactions.
•Inform patient of need for frequent laboratory tests and importance of complying with scheduled appointments.

isradipine
DynaCirc

Class and Category
Chemical: Dihydropyridine derivative
Therapeutic: Antihypertensive
Pregnancy category: C

Indications and Dosages
➤ *To manage essential hypertension*
CAPSULES
Adults. *Initial:* 2.5 mg b.i.d., increased by 5 mg q 2 to 4 wk, if needed. *Maximum:* 20 mg/day.

Route	Onset	Peak	Duration
P.O.	2 to 3 hr	2 to 4 wk	Unknown

Mechanism of Action
Inhibits calcium movement into coronary vascular smooth-muscle cells by blocking the slow calcium channels in their membranes. By decreasing the intracellular calcium level, isradipine inhibits smooth-muscle cell contractions. The result is relaxation of coronary and vascular smooth muscle, decreased peripheral vascular resistance, and reduced systolic and diastolic blood pressure, all of which decrease myocardial oxygen demand.

Contraindications
Hypersensitivity to isradipine or its components

Interactions
DRUGS
anesthetics (hydrocarbon inhalation), antihypertensives, hydrochlorothiazide, prazocin: Increased risk of hypotension
beta blockers: Increased adverse effects of beta blockers
cimetidine: Increased blood level and bioavailability of isradipine
digoxin: Transiently increased blood digoxin level and risk of digitalis toxicity
estrogens: Possibly increased fluid retention and decreased therapeutic effects of isradipine
lithium: Increased risk of neurotoxicity
NSAIDs, sympathomimetics: Possibly decreased therapeutic effects of isradipine
procainamide, quinidine: Increased risk of prolonged QT interval
FOODS
grapefruit juice: Doubled isradipine bioavailability
other foods: Prolonged time to achieve peak blood level

Adverse Reactions
CNS: Asthenia, dizziness, fatigue, headache, paresthesia, somnolence, syncope, weakness
CV: Angina, hypotension, orthostatic hypotension, palpitations, peripheral edema, tachycardia
EENT: Gingival hyperplasia, pharyngitis, rhinitis
GI: Abdominal cramps, constipation, diarrhea, elevated liver function test results, indigestion, nausea, vomiting
MS: Back pain
RESP: Cough
SKIN: Flushing, photosensitivity, rash

Nursing Considerations
• Monitor blood pressure and heart rate frequently during isradipine therapy.
• Monitor patient with impaired hepatic or renal function for an increased blood isradipine level.
• Avoid giving drug with food, which increases time to achieve peak effect by about 1 hour.
• Observe for mild peripheral edema caused by vasodilation of small blood vessels. Know that this type of edema doesn't result from fluid retention or heart failure.
PATIENT TEACHING
• Inform patient that isradipine therapy will be long-term and will require laboratory tests and follow-up visits to monitor drug effects.

• Instruct patient to take drug exactly as prescribed and to swallow capsules whole, not crush or chew them.
• Advise patient to take drug on an empty stomach 1 hour before or 2 hours after meals.
• Instruct patient to take a missed dose as soon as remembered unless it's nearly time for the next dose. If it is, advise him to wait and take the next scheduled dose, but not to double the dose. If more than one dose is missed, tell him to contact prescriber.
• **WARNING** Urge patient not to stop taking drug suddenly. Doing so may lead to life-threatening problems.
• Inform patient that fragments of capsules may be visible in stool.
• Caution patient not to drink grapefruit juice during isradipine therapy.
• Advise patient to avoid potentially hazardous activities until drug's CNS effects are known.
• Caution patient to change position slowly to minimize effects of orthostatic hypotension.
• Urge patient to contact prescriber if he experiences chest pain, fainting, irregular heartbeat, rash, or swollen ankles.
• Instruct patient to maintain good oral hygiene, perform gum massage, and see his dentist every 6 months to prevent gum bleeding and gum disorders.
• To help prevent photosensitivity reactions, caution patient to avoid direct sunlight and to wear protective clothing and apply sunscreen when outdoors.
• Instruct patient to store drug at room temperature in a dry place.

itraconazole

Sporanox

Class and Category
Chemical: Triazole derivative
Therapeutic: Antifungal
Pregnancy category: C

Indications and Dosages
➤ *To treat blastomycosis caused by* Blastomyces dermatitidis *and histoplasmosis caused by* Histoplasma capsulatum
CAPSULES
Adults and adolescents. *Initial:* 200 mg q.d., increased by 100 mg/day, if needed. *Maximum:* 400 mg/day, with dosage greater than 200 mg given in divided doses b.i.d.

➤ *To treat aspergillosis unresponsive to amphotericin B*
CAPSULES
Adults and adolescents. 200 to 400 mg/day, with dosage greater than 200 mg/day given in divided doses b.i.d.

➤ *To treat pulmonary and extrapulmonary blastomycosis, histoplasmosis, and refractory aspergillosis*
I.V. INFUSION
Adults and adolescents. 200 mg infused over 1 hr q 12 hr for 4 doses; then 200 mg q.d. Drug changed to P.O. form within 14 days and therapy continued for at least 3 mo.
DOSAGE ADJUSTMENT In life-threatening situations, loading dose adjusted to 200 mg P.O. or I.V. t.i.d. for 3 days. Be aware that I.V. itraconazole shouldn't be used in patients with creatinine clearance less than 30 ml/min/1.73 m².

➤ *To treat oropharyngeal candidiasis*
ORAL SOLUTION
Adults and adolescents. 100 mg b.i.d. for 7 to 14 days.

➤ *To treat esophageal candidiasis*
ORAL SOLUTION
Adults and adolescents. 100 mg q.d. for at least 3 wk and continued for 2 wk after symptoms resolve.

➤ *To treat onychomycosis of toenails only or of toenails and fingernails*
CAPSULES
Adults and adolescents. 200 mg q.d. for 12 wk.

➤ *To treat onychomycosis of fingernails only*
CAPSULES
Adults and adolescents. 200 mg b.i.d. for 7 days, then repeated after 3 wk.

Mechanism of Action

Inhibits the synthesis of ergosterol, an essential component of fungal cell membranes, by binding with a cytochrome P-450 enzyme needed to convert lanosterol to ergosterol. The lack of ergosterol results in increased cellular permeability and leakage of cell contents. Itraconazole also may lead to fungal cell death by inhibiting fungal respiration under aerobic conditions.

Incompatibilities

Don't administer itraconazole through same I.V. line with other drugs. Don't mix I.V. itra-conazole with D_5W or solutions that contain LR.

Contraindications

Concurrent therapy with cisapride, dofetilide, HMG-CoA inhibitors (lovastatin and simvastatin), oral midazolam, pimozide, quinidine, or triazolam; evidence of ventricular dysfunction, such as with congestive heart failure or a history of congestive heart failure (onychomycosis treatment); hypersensitivity to itraconazole or its components; planning for pregnancy during onychomycosis treatment

Interactions
DRUGS
alfentanil, buspirone, busulfan, carbamazepine, cyclosporine, digoxin, docetaxel, dofetilide, indinavir, methylprednisolone, phenytoin, pimozide, quinidine, rifabutin, ritonavir, saquinavir, sirolimus, tacrolimus, trimetrexate, vinca alkaloids: Possibly increased blood levels of these drugs
alprazolam, diazepam, oral midazolam, triazolam: Elevated blood levels and possibly prolonged sedative effects of these drugs
antacids, anticholinergics, H_2-receptor antagonists, omeprazole, sucralfate: Possibly decreased itraconazole absorption
atorvastatin, lovastatin, simvastatin: Increased blood levels of these drugs; possibly rhabdomyolysis
calcium channel blockers: Possibly edema and increased blood levels of these drugs
carbamazepine, isoniazid, nevirapine, phenobarbital, phenytoin, rifabutin, rifampin: Possibly decreased blood itraconazole level
cisapride: Possibly inhibited cisapride metabolism, which may lead to life-threatening cardiovascular complications as well as sudden death
clarithromycin, erythromycin, indinavir, ritonavir: Possibly increased blood itraconazole level
didanosine: Possibly decreased therapeutic effects of itraconazole
oral antidiabetic drugs: Possibly increased blood levels of these drugs and risk of hypoglycemia
warfarin: Increased anticoagulant effect of warfarin

Adverse Reactions

CNS: Dizziness, drowsiness, fatigue, fever, headache, vertigo

CV: Congestive heart failure, hypertension
GI: Abdominal pain, anorexia, constipation, diarrhea, elevated liver function test results, flatulence, hepatotoxicity, hyperbilirubinemia, indigestion, nausea, vomiting
RESP: Cough, dyspnea
SKIN: Diaphoresis, pruritus, rash
Other: Hypokalemia

Nursing Considerations
• Because itraconazole has been linked to serious adverse cardiac and hepatic effects, expect to send appropriate nail specimens for laboratory testing to confirm onychomycosis before beginning therapy.
• Be aware that I.V. itraconazole is for infusion only. Don't administer by bolus.
• **WARNING** Keep in mind that itraconazole is a potent inhibitor of the cytochrome P-450 3A4 (CYP3A4) isoenzyme system, which may increase blood levels of drugs metabolized by this system. Patients using such drugs as cisapride with itraconazole or other CYP3A4 inhibitors have experienced life-threatening cardiovascular complications, such as prolonged QT interval, torsades de pointes, and ventricular tachycardia, as well as sudden death.
• Administer itraconazole capsules (but not oral solution) with a meal to ensure maximal absorption.
• Infuse each I.V. dose over 1 hour.
• Keep in mind that a patient with AIDS may have hypochlorhydria, which reduces drug absorption. For such a patient, expect to administer higher doses of itraconazole.
• Monitor liver function test results in patients with impaired hepatic function and those who have experienced hepatotoxicity with other drugs.
• If patient develops signs and symptoms of congestive heart failure, such as fatigue, dyspnea, and peripheral edema, expect to discontinue drug.
• Assess patient for rash every 8 hours during therapy; notify prescriber if rash occurs.
• If patient also receives warfarin, monitor PT and assess patient for signs and symptoms of bleeding.
• If patient also receives digoxin, monitor blood digoxin level as appropriate to detect toxic level, and assess patient for signs and symptoms of digitalis toxicity, such as nausea and yellow vision.

• Instruct patient to take itraconazole capsules with a meal, but oral solution without food.
• If patient also takes an oral antidiabetic drug, instruct him to monitor his blood glucose level frequently because of the increased risk of hypoglycemia.
• Advise patient to avoid taking antacids with oral itraconazole.
• Advise patient to notify prescriber immediately of changes in other drugs, such as new drugs and dosage changes.
• Advise patient to notify prescriber immediately about abdominal pain, diarrhea, headache, nausea, rash, or vomiting.
• Instruct patient to notify prescriber if he experiences signs of liver problems, such as abdominal pain, dark urine, fatigue, loss of appetite, pale stools, weakness, or yellow eyes or skin.
• Caution breast-feeding patient to consult prescriber about continuation of breast-feeding during itraconazole therapy.

J·K·L

kanamycin sulfate
Kantrex

Class and Category
Chemical: Aminoglycoside
Therapeutic: Antibiotic
Pregnancy category: D

Indications and Dosages
➤ *To treat infections caused by gram-negative organisms (including* Acinetobacter *sp.,* Enterobacter aerogenes, Escherichia coli, Haemophilus influenzae, Klebsiella pneumoniae, Neisseria *sp.,* Proteus *sp.,* Providencia *sp.,* Salmonella *sp.,* Serratia marcescens, Shigella *sp., and* Yersinia *sp.) and gram-positive organisms (including* Staphylococcus aureus *and* Staphylococcus epidermidis)

I.V. INFUSION
Adults and children. 5 mg/kg q 8 hr or 7.5 mg/kg q 12 hr for 7 to 10 days. *Maximum:* 1.5 g/day.

I.M. INJECTION
Adults and children. 3.75 mg/kg q 6 hr, 5 mg/kg q 8 hr, or 7.5 mg/kg q 12 hr for 7 to 10 days. *Maximum:* 1.5 g/day.
➤ *As adjunct to suppress intestinal bacterial growth*

CAPSULES
Adults. 1 g/hr for 4 hr and then 1 g q 6 hr for 36 to 72 hr.
➤ *To treat hepatic coma*

CAPSULES
Adults. 8 to 12 g/day administered in divided doses.
➤ *To treat respiratory tract infection*

INHALATION NEBULIZER
Adults. 250 mg b.i.d. to q.i.d. *Maximum:* 1.5 g/day.
DOSAGE ADJUSTMENT For elderly patients and those with renal failure, dosage reduced and blood kanamycin level and renal function test results monitored.

Route	Onset	Peak	Duration
P.O.	Slow	Unknown	Unknown
I.V.	Rapid	Unknown	Unknown
I.M.	Unknown	1 to 2 hr	Unknown

Mechanism of Action
Binds to negatively charged sites on bacterial outer cell membranes, which disrupts cell membrane integrity. Kanamycin also binds to bacterial ribosomal subunits and inhibits protein synthesis; these actions lead to cell death.

Contraindications
Hypersensitivity to kanamycin, other aminoglycosides, or their components; intestinal obstruction (oral form)

Incompatibilities
Don't mix kanamycin in same syringe or administer through same I.V. line as other antibiotics.

Interactions
DRUGS
cephalosporins, vancomycin: Increased risk of nephrotoxicity
digoxin, loop diuretics: Increased ototoxic and nephrotoxic effects of kanamycin
general anesthetics, neuromuscular blockers: Increased risk of neuromuscular blockade
penicillins: Inactivation of kanamycin or synergistic effects

Adverse Reactions
CNS: Ataxia, dizziness, headache
EENT: Hearing loss
GI: Diarrhea
GU: Elevated BUN and serum creatinine levels, oliguria, proteinuria
MS: Muscle paralysis
RESP: Apnea
SKIN: Injection site irritation or pain

Nursing Considerations
•Obtain body fluid or tissue specimen for culture and sensitivity testing before kanamycin therapy begins, as indicated. Therapy may begin before test results are available.
•Administer I.M. injection deep into upper outer quadrant of gluteus maximus. Rotate injection sites.
•Be aware that oral kanamycin is minimally absorbed from intact GI mucosa but may be more extensively absorbed from mechanically irrigated areas of the GI tract.
•For I.V. use, dilute 500-mg vial with 100 to 200 ml of NS or D_5W, or 1-g vial with 200 to 400 ml of NS or D_5W, and infuse over 30 to 60

min. Be aware that vial contents may darken during storage but potency isn't affected.
• Keep patient well hydrated before and during therapy.
• Monitor blood kanamycin level periodically during therapy, as appropriate.
• Be aware that prolonged treatment increases the risk of ototoxicity and nephrotoxicity. Monitor hearing and renal function if therapy lasts longer than 10 days.

PATIENT TEACHING
• Explain the need to take kanamycin at prescribed intervals around the clock until patient completes full course of therapy.
• Advise patient to report dizziness, hearing loss, and severe diarrhea or headache to prescriber.

ketoprofen

Actron, Apo-Keto (CAN), Orudis, Orudis KT, Orudis-SR (CAN), Oruvail, Rhodis

Class and Category

Chemical: Propionic acid derivative
Therapeutic: Analgesic, anti-inflammatory
Pregnancy category: B

Indications and Dosages

➤ *To treat symptoms of rheumatoid arthritis*

CAPSULES, TABLETS
Adults. *Initial:* 75 mg t.i.d. or 50 mg q.i.d. *Maximum:* 300 mg/day.

E.R. CAPSULES
Adults. *Maintenance:* 150 to 200 mg q.d. *Maximum:* 300 mg/day.

➤ *To relieve pain associated with dysmenorrhea*

TABLETS
Adults. *Initial:* 25 to 50 mg q 6 to 8 hr p.r.n. *Maximum:* 300 mg/day.
DOSAGE ADJUSTMENT Dosage reduced by 33% to 50% for patients with renal impairment.

Mechanism of Action

Blocks the activity of cyclooxygenase, the enzyme needed for prostaglandin synthesis. Prostaglandins, important mediators of the inflammatory response, cause local vasodilation with swelling and pain. By blocking cyclooxygenase and inhibiting prostaglandins, this NSAID reduces inflammatory symptoms and relieves pain.

Contraindications

Angioedema; aspirin-, iodide-, or NSAID-induced asthma, bronchospasm, nasal polyps, rhinitis, or urticaria; hypersensitivity to ketoprofen or its components

Interactions

DRUGS
acetaminophen: Possibly increased adverse renal effects with long-term acetaminophen use
ACE inhibitors: Possibly decreased hypotensive effect of ACE inhibitors
aspirin, other NSAIDs: Increased risk of bleeding and adverse GI effects, increased and prolonged blood ketoprofen levels
cefamandole, cefoperazone, cefotetan: Increased risk of hypoprothrombinemia and bleeding
colchicine, platelet aggregation inhibitors: Increased risk of GI bleeding, hemorrhage, and ulcers
corticosteroids, potassium supplements: Increased risk of adverse GI effects
cyclosporine: Increased risk of nephrotoxicity from both drugs, increased blood cyclosporine level
diuretics (loop, potassium-sparing, and thiazide): Decreased diuretic and antihypertensive effects
gold compounds, nephrotoxic drugs: Increased risk of adverse renal effects
heparin, oral anticoagulants, thrombolytics: Increased anticoagulant effects, increased risk of hemorrhage
insulin, oral antidiabetic drugs: Possibly increased hypoglycemic effects of these drugs
lithium: Increased blood lithium level and possibly toxicity
methotrexate: Decreased methotrexate clearance, increased risk of methotrexate toxicity
plicamycin, valproic acid: Increased risk of hypoprothrombinemia and GI bleeding, hemorrhage, and ulcers
probenecid: Possibly increased blood level, effectiveness, and risk of toxicity of ketoprofen

ACTIVITIES
alcohol use: Increased risk of adverse GI effects

Adverse Reactions

CNS: Headache, irritability, nervousness
CV: Edema, fluid retention, hypertension
EENT: Tinnitus, vision changes
GI: Abdominal pain, constipation, diarrhea, flatulence, GI bleeding, indigestion, nausea, vomiting

GU: Decreased urine output
SKIN: Rash
Other: Rapid weight gain

Nursing Considerations
• Administer ketoprofen with food to decrease GI upset.
• If patient also takes acetaminophen, monitor fluid intake and output, BUN level, and serum creatinine level for evidence of adverse renal effects.

PATIENT TEACHING
• Instruct patient to take ketoprofen with food or after meals to prevent GI upset. Advise him to take drug with a full glass of water and to avoid lying down for 15 to 30 minutes afterward to prevent drug from lodging in esophagus and causing irritation.
• Advise patient to swallow drug whole and not to crush, break, chew, or open capsules.
• Instruct patient to avoid aspirin, aspirin-containing products, and alcohol while taking ketoprofen to decrease the risk of adverse GI effects.
• If patient also takes an anticoagulant, advise him to watch for and immediately report bleeding problems, such as bloody or tarry stools and bloody vomitus.
• If patient also takes insulin or an oral antidiabetic drug, advise him to be on the alert for hypoglycemia and to monitor his blood glucose levels closely. Encourage him to carry candy or other simple sugars to treat mild hypoglycemia. If he experiences frequent or severe episodes, instruct him to notify prescriber.
• Inform patient that he may experience nervousness and irritability while taking ketoprofen.
• Instruct patient to notify prescriber immediately if he develops a rash, signs of GI bleeding, decreased urine output, dark yellow or brown urine, or signs of fluid retention, including swelling of extremities and unexplained rapid weight gain.

ketorolac tromethamine

Toradol

Class and Category
Chemical: Acetic acid derivative
Therapeutic: Analgesic, anti-inflammatory
Pregnancy category: C

Indications and Dosages
➤ *To treat moderate to severe pain*

TABLETS
Adults ages 16 to 64. *Initial:* 20 mg as a single dose, followed by 10 mg q 4 to 6 hr p.r.n., up to 4 times a day. *Maximum:* 40 mg/day for no more than 5 days.
DOSAGE ADJUSTMENT For patients who weigh less than 50 kg, elderly patients, and patients with impaired renal function, initial dose reduced to 10 mg.

I.M. INJECTION
Adults ages 16 to 64. *Initial:* 60 mg as a single dose, followed by oral ketorolac if needed; or 30 mg q 6 hr p.r.n. *Maximum:* 120 mg/day for no more than 5 days.
DOSAGE ADJUSTMENT For patients who weigh less than 50 kg, elderly patients, and patients with impaired renal function, initial dose reduced to 30 mg, followed by oral ketorolac if needed; or 15 mg q 6 hr p.r.n., up to maximum of 60 mg/day for no more than 5 days.

I.V. INJECTION
Adults ages 16 to 64. *Initial:* 30 mg as a single dose, followed by oral ketorolac if needed; or 30 mg q 6 hr p.r.n. *Maximum:* 120 mg/day for no more than 5 days.
DOSAGE ADJUSTMENT For patients who weigh less than 50 kg, elderly patients, and patients with impaired renal function, initial dose reduced to 15 mg, followed by oral ketorolac if needed; or 15 mg q 6 hr p.r.n., up to maximum of 60 mg/day for no more than 5 days.

Route	Onset	Peak	Duration
P.O.	30 to 60 min	2 to 3 hr	5 to 6 hr
I.M., I.V.	30 to 60 min	1 to 2 hr	4 to 6 hr

Mechanism of Action
Blocks the activity of cyclooxygenase, the enzyme needed to synthesize prostaglandins. Prostaglandins mediate the inflammatory response and cause local vasodilation, swelling, and pain. They also promote pain transmission from the periphery to the spinal cord. By blocking cyclooxygenase and inhibiting prostaglandins, this NSAID reduces inflammatory symptoms and relieves pain.

Contraindications
Advanced renal impairment or risk of renal impairment due to volume depletion; before or during surgery if hemostasis is critical; breast-feeding; cerebrovascular bleeding; concurrent use of aspirin or other salicylates,

other NSAIDs, or probenecid; hemorrhagic diathesis; history of GI bleeding, GI perforation, or peptic ulcer disease; hemophilia or other bleeding problems, including coagulation or platelet function disorders; hypersensitivity to ketorolac tromethamine, aspirin, other NSAIDs, or their components; incomplete hemostasis; labor and delivery

Interactions
DRUGS
ACE inhibitors: Increased risk of renal function impairment
acetaminophen, gold compounds: Increased risk of adverse renal effects
amphotericin, penicillamine, and other nephrotoxic drugs: Increased risk or severity of adverse renal reactions
corticosteroids, potassium supplements: Increased risk of gastric ulcers or hemorrhage
antihypertensives, diuretics: Possibly reduced effects of these drugs
aspirin and other salicylates, other NSAIDs: Additive toxicity
cefamandole, cefoperazone, cefotetan: Possibly hypoprothrombinemia
furosemide: Decreased effects of furosemide
heparin, oral anticoagulants, platelet aggregation inhibitors, thrombolytics: Increased risk of GI bleeding and I.M. hematoma formation
lithium: Possibly increased blood lithium level and increased risk of lithium toxicity
methotrexate: Possibly methotrexate toxicity
plicamycin, valproic acid: Possibly hypoprothrombinemia and increased risk of bleeding
probenecid: Decreased elimination of ketorolac, increased risk of adverse effects
ACTIVITIES
alcohol use: Increased risk of adverse GI effects

Adverse Reactions
CNS: Dizziness, drowsiness, headache
CV: Edema, fluid retention, hypertension
EENT: Stomatitis
GI: Abdominal pain; bloating; constipation; diarrhea; flatulence; GI bleeding, perforation, or ulceration; hepatic failure; indigestion; nausea; vomiting
SKIN: Diaphoresis, pruritus, rash
Other: Anaphylaxis, injection site pain, unusual weight gain

Nursing Considerations
•Read ketorolac label carefully. Don't use I.M. form for I.V. administration. Be aware that ketorolac isn't for intrathecal or epidural use.

•Inject I.M. ketorolac slowly, deep into a large muscle mass. Monitor site for bleeding, bruising, or hematoma.
•Administer I.V. injection over at least 15 seconds.
•Notify prescriber if pain relief is inadequate or if breakthrough pain occurs between doses because supplemental doses of an opioid analgesic may be required.
•**WARNING** Monitor liver function test results for possible elevations. If elevated levels persist or worsen, notify prescriber and expect to discontinue drug, as ordered, to prevent hepatic impairment.
•**WARNING** Monitor patients with a history of peripheral edema, heart failure, or hypertension for adequate fluid balance because drug can promote fluid retention and exacerbate these conditions. Assess for dyspnea, edema, unexplained rapid weight gain, and decreased activity tolerance. Notify prescriber if such symptoms develop.
PATIENT TEACHING
•Instruct patient to take ketorolac tablets with a meal, snack, or antacid to prevent stomach upset. Advise him to take drug with a full glass of water and to remain upright for at least 15 minutes after taking tablet.
•Advise patient not to use aspirin, other salicylates, or other NSAIDs while taking ketorolac without consulting prescriber. Encourage patient to limit use of acetaminophen to only a few days during ketorolac therapy and to notify prescriber of use.
•Caution patient to avoid hazardous activities until drug's CNS effects are known.
•Urge patient to avoid alcohol during ketorolac therapy.
•Encourage patient to have dental procedures performed before starting drug therapy because of increased risk of bleeding.
•Teach patient proper oral hygiene measures, and encourage him to use a soft-bristled toothbrush while taking ketorolac.

labetalol hydrochloride
Normodyne, Trandate

Class and Category
Chemical: Benzamine derivative
Therapeutic: Antihypertensive
Pregnancy category: C

Indications and Dosages
➤ *To manage hypertension*

TABLETS

Adults. *Initial:* 100 mg b.i.d., increased by 100 mg b.i.d. as needed and tolerated q 2 to 3 days. *Maintenance:* 200 to 400 mg b.i.d. For severe hypertension, 1.2 to 2.4 g/day in divided doses b.i.d. or t.i.d.

➤ *To manage severe hypertension and treat hypertensive emergencies*

I.V. INFUSION

Adults. 200 mg diluted in 160 ml of D_5W and infused at 2 mg/min until desired response occurs.

I.V. INJECTION

Adults. 20 mg given over 2 min; additional doses given in increments of 40 to 80 mg q 10 min as indicated until desired response occurs. *Maximum:* 300 mg.

Route	Onset	Peak	Duration
P.O.	20 min to 2 hr	1 to 4 hr	8 to 24 hr
I.V.	2 to 5 min	5 to 15 min	2 to 4 hr

Mechanism of Action

Selectively blocks $alpha_1$ and $beta_2$ receptors in vascular smooth muscle and $beta_1$ receptors in the heart. These actions reduce peripheral vascular resistance and blood pressure. Potent beta blockade prevents reflex tachycardia, which commonly occurs when alpha blockers reduce the resting heart rate, cardiac output, or stroke volume.

Incompatibilities

Don't dilute labetalol in sodium bicarbonate solution or administer through same I.V. line as alkaline drugs, such as furosemide; doing so may cause white precipitate to form.

Contraindications

Asthma, cardiogenic shock, heart failure, hypersensitivity to labetalol or its components, second- or third-degree heart block, severe bradycardia

Interactions

DRUGS

allergen immunotherapy, allergenic extracts for skin testing: Increased risk of serious systemic reaction or anaphylaxis
calcium channel blockers, clonidine, diazoxide, guanabenz, reserpine: Possibly hypotension

cimetidine: Possibly increased labetalol effects
estrogens, NSAIDs: Possibly reduced antihypertensive effect of labetalol
general anesthetics: Increased risk of hypotension and myocardial depression
insulin, oral antidiabetic drugs: Increased risk of hyperglycemia
nitroglycerin: Possibly hypertension
phenoxybenzamine, phentolamine: Possibly additive $alpha_1$-blocking effects
sympathomimetics with alpha- and beta-adrenergic effects (such as pseudoephedrine): Possibly hypertension, excessive bradycardia, or heart block
xanthines (aminophylline and theophylline): Possibly decreased therapeutic effects of both drugs

FOODS

all food: Increased blood labetalol level

ACTIVITIES

alcohol use: Increased labetalol effects

Adverse Reactions

CNS: Anxiety, confusion, depression, dizziness, drowsiness, fatigue, paresthesia, syncope, vertigo, weakness, yawning
CV: Bradycardia, chest pain, edema, heart block, heart failure, hypotension, orthostatic hypotension, ventricular arrhythmias
EENT: Nasal congestion, taste perversion
GI: Elevated liver function test results, hepatic necrosis, hepatitis, indigestion, nausea, vomiting
GU: Ejaculation failure, impotence
RESP: Dyspnea, wheezing
SKIN: Jaundice, pruritus, rash, scalp tingling

Nursing Considerations

• During I.V. labetalol administration, monitor blood pressure according to facility policy, usually every 5 minutes for 30 minutes, then every 30 minutes for 2 hours, and then every hour for 6 hours.
• Keep patient in supine position for 3 hours after I.V. administration.
• **WARNING** Be aware that labetalol masks common signs of shock.
• Monitor blood glucose level in diabetic patient because labetalol may conceal symptoms of hypoglycemia.
• Be aware that stopping labetalol tablets abruptly after long-term therapy could result in angina, MI, or ventricular arrhythmias. Expect to taper dosage over 2 weeks while monitoring response.

PATIENT TEACHING
•Advise patient to report confusion, difficulty breathing, rash, slow pulse, and swelling in arms or legs.
•Caution patient not to discontinue drug abruptly because doing so could cause angina and rebound hypertension.
•Suggest that patient minimize effects of orthostatic hypotension by rising slowly, avoiding sudden position changes, and taking drug at bedtime, if approved by prescriber.
•Instruct diabetic patient to monitor blood glucose level frequently and to be alert for signs of hypoglycemia.
•Inform patient that scalp tingling may occur during the early phase of treatment but is transient.
•Urge patient to avoid alcohol during labetalol therapy.

lactulose

Acilac (CAN), Cephulac, Cholac, Chronulac, Constilac, Constulose, Duphalac, Enulose, Evalose, Heptalac, Lactulax (CAN), Laxilose (CAN), PMS-Lactulose (CAN), Portalac

Class and Category
Chemical: Synthetic disaccharide sugar
Therapeutic: Ammonia reducer, laxative
Pregnancy category: B

Indications and Dosages
➤ *To treat constipation*
POWDER, SYRUP
Adults. *Initial:* 10 to 20 g/day, increased p.r.n. *Maximum:* 40 g/day.
➤ *To prevent and treat hepatic encephalopathy*
POWDER, SYRUP
Adults. *Initial:* 20 to 30 g t.i.d. or q.i.d. until two or three soft stools occur daily. *Usual:* 60 to 100 g/day in divided doses. For acute episodes, 20 to 30 g q 2 hr initially to achieve rapid laxative effect and then reduced to usual dosage.
RETENTION ENEMA
Adults. 200 g (300 ml) diluted in 700 ml of water or NS and given q 4 to 6 hr, as needed.

Route	Onset	Peak	Duration
P.O.	24 to 48 hr	Unknown	Unknown

Mechanism of Action
Arrives unchanged in the colon, where it breaks down into lactic acid and small amounts of formic and acetic acids, acidifying fecal contents. Acidification leads to increased osmotic pressure in the colon, which, in turn, increases stool water content and softens stool.

Also, lactulose makes the intestinal contents more acidic than blood. This prevents ammonia diffusion from the intestines into the blood, as occurs in hepatic encephalopathy. The trapped ammonia is converted into ammonia ions and, by lactulose's cathartic effect, is expelled in the feces (with other nitrogenous wastes).

Contraindications
Hypersensitivity to lactulose or its components, low-galactose diet

Interactions
DRUGS
antacids, antibiotics (especially oral neomycin), other laxatives: Decreased effectiveness of lactulose

Adverse Reactions
GI: Abdominal cramps and distention, diarrhea, flatulence
ENDO: Hyperglycemia
Other: Hypernatremia, hypokalemia, hypovolemia

Nursing Considerations
•When giving lactulose by retention enema, use a rectal tube with a balloon to help patient retain enema for 30 to 60 minutes. If not retained for at least 30 minutes, repeat dose. Be sure to deflate the balloon and remove the rectal tube after administration has been completed.
•Expect to periodically check serum electrolyte levels of elderly or debilitated patient who uses oral drug longer than 6 months.
•Monitor blood ammonia level in patient with hepatic encephalopathy. Also monitor for dehydration, hypernatremia, and hypokalemia when giving higher lactulose doses to treat this condition.
•Monitor diabetic patient for hyperglycemia because lactulose contains galactose and lactose.
•Plan to replace fluids if frequent bowel movements cause hypovolemia.

PATIENT TEACHING

• Advise patient to take lactulose with food or to dilute it with juice to minimize sweet taste.
• Direct patient not to use other laxatives while taking lactulose.
• Instruct patient to report abdominal distention or severe diarrhea.
• Advise diabetic patient to monitor blood glucose level frequently and to report hyperglycemia.
• Instruct patient to increase fluid intake if frequent bowel movements occur.
• Teach patient with chronic constipation the importance of exercising, increasing fiber in her diet, and increasing fluid intake.
• Inform patient that because oral lactulose must reach the colon to work, bowel movement may not occur for 24 to 48 hours after taking drug.

lamotrigine

Lamictal

Class and Category

Chemical: Phenyltriazine
Therapeutic: Anticonvulsant
Pregnancy category: C

Indications and Dosages

➤ *As adjunct to treat partial seizures and Lennox-Gastaut syndrome*

CHEWABLE TABLETS, TABLETS

Adults and children age 12 and older also taking enzyme-inducing anticonvulsants.
50 mg q.d. for 2 wk and then 100 mg/day in divided doses b.i.d. for 2 wk. Increased by 100 mg q 1 to 2 wk, if needed. *Maintenance:* 300 to 500 mg/day in divided doses b.i.d. *Maximum:* 700 mg/day in divided doses b.i.d.
Children ages 2 to 12 also taking enzyme-inducing anticonvulsants. 0.6 mg/kg/day in divided doses b.i.d. for 2 wk and then 1.2 mg/kg/day in divided doses b.i.d. for 2 wk. Increased by 1.2 mg/kg q 1 to 2 wk, if needed to reach maintenance dosage. *Maintenance:* 5 to 15 mg/kg/day in divided doses b.i.d. *Maximum:* 400 mg/day.
Adults and children age 12 and older also taking enzyme-inducing anticonvulsants and valproic acid. 25 mg q.o.d. for 2 wk, followed by 25 mg q.d. for 2 wk. Increased by 25 to 50 mg q 1 to 2 wk, if needed. *Maintenance:* 100 to 400 mg/day as a single dose or in divided doses b.i.d. *Maximum:* 400 mg/day.

Children ages 2 to 12 also taking enzyme-inducing anticonvulsants and valproic acid.
0.15 mg/kg/day as a single dose or in divided doses b.i.d. for 2 wk and then 0.3 mg/kg/day as a single dose or in divided doses b.i.d. for next 2 wk. Increased by 0.3 mg/kg q 1 to 2 wk, if needed to reach maintenance dosage. *Maintenance:* 1 to 5 mg/kg/day as a single dose or in divided doses b.i.d. *Maximum:* 200 mg/day.

➤ *To treat partial seizures after conversion from an enzyme-inducing anticonvulsant*

CHEWABLE TABLETS, TABLETS

Adults. With enzyme-inducing anticonvulsant, 50 mg q.d. for 2 wk, followed by 100 mg q.d. for next 2 wk. Increased by 100 mg q 1 to 2 wk (while continuing to take enzyme-inducing anticonvulsant), if needed until usual maintenance dosage—500 mg/day in divided doses b.i.d.—is achieved. Then, enzyme-inducing anticonvulsant is tapered over 4 wk and discontinued.

Route	Onset	Peak	Duration
P.O.	Days to wks	Unknown	Unknown

Mechanism of Action

May stabilize neuron membranes by blocking sodium channels in the membranes. This action inhibits the release of excitatory neurotransmitters, such as glutamate and aspartate, through these channels. By blocking the release of neurotransmitters, lamotrigine inhibits the spread of seizure activity in the brain and reduces seizure frequency.

Contraindications

Hypersensitivity to lamotrigine or its components

Interactions

DRUGS

acetaminophen (long-term use): Possibly decreased blood lamotrigine level
carbamazepine, phenobarbital, phenytoin, primidone: Decreased blood lamotrigine level, possibly increased CNS depression
folate inhibitors, such as co-trimoxazole and methotrexate: Increased blood lamotrigine level
valproic acid: Increased blood lamotrigine level, decreased lamotrigine clearance, decreased blood valproic acid level

ACTIVITIES
alcohol use: Possibly increased CNS depression

Adverse Reactions
CNS: Amnesia, anxiety, ataxia, confusion, depression, dizziness, drowsiness, emotional lability, fever, headache, increased seizure activity, lack of coordination
CV: Chest pain
EENT: Blurred vision, diplopia, dry mouth, nystagmus
GI: Abdominal pain, anorexia, constipation, diarrhea, vomiting
HEME: Anemia, eosinophilia, leukopenia, thrombocytopenia
SKIN: Petechiae, photosensitivity, pruritus, rash, Stevens-Johnson syndrome
Other: Angioedema, flulike symptoms, lymphadenopathy

Nursing Considerations
•**WARNING** Lamotrigine may cause severe, potentially life-threatening rashes. Notify prescriber at first sign of rash and expect to discontinue drug.
•Monitor for seizure activity during therapy.
•Be aware that abrupt discontinuation of lamotrigine may cause increased seizure activity. Expect to taper dosage over at least 2 weeks.

PATIENT TEACHING
•Advise patient to take lamotrigine exactly as prescribed and not to discontinue drug abruptly because doing so may increase seizure activity.
•Advise patient to notify prescriber immediately if rash occurs.
•Instruct patient to report increased seizure activity, vision changes, and vomiting.
•Caution patient to avoid potentially hazardous activities until drug's CNS effects are known.
•Advise patient to avoid direct sunlight and to wear protective clothing to minimize the risk of photosensitivity.
•Instruct patient to wear medical identification stating that she takes an anticonvulsant.

lansoprazole
Prevacid

Class and Category
Chemical: Substituted benzimidazole
Therapeutic: Antisecretory, antiulcer
Pregnancy category: B

Indications and Dosages
➤ *To treat duodenal ulcers and maintain healed duodenal ulcers*

DELAYED-RELEASE CAPSULES
Adults. 15 to 30 mg q.d. a.c. in the morning for 4 wk. *Maximum:* 30 mg/day.
➤ *To treat gastric ulcers*

DELAYED-RELEASE CAPSULES
Adults. 15 to 30 mg q.d. a.c. in the morning for up to 8 wk.
➤ *To treat gastroesophageal reflux disease*

DELAYED-RELEASE CAPSULES
Adults. 15 mg q.d. a.c. in the morning for up to 8 wk.
➤ *To treat erosive esophagitis*

DELAYED-RELEASE CAPSULES
Adults. *Initial:* 30 mg q.d. a.c. in the morning for up to 8 wk. Continued an additional 8 wk if indicated. *Maintenance:* 15 mg q.d.
➤ *To treat pathological hypersecretory conditions, such as Zollinger-Ellison syndrome*

DELAYED-RELEASE CAPSULES
Adults. *Initial:* 60 mg q.d. a.c. in the morning, increased as needed according to patient's condition. Doses exceeding 120 mg/day administered in divided doses. *Maximum:* 180 mg/day.
➤ *To eradicate* Helicobacter pylori *and reduce the risk of duodenal ulcer recurrence*

DELAYED-RELEASE CAPSULES
Adults. 30 mg plus 1 g of amoxicillin and 500 mg of clarithromycin q 12 hr a.c. for 10 to 14 days. Alternatively, 30 mg plus 1 g of amoxicillin t.i.d. a.c. for 14 days.
➤ *To treat symptomatic pediatric gastroesophageal reflux disease or erosive esophagitis*

DELAYED-RELEASE CAPSULES, DELAYED-RELEASE SUSPENSION
Children age 1 to 11 weighing 30 kg (66 lb) or less. 15 mg q.d. for up to 12 wk.
Children age 1 to 11 weighing more than 30 kg. 30 mg q.d. for up to 12 wk.

Route	Onset	Peak	Duration
P.O.	1 to 3 hr	Unknown	Over 24 hr

Mechanism of Action
Binds to and inactivates the hydrogen-potassium adenosine triphosphate enzyme system (also called the proton pump) in gastric parietal cells. This action blocks the final step of gastric acid production.

Contraindications
Hypersensitivity to lansoprazole or its components

Interactions
DRUGS
ampicillin, digoxin, iron salts, ketoconazole, other drugs that depend on low gastric pH for bioavailability: Inhibited absorption of these drugs
sucralfate: Delayed lansoprazole absorption
theophylline: Slightly decreased blood theophylline level

Adverse Reactions
CNS: Dizziness, headache
GI: Abdominal pain, anorexia, diarrhea, increased appetite, nausea, pseudomembranous colitis, vomiting
MS: Arthralgia
SKIN: Pruritus, rash

Nursing Considerations
• Give patient delayed-release lansoprazole capsules before meals. Antacids may be used concomitantly if needed.
• Open capsule and sprinkle granules on applesauce if patient has difficulty swallowing capsule. Don't crush granules.
• For patient with NG tube, open capsule, mix granules in 40 ml of apple juice, and inject through tube. Flush tube with apple juice afterward.
• Expect to use lansoprazole with antibiotics because decreased gastric acid secretion helps antibiotics eradicate *H. pylori.*
• If lansoprazole is used with antibiotics, monitor for diarrhea, which may be caused by pseudomembranous colitis.
PATIENT TEACHING
• Instruct patient to take lansoprazole as prescribed, usually before a meal (preferably breakfast) to decrease food-stimulated gastric acid output.
• Instruct patient who has difficulty swallowing to open capsules and sprinkle granules on applesauce. Direct her not to chew granules.
• Inform patient that she may take antacids with lansoprazole.
• Advise patient to report diarrhea, severe headache, or worsening of symptoms immediately to prescriber.

leflunomide

Arava

Class and Category
Chemical: Malonitrilamide immunomodulator
Therapeutic: Antirheumatic
Pregnancy category: X

Indications and Dosages
➤ *To relieve symptoms of active rheumatoid arthritis and to slow disease progression*
TABLETS
Adults. *Loading:* 100 mg q.d. for 3 days. *Maintenance:* 20 mg q.d., reduced to 10 mg q.d. if poorly tolerated. *Maximum:* 20 mg/day.

Mechanism of Action
Inhibits dihydroorotate dehydrogenase, the enzyme in the autoimmune process that leads to rheumatoid arthritis. This action relieves inflammation and prevents alteration of the autoimmune process.

Contraindications
Hypersensitivity to leflunomide or its components, pregnancy

Interactions
activated charcoal, cholestyramine: Decreased blood leflunomide level
methotrexate: Increased risk of hepatotoxicity
NSAIDs: Possibly impaired metabolism of NSAIDs
rifampin, tolbutamide: Increased blood leflunomide level
vaccines (live): Possibly adverse reactions to vaccines caused by leflunomide-induced immunosuppression

Adverse Reactions
CNS: Anxiety, dizziness, drowsiness, fatigue, fever, headache, paresthesia
CV: Chest pain, hypertension, palpitations, tachycardia
EENT: Blurred vision, conjunctivitis, dry mouth, mouth ulcers, pharyngitis, rhinitis, sinusitis
GI: Abdominal pain, constipation, diarrhea, flatulence, gastritis, gastroenteritis, hepatotoxicity, nausea, vomiting
GU: UTI
HEME: Anemia
MS: Back pain, synovitis, tendinitis
RESP: Bronchitis, dyspnea, respiratory tract infection
SKIN: Alopecia (transient), erythematous rash, pruritus, urticaria
Other: Weight loss

J
K
L

Nursing Considerations
- Be aware that patient should have regular medical follow-up to monitor hepatic function and response to leflunomide.
- Expect to discontinue drug if hepatic dysfunction develops.

PATIENT TEACHING
- Advise patient that leflunomide doesn't cure arthritis but may relieve its symptoms.
- Inform patient that reversible hair loss may occur.
- Caution female patient of childbearing age not to become pregnant while taking drug because of the high risk of birth defects.
- Instruct patient to report signs of hepatotoxicity, such as mouth ulcers, unusual bleeding or bruising, and yellow skin or eyes.
- Advise patient to avoid live vaccines during leflunomide therapy.

lepirudin

Refludan

Class and Category
Chemical: Yeast-derived recombinant form of hirudin
Therapeutic: Anticoagulant
Pregnancy category: B

Indications and Dosages
➤ *To prevent thromboembolic complications in patients with heparin-induced thrombocytopenia and associated thromboembolic disease*

I.V. INFUSION AND INJECTION
Adults. *Initial:* 0.4 mg/kg, but no more than 44 mg, given by bolus over 15 to 20 sec, followed by continuous infusion of 0.15 mg/kg/hr for 2 to 10 days or longer, as indicated. *Maximum:* 0.21 mg/kg/hr.
DOSAGE ADJUSTMENT For patients with renal insufficiency, bolus dose decreased to 0.2 mg/kg and infusion rate adjusted as follows: for creatinine clearance of 45 to 60 ml/min/1.73 m², 50% of standard infusion rate; for creatinine clearance of 30 to 44 ml/min/1.73 m², 30% of standard infusion rate; for creatinine clearance of 15 to 29 ml/min/1.73 m², 15% of standard infusion rate; for creatinine clearance of less than 15 ml/min/1.73 m², drug probably discontinued.

Route	Onset	Peak	Duration
I.V.	Immediate	Unknown	Unknown

Mechanism of Action
Forms a tight bond with thrombin, neutralizing this enzyme's actions, even when the enzyme is trapped within clots. One molecule of lepirudin binds with one molecule of thrombin. Thrombin causes fibrinogen to convert to fibrin, which is essential for clot formation.

Incompatibilities
Don't mix lepirudin in same I.V. line with other drugs.

Contraindications
Hypersensitivity to lepirudin or other hirudins

Interactions
oral anticoagulants, platelet aggregation inhibitors, thrombolytics: Increased risk of bleeding complications and enhanced effects of lepirudin

Adverse Reactions
CNS: Chills, fever, intracranial hemorrhage
CV: Heart failure
EENT: Epistaxis
GI: GI or rectal bleeding, hepatic dysfunction
GU: Hematuria, vaginal bleeding
HEME: Anemia, easy bruising, hematoma
RESP: Hemoptysis, pneumonia
SKIN: Excessive bleeding from wounds, rash, pruritus, urticaria
Other: Injection site bleeding, sepsis

Nursing Considerations
- Be aware that patients with heparin-induced thrombocytopenia have low platelet counts, which can lead to severe bleeding and even death. Lepirudin prevents clotting without further reducing platelet count.
- To reconstitute, mix drug with NS or sterile water for injection. Warm solution to room temperature before administering.
- For I.V. bolus, reconstitute 50 mg with 1 ml of sterile water for injection or sodium chloride for injection. Then further dilute by withdrawing reconstituted solution into a 10-ml syringe and adding enough sterile water for injection, sodium chloride for injection, or D$_5$W to produce a total volume of 10 ml, or 5 mg of lepirudin/ml. Administer prescribed dose over 15 to 20 seconds.
- For I.V. infusion, reconstitute 2 vials of drug and transfer to infusion bag that contains 250 or 500 ml of NS or D$_5$W. Concentration will be 0.4 or 0.2 mg/ml.

• Adjust infusion rate as prescribed, according to patient's APTT ratio, which is APTT divided by a control value. Target APTT ratio during treatment is 1.5 to 2.5.

• Expect to obtain first APTT 4 hours after starting infusion and to obtain follow-up APTT daily (more often for patients with hepatic or renal impairment).

• Stop infusion for 2 hours, as ordered, if APTT is above target range. Expect to decrease infusion rate by one-half when restarting. If APTT is below target range, expect to increase rate in 20% increments and recheck APTT in 4 hours.

• Avoid I.M. injections or needle sticks during therapy to minimize the risk of hematoma.

• Observe I.M. injection sites, I.V. infusion sites, and wounds for bleeding.

• Monitor for ecchymoses on arms and legs, epistaxis, hematemesis, hematuria, melena, and vaginal bleeding.

PATIENT TEACHING

• Instruct patient to report unusual or unexpected bleeding, such as blood in urine, easy bruising, nosebleeds, tarry stools, and vaginal bleeding.

• Advise patient to avoid bumping arms and legs and to use an electric razor and a soft-bristled toothbrush to minimize risk of bruising and bleeding.

leuprolide acetate

Eligard 7.5 mg, Eligard 22.5 mg, Lupron, Lupron Depot, Lupron Depot-3 Month 11.25 mg, Lupron Depot-3 Month 22.5 mg, Lupron Depot-4 Month 30 mg, Lupron Depot-Ped, Lupron-3 Month SR Depot 22.5 mg

Class and Category

Chemical: Synthetic peptide gonadotropin-releasing hormone analogue
Therapeutic: Antianemic, antiendometrionic agent, antineoplastic, gonadotropin inhibitor
Pregnancy category: X

Indications and Dosages

➤ *To treat prostate cancer*
S.C. INJECTION (LEUPROLIDE ACETATE INJECTION)
Adults. 1 mg q.d.
S.C. INJECTION (LEUPROLIDE ACETATE FOR INJECTABLE SUSPENSION)
Adult males. 7.5 mg/mo.
I.M. INJECTION (LEUPROLIDE ACETATE FOR INJECTION)
Adults. 7.5 mg/mo, 22.5 mg q 3 mo or 30 mg q 4 mo.

➤ *To treat precocious central puberty*
S.C. injection (leuprolide acetate injection)
Children. 50 mcg/kg/day. Dosage increased in increments of 10 mcg/kg/day.
I.M. INJECTION (LEUPROLIDE ACETATE FOR INJECTION)
Children who weigh more than 37.5 kg (83 lb). *Initial:* 15 mg q 4 wk. *Maintenance:* Dosage increased as needed in increments of 3.75 mg q 4 wk. *Maximum:* 15 mg q 4 wk.
Children who weigh 25 to 37.5 kg (55 to 83 lb). *Initial:* 11.25 mg q 4 wk. *Maintenance:* Dosage increased as needed in increments of 3.75 mg q 4 wk. *Maximum:* 15 mg q 4 wk.
Children who weigh less than 25 kg. *Initial:* 7.5 mg q 4 wk. *Maintenance:* Dosage increased as needed in increments of 3.75 mg q 4 wk. *Maximum:* 15 mg q 4 wk.

➤ *To treat endometriosis*
I.M. INJECTION (LEUPROLIDE ACETATE FOR INJECTION)
Adults. 3.75 mg q mo or 11.25 mg q 3 mo for up to 6 mo. *Maximum:* 33.75 mg total dose.

➤ *As adjunct to treat anemia due to uterine leiomyomas*
I.M. INJECTION (LEUPROLIDE ACETATE FOR INJECTION)
Adults. 3.75 mg q mo for up to 3 mo or 11.25 mg as a single dose. *Maximum:* 11.25 mg total dose.

Route	Onset	Peak	Duration
I.M., S.C.*	1 wk	Unknown	4 to 12 wk after therapy
I.M., S.C.†	2 to 4 wk	After 1 to 2 mo	60 to 90 days after therapy

Contraindications

Adult females and children (leuprolide acetate for injectable suspension); hypersensitivity to benzyl alcohol, gonadorelin, and gonadotropin-releasing hormone analogues, including leuprolide, and their components; pregnancy; undiagnosed abnormal vaginal bleeding

Adverse Reactions

CNS: Dizziness, fatigue, headache, insomnia, malaise, memory loss, paresthesia, syncope (all adults); anxiety, depression, mood changes, nervousness (adult females)

---

* Gonadotropin inhibitor.
† Antiendometrionic, antineoplastic.

CV: Arrhythmias, edema, palpitations (all adults); angina, MI, thrombophlebitis (adult males)
EENT: Blurred vision (all adults)
ENDO: Breast tenderness or swelling (all adults); amenorrhea, androgenic effects (adult females); decreased size of testicles (adult males)
GI: Nausea, vomiting (all adults); constipation, gastroenteritis (adult males)
GU: Decreased libido (all adults); endometriosis flareup, vaginitis (adult females); impotence, prostate cancer flareup (adult males); uterine bleeding, vaginal discharge (female children)
MS: Arthralgia, bone density loss, bone pain, myalgia (all adults); body pain (children)
RESP: Pulmonary embolism (adult males)
SKIN: Rash (children)
Other: Anaphylaxis, hot flashes, weight gain (all adults); injection site burning, edema, itching, pain, or redness (adults and children)

Mechanism of Action

After initially stimulating follicle-stimulating hormone (FSH) and luteinizing hormone (LH), continuous leuprolide therapy suppresses secretion of gonadotropin-releasing hormone, causing testosterone and estradiol levels to fall. In children with central precocious puberty, this results in cessation of menses and reproductive organ development.

In adult males, continuous suppression results in decreasing testosterone levels and pharmacologic castration, which slows the activity of prostatic neoplastic cells. In women with endometriosis or uterine leiomyomas, leuprolide suppresses ovarian function, causing atrophy and inactivation of endometrial tissues and resulting in amenorrhea.

Nursing Considerations

•Reconstitute leuprolide acetate depot suspension with diluent provided by manufacturer. Add diluent to powder for suspension and thoroughly shake vials to disperse particles into a uniform milky suspension. Use immediately after mixing and discard any unused portion. If using a prefilled dual-chamber syringe, follow manufacturer's instructions to release diluent into chamber containing powder. Shake gently after diluted to disperse particles evenly in solution. Be aware that no dilution or reconstitution is necessary for leuprolide acetate injection for S.C. administration. Rotate injection sites.

•**WARNING** Be aware that leuprolide acetate for injectable suspension (Eligard 7.5 mg) is approved only for use in males for the palliative treatment of prostate cancer. Use the provided syringes and delivery system, and read and follow the instructions carefully to ensure proper mixing of the product; shaking alone is inadequate to mix the product.

•**WARNING** Monitor patient for possible allergic reaction (erythema and induration) at injection site because leuprolide injections contain benzyl alcohol. Be aware that manufacturer recommends that injection be administered by physician.

•During first weeks of leuprolide therapy, monitor patient being treated for prostate cancer for initial worsening of symptoms, such as increased bone pain, difficult urination, and paresthesia or paralysis (in patients with vertebral metastasis).

•Expect to discontinue therapy before age 11 in females and age 12 in males treated for precocious central puberty.

•Monitor bone density test results, as ordered, of women at risk for osteoporosis who are receiving leuprolide because of potential for drug-induced estrogen loss, which may result in decreased bone density.

PATIENT TEACHING

•Instruct patient who is self-administering leuprolide injection to use syringe provided by manufacturer. If manufacturer's syringe is unavailable, advise her to use only a 0.5-ml disposable, low-dose, U-100 insulin syringe to ensure accurate dosage. Substitution of syringes is *not* recommended for leuprolide acetate for injectable suspension.

•Advise women to immediately report monthly menses or breakthrough bleeding.

•Instruct female patient of childbearing age to use a nonhormonal form of contraception during leuprolide therapy. Advise her to stop taking drug and notify prescriber at once if she becomes pregnant.

•Inform patient with osteoporosis or at risk for developing it that drug may increase bone density loss.

•Inform parents of child treated for central precocious puberty that they should expect normal gonadal-pituitary function to return 4 to 12 weeks after drug is discontinued.

• Advise patient to report symptoms of depression or memory problems.

levalbuterol hydrochloride

Xopenex

Class and Category
Chemical: Sympathomimetic amine
Therapeutic: Bronchodilator
Pregnancy category: C

Indications and Dosages
➤ *To prevent or treat bronchospasm in reversible obstructive airway disease*
INHALATION SOLUTION
Adults and children age 12 and older. 0.63 to 1.25 mg t.i.d. q 6 to 8 hr. *Maximum:* 1.25 mg t.i.d.
Children ages 6 to 11. 0.31 to 0.63 mg t.i.d. *Maximum:* 0.63 mg t.i.d.
DOSAGE ADJUSTMENT For elderly patients, dosage limited to 0.63 mg t.i.d. q 6 to 8 hr.

Route	Onset	Peak	Duration
Inhalation	10 to 17 min	1.5 hr	5 to 6 hr

Mechanism of Action
Attaches to beta$_2$ receptors on bronchial cell membranes, which stimulates the intracellular enzyme adenyl cyclase to convert adenosine triphosphate to cAMP. An increased intracellular cAMP level relaxes bronchial smooth muscle and inhibits histamine release from mast cells.

Contraindications
Hypersensitivity to levalbuterol, other sympathomimetic amines, or their components

Interactions
DRUGS
beta blockers: Blocked effects of both drugs
digoxin: Decreased blood digoxin level
loop or thiazide diuretics: Increased risk of hypokalemia
MAO inhibitors, sympathomimetics, tricyclic antidepressants: Increased risk of adverse cardiovascular effects

Adverse Reactions
CNS: Anxiety, chills, dizziness, hypertonia, insomnia, migraine headache, nervousness, paresthesia, syncope, tremor
CV: Chest pain, hypertension, hypotension, tachycardia
EENT: Dry mouth and throat, rhinitis, sinusitis
GI: Diarrhea, indigestion, nausea, vomiting
MS: Leg cramps, myalgia
RESP: Asthma exacerbation, cough, dyspnea, paradoxical bronchospasm
Other: Flulike symptoms, lymphadenopathy

Nursing Considerations
• Use levalbuterol cautiously in patients with arrhythmias, diabetes mellitus, hypertension, hyperthyroidism, or a history of seizures.
• Give drug only by nebulizer.
• Monitor pulse rate and blood pressure before and after nebulizer treatment.
• Because drug may provoke paradoxical bronchospasm, observe for dyspnea, wheezing, and increased coughing.
PATIENT TEACHING
• Teach patient how to use levalbuterol nebulizer and to measure correct dose.
• Instruct patient to notify prescriber if drug fails to work or if she needs more frequent treatments because her asthma is worsening.
• Instruct patient not to increase dosage or frequency unless advised to do so by prescriber.
• Advise patient to stop using drug and contact prescriber if paradoxical bronchospasm occurs.
• Instruct patient to use inhalation solution within 2 weeks of opening the foil pouch and to protect drug from light and heat.
• Urge patient to consult prescriber before using OTC or other drugs.

levetiracetam

Keppra

Class and Category
Chemical: Pyrrolidine derivative
Therapeutic: Anticonvulsant
Pregnancy category: C

Indications and Dosages
➤ *As adjunct to treat partial seizures*
TABLETS
Adults and adolescents over age 16. *Initial:* 500 mg b.i.d., increased by 1,000 mg/day q 2 wk if needed. *Maximum:* 3,000 mg/day.
DOSAGE ADJUSTMENT Maximum dosage reduced to 2,000 mg/day for patients with creatinine clearance of 50 to 80 ml/min/1.73 m^2; to 1,500 mg/day for creatinine clearance of 30 to 49 ml/min/1.73 m^2; and to 1,000 mg/day for creatinine clearance of less than 30 ml/min/1.73 m^2. For patients with end-stage renal disease who are receiving dialysis, expect to give an additional 250 to 500 mg/dose, as prescribed, after each dialysis session.

Mechanism of Action

May protect against secondary generalized seizure activity by selectively preventing the coordination of epileptiform burst firing. Levetiracetam does not appear to involve inhibitory and excitatory neurotransmission.

Contraindications

Hypersensitivity to levetiracetam or its components

Adverse Reactions

CNS: Aggression, anger, asthenia, ataxia, dizziness, headache, irritability, mental or mood changes, paresthesia, somnolence, vertigo
EENT: Diplopia, pharyngitis, rhinitis, sinusitis
GI: Anorexia
RESP: Cough
Other: Infection

Nursing Considerations

• Monitor for drug compliance during first 4 weeks of levetiracetam therapy, when adverse reactions are most common.
• Monitor patient for seizure activity during therapy. As appropriate, implement seizure precautions according to facility policy.
• Be aware that abrupt discontinuation of levetiracetam may cause increased seizure activity. Expect to taper dosage gradually.

PATIENT TEACHING

• Caution patient that levetiracetam may cause dizziness and drowsiness, especially during first 4 weeks of therapy.
• Advise patient to avoid driving and other activities that require a high level of alertness until drug's full CNS effects are known.
• Caution patient not to stop taking levetiracetam abruptly; inform her that drug dosage should be tapered under prescriber's direction to avoid breakthrough seizures.
• Advise patient to continue taking other anticonvulsants, as prescribed, while taking levetiracetam.
• Encourage patient to avoid alcohol during levetiracetam therapy because alcohol can increase incidence of drowsiness and dizziness.
• Instruct patient to see prescriber regularly so that her progress can be monitored.

levodopa

Dopar, Larodopa

Class and Category

Chemical: Dihydroxyphenylalanine isomer, metabolic precursor of dopamine
Therapeutic: Antidyskinetic
Pregnancy category: Not rated

Indications and Dosages

➤ *To manage symptoms of primary Parkinson's disease, postencephalitic parkinsonism, and parkinsonism caused by CNS injury from carbon monoxide or manganese intoxication*

CAPSULES, TABLETS

Adults and children age 12 and older. *Initial:* 250 mg/day in divided doses b.i.d. to q.i.d. Increased by 100 to 750 mg q 3 to 7 days, as indicated. *Maximum:* 8 g/day.

Route	Onset	Peak	Duration
P.O.	14 to 21 days*	Unknown	5 hr

Contraindications

Angle-closure glaucoma, history of melanoma, hypersensitivity to levodopa or its components, suspicious undiagnosed skin lesions, use within 14 days of MAO inhibitor therapy

Interactions

DRUGS

antacids: Increased blood levodopa level
antihypertensives: Risk of orthostatic hypotension
benzodiazepines: Possibly decreased therapeutic effects of levodopa
bromocriptine: Possibly additive effects of levodopa
furazolidone, MAO inhibitors, procarbazine: Risk of severe hypertension
haloperidol, loxapine, molindone, papaverine, phenothiazines, phenytoin, rauwolfia alkaloids: Decreased effects of levodopa
inhaled anesthetics, sympathomimetics: Increased risk of arrhythmias
iron salts: Possibly decreased blood level and effectiveness of levodopa
methyldopa: Possibly toxic CNS effects
metoclopramide: Possibly worsening of Parkinson's disease and decreased therapeutic effects of metoclopramide
pyridoxine (vitamin B_6): Decreased antidyskinetic effect of levodopa

---

* With multiple doses.

Mechanism of Action

By supplementing a low level of endogenous dopamine, levodopa helps control alterations in voluntary muscle movement (such as tremors and rigidity) associated with Parkinson's disease. Dopamine, a neurotransmitter that's synthesized and released by neurons leading from substantia nigra to basal ganglia, is essential for normal motor function. By stimulating peripheral and central dopaminergic$_2$ (D_2) receptors on postsynaptic cells, dopamine inhibits the firing of striatal neurons (such as cholinergic neurons). In Parkinson's disease, progressive degeneration of these neurons substantially reduces the supply of intrasynaptic dopamine. Levodopa, a dopamine precursor, increases the dopamine supply in neurons, making more available to stimulate dopaminergic receptors.

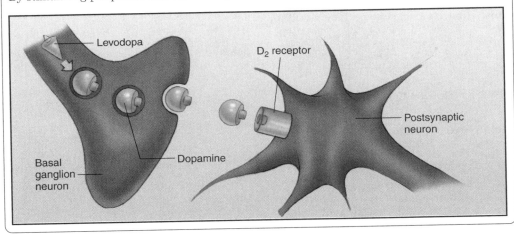

FOODS

high-protein food: Decreased levodopa absorption

ACTIVITIES

cocaine use: Increased risk of arrhythmias

Adverse Reactions

CNS: Aggressiveness, anxiety, ataxia, confusion, delusions, dizziness, dream disturbances, dyskinesia, dystonia, euphoria, hallucinations, headache, increased tremor, insomnia, malaise, mood changes, severe depression, suicidal tendencies, syncope, weakness
CV: Arrhythmias, hot flashes, orthostatic hypotension, palpitations
EENT: Bitter aftertaste, blurred vision, darkened saliva, diplopia, dry mouth, increased salivation, mydriasis, tooth clenching and grinding
GI: Abdominal pain, anorexia, constipation, diarrhea, flatulence, GI bleeding, hepatotoxicity, hiccups, indigestion, nausea, vomiting
GU: Darkened urine, priapism, urine retention
SKIN: Darkened sweat, diaphoresis, rash

Nursing Considerations

•Expect to discontinue levodopa 6 to 8 hours before surgery to avoid interactions with anesthetics.
•Observe patient for mental or behavioral changes and suicidal tendencies. Notify prescriber immediately if they occur.
•Monitor for muscle twitching and blepharospasm (eyelid spasm), which are early signs of drug overdose. Report these signs immediately.
•Expect patient to be tested for acromegaly and diabetes during long-term levodopa therapy. Also expect to monitor hematopoietic, hepatic, and renal function.

PATIENT TEACHING

•Advise patient to take levodopa with meals if she experiences adverse GI reactions.
•Because protein impairs drug absorption, instruct patient to avoid high-protein meals during levodopa therapy and to distribute protein intake equally throughout the day.
•Caution patient to avoid excessive use of vitamins and fortified cereals that contain

vitamin B$_6$ or iron, which can reduce levodopa's effects.
- Instruct patient to report fainting, increased muscle tremor, difficult urination, and severe or persistent nausea and vomiting.
- Urge patient to continue taking drug even if results of therapy aren't evident immediately.
- Inform patient that saliva, sweat, and urine may darken but that this isn't harmful.
- Direct patient to protect drug from heat, light, and moisture and to discard darkened pills because they have lost their potency.
- Advise patient to change position slowly to minimize effects of orthostatic hypotension.
- Caution male patient about risk of priapism (persistent, painful erection), and urge him to seek medical treatment immediately if it occurs.

levofloxacin

Levaquin

Class and Category

Chemical: Fluoroquinolone
Therapeutic: Antibiotic
Pregnancy category: C

Indications and Dosages

➤ *To treat acute maxillary sinusitis caused by* Haemophilus influenzae, Moraxella catarrhalis, *or* Streptococcus pneumoniae

TABLETS, I.V. INFUSION

Adults. 500 mg q.d. for 10 to 14 days.

➤ *To treat acute exacerbations of chronic bacterial bronchitis caused by* H. influenzae, Haemophilus parainfluenzae, M. catarrhalis, S. pneumoniae, *or* Staphylococcus aureus

TABLETS, I.V. INFUSION

Adults. 500 mg q.d. for 7 days.

➤ *To treat community-acquired pneumonia caused by* Chlamydia pneumoniae, H. influenzae, H. parainfluenzae, Klebsiella pneumoniae, Legionella pneumophila, M. catarrhalis, Mycoplasma pneumoniae, S. aureus, *or* S. pneumoniae

TABLETS, I.V. INFUSION

Adults. 500 mg q.d. for 7 to 14 days.

➤ *To treat uncomplicated UTIs caused by* Escherichia coli, K. pneumoniae, *or* Staphylococcus saprophyticus

TABLETS, I.V. INFUSION

Adults. 250 mg q.d. for 3 days.

➤ *To treat complicated UTIs and acute pyelonephritis caused by* E. coli

TABLETS, I.V. INFUSION

Adults. 250 mg q.d. for 10 days.

➤ *To treat mild to moderate skin and soft-tissue infections caused by* S. aureus *or* Streptococcus pyogenes

TABLETS, I.V. INFUSION

Adults. 500 mg q.d. for 7 to 10 days.

➤ *To treat complicated skin and soft-tissue infections caused by methicillin-sensitive* Enterococcus faecalis, Proteus mirabilis, S. aureus, *or* S. pyogenes

TABLETS, I.V. INFUSION

Adults. 750 mg q.d. for 7 to 14 days.

DOSAGE ADJUSTMENT For patients with impaired renal function, dosage reduced as follows: for complicated UTIs in patients with creatinine clearance of 10 to 19 ml/min/1.73 m^2, 250 mg initially and then maintenance dosage of 250 mg q 48 hr. For all other indications, in patients with creatinine clearance of 50 to 80 ml/min/1.73 m^2, 500 mg initially and then maintenance dosage of 500 mg q 24 hr; with creatinine clearance of 20 to 49 ml/min/1.73 m^2, 500 mg initially and then maintenance dosage of 250 mg q 24 hr; with creatinine clearance of 10 to 19 ml/min/1.73 m^2, 500 mg initially and then maintenance dosage of 250 mg q 48 hr.

Mechanism of Action

Interferes with bacterial cell replication by inhibiting the bacterial enzyme DNA gyrase, which is essential for replication and repair of bacterial DNA.

Contraindications

Hypersensitivity to levofloxacin, other fluoroquinolones, or their components

Interactions

DRUGS

aluminum-, calcium-, or magnesium-containing antacids; iron; sucralfate; zinc: Reduced GI absorption of levofloxacin
antineoplastics: Decreased blood levofloxacin level
cimetidine: Increased blood levofloxacin level
cyclosporine: Increased risk of nephrotoxicity
NSAIDs: Possibly increased CNS stimulation and risk of seizures
oral anticoagulants: Increased anticoagulant effect and risk of bleeding
oral antidiabetic drugs: Possibly hyperglycemia or hypoglycemia

theophylline: Increased blood theophylline level and risk of toxicity

ACTIVITIES

sun exposure: Increased risk of photosensitivity

Adverse Reactions

CNS: Anxiety, dizziness, headache, nervousness, seizures, sleep disturbance

CV: Arrhythmias, prolonged QT interval

EENT: Taste perversion

GI: Abdominal pain, anorexia, constipation, diarrhea, flatulence, indigestion, nausea, pseudomembranous colitis, vomiting

GU: Crystalluria, vaginal candidiasis

HEME: Eosinophilia, hemolytic anemia

MS: Back pain, tendon rupture

SKIN: Photosensitivity, pruritus, rash, urticaria

Other: Anaphylaxis

Nursing Considerations

• Use levofloxacin cautiously in patients with renal insufficiency. Monitor renal function test results as appropriate during treatment.

• Also use drug cautiously in patients with CNS disorders that may lower the seizure threshold, such as epilepsy.

• Expect to obtain culture and sensitivity test results before levofloxacin treatment begins.

• Avoid giving drug within 2 hours of antacids.

• Ensure that patient is well hydrated during treatment to prevent crystalluria.

• Frequently monitor blood glucose level of diabetic patient who uses an oral antidiabetic drug because oral antidiabetic drugs may interact with levofloxacin, causing hyperglycemia or hypoglycemia.

PATIENT TEACHING

• Advise patient to increase fluid intake during levofloxacin therapy.

• Direct patient to separate doses of antacid, iron, sucralfate, and zinc by at least 2 hours from levofloxacin.

• Advise patient to avoid excessive sunlight and to wear sunscreen because of increased risk of photosensitivity.

• Advise diabetic patient to monitor blood glucose level frequently and notify prescriber of significant changes.

levomethadyl acetate hydrochloride

Orlaam

Class, Category, and Schedule

Chemical: Diphenylheptane derivative

Therapeutic: Opioid abuse therapy adjunct

Pregnancy category: C

Controlled substance: Schedule II

Indications and Dosages

➤ *As adjunct to treat opioid addiction*

ORAL SOLUTION

Adults. *Initial:* 20 to 40 mg for first dose. Later doses, which may be increased by 5 to 10 mg, given q 48 to 72 hr until steady state is reached, usually in 1 to 2 wk. *Maintenance:* 60 to 80 mg three times/wk at 48- to 72-hr intervals. *Maximum:* 140 mg three times/wk, or two 130-mg doses and one 180-mg dose/wk.

DOSAGE ADJUSTMENT For methadone-dependent patients, initial dose increased—usually to 1.2 to 1.3 times the daily methadone dose, but to no more than 120 mg.

Route	Onset	Peak	Duration
P.O.	2 to 4 hr	7 to 10 days	24 to 72 hr

Mechanism of Action

Produces morphinelike effects on the CNS and smooth muscle by acting at mu opioid receptors to produce analgesia, euphoria, respiratory depression, and sedation. By cross-substituting for opioid antagonists, levomethadyl suppresses withdrawal symptoms in opioid-tolerant people.

Contraindications

Asthma, hypersensitivity to narcotics, known or suspected QT-interval prolongation (QTc interval greater than 430 milliseconds [male] or 450 milliseconds [female]), risk of QT-interval prolongation, upper airway obstruction

Interactions

DRUGS

CNS depressants: Possibly increased CNS and respiratory depression and risk of hypotension

cytochrome P-450 hepatic enzyme inducers, such as carbamazepine, phenytoin, and rifampin: Increased peak effect and decreased duration of action of levomethadyl

hepatic enzyme inhibitors, such as antifungal drugs (including ketoconazole), cimetidine, and erythromycin: Possibly delayed onset of action and prolonged duration of action of levomethadyl

opioid analgesics (mu-receptor agonists): Increased risk of overdose

opioid analgesics (partial mu-receptor agonists and agonist-antagonists), opioid antagonists: Possibly withdrawal symptoms

ACTIVITIES

alcohol use: Increased CNS effects and risk of levomethadyl toxicity

Adverse Reactions

CNS: Anxiety, depression, dream disturbances, drowsiness, euphoria, headache, insomnia, nervousness, sedation, weakness, yawning
CV: Bradycardia, edema, palpitations, prolonged QT interval, torsades de pointes
EENT: Blurred vision, dry mouth, rhinitis
GI: Abdominal pain, constipation, diarrhea, elevated liver function test results, nausea, vomiting
GU: Amenorrhea, ejaculation disorders, impotence
MS: Arthralgia
RESP: Cough
SKIN: Diaphoresis, rash
Other: Physical and psychological dependence

Nursing Considerations

•Be aware that, because levomethadyl may cause serious and possibly life-threatening arrhythmias (such as torsades de pointes), this drug should be used to treat only opiate-addicted patients who fail to show an acceptable response to other treatments for opiate addiction, either because the treatments weren't sufficiently effective or because intolerable adverse effects prevented effective doses.
•Before starting therapy, expect to obtain a 12-lead ECG to determine whether patient has a prolonged QT interval (QTc greater than 430 milliseconds [male] or 450 milliseconds [female]). If QT interval is prolonged, be aware that levomethadyl shouldn't be given. Expect to obtain an ECG before treatment starts, 12 to 14 days after it starts, and periodically thereafter, to rule out any changes in the QT interval.
•Monitor heart rate and rhythm frequently, especially if patient has a risk factor for prolonged QT syndrome, such as bradycardia, cardiac hypertrophy, congestive heart failure, hypokalemia, hypomagnesemia, or use of a diuretic.
•Be aware that levomethadyl causes dependence similar to that caused by morphine and has potential for abuse.
•Monitor patient's tolerance and reaction to drug during first week of therapy and when dosage increases.
•Monitor patient's vital signs regularly.
•Assess patient for signs and symptoms of withdrawal, such as abdominal cramps, diaphoresis, diarrhea, and dizziness. If she experiences withdrawal symptoms, expect to increase dosage or provide other treatment.

PATIENT TEACHING

•Review drug administration schedule with patient. Advise her that daily use of levomethadyl could lead to overdose.
•Caution patient to avoid alcohol and other CNS depressants while taking levomethadyl.
•**WARNING** Advise patient to seek immediate medical attention if she experiences palpitations, dizziness, light-headedness, syncope, or seizures because these problems may signal a life-threatening arrhythmia.
•**WARNING** Caution patient that the use of street drugs during levomethadyl therapy can cause serious complications and even death.
•Urge patient to keep follow-up appointments because skipping doses could cause severe adverse reactions.
•Advise patient not to engage in hazardous activities until drug's CNS effects are known.

levorphanol tartrate

Levo-Dromoran

Class, Category, and Schedule

Chemical: Morphinan derivative
Therapeutic: Analgesic, anesthesia adjunct
Pregnancy category: Not rated
Controlled substance: Schedule II

Indications and Dosages

➤ *To relieve moderate to severe pain*
TABLETS
Adults. 2 mg q 6 to 8 hr, p.r.n. Increased to 3 mg q 6 to 8 hr, if indicated.
I.V. INJECTION
Adults. Up to 1 mg q 3 to 6 hr, p.r.n. *Maximum:* 8 mg/day for non-opioid-dependent patients.
I.M. OR S.C. INJECTION
Adults. 1 to 2 mg q 6 to 8 hr, p.r.n. *Maximum:* 8 mg/day for non-opioid-dependent patients.

➤ *To provide preoperative sedation*
I.M. OR S.C. INJECTION
Adults. 1 to 2 mg 60 to 90 min before procedure.

Route	Onset	Peak	Duration
P.O.	10 to 60 min	90 to 120 min	4 to 5 hr
I.V.	Unknown	In 20 min	4 to 5 hr
I.M.	Unknown	60 min	4 to 5 hr
S.C.	Unknown	60 to 90 min	4 to 5 hr

Mechanism of Action

Decreases intracellular level of cyclic adenosine monophosphate by inhibiting adenylate cyclase, which regulates the release of pain neurotransmitters, such as substance P, gamma-aminobutyric acid, dopamine, acetylcholine, and noradrenaline. Levorphanol also stimulates mu and kappa opioid receptors, altering the perception of pain and, possibly, the emotional response to it.

Incompatibilities

Don't mix levorphanol tartrate with solutions that contain aminophylline, ammonium chloride, amobarbital sodium, chlorothiazide sodium, heparin sodium, methicillin sodium, nitrofurantoin sodium, novobiacin sodium, pentobarbital sodium, perphenazine, phenobarbital sodium, phenytoin, secobarbital sodium, sodium bicarbonate, sodium iodide, sulfadiazine sodium, sulfisoxazole diethanolamine, or thiopental sodium.

Contraindications

Acute alcoholism, acute or severe asthma, anoxia, hypersensitivity to levorphanol tartrate or its components, increased intracranial pressure, respiratory depression, upper airway obstruction

Interactions

DRUGS

alfentanil, CNS depressants, fentanyl, sufentanil: Possibly increased CNS and respiratory depression and hypotension
anticholinergics: Increased risk of severe constipation
antidiarrheals, such as difenoxin and atropine, kaolin, and loperamide: Increased risk of severe constipation and increased CNS depression
antihypertensives: Increased risk of hypotension
buprenorphine: Possibly decreased therapeutic effects of levorphanol and increased risk of respiratory depression
hydroxyzine: Increased risk of CNS depression and hypotension
metoclopramide: Possibly antagonized effects of metoclopramide
naloxone, naltrexone: Decreased therapeutic effects of levorphanol
neuromuscular blockers: Increased risk of prolonged CNS and respiratory depression

ACTIVITIES

alcohol use: Possibly increased CNS and respiratory depression and hypotension

Adverse Reactions

CNS: Amnesia, coma, confusion, delusions, depression, dizziness, drowsiness, dyskinesia, hypokinesia, insomnia, nervousness, personality disorder, seizures
CV: Bradycardia, cardiac arrest, hypotension, orthostatic hypotension, palpitations, shock, tachycardia
EENT: Abnormal vision, diplopia, dry mouth
GI: Abdominal pain, biliary tract spasm, constipation, hepatic failure, indigestion, nausea, vomiting
GU: Dysuria, urine retention
RESP: Apnea, hyperventilation
SKIN: Cyanosis, pruritus, rash, urticaria
Other: Injection site pain, redness, and swelling; physical and psychological dependence

Nursing Considerations

•**WARNING** Be aware that levorphanol may be habit-forming.
•Administer drug with food if GI distress occurs.
•If respiratory depression occurs, expect to administer naloxone to reverse it.
•Monitor supine and standing blood pressure, and notify prescriber of orthostatic hypotension.
•Carefully assess for adverse reactions in elderly patients; they are especially sensitive to drug and are at increased risk for constipation.

PATIENT TEACHING

•Advise patient to avoid potentially hazardous activities until drug's CNS effects are known.
•Instruct patient to avoid alcoholic beverages while taking levorphanol.
•Direct patient to change position slowly to minimize effects of orthostatic hypotension.
•Advise patient to notify prescriber if constipation, nausea, or vomiting occurs.
•If patient reports dry mouth, suggest that she use sugarless candy or gum or ice chips.

levothyroxine sodium

(L-thyroxine sodium, T_4, thyroxine sodium)

Eltroxin (CAN), Levo-T, Levothroid, Levoxyl, PMS-Levothyroxine Sodium (CAN), Synthroid, Unithroid

Class and Category

Chemical: Synthetic thyroxine (T_4)
Therapeutic: Thyroid hormone replacement
Pregnancy category: A

J
K
L

Indications and Dosages

➤ *To treat mild hypothyroidism*

TABLETS

Adults. *Initial:* 50 mcg q.d., increased by 25 to 50 mcg q 2 to 3 wk until desired response occurs or therapeutic blood level is reached. *Maintenance:* 75 to 125 mcg q.d.

DOSAGE ADJUSTMENT For elderly patients and those with cardiovascular disease or chronic hypothyroidism, initial dosage usually reduced to 12.5 to 25 mcg q.d. and then increased by 12.5 to 25 mcg q 3 to 4 wk until desired response occurs. For elderly patients, maintenance dosage is limited to 75 mcg q.d.

Children over age 10. 2 to 3 mcg/kg q.d. *Usual:* 150 to 200 mcg/day.

Children ages 6 to 10. 4 to 5 mcg/kg q.d. *Usual:* 100 to 150 mcg/day.

Children ages 1 to 5. 3 to 5 mcg/kg q.d. *Usual:* 75 to 100 mcg/day.

Infants ages 6 to 12 months. 5 to 6 mcg/kg q.d. *Usual:* 50 to 75 mcg q.d.

Infants under age 6 months. 5 to 6 mcg/kg q.d. *Usual:* 25 to 50 mcg q.d.

➤ *To treat severe hypothyroidism*

TABLETS

Adults. *Initial:* 12.5 to 25 mcg q.d. Increased by 25 mcg q 2 to 3 wk until desired response occurs or therapeutic blood level is reached. *Maintenance:* 75 to 125 mcg q.d. *Maximum:* 200 mcg q.d.

Children over age 10. 2 to 3 mcg/kg q.d. *Usual:* 150 to 200 mcg/day.

Children ages 6 to 10. 4 to 5 mcg/kg q.d. *Usual:* 100 to 150 mcg/day.

Children ages 1 to 5. 3 to 5 mcg/kg q.d. *Usual:* 75 to 100 mcg/day.

Infants ages 6 to 12 months. 5 to 6 mcg/kg q.d. *Usual:* 50 to 75 mcg q.d.

Infants under age 6 months. 5 to 6 mcg/kg q.d. *Usual:* 25 to 50 mcg q.d.

I.V. OR I.M. INJECTION

Adults. 50 to 100 mcg q.d. until therapeutic blood level is reached.

Children. 75% of usual P.O. dose q.d. until therapeutic blood level is reached.

➤ *To treat myxedema coma*

I.V. INJECTION

Adults. 200 to 500 mcg on day 1. If no significant improvement, 100 to 300 mcg on day 2. Daily dose continued as prescribed until therapeutic blood level is reached and P.O. administration is tolerated.

Children. 75% of usual P.O. dose q.d. until therapeutic blood level is reached and P.O. administration is tolerated.

Route	Onset	Peak	Duration
P.O.	3 to 5 days	3 to 4 wk	1 to 3 wk
I.V.	6 to 8 hr	24 hr	Unknown
I.M.	Unknown	Unknown	1 to 3 wk

Mechanism of Action

Replaces endogenous thyroid hormone, which may exert its physiologic effects by controlling DNA transcription and protein synthesis. Levothyroxine exhibits all of the following actions of endogenous thyroid hormone. The drug:

• increases energy expenditure
• accelerates the rate of cellular oxidation, which stimulates body tissue growth, maturation, and metabolism
• regulates differentiation and proliferation of stem cells
• aids in myelination of nerves and development of synaptic processes in the nervous system
• regulates growth
• decreases blood and hepatic cholesterol concentrations
• enhances carbohydrate and protein metabolism, increasing gluconeogenesis and protein synthesis.

Contraindications

Acute MI (unless caused or complicated by hyperthyroidism), hypersensitivity to levothyroxine or its components, uncorrected adrenal insufficiency, untreated thyrotoxicosis

Interactions

DRUGS

adrenocorticoids: Possibly adrenocorticoid dosage adjustments as thyroid status changes

aluminum- and magnesium-containing antacids, bile acid sequestrants, calcium carbonate, cation exchange resins, cholestyramine, colestipol, ferrous sulfate, kayexalate, sucralfate: Possibly reduced effects of levothyroxine

amiodarone, iodide: Possibly hyperthyroidism

beta blockers: Possibly impaired action of beta blockers and decreased conversion of T_4 to triiodothyronine (T_3)

cholestyramine, colestipol: Delayed or inhibited levothyroxine absorption

digoxin: Reduced therapeutic effects of digoxin

estrogen, phenylbutazone, phenytoin: Reduced binding of levothyroxine to protein, possibly requiring increased levothyroxine dosage
insulin, oral antidiabetic drugs: Possibly uncontrolled diabetes mellitus, requiring increased dosage of insulin or oral antidiabetic drug
ketamine: Possibly hypertension and tachycardia
maprotiline: Increased risk of arrhythmias
oral anticoagulants: Altered anticoagulant activity, possibly need for anticoagulant dosage adjustment
selective serotonin reuptake inhibitors, tricyclic and tetracyclic antidepressants: Increased therapeutic and toxic effects of both drugs
sympathomimetics: Increased risk of coronary insufficiency in patients with coronary artery disease
theophylline: Decreased theophylline clearance
Foods
dietary fiber, soybean flour (infant formula), walnuts: Possibly decreased absorption of levothyroxine from GI tract

Adverse Reactions

CNS: Fatigue, headache, insomnia, somnolence
ENDO: Hyperthyroidism (with overdose)
MS: Muscle weakness, myalgia
SKIN: Alopecia (transient), rash, urticaria
Other: Weight gain

Nursing Considerations

•Administer levothyroxine tablets as a single daily dose 30 to 60 minutes before breakfast. If patient has difficulty swallowing, crush tablet and suspend in a small amount of water or food.
•To prevent decreased drug absorption, administer oral levothyroxine at least 4 hours before or after aluminum- or magnesium-containing antacids, bile acid sequestrants, calcium carbonate, cation exchange resins, cholestyramine, colestipol, ferrous sulfate, kayexalate, or sucralfate.
•Expect to give drug I.V. or I.M. if patient can't take tablets. Be aware that drug shouldn't be given S.C.
•For I.V. use, reconstitute drug by adding 5 ml of NS.
•Monitor PT of patient receiving anticoagulants; she may require a dosage adjustment.
•Monitor blood glucose level of diabetic patient. Prescriber may reduce antidiabetic drug dosage as thyroid hormone level enters therapeutic range.
•Expect patient to undergo regular thyroid function tests during levothyroxine therapy.

PATIENT TEACHING
•Inform patient that levothyroxine replaces a hormone that is normally produced by the thyroid gland and that she'll probably need to take drug for life.
•Instruct patient to take drug before breakfast because drug absorption is increased on an empty stomach and evening doses may cause insomnia.
•Inform patient that drug may require a few weeks to take effect.
•Advise patient not to discontinue drug or change dosage unless instructed to do so by prescriber.
•Instruct patient to report signs of hyperthyroidism, such as diarrhea, excessive sweating, heat intolerance, insomnia, palpitations, and weight loss.
•Inform patient that transient hair loss may occur during first few months of therapy.
•Instruct female patient of childbearing age to notify prescriber immediately if she becomes pregnant because levothyroxine dosage may need to be increased.

lidocaine hydrochloride

J
K
L

(lignocaine hydrochloride)

Alphacaine (CAN), Anestacon, DermaFlex, Dilocaine, L-Caine, Xylocaine, Xylocard (CAN)

Class and Category

Chemical: Aminoacyamide
Therapeutic: Class IB antiarrhythmic, local anesthetic
Pregnancy category: B

Indications and Dosages

➤ *To treat ventricular tachycardia or ventricular fibrillation*
I.V. INFUSION AND INJECTION
Adults. *Loading:* 50 to 100 mg (or 1 to 1.5 mg/kg), administered at 25 to 50 mg/min. If desired response isn't achieved after 5 to 10 min, second dose of 25 to 50 mg (or 0.5 to 0.75 mg/kg) is given q 5 to 10 min until maximum loading dose (300 mg in 1 hr) has been given. *Maintenance:* 20 to 50 mcg/kg/ min (1 to 4 mg/min) by continuous infusion. Smaller bolus dose repeated 15 to 20 min after start of infusion if needed to maintain therapeutic blood level. *Maximum:* 300 mg (or 3 mg/kg) over 1 hr. **Children.** *Loading:* 1 mg/kg. *Maintenance:* 30 mcg/kg/min by continuous infusion. *Maximum:* 3 mg/kg.

DOSAGE ADJUSTMENT For elderly patients receiving I.V. lidocaine to treat arrhythmias and for patients with acute hepatitis or decompensated cirrhosis, loading dose and continuous infusion rate reduced by 50%.

I.M. INJECTION

Adults. 300 mg, repeated after 60 to 90 min, if needed.

➤ *To provide topical anesthesia for skin or mucous membranes*

FILM-FORMING GEL, JELLY, OR OINTMENT

Adults. Thin layer applied to skin or mucous membranes as needed before procedure.

Route	Onset	Peak	Duration
I.V.	45 to 90 sec	Immediate	10 to 20 min
I.M.	5 to 15 min	Unknown	60 to 90 min
Topical	2 to 5 min	Unknown	0.5 to 1 hr

Mechanism of Action

Combines with fast sodium channels in myocardial cell membranes, which inhibits sodium influx into cells and decreases ventricular depolarization, automaticity, and excitability during diastole. Lidocaine also blocks nerve impulses by decreasing the permeability of neuronal membranes to sodium. This action produces local anesthesia.

Contraindications

Adams-Stokes syndrome; hypersensitivity to lidocaine, amide anesthetics, or their components; severe heart block (without artificial pacemaker); Wolff-Parkinson-White syndrome

Interactions

DRUGS

beta blockers, cimetidine: Increased blood lidocaine level and risk of toxicity

MAO inhibitors, tricyclic antidepressants: Risk of severe, prolonged hypertension

mexiletine, tocainide: Additive cardiac effects

neuromuscular blockers: Possibly increased neuromuscular blockade

phenytoin, procainamide: Increased cardiac depression

Adverse Reactions

CNS: Anxiety, confusion, difficulty speaking, dizziness, hallucinations, lethargy, paresthesia, seizures

CV: Bradycardia, cardiac arrest, hypotension, new or worsening arrhythmias

EENT: Blurred vision, diplopia, tinnitus

GI: Nausea

MS: Muscle twitching

RESP: Respiratory arrest or depression

Other: Injection site burning, irritation, stinging, swelling, and tenderness

Nursing Considerations

•Observe for respiratory depression after bolus injection and during I.V. infusion of lidocaine.

•Keep life-support equipment and vasopressors nearby during I.V. administration in case respiratory depression or other reactions occur.

•Carefully check prefilled syringes before using. Use only syringes labeled "for cardiac arrhythmias" for I.V. administration.

•As prescribed, titrate I.V. dose to minimum amount needed to prevent arrhythmias.

•During I.V. administration, place patient on cardiac monitor, as ordered, and closely observe her at all times. Monitor for worsening arrhythmias, widening QRS complex, and prolonged PR interval—possible signs of drug toxicity.

•Monitor blood lidocaine level, as ordered. Check for therapeutic level of 2 to 5 mcg/ml.

•If signs of toxicity, such as dizziness, occur, notify prescriber and expect to discontinue or slow infusion.

•Give I.M. injection in deltoid muscle only.

•Apply lidocaine jelly or ointment to gauze or bandage before applying to skin.

•Monitor vital signs as well as BUN and serum creatinine and electrolyte levels during and after therapy.

PATIENT TEACHING

•Inform patient who receives lidocaine as an anesthetic that she will experience numbness.

•Advise patient to report difficulty speaking, dizziness, injection site pain, nausea, numbness or tingling, and vision changes.

lincomycin hydrochloride

Lincocin

Class and Category

Chemical: Lincosamide

Therapeutic: Bacteriostatic or bactericidal antibiotic

Pregnancy category: C

Indications and Dosages

➤ *To treat serious respiratory, skin, and soft-tissue infections caused by suscepti-*

ble strains of streptococci, pneumococci, and staphylococci

CAPSULES

Adults and adolescents. 500 mg q 6 to 8 hr.

Children over age 1 month. 7.5 to 15 mg/kg q 6 hr; alternatively, 10 to 20 mg/kg q 8 hr.

I.V. INFUSION

Adults. 600 mg to 1 g q 8 to 12 hr. *Maximum:* 8 g/day in divided doses for life-threatening infection.

Children over age 1 month. 10 to 20 mg/kg/day in divided doses q 8 to 12 hr, depending on severity of infection.

I.M. INJECTION

Adults and adolescents. 600 mg q 12 to 24 hr.

Children over age 1 month. 10 mg/kg q 12 to 24 hr.

DOSAGE ADJUSTMENT Dosage reduced by 25% to 30% for patients with severely impaired renal function.

Mechanism of Action

Inhibits protein synthesis in susceptible bacteria by binding to the 50S subunit of bacterial ribosomes and preventing peptide bond formation, thus causing bacterial cells to die.

Incompatibilities

Don't administer lincomycin with novobiocin or kanamycin.

Contraindications

Hypersensitivity to lincomycin or clindamycin

Interactions

DRUGS

antimyasthenic drugs: Possibly antagonized effects of these drugs

chloramphenicol, clindamycin, erythromycin: Possibly blocked access of lincomycin to its site of action

hydrocarbon inhalation anesthetics, neuromuscular blockers: Increased neuromuscular blockade, possibly severe respiratory depression

opioid analgesics: Increased risk of prolonged or increased respiratory depression

Adverse Reactions

CNS: Fever, vertigo

CV: Cardiac arrest and hypotension (with rapid administration)

EENT: Glossitis, stomatitis, tinnitus

GI: Abdominal cramps, colitis, diarrhea, nausea, pseudomembranous colitis, rectal candidiasis, vomiting

GU: Vaginal candidiasis

HEME: Agranulocytosis, eosinophilia, leukopenia, neutropenia, thrombocytopenic purpura

SKIN: Erythema multiforme, rash, Stevens-Johnson syndrome, urticaria

Other: Anaphylaxis, angioedema, superinfection

Nursing Considerations

•Expect to obtain a specimen for culture and sensitivity testing before administering first dose of lincomycin.

•**WARNING** Be aware that some preparations of lincomycin contain benzyl alcohol, which can cause a fatal toxic syndrome in neonates or premature infants, characterized by CNS, respiratory, circulatory, and renal impairment and metabolic acidosis. Because lincomycin has appeared in breast milk, breast-feeding patient may be required to discontinue drug or stop breast-feeding.

•Dilute 600-mg dose in at least 100 ml of D_5W, $D_{10}W$, NS, D_5NS, or other compatible diluent recommended by manufacturer. Dilute higher doses in 100 ml of a compatible diluent for each gram being administered—for example, dilute a 3-g dose in at least 300 ml of diluent. Use diluted solution within 24 hours if stored at room temperature.

•**WARNING** Administer lincomycin over at least 1 hour for each gram being administered. For example, infuse 1 g over 1 hour and 3 g over 3 hours. Too-rapid infusion may result in cardiac arrest or hypotension.

•**WARNING** Monitor patient for a hypersensitivity reaction, such as rash, pruritus, wheezing, and dysphagia due to laryngeal edema. If such reactions occur, discontinue infusion and notify prescriber immediately. If anaphylaxis occurs, administer epinephrine, antihistamines, oxygen, and corticosteroids, as prescribed. Be aware that patients with a history of asthma or significant allergies are at increased risk for a hypersensitivity reaction.

•Observe patient for signs of superinfection, such as vaginal itching and sore mouth.

•Monitor patient for signs of pseudomembranous colitis, such as watery, loose stools. Patients with a history of GI disease, partic-

ularly colitis or regional enteritis, are at increased risk for colitis. Be aware that antibiotic-related diarrhea may be more severe and less well tolerated in elderly patients. Expect to discontinue lincomycin if diarrhea occurs.
•Monitor results of liver and renal function tests, CBC, and platelet counts periodically during lincomycin therapy.
•Before diluting drug, store it at a controlled room temperature of 20° to 25° C (68° to 77° F).

PATIENT TEACHING
•Advise patient to take lincomycin capsules with a full glass of water on an empty stomach 1 hour before or 2 hours after meals to maximize drug's effectiveness.
•Review with patient possibly serious adverse reactions associated with lincomycin use, such as difficulty breathing, rash, and chest tightness, and tell her to report any that occur.
•Inform patient that yogurt or buttermilk can help maintain intestinal flora and may decrease the risk of diarrhea.
•Stress the importance of following dosage regimen and keeping follow-up medical appointments and appointments for laboratory tests.

lindane

Bio-Well, GBH, G-well, Hexit (CAN), Kildane, Kwell, Kwellada (CAN), Kwildane, PMS-Lindane (CAN), Scabene, Thionex

Class and Category
Chemical: Benzene derivative
Therapeutic: Pediculicide, scabicide
Pregnancy category: B

Indications and Dosages
➤ *To treat scabies and pediculosis*
CREAM, LOTION
Adults and children. For scabies, thin layer applied once over entire skin surface. For pediculosis, thin layer applied once to affected skin and hair.
SHAMPOO
Adults and children. 30 ml (for short hair) or 45 ml (for long hair) applied to dry hair and worked into lather for 4 to 5 min.

Contraindications
Hypersensitivity to lindane or its components, prematurity (in neonates), seizure disorders

Mechanism of Action
Penetrates parasite skeleton and inhibits neuronal membrane function, causing seizures and death. Lindane also kills parasite eggs.

Interactions
ACTIVITIES
use of oil-based hair products: Possibly increased absorption of lindane

Adverse Reactions
CNS: Dizziness, irritability, nervousness, restlessness, seizures, unsteadiness
SKIN: Erythema, pruritus, rash, urticaria

Nursing Considerations
•Use lindane cautiously in patients at risk for CNS toxicity, such as infants and elderly patients.
•Wear gloves when applying drug. If another person will apply drug, supply gloves for use.
•For scabies, apply thin layer of preparation to dry skin and rub in thoroughly. Trim patient's nails, and apply under nails with toothbrush. Apply to body from neck down, including soles. Leave drug on for 8 to 12 hours (usually overnight), and then remove with bath or shower.
•Expect to reduce application time for infants and children to 6 to 8 hours, as prescribed, because of the risk of systemic absorption.
•Keep lindane away from mouth and eyes. Don't use on open wounds, cuts, or sores.
•Expect to administer topical steroids or oral antihistamines to reduce pruritus, which may continue for several weeks with scabies.
•For hospitalized patients, use special linen-handling precautions until treatment is completed.
•WARNING Be aware that lindane may cause seizures or other adverse CNS reactions.

PATIENT TEACHING
•Inform patient that lindane is for one-time use but may be reapplied after 1 week if she finds live lice or nits (eggs).
•Caution patient to avoid eyes, mucous membranes, and open areas of skin when applying drug and not to inhale vapors.
•Instruct patient (or parents of a child) to wear gloves when applying drug.
•For scabies, instruct patient to shake lotion bottle well before using and to apply lotion or cream in a thin layer all over body from

the neck down, avoiding face and scalp. Direct her to leave drug on for 8 to 12 hours and then wash it off in the bath or shower. Explain that itching may persist for several weeks after treatment.
• For pubic lice, instruct patient to shake lotion bottle well before using and to apply a thin layer of lotion to pubic hair and skin as well as to groin, thighs, and lower stomach if they're also affected. Direct her to leave lotion on for 12 hours and then thoroughly wash it off in the bath or shower.
• For head lice, instruct patient to shake lotion bottle well before using and to apply lotion to affected areas of head and scalp as well as nearby hairy areas and rub it in well. Tell her to leave lotion on for 12 hours and then thoroughly wash it off.
• For head or pubic lice, instruct patient to wash and dry her hair before applying lindane shampoo, especially if she uses oil-based hair products. Instruct her to shake bottle well before using and then apply shampoo to dry hair, working it in thoroughly and adding a small amount of water if needed to form good lather. Direct her to wait 4 minutes, rinse her hair well, and then dry it with a clean towel. Instruct her to use a fine-toothed comb or tweezers to remove nits or nit shells. Direct patient not to use shampoo again for 7 days and then only if she finds live lice. Caution patient not to use shampoo in the shower to avoid getting it in her eyes and mouth.
• Advise patient to wash lindane off her skin and to contact prescriber if irritation (severe itching, hives, or redness) occurs.
• Explain that if lice come back, the problem is probably reinfestation rather than treatment failure.
• Advise patient to notify family members and sexual contacts about infestation.

linezolid

Zyvox

Class and Category

Chemical: Oxazolidinone
Therapeutic: Antibiotic
Pregnancy category: C

Indications and Dosages

➤ *To treat vancomycin-resistant* Enterococcus faecium *infections, including bacteremia*

ORAL SUSPENSION, TABLETS, I.V. INFUSION
Adults. 600 mg q 12 hr for 14 to 28 days.

➤ *To treat nosocomial pneumonia caused by* Staphylococcus aureus *(methicillin-susceptible and -resistant strains) or* Streptococcus pneumoniae *(penicillin-susceptible strains only) and community-acquired pneumonia, including accompanying bacteremia, caused by* S. aureus *(methicillin-susceptible strains only) or* S. pneumoniae *(penicillin-susceptible strains only)*

ORAL SUSPENSION, TABLETS, I.V. INFUSION
Adults. 600 mg q 12 hr for 10 to 14 days.

➤ *To treat complicated skin and soft-tissue infections caused by* S. aureus *(methicillin-susceptible and -resistant strains),* Streptococcus pyogenes, *or* Streptococcus agalactiae

ORAL SUSPENSION, TABLETS, I.V. INFUSION
Adults. 600 mg q 12 hr for 10 to 14 days.

➤ *To treat uncomplicated skin and soft-tissue infections caused by* S. aureus *(methicillin-susceptible strains only) or* S. pyogenes

ORAL SUSPENSION, TABLETS
Adults. 400 mg q 12 hr for 10 to 14 days.

Incompatibilities

Don't add other drugs to linezolid solution. Don't infuse linezolid in the same I.V. line as amphotericin B, chlorpromazine hydrochloride, co-trimoxazole, diazepam, erythromycin lactobionate, pentamidine isethionate, or phenytoin sodium because these drugs are physically incompatible. Don't infuse linezolid with ceftriaxone sodium because these drugs are chemically incompatible.

Contraindications

Hypersensitivity to linezolid or its components; phenylketonuria (oral suspension)

Interactions

DRUGS
adrenergics, including pseudoephedrine and phenylpropanolamine: Enhanced vasopressor response of adrenergics, resulting in increased blood pressure
serotonergics: Possibly serotonin syndrome
FOODS
tyramine-containing foods and beverages: Possibly hypertension

J
K
L

Mechanism of Action

Linezolid inhibits bacterial protein synthesis by interfering with the translation of ribonucleic acid (RNA) to protein. In bacteria, protein synthesis begins with the binding of one 30S ribosomal subunit and one 50S ribosomal subunit to a messenger RNA (mRNA) molecule to form a 70S initiation complex. The 50S ribosomal subunit consists of 23S ribosomal RNA (rRNA) and other ribosomal subunits. Then the process of translation begins. In translation, transfer RNA (tRNA) attaches to the 50S subunit and brings specific amino acids into place. As the tRNA and amino acids fall into place, they are joined together by peptide bonds and elongate to form a polypep-

tide chain, as shown below left. This chain eventually combines with other polypeptide chains to form a complete protein molecule. After translation is complete, the ribosomal subunits fall away and are ready to combine with more mRNA to start the translation process over again.

Linezolid binds to a site on the bacterial 23S rRNA of the 50S subunit. This action prevents the formation of a functional 70S initiation complex, an essential component of the bacterial translation process. Without proper protein production, as shown below right, susceptible bacteria can't multiply. Linezolid is bacteriostatic against staphylococci and enterococci and bactericidal against most streptococci.

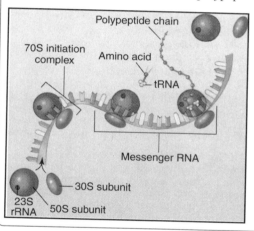

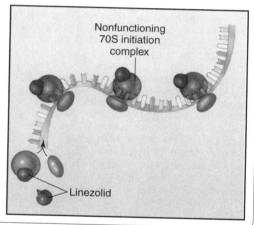

Adverse Reactions

CNS: Dizziness, fever, headache, insomnia
CV: Hypertension
EENT: Oral candidiasis, tongue discoloration
GI: Abdominal pain, constipation, diarrhea, indigestion, nausea, pseudomembranous colitis, vomiting
GU: Vaginal candidiasis
HEME: Anemia, leukopenia, pancytopenia, and thrombocytopenia
SKIN: Pruritus, rash

Nursing Considerations

• Obtain body tissue and fluid specimens for culture and sensitivity tests, as ordered, before giving first dose of linezolid. Expect to begin drug therapy before test results are known.

• Infuse I.V. solution over 30 to 120 minutes with D₅W, NS, or LR.

• **WARNING** Monitor CBC weekly, as ordered, to detect or track worsening myelosuppression in patients who need more than 2 weeks of therapy, who have pre-existing myelosuppression and are receiving drugs that produce bone marrow suppression, or who have chronic infection and are receiving or have received antibiotic therapy.

• Monitor bowel pattern daily. Assess patient for evidence of secondary infection, including oral candidiasis and profuse, watery diarrhea.

• Be aware that linezolid is a reversible non-selective monoamine oxidase inhibitor and therefore has the potential to react with adrenergics and serotonergics.

PATIENT TEACHING

• Caution patient with phenylketonuria that oral suspension contains phenylalanine.
• Advise patient not to take OTC cold remedies without consulting prescriber because medications that contain pseudoephedrine or propanolamine may cause or worsen hypertension.
• Instruct patient to avoid foods and beverages that contain large amounts of tyramine, including aged cheese, fermented or air-dried meats, sauerkraut, soy sauce, tap beers, red wines, and protein-rich foods that have been stored for long periods or poorly refrigerated.
• Instruct patient to notify prescriber immediately if severe diarrhea occurs because drug may need to be discontinued.

liothyronine sodium

(L-triiodothyronine, sodium L-triiodothyronine, T₃, thyronine sodium)

Cytomel, Triostat

Class and Category

Chemical: Synthetic triiodothyronine (T₃)
Therapeutic: Thyroid hormone replacement
Pregnancy category: A

Indications and Dosages

➤ *To treat mild hypothyroidism*

TABLETS

Adults. *Initial:* 25 mcg q.d. Increased by 12.5 to 25 mcg q 1 to 2 wk until desired response occurs. *Maintenance:* 25 to 50 mcg/day.
DOSAGE ADJUSTMENT For elderly patients and those with cardiovascular disease, initial dose reduced to 5 mcg q.d. and then increased by 5 mcg q 2 wk.

➤ *To treat congenital hypothyroidism*

TABLETS

Adults and children. *Initial:* 5 mcg q.d. Increased by 5 mcg q 3 to 4 days until desired response occurs. *Maintenance:* Highly individualized.

➤ *To treat simple nontoxic goiter*

TABLETS

Adults. *Initial:* 5 mcg q.d. Increased by 5 to 10 mcg q 1 to 2 wk up to 25 mcg/day. Then

increased by 12.5 to 25 mcg/wk, as indicated. *Maintenance:* 50 to 100 mcg/day.

➤ *To treat myxedema*

TABLETS

Adults. *Initial:* 2.5 to 5 mcg q.d. Increased by 5 to 10 mcg q 1 to 2 wk up to 25 mcg/day. Then increased by 12.5 to 25 mcg q 1 to 2 wk, as indicated. *Maintenance:* 25 to 50 mcg/day.

➤ *To treat myxedema coma or premyxedema coma (severe hypothyroidism)*

I.V. INJECTION

Adults. *Initial:* 25 to 50 mcg. Repeated q 4 to 12 hr as indicated by patient's response. Then P.O. therapy is resumed as soon as possible.
DOSAGE ADJUSTMENT When treating myxedema coma in patients with known or suspected cardiovascular disease, initial dose decreased to 10 to 20 mcg.

➤ *To differentiate hyperthyroidism from euthyroidism (T₃ suppression test)*

TABLETS

Adults. 75 to 100 mcg/day for 7 days.

Route	Onset	Peak	Duration
P.O.	24 to 72 hr	48 to 72 hr	Up to 72 hr
I.V.	2 to 4 hr	2 days	Unknown

Mechanism of Action

Replaces endogenous thyroid hormone, which may exert its physiologic effects by controlling DNA transcription and protein synthesis. Liothyronine exhibits all of the following actions of endogenous thyroid hormone. The drug:
• increases energy expenditure
• accelerates the rate of cellular oxidation, which stimulates body tissue growth, maturation, and metabolism
• regulates differentiation and proliferation of stem cells
• aids in myelination of nerves and development of synaptic processes in the nervous system
• regulates growth
• decreases blood and hepatic cholesterol concentrations
• enhances carbohydrate and protein metabolism, increasing gluconeogenesis and protein synthesis.

Contraindications

Acute MI (unless caused or complicated by hypothyroidism), hypersensitivity to liothyronine or its components, uncorrected adrenal insufficiency, untreated thyrotoxicosis

Interactions

DRUGS

adrenocorticoids: Possibly need for adrenocorticoid dosage adjustments as thyroid status changes
beta blockers: Possibly impaired action of beta blockers
cholestyramine, colestipol: Decreased liothyronine absorption
digoxin: Reduced therapeutic effects of digoxin
estrogen, phenylbutazone, phenytoin: Reduced binding of liothyronine to protein, possibly requiring increased liothyronine dosage
insulin, oral antidiabetic drugs: Possibly uncontrolled diabetes mellitus, requiring increased dosage of insulin or oral antidiabetic drug
ketamine: Possibly hypertension and tachycardia
maprotiline: Increased risk of arrhythmias
oral anticoagulants: Altered anticoagulant activity, possibly need for anticoagulant dosage adjustment
sympathomimetics: Increased risk of coronary insufficiency in patients with coronary artery disease
theophylline: Decreased theophylline clearance
tricyclic antidepressants: Increased therapeutic and toxic effects of both drugs

Adverse Reactions

CNS: Insomnia
ENDO: Hyperthyroidism (with overdose)
SKIN: Alopecia (transient), rash, urticaria

Nursing Considerations

• Be aware that liothyronine is used most often when rapid onset or rapidly reversible thyroid hormone replacement is needed.
• Administer tablet as a single daily dose before breakfast.
• Give I.V. injections more than 4 hours but less than 12 hours apart.
• Evaluate response to therapy by monitoring pulse rate and blood pressure.
• Expect patient to undergo regular thyroid function tests during liothyronine therapy.
• Monitor PT of patient receiving anticoagulants; she may require a dosage adjustment.

• Frequently monitor blood glucose level of diabetic patient. Prescriber may reduce antidiabetic drug dosage as thyroid hormone level enters therapeutic range.
• Be aware that liothyronine is used in T_3 suppression test to differentiate hyperthyroidism from euthyroidism (normal thyroid function). For this test, ^{131}I uptake test is performed before and after liothyronine administration. Suppression of ^{131}I uptake by 50% indicates normal thyroid function.

PATIENT TEACHING

• Inform patient that liothyronine usually is taken for life. Caution her not to discontinue drug or change dosage unless instructed by prescriber.
• Instruct patient to take drug before breakfast because evening doses may cause insomnia.
• Advise patient to report signs of hyperthyroidism, such as chest pain, excessive sweating, heat intolerance, increased pulse rate, nervousness, and palpitations.
• Inform patient that transient hair loss may occur during first few months of therapy.
• Instruct diabetic patient to monitor blood glucose level frequently because antidiabetic drug dosage may need to be reduced.
• Inform patient of need for periodic blood tests to monitor drug effectiveness.

liotrix

Thyrolar

Class and Category

Chemical: Levothyroxine sodium (T_4) and liothyronine sodium (T_3)
Therapeutic: Thyroid hormone replacement
Pregnancy category: A

Indications and Dosage

➤ *To treat hypothyroidism without myxedema*

TABLETS

Adults and children. *Initial:* 50 mcg of levothyroxine/12.5 mcg of liothyronine q.d., increased monthly until therapeutic effects occur. *Maintenance:* 50 to 100 mcg of levothyroxine/12.5 to 25 mcg of liothyronine q.d.

➤ *To treat myxedema or hypothyroidism in patients with cardiovascular disease, to treat congenital hypothyroidism in children*

TABLETS
Adults and children. *Initial:* 12.5 mcg of levo-thyroxine/3.1 mcg of liothyronine q.d., increased q 2 to 3 wk until therapeutic effects occur. *Maintenance:* 50 to 100 mcg of levothyroxine/12.5 to 25 mcg of liothyronine q.d.
DOSAGE ADJUSTMENT For elderly patients, initial dose usually reduced to 25% to 50% of adult dose; dosage then doubled q 6 to 8 wk until therapeutic effects occur.

Mechanism of Action
Replaces endogenous thyroid hormone, which may exert its physiologic effects by controlling DNA transcription and protein synthesis. Liotrix exhibits all of the following actions of endogenous thyroid hormone. The drug:
•Increases energy expenditure
•Accelerates the rate of cellular oxidation, which stimulates growth, maturation, and metabolism of body tissues
•Regulates differentiation and proliferation of stem cells
•Aids in myelination of nerves and development of synaptic processes in the nervous system
•Regulates growth
•Decreases blood and hepatic cholesterol concentrations
•Enhances carbohydrate and protein metabolism, increasing gluconeogenesis and protein synthesis.

Contraindications
Acute MI (unless caused or complicated by hypothyroidism), hypersensitivity to liotrix or its components, uncorrected adrenal insufficiency, untreated thyrotoxicosis

Interactions
DRUGS
adrenocorticoids: Possibly need for adrenocorticoid dosage adjustments as thyroid status changes
beta blockers: Possibly impaired action of beta blockers
cholestyramine, colestipol: Decreased liotrix absorption
digoxin: Reduced therapeutic effects of digoxin
estrogen, phenylbutazone, phenytoin: Reduced binding of liotrix to protein, possibly requiring increased liotrix dosage

insulin, oral antidiabetic drugs: Possibly uncontrolled diabetes mellitus, requiring increased dosage of insulin or oral antidiabetic drug
ketamine: Possibly hypertension and tachycardia
maprotiline: Increased risk of arrhythmias
oral anticoagulants: Altered anticoagulant activity, possibly need for anticoagulant dosage adjustment
sympathomimetics: Increased risk of coronary insufficiency in patients with coronary artery disease
theophylline: Decreased theophylline clearance
tricyclic antidepressants: Increased therapeutic and toxic effects of both drugs

Adverse Reactions
CNS: Insomnia
ENDO: Hyperthyroidism (with overdose)
SKIN: Alopecia (transient), rash, urticaria

Nursing Considerations
•Be aware that liotrix is a combination product consisting of a uniform 4:1 mixture of levothyroxine and liothyronine.
•Administer liotrix tablet as a single daily dose before breakfast.
•Expect patient to undergo periodic thyroid function tests during liotrix therapy.
•Monitor patient's response to therapy, including pulse rate and blood pressure.
•Monitor PT of patient on anticoagulants; she may require a dosage adjustment.
•Frequently monitor blood glucose level of diabetic patient. Prescriber may reduce antidiabetic drug dosage as hormone replacement is achieved.
PATIENT TEACHING
•Inform patient that liotrix usually is taken for life. Caution her not to discontinue drug or change dosage unless instructed by prescriber.
•Instruct patient to take drug before breakfast because evening doses may cause insomnia.
•Instruct patient to report signs of hyperthyroidism, such as chest pain, excessive sweating, heat intolerance, insomnia, palpitations, and weight loss.
•Advise diabetic patient to monitor blood glucose level frequently because antidiabetic drug dosage may need to be reduced.
•Inform patient that transient hair loss may occur during first few months of therapy.

J K L

•Inform patient of need for periodic blood tests to monitor drug effectiveness.

lisinopril

Prinivil, Zestril

Class and Category

Chemical: Lysine ester of enalaprilat
Therapeutic: Antihypertensive, vasodilator
Pregnancy category: C (first trimester), D (later trimesters)

Indications and Dosages

➤ *To manage uncomplicated essential hypertension*

TABLETS

Adults. *Initial:* 10 mg/day. *Maintenance:* 20 to 40 mg/day. *Maximum:* 80 mg/day.
DOSAGE ADJUSTMENT For patients with renal failure, initial dosage reduced to 5 mg/day if creatinine clearance is 10 to 30 ml/min/ 1.73 m^2, and to 2.5 mg/day if creatinine clearance is less than 10 ml/min/1.73 m^2. For patients receiving a diuretic, initial dosage reduced to 5 mg/day.

➤ *To treat heart failure, along with digoxin and diuretics*

TABLETS

Adults. *Initial:* 5 mg/day. *Maintenance:* 5 to 20 mg/day. *Maximum:* 80 mg/day.
DOSAGE ADJUSTMENT For patients with hyponatremia or creatinine clearance of 30 ml/ min/1.73 m^2 or less, initial dosage reduced to 2.5 mg/day.

➤ *To improve survival in hemodynamically stable patient after acute MI*

TABLETS

Adults. 5 mg within 24 hr after onset of symptoms, followed by 5 mg after 24 hr and 10 mg after 48 hr. *Maintenance:* 10 mg/day for 6 wk. *Maximum:* 80 mg/day.
DOSAGE ADJUSTMENT For patients with baseline systolic blood pressure of 120 mm Hg or less, initial dosage decreased to 2.5 mg/day for first 3 days after MI. If systolic blood pressure falls to 100 mm Hg or less during therapy, maintenance dosage decreased to 2.5 to 5 mg as tolerated; if systolic blood pressure is 90 mm Hg or less for more than 1 hr, drug is discontinued.

Route	Onset	Peak	Duration
P.O.	1 hr	6 to 8 hr	24 hr

Mechanism of Action

May reduce blood pressure by inhibiting the conversion of angiotensin I to angiotensin II. Angiotensin II is a potent vasoconstrictor that also stimulates the adrenal cortex to secrete aldosterone. Lisinopril may also inhibit renal and vascular production of angiotensin II. Decreased release of aldosterone reduces sodium and water reabsorption and increases their excretion, thereby reducing blood pressure.

Contraindications

Hypersensitivity to lisinopril, other ACE inhibitors, or their components

Interactions

DRUGS

allopurinol, bone marrow depressants (such as methotrexate), procainamide, systemic corticosteroids: Increased risk of potentially fatal neutropenia or agranulocytosis
cyclosporine, potassium-sparing diuretics, potassium supplements: Increased risk of hyperkalemia
diuretics, other antihypertensives: Increased hypotensive effect
lithium: Increased blood lithium level and risk of lithium toxicity
NSAIDs, sympathomimetics: Possibly reduced antihypertensive effect

FOODS

high-potassium diet, potassium-containing salt substitutes: Increased risk of hyperkalemia

ACTIVITIES

alcohol use: Possibly increased hypotensive effect

Adverse Reactions

CNS: Dizziness, fatigue, headache, syncope, vertigo
CV: Chest pain, hypotension, orthostatic hypotension
GI: Abdominal pain, anorexia, diarrhea, indigestion, nausea, vomiting
GU: Decreased libido, impotence
HEME: Agranulocytosis, anemia, neutropenia
MS: Muscle spasms, myalgia
RESP: Cough, dyspnea, upper respiratory tract infection
SKIN: Pruritus, rash
Other: Angioedema

Nursing Considerations

• Use lisinopril cautiously in patients with fluid volume deficit, heart failure, impaired renal function, or sodium depletion.

• Monitor blood pressure frequently, especially early in treatment. If excessive hypotension develops, expect to withhold drug for several days.

• **WARNING** If angioedema affects face, glottis, larynx, limbs, lips, mucous membranes, or tongue, notify prescriber immediately and expect to discontinue lisinopril and start appropriate therapy at once. If airway obstruction threatens, promptly give 0.3 to 0.5 ml of epinephrine 1:1,000 solution S.C., as prescribed.

• Notify prescriber if patient experiences persistent, nonproductive cough; this is a common adverse effect of ACE inhibitors such as lisinopril.

• Monitor for dehydration, which can lead to hypotension. Be aware that diarrhea and vomiting can cause dehydration.

PATIENT TEACHING

• Explain to patient that lisinopril helps to control but doesn't cure hypertension and that she may need lifelong therapy.

• Advise patient to take lisinopril at the same time every day.

• Emphasize the importance of taking drug as ordered, even if patient feels well; caution her not to stop taking it without consulting prescriber.

• Instruct patient to report dizziness, especially during the first few days of therapy.

• Inform patient that a persistent, nonproductive cough may develop during lisinopril therapy. Urge her to notify prescriber immediately if cough becomes difficult to tolerate.

• Advise patient to drink adequate fluid and avoid excessive sweating, which can lead to dehydration and hypotension. Make sure she understands that diarrhea and vomiting also can cause hypotension.

• Caution patient not to use salt substitutes that contain potassium.

• Instruct patient to report signs of infection, such as fever and sore throat, which may indicate neutropenia.

• Advise patient to change position slowly to minimize effects of orthostatic hypotension.

lithium carbonate

Carbolith (CAN), Duralith (CAN), Eskalith, Eskalith CR, Lithane, Lithizine (CAN), Lithobid, Lithonate, Lithotabs

lithium citrate

Cibalith-S

Class and Category

Chemical: Alkaline metal, monovalent cation
Therapeutic: Antidepressant, antimanic
Pregnancy category: D

Indications and Dosage

➤ *To treat recurrent bipolar affective disorder, to prevent bipolar disorder depression*

CAPSULES, TABLETS

Adults and children age 12 and older. *Initial:* 300 to 600 mg t.i.d. *Maintenance:* 300 mg t.i.d. or q.i.d. *Maximum:* 2,400 g/day.
Children up to age 12. 15 to 20 mg/kg/day in divided doses b.i.d. or t.i.d.

E.R. TABLETS

Adults and children age 12 and older. *Initial:* 900 to 1,800 mg/day in divided doses b.i.d. or t.i.d. *Maintenance:* 450 mg b.i.d. or 300 mg t.i.d. *Maximum:* 2,400 g/day.

SLOW-RELEASE CAPSULES

Adults and children age 12 and older. 600 to 900 mg on day 1, increased to 1,200 to 1,800 mg/day in divided doses t.i.d. *Maintenance:* 900 to 1,200 mg/day in divided doses t.i.d. *Maximum:* 2,400 g/day.

SYRUP (LITHIUM CITRATE)

Adults and children age 12 and older. 8 to 16 mEq (equivalent of 300 to 600 mg of lithium carbonate) t.i.d. *Maintenance:* Equivalent of 300 mg of lithium carbonate t.i.d. or q.i.d. *Maximum:* Equivalent of 2,400 g/day of lithium carbonate.
Children up to age 12. 0.4 to 0.5 mEq (equivalent of 15 to 20 mg of lithium carbonate)/kg/day in divided doses b.i.d. or t.i.d.

Route	Onset	Peak	Duration
P.O.	1 to 3 wk	Unknown	Unknown

Contraindications

Blood dyscrasias, bone marrow depression, brain damage, cerebrovascular disease, coma, coronary artery disease, excessive intake of other CNS depressants, hypersensitivity to lithium or its components, impaired hepatic

J
K
L

function, myeloproliferative disorders, severe depression, severe hypertension or hypotension

Mechanism of Action

May increase presynaptic degradation of the catecholamine neurotransmitters serotonin, dopamine, and norepinephrine; inhibit their release at neuronal synapses; and decrease postsynaptic receptor sensitivity. These actions may correct the overactive catecholamine systems in patients with mania.

Lithium's antidepressant action may result from enhanced serotonergic activity. The neurotransmitter serotonin is responsible for feeling of well-being.

Interactions
DRUGS

ACE inhibitors, NSAIDs, piroxicam: Possibly increased blood lithium level
acetazolamide, sodium bicarbonate, urea, xanthines: Decreased blood lithium level
calcium channel blockers, molindone: Increased risk of neurotoxicity from lithium
calcium iodide, iodinated glycerol, potassium iodide: Possibly increased hypothyroid effects of both drugs
carbamazepine: Possibly increased therapeutic effects of carbamazepine and neurotoxic effect of lithium
chlorpromazine, other phenothiazines: Possibly impaired GI absorption and decreased blood levels of these drugs; possibly masking of early signs of lithium toxicity
desmopressin, lypressin, vasopressin: Possibly impaired antidiuretic effects of these drugs
diuretics (loop and osmotic): Increased lithium reabsorption by kidneys, possibly leading to lithium toxicity
fluoxetine, methyldopa, metronidazole: Increased risk of lithium toxicity
haloperidol: Increased risk of irreversible neurotoxicity and brain damage
neuromuscular blockers: Risk of prolonged paralysis or weakness
norepinephrine: Possibly decreased therapeutic effects of norepinephrine and severe respiratory depression
thyroid hormones: Possibly hypothyroidism
tricyclic antidepressants: Possibly severe mood swings from mania to depression

FOODS

high-sodium foods: Increased excretion and possibly decreased therapeutic effects of lithium

Adverse Reactions

CNS: Ataxia, coma, confusion, depression, dizziness, drowsiness, headache, lethargy, mania, seizures, syncope, tremor (in hands), vertigo
CV: Arrhythmias (including bradycardia and tachycardia), ECG changes, edema
EENT: Dental caries, dry mouth, exophthalmos
ENDO: Diabetes insipidus, euthyroid goiter, hypothyroidism, myxedema
GI: Abdominal distention and pain, anorexia, diarrhea, nausea, thirst
GU: Stress incontinence, urinary frequency
HEME: Leukocytosis
MS: Muscle twitching and weakness
RESP: Dyspnea
SKIN: Acne; alopecia; dry, thin hair; pruritus; rash
Other: Cold sensitivity, weight gain or loss

Nursing Considerations

• Administer lithium after meals to slow absorption from GI tract and reduce adverse reactions. Dilute syrup with juice or other flavored drink before giving.
• Note that 5 ml of lithium citrate equals 8 mEq of lithium ion or 300 mg of lithium carbonate.
• Expect to monitor blood lithium level two or three times weekly during first month and then weekly to monthly during maintenance therapy. In uncomplicated cases, plan to monitor lithium level every 2 to 3 months.
• Be aware that lithium has a narrow therapeutic range. Even a slightly high blood level is dangerous, and some patients exhibit signs of toxicity at normal levels.
• Expect prescriber to decrease dosage after acute manic episode is controlled.
• WARNING Be aware that lithium affects the normal shift of intracellular and extracellular potassium ions, which can cause ECG changes, such as flattened or inverted T waves, and can increase the risk of cardiac arrest.
• Monitor ECGs, renal and thyroid function test results, and serum electrolyte levels, as appropriate, during lithium treatment.
• WARNING Be aware that lithium can cause reversible leukocytosis, which usually peaks

within 7 to 10 days of initiating therapy; WBC count typically returns to baseline within 10 days after lithium is discontinued.
• Weigh patient daily to detect sudden weight changes.
• Frequently monitor blood glucose level in diabetic patient because lithium alters glucose tolerance.
• Palpate thyroid gland to detect enlargement because drug may cause goiter.
• Ensure that patient's fluid and sodium intake is adequate during treatment.

PATIENT TEACHING
• Advise patient to take lithium with or after meals to minimize adverse reactions.
• Instruct patient to swallow E.R. or slow-release form whole.
• Direct patient to mix syrup form with juice or other flavored drink before taking.
• Inform patient that frequent urination, nausea, and thirst may occur during the first few days of treatment.
• Caution patient not to stop taking lithium or adjust dosage without first consulting prescriber.
• Instruct patient to report signs of toxicity, such as diarrhea, drowsiness, muscle weakness, tremor, uncoordinated body movements, and vomiting.
• Urge patient to avoid potentially hazardous activities until drug's CNS effects are known.
• Advise patient to maintain normal fluid and sodium intake.
• Emphasize the importance of complying with scheduled checkups and laboratory tests.

lomefloxacin hydrochloride

Maxaquin

Class and Category
Chemical: Fluoroquinolone
Therapeutic: Antibiotic
Pregnancy category: C

Indications and Dosage
➤ *To treat mild to moderate lower respiratory tract infections caused by susceptible organisms, including* Haemophilus influenzae *and* Moraxella catarrhalis

TABLETS
Adults. 400 mg q.d. for 10 days.
➤ *To treat uncomplicated cystitis caused by* Escherichia coli; *to treat uncomplicated cystitis caused by* Klebsiella pneumoniae, Proteus mirabilis, *or* Staphylococcus saprophyticus

TABLETS
Adults. 400 mg q.d. for 3 days.
➤ *To treat complicated UTIs caused by* Citrobacter diversus, Enterobacteriaceae, E. coli, K. pneumoniae, P. mirabilis, *or* Pseudomonas aeruginosa

TABLETS
Adults. 400 mg q.d. for 14 days.
➤ *To provide prophylaxis for transurethral surgery*

TABLETS
Adults. 400 mg as a single dose 2 to 6 hr before surgery.
➤ *To provide prophylaxis for transrectal biopsy*

TABLETS
Adults. 400 mg as a single dose 1 to 6 hr before surgery.
➤ *To treat gonorrhea (as alternative to ciprofloxacin or ofloxacin)*

TABLETS
Adults. 400 mg as a single dose.
DOSAGE ADJUSTMENT For patients with creatinine clearance between 11 and 39 ml/min/1.73 m², loading dose of 400 mg given on day 1 and followed by 200 mg q.d.

Mechanism of Action
Inhibits the bacterial enzyme DNA gyrase, which normally is responsible for the unwinding and supercoiling of bacterial DNA before it replicates. By inhibiting this enzyme, lomefloxacin interferes with bacterial cell replication and causes cell death.

Contraindications
History of tendinitis or tendon rupture, hypersensitivity to lomefloxacin or any quinolone derivative

Interactions
DRUGS
aluminum-, calcium-, or magnesium-containing antacids; iron salts; sucralfate; zinc: De-

creased absorption and blood level of lomefloxacin
cyclosporine: Possibly increased blood cyclosporine level, increased nephrotoxicity
probenecid: Decreased lomefloxacin excretion, increased risk of toxicity
warfarin: Possibly increased anticoagulant effect and risk of bleeding

Adverse Reactions
CNS: Dizziness, drowsiness, hallucinations, headache, insomnia, nervousness, vertigo
EENT: Oral candidiasis, taste perversion
GI: Abdominal pain, diarrhea, indigestion, nausea, pseudomembranous colitis, vomiting
GU: Vaginal candidiasis
MS: Tendinitis, tendon rupture
SKIN: Photosensitivity
Other: Anaphylaxis

Nursing Considerations
•Expect to obtain body fluid or tissue sample for culture and sensitivity testing and to review results, if possible, before lomefloxacin therapy begins.
•If patient's culture test results are positive for gonorrhea, expect to obtain serologic test for syphilis at the time of diagnosis and to repeat test 3 months after lomefloxacin therapy.
•Administer drug with meals and with a full glass of water.
•Ensure that patient maintains adequate fluid intake during therapy.
•Observe for signs of secondary infections, such as sore mouth or vaginal discharge.
•Notify prescriber if patient experiences severe or prolonged diarrhea, which may indicate pseudomembranous colitis.
•Monitor for tendon inflammation, pain, or rupture, especially in shoulders, hands, and Achilles tendons.
•Be aware that prolonged use of lomefloxacin may lead to growth of drug-resistant organisms.
PATIENT TEACHING
•Advise patient to take lomefloxacin at the same time each day with meals and with a full glass of water.
•Caution patient not to take antacids, iron, sucralfate, or zinc 1 hour before or 2 hours after taking lomefloxacin because these preparations impair drug absorption.
•Urge patient to drink plenty of fluids during treatment.

•Instruct patient to complete the full course of therapy, even if symptoms subside.
•Advise patient to notify prescriber if symptoms don't improve within a few days after starting lomefloxacin or if severe GI distress or diarrhea develops.
•Instruct patient to notify prescriber and stop taking drug if she experiences tendon inflammation or pain and to rest until tendinitis and tendon rupture have been ruled out.
•Urge patient to avoid direct sunlight, to wear protective clothing, and to use sunscreen because photosensitivity reactions can occur during therapy and for several days afterward.
•Caution patient to avoid potentially hazardous activities until drug's CNS effects are known.

loracarbef

Lorabid

Class and Category
Chemical: Carbacephem
Therapeutic: Antibiotic
Pregnancy category: B

Indications and Dosages
➤ *To treat acute bronchitis caused by* Haemophilus influenzae, Moraxella catarrhalis, *or* Streptococcus pneumoniae
CAPSULES, ORAL SUSPENSION
Adults and adolescents. 200 to 400 mg q 12 hr for 7 days.

➤ *To treat chronic bronchitis exacerbations caused by* H. influenzae, M. catarrhalis, *or* S. pneumoniae
CAPSULES, ORAL SUSPENSION
Adults and adolescents. 400 mg q 12 hr for 7 days.

➤ *To treat pneumonia caused by* H. influenzae *or* S. pneumoniae
CAPSULES, ORAL SUSPENSION
Adults and adolescents. 400 mg q 12 hr for 14 days.

➤ *To treat pharyngitis, sinusitis, or tonsillitis caused by* Streptococcus pyogenes
CAPSULES, ORAL SUSPENSION
Adults and adolescents. 200 to 400 mg q 12 hr for 10 days.
Children. 7.5 mg/kg q 12 hr for 10 days.

➤ *To treat acute otitis media caused by* H. influenzae, M. catarrhalis, S. pneumoniae, *or* S. pyogenes
ORAL SUSPENSION
Children. 15 mg/kg q 12 hr for 10 days.

➤ *To treat uncomplicated skin and soft-tissue infections caused by* Staphylococcus aureus *or* S. pyogenes
CAPSULES, ORAL SUSPENSION
Adults and adolescents. 200 mg q 12 hr for 7 days.
ORAL SUSPENSION
Children. 7.5 mg/kg q 12 hr for 7 days.

➤ *To treat uncomplicated cystitis caused by* Escherichia coli *or* Staphylococcus saprophyticus
CAPSULES, ORAL SUSPENSION
Adults and adolescents. 200 mg q.d. for 7 days.

➤ *To treat uncomplicated pyelonephritis caused by* E. coli
CAPSULES, ORAL SUSPENSION
Adults and adolescents. 400 mg q 12 hr for 14 days.
DOSAGE ADJUSTMENT For patients with creatinine clearance of 10 to 49 ml/min/1.73 m², 50% of usual dose given at normal dosing interval or usual dose given at twice the normal dosing interval; with creatinine clearance of less than 10 ml/min/1.73 m², usual adult dosage given q 3 to 5 days.

Mechanism of Action
Interferes with bacterial cell wall synthesis by inhibiting the final step in the cross-linking of peptidoglycan strands. Peptidoglycan makes the bacterial cell membrane rigid and protective. Without it, bacterial cells rupture and die.

Contraindications
Hypersensitivity to loracarbef, other cephalosporins, or their components

Interactions
DRUGS
probenecid: Inhibited renal excretion of loracarbef, resulting in increased blood level
FOODS
all foods: Inhibited drug absorption

Adverse Reactions
CNS: Dizziness, drowsiness, headache, insomnia, nervousness, seizures

EENT: Oral candidiasis
GI: Abdominal pain, anorexia, diarrhea, nausea, pseudomembranous colitis, vomiting
GU: Vaginal candidiasis
SKIN: Pruritus, rash, urticaria

Nursing Considerations
•Expect to obtain body fluid or tissue sample for culture and sensitivity testing and to review results, if possible, before giving first dose of loracarbef.
•Be aware that oral suspension is absorbed more rapidly and produces a higher peak plasma level than capsules.
•Monitor for signs of secondary infections, such as sore mouth and vaginal discharge.
•Monitor for seizures, especially if patient has impaired renal function.
PATIENT TEACHING
•Advise patient to take loracarbef at least 1 hour before or 2 hours after meals.
•Instruct patient to complete the full course of therapy as prescribed, even if symptoms decrease.
•Instruct patient to discard unused oral solution after 14 days.
•Advise patient to report diarrhea, hives, or severe rash to prescriber.

lorazepam

Apo-Lorazepam (CAN), Ativan, Lorazepam Intensol, Novo-Lorazem (CAN), Nu-Loraz (CAN)

Class, Category, and Schedule
Chemical: Benzodiazepine
Therapeutic: Amnestic, antianxiety, anticonvulsant, sedative
Pregnancy category: D (parenteral), Not rated (oral)
Controlled substance: Schedule IV

Indications and Dosages
➤ *To treat anxiety*
ORAL CONCENTRATE, TABLETS
Adults and adolescents. 1 to 3 mg b.i.d. or t.i.d. *Maximum:* 10 mg/day.
DOSAGE ADJUSTMENT For elderly or debilitated patients, initial dosage possibly reduced to 0.5 to 2 mg/day in divided doses.

➤ *To treat insomnia caused by anxiety*
ORAL CONCENTRATE, TABLETS
Adults and adolescents. 2 to 4 mg h.s.
DOSAGE ADJUSTMENT Dosage possibly reduced for elderly or debilitated patients.

> *To provide preoperative sedation*

I.V. INJECTION

Adults and adolescents. 0.044 mg/kg or 2 mg, whichever is less, given 2 hr before procedure. *Maximum:* 0.05 mg/kg or total of 4 mg.

I.M. INJECTION

Adults and adolescents. 0.05 mg/kg 2 hr before procedure. *Maximum:* 4 mg.

> *To treat status epilepticus*

I.V. INJECTION

Adults and adolescents. *Initial:* 4 mg at a rate of 2 mg/min. Repeated in 10 to 15 min if seizures don't subside. *Maximum:* 8 mg/ 24 hr.

Route	Onset	Peak	Duration
I.V.	5 min	Unknown	12 to 24 hr
I.M.	15 to 30 min	Unknown	12 to 24 hr

Mechanism of Action

May potentiate the effects of gamma-aminobutyric acid (GABA) and other inhibitory neurotransmitters by binding to specific benzodiazepine receptors in the limbic and cortical areas of the CNS. GABA inhibits excitatory stimulation, which helps control emotional behavior. The limbic system contains a highly dense area of benzodiazepine receptors, which may explain the drug's antianxiety effects. Also, lorazepam hyperpolarizes neuronal cells, thereby interfering with their ability to generate seizures.

Incompatibilities

Don't mix I.V. lorazepam in same syringe as buprenorphine.

Contraindications

Acute angle-closure glaucoma, hypersensitivity to lorazepam or its components, intra-arterial administration, psychosis

Interactions

DRUGS

CNS depressants: Additive CNS depression
digoxin: Possibly increased blood digoxin level and risk of digitalis toxicity
fentanyl: Possibly decreased therapeutic effects of fentanyl
probenecid: Possibly increased therapeutic and adverse effects of lorazepam

ACTIVITIES

alcohol use: Increased CNS depression

Adverse Reactions

CNS: Amnesia, anxiety, ataxia, confusion, delusions, depression, dizziness, drowsiness, euphoria, headache, hypokinesia, irritability, malaise, nervousness, slurred speech, tremor
CV: Chest pain, palpitations, tachycardia
EENT: Blurred vision, dry mouth, increased salivation, photophobia
GI: Abdominal pain, constipation, diarrhea, nausea, thirst, vomiting
GU: Libido changes
SKIN: Diaphoresis
Other: Injection site pain (I.M.) or phlebitis (I.V.), physical and psychological dependence, withdrawal symptoms

Nursing Considerations

• Use extreme caution when giving lorazepam to elderly patients because it can cause hypoventilation.
• Inject I.M. lorazepam deep into a large muscle mass, such as the gluteus maximus.
• Dilute I.V. drug with equal amount of sterile water for injection, sodium chloride for injection, or D₅W. Give diluted drug slowly, at a rate not to exceed 2 mg/min.
• During I.V. use, monitor respirations every 5 to 15 minutes and keep emergency resuscitation equipment readily available.
• Because abrupt drug discontinuation increases the risk of withdrawal symptoms, expect to taper dosage gradually, especially in epileptic patients.

PATIENT TEACHING

• Instruct patient to take lorazepam exactly as prescribed and not to stop drug without consulting prescriber because of the risk of withdrawal symptoms.
• Advise patient to avoid potentially hazardous activities until drug's CNS effects are known.
• Urge patient to avoid alcohol while taking lorazepam because it increases drug's CNS depressant effects.
• Instruct patient to report excessive drowsiness and nausea.

losartan potassium

Cozaar

Class and Category

Chemical: Angiotensin II receptor antagonist
Therapeutic: Antihypertensive

Pregnancy category: C (first trimester), D (later trimesters)

Indications and Dosages

➤ *To manage hypertension*

TABLETS

Adults. *Initial:* 50 mg q.d. *Maintenance:* 25 to 100 mg as a single dose or in divided doses b.i.d.

Route	Onset	Peak	Duration
P.O.	Unknown	6 hr	Over 24 hr

Mechanism of Action

Blocks binding of angiotensin II to receptor sites in many tissues, including vascular smooth muscle and adrenal glands. Angiotensin II is a potent vasoconstrictor that also stimulates the adrenal cortex to secrete aldosterone. The inhibiting effects of angiotensin II reduce blood pressure.

Contraindications

Hypersensitivity to losartan or its components

Interactions

DRUGS

cyclosporine, potassium-sparing diuretics, potassium supplements: Increased risk of hyperkalemia
diuretics, other antihypertensives: Possibly hypotension
indomethacin, NSAIDs, sympathomimetics: Possibly decreased antihypertensive effect of losartan

FOODS

high-potassium diet, potassium-containing salt substitutes: Increased risk of hyperkalemia

Adverse Reactions

CNS: Dizziness, fatigue, headache, insomnia
CV: Hypotension
EENT: Nasal congestion
GI: Diarrhea, indigestion, nausea, vomiting
MS: Back pain, leg pain, muscle spasms
RESP: Cough, upper respiratory tract infection
Other: Hyperkalemia

Nursing Considerations

• Be aware that losartan is more effective in some patients when given in two divided doses daily and that it may be used with other antihypertensives.

• **WARNING** Be aware that patients with severe heart failure or renal artery stenosis may experience acute renal failure because losartan inhibits the angiotensin-aldosterone system, on which renal function depends. Monitor such patients closely.
• Frequently monitor blood pressure to evaluate drug effectiveness.
• Periodically monitor serum potassium level, as appropriate, to detect hyperkalemia.

PATIENT TEACHING

• Instruct patient taking losartan to avoid potassium-containing salt substitutes, which can increase the risk of hyperkalemia.
• To reduce the risk of dehydration and hypotension, advise patient to avoid exercise in hot weather and excessive alcohol use. Also instruct her to notify prescriber if she experiences prolonged diarrhea, nausea, or vomiting.
• Caution patient to avoid potentially hazardous activities until drug's CNS effects are known.
• Explain the importance of regular exercise, proper diet, and other lifestyle changes in controlling hypertension.

lovastatin

(mevinolin)

Mevacor

Class and Category

Chemical: Mevinic acid derivative
Therapeutic: Antihyperlipidemic
Pregnancy category: X

Indications and Dosages

➤ *To reduce LDL and total cholesterol levels in patients with primary hypercholesterolemia*

TABLETS

Adults. *Initial:* 20 mg as a single dose with evening meal. *Maintenance:* 20 to 80 mg/day as a single dose or in divided doses with meals. *Maximum:* 80 mg/day.

DOSAGE ADJUSTMENT For patients who also take immunosuppressants, initial dosage decreased to 10 mg q.d. and maximum dosage limited to 20 mg q.d. For patients with creatinine clearance of less than 30 ml/min/1.73 m², maximum dosage limited to 20 mg q.d.

➤ *To reduce LDL, total cholesterol, and apolipoprotein B levels in adolescents with heterozygous familial hypercholesterolemia*

TABLETS

Adolescents 1 yr post-menarche (ages 10 to 17). *Initial:* 20 mg/day for LDL reduction of 20% or more, 10 mg/day for LDL reduction of less than 20%; dosage adjusted after at least 4 wk. *Maintenance:* 10 to 40 mg/day. *Maximum:* 40 mg/day.

Route	Onset	Peak	Duration
P.O.	In 2 wk	Unknown	4 to 6 wk

Mechanism of Action

Interferes with the hepatic enzyme hydroxymethylglutaryl-coenzyme A reductase. By doing so, lovastatin reduces the formation of mevalonic acid (a cholesterol precursor), thus interrupting the pathway by which cholesterol is synthesized. When the cholesterol level declines in hepatic cells, LDLs are consumed, which also reduces the amount of circulating total cholesterol and serum triglycerides. The decrease in LDLs may result in a decreased level of apolipoprotein B, which is found within each LDL particle.

Contraindications

Acute hepatic disease, breast-feeding, hypersensitivity to lovastatin or its components, pregnancy, unexplained elevated liver function test results

Interactions

DRUGS

bile acid sequestrants, cholestyramine, colestipol: Decreased lovastatin bioavailability
cyclosporine, erythromycin, fibric acid derivatives, immunosuppressants, niacin: Increased risk of severe myopathy or rhabdomyolysis
isradipine: Increased hepatic clearance of lovastatin
itraconazole, ketoconazole: Increased blood lovastatin level
oral anticoagulants: Increased anticoagulant effect and risk of bleeding

FOODS

all foods: Increased lovastatin absorption

ACTIVITIES

alcohol use: Increased blood lovastatin level

Adverse Reactions

CNS: Dizziness, fatigue, headache, insomnia
EENT: Blurred vision, cataracts, pharyngitis, rhinitis, sinusitis
GI: Abdominal cramps and pain, constipation, diarrhea, flatulence, indigestion, nausea, vomiting
MS: Arthritis, back pain, myalgia, myositis, rhabdomyolysis
RESP: Cough, upper respiratory tract infection
SKIN: Pruritus, rash

Nursing Considerations

• Monitor liver function test results before and during lovastatin therapy.
• Administer lovastatin 1 hour before or 4 hours after giving bile acid sequestrant, cholestyramine, or colestipol.
• Expect patient to follow a standard low-cholesterol diet during therapy.
• Be aware that drug exerts effects mainly on total cholesterol and LDL levels and has only slight effects on HDL and triglyceride levels.

PATIENT TEACHING

• Instruct patient who takes lovastatin once daily to take it with the evening meal to enhance absorption.
• Advise patient to report muscle aches and pains, severe GI distress, and vision changes.
• Urge patient to avoid alcohol while taking drug.
• Direct patient to follow low-cholesterol diet as adjunct to therapy. Recommend weight loss and exercise programs as appropriate.
• Stress the importance of periodic eye examinations during therapy.
• Teach adolescent female patients appropriate contraceptive methods.

loxapine hydrochloride

Loxapac (CAN), Loxitane, Loxitane C, Loxitane IM

loxapine succinate

Loxapac (CAN), Loxitane

Class and Category

Chemical: Dibenzoxazepine derivative
Therapeutic: Antipsychotic
Pregnancy category: C

Indications and Dosages
➤ *To treat psychotic disorders and schizo-*
  phrenia
CAPSULES, ORAL SOLUTION
Adults. *Initial:* 10 mg b.i.d., increased over 7
days. *Maintenance:* 15 to 25 mg b.i.d. to
q.i.d. *Maximum:* 250 mg/day.
DOSAGE ADJUSTMENT For elderly patients,
dosage reduced to 3 to 5 mg b.i.d.
➤ *To treat acute exacerbations of psychot-*
  ic disorders
I.M. INJECTION
Adults. 12.5 to 50 mg q 4 to 6 hr or longer.
Maximum: 250 mg/day.

Route	Onset	Peak	Duration
P.O.	20 to 30 min	1.5 to 3 hr	12 hr

Mechanism of Action
May treat psychotic disorders by blocking
dopamine at postsynaptic receptors in the
brain. With prolonged use, loxapine enhances antipsychotic effects by causing
depolarization blockade of dopamine
tracts, resulting in decreased dopamine
neurotransmission.

Contraindications
Blood dyscrasias, bone marrow depression,
cerebrovascular disease, coma, coronary artery disease, hypersensitivity to loxapine or
its components, impaired hepatic function,
myeloproliferative disorders, severe drug-
induced CNS depression, severe hypertension
or hypotension

Interactions
DRUGS
amphetamines, ephedrine: Decreased effects
of these drugs
antacids, antidiarrheals (adsorbent): Possibly
decreased absorption of oral loxapine
anticholinergics: Possibly increased anticholinergic effects
anticonvulsants: Lowered seizure threshold,
increased risk of seizures
antidyskinetics: Possibly antagonized therapeutic effects of these drugs
bromocriptine: Possibly decreased therapeutic effects of bromocriptine
CNS depressants: Increased CNS depression

dopamine: Possibly decreased alpha-adrenergic
effects of dopamine
epinephrine: Possibly severe hypotension or
tachycardia, decreased effects of epinephrine
guanadrel, guanethidine, levodopa: Possibly
decreased therapeutic effects of these drugs
MAO inhibitors, tricyclic antidepressants:
Possibly increased blood levels of these drugs
and increased CNS depressant and anticholinergic effects of these drugs and loxapine
metaraminol: Possibly decreased vasopressor
effect of metaraminol
methoxamine: Possibly decreased vasopressor effect and duration of action of methoxamine
ACTIVITIES
alcohol use: Increased CNS depression

Adverse Reactions
CNS: Confusion, drowsiness, dystonia, invol-
untary motor activity, neuroleptic malignant
syndrome, pseudoparkinsonism, sleep distur-
bance, tardive dyskinesia
CV: Orthostatic hypotension
EENT: Blurred vision, dry mouth
ENDO: Galactorrhea, gynecomastia
GI: Constipation, ileus, nausea, vomiting
GU: Menstrual irregularities, sexual dysfunc-
tion, urine retention
SKIN: Photosensitivity (mild), rash
Other: Weight gain

Nursing Considerations
•Be aware that loxapine's full antipsychotic
effect may require weeks.
•Assess for signs of tardive dyskinesia, including involuntary protrusion of tongue and
chewing movements. These signs may appear
months or years after loxapine therapy begins
and may not disappear with dosage reduction.
•Observe for extrapyramidal reactions or
parkinsonian symptoms, such as excessive
salivation, masklike facies, rigidity, and
tremor, especially in first few days of treatment. Prescriber may reduce dosage to control these symptoms.
•WARNING Monitor for neuroleptic malignant
syndrome, a rare but possibly fatal adverse
reaction. Early signs include altered mental
status, arrhythmias, fever, and muscle rigidity.
PATIENT TEACHING
•Instruct patient to dilute loxapine oral solution with orange or grapefruit juice just
before taking. Advise her to use the cali-

brated dropper that accompanies the solution to ensure correct dosage.
•Direct patient to avoid taking antacids and antidiarrheals 2 hours before or after taking loxapine.
•Caution patient to avoid alcohol while taking loxapine.
•Advise patient to change position slowly to minimize effects of orthostatic hypotension.
•Urge patient to avoid potentially hazardous activities until drug's CNS effects are known.
•Advise patient to avoid prolonged exposure to sun and to use sunscreen to minimize the risk of photosensitivity.
•Encourage patient to have periodic eye examinations during therapy.

lypressin

Diapid

Class and Category
Chemical: Synthetic vasopressin analogue
Therapeutic: Antidiuretic
Pregnancy category: C

Indications and Dosages
➤ *To control and prevent dehydration, polydipsia, and polyuria in patients with neurogenic diabetes insipidus that is unresponsive to other therapy*
NASAL SOLUTION
Adults and adolescents. 1 or 2 sprays q.i.d. If more drug is needed, interval between doses is decreased rather than increasing number of sprays/dose.

Route	Onset	Peak	Duration
Intranasal	In 1 hr	0.5 to 2 hr	3 to 4 hr

Mechanism of Action
Increases cellular permeability of collecting ducts in kidneys, leading to increased urine osmolality and decreased urine output.

Contraindications
Hypersensitivity to lypressin or its components

Interactions
DRUGS
carbamazepine, chlorpropamide, clofibrate: Possibly increased antidiuretic effect
demeclocycline, lithium, norepinephrine: Decreased antidiuretic effect of lypressin

Adverse Reactions
CNS: Headache
EENT: Conjunctivitis; nasal congestion, irritation, and itching; periorbital edema and itching; rhinorrhea
GI: Abdominal cramps, diarrhea, heartburn (if excessive intranasal use causes dripping into pharynx)
RESP: Cough, transient dyspnea (if drug is accidentally inhaled)
Other: Water intoxication

Nursing Considerations
•Assess patient for nasal congestion or upper respiratory tract infection, which can reduce lypressin absorption and require larger doses or adjunct therapy.
•Administer final spray of drug at bedtime to help control nocturia.
•WARNING Be aware that inadvertent inhalation, although rare, may cause chest tightness, continuous cough, and dyspnea.
•Observe for nasal irritation during long-term therapy.
•Monitor for signs and symptoms of water intoxication, including coma, confusion, drowsiness, persistent headache, seizures, urine retention, and weight gain.
PATIENT TEACHING
•Teach patient how to administer lypressin correctly by holding head upright and bottle in a vertical position and spraying 1 or 2 sprays in each nostril with each dose.
•Instruct patient to take last dose of day at bedtime to control nocturia.
•Instruct patient to use drug exactly as prescribed. Explain that using extra sprays wastes drug.
•Advise patient to report abdominal cramps, heartburn, persistent headache, severe nasal irritation, and shortness of breath.

M

magnesium chloride

(contains 64 mg of elemental magnesium per tablet, 100 mg of elemental magnesium per enteric-coated tablet, 64 mg of elemental magnesium per E.R. tablet, and 200 mg of elemental magnesium per 1 ml of injection)

Chloromag, Mag-L-100, Slow-Mag

magnesium citrate (citrate of magnesia)

(contains 40.5 to 47 mg of elemental magnesium per 5 ml of oral solution)

Citroma, Citro-Mag (CAN)

magnesium gluconate

(contains 54 mg of elemental magnesium per 5 ml of oral solution and 27 to 29.3 mg of elemental magnesium per tablet)

Almora, Maglucate (CAN), Magonate, Magtrate

magnesium hydroxide (milk of magnesia)

(contains 135 mg of elemental magnesium per tablet, 129 to 130 mg of elemental magnesium per chewable tablet, and 164 to 328 mg of elemental magnesium per 5 ml of liquid, liquid concentrate, or oral solution)

Phillips' Chewable Tablets, Phillips' Magnesia Tablets (CAN), Phillips' Milk of Magnesia, Phillips' Milk of Magnesia Concentrate

magnesium lactate

(contains 84 mg of elemental magnesium per E.R. tablet)

Mag-Tab SR Caplets

magnesium oxide

(contains 84.5 mg of elemental magnesium per capsule and 50 to 302 mg of elemental magnesium per tablet)

Mag-200, Mag-Ox 400, Maox, Uro-Mag

magnesium sulfate

(contains 100 to 500 mg of elemental magnesium per 1 ml of injection, 1 to 5 g of elemental magnesium per 10 ml of injection, and 40 mEq per 5 mg of crystals)

Class and Category

Chemical: Cation, electrolyte
Therapeutic: Antacid, antiarrhythmic, anticonvulsant, electrolyte replacement, laxative
Pregnancy category: A (parenteral magnesium sulfate), Not rated (others)

Indications and Dosages

➤ *To correct magnesium deficiency caused by alcoholism, magnesium-depleting drugs, malnutrition, or restricted diet; to prevent magnesium deficiency based on U.S. and Canadian recommended daily allowances*

CAPSULES, CHEWABLE TABLETS, CRYSTALS, ENTERIC-COATED TABLETS, E.R. TABLETS, LIQUID, LIQUID CONCENTRATE, ORAL SOLUTION, TABLETS (MAGNESIUM CHLORIDE, CITRATE, GLUCONATE, HYDROXIDE, LACTATE [EXCEPT IN CHILDREN], OXIDE, SULFATE)

Dosage individualized based on severity of deficiency and normal recommended daily allowances listed below.

Male adults and children over age 10. 270 to 400 mg/day (130 to 250 mg/day Canadian).

Female adults and children over age 10. 280 to 300 mg/day (135 to 210 mg/day Canadian).

Pregnant females. 320 mg/day (195 to 245 mg/day Canadian).

Breast-feeding females. 340 to 355 mg/day (245 to 265 mg/day Canadian).

Children ages 7 to 10. 170 mg/day (100 to 135 mg/day Canadian).

Children ages 4 to 6. 120 mg/day (65 mg/day Canadian).

Children from birth to age 3. 40 to 80 mg/day (20 to 50 mg/day Canadian).

➤ *To treat mild magnesium deficiency*

I.M. INJECTION (MAGNESIUM SULFATE)

Adults and adolescents. 1 g q 6 hr for 4 doses.

➤ *To treat severe hypomagnesemia*

I.V. INFUSION (MAGNESIUM CHLORIDE)

Adults. 4 g diluted in 250 ml of D_5W and infused at a rate not to exceed 3 ml/min. *Maximum:* 40 g/day.

I.V. INFUSION (MAGNESIUM SULFATE)

Adults and adolescents. 5 g diluted in 1 L of I.V. solution and infused over 3 hr.

➤ *To provide supplemental magnesium in total parenteral nutrition*

I.V. INFUSION (MAGNESIUM SULFATE)

Adults. 1 to 3 g/day.

Children. 0.25 mg to 1.25 g/day.

DOSAGE ADJUSTMENT Adult dosage may be increased to 6 g/day for certain conditions, such as short-bowel syndrome.

I.M. INJECTION (MAGNESIUM SULFATE)

Adults and adolescents. Up to 250 mg/kg q 4 hr, p.r.n.

➤ *To prevent and control seizures in preeclampsia or eclampsia as well as seizures caused by epilepsy, glomerulonephritis, or hypothyroidism*

I.V. INFUSION OR INJECTION (MAGNESIUM SULFATE)

Adults. *Loading:* 4 g diluted in 250 ml of compatible solution and infused over 30 min. *Maintenance:* 1 to 2 g/hr by continuous infusion.

I.M. INJECTION (MAGNESIUM SULFATE)

Adults. 4 to 5 g q 4 hr, p.r.n.

Children. 20 to 40 mg/kg, repeated p.r.n.

➤ *To relieve indigestion associated with hyperacidity*

CHEWABLE TABLETS, LIQUID, LIQUID CONCENTRATE, ORAL SOLUTION TABLETS (MAGNESIUM HYDROXIDE)

Adults and adolescents. 400 to 1,200 mg (5 to 15 ml liquid or 2.5 to 7.5 ml liquid concentrate) up to 4 times/day with water, or 622 to 1,244 mg (tablets or chewable tablets) up to 4 times/day.

CAPSULES, TABLETS (MAGNESIUM OXIDE)

Adults and adolescents. 140 mg (capsules) t.i.d. or q.i.d. with water or milk, or 400 to 800 mg/day (tablets).

➤ *To relieve constipation, to evacuate colon for rectal or bowel examination*

LIQUID, LIQUID CONCENTRATE (MAGNESIUM HYDROXIDE)

Adults and children age 12 and older. 2.4 to 4.8 g (30 to 60 ml)/day as a single dose or in divided doses.

Children ages 6 to 11. 1.2 to 2.4 g (15 to 30 ml)/day as a single dose or in divided doses.

Children ages 2 to 5. 0.4 to 1.2 g (5 to 15 ml)/day as a single dose or in divided doses.

ORAL SOLUTION (MAGNESIUM CITRATE)

Adults and children age 12 and older. 11 to 25 g/day as a single dose or in divided doses.

Children ages 6 to 11. 5.5 to 12.5 g/day as a single dose or in divided doses.

Children ages 2 to 5. 2.7 to 6.25 g/day as a single dose or in divided doses.

CRYSTALS (MAGNESIUM SULFATE)

Adults and children age 12 and older. 10 to 30 g/day as a single dose or in divided doses.

DOSAGE ADJUSTMENT Dosage limited to 20 g of magnesium sulfate q 48 hr for patients with severe renal impairment.

Children ages 6 to 11. 5 to 10 g/day as a single dose or in divided doses.

Children ages 2 to 5. 2.5 to 5 g/day as a single dose or in divided doses.

CAPSULES, TABLETS (MAGNESIUM OXIDE)

Adults. 2 to 4 g with a full glass of water or milk, usually h.s.

Route	Onset	Peak	Duration
P.O.*	0.5 to 3 hr	Unknown	Unknown
P.O.†	20 min	Unknown	20 to 180 min
I.M.‡	1 hr	Unknown	3 to 4 hr
I.V.‡	Immediate	Unknown	About 30 min

Mechanism of Action

Assists all enzymes involved in phosphate transfer reactions that use adenosine triphosphate (ATP). Magnesium is required for normal function of the ATP-dependent sodium-potassium pump in muscle membranes. It may effectively treat digitalis glycoside–induced arrhythmias because correction of hypomagnesemia improves the sodium-potassium pump's ability to distribute potassium into intracellular spaces and because magnesium decreases calcium uptake and potassium outflow through myocardial cell membranes.

As a laxative, magnesium exerts a hyperosmotic effect in the small intestine. It causes water retention that distends the bowel and causes the duodenum to secrete cholecystokinin. This substance stimulates fluid secretion and intestinal motility.

As an antacid, magnesium reacts with water, converting magnesium oxide to magnesium hydroxide. Magnesium hydroxide rapidly reacts with gastric acid to form water and magnesium chloride, which increases gastric pH.

As an anticonvulsant, magnesium depresses the CNS and blocks peripheral neuromuscular impulse transmission by decreasing the amount of available acetylcholine.

Incompatibilities

Don't combine magnesium sulfate with alkali carbonates and bicarbonates, alkali hydroxides, arsenates, calcium, clindamycin phosphate, dobutamine, fat emulsions, heavy

---

* For laxative effect.
† For antacid effect.
‡ For anticonvulsant effect.

metals, hydrocortisone sodium succinate, phosphates, polymyxin B, procaine hydrochloride, salicylates, sodium bicarbonate, strontium, and tartrates.

Contraindications
Hypersensitivity to magnesium salts or any component of magnesium-containing preparations
For magnesium chloride: Coma, heart disease, renal impairment
For magnesium sulfate: Heart block, MI, preeclampsia 2 hours or less before delivery (I.V. form)
For magnesium used as laxative: Acute abdominal problem (as indicated by abdominal pain, nausea, or vomiting), diverticulitis, fecal impaction, intestinal obstruction or perforation, presence of colostomy or ileostomy, severe renal impairment, ulcerative colitis

Interactions
DRUGS
amphotericin B, cisplatin, cyclosporine, gentamicin: Possibly magnesium wasting and need for magnesium dosage adjustment
anticholinergics: Possibly decreased absorption and therapeutic effects of these drugs
calcium salts (I.V.): Possibly neutralization of magnesium sulfate's effects
cellulose sodium phosphate: Possibly binding with magnesium, possibly decreased therapeutic effectiveness of cellulose
CNS depressants: Possibly increased CNS depression
digoxin (I.V.): Possibly heart block and conduction changes, especially when calcium salts are also administered
digoxin, fluoroquinolones, folic acid, H₂-receptor blockers, iron preparations, isoniazid, ketoconazole, penicillamine, phenothiazines, phenytoin, phosphates (oral), tetracyclines: Possibly decreased absorption and blood levels of these drugs
diuretics (loop or thiazide): Possibly hypomagnesemia
edetate sodium, sodium polystyrene sulfonate: Possibly binding with magnesium
enteric-coated drugs: Possibly quicker dissolution of these drugs and increased risk of adverse GI reactions
etidronate (oral): Decreased etidronate absorption
mecamylamine: Possibly prolonged effects of mecamylamine
methenamine, streptomycin, sucralfate, tetracyclines, tobramycin (oral), urinary acidifiers:

Possibly decreased therapeutic effects of these drugs
misoprostol: Increased misoprostol-induced diarrhea
neuromuscular blockers: Possibly increased neuromuscular blockade
nifedipine: Possibly increased hypotensive effects when taken with magnesium sulfate
potassium-sparing diuretics: Increased risk of hypermagnesemia
salicylates: Possibly increased excretion and lower blood levels of salicylates
sodium polystyrene sulfonate resin: Possibly metabolic alkalosis
FOODS
high-glucose intake: Increased urinary excretion of magnesium
ACTIVITIES
alcohol use: Increased urinary excretion of magnesium

Adverse Reactions
CNS: Confusion, decreased reflexes, dizziness, syncope
CV: Arrhythmias, Hypotension
GI: Flatulence, vomiting
MS: Muscle cramps
RESP: Dyspnea, respiratory depression or paralysis
SKIN: Diaphoresis
Other: Allergic reaction, hypermagnesemia, injection site pain or irritation (I.M. form), laxative dependence, magnesium toxicity

Nursing Considerations
• Be aware that magnesium sulfate is the elemental form of magnesium. Oral preparations aren't all equivalent.
• Be aware that drug isn't metabolized. Drug remaining in the GI tract produces watery stool within 30 minutes to 3 hours.
• Make sure patient chews magnesium chewable tablets thoroughly before swallowing.
• Avoid giving other oral drugs within 2 hours of a magnesium-containing antacid.
• Before administering drug as a laxative, shake oral solution, liquid, or liquid concentrate well and give with a large amount of water.
• WARNING Observe for and report to prescriber early signs of hypermagnesemia: bradycardia, depressed deep tendon reflexes, diplopia, dyspnea, flushing, hypotension, nausea, slurred speech, vomiting, and weakness.
• WARNING Be aware that magnesium may precipitate myasthenic crisis by decreasing patient's sensitivity to acetylcholine.

M

• Frequently assess cardiac status of patient taking drugs that lower heart rate, such as beta blockers, because magnesium may aggravate symptoms of heart block.
• **WARNING** Be aware that magnesium chloride for injection contains the preservative benzyl alcohol, which may cause fatal toxic syndrome in neonates and premature infants.
• Provide adequate diet, exercise, and fluids for patient being treated for constipation.
• Monitor serum electrolyte levels in patients with renal insufficiency because they're at risk for magnesium toxicity.
• Be aware that magnesium salts aren't intended for long-term use.

PATIENT TEACHING
• Advise patient to chew magnesium chewable tablets thoroughly before swallowing and to follow with a full glass of water. Mention that these tablets have a chalky taste.
• Instruct patient to take magnesium-containing antacid between meals and at bedtime. Urge him not to take other drugs within 2 hours of a magnesium-containing antacid.
• Tell patient to notify prescriber and avoid using a magnesium-containing laxative if he experiences abdominal pain, nausea, or vomiting.
• Instruct patient to refrigerate magnesium citrate solution.
• Caution patient about the risk of dependence with long-term laxative use.
• Teach patient to prevent constipation by increasing dietary fiber and fluid intake and exercising regularly.
• Inform patient that magnesium supplements used to replace electrolytes can cause diarrhea.

mannitol

Osmitrol, Resectisol

Class and Category

Chemical: Hexahydroxy alcohol
Therapeutic: Antiglaucoma, diagnostic agent, osmotic diuretic, urinary irrigant
Pregnancy category: B

Indications and Dosages

➤ *To reduce intracranial or intraocular pressure*
I.V. INFUSION
Adults and adolescents. 0.25 to 2 g/kg as 15% to 25% solution given over 30 to 60 min. If used before eye surgery, 1.5 to 2 g/kg 60 to 90 min before procedure. *Maximum:* 6 g/kg/day.

DOSAGE ADJUSTMENT For small or debilitated patients, dosage reduced to 0.5 g/kg.
➤ *To diagnose oliguria or inadequate renal function*
I.V. INFUSION
Adults and adolescents. 200 mg/kg or 12.5 g as 15% to 20% solution given over 3 to 5 min. Second dose given only if patient fails to excrete 30 to 50 ml of urine in 2 to 3 hr. Drug discontinued if no response after second dose. Alternatively, 100 ml of 20% solution diluted in 180 ml of NS (forming 280 ml of 7.2% solution) and infused at 20 ml/min; followed by measurement of urine output. *Maximum:* 6 g/kg/day.
➤ *To prevent oliguria or acute renal failure*
I.V. INFUSION
Adults and adolescents. 50 to 100 g as 5% to 25% solution. *Maximum:* 6 g/kg/day.
➤ *To treat oliguria*
I.V. INFUSION
Adults and adolescents. 50 to 100 g as 15% to 25% solution given over 90 min to several hr. *Maximum:* 6 g/kg/day.
➤ *To promote diuresis in drug toxicity*
I.V. INFUSION
Adults and adolescents. *Loading:* 25 g. *Maintenance:* Up to 200 g as 5% to 25% solution given continuously to maintain urine output of 100 to 500 ml/hr with positive fluid balance of 1 to 2 L. *Maximum:* 6 g/kg/day.
➤ *To promote diuresis in hemolytic transfusion reaction*
I.V. INFUSION
Adults. 20 g given over 5 min and repeated if needed. *Maximum:* 6 g/kg/day.
➤ *To provide irrigation during transurethral resection of prostate gland*
IRRIGATION SOLUTION
Adults. 2.5% or 5% solution, as needed.

Route	Onset	Peak	Duration
I.V.*	1 to 3 hr	Unknown	Up to 8 hr
I.V.†	30 to 60 min	Unknown	4 to 8 hr
I.V.‡	In 15 min	Unknown	3 to 8 hr

* To produce diuresis.
† To decrease intraocular pressure.
‡ To decrease intracranial pressure.

Mechanism of Action
Elevates plasma osmolality, causing water to flow from tissues, such as the brain and eyes, and from CSF, into extracellular fluid, thereby decreasing intracranial and intraocular pressure.

As an osmotic diuretic, mannitol increases the osmolarity of glomerular filtrate, which decreases water reabsorption. This leads to increased excretion of water, sodium, chloride, and toxic substances.

As an irrigant, mannitol minimizes the hemolytic effects of water used as an irrigant and reduces the movement of hemolyzed blood from the urethra to the systemic circulation, which prevents hemoglobinemia and serious renal complications.

Incompatibilities
Don't administer mannitol through same I.V. line as blood or blood products.

Contraindications
Active intracranial bleeding (except during craniotomy), anuria, hepatic failure, hypersensitivity to mannitol or its components, pulmonary edema, severe dehydration, severe heart failure, severe pulmonary congestion, severe renal insufficiency

Interactions
DRUGS
digoxin: Increased risk of digitalis toxicity from hypokalemia
diuretics: Possibly increased therapeutic effects of mannitol

Adverse Reactions
CNS: Chills, dizziness, fever, headache, seizures
CV: Chest pain, heart failure, hypertension, tachycardia, thrombophlebitis
EENT: Blurred vision, dry mouth, rhinitis
GI: Diarrhea, nausea, thirst, vomiting
GU: Polyuria, urine retention
RESP: Pulmonary edema
SKIN: Extravasation with edema and tissue necrosis, rash, urticaria
Other: Dehydration, hyperkalemia, hypernatremia, hypervolemia, hypokalemia, hyponatremia (dilutional), metabolic acidosis, water intoxication

Nursing Considerations
• If crystals form in mannitol solution exposed to low temperature, place solution in hot-water bath to redissolve crystals.

• Use a 5-micron in-line filter when administering drug solution of 15% or greater.
• During I.V. infusion of mannitol, monitor vital signs, central venous pressure, and fluid intake and output every hour. Measure urine output with indwelling urinary catheter, as appropriate.
• Check weight and monitor BUN and serum creatinine electrolyte levels daily.
• Provide frequent mouth care to relieve thirst and dry mouth.
PATIENT TEACHING
• Inform patient that he may experience dry mouth and thirst during mannitol therapy.
• Instruct patient to report chest pain, difficulty breathing, or pain at I.V. site.

maprotiline hydrochloride
Ludiomil

Class and Category
Chemical: Dibenzobicyclooctadiene derivative
Therapeutic: Antidepressant, tricyclic antidepressant
Pregnancy category: B

Indications and Dosages
➤ *To treat mild to moderate depression*
TABLETS
Adults and adolescents. *Initial:* 75 mg/day in divided doses for 2 wk. Increased in 25-mg increments as needed and tolerated. *Maintenance:* 150 to 225 mg/day in divided doses; for prolonged therapy, possibly 75 to 150 mg/day in divided doses.

➤ *To treat severe depression in hospitalized patients*
TABLETS
Adults and adolescents. *Initial:* 100 to 150 mg/day in divided doses, increased as needed and tolerated. *Maintenance:* 150 to 225 mg/day in divided doses; for prolonged therapy, possibly 75 to 150 mg/day in divided doses.
DOSAGE ADJUSTMENT For patients over age 60, initial dosage reduced to 25 mg/day and then increased by 25 mg/wk up to maintenance dosage of 50 to 75 mg/day in divided doses.

Route	Onset	Peak	Duration
P.O.	1 to 3 wk	3 to 6 wk	Unknown

Mechanism of Action
Blocks norepinephrine's reuptake at adrenergic nerve fibers. Normally, when a nerve impulse reaches an adrenergic nerve fiber, norepinephrine is released from its storage sites and metabolized in the nerve or at the synapse. Some norepinephrine reaches receptor sites on target organs and tissues, but most is taken back into the nerve and stored by way of the reuptake mechanism. By blocking norepinephrine reuptake, maprotiline increases its level at nerve synapses. An elevated norepinephrine level may improve mood and, consequently, decrease depression.

Contraindications
Hypersensitivity to maprotiline, mirtazapine, or their components; use within 14 days of MAO inhibitor therapy

Interactions
DRUGS
anticholinergics, antihistamines: Increased atropine-like adverse effects, such as blurred vision, constipation, dizziness, and dry mouth
anticonvulsants: Increased risk of CNS depression, possibly lower seizure threshhold and increased risk of seizures
bupropion, clozapine, haloperidol, loxapine, molindone, other tricyclic antidepressants, phenothiazines, pimozide, thioxanthenes, trazodone: Possibly increased anticholinergic effects, possibly lowered seizure threshhold and increased risk of seizures
cimetidine: Possibly increased blood maprotiline level
clonidine, guanadrel, guanethidine: Possibly decreased antihypertensive effects of these drugs, possibly increased CNS depression (with clonidine)
CNS depressants: Increased risk of CNS depression
estrogens, oral contraceptives containing estrogen: Possibly decreased therapeutic effects and increased adverse effects of maprotiline
MAO inhibitors: Increased risk of hyperpyrexia, hypertensive crisis, severe seizures, or death
sympathomimetics: Increased risk of arrhythmias, hyperpyrexia, hypertension, or tachycardia
thyroid hormones: Increased risk of arrhythmias

ACTIVITIES
alcohol use: Increased risk of CNS depression

Adverse Reactions
CNS: Agitation, dizziness, drowsiness, fatigue, headache, insomnia, seizures, tremor, weakness
EENT: Blurred vision, dry mouth, increased intraocular pressure
ENDO: Gynecomastia
GI: Constipation, diarrhea, epigastric distress, increased appetite, nausea, vomiting
GU: Impotence, libido changes, testicular swelling, urinary hesitancy, urine retention
HEME: Agranulocytosis
SKIN: Diaphoresis, photosensitivity, pruritus, rash
Other: Weight loss

Nursing Considerations
•Give largest dose of maprotiline at bedtime if daytime drowsiness occurs.
•Check CBC as ordered, if fever, sore throat, or other signs of agranulocytosis develop.
•Take seizure precautions according to facility policy.
•Expect to taper drug dosage gradually because abrupt drug discontinuation may produce withdrawal symptoms.

PATIENT TEACHING
•Advise patient to take maprotiline exactly as prescribed. Caution him not to stop taking drug abruptly because of the risk of withdrawal symptoms, including headache, nausea, nightmares, and vertigo.
•Inform patient that he may not feel drug's effects for several weeks.
•Suggest that patient take drug with food if adverse GI reactions develop.
•Urge patient to report difficulty urinating, excessive drowsiness, fever, or sore throat.
•Advise patient to avoid potentially hazardous activities until drug's CNS effects are known.
•Urge patient to avoid alcohol and other CNS depressants while taking drug.

mecamylamine hydrochloride

Inversine

Class and Category
Chemical: Ganglionic blocker, secondary amine
Therapeutic: Antihypertensive
Pregnancy category: C

Indications and Dosages

➤ *To manage moderately severe to severe hypertension, to treat uncomplicated malignant hypertension*

TABLETS

Adults. *Initial:* 2.5 mg b.i.d. Total dosage increased by 2.5 mg q 2 days until desired response occurs. *Maintenance:* 25 mg/day in divided doses t.i.d.

Route	Onset	Peak	Duration
P.O.	0.5 to 2 hr	3 to 5 hr	6 to 12 hr

Mechanism of Action

Reduces blood pressure by blocking acetylcholine's effects at autonomic ganglia. This action decreases the effects of the sympathetic and parasympathetic nervous systems, reduces sympathetic tone in blood vessels, and causes vasodilation.

Contraindications

Chronic pyelonephritis; concurrent use of antibiotics or sulfonamides; coronary insufficiency; glaucoma; hypersensitivity to mecamylamine; mild, moderate, or labile hypertension; organic pyloric stenosis; recent MI; uncooperative behavior; uremia

Interactions

DRUGS

diuretics, other antihypertensives: Increased antihypertensive effects
urinary alkalinizers: Increased risk of mecamylamine toxicity

ACTIVITIES

alcohol use: Possibly increased effects of mecamylamine
vigorous exercise: Increased effects of mecamylamine

Adverse Reactions

CNS: Choreiform movements, confusion, dizziness, fatigue, headache, nervousness, paresthesia, seizures, syncope, tremor, weakness
CV: Hypotension, orthostatic hypotension
EENT: Blurred vision, dry mouth, mydriasis
GI: Anorexia, constipation, diarrhea, ileus, nausea, vomiting
GU: Decreased libido, impotence, urine retention
RESP: Interstitial pulmonary edema and fibrosis

Nursing Considerations

• Use mecamylamine cautiously in patients with coronary artery disease and those who have had a CVA because drug may reduce blood flow to heart and brain.
• Also use drug cautiously in patients with renal insufficiency because drug may further impair renal function and may accumulate in blood.
• Give drug after meals for more gradual absorption and more constant blood pressure control.
• Give largest doses of drug at noon and in the evening.
• Monitor blood pressure with patient standing at start of treatment to determine drug's effectiveness and need for increased dosage. Check blood pressure 3 to 5 hours after dose, during drug's peak effect.
• Expect to reduce dosage for patients with conditions that may decrease drug requirements, such as fever, infection, and sodium depletion.
• Monitor for orthostatic hypotension, especially in the morning, during hot weather, and after exercise.
• Assess bowel function and be alert for signs of ileus (abdominal cramps and distention, constipation, and diarrhea).
• Expect to discontinue drug gradually to prevent rebound hypertension.

PATIENT TEACHING

• Instruct patient to take mecamylamine after meals and at the same time every day.
• Urge patient not to use alcohol while taking drug.
• Instruct patient to change position slowly to minimize effects of orthostatic hypotension.
• Inform patient that excessive sweating, vigorous exercise, hot weather, and salt depletion can cause dizziness and hypotension.
• Caution patient to avoid potentially hazardous activities until drug's CNS effects are known.
• Instruct patient to report abdominal cramps or distention, blurred vision, persistent constipation or liquid stools, severe dizziness, shortness of breath, or tremor.
• Inform male patient that drug may cause decreased libido and impotence.
• If possible, teach patient how to monitor his blood pressure daily at home and provide guidelines for calling prescriber.

M

meclizine hydrochloride

(meclozine hydrochloride)

Antivert, Bonamine (CAN), Bonine, Dizmiss, Dramamine II, Meclicot, Medivert, Meni-D

Class and Category

Chemical: Piperazine derivative
Therapeutic: Antiemetic, antivertigo
Pregnancy category: B

Indications and Dosages

➤ *To prevent and treat vertigo*

CAPSULES, CHEWABLE TABLETS, TABLETS
Adults and adolescents. 25 to 100 mg/day, p.r.n., in divided doses.

➤ *To treat motion sickness*

CAPSULES, TABLETS
Adults. 25 to 50 mg 1 hr before travel and then q 24 hr, p.r.n., for duration of trip.

Route	Onset	Peak	Duration
P.O.	1 hr	Unknown	8 to 24 hr

Mechanism of Action

May inhibit nausea and vomiting by reducing the sensitivity of the labyrinthine apparatus and blocking cholinergic synapses in the brain's vomiting center.

Contraindications

Hypersensitivity to meclizine or its components

Interactions

DRUGS
anticholinergics: Possibly potentiated anticholinergic effects
apomorphine: Possibly decreased emetic response to apomorphine
CNS depressants: Possibly potentiated CNS depression

ACTIVITIES
alcohol use: Possibly potentiated CNS depression

Adverse Reactions

CNS: Dizziness, drowsiness, euphoria, excitement, fatigue, hallucinations, headache, insomnia, nervousness, restlessness, vertigo
CV: Hypotension, palpitations, tachycardia
EENT: Blurred vision; diplopia; dry mouth, nose, and throat; tinnitus
GI: Abdominal pain, anorexia, constipation, diarrhea, nausea, vomiting
GU: Urinary frequency and hesitancy, urine retention
RESP: Bronchospasm, thickening of respiratory secretions
SKIN: Jaundice, rash, urticaria

Nursing Considerations

•Use meclizine cautiously in patients with asthma, glaucoma, or prostate enlargement.
•Be aware that drug may mask signs of brain tumor, intestinal obstruction, or ototoxicity.

PATIENT TEACHING
•Inform patient that drug works best for motion sickness when taken before travel.
•Instruct patient to chew meclizine chewable tablets thoroughly before swallowing.
•Instruct patient to report blurred vision or drowsiness.
•Urge patient to avoid alcohol while taking drug.
•Caution patient to avoid potentially hazardous activities until drug's CNS effects are known.
•Advise patient to have regular eye examinations during long-term therapy.

meclofenamate sodium

Meclomen

Class and Category

Chemical: Fenamate (anthranilic acid) derivative
Therapeutic: Analgesic, antidysmenorrheal, anti-inflammatory, antirheumatic
Pregnancy category: Not rated

Indications and Dosages

➤ *To relieve pain and inflammation in rheumatoid arthritis and osteoarthritis*

CAPSULES
Adults and adolescents over age 14. 50 to 100 mg q 6 to 8 hr, p.r.n. *Maximum:* 400 mg/day.

➤ *To relieve mild to moderate pain*

CAPSULES
Adults and adolescents over age 14. 50 mg q 4 to 6 hr, p.r.n. Increased to 100 mg q 4 to 6 hr, if needed. *Maximum:* 400 mg/day.

➤ *To treat hypermenorrhea and primary dysmenorrhea*

CAPSULES
Adults and adolescents over age 14. 100 mg
t.i.d. for up to 6 days.

Route	Onset	Peak	Duration
P.O.*	1 hr	0.5 to 2 hr	4 to 6 hr
P.O.†	Few days	2 to 3 wk	Unknown

Mechanism of Action
Blocks the activity of cyclooxygenase, the
enzyme needed to synthesize prostaglandins, which mediate the inflammatory response and cause local vasodilation,
swelling, and pain. By blocking cyclooxygenase and inhibiting prostaglandins, this
NSAID reduces inflammatory symptoms.
This mechanism also relieves pain because prostaglandins promote pain transmission from the periphery to the spinal
cord.

Contraindications
Hypersensitivity to aspirin, iodides, meclofenamate, other NSAIDs, or their components

Interactions
DRUGS
acetaminophen: Increased risk of adverse
renal effects with long-term use of both
drugs
anticoagulants, thrombolytics: Prolonged PT
and increased risk of bleeding
antihypertensives: Decreased effectiveness of
antihypertensives
beta blockers: Impaired antihypertensive effect of beta blockers
*cefamandole, cefoperazone, cefotetan, plica-
mycin, valproic acid:* Hypoprothrombinemia
and increased risk of bleeding
cimetidine: Altered blood meclofenamate
level
*colchicine, glucocorticoids, potassium supple-
ments:* Increased GI irritability and bleeding
*cyclosporine, gold compounds, nephrotoxic
drugs:* Increased risk of nephrotoxicity
digoxin: Increased blood digoxin level
insulin, oral antidiabetic drugs: Decreased
effectiveness of these drugs
lithium: Increased risk of lithium toxicity

loop diuretics: Decreased effectiveness of
loop diuretics
methotrexate: Increased risk of methotrexate
toxicity
NSAIDs, salicylates: Increased GI irritability
and risk of bleeding, decreased meclofenamate effectiveness
phenytoin: Increased blood phenytoin level
probenecid: Increased risk of meclofenamate
toxicity
ACTIVITIES
alcohol use: Increased GI irritability and
bleeding

Adverse Reactions
CNS: Dizziness, drowsiness, fatigue, head-
ache, insomnia
CV: Peripheral edema
EENT: Stomatitis, tinnitus
GI: Abdominal pain; anorexia; constipation;
diarrhea; elevated liver function test results;
flatulence; GI bleeding, perforation, and ul-
ceration; indigestion; nausea; vomiting
GU: Dysuria, elevated BUN and serum cre-
atinine levels
HEME: Decreased hematocrit and hemoglo-
bin level
SKIN: Jaundice, pruritus, rash, urticaria

Nursing Considerations
•To minimize GI irritation, administer drug
with milk, food, or antacids that contain
aluminum or magnesium hydroxide.
•Give drug with a full glass of water.
•Expect lower doses of meclofenamate to be
used for long-term therapy.
PATIENT TEACHING
•Advise patient to take meclofenamate with
a full glass of water to prevent drug from
lodging in esophagus and causing irritation.
Also suggest taking drug with food or milk
to avoid GI distress.
•Instruct patient to report itching, rash, severe
diarrhea, and swelling in ankles or fingers.
•Caution patient to avoid potentially hazardous
activities until drug's CNS effects are known.

meloxicam

Mobic

Class and Category
Chemical: Oxicam derivative
Therapeutic: Anti-inflammatory
Pregnancy category: C

---

* For analgesic effect.
† For antirheumatic effect.

Indications and Dosages
➤ *To relieve pain due to osteoarthritis*
TABLETS
Adults. 7.5 mg q.d. *Maximum:* 15 mg/day.

Mechanism of Action
Blocks activity of cyclooxygenase, the enzyme needed to synthesize prostaglandins, which mediate the inflammatory response and cause local vasodilation, swelling, and pain. Prostaglandins also promote pain transmission from the periphery to the spinal cord. By blocking cyclooxygenase and inhibiting prostaglandins, the NSAID meloxicam reduces inflammatory symptoms and relieves pain.

Contraindications
Angioedema, asthma, bronchospasm, nasal polyps, rhinitis, or urticaria induced by hypersensitivity to aspirin, meloxicam, other NSAIDs, or their components

Interactions
DRUGS
ACE inhibitors: Decreased antihypertensive effect, increased risk of renal failure
aspirin: Increased risk of GI ulceration
furosemide: Decreased diuretic effect of furosemide, possibly renal impairment
lithium: Elevated blood lithium level, possibly lithium toxicity
warfarin and other oral anticoagulants: Increased risk of bleeding
ACTIVITIES
alcohol use, smoking: Increased risk of GI bleeding

Adverse Reactions
GI: Diarrhea, elevated liver function test results, flatulence, indigestion

Nursing Considerations
• Monitor patient for adequate hydration before beginning meloxicam therapy to decrease risk of renal dysfunction.
• **WARNING** Monitor BUN, serum creatinine, and serum electrolyte levels for early signs of impaired renal function, especially in elderly patients, patients taking diuretics, and those with heart failure or renal or hepatic dysfunction.
PATIENT TEACHING
• Instruct patient to take meloxicam with food or after meals if stomach upset occurs.

• Caution patient to avoid using other NSAIDs, aspirin, or products containing aspirin while taking meloxicam.
• Advise patient to refrain from smoking and alcohol use because these activities may increase the risk of adverse GI reactions.
• Instruct patient to notify prescriber if he develops signs or symptoms of hepatic dysfunction, such as dark yellow or brown urine, fatigue, fever, itching, lethargy, nausea, or yellowing of eyes or skin.
• Advise patient, especially if he's taking an oral anticoagulant such as warfarin, to report immediately signs of bleeding, such as easy bruising, stomach pain, blood in urine, or black tarry stools.

meperidine hydrochloride
(pethidine hydrochloride)
Demerol

Class, Category, and Schedule
Chemical: Phenylpiperidine derivative opioid
Therapeutic: Analgesic
Pregnancy category: Not rated
Controlled substance: Schedule II

Indications and Dosages
➤ *To relieve moderate to severe pain*
SYRUP, TABLETS, I.M. OR S.C. INJECTION
Adults. 50 to 150 mg q 3 to 4 hr, p.r.n.
Children. 1.1 to 1.8 mg/kg q 3 to 4 hr, p.r.n.
➤ *To provide preoperative sedation*
I.V. INJECTION
Adults. 15 to 35 mg/hr, p.r.n.
I.M. OR S.C. INJECTION
Adults. 50 to 100 mg 30 to 90 min before surgery.
Children. 1 to 2 mg/kg 30 to 90 min before surgery. *Maximum:* 100 mg q 3 to 4 hr.
➤ *As adjunct to anesthesia*
I.V. INFUSION OR INJECTION
Adults. Individualized. Repeated slow injections of 10 mg/ml solution or continuous infusion of dilute solution (1 mg/ml) titrated as needed.
➤ *To provide obstetric analgesia*
I.M. OR S.C. INJECTION
Adults. 50 to 100 mg given with regular, painful contractions; repeated q 1 to 3 hr.
DOSAGE ADJUSTMENT For patients with creatinine clearance of 10 to 50 ml/min/1.73 m^2,

75% of usual dose is used; with creatinine clearance of less than 10 ml/min/1.73 m², 50% of usual dose is used.

Route	Onset	Peak	Duration
P.O.	15 min	1 to 1.5 hr	2 to 4 hr
I.V.	1 min	5 to 7 min	2 to 4 hr
I.M., S.C.	10 to 15 min	30 to 50 min	2 to 4 hr

Mechanism of Action
Binds with opiate receptors in the spinal cord and higher levels of the CNS. In this way, meperidine stimulates mu and kappa receptors, which alters the perception of and emotional response to pain.

Incompatibilities
Don't mix meperidine in same syringe with aminophylline, barbiturates, heparin, iodides, methicillin, morphine sulfate, phenytoin, sodium bicarbonate, sulfadiazine, or sulfisoxazole.

Contraindications
Acute asthma; hypersensitivity to meperidine, narcotics, or their components; increased intracranial pressure; severe respiratory depression; upper respiratory tract obstruction; use within 14 days of MAO inhibitor therapy

Interactions
DRUGS
alfentanil, CNS depressants, fentanyl, sufentanil: Increased risk of CNS and respiratory depression and hypotension
amphetamines, MAO inhibitors: Risk of increased CNS excitation or depression with possibly fatal reactions
anticholinergics: Increased risk of severe constipation
antidiarrheals (such as loperamide and difenoxin and atropine): Increased risk of severe constipation and increased CNS depression
antihypertensives: Increased risk of hypotension
buprenorphine: Possibly decreased therapeutic effects of meperidine and increased risk of respiratory depression
hydroxyzine: Increased risk of CNS depression and hypotension

metoclopramide: Possibly decreased effects of metoclopramide
naloxone, naltrexone: Decreased pharmacologic effects of meperidine
neuromuscular blockers: Increased risk of prolonged respiratory and CNS depression
oral anticoagulants: Possibly increased anticoagulant effect and risk of bleeding
ACTIVITIES
alcohol use: Possibly increased CNS and respiratory depression and hypotension

Adverse Reactions
CNS: Confusion, depression, dizziness, drowsiness, euphoria, headache, increased intracranial pressure, lack of coordination, malaise, nervousness, nightmares, restlessness, seizures, syncope, tremor
CV: Hypotension, orthostatic hypotension, tachycardia
EENT: Blurred vision, diplopia, dry mouth
GI: Abdominal cramps or pain, anorexia, constipation, ileus, nausea, vomiting
GU: Dysuria, urinary frequency, urine retention
RESP: Dyspnea, respiratory arrest or depression, wheezing
SKIN: Diaphoresis, flushing, pruritus, rash, urticaria
Other: Injection site pain, redness, and swelling; physical and psychological dependence

Nursing Considerations
•Use meperidine with extreme caution in patients with acute abdominal conditions, hepatic or renal disorders, hypothyroidism, prostatic hyperplasia, seizures, or supraventricular tachycardia.
•To minimize local anesthetic effect, dilute syrup with water before administration.
•Give I.V. dose slowly by direct injection or as a slow continuous infusion. Mix with D₅W, NS, or Ringer's or LR solution.
•Keep naloxone available when giving I.V. meperidine.
•Be aware that S.C. injection is painful and isn't recommended.
•Be aware that oral form of meperidine is less than half as effective as parenteral meperidine. Give I.M. form when possible, and expect to increase dosage when switching patient to oral form.
•Monitor respiratory and cardiovascular status during treatment. Notify prescriber

M

immediately and expect to discontinue drug if respiratory rate falls below 12 breaths/minute or if respiratory depth decreases.
• Monitor bowel function to detect constipation, and assess the need for stool softeners.
• Assess for signs of physical dependence and abuse.
• Expect withdrawal symptoms to occur if drug is abruptly withdrawn after long-term use.

PATIENT TEACHING
• Inform patient that meperidine is a controlled substance and that he'll need identification to purchase it.
• Advise patient to take drug exactly as prescribed.
• Instruct patient to report constipation, severe nausea, and shortness or breath.
• Advise patient to avoid potentially hazardous activities until drug's CNS effects are known. Caution ambulatory patient to take extra precautions because of the risk of drowsiness.
• Instruct patient to prevent postoperative atelectasis by turning, coughing, and deep-breathing.
• Urge patient to avoid alcohol, sedatives, and tranquilizers during meperidine therapy.

mephentermine sulfate

Wyamine

Class and Category

Chemical: Sympathomimetic amine
Therapeutic: Vasopressor
Pregnancy category: C

Indications and Dosages

➤ *To treat hypotension secondary to spinal anesthesia*

I.V. INJECTION
Adults. 30 to 45 mg (15 mg for obstetric patients); may be repeated, as needed, to maintain blood pressure.

I.V. INFUSION
Adults. Dosage individualized based on patient response to therapy. Average dose is 1 to 5 mg/min.

Route	Onset	Peak	Duration
I.V.	Almost immediate	Unknown	15 to 30 min

Mechanism of Action

Stimulates alpha-adrenergic receptors directly and indirectly, resulting in positive inotropic and chronotropic effects. Indirect stimulation occurs by the release of norepinephrine from its storage sites in the heart and other tissues. By enhancing cardiac contraction, mephentermine improves cardiac output, thereby increasing blood pressure. Increased peripheral resistance from peripheral vasoconstriction may also contribute to increased blood pressure. Mephentermine can affect the heart rate but the change is variable, based on vagal tone. It may also stimulate beta-adrenergic receptors.

Contraindications

Hypersensitivity to mephentermine, phenothiazine-induced hypotension, use within 14 days of MAO inhibitor therapy

Interactions

DRUGS
alpha blockers and other drugs with alpha-blocking effects: Possibly decreased peripheral vasoconstrictive and hypertensive effects of mephentermine
beta blockers (ophthalmic): Decreased effects of mephentermine; increased risk of bronchospasm, wheezing, decreased pulmonary function, and respiratory failure
beta blockers (systemic): Increased risk of bronchospasm, decreased effects of both drugs
diuretics and other antihypertensives: Possibly reduced effectiveness of these drugs
doxapram: Possibly increased vasopressor effects of either drug
ergot alkaloids: Increased vasopressor effects
guanadrel, guanethidine, mecamylamine, methyldopa, reserpine: Possibly decreased effects of these drugs and increased risk of adverse effects
hydrocarbon inhalation anesthetics: Increased risk of atrial and ventricular arrhythmias
MAO inhibitors: Intensified and extended cardiac stimulation and vasopressor effects, possibly severe headache and hypertensive crisis
maprotiline, tricyclic antidepressants: Increased vasopressor response; increased risk

of prolonged QTc interval, arrhythmias, hypertension, and hyperpyrexia
methylphenidate: Possibly increased vasopressor effect of mephentermine
nitrates: Possibly reduced antianginal effects of nitrates and decreased vasopressor effect
other sympathomimetics (such as dopamine): Possibly increased cardiac effects and adverse reactions
oxytocin: Possibly severe hypertension
thyroid hormones: Increased effects of both drugs, increased risk of coronary insufficiency in patients with coronary artery disease

Adverse Reactions
CNS: Anxiety, dizziness, drowsiness, euphoria, headache, incoherence, nervousness, psychosis, restlessness, seizures, weakness
CV: Angina, arrhythmias (including bradycardia, tachycardia, and ventricular arrhythmias), hypertension, hypotension, palpitations, peripheral vasoconstriction
GI: Nausea, vomiting
RESP: Dyspnea
SKIN: Peripheral necrosis

Nursing Considerations
• Before administering mephentermine, expect to intervene, as ordered, to correct hemorrhage, hypovolemia, metabolic acidosis, or hypoxia.
• Discard vial if you observe discoloration or precipitate.
• Using D_5W or NS, prepare a 1-mg/ml concentration solution for infusion.
• Administer drug using an infusion pump to provide a controlled rate.
• Monitor blood pressure, cardiac rate and rhythm, central venous pressure (if appropriate), and urine output during administration. Adjust infusion rate according to patient response, as ordered. Be aware that patients with a history of cardiovascular disease (including hypertension) or hyperthyroidism and chronically ill patients are at increased risk for mephentermine's adverse cardiovascular effects.
• Assess patients with angle-closure glaucoma for signs of an exacerbation, such as eye pain or blurred vision.
• Assess circulation in patients with a history of occlusive vascular disease, such as athero-

sclerosis and Raynaud's disease, because mephentermine may cause decreased circulation and increase the risk of necrosis or gangrene. Inspect I.V. site periodically for signs of extravasation.
• **WARNING** Be aware that weeping, excitability, seizures, and hallucinations are some of the symptoms of mephentermine overdose. Contact prescriber immediately if patient experiences such symptoms, and expect to provide supportive treatment.
• Be aware that mephentermine can increase contractions in pregnant women, especially during the third trimester. Expect drug to be prescribed only when benefits outweigh potential adverse effects.
• Store drug at 15° to 30° C (59° to 86° F); don't freeze.
PATIENT TEACHING
• Instruct patient receiving mephentermine to report adverse reactions, including chest pain, difficulty breathing, dizziness, irregular heartbeat, headache, and weakness.

mephenytoin
Mesantoin

Class and Category
Chemical: Hydantoin derivative
Therapeutic: Anticonvulsant
Pregnancy category: Not rated

Indications and Dosages
➤ *To control generalized tonic-clonic, focal, and jacksonian seizures when other drugs are ineffective*
TABLETS
Adults. *Initial:* 50 to 100 mg/day during first wk. Increased by 50 to 100 mg at 1-wk intervals until desired response is reached. *Maintenance:* 200 to 600 mg/day in equally divided doses. *Maximum:* 1.2 g/day.
Children. *Initial:* 20 to 50 mg/day. Increased by 25 to 50 mg at 1-wk intervals until desired response occurs. *Maintenance:* 100 to 400 mg/day in equally divided doses. *Maximum:* 400 mg/day.
➤ *To replace other anticonvulsants*
TABLETS
Adults. 50 to 100 mg q.d. during first wk. Dosage gradually increased while decreasing dosage of other drug over 3 to 6 wk.

Route	Onset	Peak	Duration
P.O.	30 min	Unknown	24 to 48 hr

Mechanism of Action

Limits the spread of seizure activity and the start of new seizures by:
• regulating voltage-dependent sodium and calcium channels in neurons
• inhibiting calcium movement across neuronal membranes
• enhancing sodium-potassium-adenosine triphosphatase activity in neurons and glial cells.

These actions may result from mephenytoin's ability to slow the recovery rate of inactivated sodium channels.

Contraindications

Hypersensitivity to mephenytoin, phenytoin, other hydantoins, or their components

Interactions

DRUGS

acetaminophen: Increased risk of hepatotoxicity with long-term acetaminophen use
amiodarone: Possibly increased blood mephenytoin level and risk of toxicity
antacids: Possibly decreased mephenytoin effectiveness
antineoplastics: Increased mephenytoin metabolism
bupropion, clozapine, loxapine, MAO inhibitors, maprotiline, phenothiazines, pimozide, thioxanthenes: Possibly lowered seizure threshold and decreased therapeutic effects of mephenytoin, possibly intensified CNS depressant effects of these drugs
calcium channel blockers, fluconazole, itraconazole, ketoconazole, miconazole, omeprazole: Possibly increased blood phenytoin level
carbamazepine: Decreased blood carbamazepine level, possibly increased blood phenytoin level and risk of toxicity
chloramphenicol, cimetidine, disulfiram, isoniazid, methylphenidate, metronidazole, phenylbutazone, ranitidine, salicylates, sulfonamides, trimethoprim: Possibly impaired metabolism of these drugs and increased risk of mephenytoin toxicity
corticosteroids, cyclosporine, digoxin, disopyramide, doxycycline, furosemide, levodopa, mexiletine, quinidine: Decreased therapeutic effects of these drugs

diazoxide: Possibly decreased therapeutic effects of both drugs
estrogens, progestins: Decreased therapeutic effects of these drugs, increased blood phenytoin level
felbamate: Possibly impaired metabolism and increased blood level of phenytoin
fluoxetine: Possibly increased blood phenytoin level and risk of toxicity
folic acid: Increased mephenytoin metabolism, decreased seizure control
haloperidol: Possibly lowered seizure threshold and decreased therapeutic effects of mephenytoin; possibly decreased blood haloperidol level
insulin, oral antidiabetic drugs: Possibly increased blood glucose level and decreased therapeutic effects of these drugs
lamotrigine: Possibly decreased therapeutic effects of lamotrigine
lithium: Increased risk of lithium toxicity
methadone: Possibly increased methadone metabolism, leading to withdrawal symptoms
molindone: Possibly lowered seizure threshold, impaired absorption, and decreased therapeutic effects of mephenytoin
oral anticoagulants: Possibly impaired metabolism of these drugs and increased risk of mephenytoin toxicity; possibly increased anticoagulant effect initially, but decreased effect with prolonged therapy
oral contraceptives containing estrogen and progestin: Possibly breakthrough bleeding and decreased contraceptive effectiveness
rifampin: Possibly decreased therapeutic effects of mephenytoin
streptozocin: Possibly decreased therapeutic effects of streptozocin
sucralfate: Possibly decreased mephenytoin absorption
tricyclic antidepressants: Possibly lowered seizure threshold and decreased therapeutic effects of mephenytoin; possibly decreased blood level of tricyclic antidepressants
valproic acid: Decreased blood phenytoin level, increased blood valproic acid level
vitamin D analogues: Decreased vitamin D analogue activity, risk of anticonvulsant-induced rickets and osteomalacia
xanthines: Possibly inhibited mephenytoin absorption and increased clearance of xanthines
zaleplon: Increased clearance and decreased effectiveness of zaleplon

ACTIVITIES
alcohol use: Possibly decreased mephenytoin effectiveness

Adverse Reactions
CNS: Ataxia, choreoathetoid movements, confusion, dizziness, drowsiness, excitement, fatigue, fever, headache, peripheral neuropathy, sedation, slurred speech, stuttering, tremor
EENT: Gingival hyperplasia, nystagmus
GI: Constipation, diarrhea, nausea, vomiting
HEME: Agranulocytosis, leukopenia, thrombocytopenia
MS: Muscle twitching
SKIN: Rash, Stevens-Johnson syndrome, toxic epidermal necrolysis
Other: Lymphadenopathy, systemic lupus erythematosus

Nursing Considerations
•Because of mephenytoin's potentially dangerous adverse effects, expect to use it only when other drugs are ineffective.
•Keep in mind that mephenytoin doesn't control absence seizures.
•**WARNING** Be aware that drug shouldn't be abruptly discontinued because doing so may cause status epilepticus. Plan to reduce dosage gradually or substitute another drug, as prescribed, when discontinuing mephenytoin.
•Obtain CBC and differential before treatment, after 2 weeks of treatment, and then monthly during first year of treatment, as ordered.
•Notify prescriber immediately and expect to discontinue mephenytoin and substitute another drug if depressed blood counts, enlarged lymph nodes, or rash develops.
PATIENT TEACHING
•Instruct patient to take mephenytoin exactly as prescribed and not to discontinue drug abruptly.
•Advise patient to take drug with food to enhance absorption and reduce adverse GI reactions.
•Caution patient on once-a-day therapy to be especially careful not to miss a dose.
•Advise patient to report impaired coordination, persistent headache, rash, severe GI distress, swollen gums or lymph nodes, or unusual bleeding or bruising.
•Encourage patient to maintain good oral hygiene and to have regular dental checkups to reduce the risk of gum disease.
•Instruct patient to keep medical appointments to monitor drug effectiveness and check for adverse reactions. Explain the need for periodic laboratory tests.
•Advise patient to wear medical identification stating that he has epilepsy and takes mephenytoin to prevent seizures.

mephobarbital

Mebaral

Class, Category, and Schedule
Chemical: Barbiturate derivative
Therapeutic: Anticonvulsant, sedative
Pregnancy category: D
Controlled substance: Schedule IV

Indications and Dosages
➤ *To treat seizures*
TABLETS
Adults. 400 to 600 mg/day as a single dose or in divided doses, usually beginning with low dose and increasing over 4 to 5 days until optimum dosage is determined.
Children over age 5. 32 to 64 mg t.i.d. or q.i.d.
Children under age 5. 16 to 32 mg t.i.d. or q.i.d.

➤ *To provide sedation*
TABLETS
Adults. 32 to 100 mg t.i.d. or q.i.d.
Children. 16 to 32 mg t.i.d. or q.i.d.

Route	Onset	Peak	Duration
P.O.	30 to 60 min	Unknown	10 to 16 hr

Mechanism of Action
May reduce seizure activity by reducing transmission of monosynaptic and polysynaptic nerve impulses, which causes decreased excitability in nerve cells. As a sedative, mephobarbital inhibits upward conduction of nerve impulses to the reticular formation of the brain, which disrupts impulse transmission to the cortex. As a result, mephobarbital depresses the CNS and produces drowsiness, hypnosis, and sedation.

Contraindications
Hepatic disease or failure; history of addiction to sedatives or hypnotics; hypersensitivity to mephobarbital, other barbiturates, or their

components; nephritis; porphyria; severe respiratory disease with obstruction or dyspnea

Interactions
DRUGS
acetaminophen: Possibly decreased effects of acetaminophen (with long-term mephobarbital use)
anesthetics (halogenated hydrocarbon): Increased risk of hepatotoxicity (with long-term mephobarbital use)
carbamazepine, chloramphenicol, corticosteroids, cyclosporine, dacarbazine, digoxin, disopyramide, doxycycline, griseofulvin, metronidazole, oral contraceptives, phenylbutazone, quinidine, theophyllines, vitamin D: Decreased effectiveness of these drugs
CNS depressants: Increased CNS depression
divalproex sodium, valproic acid: Increased risk of CNS depression and neurotoxicity
guanadrel, guanethidine: Increased risk of orthostatic hypotension
haloperidol: Possibly decreased blood haloperidol level and change in seizure pattern
hydantoins: Possibly interference with hydantoin metabolism
leucovorin: Possibly decreased anticonvulsant effect of mephobarbital
maprotiline: Possibly increased CNS depression and decreased therapeutic effects of mephobarbital
mexiletine: Possibly decreased blood mexiletine level
oral anticoagulants: Possibly decreased therapeutic effects of anticoagulants, possibly increased risk of bleeding when mephobarbital is discontinued
tricyclic antidepressants: Possibly decreased therapeutic effects of tricyclic antidepressants
ACTIVITIES
alcohol use: Increased CNS depression

Adverse Reactions
CNS: Agitation, anxiety, ataxia, confusion, delusions, depression, dizziness, drowsiness, fever, hallucinations, headache, insomnia, irritability, nervousness, nightmares, paradoxical stimulation, seizures, syncope, tremor
CV: Orthostatic hypotension
EENT: Vision changes
GI: Anorexia, constipation, hepatic dysfunction, nausea, vomiting
HEME: Agranulocytosis

MS: Arthralgia, bone pain, muscle twitching or weakness
RESP: Respiratory depression
SKIN: Exfoliative dermatitis, rash, Stevens-Johnson syndrome
Other: Physical and psychological dependence, weight loss

Nursing Considerations
• Observe for signs of physical and psychological dependence, especially with prolonged use of mephobarbital at high doses.
• Observe for signs of chronic barbiturate intoxication, including confusion, insomnia, poor judgment, slurred speech, and unsteady gait.
• Assess for paradoxical stimulation in patient who receives drug for acute or chronic pain.
• WARNING Expect to taper dosage gradually when discontinuing drug. Be aware that withdrawal symptoms can be severe and may cause death. Mild signs and symptoms, including anxiety, muscle twitching, nausea, orthostatic hypotension, and progressive weakness, may appear 8 to 12 hours after last drug dose. More severe signs include delirium and seizures.
PATIENT TEACHING
• Advise patient to take mephobarbital exactly as prescribed. Caution him not to stop taking drug abruptly because of the risk of withdrawal symptoms and, for epileptic patients, seizures.
• Instruct patient to avoid alcohol, sleeping pills, and other sedatives while taking mephobarbital because of the risk of increased CNS depression.
• Advise patient to avoid potentially hazardous activities until drug's CNS effects are known.
• Advise patient to change position slowly to minimize effects of orthostatic hypotension.
• Urge patient to report confusion, fever, rash, or severe dizziness.

meprobamate

Apo-Meprobamate (CAN), Equanil, MB-Tab, Meprospan, Miltown, Neuramate

Class, Category, and Schedule
Chemical: Carbamate derivative
Therapeutic: Antianxiety
Pregnancy category: Not rated
Controlled substance: Schedule IV

Indications and Dosages
➤ *To treat anxiety*
S.R. CAPSULES
Adults and adolescents. 400 to 800 mg q morning and h.s. *Maximum:* 2,400 mg/day.
Children ages 6 to 12. 200 mg q morning and h.s.
TABLETS
Adults and adolescents. 1,200 to 1,600 mg/day in divided doses t.i.d. or q.i.d. *Maximum:* 2,400 mg/day.
DOSAGE ADJUSTMENT For patients with creatinine clearance of 10 to 50 ml/min/1.73 m^2, drug administered q 12 hr; with creatinine clearance of less than 10 ml/min/1.73 m^2, drug administered q 18 hr.
Children ages 6 to 12. 200 to 600 mg/day in divided doses b.i.d. or t.i.d.

Route	Onset	Peak	Duration
P.O.	In 1 hr	Unknown	Unknown

Mechanism of Action
May act at multiple sites in the CNS, including the thalamus and limbic system. Meprobamate inhibits spinal reflexes, causing CNS relaxation; its sedative effects may account for its anticonvulsant action. It also has muscle relaxant properties.

Contraindications
Hypersensitivity to meprobromate or related drugs, such as carisoprodol; porphyria

Interactions
DRUGS
CNS depressants: Increased CNS depression
ACTIVITIES
alcohol use: Increased CNS depression

Adverse Reactions
CNS: Ataxia, dizziness, drowsiness, euphoria, headache, paradoxical stimulation, paresthesia, slurred speech, syncope, vertigo, weakness
CV: Arrhythmias, including tachycardia; hypotension; palpitations
EENT: Impaired visual accommodation
GI: Diarrhea, nausea, vomiting
SKIN: Erythematous maculopapular rash, pruritus, urticaria
Other: Physical dependence

Nursing Considerations
• Use meprobamate cautiously in patients with impaired hepatic or renal function, seizure disorders, or suicidal tendencies.

• Also use drug cautiously in patients with a history of drug dependence or abuse because meprobamate use can lead to physical dependence and abuse.
• Observe for signs of chronic drug intoxication, such as ataxia, slurred speech, and vertigo.
• **WARNING** Expect to taper dosage gradually over 2 weeks when discontinuing meprobamate because abrupt drug discontinuation can exacerbate previous symptoms, such as anxiety, or cause withdrawal symptoms, such as confusion, hallucinations, muscle twitching, tremor, and vomiting.

PATIENT TEACHING
• Instruct patient to take meprobamate exactly as directed and not to stop taking it abruptly.
• Advise patient not to crush or chew S.R. capsules.
• Instruct patient to avoid hazardous activities until drug's CNS effects are known.
• Direct patient to avoid alcohol, sedatives, and other CNS depressants while taking meprobamate.
• Inform patient that drug may become less effective after several months of treatment.
• Instruct patient to report rash.

meropenem
Merrem I.V.

Class and Category
Chemical: Carbapenem
Therapeutic: Antibiotic
Pregnancy category: B

Indications and Dosages
➤ *To treat complicated appendicitis and peritonitis caused by susceptible strains of alpha-hemolytic streptococci,* Bacteroides fragilis, Bacteroides thetaiotaomicron, Escherichia coli, Klebsiella pneumoniae, Peptostreptococcus *sp., or* Pseudomonas aeruginosa
I.V. INFUSION OR INJECTION
Adults and children weighing more than 50 kg (110 lb). 1 g q 8 hr infused over 15 to 30 min or given as a bolus over 3 to 5 min.
Children over age 3 months weighing less than 50 kg. 20 mg/kg q 8 hr infused over 15 to 30 min or given as a bolus over 3 to 5 min.
DOSAGE ADJUSTMENT For patients with creatinine clearance of 26 to 50 ml/min/1.73 m^2, dosage reduced to 1 g q 12 hr. With creati-

M

nine clearance of 10 to 25 ml/min/1.73 m^2, dosage reduced to 500 mg q 12 hr. With creatinine clearance of less than 10 ml/min/1.73 m^2, dosage reduced to 500 mg q 24 hr.

➤ To treat bacterial meningitis caused by Haemophilus influenzae, Neisseria meningitidis, or Streptococcus pneumoniae in children

I.V. INFUSION OR INJECTION
Children weighing more than 50 kg. 2 g q 8 hr infused over 15 to 30 min or given as a bolus over 3 to 5 min.
Children over age 3 months weighing less than 50 kg. 40 mg/kg q 8 hr infused over 15 to 30 min or given as a bolus over 3 to 5 min. *Maximum:* 2 g q 8 hr.

Mechanism of Action
Penetrates cell walls of most gram-negative and gram-positive bacteria, inactivating penicillin-binding proteins. This action inhibits bacterial cell wall synthesis and causes cell death.

Incompatibilities
Don't mix meropenem in same solution with other drugs.

Contraindications
Hypersensitivity to meropenem, other carbapenem drugs, beta lactams, or their components

Interactions
DRUGS
probenecid: Inhibited renal excretion of meropenem
valproic acid: Possibly subtherapeutic blood level of valproic acid

Adverse Reactions
CNS: Headache, seizures
CV: Shock
EENT: Epistaxis, glossitis, oral candidiasis
GI: Anorexia, constipation, diarrhea, elevated liver function test results, nausea, pseudomembranous colitis, vomiting
GU: Elevated BUN and serum creatinine levels, hematuria, renal failure
HEME: Agranulocytosis, leukopenia, neutropenia
RESP: Apnea, dyspnea
SKIN: Diaper rash from candidiasis (children), erythema multiforme, pruritus, rash, Stevens-Johnson syndrome, toxic epidermal necrolysis

Other: Anaphylaxis; angioedema; injection site inflammation, pain, phlebitis, or thrombophlebitis; sepsis

Nursing Considerations
• Obtain body fluid and tissue samples, as ordered, for culture and sensitivity testing. Expect to review test results, if possible, before giving first dose of meropenem.
• For I.V. bolus, add 10 ml of sterile water for injection to 500 mg/20-ml vial, or 20 ml of diluent to 1 g/30-ml vial of drug. Shake to dissolve.
• **WARNING** Be aware that fatal hypersensitivity reactions have occurred with meropenem. Determine whether patient has had previous reactions to antibiotics or other allergens.
• Be prepared to administer emergency treatment for anaphylaxis.
• Institute seizure precautions, according to facility policy, for patients with bacterial meningitis or CNS or renal disorders because they're at increased risk for seizures with meropenem.
• Monitor patient with creatinine clearance of 10 to 26 ml/min/1.73 m^2 for signs and symptoms of seizures, heart failure, renal failure, or shock.
PATIENT TEACHING
• Advise patient to report diarrhea, difficulty breathing, injection site pain, or mouth soreness.

mesalamine

Asacol, Canasa, Mesasal (CAN), Pentasa, Rowasa, Salofalk (CAN)

Class and Category
Chemical: 5-Aminosalicylic acid derivative
Therapeutic: Anti-inflammatory
Pregnancy category: B

Indications and Dosages
➤ To treat and maintain remission of ulcerative colitis
DELAYED-RELEASE TABLETS (ASACOL)
Adults. *Initial:* 0.8 g t.i.d. for 6 wk. *Maintenance:* 1.6 g/day in divided doses.
DELAYED-RELEASE TABLETS (MESASAL)
Adults. 1.5 to 3 g/day in divided doses for 6 wk.
DELAYED-RELEASE TABLETS (SALOFALK)
Adults. 1 g t.i.d. or q.i.d. for 6 wk.
E.R. CAPSULES
Adults. 1 g q.i.d. for up to 8 wk.

➤ *To treat mild to moderate distal ulcerative colitis, proctitis, and proctosigmoiditis*
RECTAL SUSPENSION
Adults. 4 g (60 ml) q.d. h.s. for 3 to 6 wk.
➤ *To treat active ulcerative proctitis*
SUPPOSITORIES (CANASA)
Adults. 0.5 g b.i.d. or t.i.d. for 3 to 6 wk.

Mechanism of Action
May reduce inflammation by inhibiting the enzyme cyclooxygenase and decreasing the production of arachidonic acid metabolites, which may be increased in patients with inflammatory bowel disease. Cyclooxygenase is needed to form prostaglandin from arachidonic acid. Prostaglandin mediates inflammatory activity and produces signs and symptoms of inflammation. By inhibiting prostaglandin synthesis, mesalamine may reduce signs and symptoms of inflammation in inflammatory bowel disease. Mesalamine also may reduce inflammation by interfering with leukotriene synthesis and by inhibiting the enzyme lipoxygenase. These substances also are involved in the inflammatory response.

Contraindications
Hypersensitivity to mesalamine, salicylates, or their components

Interactions
DRUGS
digoxin: Possibly decreased absorption and bioavailability of digoxin
lactulose: Possibly interference with delayed-release tablets or E.R. capsules
omeprazole: Increased mesalamine absorption

Adverse Reactions
CNS: Chills, dizziness, fatigue, fever, headache (severe), weakness
EENT: Rhinitis
GI: Abdominal cramps or pain (severe), anorexia, bloody diarrhea, diarrhea, flatulence, indigestion, nausea, vomiting
GU: Nephrotoxicity
HEME: Agranulocytosis
MS: Back pain, dysarthria
SKIN: Acne, alopecia, pruritus, rash

Nursing Considerations
•Use mesalamine cautiously in patients with sulfite sensitivity. Some drug formulations contain sulfites, which may cause hypersensitivity reactions in these patients.
•Ensure that suppository is firm before inserting it. If it's too soft, chill in refrigerator for 30 minutes or run under cold water before removing wrapper. Moisten it with water-soluble lubricant or tap water before insertion. Have patient retain suppository for 1 to 3 hours, as directed.
•Administer rectal suspension at bedtime, and have patient retain it for the prescribed time—about 8 hours, if possible. Retention time ranges from 3.5 to 12 hours.
•Be aware that rectal suspension may darken slightly over time but that this change doesn't affect potency. Discard rectal suspension that turns dark brown.
•Assess patient for evidence of acute intolerance similar to flare-up of inflammatory bowel disease: acute abdominal cramps and pain, bloody diarrhea, and, possibly, fever, headache, and rash.
•For patients with impaired renal function, expect to monitor renal function test results periodically during long-term therapy because drug may cause nephrotoxicity.
•Monitor patient's CBC with differential for eosinophilia, which may indicate an allergic reaction.
PATIENT TEACHING
•Instruct patient taking oral drug to swallow tablets or capsules whole and not to break outer coating.
•Teach patient how to administer rectal suspension or suppositories correctly. Emphasize shaking suspension bottle well before using.
•Advise patient to notify prescriber immediately about abdominal cramps or pain, bloody diarrhea, fever, headache, or rash.

mesoridazine besylate
Serentil

Class and Category
Chemical: Alkylpiperidine phenothiazine derivative
Therapeutic: Antipsychotic
Pregnancy category: Not rated

Indications and Dosages
➤ *To treat schizophrenia in patients who failed to respond to other antipsychotic*

drugs, either because those drugs were ineffective or because intolerable adverse effects prevented attainment of an effective dose

ORAL SOLUTION, TABLETS

Adults and adolescents. 50 mg t.i.d., increased as needed and tolerated. *Maximum:* 400 mg/day.

I.M. INJECTION

Adults and adolescents. 25 mg, repeated in 30 to 60 min, as needed. *Maximum:* 200 mg/day.

Route	Onset	Peak	Duration
P.O., I.M.	Up to several wk	6 wk to 6 mo	4 to 8 hr

Mechanism of Action

Depresses brain areas that control activity and aggression—including the cerebral cortex, hypothalamus, and limbic system—by an unknown mechanism.

Contraindications

Blood dyscrasias; bone marrow depression; cerebral arteriosclerosis; coma; concurrent use of high doses of CNS depressants; concurrent use of other drugs that prolong the QTc interval, such as disopyramide, procainamide, and quinidine; congenital long-QT syndrome; coronary artery disease; hepatic dysfunction; history of arrhythmias; hypersensitivity to mesoridazine, other phenothiazines, or their components; myeloproliferative disorders; severe CNS depression; severe hypertension or hypotension; subcortical brain damage

Interactions

DRUGS

aluminum- or magnesium-containing antacids, antidiarrheals (adsorbent): Decreased mesoridazine absorption

amantadine, anticholinergics: Increased anticholinergic effects, and possibly decreased therapeutic effects of mesoridazine

aminoglycosides, ototoxic drugs: Masked symptoms of ototoxicity, such as dizziness, tinnitus, and vertigo

anticonvulsants: Possibly lowered seizure threshold

antithyroid drugs: Increased risk of agranulocytosis

appetite suppressants: Possibly antagonized anorectic effect

astemizole, cisapride, disopyramide, erythromycin, pimozide, probucol, procainamide, quinidine: Increased risk of prolonged QT interval and life-threatening arrhythmias

beta blockers: Increased blood levels of both drugs, possibly resulting in additive hypotension, retinopathy, arrhythmias, and tardive dyskinesia

CNS depressants, general anesthetics: Increased CNS depression

dextroamphetamine: Possibly interference with action of either drug

levodopa: Possibly inhibited effects of levodopa

lithium: Possibly decreased absorption of mesoridazine

opioid analgesics: Possibly decreased mesoridazine effects; increased CNS and respiratory depression and orthostatic hypotension; increased risk of severe constipation

oral anticoagulants: Possibly decreased therapeutic effects of anticoagulants

sympathomimetics: Possibly decreased therapeutic effects of these drugs and increased risk of hypotension

thiazide diuretics: Possibly orthostatic hypotension, hyponatremia, and water intoxication

tricyclic antidepressants: Increased tricyclic antidepressant levels, inhibited mesoridazine metabolism, increased risk of neuroleptic malignant syndrome

ACTIVITIES

alcohol use: Increased CNS depression

Adverse Reactions

CNS: Ataxia, dizziness, drowsiness, extrapyramidal reactions (tardive dyskinesia, pseudoparkinsonism), fever, neuroleptic malignant syndrome, restlessness, seizures, slurred speech, syncope, tremor, weakness

CV: Hypotension, orthostatic hypotension, prolonged QTc interval, torsades de pointes

EENT: Blurred vision, dry mouth, hypertrophic papillae of tongue, increased salivation, photophobia

ENDO: Galactorrhea, gynecomastia

GI: Constipation, hepatotoxicity, nausea, vomiting

GU: Dysuria, ejaculation disorders, impotence, menstrual irregularities, priapism

HEME: Agranulocytosis, leukopenia, thrombocytopenia
SKIN: Contact dermatitis, decreased sweating, jaundice, photosensitivity, rash
Other: Injection site pain, weight gain

Nursing Considerations
•Before beginning mesoridazine therapy, expect to perform a 12-lead ECG to detect prolonged QTc interval. If patient's QTc interval is greater than 450 msec, expect to withhold drug because of the risk of life-threatening torsades de pointes.
•Wear gloves when working with liquid and parenteral forms of mesoridazine, and avoid contact with clothing or skin; drug may cause contact dermatitis.
•Discard injection solution if it's frankly discolored or contains precipitate; slightly yellow color is acceptable.
•Inject I.M. drug deep into upper outer quadrant of buttocks; massage area afterward to prevent sterile abscess.
•Implement continuous ECG monitoring, as ordered, to detect arrhythmias. Expect to discontinue mesoridazine if the QTc interval exceeds 500 msec.
•Monitor serum potassium level before and during therapy, and administer potassium supplements as prescribed.
•Assess patient for hypotension and orthostatic hypotension, especially during I.M. therapy. Notify prescriber if either develops.
•**WARNING** Monitor patient for evidence of neuroleptic malignant syndrome, a potentially fatal reaction to antipsychotic drugs, and notify prescriber if they develop. Early signs include altered mental status, fever, hypertension or hypotension, muscle rigidity, and tachycardia.
•Assess patient for signs of blood dyscrasias, including cellulitis, fever, and pharyngitis. If they develop, discontinue drug, as directed.
•Monitor patient for signs of tardive dyskinesia, even after treatment stops. Notify prescriber if they develop.
•Expect to taper drug dosage before discontinuation to avoid adverse reactions, such as dizziness, nausea, tremor, and vomiting.
PATIENT TEACHING
•Instruct patient to take mesoridazine exactly as prescribed and not to stop it abruptly.
•Inform patient that I.M. injection may be painful.

•Caution patient to avoid potentially hazardous activities until drug's CNS effects are known.
•Advise patient to change position slowly to minimize effects of orthostatic hypotension.
•Instruct patient to report fever, involuntary facial movements, sore throat, unusual bleeding or bruising, and yellowing of eyes or skin.
•Urge patient to avoid alcohol and prolonged sun exposure during therapy.
•If patient requires long-term therapy, explain the risk of tardive dyskinesia. Also advise him to have regular eye examinations.

metaproterenol sulfate
Alupent, Arm-a-Med Metaproterenol, Dey-Lute Metaproterenol

Class and Category
Chemical: Sympathomimetic amine
Therapeutic: Antiasthmatic, bronchodilator
Pregnancy category: C

Indications and Dosages
➤ *To treat bronchospasm*
SYRUP, TABLETS
Adults and children age 9 or older who weigh more than 27 kg (59 lb). 20 mg q 6 to 8 hr.
Children ages 6 to 9 who weigh 27 kg or less. 10 mg q 6 to 8 hr.
INHALATION AEROSOL
Adults and adolescents. 2 to 3 inhalations (1.3 to 1.95 mg) q 3 to 4 hr. *Maximum:* 12 inhalations/day.
Children ages 6 to 12. 1 to 3 inhalations (0.65 to 1.95 mg) q 3 to 4 hr. *Maximum:* 12 inhalations/day.
INHALATION NEBULIZER
Adults and adolescents. 0.2 to 0.3 ml of 5% solution diluted in 2.5 ml of NS t.i.d. or q.i.d., p.r.n., but not more frequently than q 4 hr.
Children ages 6 to 12. 0.1 to 0.2 ml of 5% solution diluted in NS to a total volume of 3 ml t.i.d. or q.i.d., p.r.n., but not more frequently than q 4 hr.

Route	Onset	Peak	Duration
P.O.	15 min	1 hr	4 hr or longer
Inhalation (aerosol)	1 min	1 hr	4 hr or longer
Inhalation (nebulizer)	5 to 30 min	Unknown	4 hr or longer

M

Mechanism of Action
Attaches to beta$_2$ receptors on bronchial cell membranes. This stimulates the intracellular enzyme adenyl cyclase to convert adenosine triphosphate to cyclic adenosine monophosphate (cAMP). An increased intracellular level of cAMP relaxes bronchial smooth-muscle cells and inhibits histamine release.

Contraindications
Angina, cerebral arteriosclerosis, dilated heart failure, heart block from digitalis toxicity, hypersensitivity to metaproterenol or its components, labor, local anesthesia, organic brain damage, tachyarrhythmias

Interactions
DRUGS
beta blockers: Increased risk of bronchospasm
MAO inhibitors, tricyclic antidepressants: Possibly potentiated cardiovascular effects of metaproterenol
other sympathomimetics: Possibly additive effects of both drugs and risk of toxicity
theophylline: Increased risk of arrhythmias

Adverse Reactions
CNS: Dizziness, fatigue, headache, insomnia, malaise, nervousness, tremor
CV: ECG changes, hypertension, palpitations, tachycardia
EENT: Dry mouth, pharyngitis, taste perversion
GI: Diarrhea, nausea, vomiting
RESP: Asthma exacerbation, cough

Nursing Considerations
•Anticipate that a single dose of nebulized metaproterenol may not completely stop an acute asthma attack.
•Monitor for adverse reactions and signs of toxicity, especially if patient uses tablets and aerosol. Notify prescriber if they develop.
•Be aware that tolerance may occur with continued use.
PATIENT TEACHING
•Caution patient not to use metaproterenol inhaler or nebulizer more often than prescribed.
•Teach patient to use inhaler correctly, to hold breath during second half of inhalation, and to wait 2 minutes between inhalations.
•Instruct parents to use spacer with their child's metered-dose inhaler.
•Advise patient to use metaproterenol 5 minutes before using corticosteroid inhaler, if prescribed, to maximize airway opening.

•Instruct patient to notify prescriber immediately if diarrhea, increased shortness of breath, insomnia, or irregular heartbeat occurs.
•Instruct patient to notify prescriber if drug becomes less effective.

metaraminol bitartrate
Aramine

Class and Category
Chemical: Sympathomimetic amine
Therapeutic: Vasopressor
Pregnancy category: C

Indications and Dosages
➤ *To treat hypotension secondary to spinal anesthesia or as adjunct to treat hypotension caused by hemorrhage, adverse drug reactions, surgical complications, or shock resulting from brain damage secondary to trauma or tumor*
I.V. INFUSION
Adults. 15 to 100 mg (base) mixed in 500 ml of NS or D$_5$W; dosage individualized to maintain desired blood pressure.

➤ *To treat severe shock*
I.V. INJECTION
Adults. 500 mcg (0.5 mg) to 5 mg (base), followed by I.V. infusion individualized to maintain desired blood pressure.

Route	Onset	Peak	Duration
I.V.	1 to 2 min	Unknown	20 to 60 min

Mechanism of Action
Thought to directly stimulate alpha-adrenergic receptors and inhibit activity of the intracellular enzyme adenyl cyclase, which then inhibits production of cAMP. Inhibition of cAMP causes arterial and venous constriction and increases peripheral vascular resistance and systolic blood pressure. Metaraminol also directly stimulates beta-adrenergic receptors in the myocardium and increases adenyl cyclase activity, producing positive inotropic and chronotropic effects.

Incompatibilities
Don't mix metaraminol with barbiturates, penicillins, phenytoin, sodium salts, or other

drugs that have poor solubility in acidic solutions.

Contraindications
Hypersensitivity to metaraminol or its components, including sulfites; use with cyclopropane or halothane anesthesia unless clinically warranted

Interactions
DRUGS
alpha blockers and other drugs with alpha-blocking effects: Possibly decreased peripheral vasoconstrictive and hypertensive effects of metaraminol
beta blockers (ophthalmic): Decreased effects of metaraminol; increased risk of bronchospasm, wheezing, decreased pulmonary function, and respiratory failure
beta blockers (systemic): Increased risk of bronchospasm, decreased effects of both drugs
digoxin: Increased risk of arrhythmias
diuretics and other antihypertensives: Possibly reduced effectiveness of these drugs
doxapram: Possibly increased vasopressor effects of both drugs
ergot alkaloids: Increased vasopressor effects
guanadrel, guanethidine, mecamylamine, methyldopa: Possibly decreased effects of these drugs and increased risk of adverse effects
hydrocarbon inhalation anesthetics: Increased risk of atrial and ventricular arrhythmias
MAO inhibitors: Intensified and extended cardiac stimulation and vasopressor effects, possibly severe hypertension
maprotiline, tricyclic antidepressants: Increased vasopressor response; increased risk of prolonged QTc interval, arrhythmias, hypertension, and hyperpyrexia
methylphenidate: Possibly increased vasopressor effect of metaraminol
nitrates: Possibly reduced antianginal effects of nitrates, decreased vasopressor effect
other sympathomimetics (such as dopamine): Possibly increased cardiac effects and adverse reactions
oxytocin: Possibly severe hypertension
thyroid hormones: Increased effects of both drugs, increased risk of coronary insufficiency in patients with coronary artery disease

Adverse Reactions
CNS: Anxiety, dizziness, headache, nervousness, seizures, weakness

CV: Angina, arrhythmias (including bradycardia, tachycardia, and ventricular arrhythmias), hypertension, hypotension, palpitations, peripheral vasoconstriction
GI: Nausea, vomiting
RESP: Dyspnea
SKIN: Extravasation with tissue necrosis and sloughing
Other: Injection site abscess

Nursing Considerations
•Before starting metaraminol therapy, expect to administer blood, plasma volume expanders, I.V. fluids, and electrolyte replacement therapy, as ordered, to correct conditions that caused hypotension, such as hemorrhage or hypovolemia.
•Discard vial if you observe discoloration or precipitates.
•To prepare an I.V. infusion, add 15 to 100 mg of metaraminol to 500 ml of appropriate solution, such as NS or D_5W. (You may use a smaller or larger amount of solution, depending on patient's fluid needs.) Use within 24 hours.
•Expect to use large veins for I.V. administration, such as antecubital fossa or a vein in the thigh. Administer infusion using an infusion pump to provide a controlled rate.
•Monitor blood pressure, cardiac rate and rhythm, central venous pressure, and urine output during administration. Be aware that vasoconstrictive effects of prolonged metaraminol administration may prevent volume expansion and prolong shock state. If this occurs, expect to administer blood and plasma volume expanders, as ordered.
•Allow at least 10 minutes between dosage adjustments to achieve maximum effect. Adjust infusion rate to patient response, as ordered.
•**WARNING** Assess for allergic reactions—including anaphylaxis and, possibly, life-threatening asthmatic episodes—because drug contains sodium bisulfite.
•Expect to discontinue metaraminol infusion gradually. Continue to monitor patient's blood pressure after infusion has stopped; elevated blood pressure may persist from drug's cumulative effects. Expect to restart metaraminol, as prescribed, if hypotension recurs.
•Be aware that patients with a history of cardiovascular disease (including hypertension) or hyperthyroidism and chronically ill patients are at increased risk for drug's adverse cardiovascular effects. Monitor patients with acute MI for

worsening of condition because metaraminol can intensify or prolong myocardial ischemia.

•Monitor patients with cirrhosis for arrhythmias and diuresis. Expect to administer electrolytes, as prescribed, if diuresis occurs.

•Assess patients with angle-closure glaucoma for signs of an exacerbation, such as eye pain or blurred vision.

•Assess circulation in patients with a history of occlusive vascular disease, such as atherosclerosis, diabetic endarteritis, and Raynaud's disease, because metaraminol may cause decreased circulation and increase the risk of necrosis or gangrene. Inspect I.V. site periodically for signs of extravasation.

•WARNING Be aware that headache, euphoria, arrhythmias, severe hypertension, and MI are some of the symptoms of metaraminol overdose. Contact prescriber immediately if patient experiences such symptoms, and expect to provide supportive treatment.

•Monitor patients with a history of malaria for signs of a metaraminol-induced relapse, such as fever, chills, and muscle aches.

•Store drug at 15° to 30° C (59° to 86° F); protect from freezing and light.

PATIENT TEACHING

•Advise patient to immediately report any discomfort at metaraminol infusion site, such as pain, swelling, or redness.

•Instruct patient to report adverse reactions, including chest pain, difficulty breathing, dizziness, irregular heartbeat, headache, and weakness.

metaxalone

Skelaxin

Class and Category

Chemical: Oxazolidinone derivative
Therapeutic: Skeletal muscle relaxant
Pregnancy category: Not rated

Indications and Dosages

➤ *To relieve discomfort caused by acute, painful musculoskeletal conditions*

TABLETS

Adults and children over age 12. 800 mg t.i.d. or q.i.d.

Route	Onset	Peak	Duration
P.O.	Usually in 1 hr	Unknown	4 to 6 hr

Mechanism of Action

May depress the CNS, resulting in sedation, which in turn may reduce skeletal muscle spasms to provide pain relief. Metaxalone does not directly relax tense skeletal muscles.

Contraindications

Hypersensitivity to metaxalone or its components, significant renal or hepatic disease, tendency to develop drug-induced, hemolytic, or other anemias

Interactions

DRUGS

CNS depressants: Increased CNS depression

ACTIVITIES

alcohol use: Increased CNS depression

Adverse Reactions

CNS: Dizziness, drowsiness, excitement, headache, insomnia, irritability, nervousness, restlessness

GI: Abdominal cramps or pain, GI upset, jaundice, hepatotoxicity, nausea, vomiting

HEME: Hemolytic anemia, leukopenia

SKIN: Pruritus, rash

Nursing Considerations

•Be aware that metaxalone may not be prescribed for women who are or may become pregnant unless the potential benefits outweigh the risks because drug's effect on fetus is unknown.

•Monitor patient for excessive drowsiness, which may lead to respiratory depression.

•Caution patient to consult prescriber before taking other drugs, such as sleeping pills, cold or allergy preparations, narcotic analgesics, and antidepressants.

•Monitor liver function test results for elevations, especially in patients with preexisting hepatic disease.

•Monitor renal function test results, as prescribed, for signs of impaired renal function because drug is excreted by the kidneys.

•Provide rest and other pain-relief measures.

•Store drug at 15° to 30° C (59° to 86° F).

PATIENT TEACHING

•Advise patient to take metaxalone tablets exactly as prescribed and not to increase dosage or frequency.

•Caution patient to avoid potentially hazardous activities, such as driving or operating machinery, until drug's CNS effects are known.

•Instruct patient to avoid alcohol and other CNS depressants during metaxalone therapy.

•Urge patient to notify prescriber if he notices a rash or itching, which may signify a hypersensitivity reaction, or if he develops signs of hepatotoxicity, such as tiredness, nausea, yellow skin, or flulike symptoms.

metformin hydrochloride

Gen-Metformin (CAN), Glucophage, Glucophage XR, Glycon (CAN), Novo-Metformin (CAN)

Class and Category

Chemical: Dimethylbiguanide
Therapeutic: Antidiabetic
Pregnancy category: B

Indications and Dosages

➤ *To reduce blood glucose level in type 2 diabetes mellitus*

TABLETS

Adults and children age 10 and older. *Initial:* 500 mg b.i.d. or 850 mg q.d. Increased as prescribed by 500 mg/wk or by 850 mg q 2 wk until desired response occurs. *Usual:* 500 to 850 mg b.i.d. or t.i.d. *Maximum:* 2,550 mg/day (adults and adolescents age 17 and older); 2,000 mg/day (children ages 10 to 16).

DOSAGE ADJUSTMENT For patients who also take insulin, initial dosage reduced to 500 mg q.d. and then increased as prescribed by 500 mg q wk until blood glucose level is controlled.

E.R. TABLETS

Adults and adolescents age 17 and older. Dosage highly individualized; treatment started with lowest possible dosage needed to achieve glucose control. *Maximum:* 2,000 mg/day.

Route	Onset	Peak	Duration
P.O. (tablets)	Unknown	Up to 2 wk	2 wk after drug discontinued

Contraindications

Hypersensitivity to metformin or its components, impaired renal function, metabolic acidosis, use of iodinated contrast media within preceding 48 hours

Mechanism of Action

May promote the storage of excess glucose as glycogen in the liver, which reduces glucose production. Metformin also may improve glucose use by skeletal muscle and adipose tissue by increasing glucose transport across cell membranes. It also may increase the number of insulin receptors on cell membranes and make them more sensitive to insulin. In addition, metformin modestly decreases blood triglyceride and total cholesterol levels.

Interactions

DRUGS

cationic drugs (such as amiloride, cimetidine, digoxin, morphine, procainamide, quinidine, quinine, ranitidine, triamterene, trimethoprim, vancomycin), nifedipine: Increased blood metformin level

calcium channel blockers, corticosteroids, estrogens, isoniazid, nicotinic acid, oral contraceptives, phenothiazines, phenytoin, sympathomimetics, thiazide and other diuretics, thyroid drugs: Possibly hyperglycemia

clofibrate, MAO inhibitors, probenecid, propranolol, rifabutin, rifampin, salicylates, sulfonamides, sulfonylureas: Increased risk of hypoglycemia

FOODS

all foods: Possibly delayed metformin absorption

ACTIVITIES

alcohol use: Increased risk of hypoglycemia and lactate formation

Adverse Reactions

CNS: Headache
EENT: Metallic taste
ENDO: Hypoglycemia
GI: Abdominal distention, anorexia, constipation, diarrhea, flatulence, indigestion, nausea, vomiting
HEME: Aplastic anemia, megaloblastic anemia, thrombocytopenia
SKIN: Photosensitivity, rash
Other: Lactic acidosis, weight loss

Nursing Considerations

•Administer metformin tablets with food, which decreases and slightly delays absorption, thus reducing the risk of adverse GI reactions. Administer E.R. tablets with evening meal; don't break or crush them.

• Expect prescriber to alter dosage if patient has a condition that decreases or delays gastric emptying, such as diarrhea, gastroparesis, GI obstruction, ileus, or vomiting.

• Assess BUN and serum creatinine level, as appropriate, before and during long-term therapy in patients at increased risk for lactic acidosis.

• Monitor blood glucose level to evaluate drug effectiveness. Assess for hyperglycemia and the need for insulin during times of increased stress, such as infection and surgery.

• Withhold drug, as ordered, if patient becomes dehydrated because dehydration increases the risk of lactic acidosis.

• Be aware that iodinated contrast media used in radiographic studies increase the risk of renal failure and lactic acidosis during metformin therapy. Expect to withhold metformin for 48 hours before and after testing.

PATIENT TEACHING

• Instruct patient to take metformin tablets with meals: at breakfast if taking drug once a day, or at breakfast and dinner if taking drug twice a day. Instruct him to take E.R. tablets once daily with evening meal and to swallow them whole, not crush or chew them.

• Direct patient to take drug exactly as prescribed and not to change the dosage or frequency unless instructed.

• Stress the importance of following prescribed diet, exercising regularly, controlling weight, and frequently checking blood glucose level.

• Teach patient how to measure his blood glucose level and recognize signs of hyperglycemia and hypoglycemia. Urge him to notify prescriber if blood glucose level is abnormal.

• Caution patient to avoid alcohol, which can increase the risk of hypoglycemia.

• Instruct patient to watch for early signs of lactic acidosis, including drowsiness, hyperventilation, malaise, and muscle pain. Urge him to discontinue drug and notify prescriber if such signs develop.

• Advise patient to expect laboratory monitoring of glycosylated hemoglobin level every 3 months until blood glucose level is controlled.

methadone hydrochloride

Dolophine, Methadose

Class, Category, and Schedule

Chemical: Phenylheptylamine
Therapeutic: Synthetic opiate agonist
Pregnancy category: Not rated
Controlled substance: Schedule II

Indications and Dosages

➤ *To manage narcotic detoxification*

DISPERSIBLE TABLETS, ORAL CONCENTRATE, I.M. OR S.C. INJECTION

Adults. *Initial:* 15 to 40 mg q.d. or as needed. *Usual:* Dosage individualized based on clinical response. *Maximum:* 120 mg/day.

Children. Dosage individualized based on age and size. *Maximum:* 120 mg/day.

➤ *To maintain narcotic abstinence*

DISPERSIBLE TABLETS, ORAL CONCENTRATE

Adults. Dosage individualized based on clinical response. *Maximum:* 120 mg/day.

Children. Dosage individualized based on age and size. *Maximum:* 120 mg/day.

➤ *To treat severe or chronic pain*

ORAL CONCENTRATE, ORAL SOLUTION

Adults. 5 to 20 mg q 4 to 8 hr. Dosage increased or dosing interval decreased, as prescribed and as needed. *Maximum:* 120 mg/day.

Children. Dosage individualized based on age and size.

TABLETS, I.M. OR S.C. INJECTION

Adults. 2.5 to 10 mg q 3 to 4 hr as needed. For chronic pain, dosage and dosing interval adjusted, as prescribed and as needed.

Children. Dosage individualized based on age and size.

Route	Onset	Peak	Duration
P.O.	30 to 60 min	1.5 to 2 hr	4 to 6 hr
I.M.	10 to 20 min	1 to 2 hr	4 to 5 hr

Mechanism of Action

Binds with and activates opioid receptors (primarily mu receptors) in the spinal cord and in higher levels of the CNS to produce analgesia and euphoric effects.

Contraindications

Acute or postoperative pain, acute or severe asthma, chronic respiratory disease, diarrhea associated with pseudomembranous colitis or poisoning, hypersensitivity to methadone or its components, respiratory depression, severe inflammatory bowel disease

Interactions

DRUGS

ammonium chloride, ascorbic acid, potassium, sodium phosphate: May precipitate methadone withdrawal symptoms

amitriptyline, chloripramine, nortriptyline: Increased CNS and respiratory depression

anticholinergics: Possibly severe constipation leading to ileus; urine retention

antiemetics, general anesthetics, hypnotics, phenothiazines, sedatives, tranquilizers: Possibly coma, hypotension, respiratory depression, and severe sedation

antihistamines, choral hydrate, glutethimide, MAO inhibitors, methocarbamol: Increased CNS and respiratory depressant effects of methadone

antihypertensives, hypotension-producing drugs: Increased hypotension, risk of orthostatic hypotension

buprenorphine: Decreased therapeutic effect of methadone, increased respiratory depression, possibly withdrawal symptoms

cimetidine: Increased analgesic and CNS and respiratory depressant effects of methadone

diuretics: Decreased diuresis

hydroxyzine: Increased analgesic, CNS depressant, and hypotensive effects of methadone

loperamide, paregoric: Increased CNS depression, possibly severe constipation

metoclopramide: Possibly antagonized metoclopramide effects on GI motility

mixed agonist-antagonist analgesics: Possibly withdrawal symptoms

naloxone: Antagonized analgesic and CNS and respiratory depressant effects of methadone, possibly withdrawal symptoms

naltrexone: Possibly induction or worsening of withdrawal symptoms if methadone given within 7 days before naltrexone

neuromuscular blockers: Increased or prolonged respiratory depression

opioid analgesics (such as alfentanil and sufentanil): Increased CNS and respiratory depression, increased hypotension

phenytoin, rifampin: May precipitate withdrawal symptoms

ACTIVITIES

alcohol use: Increased CNS and respiratory depression, possibly hypotension

Adverse Reactions

CNS: Amnesia, anxiety, coma, confusion, decreased concentration, delirium, delusions, depression, dizziness, drowsiness, euphoria, fever, hallucinations, headache, insomnia, lethargy, light-headedness, malaise, psychosis, restlessness, sedation, seizures, syncope, tremor

CV: Bradycardia, cardiac arrest, hypotension, orthostatic hypotension, palpitations, shock, tachycardia

EENT: Blurred vision, diplopia, dry mouth, laryngeal edema or laryngospasm (allergic), miosis, nystagmus, rhinitis

GI: Abdominal cramps or pain, anorexia, biliary tract spasm, constipation, diarrhea, dysphagia, elevated liver function test results, gastroesophageal reflux, hiccups, ileus and toxic megacolon (in patients with inflammatory bowel disease), indigestion, nausea, vomiting

GU: Decreased ejaculate potency, difficult ejaculation, impotence, prolonged labor, urinary hesitancy, urine retention

HEME: Anemia, leukopenia, thrombocytopenia

MS: Arthralgia

RESP: Apnea, asthma exacerbation, atelectasis, bronchospasm, depressed cough reflex, hypoventilation, pulmonary edema, respiratory arrest and depression, wheezing

SKIN: Diaphoresis, flushing, pallor, pruritus

Other: Allergic reaction; facial edema; injection site edema, pain, rash, or redness; physical and psychological dependence; withdrawal symptoms

Nursing Considerations

•Before giving methadone, make sure opioid antagonist and equipment for administering oxygen and controlling respiration are nearby.

•Before therapy begins, assess patient's current drug use, including all prescription and OTC drugs.

•Dilute oral concentrate with water or another liquid to a volume of at least 30 ml, but preferably to 90 ml or more, before administration. Dissolve dispersible tablets in

M

water or another liquid before administration.
•Monitor patient for expected excessive drowsiness, unsteadiness, or confusion during first 3 to 5 days of therapy, and notify prescriber if effects continue to worsen or persist beyond this time.
•**WARNING** Monitor respiratory and circulatory status carefully and at frequent intervals during methadone therapy because respiratory depression, circulatory depression, respiratory arrest, shock, hypotension, and cardiac arrest are potential hazards of therapy. Monitor children frequently for respiratory depression and paradoxical CNS excitation because of their increased sensitivity to drug. Assess for excessive or persistent sedation; dosage may need to be adjusted.
•Monitor for drug tolerance, especially in patients with a history of chronic drug abuse, because methadone can cause physical and psychological dependence.
•Monitor patient for pain because maintenance dosage doesn't provide pain relief; patients who have developed a tolerance to opiate agonists, including those with chronic cancer pain, may require higher-than-usual dosage.
•Monitor patients who are pregnant or who have liver or renal impairment for increased adverse effects from methadone because drug may have a prolonged duration and cumulative effect in these patients. Methadone may prolong labor by reducing strength, duration, and frequency of uterine contractions, so expect dosage to be tapered before third trimester of pregnancy. Breast-feeding mothers on maintenance therapy put their infants at risk of withdrawal symptoms if they abruptly stop breast-feeding or discontinue methadone therapy. Methadone also accumulates in CNS tissue, increasing the risk of seizures in infants.
•Monitor plasma amylase and lipase levels in patients who develop biliary tract spasms because levels may increase up to 2 to 15 times normal. Notify prescriber immediately of any significant or sustained increase.
•Monitor patient for withdrawal symptoms and tolerance to therapy because physiologic dependence can occur with long-term methadone use. Avoid abrupt discontinuation because withdrawal symptoms will occur within 3 to 4 days after last dose.

•Monitor patients, especially the elderly, for cardiac arrhythmias, hypotension, hypovolemia, orthostatic hypotension, and vasovagal syncope because drug may produce cholinergic adverse reactions in patients with cardiac disease, resulting in bradycardia and peripheral vasodilation; dosage decrease may be indicated.
•Monitor patients with prostatic hypertrophy, urethral stricture, or renal disease for urine retention and oliguria because drug can increase tension of detrusor muscle.
•Be prepared to treat symptoms of anxiety if they occur. Be aware that anxiety may be confused with symptoms of opiate abstinence and that methadone doesn't have antianxiety effects.

PATIENT TEACHING
•Instruct patient taking oral concentrate form of methadone to dilute it with water or another liquid to a volume of at least 30 ml and preferably to 90 ml or more before administration.
•Instruct patient to dissolve dispersible tablets in water or other liquid before administration.
•Advise patient to notify prescriber of all other drugs he's currently taking and to avoid alcohol and other depressants, such as sleeping pills and tranquilizers, because they may increase drug's CNS depressant effects.
•Instruct patient to take drug only as prescribed and not to change dosage without prescriber approval. Inform patient that abrupt cessation of methadone therapy can precipitate withdrawal symptoms. Urge him to notify prescriber if he develops any concerns over therapy.
•Instruct patient to avoid activities that require mental alertness because methadone therapy may cause drowsiness or sleepiness.
•Teach patient to change positions slowly to minimize effects of orthostatic hypotension.
•Instruct patient to notify prescriber of worsening or breakthrough pain because dosage may need to be adjusted.
•Inform parents of child on methadone maintenance therapy that child may experience unusual excitement or restlessness; advise them to notify prescriber of any change in child's behavior.
•Instruct female patient to notify prescriber immediately if she becomes pregnant during methadone therapy because drug may cause physical dependence in fetus and withdrawal symptoms in neonate.

- Caution patient who is breast-feeding not to stop doing so abruptly and not to stop taking methadone without prescriber's approval because infant may experience withdrawal symptoms.

methamphetamine hydrochloride

Desoxyn, Desoxyn Gradumet

Class, Category, and Schedule

Chemical: Amphetamine
Therapeutic: CNS stimulant
Pregnancy category: C
Controlled substance: Schedule II

Indications and Dosages

➤ *To treat attention-deficit hyperactivity disorder (ADHD)*

E.R. TABLETS

Children age 6 and older. 20 to 25 mg q.d.

TABLETS

Children age 6 and older. *Initial:* 5 mg q.d. or b.i.d. Increased by 5 mg q wk. *Maintenance:* 20 to 25 mg/day in divided doses b.i.d.

Route	Onset	Peak	Duration
P.O.	Unknown	Unknown	6 to 24 hr

Mechanism of Action

May produce CNS stimulation by facilitating norepinephrine's release and blocking its reuptake at adrenergic nerve terminals and by directly stimulating alpha and beta receptors in the peripheral nervous system. Methamphetamine also promotes dopamine release and blocks its reuptake in the brain's limbic regions. The drug appears to act mainly in the cerebral cortex and, possibly, the reticular activating system. These actions decrease motor restlessness, increase alertness, and diminish drowsiness and fatigue. The drug's peripheral actions include increased blood pressure and mild bronchodilation and respiratory stimulation.

Contraindications

Advanced arteriosclerosis; glaucoma; hypersensitivity to methamphetamine, sympathomimetic amines, or their components; hyperthyroidism; history of drug abuse; moderate to severe hypertension; severe agitation; symptomatic cardiovascular disease; use within 14 days of MAO inhibitor therapy

Interactions

DRUGS

ascorbic acid: Decreased methamphetamine absorption and therapeutic effect
beta blockers: Increased risk of heart block, hypotension, and severe bradycardia
CNS stimulants: Increased CNS stimulation and risk of adverse reactions
digoxin, levodopa: Increased risk of arrhythmias
diuretics, other antihypertensives: Possibly decreased antihypertensive effect
ethosuximide, phenobarbital, phenytoin: Possibly delayed absorption of these drugs
haloperidol, phenothiazines: Possibly interference with these drugs' therapeutic effects and with methamphetamine's CNS stimulant effects
inhalation anesthetics: Increased risk of ventricular arrhythmias
insulin: Altered insulin requirements
lithium: Possibly antagonized CNS stimulant effects of methamphetamine
MAO inhibitors: Possibly severe hypertension, risk of hypertensive crisis, increased vasopressor effect of methamphetamine
meperidine: Increased risk of hypotension and life-threatening interactions, such as severe respiratory depression and coma
metrizamide (intrathecal): Increased risk of seizures
thyroid hormones: Enhanced effects of both drugs
tricyclic antidepressants: Increased risk of arrhythmias and severe hypertension
urinary acidifiers: Increased metabolism and shortened pharmacologic effects of methamphetamine
urinary alkalinizers: Decreased metabolism and prolonged pharmacologic effects of methamphetamine

FOODS

caffeine: Increased methamphetamine effects

Adverse Reactions

CNS: Dizziness, euphoria, headache, hyperactivity, insomnia, irritability, nervousness, psychotic episodes, restlessness, talkativeness, tremor
CV: Arrhythmias, chest pain, hypertension, hypotension, palpitations, tachycardia
EENT: Blurred vision, dry mouth, taste perversion
GI: Abdominal cramps, anorexia, constipation, diarrhea, nausea, vomiting

M

GU: Impotence, libido changes
SKIN: Diaphoresis, urticaria
Other: Physical and psychological dependence

Nursing Considerations

• Use methamphetamine cautiously in patients with a history of psychiatric problems or suicidal or homicidal tendencies.
• Assess for seizures in patients with a history of seizure disorders because drug may lower seizure threshold.
• Observe for signs of drug tolerance and, possibly, extreme dependence, which may develop after a few weeks. Be aware that methamphetamine abuse may occur.
• Expect treatment for ADHD to include psychological, educational, and social measures in addition to drug therapy.
• Watch for signs of chronic methamphetamine intoxication, including hyperactivity, insomnia, irritability, and personality changes. Notify prescriber if such signs occur.

PATIENT TEACHING

• Instruct parent of patient to give methamphetamine at least 6 hours before bedtime to prevent insomnia.
• Explain the high risk of abuse with this drug. Instruct parent of patient not to increase dosage unless advised to do so by prescriber and not to give drug to prevent fatigue.
• Caution parent that patient should not crush or chew E.R. tablets.
• Advise parent that patient should avoid caffeine, which increases drug's effects.
• Instruct parent of patient to report signs of overstimulation, such as diarrhea, hyperactivity, insomnia, and irritability.

methazolamide

MZM, Neptazane

Class and Category

Chemical: Sulfonamide derivative
Therapeutic: Antiglaucoma
Pregnancy category: C

Indications and Dosages

➤ *To treat open-angle glaucoma*
TABLETS
Adults. 50 to 100 mg b.i.d. or t.i.d.

Route	Onset	Peak	Duration
P.O.	2 to 4 hr	6 to 8 hr	10 to 18 hr

Mechanism of Action

Inhibits the enyzme carbonic anhydrase, which normally appears in renal proximal tubule cells, choroid plexus of the brain, and ciliary processes of the eye. By inhibiting this enzyme in the eyes, methazolamide decreases aqueous humor secretion, which reduces intraocular pressure.

Contraindications

Cirrhosis; hyperchloremic acidosis; hypersensitivity to methazolamide, other carbonic anhydrase inhibitors, or their components; hypokalemia; hyponatremia; severe adrenocortical, hepatic, or renal impairment

Interactions
DRUGS

amphetamines, anticholinergics, mecamylamine, procainamide, quinidine: Decreased renal clearance of these drugs, increased risk of toxicity
amphotericin B, corticosteroids: Increased risk of severe hypokalemia
barbiturates, carbamazepine, phenytoin, primidone: Increased risk of osteopenia
digoxin: Increased risk of hypokalemia and digitalis toxicity
ephedrine: Possibly prolonged duration of action of ephedrine
insulin, oral antidiabetic drugs: Increased risk of glycosuria and hyperglycemia
lithium: Increased lithium excretion
mannitol: Increased diuresis and further reduction of intraocular pressure
methenamine compounds: Decreased methenamine effectiveness
mexiletine: Possibly impaired renal excretion of mexiletine
neuromuscular blockers: Possibly prolonged duration of action of blockers from methazolamide-induced hypokalemia, increased risk of prolonged respiratory paralysis and depression
salicylates: Possibly CNS depression and metabolic acidosis, increased risk of methazolamide toxicity

Adverse Reactions

CNS: Confusion, depression, drowsiness, fatigue, fever, malaise, paresthesia, seizures, weakness
EENT: Hearing loss, myopia (transient), taste perversion, tinnitus

GI: Anorexia, diarrhea, nausea, vomiting
GU: Crystalluria, nephrotoxicity, renal calculi
SKIN: Photosensitivity, pruritus, rash, Stevens-Johnson syndrome, urticaria
Other: Metabolic acidosis

Nursing Considerations
• Use methazolamide cautiously in patients with obstructive pulmonary disease.
• Monitor fluid intake and output, weight, and serum electrolyte levels during methazolamide therapy.

PATIENT TEACHING
• Direct patient to take methazolamide exactly as prescribed because increasing dosage may lead to metabolic acidosis.
• Advise patient to take drug with food if GI distress occurs.
• Instruct patient to notify prescriber if rash develops.
• Caution patient to avoid potentially hazardous activities until drug's CNS effects are known.
• Stress the importance of regular eye examinations during methazolamide therapy.

methenamine hippurate

Hiprex, Urex

methenamine mandelate

Mandelamine

Class and Category
Chemical: Formaldehyde precursor, hexamethylenetetramine
Therapeutic: Antibiotic
Pregnancy category: C

Indications and Dosages
➤ *To prevent or suppress frequently recurring UTIs caused by a wide variety of gram-negative and gram-positive bacteria (including enterococci,* Escherichia coli, Micrococcus pyogenes, *and staphylococci) in intermittently catheterized patients with neurogenic bladder*

ENTERIC-COATED TABLETS, ORAL SUSPENSION (METHENAMINE MANDELATE)
Adults and adolescents. 1 g q.i.d. a.c. and h.s.
Children ages 6 to 12. 500 mg q.i.d., or 50 mg/kg/day in divided doses.
Children under age 6. 18.4 mg/kg q.i.d.

TABLETS (METHENAMINE HIPPURATE)
Adults and adolescents. 1 g b.i.d.
Children ages 6 to 12. 0.5 to 1 g q 12 hr.

Mechanism of Action
Hydrolyzes to formaldehyde and ammonia in an acidic environment, such as urine, producing greater amounts of formaldehyde as pH decreases. Formaldehyde exerts a bactericidal action, possibly by denaturing proteins. To facilitate hydrolysis, methenamine is formulated with a weak organic acid, such as hippuric acid or mandelic acid.

Contraindications
Concurrent therapy with sulfonamides, hypersensitivity to methenamine, renal insufficiency, severe dehydration, severe hepatic disease

Interactions
DRUGS
bicarbonate-containing antacids, urinary alkalinizers: Decreased methenamine effectiveness
sulfonamides, such as sulfamethizole: Possibly formation of insoluble precipitate in urine
FOODS
milk, milk products, most fruits: Possibly decreased effectiveness of methenamine

Adverse Reactions
CNS: Headache
CV: Edema
EENT: Stomatitis
GI: Abdominal cramps, anorexia, diarrhea, nausea, vomiting
GU: Bladder irritation, crystalluria, dysuria, hematuria, proteinuria, urinary frequency
RESP: Pulmonary hypersensitivity (dyspnea, pneumonitis)
SKIN: Pruritus, rash, urticaria

Nursing Considerations
• Be aware that methenamine is used for prophylaxis; it isn't recommended as primary treatment for UTI.
• Be aware that drug shouldn't be given to patients whose creatinine clearance is less than 50 ml/min/1.73 m^2.
• Before giving first dose, expect to obtain urine specimen for culture and sensitivity tests, as ordered, and to review test results if available.
• Plan to give methenamine mandelate around the clock to maintain a therapeutic blood level.
• Make sure patient receives adequate fluids.

M

•Expect to repeat culture and sensitivity tests if patient fails to improve.

PATIENT TEACHING
•Instruct patient to take methenamine with food to avoid GI distress.
•Direct patient to drink extra fluids; avoid alkaline foods, such as milk, milk products, and most fruits; and avoid antacids that contain sodium bicarbonate or carbonate during methenamine therapy.
•Instruct patient to report painful urination, rash, or severe GI distress.
•Urge patient to comply with order for urine testing before and during long-term therapy.

methicillin sodium

Staphcillin

Class and Category
Chemical: Penicillinase-resistant penicillin
Therapeutic: Antibiotic
Pregnancy category: B

Indications and Dosages
➤ *To treat general infections, such as sepsis, sinusitis, and skin and soft-tissue infections, caused by susceptible organisms (including penicillinase-producing and non-penicillinase-producing strains of* Staphylococcus epidermidis, Staphylococcus saprophyticus, *and* Streptococcus pneumoniae)

I.V. INFUSION, I.M. INJECTION
Adults and children weighing 40 kg (88 lb) or more. 1 g q 4 to 6 hr (I.M.) or 1 g q 6 hr (I.V.). *Maximum:* 24 g/day.
Children weighing less than 40 kg. 25 mg/kg q 6 hr.
DOSAGE ADJUSTMENT For adults and children with cystic fibrosis, dosage adjusted to 50 mg/kg q 6 hr.
➤ *To treat bacterial meningitis*
I.V. INFUSION, I.M. INJECTION
Neonates weighing 2 kg (4.4 lb) or more. 50 mg/kg q 8 hr for first wk after birth and then 50 mg/kg q 6 hr.
Neonates weighing less than 2 kg. 25 to 50 mg/kg q 12 hr for first wk after birth and then 50 mg/kg q 8 hr.

Incompatibilities
Don't mix methicillin in same syringe or I.V. solution with other drugs. Don't mix methi-cillin with dextrose solutions because their low acidity may damage drug. Administer methicillin at least 1 hour before or after aminoglycosides and at different sites; otherwise, mutual inactivation can occur.

Mechanism of Action
Kills bacterial cells by inhibiting bacterial cell wall synthesis. In susceptible bacteria, the rigid, cross-linked cell wall is assembled in several steps. In the final stage of cross-linking, methicillin binds with and inactivates penicillin-binding proteins (enzymes responsible for linking cell wall strands), resulting in bacterial cell lysis and death. *Staphylococcus aureus* has developed resistance to methicillin by altering its penicillin-binding proteins.

Contraindications
Hypersensitivity to methicillin sodium, other penicillins, or their components

Interactions
DRUGS
aminoglycosides: Substantial aminoglycoside inactivation
chloramphenicol, erythromycins, sulfonamides, tetracyclines: Possibly decreased therapeutic effects of methicillin
methotrexate: Increased risk of methotrexate toxicity
probenecid: Possibly decreased renal clearance, increased blood level, and increased risk of toxicity of methicillin

Adverse Reactions
CNS: Aggressiveness, agitation, anxiety, confusion, depression, headache, seizures
EENT: Oral candidiasis
GI: Abdominal pain, diarrhea, hepatotoxicity, nausea, pseudomembranous colitis, vomiting
GU: Interstitial nephritis, vaginitis
HEME: Leukopenia, neutropenia, thrombocytopenia
SKIN: Exfoliative dermatitis, pruritus, rash, urticaria
Other: Anaphylaxis; infusion site redness, swelling, and tenderness; injection site pain, redness, and swelling; serum sickness–like reaction

Nursing Considerations

• **WARNING** Be aware that methicillin is not a first-line treatment for the indications above because of the prevalence of methicillin-resistant *Staphylococcus aureus.*

• Before giving first dose, obtain appropriate body fluid or tissue specimens for culture and sensitivity tests, as ordered, and review test results if available.

• Inject I.M. form deep into gluteal muscle.

• During I.V. use, observe infusion site closely for redness, swelling, and tenderness.

• Monitor fluid intake and output and renal function test results during methicillin therapy.

• Observe for signs of superinfection, such as diarrhea, vaginal itching, and white patches or sores in mouth or on tongue. Notify prescriber if they occur.

• Closely monitor renal function test results, including serum creatinine level; about one-third of patients experience interstitial nephritis after 10 days of methicillin therapy.

• Monitor liver function test results, and observe for signs of hepatotoxicity, such as fever and nausea. Notify prescriber if they develop.

PATIENT TEACHING

• Inform patient that I.M. injection may be painful.

• Unless contraindicated, instruct patient to drink extra fluids during methicillin therapy.

• Advise patient to report diarrhea, injection site pain, mouth sores, or rash.

methimazole

Tapazole

Class and Category

Chemical: Thioimidazole derivative
Therapeutic: Antithyroid
Pregnancy category: D

Indications and Dosages

➤ *To treat mild hyperthyroidism*

TABLETS

Adults and adolescents. *Initial:* 15 mg/day as a single dose or in divided doses b.i.d. for 6 to 8 wk or until euthyroid level is reached. *Maintenance:* 5 to 30 mg/day as a single dose or in divided doses b.i.d.

Children. *Initial:* 0.4 mg/kg/day as a single dose or in divided doses b.i.d. *Maintenance:* 0.2 mg/kg/day as a single dose or in divided doses b.i.d.

➤ *To treat moderate hyperthyroidism*

TABLETS

Adults and adolescents. *Initial:* 30 to 40 mg/day as a single dose or in divided doses b.i.d. for 6 to 8 wk or until euthyroid level is reached. *Maintenance:* 5 to 30 mg/day as a single dose or in divided doses b.i.d.

Children. *Initial:* 0.4 mg/kg/day as a single dose or in divided doses b.i.d. *Maintenance:* 0.2 mg/kg/day as a single dose or in divided doses b.i.d.

➤ *To treat severe hyperthyroidism*

TABLETS

Adults and adolescents. *Initial:* 60 mg/day as a single dose or in divided doses b.i.d. for 6 to 8 wk or until euthyroid level is reached. *Maintenance:* 5 to 30 mg/day as a single dose or in divided doses b.i.d.

Children. *Initial:* 0.4 mg/kg/day as a single dose or in divided doses b.i.d. *Maintenance:* 0.2 mg/kg/day as a single dose or in divided doses b.i.d.

➤ *As adjunct to treat thyrotoxicosis*

SUPPOSITORIES

Adults and adolescents. 15 to 20 mg q 4 hr on first day and then adjusted based on patient response.

Children. 0.4 mg/kg/day as a single dose or in divided doses b.i.d.

Route	Onset	Peak	Duration
P.O.	5 days	7 wk	Unknown

Mechanism of Action

Directly interferes with thyroid hormone synthesis in the thyroid gland by inhibiting iodide incorporation into thyroglobulin. Iodination of thyroglobulin is an important step in synthesizing the thyroid hormones thyroxine and triiodothyronine. Eventually, thyroglobulin is depleted and the circulating thyroid hormone level drops.

Contraindications

Breast-feeding; hypersensitivity to methimazole, other antithyroid drugs, or their components

Interactions

DRUGS

amiodarone, iodine, potassium iodide: Decreased response to methimazole
digoxin: Possibly increased blood digoxin level

oral anticoagulants: Possibly a need for altered anticoagulant dosage

Adverse Reactions

CNS: Drowsiness, headache, paresthesia, vertigo
CV: Edema
EENT: Loss of taste
ENDO: Hypothyroidism
GI: Diarrhea, indigestion, nausea, vomiting
HEME: Agranulocytosis, aplastic anemia, leukopenia, thrombocytopenia
MS: Arthralgia, myalgia
SKIN: Alopecia, jaundice, pruritus, rash, skin discoloration, urticaria
Other: Lupus-like symptoms, lymphadenopathy

Nursing Considerations

• Closely monitor thyroid function test results during methimazole therapy.
• Check CBC results to detect abnormalities caused by inhibition of myelopoiesis.
• Observe patient for signs of hypothyroidism, such as cold intolerance, depression, and edema.
• Be aware that hyperthyroidism may increase metabolic clearance of beta blockers and theophylline and that dosages of these drugs may need to be reduced as the patient's thyroid condition becomes corrected.

PATIENT TEACHING
• Instruct patient to take drug with meals to avoid adverse GI reactions.
• Advise patient that temporary hair loss or thinning may occur during therapy and for months afterward.
• Instruct patient to notify prescriber immediately about cold intolerance, fever, sore throat, tiredness, and unusual bleeding or bruising.

methocarbamol

Carbacot, Robaxin, Robaxin 750, Skelex
Class and Category
Chemical: Carbamate derivative of guaifenesin
Therapeutic: Skeletal muscle relaxant
Pregnancy category: C

Indications and Dosages

➤ *To relieve discomfort caused by acute, painful musculoskeletal conditions*
TABLETS
Adults and adolescents. *Initial:* 1,500 mg q.i.d. for 2 to 3 days; for severe discomfort,

8,000 mg/day. *Maintenance:* 750 mg q 4 hr, 1,000 mg q.i.d., or 1,500 mg t.i.d.
I.V. INJECTION (100 MG/ML)
Adults and adolescents. Up to 3,000 mg/day administered at 8-hr intervals for 3 consecutive days. Regimen repeated as prescribed after patient is drug-free for 48 hr.
I.M. INJECTION (100 MG/ML)
Adults and adolescents. 1,000 to 3,000 mg/day administered at 8-hr intervals for 3 consecutive days. Regimen repeated as prescribed after patient is drug-free for 48 hr.
➤ *To provide supportive therapy for tetanus*
TABLETS
Adults and adolescents. 24,000 mg/day given by NG tube.
I.V. INFUSION OR INJECTION (100 MG/ML)
Adults and adolescents. 1,000 to 3,000 mg by infusion or 1,000 to 2,000 mg by direct injection q 6 hr. *Maximum:* 300 mg (3 ml)/min.
Children. 15 mg/kg q 6 hr.

Route	Onset	Peak	Duration
P.O.	30 min	Unknown	Unknown
I.V.	Immediate	Unknown	Unknown

Mechanism of Action

May depress the CNS, which leads to sedation and reduced skeletal muscle spasms. Methocarbamol also alters the perception of pain.

Contraindications

Hypersensitivity to methocarbamol or its components, renal disease (injectable form)

Interactions

DRUGS
CNS depressants: Increased CNS depression
ACTIVITIES
alcohol use: Increased CNS depression

Adverse Reactions

CNS: Dizziness, drowsiness, fever, headache, light-headedness, seizures (I.V.), syncope, vertigo, weakness
CV: Bradycardia, hypotension, and thrombophlebitis (parenteral)
EENT: Blurred vision, conjunctivitis, diplopia, metallic taste, nasal congestion, nystagmus
GI: Nausea
GU: Black, brown, or green urine
SKIN: Flushing, pruritus, rash, urticaria

Other: Anaphylaxis (parenteral), injection site irritation or pain (I.M.), injection site sloughing (I.V.)

Nursing Considerations
•If needed, crush tablets and mix with water for administration by NG tube.
•Administer I.V. form of methocarbamol directly through I.V. infusion line at 3 ml/min. To prepare solution for I.V. infusion, add 10 ml to no more than 250 ml of D_5W or NS. Infuse at no more than 300 mg (3 ml)/min to avoid hypotension and seizures.
•Keep patient recumbent during I.V. administration and for at least 15 minutes afterward. Then have him rise slowly.
•Monitor I.V. site regularly for signs of phlebitis.
•Inject I.M. form deep into large muscle mass, such as gluteal muscle. Administer no more than 5 ml/dose every 8 hours. One dose is usually adequate.
•Don't give drug by S.C. route.
•Keep epinephrine, antihistamines, and corticosteroids available in case patient experiences anaphylactic reaction to parenterally administered drug.

PATIENT TEACHING
•Instruct patient to take methocarbamol tablets exactly as prescribed and not to increase dosage or frequency.
•Advise patient to take drug with food or milk to avoid nausea.
•Inform patient that urine may turn green, black, or brown but that this will resolve when drug is discontinued.
•Advise patient to avoid potentially hazardous activities until drug's CNS effects are known.
•Instruct patient to avoid alcohol and other CNS depressants during methocarbamol therapy.

methotrexate
(amethopterin)
Rheumatrex

methotrexate sodium
Folex, Folex PFS, Mexate, Mexate-AQ

Class and Category
Chemical: Folic acid analogue
Therapeutic: Antipsoriatic, antirheumatic
Pregnancy category: X

Indications and Dosages
➤ *To treat severe psoriasis unresponsive to other therapy*

TABLETS (METHOTREXATE)
Adults. 2.5 to 5 mg q 12 hr for 3 doses/wk, increased as ordered by 2.5 mg/wk. *Maximum:* 20 mg/wk.

I.V. OR I.M. INJECTION (METHOTREXATE SODIUM)
Adults. 10 mg/wk. *Maximum:* 25 mg/wk.

➤ *To treat severe rheumatoid arthritis unresponsive to other therapy*

TABLETS (METHOTREXATE)
Adults. 2.5 to 5 mg q 12 hr for 3 doses/wk, increased as ordered by 2.5 mg/wk. *Maximum:* 20 mg/wk.

Route	Onset	Peak	Duration
P.O., I.V., I.M.	3 to 6 wk	Unknown	Unknown

Mechanism of Action
May exert its immunosuppressive effects by inhibiting the replication and function of T lymphocytes and, possibly, B lymphocytes, which are involved in immune and inflammatory processes. Methotrexate also slows the growth of rapidly proliferating cells, such as epithelial skin cells associated with psoriasis. This action may result from the drug's ability to inhibit dihydrofolate reductase, the enzyme that reduces folic acid to tetrahydrofolic acid. Inhibition of tetrahydrofolic acid interferes with DNA synthesis and cell reproduction in rapidly proliferating cells.

Contraindications
Breast-feeding, hypersensitivity to methotrexate or its components, pregnancy

Interactions
DRUGS
bone marrow depressants: Possibly increased bone marrow depression
folic acid: Possibly decreased effectiveness of methotrexate
hepatotoxic drugs: Increased risk of hepatotoxicity
neomycin: Possibly decreased absorption of methotrexate
NSAIDs, probenecid, salicylates: Increased risk of methotrexate toxicity
oral anticoagulants: Increased risk of bleeding
sulfonamides: Increased risk of hepatotoxicity

vaccines: Risk of disseminated infection with live-virus vaccines, risk of suppressed response to killed-virus vaccines

ACTIVITIES

alcohol use: Increased risk of hepatotoxicity

Adverse Reactions

CNS: Cerebral thrombosis, chills, drowsiness, fatigue, fever, headache

CV: Chest pain, deep vein thrombosis, hypotension, pericardial effusion, pericarditis, thromboembolism

EENT: Blurred vision, conjunctivitis, gingivitis, glossitis, pharyngitis, stomatitis, tinnitus

GI: Anorexia, diarrhea, enteritis, GI bleeding, hepatotoxicity, nausea, pancreatitis, vomiting

GU: Cystitis, hematuria, nephropathy, renal failure, tubular necrosis

HEME: Anemia, leukopenia, thrombocytopenia

MS: Arthralgia, myalgia

RESP: Dry cough, dyspnea, pulmonary fibrosis, pulmonary infiltrates

SKIN: Acne, alopecia, ecchymosis, photosensitivity, pruritus, psoriatic lesions, rash, Stevens-Johnson syndrome, urticaria

Other: Increased risk of infection

Nursing Considerations

• Follow facility policy for handling methotrexate; preparing and handling parenteral form poses a risk of carcinogenicity, mutagenicity, or teratogenicity. Avoid skin contact with parenteral form.

• Monitor results of CBC, chest X-ray, liver and renal function tests, and urinalysis before and during treatment.

• Unless contraindicated, increase patient's fluid intake to 2 to 3 L/day to reduce the risk of adverse GU reactions.

• Assess for signs of bleeding and infection.

• **WARNING** Expect renal impairment to severely alter drug elimination.

• Be aware that high doses of methotrexate can impair renal elimination by forming crystals that obstruct urine flow. To prevent drug precipitation, alkalinize patient's urine with sodium bicarbonate tablets, as ordered.

• Follow standard precautions when caring for patient because drug can cause immunosuppression.

• If patient becomes dehydrated from vomiting, notify prescriber and expect to withhold drug until patient recovers.

• If patient receives high doses of drug, keep leucovorin readily available to use as antidote.

• Be aware that methotrexate resistance may develop with prolonged use.

PATIENT TEACHING

• Prepare a calendar of treatment days for patient, and stress the importance of following instructions exactly.

• Instruct patient to avoid alcohol during methotrexate therapy.

• Encourage frequent mouth care to reduce the risk of mouth sores.

• Instruct patient to use sunblock when exposed to sunlight.

• Advise patient to notify prescriber about bruising, chills, cough, fever, dark or bloody urine, mouth sores, shortness of breath, sore throat, and yellow skin or eyes.

• Urge women of childbearing age to use contraception during methotrexate therapy.

methsuximide

Celontin

Class and Category

Chemical: Succinimide derivative
Therapeutic: Anticonvulsant
Pregnancy category: Not rated

Indications and Dosages

➤ *To treat absence seizures unresponsive to other drugs*

CAPSULES

Adults and children. *Initial:* 300 mg q.d. Increased by 150 to 300 mg/day q 1 to 2 weeks until control is achieved with minimal adverse reactions. *Maximum:* 1.2 g/day in divided doses.

Mechanism of Action

Elevates seizure threshold and reduces frequency of seizures by depressing the motor cortex and elevating the threshold of CNS response to convulsive stimuli. Methsuximide is metabolized to the active metabolite *N*-demethylmethsuximide, which may add to the anticonvulsant effects of the drug.

Contraindications

Hypersensitivity to methsuximide, succinimides, or their components

Interactions

DRUGS

carbamazepine, phenobarbital, phenytoin, primidone: Possibly decreased blood methsuximide level

CNS depressants: Possibly increased CNS depression

haloperidol: Altered seizure pattern; possibly decreased blood haloperidol level

loxapine, MAO inhibitors, maprotiline, molindone, phenothiazines, pimozide, thioxanthenes, tricyclic antidepressants: Possibly lowered seizure threshold and reduced therapeutic effect of methsuximide

ACTIVITIES

alcohol use: Possibly increased CNS depression

Adverse Reactions

CNS: Aggressiveness, ataxia, decreased concentration, dizziness, drowsiness, fatigue, fever, headache, insomnia, irritability, mental depression, nightmares, seizures

EENT: Periorbital edema, pharyngitis

GI: Abdominal and epigastric pain, abdominal cramps, abnormal liver function test results, anorexia, diarrhea, hiccups, nausea, vomiting

GU: Microscopic hematuria, proteinuria

HEME: Agranulocytosis, aplastic anemia, eosinophilia, leukopenia, pancytopenia

MS: Muscle pain

SKIN: Erythematous and pruritic rash, Stevens-Johnson syndrome, systemic lupus erythematosus, urticaria

Other: Lymphadenopathy

Nursing Considerations

• Monitor CBC and platelet count and assess patient for signs of infection, such as cough, fever, and pharyngitis, because methsuximide may cause blood dyscrasias.

• Monitor liver function test results and urinalysis results in patients with a history of hepatic or renal disease because methsuximide may cause functional changes in the liver and kidneys.

• When administering drug to patient with a history of mixed-type epilepsy, institute seizure precautions according to facility protocol because drug may increase frequency of generalized tonic-clonic seizures.

• Expect the dosage to be carefully and slowly adjusted according to patient's response and needs and withdrawn slowly to avoid precipitating seizures.

• Plan to use the 150-mg capsule when making dosage adjustments for small children.

• Notify prescriber if patient develops depression or aggressiveness. Expect to have drug withdrawn slowly if these behavioral changes occur.

PATIENT TEACHING

• Stress the importance of complying with methsuximide regimen.

• Advise patient to take a missed dose as soon as he remembers unless it's nearly time for the next dose. Warn him not to double the dose.

• Instruct patient not to take capsules that are melted or not full because drug effectiveness will be reduced.

• Instruct patient to take the drug with milk or food to reduce gastric irritation.

• Advise patient to notify prescriber if he develops cough, fever, or pharyngitis.

• Urge patient to avoid alcohol because of the increased risk of CNS depression.

• Instruct patient not to engage in potentially hazardous activities until drug's adverse effects are known.

• Caution patient not to stop taking drug abruptly because doing so increases the risk of absence seizures.

• Instruct patient to avoid excessive heat when storing or transporting drug, such as near an oven or in a closed car, because the capsules can melt easily.

methyldopa

Aldomet, Apo-Methyldopa (CAN), Dopamet (CAN), Nu-Medopa (CAN)

methyldopate hydrochloride

Aldomet

Class and Category

Chemical: 3,4-dihydroxyphenylalanine (DOPA) analogue

Therapeutic: Antihypertensive

Pregnancy category: B (oral form), C (parenteral form)

Indications and Dosages

➤ *To manage hypertension, to treat hypertensive crisis*

ORAL SUSPENSION, TABLETS (METHYLDOPA)

Adults. *Initial:* 250 mg b.i.d. or t.i.d. for first 48 hr, increased as ordered after 2 days. *Maintenance:* 500 to 2,000 mg/day in divided doses b.i.d. to q.i.d. *Maximum:* 3,000 mg/day.

Children. *Initial:* 10 mg/kg/day in divided doses b.i.d. to q.i.d. for first 48 hr, increased as ordered after 2 days. *Maximum:* 65 mg/kg or 3,000 mg/day.

I.V. INFUSION (METHYLDOPATE HYDROCHLORIDE)

Adults. 250 to 500 mg diluted in D_5W and infused over 30 to 60 min q 6 hr. *Maximum:* 1,000 mg q 6 hr.

Children. 20 to 40 mg/kg infused over 30 to 60 min q 6 hr. *Maximum:* 65 mg/kg or 3,000 mg/day.

Route	Onset	Peak	Duration
P.O.	Unknown	4 to 6 hr*	12 to 24 hr†
I.V.	Unknown	4 to 6 hr	10 to 16 hr

Mechanism of Action

Is decarboxylated in the body to produce alpha-methylnorepinephrine, a metabolite that stimulates central inhibitory alpha-adrenergic receptors. This action may reduce blood pressure by decreasing sympathetic stimulation of the heart and peripheral vascular system.

Incompatibilities

Don't administer methyldopa through same I.V. line as barbiturates or sulfonamides.

Contraindications

Active hepatic disease, hypersensitivity to methyldopa or its components, impaired hepatic function from previous methyldopa therapy, use within 14 days of MAO inhibitor therapy

Interactions

DRUGS

antihypertensives: Increased hypotension
appetite suppressants, NSAIDs, tricyclic antidepressants: Possibly decreased therapeutic effects of methyldopa
central anesthetics: Possibly need for reduced anesthetic dosage
CNS depressants: Possibly increased CNS depression
haloperidol: Increased risk of adverse CNS effects

levodopa: Possibly decreased therapeutic effects of levodopa and increased risk of adverse CNS effects
lithium: Increased risk of lithium toxicity
MAO inhibitors: Possibly hallucinations, headaches, hyperexcitability, and severe hypertension
oral anticoagulants: Possibly increased therapeutic effects of anticoagulants
sympathomimetics: Possibly decreased therapeutic effects of methyldopa and increased vasopressor effects of sympathomimetics

ACTIVITIES

alcohol use: Possibly increased CNS depression

Adverse Reactions

CNS: Decreased concentration, depression, dizziness, drowsiness, fever, headache, involuntary motor activity, memory loss (transient), nightmares, paresthesia, parkinsonism, sedation, vertigo, weakness
CV: Angina, bradycardia, edema, heart failure, myocarditis, orthostatic hypotension
EENT: Black or sore tongue, dry mouth, nasal congestion
ENDO: Gynecomastia
GI: Constipation, diarrhea, flatulence, hepatic necrosis, hepatitis, nausea, pancreatitis, vomiting
GU: Decreased libido, impotence
HEME: Agranulocytosis, hemolytic anemia, leukopenia, positive Coombs' test, positive tests for ANA and rheumatoid factor, thrombocytopenia
SKIN: Eczema, rash, urticaria
Other: Weight gain

Nursing Considerations

•For I.V. infusion, add methyldopate to 100 ml of D_5W and administer over 30 to 60 minutes.
•Expect to monitor CBC and differential results before and periodically during methyldopa therapy.
•Monitor blood pressure regularly during therapy.
•Monitor results of Coombs' test; a positive result after several months of treatment indicates that patient has hemolytic anemia. Expect prescriber to discontinue drug.
•Assess for weight gain and edema. If they develop, administer a diuretic, as prescribed.
•Notify prescriber if patient experiences signs of heart failure (dyspnea, edema, hy-

---

* For single dose; 2 to 3 days for multiple doses.
† For single dose; 24 to 48 hr for multiple doses.

pertension) or involuntary, rapid, jerky movements.
•Be aware that hypertension may return within 48 hours after stopping drug.

PATIENT TEACHING
•Instruct patient to take methyldopa exactly as prescribed and not to skip a dose. Explain that hypertension can return within 48 hours after stopping drug.
•Suggest that patient take drug at bedtime to minimize daytime drowsiness.
•Instruct patient to weigh himself daily and to report a gain of more than 5 lb (2.3 kg) in 2 days.
•Advise patient to change position slowly to minimize effects of orthostatic hypotension.
•Direct patient to notify prescriber about bruising, chest pain, fever, involuntary jerky movements, prolonged dizziness, rash, and yellow eyes or skin.
•Caution patient not to discontinue drug abruptly; doing so may precipitate withdrawal symptoms, such as headache, hypertension, increased sweating, nausea, and tremor.

methylphenidate hydrochloride

Concerta, Metadate, Metadate CD, Metadate ER, Methylin, Methylin ER, PMS-Methylphenidate (CAN), Riphenidate (CAN), Ritalin, Ritalin-LA, Ritalin SR (CAN), Ritalin-SR

Class, Category, and Schedule
Chemical: Piperidine derivative
Therapeutic: CNS stimulant
Pregnancy category: C
Controlled substance: Schedule II

Indications and Dosages
➤ *To treat attention-deficit hyperactivity disorder (ADHD)*
CAPSULES, E.R. TABLETS, S.R. TABLETS, TABLETS
Adults and adolescents. 5 to 20 mg b.i.d. or t.i.d. *Maximum:* 90 mg/day.
Children ages 6 to 12. 5 mg b.i.d. before breakfast and lunch; increased as ordered by 5 to 10 mg/day at 1–wk intervals. *Maximum:* 60 mg/day.
E.R. ONCE-DAILY TABLETS (CONCERTA)
Adults and children age 6 and over. 18 mg q.d.; increased in 18-mg increments at 1-wk intervals. *Maximum:* 54 mg/day.

E.R. ONCE-DAILY CAPSULES (METADATE CD)
Children age 6 and over. 20 mg q.d. Dosage titrated to 40 or 60 mg q.d. based on individual response. *Maximum:* 60 mg/day.
DOSAGE ADJUSTMENT Dosage reduced or drug discontinued if no improvement in symptoms achieved within 1 mo. When maintenance dosage is achieved with tablets, regimen may be switched to E.R. or S.R. tablets.
➤ *To treat narcolepsy*
TABLETS
Adults and adolescents. 5 to 20 mg b.i.d. or t.i.d. *Maximum:* 90 mg/day.

Route	Onset	Peak	Duration
P.O. (tablets)	Unknown	Unknown	3 to 6 hr
P.O. (E.R., S.R.)	Unknown	Unknown	About 8 hr
P.O. (E.R. once-daily)	Unknown	Unknown	About 12 hr

Mechanism of Action
Blocks the reuptake mechanism of dopaminergic neurons in the cerebral cortex and subcortical structures of the brain, including the thalamus. This activity decreases motor restlessness and improves concentration in children with ADHD.
Methylphenidate also may trigger sympathomimetic activity. This action produces increased motor activity, alertness, mild euphoria, and decreased fatigue in patients with narcolepsy.

Contraindications
Anxiety, depression, glaucoma, hypersensitivity to methylphenidate or its components, motor tics, severe agitation, tension, Tourette syndrome, use within 14 days of MAO inhibitor therapy

Interactions
DRUGS
anticholinergics: Possibly increased anticholinergic effects of both drugs
anticonvulsants, oral anticoagulants, phenylbutazone, tricyclic antidepressants: Inhibited metabolism and increased blood levels of these drugs
diuretics, antihypertensives: Decreased therapeutic effects of these drugs

MAO inhibitors: Possibly increased adverse effects of methylphenidate, possibly severe hypertension

FOODS

caffeine: Increased methylphenidate effects

Adverse Reactions

CNS: Dizziness, fever, headache, hyperactivity, insomnia, nervousness, psychosis, Tourette syndrome
CV: Angina, bradycardia, hypertension, hypotension, palpitations, tachycardia
EENT: Dry throat, vision changes
ENDO: Growth suppression in children (with long-term use)
GI: Abdominal pain, anorexia, hepatotoxicity, nausea, vomiting
HEME: Anemia, leukopenia, thrombocytopenia, thrombocytopenic purpura
MS: Arthralgia
SKIN: Erythema multiforme, exfoliative dermatitis, rash, urticaria
Other: Physical and psychological dependence, weight loss

Nursing Considerations

•WARNING Be aware that methylphenidate may induce CNS stimulation and psychosis and may worsen behavior disturbances and thought disorders. Use drug cautiously in children with psychosis.
•WARNING Know that the E.R. tablet form (Concerta) shouldn't be administered to patients with esophageal motility disorders; drug may cause GI obstruction because the tablet doesn't change shape in GI tract.
•Monitor blood pressure and pulse rate to detect hypertension and signs of excessive stimulation. Notify prescriber if you detect such signs. For patient with hypertension, expect to increase antihypertensive dosage or add another antihypertensive to existing regimen.
•WARNING Monitor for signs of physical or psychological dependence. Methylphenidate's abuse potential is similar to that of amphetamines; use cautiously in patients with a history of drug abuse.
•Be aware that drug shouldn't be abruptly discontinued after long-term therapy; doing so may unmask dysphoria, paranoia, severe depression, or suicidal thoughts.
•Expect patient currently taking methylphenidate tablets b.i.d. or t.i.d., or E.R. tablets at doses of 20 to 60 mg/day, to be switched to E.R. once-daily tablets, as prescribed.

PATIENT TEACHING
•Instruct patient not to chew or crush E.R. tablets.
•Suggest that patient take tablets at least 6 hours before bedtime to avoid insomnia. Instruct him to take E.R. once-daily tablets in the morning.
•Advise patient taking E.R. once-daily tablets (Concerta) not to be alarmed if he notices intact tablet in stool. Inform him that drug is slowly released from nonabsorbable tablet shell.
•Inform patient taking capsule form to swallow it whole or sprinkle the capsule contents onto a tablespoon of applesauce and take immediately, followed by a liquid such as water.
•Direct patient to notify prescriber about excessive nervousness, fever, insomnia, palpitations, rash, or vomiting.
•Warn patient with seizure disorder that drug may cause seizures.
•Inform parents of children on long-term therapy that drug has the potential to delay growth.

methylprednisolone

Medrol, Meprolone

methylprednisolone acetate

depMedalone, Depoject, Depo-Medrol, Depopred, Depo-Predate, Methylcotolone

methylprednisolone sodium succinate

A-methaPred, Solu-Medrol

Class and Category

Chemical: Synthetic glucocorticoid
Therapeutic: Anti-inflammatory, immunosuppressant
Pregnancy category: Not rated

Indications and Dosages

➤ *To treat ulcerative colitis*
I.V. INFUSION (METHYLPREDNISOLONE SODIUM SUCCINATE)
Adults. 40 to 120 mg 3 to 7 times/wk for 2 or more wk. Later doses given I.V. or I.M., based on patient's condition and response.
Children. 0.14 to 0.84 mg/kg/day in divided doses q 12 to 24 hr.
➤ *To treat a wide range of immune and inflammatory disorders, including allergic*

rhinitis, asthma, Crohn's disease, and systemic lupus erythematosus

TABLETS (METHYLPREDNISOLONE)
Adults. 4 to 48 mg/day as a single dose or in divided doses.
Children. 0.42 to 1.67 mg/kg/day in divided doses t.i.d. or q.i.d.

I.V. INFUSION, I.M. INJECTION (METHYLPREDNISOLONE SODIUM SUCCINATE)
Adults. *Initial:* 10 to 40 mg infused over several min. Later doses given I.V. or I.M., based on patient's condition and response.
Children. 0.14 to 0.84 mg/kg q 12 to 24 hr.

I.M. INJECTION (METHYLPREDNISOLONE ACETATE)
Adults. 40 to 120 mg q.d. to q 2 wk, according to clinical response.
Children. 0.14 to 0.84 mg/kg 12 to 24 hr.

INTRA-ARTICULAR, INTRALESIONAL, OR SOFT-TISSUE INJECTION (METHYLPREDNISOLONE ACETATE)
Adults. 4 to 80 mg q 1 to 5 wk, according to clinical response.

➤ *To treat adrenal hyperplasia*
I.M. INJECTION (METHYLPREDNISOLONE ACETATE)
Adults. 40 mg q 2 wk.
Children. 0.14 to 0.84 mg/kg q 12 to 24 hr.

➤ *To treat acute exacerbations of multiple sclerosis*
TABLETS (METHYLPREDNISOLONE)
Adults. 160 mg q.d. for 7 days followed by 64 mg q.o.d. for 1 mo.
I.V. OR I.M. INJECTION (METHYLPREDNISOLONE ACETATE, METHYLPREDNISOLONE SODIUM SUCCINATE)
Adults. 160 mg q.d. for 1 wk followed by 64 mg q.o.d. for 1 mo.

➤ *To treat adrenocortical insufficiency*
TABLETS (METHYLPREDNISOLONE), I.M. INJECTION (METHYLPREDNISOLONE SODIUM SUCCINATE)
Children. 0.18 mg/kg/day in divided doses t.i.d.
I.M. INJECTION (METHYLPREDNISOLONE ACETATE)
Children. 0.12 mg/kg q 3 days or 0.039 to 0.059 mg/kg q.d.

Route	Onset	Peak	Duration
P.O.	In 60 min	1 to 2 hr	1.25 to 1.5 days
I.V.	Rapid	30 min	Unknown
I.M.	6 to 48 hr	4 to 8 days	1 to 4 wk

Incompatibilities

Don't mix methylprednisolone with any drug without first consulting pharmacist. Don't dilute methylprednisolone acetate with any other drug.

Mechanism of Action

Binds to intracellular glucocorticoid receptors and suppresses inflammatory and immune responses by:
• inhibiting the accumulation of neutrophils and monocytes at inflammation sites
• stabilizing lysosomal membranes
• suppressing the antigen response of macrophages and helper T cells
• inhibiting the synthesis of inflammatory response mediators, such as cytokines, interleukins, and prostaglandins.

Contraindications

Fungal infection, hypersensitivity to methylprednisolone or its components, idiopathic thrombocytopenic purpura (I.M.)

Interactions

DRUGS
acetaminophen: Increased risk of hepatotoxicity
amphotericin B, carbonic anhydrase inhibitors: Possibly severe hypokalemia
anabolic steroids, androgens: Increased risk of edema and worsening of acne
anticholinergics: Possibly increased intraocular pressure
asparaginase: Increased risk of hyperglycemia and toxicity
aspirin, NSAIDs: Increased risk of adverse GI effects and bleeding
cyclosporine: Increased risk of seizures
digoxin: Possibly hypokalemia-induced arrhythmias and digitalis toxicity
ephedrine, phenobarbital, phenytoin, rifampin: Decreased blood methylprednisolone level
estrogens, oral contraceptives: Possibly increased therapeutic and toxic effects of methylprednisolone
insulin, oral antidiabetic drugs: Possibly increased blood glucose level
isoniazid: Possibly decreased therapeutic effects of isoniazid
mexiletine: Possibly decreased blood mexiletine level
neuromuscular blockers: Possibly increased neuromuscular blockade, causing respiratory depression or apnea
oral anticoagulants, thrombolytics: Increased risk of GI ulceration and hemorrhage, possibly decreased therapeutic effects of these drugs
potassium-depleting drugs, such as thiazide diuretics: Possibly severe hypokalemia

potassium supplements: Possibly decreased effects of these supplements

somatrem, somatropin: Possibly decreased therapeutic effects of these drugs

streptozocin: Increased risk of hyperglycemia

troleandomycin: Increased blood methylprednisolone level

vaccines: Decreased antibody response and increased risk of neurologic complications

ACTIVITIES

alcohol use: Increased risk of adverse GI effects and bleeding

Adverse Reactions

CNS: Ataxia, behavioral changes, depression, dizziness, euphoria, fatigue, headache, increased intracranial pressure with papilledema, insomnia, malaise, mood changes, paresthesia, restlessness, seizures, steroid psychosis, syncope, vertigo

CV: Arrhythmias (from hypokalemia), edema, fat embolism, heart failure, hypertension, hypotension, thromboembolism, thrombophlebitis

EENT: Exophthalmos, glaucoma, increased intraocular pressure, nystagmus, posterior subcapsular cataracts

ENDO: Adrenal insufficiency, cushingoid symptoms (moon face, buffalo hump, central obesity, supraclavicular fat pad enlargement), diabetes mellitus, growth suppression in children, hyperglycemia, negative nitrogen balance from protein catabolism

GI: Abdominal distention, hiccups, increased appetite, melena, nausea, pancreatitis, peptic ulcer, ulcerative esophagitis, vomiting

GU: Amenorrhea, glycosuria, menstrual irregularities, perineal burning or tingling

HEME: Easy bruising, leukocytosis

MS: Arthralgia; aseptic necrosis of femoral and humeral heads; compression fractures; muscle atrophy, twitching, or weakness; myalgia; osteoporosis; spontaneous fractures; steroid myopathy; tendon rupture

SKIN: Acne; altered skin pigmentation; diaphoresis; erythema; hirsutism; necrotizing vasculitis; petechiae; purpura; rash; scarring; sterile abscess; striae; subcutaneous fat atrophy; thin, fragile skin; urticaria

Other: Anaphylaxis, hypocalcemia, hypokalemia, hypokalemic alkalosis, impaired wound healing, masking of signs of infection, metabolic alkalosis, suppressed skin test reaction, weight gain

Nursing Considerations

•Give methylprednisolone tablets with food to minimize indigestion and GI irritation. For once-daily dosing, administer in the morning to coincide with normal cortisol secretion. Expect prescriber to add an antacid or H_2-receptor antagonist to regimen.

•Discard parenteral products that are discolored or contain particles.

•Inject I.M. form deep into gluteal muscle.

•Arrange for low-sodium diet with added potassium, as prescribed.

•Protect patient from falling, especially elderly patient at risk for fractures from osteoporosis.

•Closely monitor for signs of infection because drug may mask them.

•Assess for possible depression or psychotic episodes during therapy.

•Monitor blood glucose level; dosage of insulin or oral antidiabetic drug may need to be adjusted in diabetic patient.

•**WARNING** To avoid possibly fatal acute adrenocortical insufficiency, expect to taper long-term therapy when it must be discontinued.

PATIENT TEACHING

•Caution patient not to stop taking methylprednisolone abruptly or to change dosage without consulting prescriber.

•Instruct patient to take a missed dose as soon as he remembers unless it's nearly time for the next dose. Caution against double-dosing.

•Urge patient to notify prescriber immediately about dark or tarry stools; signs of impending adrenocortical insufficiency, such as anorexia, dizziness, fainting, fatigue, fever, joint pain, muscle weakness, or nausea; and sudden weight gain or swelling.

•Instruct patient not to obtain vaccinations unless approved by prescriber.

•Urge patient to take vitamin D, calcium supplements, or both if recommended by prescriber.

•Inform patient that insomnia and restlessness usually resolve after 1 to 3 weeks of therapy.

•Caution patient to avoid people with contagious diseases.

•Discuss the need for regular exercise or physical therapy to maintain muscle mass.

•Advise patient to carry medical identification that documents his need for long-term corticosteroid therapy.

methysergide maleate

Sansert

Class and Category

Chemical: Synthetic ergot alkaloid
Therapeutic: Antimigraine
Pregnancy category: X

Indications and Dosages

➤ *To prevent or reduce intensity and frequency of vascular headaches, including cluster headaches, migraines, severe vascular headaches that occur at least once per week, and vascular headaches that are uncontrollable or so severe that prophylaxis is indicated regardless of frequency*

TABLETS

Adults. 4 to 8 mg/day in divided doses for up to 6 mo.

DOSAGE ADJUSTMENT After each 6-mo course of treatment, a 3- to 4-wk drug-free interval is prescribed to prevent fibrosis. To prevent rebound headaches, dosage tapered gradually, as ordered, over 2 to 3 wk before starting drug-free interval.

Route	Onset	Peak	Duration
P.O.	1 to 2 days	Unknown	1 to 2 days

Mechanism of Action

May prevent migraine headaches by inhibiting the effects of serotonin, a potent vasoconstrictor that may lower the pain threshold. Methysergide also inhibits histamine release from mast cells and stabilizes platelets. This action prevents serotonin-induced platelet aggregation, inflammation, and vasoconstriction.

Contraindications

Cellulitis or phlebitis of legs, collagen disease, coronary artery disease, debilitation, hypersensitivity to methysergide, peptic ulcer disease, peripheral vascular disease, pregnancy, pulmonary disease, renal or hepatic disease, severe arteriosclerosis or hypertension, severe infection, valvular heart disease

Interactions

DRUGS

*epinephrine (parenteral), metaraminol, methoxamine, norepinephrine, other ergot alka-*loids, *phenylephrine (parenteral), sumatriptan:* Increased vasoconstriction
opioid analgesics: Possibly reversed effects of opioids

FOODS

caffeine: Additive vasoconstriction

ACTIVITIES

alcohol use: Additive vasoconstriction
smoking: Increased risk of peripheral vascular ischemia

Adverse Reactions

CNS: Anxiety, ataxia, depression, dizziness, drowsiness, euphoria, feeling of dissociation, hallucinations, headache, insomnia, light-headedness, paresthesia, seizures, tremor, weakness
CV: Chest pain; claudication; fibrosis of aorta, common iliac vessels, heart valves, and inferior vena cava; orthostatic hypotension; peripheral edema; peripheral vascular insufficiency; tachycardia
EENT: Vision changes
GI: Abdominal pain, constipation, diarrhea, epigastric pain, nausea, vomiting
HEME: Leukopenia
RESP: Pulmonary fibrosis
SKIN: Alopecia, diaphoresis, flushing, pruritus, rash, telangiectasia
Other: Weight gain

Nursing Considerations

•Expect to obtain 12-lead ECG tracing to monitor cardiac status and results of CBC and erythrocyte sedimentation rate to monitor renal status before beginning therapy.
•Administer methysergide with meals to avoid GI distress.
•Monitor for early signs of peripheral vascular insufficiency, such as claudication, diminished peripheral pulses, and cold or pale feet or hands, especially in elderly patients.

PATIENT TEACHING

•Instruct patient to take methysergide with meals to avoid GI distress.
•Caution patient against consuming alcoholic and caffeinated beverages during therapy because they may aggravate headaches.
•Urge patient to avoid smoking during therapy because nicotine constricts blood vessels, which increases the risk of peripheral vascular insufficiency.
•Advise patient to change position slowly to minimize effects of orthostatic hypotension.

M

• Caution patient not to stop taking drug abruptly to avoid rebound headaches.
• Urge women of childbearing age to use contraception during methysergide therapy.

metoclopramide hydrochloride

Apo-Metoclop (CAN), Maxeran (CAN), Metoclopramide Intensol, Octamide, PMS-Metoclopramide (CAN), Reglan

Class and Category

Chemical: Benzamide
Therapeutic: Antiemetic, upper GI stimulant
Pregnancy category: B

Indications and Dosages

➤ *To treat diabetic gastroparesis*
ORAL SOLUTION, ORAL SOLUTION CONCENTRATE, TABLETS
Adults and adolescents. 10 mg 30 min a.c. and h.s. up to q.i.d.
I.V. OR I.M. INJECTION
Adults and adolescents. 10 mg t.i.d. or q.i.d. for severe symptoms; dosage adjusted as needed.
➤ *To treat gastroesophageal reflux disease*
ORAL SOLUTION, ORAL SOLUTION CONCENTRATE, TABLETS
Adults and adolescents. 10 to 15 mg 30 min a.c. and h.s.
➤ *To prevent chemotherapy-induced vomiting*
I.V. INFUSION
Adults and adolescents. 3 mg/kg before chemotherapy and then 0.5 mg/kg/hr for 8 hr.
I.V. INJECTION
Adults and adolescents. 1 to 2 mg/kg 30 min before chemotherapy and then repeated q 2 to 3 hr, as needed.
Children. 1 mg/kg as a single dose, repeated in 1 hr. *Maximum:* 2 mg/kg.
➤ *To prevent postoperative nausea and vomiting*
I.M. INJECTION
Adults and adolescents. 10 to 20 mg near end of procedure.
DOSAGE ADJUSTMENT Usual dose reduced by one-half if creatinine clearance is less than 40 ml/min/1.73 m².

Route	Onset	Peak	Duration
P.O.	30 to 60 min	Unknown	1 to 2 hr
I.V.	1 to 3 min	Unknown	1 to 2 hr
I.M.	10 to 15 min	Unknown	1 to 2 hr

Mechanism of Action

May enhance gastric motility by antagonizing the inhibitory neurotransmitter effect of dopamine on GI smooth muscle. This results in gastric contraction, promoting gastric emptying and increased peristalsis. By altering the mechanical activity of GI smooth muscle and increasing gastric emptying, metoclopramide reduces gastroesophageal reflux. Metoclopramide also blocks dopaminergic receptors in the chemoreceptor trigger zone, thereby preventing nausea and vomiting.

Incompatibilities

Don't administer metoclopramide through same I.V. line as calcium gluconate, cephalothin sodium, chloramphenicol sodium, cisplatin, erythromycin lactobionate, furosemide, methotrexate, penicillin G potassium, or sodium bicarbonate.

Contraindications

Concurrent use of butyrophenones, phenothiazines, or other drugs that may cause extrapyramidal reactions; GI hemorrhage, mechanical obstruction, or perforation; hypersensitivity to metoclopramide or its components; pheochromocytoma; seizure disorders

Interactions

DRUGS
anticholinergics, opioid analgesics: Possibly decreased therapeutic effects of metoclopramide
apomorphine: Possibly decreased antiemetic effect of apomorphine, possibly increased CNS depression
bromocriptine, pergolide: Possibly decreased therapeutic effects of these drugs
cimetidine: Possibly decreased absorption and therapeutic effects of cimetidine
CNS depressants: Possibly increased CNS depression
cyclosporine: Increased blood cyclosporine level
digoxin: Decreased gastric absorption of digoxin
levodopa: Possibly decreased levodopa effectiveness
MAO inhibitors: Increased risk of severe hypertension in patients with essential hypertension
mexiletine: Possibly faster mexiletene absorption

succinylcholine: Possibly prolonged therapeutic action of succinylcholine

ACTIVITIES

alcohol use: Increased risk of excessive sedation

Adverse Reactions

CNS: Agitation, anxiety, depression, dizziness, drowsiness, extrapyramidal reactions (motor restlessness, parkinsonism, tardive dyskinesia), fatigue, headache, insomnia, irritability, lassitude, panic reaction, restlessness
CV: AV block, fluid retention, heart failure, hypertension, hypotension, supraventricular tachycardia
EENT: Dry mouth
ENDO: Galactorrhea, gynecomastia
GI: Constipation, diarrhea, nausea
GU: Menstrual irregularities
HEME: Agranulocytosis
SKIN: Rash
Other: Restless leg syndrome

Nursing Considerations

•Assess patient for signs of intestinal obstruction, such as abnormal bowel sounds, diarrhea, nausea, and vomiting, before administering metoclopramide. Notify prescriber if you detect them.
•For I.V. administration, you needn't dilute doses of 10 mg or less. Give drug over 1 to 2 minutes. For doses larger than 10 mg, dilute in 50 ml of NS, 0.45NS, D_5W, or LR solution and infuse over at least 15 minutes.
•Avoid rapid I.V. administration because it may cause intense anxiety, restlessness, and then drowsiness.
•**WARNING** Notify prescriber if patient displays signs of toxicity, such as disorientation, drowsiness, and extrapyramidal reactions.
•Monitor patient, especially one with heart failure or cirrhosis, for possible signs of fluid retention or volume overload due to transient increase in plasma aldosterone level.
•Store drug in a light-resistant container; discard if solution is discolored or contains particulate.

PATIENT TEACHING

•Advise patient to avoid activities that require alertness for about 2 hours after each dose of metoclopramide.
•Urge patient to avoid alcohol and CNS depressants while taking metoclopramide because they may increase CNS depression.
•Instruct patient to notify prescriber immediately if involuntary movements of the face, eyes, tongue, or hands occur.

metolazone

Diulo, Mykrox, Zaroxolyn

Class and Category

Chemical: Quinazoline derivative
Therapeutic: Antihypertensive, diuretic
Pregnancy category: B

Indications and Dosages

➤ *To manage mild to moderate hypertension*

EXTENDED TABLETS

Adults. 2.5 to 5 mg q.d.

PROMPT TABLETS (MYKROX)

Adults. 0.5 mg q.d. *Maintenance:* 0.5 to 1 mg q.d. *Maximum:* 1 mg/day.

➤ *To manage edema from heart failure or renal disease*

EXTENDED TABLETS

Adults. 5 to 20 mg q.d.

Route	Onset	Peak	Duration
P.O.	1 hr	2 hr	12 to 24 hr

Mechanism of Action

Promotes renal excretion of water and sodium by inhibiting their reabsorption in distal convoluted tubules. The resulting reduction in plasma and extracellular fluid volume reduces blood pressure. Metolazone also helps reduce blood pressure by decreasing peripheral vascular resistance.

M

Contraindications

Anuria; hepatic coma; hypersensitivity to metolazone, other sulfonamide derivatives, or their components; renal failure

Interactions

DRUGS

allopurinol: Increased risk of hypersensitivity to allopurinol
amiodarone: Increased risk of arrhythmias from hypokalemia
amphotericin B: Increased risk of electrolyte imbalances
anesthetics: Increased effects of anesthetics
antigout drugs: Increased blood uric acid level and risk of gout attack
antihypertensives: Increased risk of hypotension
antineoplastics: Prolonged antineoplastic-induced leukopenia
calcium salts: Increased risk of hypercalcemia
cholestyramine, colestipol: Decreased metolazone absorption

diazoxide: Increased risk of hyperglycemia
digoxin: Increased risk of electrolyte imbalances and digoxin-induced arrhythmias
diuretics: Additive effects of both drugs, possibly leading to severe hypovolemia and electrolyte imbalances
dopamine: Increased diuretic effect of both drugs
insulin, oral antidiabetic drugs: Decreased effectiveness of these drugs, increased risk of hyperglycemia
lithium: Increased risk of lithium toxicity
methenamine: Decreased metolazone effectiveness from urinary alkalinization
methyldopa: Possibly hemolytic anemia
neuromuscular blockers: Increased risk of hypokalemia and subsequent increased neuromuscular blockade, increased risk of respiratory depression
NSAIDs, sympathomimetics: Possibly decreased metolazone effectiveness
oral anticoagulants: Decreased anticoagulant effect
vitamin D: Increased vitamin D action, increased risk of hypercalcemia

Adverse Reactions

CNS: Anxiety, chills, depression, dizziness, drowsiness, headache, insomnia, neuropathy, paresthesia, restlessness, syncope, weakness
CV: Chest pain, cold extremities, orthostatic hypotension, palpitations, peripheral edema, vasculitis, venous thrombosis
EENT: Bitter taste, blurred vision, dry mouth, epistaxis, pharyngitis, sinus congestion, tinnitus
ENDO: Hyperglycemia
GI: Abdominal pain, anorexia, cholecystitis, constipation, diarrhea, hepatic dysfunction, hepatitis, indigestion, nausea, pancreatitis, vomiting
GU: Decreased libido, glycosuria, impotence
HEME: Agranulocytosis, aplastic anemia, leukopenia, thrombocytopenia
MS: Arthralgia, gout, myalgia
RESP: Cough
SKIN: Dry skin, photosensitivity, rash, urticaria
Other: Hypochloremia, hypokalemia, hyponatremia, hypovolemia, metabolic alkalosis

Nursing Considerations

•WARNING Be aware that Mykrox prompt tablets shouldn't be substituted for Diulo or Zaroxolyn extended tablets because they aren't equivalent.

•Anticipate giving metolazone with a loop diuretic if patient responds poorly to loop diuretic alone.
•To monitor drug's diuretic effect, measure fluid intake and output and daily weight.
•If response to 1 mg of Mykrox is inadequate, expect to add another drug rather than increase dosage.
•Monitor blood chemistry test results and assess for signs and symptoms of hypochloremia, hypokalemia, and, possibly, mild metabolic alkalosis.
•Monitor serum calcium and uric acid levels, especially if patient has a history of gout or renal calculi. Metolazone may slightly increase calcium reabsorption and decrease uric acid excretion.

PATIENT TEACHING

•Inform patient that metolazone controls but doesn't cure hypertension. Discuss possible need for lifelong therapy and consequences of uncontrolled hypertension.
•Instruct patient to take drug at the same time each day.
•Direct patient to take drug with food or milk to minimize adverse GI reactions.
•Advise patient to change position slowly to minimize effects of orthostatic hypotension.
•Urge patient to notify prescriber about persistent, severe diarrhea, nausea, or vomiting, which can cause dehydration and increase the risk of orthostatic hypotension.
•Stress the importance of weight and diet control, especially limiting sodium intake.
•Inform diabetic patient that drug may increase blood glucose level and that he should check his blood glucose level frequently.

metoprolol succinate

Toprol-XL

metoprolol tartrate

Apo-Metoprolol (CAN), Betaloc (CAN), Betaloc Durules (CAN), Lopresor (CAN), Lopresor SR (CAN), Lopressor, Novometoprol (CAN)

Class and Category

Chemical: Beta$_1$-adrenergic antagonist
Therapeutic: Antianginal, antihypertensive, MI prophylaxis and treatment
Pregnancy category: C

Indications and Dosages

➤ *To manage hypertension, alone or with other antihypertensives*

E.R. TABLETS (METOPROLOL SUCCINATE)

Adults. *Initial:* 50 to 100 mg q.d., adjusted weekly as prescribed. *Maximum:* 400 mg q.d.

E.R. TABLETS (METOPROLOL TARTRATE)

Adults. *Maintenance:* 100 to 400 mg q.d. to maintain blood pressure control after therapeutic level has been achieved with immediate-release tablets.

TABLETS (METOPROLOL TARTRATE)

Adults. *Initial:* 100 mg q.d., adjusted weekly as prescribed. *Maximum:* 450 mg/day as a single dose or in divided doses.

➤ *To treat acute MI or evolving acute MI*

TABLETS (METOPROLOL TARTRATE), I.V. INJECTION (METOPROLOL TARTRATE)

Adults. *Initial:* 5 mg by I.V. bolus q 2 min for 3 doses followed by 50 mg P.O. for patients who tolerate total I.V. dose (or 25 to 50 mg P.O. for patients who can't tolerate total I.V. dose) q 6 hr for 48 hr, starting 15 min after final I.V. dose; after 48 hr, 100 mg b.i.d. followed by maintenance dosage. *Maintenance:* 100 mg P.O. b.i.d. for at least 3 mo.

➤ *To treat angina pectoris and chronic stable angina*

E.R. TABLETS (METOPROLOL SUCCINATE)

Adults. 100 mg q.d., increased weekly as prescribed. *Maximum:* 400 mg/day as a single dose or in divided doses.

E.R. TABLETS (METOPROLOL TARTRATE)

Adults. *Initial:* 100 mg q.d., adjusted weekly as prescribed. *Maximum:* 450 mg/day.

TABLETS (METOPROLOL TARTRATE)

Adults. *Initial:* 50 mg b.i.d., adjusted weekly as prescribed. *Maximum:* 450 mg/day.

➤ *To treat stable, symptomatic (New York Heart Association [NYHA] Class II or III), ischemic, hypertensive, or cardiomyopathic heart failure*

E.R. TABLETS (METOPROLOL SUCCINATE)

Adults. *Initial:* 25 mg q.d. (NYHA Class II) or 12.5 mg q.d. (NYHA Class III or more severe heart failure) for 2 wk. Then dosage doubled every 2 wk as tolerated. *Maximum:* 200 mg/day.

Contraindications

Acute heart failure, bradycardia below 45 beats/minute, cardiogenic shock, hypersensitivity to metoprolol or its components, second- or third-degree AV block

Route	Onset	Peak	Duration
P.O.	60 min	1 to 2 hr	Unknown
P.O. (E.R.)	Unknown	6 to 12 hr	Unknown
I.V.	Unknown	20 min	Unknown

Mechanism of Action

Inhibits stimulation of beta$_1$-receptor sites, located primarily in the heart, resulting in decreased cardiac excitability, cardiac output, and myocardial oxygen demand. These effects help relieve angina. Metoprolol also helps reduce blood pressure by decreasing release of renin from the kidneys.

Interactions

DRUGS

aluminum salts, barbiturates, calcium salts, cholestyramine, colestipol, NSAIDs, rifampin, salicylates, sulfinpyrazone: Decreased therapeutic effects of metoprolol

amiodarone, digoxin, diltiazem, verapamil: Increased risk of complete AV block

calcium channel blockers: Increased risk of heart failure, increased therapeutic effects of both drugs

cimetidine: Increased blood metoprolol level

clonidine, diazoxide, guanabenz: Increased risk of hypotension

estrogens: Possibly decreased antihypertensive effect of metoprolol

general anesthetics: Increased risk of hypotension and heart failure

insulin, oral antidiabetic drugs: Decreased blood glucose control, possibly masking of signs and symptoms of hypoglycemia (by metoprolol)

lidocaine: Increased risk of lidocaine toxicity

MAO inhibitors: Increased risk of hypertension

neuromuscular blockers: Possibly enhanced and prolonged neuromuscular blockade

other antihypertensives: Additive hypotensive effect

phenothiazines: Possibly increased blood levels of both drugs

propafenone: Increased blood level and half-life of metoprolol

sympathomimetics, xanthines: Possibly decreased therapeutic effects of these drugs or metoprolol

M

Foods
all foods: Increased bioavailability of metoprolol

Adverse Reactions

CNS: Anxiety, confusion, depression, dizziness, drowsiness, fatigue, hallucinations, headache, insomnia, weakness
CV: Arrhythmias (including AV block and bradycardia), chest pain, heart failure, orthostatic hypotension
EENT: Nasal congestion
GI: Constipation, diarrhea, nausea, vomiting
GU: Impotence
HEME: Leukopenia, thrombocytopenia
MS: Back pain, myalgia
RESP: Bronchospasm, dyspnea
SKIN: Rash

Nursing Considerations

•For patient with acute MI who can't tolerate initial dosage or who delays treatment, start with maintenance dosage, as prescribed and tolerated.
•Before starting therapy for heart failure, expect to give a diuretic, an ACE inhibitor, and digoxin to stabilize patient.
•Be aware that the metoprolol dosage for heart failure is highly individualized. Monitor patient for signs and symptoms of worsening heart failure during dosage increases. If heart failure worsens, expect to increase the diuretic dosage and possibly decrease the metoprolol dosage or temporarily discontinue drug, as prescribed. Be aware that the metoprolol dosage shouldn't be increased until signs and symptoms of worsening heart failure have been stabilized.
•If patient with heart failure develops symptomatic bradycardia, expect to decrease the metoprolol dosage.
•WARNING If dosage exceeds 400 mg/day, monitor patient for bronchospasm and dyspnea because metoprolol competitively blocks beta$_2$-adrenergic receptors in bronchial and vascular smooth muscles.
•WARNING When substituting metoprolol for clonidine, expect to gradually reduce clonidine dosage and increase metoprolol dosage over several days, as prescribed. Giving these drugs together causes additive hypotensive effects.
•Be aware that patients who take metoprolol may be at risk for AV block. If AV block results from depressed AV node conduction, pre-

pare to administer appropriate drug, as prescribed, or assist with insertion of temporary pacemaker.
•Check for signs of poor glucose control in patient with diabetes mellitus. Metoprolol may interfere with therapeutic effects of insulin and oral antidiabetic drugs. It also may mask evidence of hypoglycemia, such as palpitations, tachycardia, and tremor.
•Be aware that abrupt withdrawal of drug can precipitate thyroid storm in patient with hyperthyroidism or thyrotoxicosis.
•WARNING Expect to taper metoprolol dosage when drug is discontinued; abrupt discontinuation can cause myocardial ischemia, MI, ventricular arrhythmias, or severe hypertension, especially in patients with cardiac disease.

Patient Teaching
•Instruct patient to take metoprolol with food at the same time each day—once daily for E.R. tablets. Inform him that he may halve tablets but not chew or crush them.
•Advise patient to notify prescriber if pulse rate falls below 60 beats/minute or is significantly lower than usual.
•Urge diabetic patient to check blood glucose level frequently during metoprolol therapy.
•Caution patient not to stop taking metoprolol abruptly.

metronidazole

Apo-Metronidazole (CAN), Flagyl, Flagyl I.V. RTU, Metric 21, MetroGel, MetroGel-Vaginal, Nidagel (CAN), Novonidazol (CAN), Protostat, Trikacide (CAN)

metronidazole hydrochloride

Flagyl I.V.

Class and Category

Chemical: Nitroimidazole derivative
Therapeutic: Antibiotic, antiprotozoal
Pregnancy category: B

Indications and Dosages

➤ *To treat systemic anaerobic infections caused by* Bacteroides fragilis, Clostridium difficile, Clostridium perfringens, Eubacterium, Fusobacterium, Peptococcus, Peptostreptococcus, *and* Veillonella *sp.*

CAPSULES, TABLETS
Adults and adolescents. 7.5 mg/kg up to
1,000 mg q 6 hr for 7 days or longer. *Maximum:* 4,000 mg/day.
Children. 7.5 mg/kg q 6 hr or 10 mg/kg q
8 hr.
I.V. INFUSION
Adults and adolescents. *Initial:* 15 mg/kg and
then 7.5 mg/kg up to 1,000 mg q 6 hr for 7
days or longer. *Maximum:* 4,000 mg/day.
Children. 7.5 mg/kg q 6 hr or 10 mg/kg q 8 hr.
➤ *To treat amebiasis (*Entamoeba histolytica)
CAPSULES, TABLETS
Adults. 500 to 750 mg t.i.d. for 5 to 10 days.
Children. 11.6 to 16.7 mg/kg t.i.d. for 10
days.
➤ *To treat trichomoniasis (*Trichomonas
   vaginalis)
CAPSULES, TABLETS
Adults. 2,000 mg as a single dose, 1,000 mg
b.i.d. for 24 hr, or 250 mg t.i.d. for 7 days.
Children. 5 mg/kg t.i.d. for 7 days.
➤ *To prevent perioperative bowel infection*
I.V. INFUSION
Adults and adolescents. 15 mg/kg 1 hr before
surgery and then 7.5 mg/kg 6 and 12 hr after
initial dose.
➤ *To treat acne in patients with rosacea*
TOPICAL GEL
Adults. Thin film applied to affected area
b.i.d. for 9 wk.
➤ *To treat bacterial vaginosis*
VAGINAL CREAM
Adults. 500 mg (1 applicatorful) q.d. or b.i.d.
for 10 to 20 days.
VAGINAL GEL
Adults. 37.5 mg (1 applicatorful) q.d. or b.i.d.
for 5 days.
VAGINAL TABLETS
Adults. 500 mg h.s. for 10 to 20 days.

Mechanism of Action
Undergoes intracellular chemical reduction during anaerobic metabolism. After
metronidazole is reduced, it damages
DNA's helical structure and breaks its
strands, which inhibits bacterial nucleic
acid synthesis and causes cell death.

Incompatibilities
Don't administer I.V. metronidazole with aluminum needles or hubs or through same I.V.
line as other drugs.

Contraindications
Breast-feeding, hypersensitivity to metronidazole or its components, trichomoniasis
during first trimester of pregnancy

Interactions
DRUGS
cimetidine: Possibly delayed elimination and
increased blood level of metronidazole
disulfiram: Possibly combined toxicity, resulting in confusion and psychotic reactions
neurotoxic drugs: Increased risk of neurotoxicity
oral anticoagulants: Possibly increased anticoagulant effect
phenobarbital: Increased metabolism and decreased blood level and half-life of metronidazole
phenytoin: Decreased phenytoin clearance
ACTIVITIES
alcohol use: Possibly disulfiram-like effects

Adverse Reactions
CNS: Ataxia, dizziness, encephalopathy,
fever, headache, light-headedness, peripheral
neuropathy, seizures (high doses)
EENT: Dry mouth, lacrimation (topical form),
metallic taste, pharyngitis
GI: Abdominal cramps or pain, anorexia, diarrhea, nausea, pancreatitis, vomiting
GU: Darkened urine, vaginal candidiasis
(oral, parenteral, and topical forms); burning
or irritation of sexual partner's penis, candidal cervicitis or vaginitis, dysuria, urinary
frequency, vulvitis (vaginal form)
HEME: Leukopenia
MS: Back pain
SKIN: Burning sensation, stinging sensation,
dry skin (topical form); erythema, pruritus,
rash, urticaria (oral and parenteral forms)
Other: Injection site edema, pain, or tenderness

Nursing Considerations
•Administer I.V. metronidazole by slow infusion over 1 hour; don't give by direct I.V. injection.
•Discontinue primary I.V. infusion during
metronidazole infusion.
•WARNING If patient experiences adverse
CNS reactions, such as seizures or peripheral
neuropathy, notify prescriber and stop drug
immediately.
•If skin irritation occurs, apply topical gel
less frequently or discontinue it, as ordered.

•Monitor CBC and culture and sensitivity test results if therapy lasts longer than 10 days or if second course of treatment is needed.

PATIENT TEACHING
•Instruct female patient to notify prescriber if she is pregnant, intends to get pregnant, or is breast-feeding.
•Direct patient to take metronidazole at evenly spaced intervals throughout the day and with food to minimize adverse GI reactions.
•Urge patient to complete the entire course of therapy.
•Caution patient to avoid alcohol during therapy and for at least 1 day afterward.
•Advise patient to avoid potentially hazardous activities until drug's CNS effects are known.
•If patient reports dry mouth, suggest ice chips or sugarless hard candy or gum; suggest a dental visit if dryness lasts longer than 2 weeks.
•Instruct patient to notify prescriber if no improvement occurs within a few days of taking tablets or capsules.
•Direct patient using topical gel to wash hands and affected area with a mild, nonirritating cleaner; to rinse well and pat dry; and then to apply a thin film of drug and wash hands again.
•Advise patient with rosacea to keep topical gel away from eyes. If drug gets into eyes, urge him to wash his eyes immediately with large amounts of cool tap water and to call prescriber if eyes continue to hurt or burn.
•Instruct patient with rosacea to notify prescriber if no improvement occurs after 3 weeks of topical use; full therapeutic effect may take 9 weeks.
•Teach patient how to fill, insert, and clean vaginal cream or gel applicator after use. Instruct her to wash her hands before and after administration.
•To help vaginal tablets dissolve, instruct patient to run tap water over unwrapped tablet for a few seconds before insertion.
•Inform patient with trichomoniasis that male sexual partners should wear condoms during her treatment and may need treatment themselves to prevent reinfection.
•Caution patient that vaginal cream and tablets (not gel) may contain oils that damage latex condoms.
•Urge patient to follow up with prescriber to make sure infection is gone.

metyrosine
Demser

Class and Category
Chemical: Alpha-methyl tyrosine
Therapeutic: Antipheochromocytoma agent
Pregnancy category: C

Indications and Dosages
➤ *To control hypertension and related symptoms until pheochromocytomectomy is performed, to treat chronic malignant pheochromocytoma*

CAPSULES
Adults and adolescents. *Initial:* 250 mg q.i.d., increased as ordered by 250 to 500 mg/day. *Maintenance:* 2,000 to 3,000 mg/day in divided doses q.i.d. Preoperative dosage given for at least 7 days. *Maximum:* 4,000 mg/day in divided doses.

Mechanism of Action
Blocks the activity of tyrosine hydroxylase, the enzyme that controls the rate of catecholamine synthesis. This action decreases production of the catecholamines epinephrine and norepinephrine, which, in patients with pheochromocytoma, are produced in excessive amounts.

Contraindications
Hypersensitivity to metyrosine or its components

Interactions
DRUGS
CNS depressants: Increased sedation
haloperidol, phenothiazines: Increased extrapyramidal effects
ACTIVITIES
alcohol use: Increased sedation

Adverse Reactions
CNS: Anxiety, confusion, depression, disorientation, extrapyramidal reactions (difficulty speaking, drooling, parkinsonism, tremor, trismus), hallucinations, headache, sedation
CV: Peripheral edema
EENT: Dry mouth, nasal congestion, pharyngeal edema
ENDO: Galactorrhea, gynecomastia
GI: Abdominal pain, diarrhea, elevated serum AST level, nausea, vomiting

GU: Crystalluria, dysuria (transient), ejaculation failure, hematuria, impotence, urolithiasis
HEME: Anemia, eosinophilia, thrombocytopenia, thrombocytosis
SKIN: Urticaria

Nursing Considerations
•Expect patient taking metyrosine to experience moderate to severe sedation at low and high dosages. Sedation begins during first 24 hours, peaks after 2 to 3 days, and tends to wane during next few days. It usually subsides after 1 week unless dosage is increased or exceeds 2 g/day.
•Obtain urine specimens as ordered to check for crystalluria and urolithiasis. If crystalluria develops, increase fluid intake to achieve daily urine output of 2,000 ml or more with doses above 2 g/day. If crystalluria persists, reduce dosage or stop drug, as ordered.
•Expect to adjust dosage, as prescribed, based on clinical response and urine catecholamine level.
•If signs and symptoms aren't adequately controlled by metyrosine, expect to add an alpha-adrenergic blocker, such as phenoxybenzamine, as prescribed.
PATIENT TEACHING
•Inform patient about metyrosine's sedative effects. Advise him to avoid alcohol and CNS depressants, which may increase sedation.
•Instruct patient to increase fluid intake, as appropriate.
•Urge patient to notify prescriber about drooling, severe diarrhea, trembling and shaking of hands and fingers, or trouble speaking.
•Inform patient that he may experience changes in sleep pattern for 2 to 3 days after stopping drug.
•Advise patient to keep regular visits with prescriber to monitor progress.

mexiletine hydrochloride
Mexitil

Class and Category
Chemical: Lidocaine analogue
Therapeutic: Class IB antiarrhythmic
Pregnancy category: C

Indications and Dosages
➤ *To treat life-threatening ventricular arrhythmias*
CAPSULES
Adults. *Initial:* 200 mg q 8 hr, adjusted, as ordered, by 50 to 100 mg/dose q 2 to 3 days, as tolerated. If patient tolerates 300 mg or less q 8 hr, total dosage may be divided and given q 12 hr. If patient continues to experience arrhythmias, dosage frequency may be changed to q.i.d. *Maximum:* 1,200 mg/day when given q 8 hr (400 mg/dose); 900 mg/day when given q 12 hr (450 mg/dose).
➤ *To rapidly control life-threatening ventricular arrhythmias*
CAPSULES
Adults. *Initial:* 400 mg followed by 200 mg after 8 hr. *Maintenance:* 200 mg q 8 hr, adjusted, as ordered, by 50 to 100 mg/dose q 2 to 3 days, as tolerated. If patient tolerates 300 mg or less q 8 hr, total dosage may be divided and given q 12 hr. If patient continues to experience arrhythmias, dosage frequency may be changed to q.i.d.
DOSAGE ADJUSTMENT For patients with severe hepatic disease or heart failure, dosage reduced and adjusted q 2 or 3 days.

Route	Onset	Peak	Duration
P.O.	0.5 to 2 hr	2 to 3 hr	8 to 12 hr

M

Mechanism of Action
Produces antiarrhythmic effect by inhibiting fast sodium channels in myocardial cell membranes, especially in the His-Purkinje system. This action decreases the duration of the action potential and effective refractory period of the His-Purkinje system. The myocardium, which becomes refractory again after the resting membrane potential is restored, is less likely to generate and respond to ectopic ventricular impulses.

Contraindications
Cardiogenic shock, second- or third-degree AV block without a pacemaker

Interactions
DRUGS
aluminum- or magnesium-containing antacids: Delayed mexiletine absorption
cimetidine: Possibly increased or decreased blood mexiletine level

hepatic enzyme inducers: Accelerated metabolism and decreased blood level of mexiletine
metoclopramide: Accelerated mexiletine absorption
other antiarrhythmics: Increased cardiac effects
rifampin: Decreased blood mexiletine level
theophylline: Increased blood theophylline level
urinary acidifiers: Accelerated renal excretion of mexiletine
urinary alkalinizers: Delayed renal excretion of mexiletine

FOODS
foods that may acidify urine (such as cheese, cranberries, eggs, fish, grains, meats, plums, poultry, and prunes): Accelerated renal excretion of mexiletine
foods that may alkalinize urine (such as milk and all vegetables and fruits except cranberries, plums, and prunes): Delayed renal excretion of mexiletine

ACTIVITIES
smoking: Reduced mexiletine half-life

Adverse Reactions
CNS: Confusion, dizziness, fatigue, headache, lack of coordination, light-headedness, nervousness, paresthesia, seizures, sleep disturbance, syncope, tremor, weakness
CV: Atrial arrhythmias, AV conduction disorders, bradycardia, cardiogenic shock, chest pain, heart failure, hypotension, palpitations, PVCs, ventricular arrhythmias (increased)
EENT: Blurred vision, dry mouth, tinnitus
GI: Constipation, diarrhea, heartburn, nausea, vomiting
HEME: Agranulocytosis, leukopenia, thrombocytopenia
RESP: Dyspnea
SKIN: Rash

Nursing Considerations
• If mexiletine is replacing another antiarrhythmic, expect to give the first dose 6 to 12 hours after the last dose of quinidine sulfate or disopyramide, 3 to 6 hours after the last dose of procainamide, or 8 to 12 hours after the last dose of tocainide, as prescribed.
• If mexiletine is replacing parenteral lidocaine, expect to reduce or withdraw lidocaine 1 to 2 hours after starting mexiletine, as prescribed.
• Monitor continuous ECG and serum mexiletine level.

• Assess for signs of thrombocytopenia, which may occur within a few days after mexiletine therapy starts. Expect platelet count to return to normal within 1 month after mexiletine therapy stops.

PATIENT TEACHING
• Instruct patient to take mexiletine at evenly spaced intervals, to avoid missing doses, and to take drug as prescribed, even if he's feeling well.
• Advise patient to take drug with food to reduce adverse GI reactions.
• Inform patient that nausea and vomiting may occur within 2 hours after dose but tend to lessen as treatment continues.
• Advise patient to avoid potentially hazardous activities until drug's CNS effects are known.
• Teach patient how to measure pulse rate, and advise him to contact prescriber if rate falls below 50 beats/minute or if rhythm becomes irregular.
• Urge patient to notify prescriber immediately about chest pain, chills, fast or irregular heartbeat, fever, shortness of breath, and unusual bleeding or bruising.
• Advise patient to avoid dramatically increasing intake of foods that may acidify urine (cheese, cranberries, eggs, fish, grains, meats, plums, poultry, prunes) or alkalinize urine (milk, all vegetables, all fruits except cranberries, plums, and prunes).
• Encourage patient to keep regular visits with prescriber to monitor progress.

mezlocillin sodium
Mezlin

Class and Category
Chemical: Acyclaminopenicillin
Therapeutic: Antibiotic
Pregnancy category: B

Indications and Dosages
➤ *To treat moderate to severe infections, including bacteremia, bone and joint infections, gynecologic infections (such as endometritis, pelvic cellulitis, and pelvic inflammatory disease), intra-abdominal infections (such as cholangitis, cholecystitis, hepatic abscess, intra-abdominal abscess, and peritonitis), lower respiratory tract infections (such as pneumonia*

and lung abscess), meningitis, septicemia caused by susceptible bacteria, or
skin and soft-tissue infections (such as
cellulitis and diabetic foot ulcer); to
manage febrile neutropenia

I.V. INFUSION, I.M. INJECTION
Adults and adolescents. 3 g q 4 hr or 4 g q
6 hr.

➤ *To treat life-threatening infections of the*
types listed above

I.V. INFUSION, I.M. INJECTION
Adults and adolescents. Up to 350 mg/kg/day.
Maximum: 24,000 mg/day.
Children and infants. 50 mg/kg q 4 hr (or in-
fused over 30 min q 4 hr).
Neonates over age 7 days weighing 2,000 g
(4.4 lb) or less. 75 mg/kg I.V. q 8 hr.
Neonates age 7 days or less weighing 2,000 g
or less. 75 mg/kg I.V. q 12 hr.
Neonates age 7 days or less weighing more
than 2,000 g. 75 mg/kg I.V. q 6 hr.

➤ *To treat uncomplicated UTI*

I.V. INFUSION, I.M. INJECTION
Adults. 1.5 to 2 g q 6 hr.

➤ *To treat complicated UTI*

I.V. INFUSION
Adults. 3 g q 6 hr.
DOSAGE ADJUSTMENT Dosing interval extended to q 6 to 8 hr if needed for patients
with creatinine clearance of 10 to 30 ml/min/
1.73 m². Dosing interval extended and dosage
reduced to 1.5 to 2 g for patients with creatinine clearance below 10 ml/min/1.73 m².

➤ *To treat uncomplicated gonorrhea*
caused by susceptible strains of Neisseria gonorrhoeae

I.V. INFUSION, I.M. INJECTION
Adults. 1 to 2 g as a single dose given with
1 g of probenecid P.O. (or probenecid given
up to 30 min before mezlocillin).

➤ *To prevent infection from potentially*
contaminated surgical procedures

I.V. INFUSION
Adults. 4 g 30 min before surgery and then
4 g q 6 hr for 2 more doses.

➤ *To prevent infection in cesarean section*

I.V. INFUSION
Adults. 4 g as soon as umbilical cord is
clamped; then 4 g q 4 hr for 2 more doses,
starting 4 hr after initial dose.

Mechanism of Action

Inhibits bacterial cell wall synthesis. In
susceptible bacteria, the rigid, cross-
linked cell wall is assembled in several
steps. Mezlocillin exerts its effects in the
final stage of the cross-linking process by
binding with and inactivating penicillin-
binding proteins (enzymes responsible for
linking cell wall strands). This action
causes bacterial cell lysis and death.

Incompatibilities

Administer mezlocillin at separate sites and
at least 1 hour before or after aminoglycosides. Don't mix mezlocillin in same I.V. bag,
bottle, or tubing as other drugs.

Contraindications

Hypersensitivity to mezlocillin, other penicillins, or their components

Interactions
DRUGS
aminoglycosides: Substantial aminoglycoside
inactivation
chloramphenicol, erythromycins, sulfon-
amides, tetracyclines: Possibly decreased
therapeutic effects of mezlocillin
methotrexate: Increased risk of methotrexate
toxicity
probenecid: Increased blood level and prolonged half-life of mezlocillin

Adverse Reactions

CNS: Depression, headache, seizures
EENT: Oral candidiasis
GI: Abdominal pain, diarrhea, pseudomem-
branous colitis, nausea, vomiting
GU: Vaginitis
HEME: Leukopenia, neutropenia
SKIN: Exfoliative dermatitis, pruritus, rash,
urticaria
Other: Anaphylaxis; hypokalemia; injection
site pain, redness, and swelling; serum sick-
ness-like reaction

Nursing Considerations

•WARNING Before starting mezlocillin therapy, make sure patient has had no previous
hypersensitivity reactions to penicillins.
•Anticipate that mezlocillin therapy will last
for at least 2 days after signs and symptoms
have resolved—typically 7 to 10 days, depending on severity of infection. Compli-

M

cated infections may need longer treatment. Group A beta-hemolytic streptococcal infections usually are treated for at least 10 days to reduce the risk of rheumatic fever or glomerulonephritis.

•For I.M. injection, reconstitute each gram of mezlocillin with 3 to 4 ml of sterile water for injection and shake vigorously. Inject no more than 2 g into a large muscle, such as the gluteus maximus, over 12 to 15 seconds to minimize discomfort.

•Although drug may be given I.M., expect to use intermittent I.V. infusion, as directed, for serious infections.

•For I.V. use, reconstitute each gram of mezlocillin with 9 to 10 ml of sterile water for injection, D_5W, or sodium chloride for injection and shake vigorously. Inject directly into I.V. tubing over 3 to 5 minutes.

•For intermittent infusion, further dilute to desired volume (50 to 100 ml) with an appropriate I.V. solution and administer over 30 minutes. Discontinue other infusions during mezlocillin administration.

•Be aware that mezlocillin powder and reconstituted solution may darken slightly but that potency isn't affected.

•Periodically monitor serum potassium level in patient receiving long-term therapy, as appropriate.

•During long-term therapy, monitor for signs and symptoms of superinfection, such as oral candidiasis and vaginitis.

PATIENT TEACHING

•Instruct patient taking mezlocillin to notify prescriber immediately if increased bruising or other bleeding tendencies develop.

•Advise patient to notify prescriber if diarrhea occurs and to check with prescriber before taking an antidiarrheal because of the risk of masking pseudomembranous colitis.

midazolam hydrochloride

Versed

Class, Category, and Schedule

Chemical: Benzodiazepine
Therapeutic: Sedative-hypnotic
Pregnancy category: D
Controlled substance: Schedule IV

Indications and Dosages

➤ *To induce preoperative sedation or amnesia, to control preoperative anxiety*

ORAL SOLUTION

Children ages 6 months to 16 years. 0.25 to 0.5 mg/kg as a single dose 30 to 45 min before surgery. *Usual:* 0.5 mg/kg. *Maximum:* 20 mg.

I.V. INJECTION

Adults age 60 and older. 1.5 mg over 2 min immediately before procedure. After 2-min waiting period, dosage adjusted to desired level in 25% increments, as ordered. *Maximum:* 1 mg in 2 min.

Adults under age 60 and adolescents. Up to 2.5 mg over 2 min immediately before procedure. After 2-min waiting period, dosage adjusted to desired level in 25% increments, as ordered. *Maximum:* 5 mg.

Children ages 6 to 12. *Initial:* 0.025 to 0.05 mg/kg, up to 0.4 mg/kg, if needed. *Maximum:* 10 mg.

Children ages 6 months to 5 years. *Initial:* 0.05 to 0.1 mg/kg, up to 0.6 mg/kg, if needed. *Maximum:* 6 mg.

I.M. INJECTION

Adults age 60 and older. 0.02 to 0.05 mg/kg as a single dose 30 to 60 min before surgery.

Adults under age 60 and adolescents. 0.07 to 0.08 mg/kg as a single dose 30 to 60 min before surgery.

Children ages 6 months to 12 years. 0.1 to 0.15 mg/kg, up to 0.5 mg/kg for more anxious patients. *Maximum:* 10 mg.

➤ *To relieve agitation and anxiety in mechanically ventilated patients*

I.V. INFUSION

Adults. *Initial:* 0.01 to 0.05 mg/kg infused over several min, repeated at 10- to 15-min intervals until adequate sedation occurs. *Maintenance:* 0.02 to 0.1 mg/kg/hr initially, adjusted to desired level in 25% to 50% increments, as ordered. After achieving desired level of sedation, infusion rate decreased by 10% to 25% every few hr, as ordered, until minimum effective infusion rate is determined.

Children. *Initial:* 50 to 200 mcg/kg over 2 to 3 min followed by 1 to 2 mcg/kg/min by continuous infusion. *Maintenance:* 0.4 to 6 mcg/kg/min.

Infants over age 32 weeks. 1 mcg/kg/min by continuous infusion.

Infants under age 32 weeks. 0.5 mcg/kg/min by continuous infusion.

Route	Onset	Peak	Duration
I.V.*	1.5 to 5 min	Rapid	2 to 6 hr
I.M.*	5 to 15 min	15 to 60 min	2 to 6 hr
I.M.†	30 to 60 min	Unknown	Unknown

Mechanism of Action
May exert its sedating effect by increasing the activity of gamma-aminobutyric acid, a major inhibitory neurotransmitter in the brain. As a result, midazolam produces a calming effect, relaxes skeletal muscles, and—at high doses—induces sleep.

Contraindications
Acute angle-closure glaucoma; alcohol intoxication; coma; hypersensitivity to midazolam, other benzodiazepines, or their components; shock

Interactions
DRUGS
antihypertensives: Increased risk of hypotension
cimetidine, diltiazem, erythromycin, fluconazole, indinavir, itraconazole, ketoconazole, ranitidine, ritonavir, saquinavir, verapamil: Intense and prolonged sedation caused by reduced midazolam metabolism
CNS depressants: Possibly increased CNS and respiratory depression and hypotension
rifampin: Decreased blood midazolam level
FOODS
grapefruit, grapefruit juice: Possibly increased blood midazolam level and risk of toxicity
ACTIVITIES
alcohol use: Possibly intense, prolonged sedative effect and increased respiratory depression and hypotension

Adverse Reactions
CNS: Agitation, delirium, or dreaming during emergence from anesthesia; anxiety; ataxia; chills; combativeness; confusion; dizziness; drowsiness; euphoria; excessive sedation; headache; insomnia; lethargy; nervousness; nightmares; paresthesia; prolonged emergence from anesthesia; restlessness; retrograde amnesia; sleep disturbance; slurred speech; weakness; yawning
CV: Cardiac arrest, hypotension, nodal rhythm, PVCs, tachycardia, vasovagal episodes
EENT: Blurred vision, diplopia, or other vision changes; increased salivation; laryngospasm; miosis; nystagmus; toothache
GI: Hiccups, nausea, retching, vomiting
RESP: Airway obstruction, bradypnea, bronchospasm, coughing, decreased tidal volume, dyspnea, hyperventilation, respiratory arrest, shallow breathing, tachypnea, wheezing
SKIN: Pruritus, rash, urticaria
Other: Injection site burning, edema, induration, pain, redness, and tenderness

Nursing Considerations
•Before administering midazolam, determine whether patient consumes alcohol or takes antihypertensives, antibiotics, or protease inhibitors because these substances can produce an intense and prolonged sedative effect when taken during midazolam therapy.
•**WARNING** Be aware that I.V. midazolam is given only in hospital or ambulatory care settings that allow continuous monitoring of respiratory and cardiac function. Keep resuscitative drugs and equipment readily available.
•As needed, combine midazolam injection with D_5W, NS, or LR solution. With D_5W and NS, solution is stable for 24 hours. With LR, solution is stable for 4 hours.
•As needed, mix injection in same syringe with atropine sulfate, meperidine hydrochloride, morphine sulfate, or scopolamine hydrobromide. The resulting solution is stable for 30 minutes.
•Assess level of consciousness frequently because the range between sedation and unconsciousness or disorientation is narrow with midazolam.
•Be aware that recovery time is usually 2 hours but may be up to 6 hours.
PATIENT TEACHING
•Inform patient that he may not remember procedure because midazolam produces amnesia.
•Advise patient to avoid potentially hazardous activities until drug's adverse CNS effects, such as dizziness and drowsiness, have worn off.

M

---

* For sedation.
† For amnesia.

•Instruct patient to avoid alcohol and other CNS depressants for 24 hours after receiving drug, unless directed otherwise by prescriber.

midodrine hydrochloride

ProAmatine

Class and Category

Chemical: Desglymidodrine prodrug
Therapeutic: Antihypotensive, vasopressor
Pregnancy category: C

Indications and Dosages

➤ *To treat symptomatic orthostatic hypotension*

TABLETS

Adults. 10 mg t.i.d. in 3- to 4-hr intervals.
DOSAGE ADJUSTMENT Initial dose possibly reduced to 2.5 mg for patients with renal impairment.

Route	Onset	Peak	Duration
P.O.	Unknown	30 min	2 to 3 hr

Mechanism of Action

Is broken down into the active metabolite desglymidodrine. Desglymidodrine directly stimulates alpha-adrenergic receptors in arteries and veins. This action increases total peripheral vascular resistance, which in turn increases systolic and diastolic blood pressure.

Contraindications

Acute renal disease, hypersensitivity to midodrine or its components, initial supine systolic pressure above 180 mm Hg, persistent and excessive supine hypertension, pheochromocytoma, severe heart disease, thyrotoxicosis, urine retention

Interactions

DRUGS

beta blockers, digoxin: Enhanced or precipitated bradycardia, AV block, arrhythmias
cimetidine, flecainide, metformin, procainamide, quinidine, ranitidine, triamterene: Possibly decreased renal clearance of these drugs
dihydroergotamine, ephedrine, phenylephrine, phenylpropanolamine, pseudoephedrine: Increased vasopressor effects

doxazosin, prazosin, terazosin: Antagonized midodrine effects
fludrocortisone acetate: Increased risk of supine hypertension

Adverse Reactions

CNS: Anxiety, asthenia, chills, confusion, delusions, dizziness, feeling of pressure or fullness in head, headache, hyperesthesia, insomnia, nervousness, paresthesia, somnolence
CV: Hypertension (sitting and supine), vasodilation
EENT: Canker sore, dry mouth, vision changes
GI: Flatulence, indigestion, nausea
GU: Dysuria, urinary frequency and urgency, urine retention
MS: Back pain, leg cramps
SKIN: Dry skin, erythema multiforme, facial flushing, piloerection, rash, scalp pruritus

Nursing Considerations

•Monitor hepatic and renal function, as ordered, before and during midodrine therapy.
•Administer drug at 3- to 4-hour intervals, if needed and ordered, to control symptoms. Don't give after evening meal, less than 4 hours before bed, or more often than every 3 hours.
•**WARNING** Monitor for severe, persistent systolic supine hypertension, which may develop with single doses up to 20 mg.
•Avoid placing patient flat in bed for any length of time. Elevate head of bed when he's supine.
•Monitor supine and sitting blood pressure frequently during midodrine therapy.

PATIENT TEACHING

•Instruct patient to take midodrine every 3 to 4 hours during daytime but not to take final dose after evening meal or within 4 hours of going to bed.
•Advise patient to elevate head of bed when he lies supine. Caution him not to remain flat for any length of time.
•Direct patient to notify prescriber immediately about headache, increased dizziness, urine retention, or vision changes.
•Encourage patient to keep follow-up appointments to monitor blood pressure and hepatic and renal function.

miglitol

Glyset

Class and Category
Chemical: Desoxynojirimycin derivative
Therapeutic: Alpha-glucosidase inhibitor, antidiabetic drug
Pregnancy category: B

Indications and Dosages
➤ *To manage type 2 diabetes mellitus*
TABLETS
Adults. *Initial:* 25 mg t.i.d. with first bite of each meal. Alternatively, 25 mg q.d., gradually increased to 25 mg t.i.d. *Maximum:* 100 mg t.i.d.
DOSAGE ADJUSTMENT After 4 to 8 wk, dosage increased, if ordered, to 50 mg t.i.d. for about 3 mo; then dosage adjusted based on glycosylated hemoglobin (HbA$_{1C}$) level.

Route	Onset	Peak	Duration
P.O.	Rapid	2 to 3 hr	Unknown

Mechanism of Action
Inhibits intestinal glucoside hydrolase enzymes, which normally hydrolyze oligosaccharides and disaccharides to glucose and other monosaccharides. This action delays carbohydrate digestion and absorption and reduces the postprandial blood glucose level.

Contraindications
Acute or chronic bowel disorder, diabetic ketoacidosis, hypersensitivity to miglitol or its components

Interactions
DRUGS
digestive enzyme preparations, intestinal adsorbents (activated charcoal): Decreased miglitol effects
digoxin: Decreased blood digoxin level
propranolol, ranitidine: Decreased bioavailability of these drugs

Adverse Reactions
GI: Abdominal pain, diarrhea, flatulence, hepatotoxicity
HEME: Low serum iron level
SKIN: Rash (transient)

Nursing Considerations
• Use miglitol cautiously in patient with serum creatinine level above 2 mg/dl.
• Be aware that some patients with type 2 diabetes also may receive a sulfonylurea as an adjunct to miglitol therapy.

• Give miglitol with first bite of each meal. Drug must be at site of enzymatic action when carbohydrates reach small intestine.
• Review patient's HbA$_{1C}$ level, as appropriate, to monitor long-term glucose control.
• Monitor for signs of overdose, such as transient increases in abdominal discomfort, diarrhea, and flatulence (but not hypoglycemia).
PATIENT TEACHING
• Explain that miglitol is an adjunct to diet, which is the primary treatment for type 2 diabetes mellitus.
• Instruct patient to take drug with first bite of each meal.
• Describe signs and symptoms of hypoglycemia and pathophysiology of diabetes to patient and family members.
• If miglitol is the only drug patient takes to control blood glucose level, explain that it won't cause hypoglycemia.
• If patient takes a sulfonylurea or insulin with miglitol, suggest that he keep a source of glucose readily available to reverse hypoglycemia.
• Explain the importance of monitoring blood and urine glucose levels.
• Inform patient that adverse GI reactions usually decrease in frequency and intensity over time.
• Teach obese patient about weight loss, calorie restriction, diet, and regular exercise, as indicated.

milrinone lactate
Primacor

Class and Category
Chemical: Bipyridine derivative
Therapeutic: Inotropic, vasodilator
Pregnancy category: C

Indications and Dosages
➤ *To provide short-term treatment of acute heart failure*
I.V. INFUSION
Adults. *Loading:* 50 mcg/kg over 10 min (at least 0.375 mcg/kg/min). *Usual:* 0.375 to 0.75 mcg/kg/min. *Maximum:* 1.13 mg/kg/day.
DOSAGE ADJUSTMENT Dosage adjusted according to cardiac output, pulmonary artery wedge pressure (PAWP), and clinical response. For patients with creatinine clearance of 30 to 39 ml/min/1.73 m^2, infusion rate re-

duced to 0.33 mcg/kg/min; of 20 to 29 ml/min/1.73 m², to 0.28 mcg/kg/min; of 10 to 19 ml/min/1.73 m², to 0.23 mcg/kg/min; and of less than 9 ml/min/1.73 m², to 0.20 mcg/kg/min.

Route	Onset	Peak	Duration
I.V.	5 to 15 min	Unknown	3 to 6 hr

Incompatibilities

Don't administer milrinone through same I.V. line as furosemide because precipitate will form. Don't add other drugs to premixed milrinone flexible containers.

Contraindications

Hypersensitivity to milrinone or its components

Interactions

DRUGS

antihypertensives: Possibly hypotension

Adverse Reactions

CNS: Headache, tremor

CV: Angina, hypotension, supraventricular arrhythmias, ventricular ectopic activity, ventricular fibrillation, ventricular tachycardia
HEME: Thrombocytopenia
RESP: Bronchospasm
Other: Hypokalemia

Nursing Considerations

• Make sure ECG equipment is available for continuous monitoring during milrinone therapy.
• Discard drug if it's discolored or contains particles.
• For loading dose, directly infuse undiluted drug into I.V. line with a compatible infusing solution. For continuous infusion, dilute drug with 0.45NS, NS, or D₅W. Dilution isn't needed when using premixed milrinone flexible containers.
• Check platelet count before and periodically during infusion, as ordered. Expect to discontinue drug if platelet count falls below 150,000/mm³.

Mechanism of Action

An inotropic drug, milrinone increases the force of myocardial contraction—and cardiac output—by blocking the enzyme phosphodiesterase. Normally, this enzyme is activated by hormones binding to cell membrane receptors. As shown below left, phosphodiesterase normally degrades intracellular cAMP, which restricts calcium movement into myocardial cells. By inhibiting phosphodiesterase, as shown below right, milrinone slows the rate of cAMP degradation, increasing the intracellular cAMP level and the amount of calcium that enters myocardial cells. In blood vessels, increased cAMP causes smooth-muscle relaxation, which improves cardiac output by reducing preload and afterload.

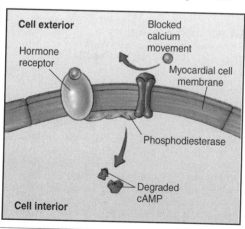

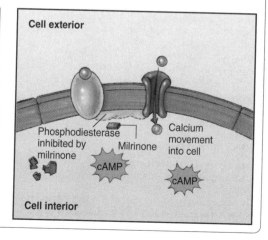

- Administer loading dose using a controlled-rate infusion device. For continuous infusion, use a calibrated electronic infusion device.
- Monitor cardiac output, pulmonary artery wedge pressure, blood pressure, heart rate, weight, and fluid status during therapy to determine drug effectiveness.
- Monitor renal function test results and serum electrolyte levels. Notify prescriber of abnormalities.
- If severe hypotension develops, notify prescriber immediately and expect to discontinue drug.
- Anticipate that patient also will receive digoxin before starting milrinone because milrinone can increase the ventricular response rate.

PATIENT TEACHING
- Reassure patient that you'll be present and that he'll be monitored constantly during milrinone therapy.

minocycline

Minocin

minocycline hydrochloride

Alti-Minocycline (CAN), Apo-Minocycline (CAN), Dynacin, Gen-Minocycline (CAN), Minocin, Novo-Minocycline (CAN), Vectrin

Class and Category
Chemical: Tetracycline
Therapeutic: Antibiotic, antiprotozoal
Pregnancy category: D

Indications and Dosages
➤ *To treat bartonellosis, brucellosis, chancroid, granuloma inguinale, inclusion conjunctivitis, lymphogranuloma venereum, nongonococcal urethritis, plague, psittacosis, Q fever, relapsing fever, respiratory tract infections (including pneumonia), rickettsial pox, Rocky Mountain spotted fever, tularemia, typhus, and UTIs caused by gramnegative organisms (including* Bartonella bacilliformis, Brucella *sp.,* Haemophilus ducreyi, Haemophilus influenzae, Vibrio cholerae, *and* Yersinia pestis), *susceptible gram-positive organisms (including certain strains of* Streptococcus pneumoniae), *and other organ-*

isms (including Actinomyces *sp.,* Bacillus anthracis, Borrelia recurrentis, Chlamydia *sp.,* Mycoplasma pneumoniae, *and* Rickettsiae); *as adjunct to treat intestinal amebiasis and as alternative to treat listeriosis caused by* Listeria monocytogenes, *syphilis caused by* Treponema pallidum, *and yaws caused by* Treponema pertenue *for nonpregnant patients allergic to penicillin*

CAPSULES, ORAL SUSPENSION
Adults and adolescents. *Initial:* 200 mg. *Maintenance:* 100 mg q 12 hr. Alternatively, 100 to 200 mg initially followed by 50 mg q 6 hr.
Children over age 8. *Initial:* 4 mg/kg. *Maintenance:* 2 mg/kg q 12 hr.

I.V. INJECTION
Adults and adolescents. *Initial:* 200 mg. *Maintenance:* 100 mg q 12 hr. *Maximum:* 400 mg q.d.
Children over age 8. *Initial:* 4 mg/kg. *Maintenance:* 2 mg/kg q 12 hr.

➤ *As adjunct to treat inflammatory acne vulgaris that's unresponsive to oral tetracycline or erythromycin*

CAPSULES, ORAL SUSPENSION
Adults and adolescents. 50 mg q.d. to t.i.d.

➤ *To treat uncomplicated gonorrhea caused by* Neisseria gonorrhoeae *in nonpregnant patients allergic to penicillin*

CAPSULES, ORAL SUSPENSION
Adults and adolescents. *Initial:* 200 mg. *Maintenance:* 100 mg q 12 hr for at least 4 days.

➤ *To treat uncomplicated gonococcal urethritis in men*

CAPSULES, ORAL SUSPENSION
Adults and adolescents. 100 mg b.i.d. for 5 days.

➤ *To treat asymptomatic meningococcal carriers with* Neisseria meningitidis *in nasopharynx*

CAPSULES, ORAL SUSPENSION
Adults and adolescents. 100 mg q 12 hr for 5 days.
Children over age 8. *Initial:* 4 mg/kg. *Maintenance:* 2 mg/kg q 12 hr for 5 days.

➤ *To treat infections caused by* Mycobacterium marinum

CAPSULES, ORAL SUSPENSION
Adults. 100 mg q 12 hr for 6 to 8 wk.

M

Route	Onset	Peak	Duration
P.O.	Unknown	2 to 4 hr	6 to 12 hr
I.V.	Unknown	Unknown	6 to 12 hr

Mechanism of Action

Inhibits bacterial protein synthesis by competitively binding to the 30S ribosomal subunit of the mRNA-ribosome complex of certain organisms.

Incompatibilities

Don't mix minocycline in same syringe with solution that contains calcium because precipitate will form.

Contraindications

Hypersensitivity to minocycline, other tetracyclines, or their components

Interactions

DRUGS

aluminum-, calcium-, or magnesium-containing antacids; calcium supplements; choline and magnesium salicylates; iron-containing preparations; magnesium-containing laxatives; sodium bicarbonate: Possibly formation of nonabsorbable complex, impaired minocycline absorption

cholestyramine, colestipol: Possibly impaired cholestyramine or colestipol absorption

cimetidine: Possibly decreased GI absorption and effectiveness of minocycline

digoxin: Possibly increased blood digoxin level and risk of digitalis toxicity

insulin: Possibly decreased need for insulin

iron salts: Possibly decreased GI absorption and antimicrobial effect of minocycline

lithium: Possibly increased or decreased blood lithium level

methoxyflurane: Increased risk of nephrotoxicity

oral anticoagulants: Possibly potentiated anticoagulant effects

oral contraceptives containing estrogen: Decreased contraceptive effectiveness, increased risk of breakthrough bleeding

penicillin: Interference with bactericidal action of penicillin

vitamin A: Possibly benign intracranial hypertension

Adverse Reactions

CNS: Dizziness, fever, headache, light-headedness, unsteadiness, vertigo

CV: Pericarditis

EENT: Blurred vision, darkened or discolored tongue, glossitis, papilledema, tooth discoloration (children), vision changes

GI: Abdominal cramps or pain, anorexia, diarrhea, dysphagia, enterocolitis, esophageal irritation and ulceration, hepatitis, hepatotoxicity, indigestion, nausea, pancreatitis, vomiting

GU: Genital candidiasis, nephrotoxicity

HEME: Eosinophilia, hemolytic anemia, neutropenia, thrombocytopenia, thrombocytopenic purpura

MS: Arthralgia, myopathy (transient)

RESP: Pulmonary infiltrates (with eosinophilia)

SKIN: Erythema multiforme, exfoliative dermatitis, brown pigmentation of skin and mucous membranes, erythematous and maculopapular rash, jaundice, onycholysis, photosensitivity, pruritus, purpura (anaphylactoid), Stevens-Johnson syndrome, urticaria

Other: Anaphylaxis, angioedema, serum sickness-like reaction, systemic lupus erythematosus exacerbation

Nursing Considerations

•WARNING Notify prescriber if patient is breast-feeding because minocycline appears in breast milk and may have toxic effects.

•Monitor results of blood, renal, and hepatic tests before and periodically during long-term therapy.

•Shake oral suspension bottle well before administering.

•To prepare drug for I.V. use, reconstitute each 100-mg vial with 5 to 10 ml of sterile water for injection. Further dilute in 500 to 1,000 ml of NS, D₅W, D₅NS, or Ringer's or LR solution. Administer final dilution immediately, but avoid rapid administration.

•Store reconstituted drug at room temperature and use within 24 hours.

•Assess patient for signs of superinfection; if they appear, notify prescriber, discontinue minocycline, and start appropriate therapy, as ordered.

•Monitor PT in patient who also takes an anticoagulant during minocycline therapy.

PATIENT TEACHING

•Instruct patient to shake oral suspension bottle well and to use calibrated liquid-measuring device.

•Advise patient to take minocycline with a full glass of water, with food or milk, and in

an upright position to minimize esophageal and GI irritation.
• Direct patient to take a missed dose as soon as he remembers unless it's nearly time for the next dose. Caution against double-dosing.
• Instruct patient not to take minocycline within 2 hours of taking an antacid or 3 hours of taking an iron preparation.
• Urge patient to complete full course of treatment even if he feels better beforehand.
• Instruct patient to notify prescriber if no improvement occurs in a few days.
• Advise patient to avoid prolonged exposure to sun or sunlamps during therapy.
• Counsel female patient to avoid becoming pregnant because minocycline should be avoided, if possible, during tooth development (last half of gestation up to age 8). Drug may permanently turn teeth yellow, gray, or brown and cause enamel hypoplasia. It also may slow skeletal growth rate.
• Encourage patient who uses an oral contraceptive to use additional contraceptive method during minocycline therapy.
• Instruct patient to notify prescriber immediately about blurred vision, dizziness, headache, known or suspected pregnancy, and unsteadiness.

minoxidil (oral)

Loniten

minoxidil (topical)

Apo-Gain (CAN), Gen-Minoxidil (CAN), Minox (CAN), Minoxigaine (CAN), Rogaine (CAN), Rogaine ES for Men, Rogaine for Men, Rogaine for Women

Class and Category

Chemical: Piperidinopyrimidine derivative
Therapeutic: Antihypertensive (oral), hair-growth stimulant (topical)
Pregnancy category: C

Indications and Dosages

➤ *To manage severe symptomatic hypertension or hypertension with target organ damage that's unresponsive to other treatment*

TABLETS

Adults and adolescents. *Initial:* 5 mg as a single dose or in divided doses b.i.d. Increased, as directed, after at least 3 days. *Maintenance:* 10 to 40 mg/day. *Maximum:* 100 mg/day.

Children. *Initial:* 0.2 mg/kg q.d. Increased, as directed, after at least 3 days. *Maintenance:* 0.25 to 1 mg/kg/day as a single dose or in divided doses b.i.d. *Maximum:* 50-mg starting dose, 50 mg/day.

DOSAGE ADJUSTMENT Dosage possibly reduced for elderly patients and patients who have renal failure or are undergoing dialysis.
➤ *To treat alopecia*

TOPICAL 2%

Adults up to age 65. 1 ml applied b.i.d. to area of desired hair growth.

TOPICAL 5%

Adult men up to age 65. 1 ml applied b.i.d. to area of desired hair growth.

Route	Onset	Peak	Duration
P.O.	30 min	2 to 3 hr	24 to 48 hr
Topical 2%	4 mo	1 yr	Unknown
Topical 5%	2 mo	1 yr	Unknown

Mechanism of Action

Reduces blood pressure by inhibiting intracellular phosphodiesterase, an enzyme that normally facilitates the hydrolysis of cAMP and cGMP. This action decreases the intracellular cAMP level, resulting in arterial smooth-muscle relaxation and, consequently, lower blood pressure. Oral minoxidil produces greater dilation in arteries than in veins. It also reduces peripheral resistance and increases the heart rate, cardiac output, and stroke volume.

Topical minoxidil may produce hair regrowth by increasing cutaneous blood flow through vasodilation. Increased blood flow may stimulate resting hair follicles into active epithelial growth.

Contraindications

Acute MI; dissecting aortic aneurysm; hypersensitivity to minoxidil or its components, including propylene glycol; pheochromocytoma; skin irritation or abrasions (topical)

Interactions

DRUGS

guanethidine: Possibly severe hypotension, increased risk of orthostatic hypotension (oral)
nitrates, other hypotension-producing drugs, potent parenteral antihypertensives: Possibly severe hypotension

NSAIDs, sympathomimetics: Decreased antihypertensive effects
topical petrolatum, topical steroids: Increased absorption of topical minoxidil if used on same area
topical retinoids: Increased absorption of topical minoxidil and, possibly, formation of granulation tissue

Adverse Reactions
CNS: Fatigue, paresthesia (oral); lightheadedness, neuritis (topical); headache (both)
CV: ECG changes, heart failure, pericardial tamponade, pericarditis, rebound hypertension (oral); cardiac tamponade, hypotension, palpitations, reflex hypertension (topical); angina, edema, fast or irregular heartbeat, pericardial effusion (both)
EENT: Vision changes (topical)
ENDO: Breast tenderness (oral)
GI: Abdominal distention, ascites, nausea, vomiting (oral)
GU: Elevated BUN and serum creatinine levels (oral); sexual dysfunction (topical)
HEME: Leukopenia; thrombocytopenia; transient decrease in hematocrit, hemoglobin, and erythrocyte counts (oral)
RESP: Dyspnea, pulmonary hypertension (oral)
SKIN: Flushing, hyperpigmentation, Stevens-Johnson syndrome (oral); allergic contact dermatitis, alopecia, dry or flaky skin, eczema, erythema, folliculitis, scalp burning (topical); hypertrichosis, rash (both)
Other: Facial edema (topical); sodium and water retention, weight gain (both)

Nursing Considerations
• WARNING Be aware that patient who receives guanethidine should be hospitalized before starting oral minoxidil therapy so that his blood pressure can be monitored.
• Be aware that drug isn't usually prescribed for mild hypertension.
• For rapid management of hypertension, expect to adjust dosage up to every 6 hours and to monitor patient as prescribed. Also expect to administer a beta blocker and diuretic.
• Monitor patient's progress by measuring blood pressure frequently and weight daily. Evaluate for signs of fluid and sodium retention and for other systemic adverse reactions.

• Monitor for signs of pericardial effusion. Be prepared to stop oral minoxidil therapy, if ordered.
• Expect to discontinue oral minoxidil gradually because abrupt discontinuation may lead to rebound hypertension.
• Apply topical minoxidil only on healthy scalp. Avoid using on sunburned or abraded scalp.
• Use gloves when applying solution.
• When using spray applicator, avoid inhaling mist.
• Expect minoxidil to be least effective in men with mainly frontal hair loss.
• Expect topical form to have little effect on blood pressure in patients who don't have hypertension.

PATIENT TEACHING
• Inform patient that oral minoxidil controls but doesn't cure hypertension.
• Advise him to take tablets at the same time every day.
• Teach patient how to take his radial pulse, and advise him to measure it daily. Instruct him to notify prescriber if it exceeds normal rate by 20 beats/minute or more.
• Stress the importance of daily blood pressure and weight measurements.
• Instruct patient to notify prescriber immediately if he experiences bloating, breathing problems, a fast or irregular heartbeat, flushed or red skin, swelling of feet or lower legs, or weight gain of more than 5 lb (2.3 kg) in 1 day.
• Advise patient to have regular checkups with prescriber to monitor progress.
• Urge patient to consult prescriber before taking other prescription or OTC drugs.
• Reassure patient that body hair thickening and darkening reverses after oral minoxidil is discontinued.
• For patient using topical minoxidil, teach proper application technique and provide manufacturer's written instructions. Advise him to wear gloves when applying drug and to make sure hair and scalp are dry first.
• Instruct patient to start applying drug at center of balding area, to let drug dry for 2 to 4 hours, and not to use hairdryer to help it dry faster.
• Warn patient to avoid applying drug to abraded, irritated, or sunburned areas of scalp; to avoid inhaling mist when using a spray applicator; and to avoid getting drug

in his eyes, nose, or mouth. If accidental contact does occur, advise him to flush the area with large amounts of cool tap water.
•Instruct patient not to shampoo his hair for at least 4 hours after application and to avoid using other skin products on treated skin. Direct him to avoid using minoxidil 24 hours before and after applying chemical hair products, such as dyes and relaxers.
•Caution patient not to use more drug or apply it more often than prescribed and not to apply it to other body areas. Explain the risk of adverse systemic reactions with excessive topical use.
•Inform patient that minoxidil may stain clothing, hats, or bed linens before it's fully dry.
•Instruct patient to notify prescriber if burning, itching, or redness develops after application. For severe reactions, advise patient to wash drug off and consult prescriber before applying it again.
•Inform patient that hair loss may continue for 2 weeks after minoxidil therapy starts. Urge him to consult prescriber if hair loss continues after 2 weeks or if growth fails to increase in 4 months.
•Inform patient that new hair growth may be lost 3 to 4 months after stopping topical minoxidil and that progressive hair loss will resume.

mirtazapine

Remeron, Remeron SolTab

Class and Category
Chemical: Piperazinoazepine
Therapeutic: Antidepressant
Pregnancy category: C

Indications and Dosages
➤ *To treat major depression*
DISINTEGRATING TABLETS, TABLETS
Adults. *Initial:* 15 mg q.d., preferably h.s. Increased as needed and tolerated at 1- to 2-wk intervals. *Maximum:* 45 mg/day.

Route	Onset	Peak	Duration
P.O.	1 to 2 wk	6 wk or longer	Unknown

Contraindications
Hypersensitivity to mirtazapine or its components, use within 14 days of an MAO inhibitor

Mechanism of Action
May inhibit neuronal reuptake of norepinephrine and serotonin. By doing so, this tetracyclic antidepressant increases the action of these neurotransmitters in nerve cells. Increased neuronal levels of serotonin and norepinephrine may elevate mood.

Interactions
DRUGS
antihypertensives: Increased hypotensive effects of these drugs or enhanced mirtazapine effects
anxiolytics, hypnotics, other CNS depressants (including sedatives): Increased CNS depression
MAO inhibitors: Possibly hyperpyrexia, hypertension, seizures
ACTIVITIES
alcohol use: Increased CNS depression

Adverse Reactions
CNS: Agitation, amnesia, anxiety, apathy, asthenia, ataxia, cerebral ischemia, chills, confusion, delirium, delusions, depersonalization, depression, dizziness, dream disturbances, drowsiness, dyskinesia, dystonia, emotional lability, euphoria, extrapyramidal reactions, fever, hallucinations, hostility, hyperkinesia, hyperreflexia, hypoesthesia, hypokinesia, lack of coordination, malaise, mania, migraine headache, neurosis, paranoia, paresthesia, seizures, somnolence, syncope, tremor, vertigo
CV: Angina, bradycardia, edema, hypercholesterolemia, hypertension, hypertriglyceridemia, hypotension, MI, orthostatic hypotension, peripheral edema, PVCs, vasodilation
EENT: Accommodation disturbances, conjunctivitis, dry mouth, earache, epistaxis, eye pain, glaucoma, gingival bleeding, glossitis, hearing loss, hyperacusis, keratoconjunctivitis, lacrimation, pharyngitis, sinusitis, stomatitis
ENDO: Breast pain
GI: Abdominal distention and pain, anorexia, cholecystitis, colitis, constipation, elevated ALT level, eructation, increased appetite, nausea, thirst, vomiting
GU: Amenorrhea, cystitis, dysmenorrhea, dysuria, hematuria, impotence, increased libido, leukorrhea, renal calculi, urinary frequency and incontinence, urine retention, UTI, vaginitis
HEME: Agranulocytosis, neutropenia

M

MS: Arthralgia, back pain, dysarthria, muscle twitching, myalgia, myasthenia, neck pain and rigidity
RESP: Asthma, bronchitis, cough, dyspnea, pneumonia
SKIN: Acne, alopecia, dry skin, exfoliative dermatitis, photosensitivity, pruritus, rash
Other: Dehydration, facial edema, flulike symptoms, herpes simplex, weight gain or loss

Nursing Considerations
• Administer mirtazapine before bedtime.
• Expect disintegrating tablet to dissolve on patient's tongue within 30 seconds.
• **WARNING** Don't give drug within 14 days of an MAO inhibitor to avoid serious, possibly fatal, reaction.
• Supervise suicidal patient closely, especially early in treatment when drug hasn't yet produced full therapeutic effect.
• Monitor patient closely for signs of infection (fever, pharyngitis, stomatitis), which may be linked to a low WBC count. If these signs occur, notify prescriber and expect to stop drug.
• Expect mirtazapine therapy to last 6 months or longer for acute depression.

PATIENT TEACHING
• Instruct patient not to swallow disintegrating tablet. Tell him to hold tablet on tongue and allow it to dissolve. Inform him that tablet will dissolve within 30 seconds.
• Inform phenylketonuric patient that mirtazapine disintegrating tablets contain 2.6 mg phenylalanine per 15-mg tablet, 5.2 mg per 30-mg tablet, and 7.8 mg per 45-mg tablet.
• Instruct patient to avoid alcohol and other CNS depressants during mirtazapine therapy and for up to 7 days after drug is discontinued.
• Advise patient to avoid potentially hazardous activities until drug's CNS effects are known.
• Direct patient to change position slowly to minimize effects of orthostatic hypotension.
• Instruct patient to notify prescriber immediately about chills, fever, mouth irritation, sore throat, and other signs of infection.
• Encourage patient to visit prescriber regularly during therapy to monitor progress.

misoprostol
Cytotec

Class and Category
Chemical: Prostaglandin E_1 analogue
Therapeutic: Antiulcer, gastric antisecretory
Pregnancy category: X

Indications and Dosages
➤ *To prevent NSAID-induced gastric ulcers*
TABLETS
Adults. 200 mcg q.i.d. or 400 mcg b.i.d. with food, with last dose h.s. every day.
DOSAGE ADJUSTMENT Dosage reduced to 100 mcg q.i.d. if patient can't tolerate 200-mcg dose.

Route	Onset	Peak	Duration
P.O.	30 min	60 to 90 min	3 to 6 hr

Mechanism of Action
May protect the stomach from NSAID-induced mucosal damage by increasing gastric mucus production and mucosal bicarbonate secretion. Misoprostol also inhibits gastric acid secretion caused by such stimuli as food, coffee, and histamine.

Contraindications
Breast-feeding, hypersensitivity to prostaglandins or prostaglandin analogues, in pregnant women (to prevent NSAID-induced gastric ulcers)

Interactions
DRUGS
magnesium-containing antacids: Increased misoprostol-induced diarrhea

Adverse Reactions
CNS: Headache
GI: Abdominal pain, constipation, diarrhea, flatulence, indigestion, nausea, vomiting
GU: Dysmenorrhea, hypermenorrhea, menstrual irregularities, vaginal bleeding

Nursing Considerations
• **WARNING** Ask patient if she is or may be pregnant. If so, notify prescriber because misoprostol may cause uterine bleeding, contractions, and spontaneous abortion in pregnant woman as well as teratogenic effects in the fetus.
• Use drug cautiously in patients with cerebrovascular disease, coronary artery disease, or uncontrolled epilepsy because of the risk of severe complications.
• Also use misoprostol cautiously in patients with inflammatory bowel disease because drug may worsen intestinal inflammation

and cause diarrhea. If diarrhea causes severe dehydration, drug may be discontinued.

PATIENT TEACHING

• Caution female patient about the risk of taking misoprostol during pregnancy, and urge her to use reliable contraception during therapy. Urge her to notify prescriber immediately if she is or might be pregnant.

• Instruct patient to take misoprostol with meals and at bedtime.

• Advise patient that he may continue to take NSAIDs, if prescribed, during misoprostol therapy.

• Inform patient that diarrhea is dose-related and usually resolves after 8 days. Instruct him to avoid magnesium-containing antacids because they may worsen diarrhea and to contact prescriber if diarrhea persists longer than 8 days.

• Urge female patient to notify prescriber immediately about postmenopausal bleeding; she may need diagnostic tests to rule out a gynecologic disorder.

mitoxantrone hydrochloride

Novantrone

Class and Category

Chemical: Anthracenedione
Therapeutic: Antineoplastic
Pregnancy category: D

Indications and Dosages

➤ *To reduce neurologic disability and frequency of relapses in patients with secondary (chronic) progressive, progressive relapsing, or worsening relapsing-remitting multiple sclerosis (patients whose neurologic status is significantly abnormal between relapses)*

I.V. INFUSION

Adults. 12 mg/m^2 over 5 to 15 min q 3 mo. *Maximum:* Cumulative dose of 140 mg/m^2.

➤ *As adjunct to treat pain related to advanced hormone-refractory prostate cancer*

I.V. INFUSION

Adults. 12 to 14 mg/m^2 over 5 to 15 min q 21 days.

➤ *As adjunct to treat acute nonlymphocytic leukemia (ANLL)*

I.V. INFUSION

Adults. *Initial:* 12 mg/m^2 over at least 3 min on days 1 to 3 with 100 mg/m^2 of cytarabine as a continuous 24-hr infusion on days 1 to 7. If patient's antileukemic response is inadequate or incomplete, a second induction course is given at the same dosage. *Maintenance:* 6 wk after induction, 12 mg/m^2 over at least 3 min on days 1 and 2 with 100 mg/m^2 of cytarabine as a continuous 24-hr infusion on days 1 to 5. A second maintenance course is given 4 wk after the first if needed and tolerated.

Mechanism of Action

Binds to DNA, causing cross-linkage and strand breakage, interfering with RNA synthesis, and inhibiting topoisomerase II, an enzyme responsible for uncoiling and repairing damaged DNA. Mitoxantrone produces a cytocidal effect on proliferating and nonproliferating cells and doesn't appear to be cell-cycle specific. The drug's role in multiple sclerosis is unknown, but it's known to inhibit B-cell, T-cell, and macrophage proliferation and impair antigen function.

Incompatibilities

Don't mix mitoxantrone in the same infusion as heparin (because a precipitate may form); don't mix with any other drugs.

Contraindications

Hypersensitivity to mitoxantrone or its components

Interactions

DRUGS

allopurinol, colchicine, probenecid, sulfinpyrazone: Possibly interference with antihyperuricemic action of these drugs
blood-dyscrasia–causing drugs (such as cephalosporins and sulfasalazine): Increased risk of leukopenia and thrombocytopenia
bone marrow depressants, such as carboplatin and lomustine: Possibly additive bone marrow depression
daunorubicin, doxorubicin: Increased risk of cardiotoxicity
methotrexate and other antineoplastics: Risk of developing leukemia
vaccines, killed virus: Decreased antibody response to vaccine

M

vaccines, live virus: Increased risk of replication of and adverse effects of vaccine virus, decreased antibody response to vaccine

Adverse Reactions
CNS: Headache, seizures
CV: Arrhythmias, chest pain, congestive heart failure, decreased left ventricular ejection fraction, ECG changes
EENT: Blue-colored cornea, conjunctivitis, mucositis, stomatitis
GI: Abdominal pain, diarrhea, GI bleeding, nausea, vomiting
GU: Blue-green urine, renal failure
HEME: Leukopenia, thrombocytopenia
RESP: Cough, dyspnea
SKIN: Alopecia, extravasation, jaundice
Other: Allergic reaction, anaphylaxis, hyperuricemia, infection, infusion site pain or redness

Nursing Considerations
• Before and periodically during mitoxantrone therapy, expect patient to undergo an echocardiogram, ECG studies, and radionuclide angiography to evaluate cardiac status, and expect to obtain hematocrit, hemoglobin level, and CBC with platelet count.
• Be aware that drug shouldn't be given to patient with multiple sclerosis whose neutrophil count is less than 1,500/mm³.
• Obtain liver function test results, as ordered, before beginning each course of therapy. Be aware that drug shouldn't be given to patient with multiple sclerosis whose liver function is abnormal.
• Anticipate obtaining pregnancy test before each course of therapy for women of childbearing age who have multiple sclerosis. Notify prescriber about test results.
• Follow facility policy for handling antineoplastics. Be aware that manufacturer recommends the use of goggles, gloves, and protective gowns during drug preparation and administration.
• Before infusing drug, dilute it in at least 50 ml of NS or D₅W.
• **WARNING** Be aware that drug shouldn't be given intrathecally because paralysis may occur.
• If mitoxantrone solution comes in contact with your skin or mucosa, wash it off thoroughly with warm water. If drug comes in contact with your eyes, irrigate them thoroughly with water or NS.
• Discard unused diluted solution because it contains no preservatives. After penetration

of the stopper, store undiluted drug for up to 7 days at room temperature or 14 days under refrigeration. Avoid freezing drug.
• If extravasation occurs, stop the infusion immediately and notify prescriber. Reinsert the I.V. line in another vein and resume the infusion. Although mitoxantrone is a nonvesicant, observe the extravasation site for signs of necrosis or phlebitis.
• Monitor patients with chickenpox or recent exposure to it and patients with herpes zoster for evidence of severe, generalized disease.
• Monitor patients with heart disease for signs and symptoms of cardiotoxicity, such as arrhythmias and chest pain. The risk of cardiotoxicity increases when the cumulative dose reaches 140 mg/m² in cancer patients or 100 mg/m² in multiple sclerosis patients.
• Monitor blood uric acid level for hyperuricemia in patients with a history of gout or renal calculi. Expect to give allopurinol, as prescribed, to patients with leukemia or lymphoma who have elevated blood uric acid level to prevent uric acid nephropathy.
• **WARNING** If severe or life-threatening nonhematologic toxicity or hematologic toxicity occurs during the first induction course, expect to withhold the second induction course until toxicity resolves.
• If patient develops thrombocytopenia, implement protective precautions according to facility policy.
• Assess patient for evidence of infection, such as fever, if leukopenia occurs. Expect to obtain appropriate specimens for culture and sensitivity testing.
• Be aware that patients receiving mitoxantrone in combination with other antineoplastics or radiation therapy are at risk for developing secondary leukemia.

PATIENT TEACHING
• Advise patient to have dental work completed, if possible, before treatment begins or deferred until blood counts return to normal because mitoxantrone may delay healing and cause gingival bleeding. Teach patient proper oral hygiene, and recommend use of a toothbrush with soft bristles.
• Encourage patient to drink plenty of fluid to increase urine output and help excrete uric acid.
• Advise patient to contact prescriber imme-

diately if GI upset occurs, but to continue taking drug unless otherwise directed.
•Stress the importance of complying with the dosage regimen and keeping follow-up medical and laboratory appointments.
•Explain that urine may appear blue-green for 24 hours after treatment and that the whites of the eyes may appear blue. Stress that these effects are temporary and harmless. Explain that hair loss is possible, but that hair should return after therapy ends.
•Caution patient to avoid receiving immunizations unless approved by prescriber. Also advise persons who live in same household as patient to avoid receiving immunizations with oral polio vaccine. Tell patient to avoid people who have recently received the oral polio vaccine or to wear a protective mask over his nose and mouth when he's around them.
•Instruct patient to avoid persons with infections if bone marrow depression occurs. Advise patient to contact prescriber if fever, chills, cough, hoarseness, lower back or side pain, or painful or difficult urination occurs; these changes may signal an infection.
•Advise patient to contact prescriber immediately if he notices unusual bleeding or bruising, black or tarry stools, blood in urine or stool, or pinpoint red spots on his skin.
•Teach patient to avoid touching his eyes or inside of his nose unless he has washed his hands immediately before.
•Stress the importance of avoiding accidental cuts from sharp objects, such as a razor or fingernail clippers, because excessive bleeding or infection may occur.
•Caution patient to avoid contact sports or other situations that may cause bruising or injury.

modafinil

Provigil

Class, Category, and Schedule
Chemical: Benzhydryl sulfinylacetamide derivative
Therapeutic: CNS stimulant
Pregnancy category: C
Controlled substance: Schedule IV

Indications and Dosages
➤ *To improve daytime wakefulness in patients with narcolepsy*

TABLETS
Adults and adolescents age 16 and older.
200 mg q.d. *Maximum:* 400 mg/day.

> ### Mechanism of Action
> May inhibit the release of gamma-amino-butyric acid (GABA), the most common inhibitory neurotransmitter, or CNS depressant, in the brain. Modafinil also increases the release of glutamate, an excitatory neurotransmitter, or CNS stimulant, in the thalamus and hippocampus. These two actions may improve wakefulness.

Contraindications
Hypersensitivity to modafinil or its components

Interactions
DRUGS
amitriptyline, citalopram, clomipramine, diazepam, imipramine, propranolol, tolbutamide, topiramate: Possibly prolonged elimination time and increased blood levels of these drugs
carbamazepine: Possibly decreased modafinil effectiveness and decreased blood carbamazepine level
cimetidine, clarithromycin, erythromycin, fluconazole, fluoxetine, fluvoxamine, itraconazole, ketoconazole, nefazodone, sertraline: Possibly inhibited metabolism, decreased clearance, and increased blood level of modafinil
contraceptive-containing implants or devices, oral contraceptives: Possibly contraceptive failure
cyclosporine: Possibly decreased blood cyclosporine level and increased risk of organ transplant rejection
dexamethasone, phenobarbital and other barbiturates, primidone, rifabutin, rifampin: Possibly decreased blood level and effectiveness of modafinil
dextroamphetamine: Possibly increased risk of adverse CNS stimulant effects
fosphenytoin, mephenytoin, phenytoin: Possibly decreased effectiveness of modafinil, increased blood phenytoin level, and increased risk of phenytoin toxicity
methylphenidate: Possibly 1-hour delay in modafinil absorption when these drugs are administered together
theophylline: Possibly decreased blood level and effectiveness of theophylline
warfarin: Possibly decreased warfarin metabolism and increased risk of bleeding

M

Foods

all foods: 1-hour delay in modafinil absorption and possibly delayed onset of action
caffeine: Increased CNS stimulation
grapefruit juice: Possibly decreased modafinil metabolism

Adverse Reactions

CNS: Anxiety, depression, headache, insomnia, nervousness
GI: Nausea
Other: Infection

Nursing Considerations

•**WARNING** Monitor patient with a history of alcoholism, stimulant abuse, or other substance abuse for proper drug compliance during modafinil therapy. Observe for signs of misuse or abuse, including frequent prescription refill requests, increased frequency of dosing, or drug-seeking behavior. Monitor patient for signs and symptoms of excessive modafinil dosage, including aggressiveness, anxiety, confusion, decreased prothrombin time, diarrhea, irritability, nausea, nervousness, palpitations, sleep disturbances, and tremor.
•Be aware that modafinil, like other CNS stimulants, may produce alterations in mood, perception, thinking, judgment, feelings, and motor skills. It may also mask signs that the patient needs sleep.
•If administering drug to patient with a known history of psychosis, emotional instability, or psychological illness with psychotic features, be prepared to perform baseline behavioral assessments or frequent clinical observation.

Patient Teaching

•Inform patient that modafinil can help, but not cure, narcolepsy and that drug's full effects may not be seen right away.
•Advise patient to avoid taking modafinil within 1 hour of eating because food may delay drug's absorption and onset of action. If he drinks grapefruit juice, encourage him to drink a consistent amount daily.
•Inform patient that drug can affect his concentration and function and can hide signs of fatigue. Urge him not to drive or perform activities that require mental alertness until drug's full CNS effects are known.
•Because alcohol may decrease alertness, advise patient to avoid it while taking modafinil.
•Encourage patient to maintain a regular sleeping pattern.
•Caution patient to avoid excessive intake of foods, beverages, and over-the-counter drugs that contain caffeine because caffeine may lead to increased CNS stimulation.
•Inform female patient that modafinil can decrease the effectiveness of certain contraceptives, including birth control pills and implantable hormonal contraceptives. If she uses such contraceptives, urge her to use an alternate birth control method during modafinil therapy and for up to 1 month after she stops taking the drug.
•Advise patient to keep follow-up appointments with prescriber so that her progress can be monitored.

moexipril hydrochloride

Univasc

Class and Category

Chemical: Prodrug of moexiprilat
Therapeutic: Antihypertensive
Pregnancy category: C (first trimester), D (later trimesters)

Indications and Dosages

➤ *To manage hypertension without diuretic therapy*

TABLETS

Adults. *Initial:* 7.5 mg q.d. 1 hr a.c. *Maintenance:* 7.5 to 30 mg as a single dose or in divided doses b.i.d. 1 hr a.c. *Maximum:* 30 mg/day.

DOSAGE ADJUSTMENT For patients with creatinine clearance of less than 40 ml/min/1.73 m^2, initial dosage reduced to 3.75 mg q.d. and increased, as ordered, to maximum of 15 mg/day.

➤ *To manage hypertension with diuretic therapy*

TABLETS

Adults. *Initial:* 3.75 mg q.d. 1 hr a.c. Increased gradually, as ordered, until blood pressure is controlled.

Route	Onset	Peak	Duration
P.O.	1 hr	3 to 6 hr	24 hr

Contraindications

History of angioedema with previous ACE inhibitor use, hypersensitivity to moexipril or its components

Mechanism of Action

Is converted to the active metabolite moexiprilat, which reduces blood pressure by inhibiting ACE activity. ACE normally catalyzes the conversion of angiotensin I to angiotensin II—a vasoconstrictor that stimulates aldosterone secretion by the adrenal cortex and directly suppresses renin release. Inhibited ACE activity results in decreased peripheral arterial resistance, increased plasma renin activity, and decreased aldosterone secretion. Decreased aldosterone secretion causes water and sodium excretion.

Interactions

DRUGS

allopurinol, bone marrow depressants, corticosteroids (systemic), cytostatic drugs, procainamide: Increased risk of possibly fatal neutropenia or agranulocytosis
antacids: Possibly decreased moexipril bioavailability
cyclosporine, heparin, potassium-containing drugs, potassium-sparing diuretics, potassium supplements: Increased risk of hyperkalemia
digoxin: Possibly increased blood digoxin level
diuretics, other hypotension-producing drugs: Hypotension, risk of renal failure (from sodium or volume depletion caused by diuretics), possibly decreased secondary aldosteronism and hypokalemia caused by diuretics
lithium: Increased blood lithium level and risk of lithium toxicity
NSAIDs (especially indomethacin), sympathomimetics: Decreased antihypertensive effect of moexipril
phenothiazines: Increased pharmacologic effects of moexipril

FOODS

all foods: Decreased moexipril absorption
low-salt milk, salt substitutes: Possibly hyperkalemia

ACTIVITIES

alcohol use: Possibly hypotension

Adverse Reactions

CNS: Anxiety, chills, confusion, CVA, dizziness, drowsiness, fatigue, fever, headache, malaise, mood changes, nervousness, sleep disturbance, syncope
CV: Angina, arrhythmias, chest pain, hypotension, MI, orthostatic hypotension, palpitations, peripheral edema
EENT: Dry mouth, hoarseness, laryngeal edema, mouth or tongue swelling, pharyngitis, rhinitis, sinusitis, taste perversion, tinnitus
GI: Abdominal distention or pain, anorexia, constipation, diarrhea, dysphagia, elevated liver function test results, hepatitis, increased appetite, nausea, pancreatitis, vomiting
GU: Azotemia, elevated BUN and serum creatinine and uric acid levels, interstitial nephritis, oliguria, proteinuria, renal insufficiency, urinary frequency
HEME: Agranulocytosis, bone marrow depression, elevated erythrocyte sedimentation rate, hemolytic anemia, leukocytosis, leukopenia, neutropenia, thrombocytopenia
MS: Arthralgia, leg heaviness or weakness, myalgia, myositis
RESP: Bronchospasm, cough, dyspnea, upper respiratory tract infection
SKIN: Alopecia, diaphoresis, flushing, onycholysis, pallor, pemphigus, photosensitivity, pruritus, rash, Stevens-Johnson syndrome, urticaria
Other: Anaphylaxis, angioedema (of arms, face, larynx, legs, lips, mucous membranes, tongue), flulike symptoms, hyperkalemia, hyponatremia, positive ANA titer

Nursing Considerations

•**WARNING** Contact prescriber if patient is or may be pregnant. Moexipril may cause fetal or neonatal harm or death if used during second or third trimester.
•Be aware that patient who already takes a diuretic should be medically supervised for several hours after first dose of moexipril.
•Administer drug 1 hour before meals.
•Monitor blood pressure, leukocyte count, and liver and renal function test results during moexipril therapy.
•Be aware that black patients may be less responsive to drug's antihypertensive effect if moexipril is used alone to control blood pressure.

PATIENT TEACHING

•Urge female patient to notify prescriber immediately if she is or may be pregnant.

•Instruct patient to take moexipril at the same time each day, 1 hour before meals.

•Direct patient to take a missed dose as soon as he remembers unless it's nearly time for the next dose. Caution against doubling the dose.

•**WARNING** Instruct patient to stop drug and seek immediate medical attention for hoarseness; swelling of tongue, glottis, larynx, face, hands, or feet; or sudden difficulty swallowing or breathing.

•Caution patient not to stop drug without consulting prescriber even if he feels better.

•Inform patient about possible dizziness, especially after first dose and if he takes a diuretic.

•Advise patient to change position slowly to minimize effects of orthostatic hypotension.

•Caution patient to avoid potentially hazardous activities until drug's CNS effects are known.

•Instruct patient to notify prescriber if he faints or experiences persistent dizziness.

•Instruct patient to report evidence of infection (such as chills, fever, and sore throat) as well as diarrhea, nausea, or vomiting, which may lead to dehydration-induced hypotension.

•Advise patient to avoid alcohol during moexipril therapy because it may cause hypotension.

•Instruct patient to check with prescriber before taking OTC drugs.

•Urge patient to avoid potassium supplements and potassium-containing salt substitutes unless prescriber allows them.

•Advise patient to visit prescriber regularly to monitor progress.

•Discuss the importance of weight control and low-salt diet in managing hypertension.

molindone hydrochloride

Moban, Moban Concentrate

Class and Category

Chemical: Dihydroindolone derivative
Therapeutic: Antipsychotic drug
Pregnancy category: Not rated

Indications and Dosages

➤ *To manage symptoms of psychotic disorders*

ORAL SOLUTION, TABLETS

Adults and children age 12 and older. *Initial:* 50 to 75 mg q.d. in divided doses t.i.d. or

q.i.d. Dosage increased to 100 mg/day in 3 to 4 days as needed. *Maintenance:* For mild psychosis, 5 to 15 mg t.i.d. or q.i.d.; for moderate psychosis, 10 to 25 mg t.i.d. or q.i.d.; for severe psychosis, 225 mg/day in divided doses. *Maximum:* 225 mg/day.

DOSAGE ADJUSTMENT Initial dosage reduced for elderly or debilitated patients.

Route	Onset	Peak	Duration
P.O.	Unknown	Unknown	24 to 36 hr

Mechanism of Action

Occupies dopamine receptor sites in the reticular activating and limbic systems in the CNS. By blocking dopamine activity in these areas, molindone reduces the symptoms of psychosis, helping the patient to think and behave more coherently.

Contraindications

Hypersensitivity to molindone, its components, or other antipsychotic drugs, including haloperidol, loxapine, phenothiazines, and thioxanthenes

Interactions

DRUGS

amphetamines: Decreased amphetamine effectiveness, decreased antipsychotic effectiveness of molindone

anesthetics, barbiturates, benzodiazepines, CNS depressants, opioid analgesics: Possibly prolonged and intensified CNS depressant effects

antacids, antidiarrheals: Decreased molindone absorption

anticholinergics, antidyskinetics, antihistamines: Possibly increased anticholinergic effects

beta blockers: Possibly increased effect of beta blocker

bromocriptine: Possibly decreased therapeutic effects of bromocriptine and increased serum prolactin level

extrapyramidal reaction–causing drugs, such as amoxapine, haloperidol, loxapine, metoclopramide, olanzapine, phenothiazines, pimozide, rauwolfia alkaloids, risperidone, tacrine, and thioxanthenes: Increased severity of extrapyramidal effects

insulin, oral antidiabetic drugs: Possibly increased serum glucose level *levodopa:* Inhibited antidyskinetic effects of levodopa, possibly decreased antipsychotic effects of molindone

lithium: Increased risk of neurotoxicity, increased extrapyramidal effects

MAO inhibitors, maprotiline, trazodone, tricyclic antidepressants: Possibly prolonged and intensified sedative or anticholinergic effects of all drugs

phenytoin, tetracycline: Interference with absorption of phenytoin and tetracycline

ACTIVITIES

alcohol use: Prolonged and intensified CNS depression

Adverse Reactions

CNS: Depression, drowsiness, euphoria, extrapyramidal reactions (such as dystonia, motor restlessness, pseudoparkinsonism, and tardive dyskinesia), headache, lack of coordination, neuroleptic malignant syndrome, tiredness

CV: Orthostatic hypotension, tachycardia, unstable blood pressure

EENT: Blinking or eyelid spasm, blurred vision, dry mouth, inability to move eyes, nasal congestion

ENDO: Breast engorgement, lactation

GI: Constipation, nausea

GU: Decreased libido, menstrual irregularities, urine retention

MS: Muscle spasms of back, face, and neck; muscle twitching; twisting movements of the body; weakness or stiffness of limbs

RESP: Dyspnea

SKIN: Diaphoresis, pallor, rash

Other: Heatstroke

Nursing Considerations

•**WARNING** Assess patient for signs and symptoms of neuroleptic malignant syndrome, such as diaphoresis, dyspnea, fatigue, fever, incontinence, pallor, severe muscle stiffness, tachycardia, and unstable blood pressure; notify prescriber immediately if they occur. Expect to discontinue drug and begin intensive medical treatment. Monitor patient carefully for recurrence if antipsychotic therapy resumes.

•Be aware that molindone shouldn't be administered to patients who have severe CNS depression or who are comatose because of drug's CNS depressant effects.

•Monitor elderly patients for orthostatic hypotension and symptoms of tardive dys-

kinesia, including blinking or eyelid spasms, involuntary movements of the limbs, and unusual facial expressions, because these patients may be sensitive to drug's anticholinergic and extrapyramidal effects. Expect to reduce dosage or discontinue drug.

•Administer oral solution undiluted or mixed with water, carbonated beverage, fruit juice, or milk.

PATIENT TEACHING

•Instruct patient to follow treatment regimen and to notify prescriber before discontinuing drug because gradual dosage reduction may be needed.

•Instruct patient not to take drug within 2 hours of taking an antacid. Advise him to take drug with food or a full glass of milk or water to reduce gastric irritation.

•Instruct patient to take oral solution undiluted or mixed with water, carbonated beverage, fruit juice, or milk.

•Warn patient of possible blurred vision, dizziness, and drowsiness, and advise him to avoid potentially hazardous activities until drug's adverse effects are known.

•Urge patient to avoid alcohol because of possible additive effects and hypotension.

•Advise patient, especially if elderly, to rise slowly from a supine or seated position to avoid dizziness, light-headedness, and fainting.

•Explain that drug may reduce the body's response to heat. Tell patient to avoid temperature extremes, such as a hot shower, hot tub, or sauna, and urge him to use caution during exercise.

•Caution patient not to take OTC drugs for colds or allergies because they can increase the risk of heatstroke and increase anticholinergic effects, such as blurred vision, constipation, dry mouth, and urine retention.

•Inform patient and family members that maximum clinical improvement in symptoms.may take several weeks or months.

montelukast sodium

Singulair

Class and Category

Chemical: Leukotriene receptor antagonist
Therapeutic: Antiasthmatic
Pregnancy category: B

Indications and Dosages
➤ *To prevent or treat asthma*
ORAL GRANULES
Children ages 12 to 23 mo. 4 mg q.d. in the evening. *Maximum:* 4 mg/day.
CHEWABLE TABLETS
Children ages 6 to 14. 5 mg q.d. in the evening. *Maximum:* 5 mg/day.
Children ages 2 to 5. 4 mg q.d. in the evening. *Maximum:* 4 mg/day.
TABLETS
Adults and adolescents age 15 and older. 10 mg q.d. in the evening. *Maximum:* 10 mg/day.

Route	Onset	Peak	Duration
P.O.	Unknown	Unknown	24 hr

Mechanism of Action
Prevents and treats asthma by antagonizing cysteinyl leukotriene receptors. Cysteinyl leukotrienes are products of arachidonic acid metabolism that are released from mast cells, eosinophils, and other cells. When cysteinyl leukotrienes bind to their receptor sites in bronchial airways, they increase endothelial membrane permeability, which leads to airway edema, smooth-muscle contraction, and altered activity of the cells involved in asthma's inflammatory process. By antagonizing cysteinyl leukotriene receptors, montelukast blocks these effects.

Contraindications
Hypersensitivity to montelukast or its components

Interactions
DRUGS
phenobarbital: Decreased amount of circulating montelukast

Adverse Reactions
CNS: Asthenia, dizziness, fatigue, headache (in all patients); fever (in children)
EENT: Dental pain, nasal congestion (in all patients); laryngitis, otitis media, pharyngitis, sinusitis (in children)
GI: Abdominal pain, elevated liver function test results, indigestion, infectious gastroenteritis (in all patients); diarrhea, nausea (in children)
GU: Pyuria
RESP: Cough

SKIN: Pruritus, rash, urticaria
Other: Anaphylaxis, angioedema (in all patients); viral infection (in children)

Nursing Considerations
•WARNING Be aware that montelukast shouldn't be administered for acute asthma attack or status asthmaticus.
•Be aware that montelukast shouldn't be abruptly substituted for inhaled or oral corticosteroids; expect to taper corticosteroid dosage gradually, as directed.
•Monitor for adverse reactions, such as cardiac and pulmonary symptoms, eosinophilia, and vasculitis, in patient undergoing corticosteroid withdrawal. Notify prescriber if such reactions occur.
PATIENT TEACHING
•Advise patient to take montelukast daily as prescribed, even when he feels well. Urge him not to decrease dosage or stop taking other prescribed asthma drugs unless instructed by prescriber.
•Caution patient not to use drug for acute asthma attack or status asthmaticus; make sure he has appropriate short-acting rescue drug available.
•Tell parents administering oral granules to pour contents directly into the child's mouth or mix with ice cream or cold or room temperature applesauce, carrots, or rice—but not liquids or other foods—just prior to administration. Liquids may be given after drug has been administered. Once packet is opened, the full dose must be administered within 15 minutes. Drug must not be stored for future use if mixed with food.
•Instruct patient to notify prescriber if he needs to use short-acting inhaled bronchodilator more often than usual, or more often than prescribed, to control symptoms.
•Teach patient to use peak flowmeter to determine personal best expiratory volume.
•Caution patient with aspirin sensitivity to avoid aspirin and NSAIDs during montelukast therapy. Montelukast may not effectively reduce bronchospasm in such a patient.
•Inform patient (or parents of child) with phenylketonuria that chewable tablet contains phenylalanine.

moricizine hydrochloride

Ethmozine

Class and Category

Chemical: Phenothiazine derivative
Therapeutic: Class I antiarrhythmic
Pregnancy category: B

Indications and Dosages

➤ *To treat life-threatening ventricular arrhythmias*

TABLETS

Adults. 200 to 300 mg q 8 hr. *Maximum:* 900 mg/day.

DOSAGE ADJUSTMENT For patients with hepatic or renal impairment, initial dosage possibly reduced to 600 mg/day or less.

Route	Onset	Peak	Duration
P.O.	2 hr	6 to 14 hr	10 to 24 hr

Mechanism of Action

Exerts potent local anesthetic activity and stabilizes myocardial cell membranes, thus reducing ventricular arrhythmias. Moricizine prolongs the PR interval, AV nodal conduction time, infranodal conduction time, and intraventricular conduction time by inhibiting sodium influx across myocardial cell membranes. These effects decrease myocardial excitability, conduction velocity, and automaticity. Prolonged conduction decreases the refractory period and increases the ratio of refractory period to action potential duration, thus preventing arrhythmias.

Contraindications

Cardiogenic shock, hypersensitivity to moricizine or its components, right bundle-branch block with left hemiblock (bifascicular block) unless pacemaker is present, second- or third-degree AV block unless pacemaker is present

Interactions

DRUGS

cimetidine: Decreased moricizine clearance, increased blood moricizine level
digoxin: Prolonged PR interval
other antiarrhythmics: Increased risk of adverse cardiac effects
propranolol: Slightly prolonged PR interval
theophylline: Increased theophylline clearance, decreased blood theophylline level

Adverse Reactions

CNS: Abnormal gait, agitation, akathisia, anxiety, asthenia, ataxia, coma, confusion, depression, dizziness, dyskinesia, euphoria, fatigue, hallucinations, headache, hypoesthesia, hypothermia, lack of coordination, memory loss, nervousness, paresthesia, seizures, sleep disturbance, somnolence, tremor, vertigo
CV: Angina, AV block, bradycardia, cardiac arrest, heart failure, hypertension, hypotension, junctional rhythm, MI, palpitations, proarrhythmias (new rhythm disturbances or worsened existing arrhythmias), pulmonary embolism, sinus pause or arrest, supraventricular arrhythmias (including atrial fibrillation and flutter), thrombophlebitis, vasodilation, ventricular tachycardia (sustained)
EENT: Bitter taste, blurred vision, diplopia, dry mouth, eye pain, lip or tongue swelling, nystagmus, periorbital edema, pharyngitis, sinusitis, tinnitus
GI: Abdominal pain, anorexia, diarrhea, dysphagia, elevated liver function test results, flatulence, hepatotoxicity, ileus, indigestion, nausea, vomiting
GU: Decreased libido, dysuria, flank pain, impotence, urinary frequency and incontinence, urine retention
MS: Myalgia
RESP: Apnea, asthma, cough, dyspnea, hyperventilation
SKIN: Diaphoresis, dry skin, pruritus, rash, urticaria
Other: Drug-induced fever

Nursing Considerations

•Expect moricizine therapy to start in hospital because of the risk of proarrhythmias.
•Expect prescriber to discontinue previous antiarrhythmic one to two plasma half-lives before starting moricizine therapy.
•If needed to increase compliance, consult prescriber about changing to 12-hour dosing interval.
•Monitor liver and renal function test results for changes; expect prescriber to lower dose for patient with hepatic or renal impairment.
•Expect proarrhythmic effects to occur during first week of therapy, regardless of dosage.
•Anticipate higher risk of ventricular tachyarrhythmias in patients with cardiomegaly, coronary artery disease, heart failure, history of MI, or sustained ventricular tachycardia.

M

•Monitor ECG during therapy because drug may cause decreased JT interval and increased PR and QRS intervals. Notify prescriber if you detect such changes.

•**WARNING** Expect to discontinue drug if second- or third-degree AV block develops and patient doesn't have a ventricular pacemaker.

•Monitor serum electrolyte levels during therapy and correct imbalances, as prescribed.

•Expect an increased risk of dizziness and nausea with higher doses.

PATIENT TEACHING

•Instruct patient to take moricizine at evenly spaced intervals, as prescribed, even if he feels well.

•Advise patient to take a missed dose as soon as he remembers if it's 4 hours or more before the next scheduled dose. Caution against double-dosing.

•Teach patient how to check his pulse rate, and direct him to do so daily. Urge him to notify prescriber about significant changes.

•Advise patient to avoid hazardous activities until drug's CNS effects are known.

•Instruct patient to notify prescriber about chest pain, fast or irregular heartbeat, shortness of breath, and swelling of feet or lower legs.

•Urge patient to visit prescriber regularly to monitor progress.

morphine sulfate

Astramorph PF, Avinza, Duramorph, Epimorph (CAN), Kadian, M-Eslon (CAN), Morphine Extra-Forte (CAN), Morphine Forte (CAN), Morphine H.P. (CAN), Morphitec (CAN), MS Contin, MSIR, MS/L, MS/L Concentrate, MS/S, OMS Concentrate, Oramorph SR, Rescudose, RMS Uniserts, Roxanol, Roxanol 100, Roxanol UD, Statex (CAN)

Class, Category, and Schedule
Chemical: Phenanthrene derivative
Therapeutic: Analgesic
Pregnancy category: C
Controlled substance: Schedule II

Indications and Dosages
➤ *To relieve acute or chronic moderate to severe pain; as adjunct to treat pulmonary edema caused by left-sided heart failure; to supplement general, local, or regional anesthesia*

CAPSULES, ORAL SOLUTION, SYRUP, TABLETS
Adults. *Initial:* 10 to 30 mg q 4 hr, p.r.n.
Children. Individualized dosage based on patient's age, size, and need.

I.V. INFUSION
Adults. *Initial:* 15 mg (or more) followed by 0.8 to 10 mg/hr, increased as needed for effectiveness. *Maintenance:* 0.8 to 80 mg/hr.
Children. 0.01 to 0.04 mg/kg/hr postoperatively, 0.025 to 2.6 mg/kg/hr for severe chronic cancer pain, or 0.03 to 0.15 mg/kg/hr for sickle cell crisis.
Neonates. *Initial:* 0.010 mg/kg/hr (10 mcg/kg/hr) postoperatively. *Maintenance:* 0.015 to 0.02 mg/kg/hr (15 to 20 mcg/kg/hr).

I.V. INJECTION
Adults. 2.5 to 15 mg injected slowly.
Children. 0.5 to 0.1 mg/kg administered slowly.

I.M. OR S.C. INJECTION
Adults. *Initial:* 10 mg (based on 70-kg [154-lb] adult) q 4 hr. *Maintenance:* 5 to 20 mg.
Children. *Initial:* 0.1 to 0.2 mg/kg q 4 hr. *Maximum:* 15 mg/dose.

EPIDURAL INFUSION (PRESERVATIVE-FREE)
Adults. *Initial:* 2 to 4 mg/24 hr, increased by 1 to 2 mg/24 hr, as directed, to achieve sufficient pain relief.

EPIDURAL INJECTION (PRESERVATIVE-FREE)
Adults. *Initial:* 5 mg into lumbar region. If pain isn't relieved after 1 hr, 1- to 2-mg doses given at appropriate intervals to relieve pain. *Maximum:* 10 mg/24 hr.

INTRATHECAL INJECTION (PRESERVATIVE-FREE)
Adults. 0.2 to 1 mg as a single dose.

SUPPOSITORIES
Adults. 10 to 30 mg q 4 hr, p.r.n.
Children. Individualized dosage based on patient's age, size, and need.

➤ *To relieve chronic moderate to severe pain that requires opioids for more than a few days*

E.R. CAPSULES
Adults. Individualized dosage given q 12 to 24 hr.

E.R. TABLETS
Adults. 30 mg q 12 hr. Dosage increased based on patient's response.

➤ *To relieve MI pain*

I.V. INJECTION
Adults. 1 to 4 mg by slow I.V. injection. Repeated up to q 5 min, if needed. *Maximum:* 2 to 15 mg.

➤ *To provide preoperative analgesia*

I.M. OR S.C. INJECTION
Adults. 5 to 20 mg given 45 to 60 min before surgery.

Children. 0.05 to 0.1 mg/kg given 45 to 60 min before surgery. *Maximum:* 10 mg.

➤ *To provide analgesia during labor*
I.M. OR S.C. INJECTION
Adults. 10 mg, with subsequent doses based on patient's response.

Route	Onset	Peak	Duration
P.O.	Unknown	1 to 2 hr	4 to 5 hr
P.O. (E.R.)	Unknown	Unknown	8 to 12 hr
I.V.	Unknown	20 min	4 to 5 hr
I.M.	10 to 30 min	30 to 60 min	4 to 5 hr
S.C.	10 to 30 min	50 to 90 min	4 to 5 hr
Epidural	15 to 60 min	Unknown	Up to 24 hr
Intrathecal	15 to 60 min	Unknown	Up to 24 hr
P.R.	20 to 60 min	Unknown	Unknown

Mechanism of Action
Binds with and activates opioid receptors (primarily mu receptors) in the brain and spinal cord to produce analgesia and euphoria.

Contraindications
For all drug forms: Asthma, hypersensitivity to morphine or its components, labor (with premature delivery), prematurity (in infants), respiratory depression, upper airway obstruction
For oral solution: Acute abdominal disorders, acute alcoholism, alcohol withdrawal syndrome, arrhythmias, brain tumor, head injuries, heart failure caused by chronic lung disease, increased intracranial or cerebrospinal pressure, recent biliary tract surgery, respiratory insufficiency, seizure disorders, severe CNS depression, surgical anastomosis, use within 14 days of MAO inhibitor therapy
For I.V., I.M., or S.C. injection: Acute alcoholism, alcohol withdrawal syndrome, arrhythmias, brain tumor, heart failure caused by chronic lung disease, seizure disorders
For epidural or intrathecal injection: Anticoagulant therapy, bleeding tendency, injection site infection, parenteral corticosteroid treatment (or other treatment or condition that prohibits drug administration by intrathecal or epidural route) within 2 weeks

Interactions
DRUGS
amitriptyline, clomipramine, nortriptyline: Increased CNS and respiratory depression
anticholinergics: Possibly severe constipation leading to ileus, urine retention
antidiarrheals (such as loperamide and paregoric): CNS depression, possibly severe constipation
antihistamines, chloral hydrate, glutethimide, MAO inhibitors, methocarbamol: Increased CNS and respiratory depressant effects of morphine
antihypertensives, hypotension-producing drugs: Increased hypotension, risk of orthostatic hypotension
buprenorphine: Decreased therapeutic effects of morphine, increased respiratory depression, possibly withdrawal symptoms
cimetidine: Increased analgesic and CNS and respiratory depressant effects of morphine
CNS depressants (antiemetics, general anesthetics, hypnotics, phenothiazines, sedatives, tranquilizers): Possibly coma, hypotension, respiratory depression, severe sedation
diuretics: Decreased diuretic efficacy
hydroxyzine: Increased analgesic, CNS depressant, and hypotensive effects of morphine
metoclopramide: Possibly antagonized metoclopramide effect on GI motility
mixed agonist-antagonist analgesics: Possibly withdrawal symptoms
naloxone: Antagonized analgesic and CNS and respiratory depressant effects of morphine, possibly withdrawal symptoms
naltrexone: Possibly induction or worsening of withdrawal symptoms if morphine given within 7 to 10 days before naltrexone
neuromuscular blockers: Increased or prolonged respiratory depression
opioid analgesics (such as alfentanil and sufentanil): Increased CNS and respiratory depression, increased hypotension
zidovudine: Decreased zidovudine clearance
ACTIVITIES
alcohol use: Increased CNS and respiratory depression, increased hypotension

Adverse Reactions
CNS: Amnesia, anxiety, coma, confusion, decreased concentration, delirium, delusions, depression, dizziness, drowsiness, euphoria, fever, hallucinations, headache, insomnia, lethargy,

light-headedness, malaise, psychosis, restlessness, sedation, seizures, syncope, tremor
CV: Bradycardia, cardiac arrest, hypotension, orthostatic hypotension, palpitations, shock, tachycardia
EENT: Blurred vision, diplopia, dry mouth, laryngeal edema or laryngospasm (allergic), miosis, nystagmus, rhinitis
GI: Abdominal cramps or pain, anorexia, biliary tract spasm, constipation, diarrhea, dysphagia, elevated liver function test results, gastroesophageal reflux, hiccups, ileus and toxic megacolon (in patients with inflammatory bowel disease), intestinal obstruction, indigestion, nausea, vomiting
GU: Decreased ejaculate potency, decreased libido, difficult ejaculation, impotence, prolonged labor, urinary hesitancy, urine retention
HEME: Anemia, leukopenia, thrombocytopenia
MS: Arthralgia
RESP: Apnea, asthma exacerbation, atelectasis, bronchospasm, depressed cough reflex, hypoventilation, pulmonary edema, respiratory arrest and depression, wheezing
SKIN: Diaphoresis, flushing, pallor, pruritus
Other: Allergic reaction; anaphylaxis; facial edema; injection site edema, pain, rash, or redness; physical and psychological dependence; withdrawal symptoms

Nursing Considerations
•Store morphine sulfate at room temperature.
•Before giving morphine, make sure opioid antagonist and equipment for administering oxygen and controlling respiration are available.
•Before therapy begins, assess patient's current drug use, including all prescription and OTC drugs.
•Expect prescriber to start patient who has never received opioids on immediate-release form and then switch to E.R. form if therapy must last longer than a few days.
•Give oral form with food or milk to minimize adverse GI reactions, if needed. If desired, mix oral solution with fruit juice to improve taste.
•If needed, open E.R. capsules and sprinkle contents on applesauce (at room temperature or cooler) just before giving to patient. Make sure patient doesn't chew or crush capsules or dissolve capsule's pellets in his mouth.
•Be aware that E.R. forms of morphine aren't interchangeable.

•Discard injection solution that is discolored or darker than pale yellow or that contains precipitates that don't disappear with shaking.
•**WARNING** Don't use highly concentrated morphine solutions (such as 10 to 25 mg/ml) for single-dose I.V., I.M., or S.C. administration. These solutions are intended for use in continuous, controlled microinfusion devices.
•For direct I.V. injection, dilute appropriate dose with 4 to 5 ml of sterile water for injection. Inject 2.5 to 15 mg directly into tubing of free-flowing I.V. solution over 4 to 5 minutes. Rapid I.V. injection may increase adverse reactions.
•For continuous I.V. infusion, dilute drug in D_5W and administer with infusion-control device. Adjust dose and rate based on patient response, as prescribed.
•Avoid I.M. route for long-term therapy because of injection site irritation.
•During S.C. injection, take care to avoid injecting drug intradermally.
•For intrathecal injection, expect prescriber to give no more than 2 ml of 0.5-mg/ml solution or 1 ml of 1-mg/ml solution. Expect intrathecal dosage to be about one-tenth of epidural dosage.
•If rectal suppository is too soft to insert, chill it in refrigerator for 30 minutes or run wrapped suppository under cold tap water.
•**WARNING** Monitor respiratory and cardiovascular status carefully and frequently during morphine therapy. Be alert for respiratory depression and hypotension.
•Monitor for excessive or persistent sedation; dosage may need to be adjusted.
•Expect morphine to cause physical and psychological dependence; monitor carefully for drug tolerance and withdrawal symptoms, such as body aches, diaphoresis, diarrhea, fever, piloerection, rhinorrhea, sneezing, and yawning.
•If tolerance to morphine develops, expect prescriber to increase dosage.
•Be aware that morphine may have a prolonged duration and cumulative effect in patients with impaired hepatic or renal function. It also may prolong labor by reducing strength, duration, and frequency of uterine contractions.
•When discontinuing morphine in patients receiving more than 30 mg/day, expect prescriber to reduce daily dose by about one-

half for 2 days and then by 25% every 2 days thereafter until total dose reaches initial amount recommended for patients who haven't previously received opioids (15 to 30 mg/day). This regimen minimizes the risk of withdrawal symptoms.

PATIENT TEACHING
•Instruct patient to take morphine exactly as prescribed and not to change dosage without consulting prescriber.
•Inform patient that he may take tablets or capsules with food or milk to relieve GI distress and may mix oral solution with juice to improve taste.
•Urge patient not to break, chew, or crush E.R. capsules and tablets to avoid rapid release and, possibly, toxicity.
•For patient who has difficulty swallowing, suggest that he open E.R. capsules and sprinkle contents on food or liquids. Urge him to take drug immediately and not let capsule contents dissolve in his mouth.
•Instruct patient to moisten rectal suppository before inserting it.
•Urge patient to avoid alcohol and other CNS depressants during morphine therapy.
•Advise patient to avoid potentially hazardous activities during morphine therapy.
•Teach patient to change position slowly to minimize effects of orthostatic hypotension.
•Instruct patient to notify prescriber about worsening or breakthrough pain.
•Inform patient that morphine may be habit-forming. Urge him to notify prescriber if he experiences anxiety, decreased appetite, excessive tearing, irritability, muscle aches or twitching, rapid heart rate, or yawning.
•Advise female patient to notify prescriber if she becomes pregnant. Regular morphine use during pregnancy may cause physical dependence in fetus and withdrawal symptoms in neonate.

moxifloxacin hydrochloride
Avelox, Avelox IV

Class and Category
Chemical: Fluoroquinolone
Therapeutic: Antibiotic
Pregnancy category: C

Indications and Dosages
➤ *To treat acute sinusitis caused by* Haemophilus influenzae, Moraxella catarrhalis, *or* Streptococcus pneumoniae; *to treat mild to moderate community-acquired pneumonia caused by* Chlamydia pneumoniae, H. influenzae, M. catarrhalis, Mycoplasma pneumoniae, *or* S. pneumoniae
TABLETS, I.V. INFUSION
Adults. 400 mg q 24 hr for 10 days.
➤ *To treat acute exacerbation of chronic bronchitis caused by* H. influenzae, H. parainfluenzae, Klebsiella pneumoniae, M. catarrhalis, S. pneumoniae, *or* Staphylococcus aureus
TABLETS, I.V. INFUSION
Adults. 400 mg q 24 hr for 5 days.
➤ *To treat uncomplicated skin and soft-tissue infections caused by* S. aureus *or* Streptococcus pyogenes
TABLETS, I.V. INFUSION
Adults. 400 mg q 24 hr for 7 days.

Mechanism of Action
Inhibits synthesis of the bacterial enzyme DNA gyrase by counteracting the excessive supercoiling of DNA during replication or transcription. Inhibition of DNA gyrase causes rapid- and slow-growing bacterial cells to die.

Incompatibilities
Do not infuse I.V. form simultaneously through the same I.V. line with other I.V. substances, additives, or drugs.

Contraindications
Hypersensitivity to moxifloxacin, other fluoroquinolones, or their components

Interactions
DRUGS
aluminum- or magnesium-containing antacids; drug formulations with divalent or trivalent cations, such as didanosine chewable buffered tablets or powder for oral solution; metal cations, such as iron; multivitamins containing iron or zinc; sucralfate: Possibly substantial interference with moxifloxacin absorption, causing low blood moxifloxacin level
class Ia antiarrhythmics, such as quinidine; class III antiarrhythmics, such as sotalol;

other drugs known to prolong QTc interval, such as disopyramide and pentamidine: Possibly prolonged QTc interval
corticosteroids: Increased risk of Achilles and other tendon ruptures
NSAIDs: Increased risk of CNS stimulation and seizures

Adverse Reactions

CNS: Dizziness, headache, seizures
CV: Hypertension, hypotension, palpitations, peripheral edema, tachycardia, vasodilation
EENT: Altered taste
GI: Abdominal pain, abnormal liver function test results, diarrhea, dyspepsia, nausea, pseudomembranous colitis, vomiting
MS: Tendon inflammation, pain, or rupture
Other: Anaphylaxis, anaphylactic shock

Nursing Considerations

• Obtain a fluid or tissue specimen for culture and sensitivity, as ordered. Expect to begin therapy before results are available.
• **WARNING** Before beginning drug therapy, determine if patient also is receiving a class Ia antiarrhythmic, such as quinidine; a class III antiarrhythmic, such as sotalol; or other drugs known to prolong the QTc interval. Be aware that these drugs should be avoided in patients taking moxifloxacin because they may prolong the QTc interval and lead to life-threatening ventricular tachycardia or torsades de pointes.
• Administer I.V. infusion over 60 minutes with ready-to-use flexible bags that contain 400 mg of moxifloxacin in 250 ml of 0.8% saline. Don't dilute further.
• If administering through Y-type tubing or piggyback method, temporarily discontinue any other solutions during the infusion of moxifloxacin, and flush the line before and after infusion with a compatible solution, such as 0.9% NaCl, 1M NaCl, 5% dextrose, sterile water for injection, 10% dextrose, or lactated Ringer's. Also flush line before and after administering other drugs via the same I.V. line.
• Don't refrigerate I.V. moxifloxacin ready-to-use bags because precipitation will occur. Discard any unused portion; premixed bags are for single-use only.
• Expect to obtain a 12-lead ECG to assess patient for a prolonged QTc interval. Ask patient if he or a blood relative has a history of prolonged QTc interval.
• If patient has hypokalemia, expect to cor-

rect it before beginning moxifloxacin therapy to prevent arrhythmias.
• Determine if patient has a history of a CNS disorder, such as cerebral arteriosclerosis or epilepsy, because drug may lower the seizure threshold. Notify prescriber before beginning therapy if patient has such a history, and institute seizure precautions according to facility policy.
• If profuse, watery diarrhea develops, contact prescriber and expect to obtain a stool specimen to rule out pseudomembranous colitis.
• Monitor serum potassium level, as ordered, during therapy to assess for hypokalemia.
• Keep emergency resuscitation equipment readily available, and observe for evidence of hypersensitivity, such as angioedema, dyspnea, and urticaria. If you suspect anaphylaxis, prepare to give epinephrine, corticosteroids, and diphenhydramine, as prescribed.

PATIENT TEACHING
• Advise patient to notify prescriber immediately if he experiences palpitations or fainting because these symptoms may indicate a serious arrhythmia.
• Teach patient to take drug at least 4 hours before and 8 hours after aluminum- or magnesium-containing antacids, didanosine chewable buffered tablets or oral solution prepared from powder, multivitamins containing iron or zinc, or sulcralfate.
• Caution patient to stop taking drug and notify prescriber immediately if he experiences difficulty breathing, a rash, or other signs of an allergic reaction.
• Advise patient to contact prescriber immediately if he experiences tendon inflammation, pain, or rupture. Also tell him to rest and refrain from exercise if this occurs.
• Caution patient to avoid activities that require mental alertness until adverse CNS effects are known.
• Urge patient to contact prescriber if diarrhea develops.
• Caution patient to complete the prescribed course of therapy even if he feels better.

mycophenolate mofetil

CellCept, CellCept Oral Suspension

mycophenolate mofetil hydrochloride

CellCept Intravenous

Class and Category
Chemical: 2-morpholinoethyl ester of mycophenolic acid
Therapeutic: Immunosuppresant
Pregnancy category: C

Indications and Dosages
➤ *To prevent organ rejection in patients receiving allogenic kidney transplants*
CAPSULES, ORAL SUSPENSION, TABLETS, I.V. INFUSION
Adults. 1 g (over 2 hr for I.V. infusion) b.i.d.
SUSPENSION
Children with body surface area less than 1.25 m². 600 mg/m² b.i.d. *Maximum:* 2 g (10 ml) daily.
CAPSULES
Children with body surface area of 1.25 m² to 1.5 m². 750 mg b.i.d.
CAPSULES, TABLETS
Children with body surface area greater than 1.5 m². 1 g b.i.d.
➤ *To prevent organ rejection in patients receiving allogenic heart transplants*
CAPSULES, ORAL SUSPENSION, TABLETS, I.V. INFUSION
Adults. 1.5 g (over 2 hr for I.V. infusion) b.i.d.
➤ *To prevent organ rejection in patients receiving allogenic liver transplants*
I.V. INFUSION
Adults. 1 g infused over 2 hr b.i.d.
CAPSULES, ORAL SUSPENSION, TABLETS
Adults. 1.5 g b.i.d.

Mechanism of Action
Hydrolyzes to form mycophenolic acid (MPA), which inhibits guanosine nucleotide synthesis and proliferation of T and B lymphocytes. MPA also suppresses antibody formation by B lymphocytes and prevents glycosylation of lymphocyte and monocyte glycoproteins that are involved in intercellular adhesion to endothelial cells. MPA also may inhibit leukocytes from sites of inflammation and graft rejection, which may explain how mycophenolate mofetil prolongs the survival of allogeneic transplants.

Incompatibilities
Don't mix or administer mycophenolate mofetil hydrochloride in the same infusion catheter with other I.V. drugs or admixtures.

Contraindications
Hypersensitivity to mycophenolate mofetil, mycophenolic acid, or any of its components; hypersensitivity to polysorbate 80 (I.V. form only)

Interactions
DRUGS
acyclovir, ganciclovir, probenecid: Increased plasma levels of both drugs
antacids with magnesium and aluminum hydroxides: Decreased absorption of oral mycophenolate mofetil
azathioprine: Increased bone marrow suppression
cholestyramine: Decreased plasma level of mycophenolate mofetil
live vaccines: Decreased effectiveness of live vaccines
oral contraceptives: Possibly decreased effectiveness of oral contraceptives

Adverse Reactions
CNS: Agitation, anxiety, chills, confusion, delirium, depression, dizziness, emotional lability, fever, hallucinations, headache, hypertonia, hypesthesia, insomnia, malaise, nervousness, neuropathy, paresthesia, psychosis, seizure, somnolence, syncope, thinking abnormality, tremor, vertigo
CV: Angina pectoris, arrhythmias, arterial thrombosis, atrial fibrillation or flutter, bradycardia, cardiac arrest, cardiovascular disorder, congestive heart failure, extrasystole, generalized edema, hemorrhage, hypercholesteremia, hyperlipemia, hypertension, hypotension, increased lactic dehydrogenase, increased SGOT and SGPT, increased venous pressure, palpitation, pericardial effusion, peripheral edema, peripheral vascular disorder, postural hypotension, pulmonary edema or hypertension, supraventricular tachycardia, thrombosis, vasodilation, vasospasm, ventricular extrasystole, ventricular tachycardia
EENT: Amblyopia, cataract, conjunctivitis, deafness, dry mouth, ear disorder or pain, epistaxis, eye hemorrhage, gingivitis, gum hyperplasia, lacrimation disorder, mouth ulceration, oral moniliasis, pharyngitis, rhinitis, sinusitis, stomatitis, tinnitus, vision abnormality, voice alteration
ENDO: Cushing's syndrome, diabetes mellitus, hypercalcemia, hypocalcemia, hypoglycemia, hypothyroid, parathyroid disorder

GI: Abdomen enlargement or pain, anorexia, ascites, cholangitis, cholestatic jaundice, constipation, diarrhea, dyspepsia, dysphagia, esophagitis, flatulence, gastritis, gastroenteritis, gastrointestinal hemorrhage, gastrointestinal infection, gastrointestinal moniliasis, hepatitis, hernia, ileus, jaundice, liver damage, liver function test abnormalities, melena, nausea, peritonitis, rectal disorder, stomach ulcer, vomiting

GU: Albuminuria; bilirubinemia; dysuria; hematuria; hydronephrosis; impotence; increased BUN or creatinine levels; kidney tubular necrosis; nocturia; oliguria; pain; prostatic disorder; pyelonephritis; renal failure; scrotal edema, urinary tract disorder or infection; urine abnormality, frequency, incontinence, or retention

HEME: anemia, coagulation disorder, hypochromic anemia, increased prothrombin time or thromboplastin time, leukocytosis, leukopenia, polyhemia, thrombocytopenia

MS: Arthralgia; back, neck or pelvic pain; joint disorder; leg cramps; myalgia; myasthenia; osteoporosis

RESP: Apnea; asthma; atelectasis; bronchitis; cough; dyspnea; hemoptysis; hyperventilation; hypoxia; lung edema; pleural effusion; pneumonia; pneumothorax; respiratory acidosis, moniliasis, neoplasm, or pain; sputum increase

SKIN: Abscess; acne; cellulite; ecchymosis; fungal dermatitis; pallor; petechia; pruritus; rash; benign neoplasm, carcinoma, disorder, hypertrophy, or ulcer; sweating; vesiculobullous rash

Other: Abnormal healing, accidental injury, acidosis, alkalosis, alopecia, cyst, dehydration, facial edema, flulike syndrome, gout, hiccup, hirsutism, hyperkalemia, hyperuricemia, hypervolemia, hypochloremia, hypokalemia, hypomagnesemia, hyponatremia, hypoproteinemia, hypophosphatemia, increased alkaline phosphatase, increased gamma glutamyl transpeptidase, infection, sepsis, thirst, weight gain or loss

Nursing Considerations

• Expect to administer I.V. form of mycophenolate mofetil within 24 hours of transplantation. Don't administer I.V. form longer than 14 days. Expect to switch patient to oral form as soon as possible, as ordered.

• Expect to administer oral form of drug as soon as possible following transplantation.

• When preparing oral suspension or I.V. form, avoid inhalation or direct contact with skin or mucous membranes. If contact occurs, wash area thoroughly with soap and water and rinse eyes with water.

• To prepare oral suspension, tap closed bottle several times to loosen powder and then measure 94 ml of water in a graduated cylinder. Add half of the water to the bottle and shake for about 1 minute. Then add reminder of water and shake again for 1 minute. Remove child-resistant cap and push bottle adapter into neck of bottle. Close bottle tightly with child-resistant cap. Be aware that the suspension bottle may become cold immediately after reconstitution.

• Know that oral suspension can be administered by 8F or larger nasogastric tube.

• When giving oral suspension, don't mix with any other drugs. Ask patient about history of phenylketonuria before initial administration because oral suspension contains aspartame.

• Don't open or crush capsules. If necessary, use the oral suspension.

• Handle I.V. form similarly to a chemotherapeutic drug because mycophenolate mofetil is genotoxic and embryotoxic and may have mutagenic properties.

• Know that I.V. form must be reconstituted and diluted to 6 mg/ml using 5% dextrose injection USP. Inject 14 ml of 5% dextrose injection USP into each vial (two vials will be needed for each 1 g dose; three vials for each 1.5 g dose), then shake gently. Further dilute a 1 g dose by adding two reconstituted vials to 140 ml of 5% dextrose injection USP; dilute a 1.5 g dose by adding three reconstituted vials to 210 ml of 5% dextrose injection USP.

• Be aware that I.V. should be administered within 4 hours of constitution as an infusion over no less than 2 hours. Never administer by rapid or bolus I.V. injection.

• Know that cyclosporine and corticosteroids should be used with mycophenolate mofetil therapy.

• Obtain CBC weekly during first month of therapy, twice monthly for the second and third months of therapy, and then monthly through the first year, as ordered.

• Monitor patient closely for adverse reactions because drug has many adverse effects, some of which can be serious or severe.

•Expect to stop drug or reduce the dose and provide supportive care, as ordered, if neutropenia develops.

PATIENT TEACHING

•Advise women of childbearing age that two forms of contraceptives should be used simultaneously before beginning mycophenolate mofetil therapy and for 6 weeks following discontinuation of therapy because of potential for fetal harm. Inform women who use oral contraceptives that drug may decrease effectiveness of oral contraceptives. Urge patient to notify prescriber immediately if pregnancy occurs.

•Tell patient to take oral form of drug on an empty stomach.

•Instruct patient not to crush tablets or capsules or open capsules.

•Inform patient not to receive live vaccines during therapy. Urge him to avoid people who have received such vaccines or to wear a protective mask when he's around them.

•Caution patient to avoid contact with people who have infections because drug causes immunosuppression.

•Tell patient to report any signs of infection, unexpected bruising or bleeding, or any other sign of bone marrow depression immediately.

•Advise patient to avoid exposure to direct sunlight and UV light and to wear sunscreen when outdoors because of increased risk for skin cancer.

•Advise patient not to take antacids at the same time as oral mycophenolate mofetil because some antacids can decrease drug's absorption.

•Stress importance of follow-up care to monitor the drug's effectiveness and possible adverse effects because of the increased risk for cancer and infections as a result of immunosuppression. Inform patient of the need for periodic laboratory tests.

M

N·O

nabumetone

Relafen

Class and Category

Chemical: Naphthylalkanone derivative
Therapeutic: Anti-inflammatory, antirheumatic
Pregnancy category: C (first trimester), Not rated (later trimesters)

Indications and Dosages

➤ *To relieve symptoms of acute and chronic osteoarthritis and rheumatoid arthritis*

TABLETS

Adult. *Initial:* 1 g/day as a single dose or in divided doses b.i.d., increased to 1.5 to 2 g/day in divided doses b.i.d. *Maintenance:* Adjusted according to clinical response. *Maximum:* 2 g/day.

Mechanism of Action

Blocks activity of cyclooxygenase, the enzyme needed to synthesize prostaglandins, which mediate the inflammatory response and cause local vasodilation, swelling, and pain. Prostaglandins also promote pain transmission from the periphery to the spinal cord. By blocking cyclooxygenase and inhibiting prostaglandins, the NSAID nabumetone reduces inflammatory symptoms and relieves pain.

Contraindications

Angioedema, asthma, bronchospasm, nasal polyps, rhinitis, or urticaria induced by aspirin, iodides, or other NSAIDs

Interactions

DRUGS

acetaminophen (long-term use): Increased risk of adverse renal effects
anticoagulants, thrombolytics: Increased risk of GI bleeding
antihypertensives: Decreased antihypertensive effectiveness
beta blockers: Decreased antihypertensive effects of beta blockers
bone marrow depressants, such as aldesleu-
kin and cisplatin: Increased risk of leukopenia and thrombocytopenia
cefamandole, cefoperazone, cefotetan, plicamycin, valproic acid: Increased risk of hypoprothrombinemia and bleeding
colchicine, other NSAIDs, salicylates: Increased GI irritability and bleeding
cyclosporine, gold compounds, nephrotoxic drugs: Increased risk of nephrotoxicity
digoxin: Increased blood digoxin level and risk of digitalis toxicity
diuretics: Decreased diuretic effectiveness
glucocorticoids, potassium supplements: Increased GI irritability and bleeding
insulin, oral antidiabetic drugs: Increased effectiveness of these drugs; risk of hypoglycemia
lithium: Increased risk of lithium toxicity
methotrexate: Increased risk of methotrexate toxicity
probenecid: Increased risk of nabumetone toxicity

ACTIVITIES

alcohol use: Increased GI irritability and bleeding

Adverse Reactions

CNS: Drowsiness, headache, fatigue, fever, nervousness, vertigo
CV: Edema
EENT: Dry mouth, pharyngitis, stomatitis, tinnitus
GI: Abdominal pain, anorexia, constipation, diarrhea, flatulence, GI bleeding and ulceration, hepatic dysfunction, indigestion, nausea, vomiting
GU: Albuminuria, azotemia, interstitial nephritis, nephrotic syndrome
HEME: Eosinophilia, granulocytopenia, leukopenia, thrombocytopenia
MS: Muscle spasms, myalgia
RESP: Pneumonitis
SKIN: Alopecia, jaundice, photosensitivity, pruritus, rash

Nursing Considerations

• Give nabumetone with food to avoid GI distress.
• **WARNING** Monitor for serious adverse GI reactions, including bleeding, which may occur without warning.
• Monitor BUN and serum creatinine and electrolyte levels for early signs of impaired renal function, especially in elderly patients; patients who take diuretics; and those who have heart failure or renal or hepatic dysfunction.

• Assess for severe hepatic reactions, including jaundice. Stop drug, as prescribed, if symptoms persist.

PATIENT TEACHING

• Instruct patient to take nabumetone with food to reduce GI distress.

• Advise patient to take drug with a full glass of water and to remain upright for 15 to 30 minutes afterward to prevent drug from lodging in the esophagus and causing irritation.

• Caution patient not to increase dosage or frequency of use without consulting prescriber.

• Urge patient to avoid alcohol to reduce risk of GI bleeding.

• Review signs of GI bleeding, such as black or tarry stools, and instruct patient to notify prescriber right away if they occur.

• Inform patient that regular laboratory tests are needed to check for drug toxicity during long-term therapy.

nadolol

Corgard, Syn-Nadolol (CAN)

Class and Category

Chemical: Nonselective beta blocker
Therapeutic: Antianginal, antihypertensive
Pregnancy category: C

Indications and Dosages

➤ *To manage hypertension, alone or with other antihypertensives*

TABLETS

Adults. *Initial:* 40 mg q.d., increased by 40 to 80 mg/day q 7 days, as prescribed. *Maintenance:* 40 to 80 mg/day. *Maximum:* 320 mg/day.

➤ *To manage angina pectoris as long-term therapy*

TABLETS

Adults. *Initial:* 40 mg q.d., increased by 40 to 80 mg/day q 3 to 7 days, as prescribed. *Maintenance:* 40 to 80 mg/day. *Maximum:* 240 mg/day.

DOSAGE ADJUSTMENT Dosage interval possibly increased to q 24 to 36 hr if creatinine clearance is 31 to 50 ml/min/1.73 m^2; to q 24 to 48 hr if it's 10 to 30 ml/min/1.73 m^2; or to q 40 to 60 hr if it's less than 10 ml/min/1.73 m^2.

Route	Onset	Peak	Duration
P.O.	Up to 5 days	4 hr	24 hr

Mechanism of Action

Selectively blocks alpha$_1$ and beta$_2$ receptors in vascular smooth muscle and beta$_1$ receptors in the heart, thereby reducing peripheral vascular resistance and blood pressure. Potent beta blockade decreases cardiac excitability, cardiac output, and myocardial oxygen demand, thus reducing angina. It also prevents reflex tachycardia, which typically occurs with most alpha blockers.

Contraindications

Asthma; bronchospasm; cardiogenic shock; heart failure; hypersensitivity to nadolol, other beta blockers, or their components; second- or third-degree AV block; severe COPD; sinus bradycardia

Interactions

DRUGS

allergen immunotherapy, allergenic extracts for skin testing: Increased risk of serious systemic reactions or anaphylaxis

amiodarone: Increased risk of conduction abnormalities and negative inotropic effects

calcium channel blockers: Increased risk of bradycardia

cimetidine: Possibly increased effects of nadolol

clonidine, guanabenz: Impaired blood pressure control

diazoxide, nitroglycerin: Increased risk of hypotension

estrogens, NSAIDs: Possibly reduced antihypertensive effect of nadolol

general anesthetics: Increased risk of hypotension and myocardial depression

insulin, oral antidiabetic drugs: Possibly increased risk of hyperglycemia and impaired recovery from hypoglycemia, masking of signs of hypoglycemia

lidocaine: Increased risk of lidocaine toxicity

neuromuscular blockers: Possibly prolonged action of these drugs

phenothiazines: Possibly increased blood levels of both drugs

reserpine: Increased risk of bradycardia and hypotension

sympathomimetics with alpha- and beta-adrenergic effects, such as pseudoephedrine:

Possibly hypertension, excessive bradycardia, and heart block
xanthines, such as theophyllines: Possibly decreased therapeutic effects of both drugs

Adverse Reactions
CNS: Anxiety, depression, dizziness, drowsiness, fatigue, headache, paresthesia, syncope, vertigo, weakness, yawning
CV: Bradycardia, chest pain, edema, heart block, heart failure, hypotension, orthostatic hypotension, ventricular arrhythmias
EENT: Nasal congestion, taste perversion
GI: Dyspepsia, elevated liver function test results, hepatic necrosis, hepatitis, nausea, vomiting
GU: Ejaculation failure, impotence
RESP: Cough, dyspnea, wheezing
SKIN: Jaundice, pruritus, scalp tingling

Nursing Complications
• Use nadolol cautiously in patients with diabetes mellitus because it may prolong or worsen hypoglycemia by interfering with glycogenolysis.
• Anticipate that drug may worsen psoriasis and, in patients with myasthenia gravis, muscle weakness and diplopia.
• **WARNING** Withdraw drug gradually over 2 weeks, or as ordered, to avoid MI caused by unopposed beta stimulation or thyroid storm caused by underlying hyperthyroidism. Expect drug to mask tachycardia caused by hyperthyroidism.

PATIENT TEACHING
• Teach patient how to take her radial pulse, and direct her to do so before each dose of nadolol.
• Instruct patient to notify prescriber if pulse rate falls below 60 beats/minute.
• Caution patient not to stop taking drug abruptly or change dosage. Direct her to take a missed dose as soon as possible unless it's within 8 hours of the next scheduled dose.
• Advise patient with diabetes to monitor blood glucose level frequently because nadolol may mask signs of hypoglycemia, such as tachycardia.
• Review signs of impending heart failure, and urge patient to notify prescriber immediately if they occur.

nafarelin acetate
Synarel

Class and Category
Chemical: Decapeptide, gonadotropin-releasing hormone analogue
Therapeutic: Antiendometriotic, gonadal hormone inhibitor
Pregnancy category: X

Indications and Dosages
➤ *To treat endometriosis*
NASAL INHALATION
Adults. 1 spray (200 mcg) into one nostril q morning and 1 spray into other nostril q evening for up to 6 mo. If amenorrhea doesn't occur in 2 mo, dosage increased, as prescribed, to 800 mcg/day in divided doses.
➤ *To treat gonadotropin-dependent precocious puberty*
NASAL INHALATION
Children at puberty. 2 sprays (400 mcg) into each nostril q morning and evening. *Maximum:* 1,800 mcg/day in divided doses t.i.d.

Route	Onset	Peak	Duration
Nasal	60 to 120 days*	20 days†	3 to 6 mo†

Mechanism of Action
Stimulates the release of the gonadotropins luteinizing hormone (LH) and follicle-stimulating hormone (FSH), which temporarily increase ovarian steroidogenesis. Within 1 month, however, repeated administration of nafarelin halts pituitary gland stimulation and decreases LH and FSH secretion. This action decreases the estrogen level, which improves symptoms of endometriosis. In children, repeated nafarelin administration returns LH and FSH to prepubescent levels, stopping development of secondary sex characteristics and slowing bone growth.

Contraindications
Breast-feeding; hypersensitivity to gonadotropin-releasing hormones, gonadotropin-releasing hormone analogues, nafarelin, or their components; pregnancy; undiagnosed vaginal bleeding

Interactions
DRUGS
nasal decongestants: Possibly impaired nafarelin absorption

* For gonadal hormone inhibitor effects, 4 wk
† For antiendometriotic effects.

Adverse Reactions

CNS: Asthenia, depression, fever, headache, mood changes, paresthesia
CV: Chest pain, edema, hot flashes, palpitations
EENT: Eye pain, rhinitis
ENDO: Galactorrhea, gynecomastia, transient increase in pubic hair growth
GU: Hypermenorrhea, hypertrophy of female genitalia, impotence, libido changes, menstrual irregularities, ovarian cysts, uterine bleeding, vaginal dryness, vaginal spotting between menses
MS: Arthralgia, decreased bone density, myalgia
RESP: Dyspnea
SKIN: Acne, hirsutism, rash, seborrhea, skin discoloration (brown)
Other: Body odor

Nursing Considerations

•Be aware that nafarelin isn't recommended for use in breast-feeding women.
•Expect to start treatment for endometriosis between days 2 and 4 of menstrual cycle. Menses should cease after 6 weeks of treatment. Continued menses may indicate lack of compliance.
•Know that bone loss may increase if endometriosis treatment lasts longer than 6 months. Safety of retreatment after 6 months is unknown.
•Avoid giving nasal decongestant within 2 hours after nafarelin administration because it may impair nafarelin absorption.
•Be aware that prescriber will regularly monitor serum hormone levels in patient with gonadotropin-dependent precocious puberty, especially during first 6 to 8 weeks of therapy, to ensure rapid suppression of pituitary function.

PATIENT TEACHING
•Instruct patient to comply with prescriber's instructions for administering nafarelin to obtain desired drug effects.
•Instruct patient to tilt her head back while administering nafarelin to enhance absorption; urge her to try not to sneeze afterward.
•Caution patient not to change dosage without consulting prescriber.
•Counsel patient to notify prescriber if she is or could be pregnant.
•Direct patient not to use nasal decongestant within 2 hours after using nafarelin. If rhinitis occurs, urge her to contact prescriber for instructions.

•Teach patient how to cope with adverse reactions to help maximize compliance.
•Inform patient with endometriosis that drug should cause menses to stop. Urge her to notify prescriber if periods fail to stop even though she's taking drug exactly as prescribed.
•Advise patient with endometriosis to avoid alcohol and tobacco during therapy because they increase bone loss.
•Inform patient with gonadotropin-dependent precocious puberty that signs of puberty will persist during first month of treatment. If they don't resolve within 2 months, advise patient or parents to notify prescriber.
•Inform patient with gonadotropin-dependent precocious puberty that prescriber will assess bone growth velocity and bone age during first 3 to 6 months of therapy.
•Reassure parents of child with precocious puberty that child will resume growing when treatment stops.

nafcillin sodium

Nafcil, Nallpen, Unipen

Class and Category

Chemical: Penicillin
Therapeutic: Antibiotic
Pregnancy category: B

Indications and Dosages

➤ *To treat infections caused by penicillinase-producing* Staphylococcus aureus

CAPSULES, TABLETS
Adults and adolescents. 250 to 1,000 mg q 4 to 6 hr. *Maximum:* 6,000 mg/day.
Children over age 1 month. 6.25 to 12.5 mg/kg q 6 hr.
Neonates. 10 mg/kg q 6 to 8 hr.

I.V. INFUSION
Adults and adolescents. 500 to 1,500 mg q 4 hr. *Maximum:* 20,000 mg/day.
Children from birth to age 12. 10 to 20 mg/kg q 4 hr, or 20 to 40 mg/kg q 8 hr.

I.M. INJECTION
Adults and adolescents. 500 mg q 4 to 6 hr. *Maximum:* 12,000 mg/day.
Children over age 1 month. 25 mg/kg q 12 hr.
Neonates. 10 mg/kg q 12 hr.

➤ *To treat streptococcal pharyngitis*

CAPSULES, TABLETS

Children. 250 mg q 8 hr.

➤ *To treat bone and joint infections, endo-carditis, meningitis, and pericarditis caused by susceptible organisms*

I.V. INFUSION

Adults and adolescents. 1,500 to 2,000 mg q 4 to 6 hr. *Maximum:* 20,000 mg/day.

I.V. INFUSION, I.M. INJECTION

Children from birth to age 12. 10 to 20 mg/kg q 4 hr or 20 to 40 mg/kg q 8 hr. For meningitis in neonates weighing up to 2 kg (4.4 lb), 25 to 50 mg/kg q 12 hr for first week after birth and then 50 mg/kg q 8 hr. For neonates weighing 2 kg or more, 50 mg/kg q 8 hr during first week after birth and then 50 mg/kg q 6 hr.

Mechanism of Action

Binds to certain penicillin-binding proteins inside bacterial cell walls, thereby inhibiting the third and final stage of bacterial cell wall synthesis. The result is cell lysis. Nafcillin's action is bolstered by its chemical composition; its unique side chain resists destruction by beta-lactamases.

Incompatibilities

Don't mix nafcillin in same I.V. bag as aminoglycosides; these drugs are chemically incompatible.

Contraindications

Hypersensitivity to nafcillin, other penicillins, or their components

Interactions

DRUGS

aminoglycosides: Substantial mutual inactivation

chloramphenicol, erythromycins, sulfonamides, tetracyclines: Possibly decreased therapeutic effects of nafcillin

hepatotoxic drugs: Increased risk of hepatotoxicity

methotrexate: Increased risk of methotrexate toxicity

probenecid: Increased blood nafcillin level

FOODS

all foods: Decreased nafcillin absorption

Adverse Reactions

CNS: Depression, headache, seizures

EENT: Oral candidiasis

GI: Abdominal pain, diarrhea, nausea, pseudomembranous colitis, vomiting

GU: Vaginitis

HEME: Leukopenia, neutropenia

SKIN: Exfoliative dermatitis, pruritus, rash, urticaria

Other: Anaphylaxis; hypokalemia; injection site pain, redness, and swelling; serum sickness–like reaction

Nursing Considerations

• Obtain body fluid or tissue samples for culture and sensitivity testing, as prescribed, and obtain test results, if possible, before giving nafcillin, as ordered.

• Give capsules or tablets at least 1 hour before meals or 2 hours afterward.

• For I.M. injection, use only reconstituted solutions from vials. Inject deep into large muscle, preferably upper outer quadrant of gluteus maximus or lateral part of thigh.

• For intermittent I.V. infusion, infuse over 30 to 60 minutes.

• Give nafcillin at least 1 hour before or after aminoglycosides, especially if patient has renal disease.

• When giving drug to patient at risk for hypertension or fluid overload, be aware that each gram of nafcillin contains 2.5 mEq of sodium.

• WARNING Avoid giving nafcillin to premature neonate if drug was reconstituted with bacteriostatic water that contains benzyl alcohol. Doing so can cause a potentially fatal condition characterized by metabolic acidosis and circulatory, CNS, renal, and respiratory dysfunction.

• Monitor for signs of superinfection, such as oral candidiasis and pseudomembranous colitis, especially in elderly, immunocompromised, or debilitated patients who receive large doses of nafcillin.

PATIENT TEACHING

• Instruct patient to take nafcillin capsules or tablets on an empty stomach.

• Urge patient to complete entire prescription, even if she feels better.

• Advise patient to notify prescriber if she experiences chills, fever, GI distress, or rash.

N
O

nalbuphine hydrochloride

Nubain

Class and Category

Chemical: Phenanthrene derivative
Therapeutic: Analgesic, anesthesia adjunct
Pregnancy category: Not rated

Indications and Dosages

➤ *To relieve moderate to severe pain*

I.V., I.M., OR S.C. INJECTION

Adults who weigh 70 kg (154 lb). 10 mg q 3 to 6 hr, p.r.n. Dosage adjusted for patients who weigh more or less.

➤ *As adjunct to anesthesia*

I.V. INJECTION

Adults. 0.3 to 3 mg/kg over 10 to 15 min followed by 0.25 to 0.5 mg/kg, as needed.

DOSAGE ADJUSTMENT For patients who have repeatedly received an opioid agonist, initial dose possibly reduced to 25% of usual dosage. For patients in whom tolerance to drug's effects hasn't developed, maximum usually is 20 mg/dose or 160 mg/day.

Route	Onset	Peak	Duration
I.V.	2 to 3 min	30 min	3 to 4 hr
I.M.	In 15 min	1 hr	3 to 6 hr
S.C.	In 15 min	Unknown	3 to 6 hr

Mechanism of Action

Binds with and stimulates mu and kappa opiate receptors in the spinal cord and higher levels in the CNS. In this way, nalbuphine alters the perception of and emotional response to pain.

Incompatibilities

Don't administer nalbuphine with diazepam or pentobarbital. Use separate I.V. line or flush line well before and after administration.

Contraindications

Hypersensitivity to nalbuphine or its components

Interactions

DRUGS

alfentanil, CNS depressants, fentanyl, sufentanil: Increased risk of hypotension and CNS and respiratory depression
anticholinergics: Increased risk of severe constipation and urine retention
antidiarrheals, such as difenoxin and atropine, loperamide, and paregoric: Increased risk of severe constipation and increased CNS depression
antihypertensives: Increased risk of hypotension
buprenorphine: Possibly decreased therapeutic effects of nalbuphine and increased risk of respiratory depression
hydroxyzine: Increased risk of CNS depression and hypotension
MAO inhibitors: Risk of possibly fatal increased CNS excitation or depression
metoclopramide: Possibly antagonized effects of metoclopramide
naloxone, naltrexone: Decreased pharmacologic effects of nalbuphine
neuromuscular blockers: Increased risk of prolonged CNS and respiratory depression

ACTIVITIES

alcohol use: Increased risk of coma, hypotension, profound sedation, and respiratory depression

Adverse Reactions

CNS: Confusion, depression, dizziness, euphoria, fatigue, hallucinations, headache, nervousness, restlessness, syncope, tiredness, weakness
CV: Hypertension, hypotension, tachycardia
EENT: Blurred vision, diplopia, dry mouth
GI: Abdominal cramps, anorexia, constipation, nausea, vomiting
GU: Decreased urine output, ureteral spasm
RESP: Dyspnea, respiratory depression, wheezing
SKIN: Diaphoresis, flushing, pruritus, rash, sensation of warmth, urticaria
Other: Injection site burning, pain, redness, swelling, and warmth

Nursing Considerations

•Use nalbuphine cautiously in patients taking other drugs that can cause respiratory depression.
•Keep resuscitation equipment and naloxone readily available to reverse nalbuphine's effects, if needed.
•For direct I.V. injection through an I.V. line with a compatible infusing solution, give drug slowly—no more than 10 mg over 3 to 5 minutes. Inject into free-flowing NS, D_5W, or LR solution.
•During prolonged use, expect to give a stool softener to minimize constipation.

•If patient is opioid-dependent, expect drug to cause withdrawal symptoms, such as abdominal cramps, anorexia, anxiety, backache, bone or joint pain, confusion, depression, diaphoresis, dysphoria, erythema, fear, fever, irritability, labile blood pressure and pulse, lacrimation, muscle spasms, myalgia, mydriasis, nasal congestion, nausea, opioid craving, piloerection, restlessness, rhinorrhea, sensation of crawling skin, sleep disturbances, tremor, uneasiness, vomiting, and yawning.
•**WARNING** Be aware that drug may obscure neurologic assessment findings if patient has a cerebral aneurysm, head injury, or increased intracranial pressure.

PATIENT TEACHING
•Advise patient to avoid potentially hazardous activities until nalbuphine's CNS effects are known.
•Counsel patient against making important decisions while receiving drug because it may cloud her judgment.

nalidixic acid

NegGram

Class and Category
Chemical: Naphthyridine derivative quinolone
Therapeutic: Antibiotic
Pregnancy category: Not rated (first trimester), B (later trimesters)

Indications and Dosages
➤ *To treat UTIs caused by gram-negative bacteria, such as most* Enterobacter *sp.,* Escherichia coli, Klebsiella *sp.,* Morganella morganii, Proteus mirabilis, Proteus vulgaris, *and* Providencia rettgeri

ORAL SUSPENSION, TABLETS
Adults and children age 12 and older. *Initial:* 1,000 mg q 6 hr for 1 to 2 wk. *Maintenance:* 500 mg q 6 hr. *Maximum:* 4,000 mg/day.
Children ages 3 months to 12 years. *Initial:* 55 mg/kg/day in divided doses q.i.d. for 1 to 2 wk. *Maintenance:* 33 mg/kg/day in divided doses q.i.d.

Contraindications
Hypersensitivity to nalidixic acid or its components, seizure disorder

Mechanism of Action
Inhibits the enzyme DNA gyrase, which is responsible for the unwinding and supercoiling of bacterial DNA before it replicates. By inhibiting this enzyme, nalidixic acid causes bacterial cells to die.

Interactions
DRUGS
aluminum-, calcium-, and magnesium-containing antacids; iron; multivitamins containing zinc; sucralfate: Possibly interference with nalidixic acid absorption
cyclosporine: Possibly increased blood cyclosporine level
nitrofurantoin: Decreased therapeutic effects of nalidixic acid
oral anticoagulants: Increased anticoagulant effects
theophylline: Possibly increased blood theophylline level
FOODS
caffeine: Decreased clearance and prolonged half-life of caffeine

Adverse Reactions
CNS: Confusion, drowsiness, hallucinations, headache, increased intracranial pressure with bulging fontanels (in infants and children), light-headedness, malaise, paresthesia, psychosis, restlessness, seizures, tremor, weakness
EENT: Altered color perception, blurred vision, diplopia, halo vision, photophobia
GI: Abdominal pain, diarrhea, nausea, pseudomembranous colitis, vomiting
HEME: Eosinophilia, hemolytic anemia, leukopenia, thrombocytopenia
SKIN: Jaundice, photosensitivity, pruritus, rash, Stevens-Johnson syndrome, urticaria
Other: Anaphylaxis, metabolic acidosis

Nursing Considerations
•Be aware that nalidixic acid shouldn't be given to patient with creatinine clearance below 10 ml/min/1.73 m^2 because of the increased risk of drug toxicity.
•Avoid giving drug within 2 hours of giving iron; multivitamin that contains zinc; sucralfate; or antacid that contains aluminum, calcium, or magnesium.
•If patient also takes cyclosporine or theophylline, monitor blood level of these drugs and adjust dosage, as prescribed.

•If patient has a history of seizures or cerebral arteriosclerosis, monitor for seizures during nalidixic acid therapy.

PATIENT TEACHING

•Advise patient to take nalidixic acid with food to avoid GI distress.

•Instruct patient to take a missed dose as soon as she remembers unless it's almost time for the next dose. Caution against double-dosing.

•Encourage patient to drink plenty of fluids during therapy unless directed otherwise by prescriber.

•Instruct patient to finish entire prescription, even if she feels better before it's finished.

•Advise patient to protect skin from sunlight.

•Urge patient to notify prescriber immediately about vision changes or such adverse CNS reactions as confusion, drowsiness, hallucinations, psychosis, and seizures.

nalmefene hydrochloride

Revex

Class and Category

Chemical: 6-Methylene analogue of naltrexone
Therapeutic: Opioid antagonist
Pregnancy category: B

Indications and Dosages

➤ *To treat known or suspected opioid overdose*

I.V. , I.M., OR S.C. INJECTION

Adults. 500 mcg/70 kg (154 lb) followed by second dose of 1,000 mcg/70 kg in 2 to 5 min, as indicated. *Maximum:* 1,500 mcg/70 kg.

➤ *To treat postoperative opioid-induced respiratory depression*

I.V. INJECTION

Adults. *Initial:* 0.25 mcg/kg q 2 to 5 min until desired degree of reversal is achieved. *Maximum:* 1 mcg/kg.

DOSAGE ADJUSTMENT Initial and subsequent doses possibly reduced to 0.1 mcg/kg for patients at increased risk for cardiovascular complications.

Route	Onset	Peak	Duration
I.V.	2 to 5 min	Unknown	30 to 60 min*
I.M., S.C.	5 to 15 min	Unknown	Several hr

Mechanism of Action

Antagonizes mu, kappa, and sigma receptors in the CNS, thus reversing the analgesia, hypotension, respiratory depression, and sedation caused by most opioids. Mu receptors are responsible for analgesia, euphoria, miosis, and respiratory depression. Kappa receptors are responsible for analgesia and sedation. Sigma receptors control dysphoria and other delusional states.

Contraindications

Hypersensitivity to nalmefene or its components

Interactions

DRUGS

opioid analgesics (including alfentanil, fentanyl, and sufentanil): Reversal of these drugs' analgesic and adverse effects, possibly withdrawal symptoms in opioid-dependent patients

Adverse Reactions

CNS: Agitation, chills, confusion, depression, dizziness, fever, hallucinations, headache, nervousness, somnolence, tremor
CV: Arrhythmias, hypertension, hypotension, tachycardia, vasodilation
EENT: Dry mouth, pharyngitis
GI: Diarrhea, nausea, vomiting
GU: Urine retention
SKIN: Pruritus
Other: Withdrawal symptoms

Nursing Considerations

•Use nalmefene cautiously in patients with hepatic or renal dysfunction because drug is metabolized by liver and excreted by kidneys.

•Also use drug cautiously in patients who have received a cardiotoxic drug and in those at increased risk for cardiovascular complications.

---

* For partial reversal of opioid effects; up to several hr for full reversal.

•**WARNING** Monitor for withdrawal symptoms, especially when giving nalmefene to opioid-dependent patient. Symptoms may include abdominal cramps, anorexia, anxiety, back-ache, bone or joint pain, confusion, depression, diaphoresis, dysphoria, erythema, fear, fever, irritability, labile blood pressure and pulse, lacrimation, muscle spasms, myalgia, mydriasis, nasal congestion, nausea, opioid craving, piloerection, restlessness, rhinorrhea, sensation of crawling skin, sleep disturbances, tremor, uneasiness, vomiting, and yawning.
•Be prepared to provide mechanical or assisted ventilation if reversal of opioid-induced respiratory depression is incomplete.

PATIENT TEACHING
•Urge opioid-dependent patient to seek drug rehabilitation.

naloxone hydrochloride

Narcan

Class and Category
Chemical: Thebaine derivative
Therapeutic: Opioid antagonist
Pregnancy category: B

Indications and Dosages
➤ *To treat known or suspected opioid overdose*
I.V. INJECTION
Adults and children age 5 and older who weigh more than 20 kg (44 lb). 0.4 to 2 mg repeated q 2 to 3 min, p.r.n. If no response after 10 mg, patient may not have narcotic-induced respiratory depression.
Infants and children under age 5. 0.01 mg/kg as a single dose; if no improvement, another 0.1 mg/kg, as prescribed. Alternatively, 0.1 mg/kg repeated q 2 to 3 min, as needed
I.V., I.M., OR S.C. INJECTION
Neonates. 0.01 mg/kg repeated I.V. q 2 to 3 min, as prescribed, until desired response occurs. Alternatively, initial I.V. dose of 0.1 mg/kg.
➤ *To treat postoperative opioid-induced respiratory depression*
I.V. INJECTION
Adults and adolescents. *Initial:* 0.1 to 0.2 mg q 2 to 3 min until desired response occurs. Additional doses given q 1 to 2 hr, if needed, based on patient response.

Children. *Initial:* 0.005 to 0.01 mg q 2 to 3 min until desired response occurs. Additional doses given q 1 to 2 hr, if needed, based on patient response.
➤ *To reverse opioid-induced asphyxia*
I.V., I.M., OR S.C. INJECTION
Neonates. *Initial:* 0.01 mg/kg q 2 to 3 min until desired response occurs. Additional doses given q 1 to 2 hr, if needed, based on patient response.
➤ *As adjunct to treat hypotension caused by septic shock*
I.V. INFUSION OR INJECTION
Adults. 0.03 to 0.2 mg/kg over 5 min followed by continuous infusion of 0.03 to 0.3 mg/kg/hr for 1 to 24 hr, as needed, based on patient response.

Route	Onset	Peak	Duration
I.V.	1 to 2 min	5 to 15 min	45 min or longer
I.M., S.C.	2 to 5 min	5 to 15 min	45 min or longer

Mechanism of Action
Briefly and competitively antagonizes mu, kappa, and sigma receptors in the CNS, thus reversing the analgesia, hypotension, respiratory depression, and sedation caused by most opioids. Mu receptors are responsible for analgesia, euphoria, miosis, and respiratory depression. Kappa receptors are responsible for analgesia and sedation. Sigma receptors control dysphoria and other delusional states.

Incompatibilities
Don't mix naloxone with any other solution unless you verify that drugs are compatible; drug is incompatible with alkaline, bisulfite, and metabisulfite solutions.

Contraindications
Hypersensitivity to naloxone or its components

Interactions
DRUGS
butorphanol, nalbuphine, pentazocine: Reversal of these drugs' analgesic and adverse effects

opioid analgesics: Reversal of these drugs' analgesic and adverse effects, possibly withdrawal symptoms in opioid-dependent patients

Adverse Reactions

CNS: Excitement, irritability, nervousness, restlessness, seizures, tremor, violent behavior
CV: Hypertension (severe), hypotension, ventricular fibrillation, ventricular tachycardia
GI: Nausea, vomiting
RESP: Pulmonary edema
SKIN: Diaphoresis
Other: Withdrawal symptoms

Nursing Considerations

• Keep resuscitation equipment readily available during naloxone administration.
• Administer drug by I.V. route whenever possible.
• Give repeat doses as prescribed, depending on patient's response.
• Anticipate that rapid reversal of opioid effects can cause diaphoresis, nausea, and vomiting.
• WARNING Monitor for withdrawal symptoms, especially when giving naloxone to opioid-dependent patient. Symptoms may include abdominal cramps, anorexia, anxiety, backache, bone or joint pain, confusion, depression, diaphoresis, dysphoria, erythema, fear, fever, irritability, labile blood pressure and pulse, lacrimation, muscle spasms, myalgia, mydriasis, nasal congestion, nausea, opioid craving, piloerection, restlessness, rhinorrhea, sensation of crawling skin, sleep disturbances, tremor, uneasiness, vomiting, and yawning.
• Expect patient with hepatic or renal dysfunction to have increased circulating blood naloxone level.

PATIENT TEACHING
• Inform patient or family that naloxone will reverse opioid-induced adverse reactions.
• Urge opioid-dependent patient to seek drug rehabilitation.

naltrexone hydrochloride

ReVia

Class and Category

Chemical: Thebaine derivative
Therapeutic: Opioid antagonist
Pregnancy category: C

Indications and Dosages

➤ *To treat opioid dependence*

TABLETS

Adults. *Initial:* 25 mg, repeated within 1 hr, if needed and if no withdrawal symptoms occur. *Maintenance:* 50 to 150 mg q.d. or 350 mg/wk by intermittent dosing regimen.

➤ *As adjunct to treat alcoholism*

TABLETS

Adults. 50 mg q.d. (up to 100 mg/day for some patients) for 12 wk.

Route	Onset	Peak	Duration
P.O.	15 to 30 min	In 12 hr	24 hr*

Mechanism of Action

Displaces opioid agonists from—or blocks them from binding with—mu, kappa, and delta receptors. Opioid receptor blockade reverses the euphoric effect of opioids. Naltrexone also inhibits the effects of endogenous opioids, thus reducing alcohol craving.

Contraindications

Acute hepatitis, acute opioid withdrawal, concurrent use of opioid analgesics (including opiate agonists, such as methadone or levo-alpha-acetyl-methadol [LAAM]), hepatic failure, hypersensitivity to naltrexone or its components, opioid dependence

Interactions

DRUGS

opioid analgesics: Reversal of the analgesic and adverse effects of these drugs, possibly withdrawal symptoms in opioid-dependent patients
thioridazine: Increased somnolence and lethargy

Adverse Reactions

CNS: Anxiety, chills, confusion, depression, dizziness, fatigue, fever, hallucinations, headache, insomnia, irritability, nervousness, restlessness
CV: Chest pain, edema, hypertension, tachycardia
EENT: Blurred vision, burning eyes, eyelid swelling, hoarseness, pharyngitis, rhinitis, sneezing, tinnitus
GI: Abdominal cramps, anorexia, constipation, diarrhea, GI ulceration, nausea, thirst, vomiting

---

* For 50 mg; 48 hr for 100 mg; 72 hr for 150 mg.

GU: Difficult ejaculation, urinary frequency
MS: Arthralgia, myalgia
RESP: Cough, dyspnea
SKIN: Pruritus, rash

Nursing Considerations
• To avoid withdrawal symptoms, wait 7 to 10 days after last opioid dose, as prescribed, before starting patient on naltrexone.
• Give drug with food or antacids to decrease adverse GI reactions.
• Anticipate that some patients may require treatment for up to 1 year.

PATIENT TEACHING
• **WARNING** Caution patient against taking opioids during naltrexone therapy or in the future because she'll be more sensitive to them. In fact, strongly warn patient that taking large doses of heroin or any other opioid (including methadone or LAAM) while taking naltrexone could lead to coma, serious injury, or death.
• Urge patient to undergo comprehensive rehabilitation in addition to receiving naltrexone.
• Inform patient about nonopioid treatments for cough, diarrhea, and pain.
• Instruct patient to carry medical identification that lists naltrexone therapy.

nandrolone decanoate

Deca-Durabolin, Hybolin Decanoate, Kabolin

Class, Category, and Schedule
Chemical: Testosterone derivative
Therapeutic: Antianemic
Pregnancy category: X
Controlled substance: Schedule III

Indications and Dosages
➤ *To manage anemia caused by chronic renal failure*

I.M. INJECTION
Adults and adolescents age 14 and older. 50 to 100 mg q 1 to 4 wk for females; 50 to 200 mg q 1 to 4 wk for males.
Children ages 2 to 13. 25 to 50 mg q 3 to 4 wk.

Mechanism of Action
Increases the production of erythropoietin, a precursor of RBCs. Nandrolone also increases the hemoglobin level and RBC volume.

Contraindications
Breast cancer in females with hypercalcemia; breast or prostate cancer in males; hypersensitivity to nandrolone, anabolic steroids, or their components; known or suspected pregnancy; nephrosis; nephrotic phase of nephritis; severe hepatic dysfunction

Interactions
DRUGS
corticosteroids: Increased risk of edema and severe acne
hepatotoxic drugs: Increased risk of hepatotoxicity
insulin, oral antidiabetic drugs: Possibly hypoglycemia
NSAIDs, oral anticoagulants, salicylates: Increased anticoagulant effects
sodium-containing drugs: Increased risk of edema
somatrem, somatropin: Possibly accelerated epiphyseal maturation

FOODS
sodium-containing foods: Increased risk of edema

Adverse Reactions
CNS: Excitement, depression, insomnia
CV: Edema, hyperlipidemia
ENDO: Feminization in postpubertal males (epididymitis, gynecomastia, impotence, oligospermia, priapism, testicular atrophy); glucose intolerance; virilism in females (acne, clitoral enlargement, decreased breast size, deepened voice, diaphoresis, emotional lability, flushing, hirsutism, hoarseness, libido changes, male-pattern baldness, menstrual irregularities, nervousness, oily hair or skin, vaginitis, weight gain); virilism in prepubertal males (acne, decreased ejaculatory volume, epididymitis, penis enlargement, prepubertal closure of epiphyseal plates, priapism, unnatural growth of body and facial hair)
GI: Diarrhea, elevated liver function test results, hepatocellular carcinoma, nausea, vomiting
GU: Urinary frequency
HEME: Unusual bleeding
SKIN: Jaundice
Other: Injection site induration and pain, physical and psychological dependence

Nursing Considerations
• Provide adequate calories and protein, as ordered, to maintain a positive nitrogen bal-

ance. Also provide adequate iron intake to ensure optimal response to nandrolone.
•Weigh patient daily to detect fluid retention, which can lead to edema. If patient retains fluid, expect to place her on sodium-restricted diet or diuretic therapy, as ordered.
•Assess boys under age 7 for secondary sexual characteristics, and notify prescriber if they develop.
•Assess for signs of virilism, and notify prescriber if they develop.
•Monitor diabetic patient for decreased blood glucose control, and notify prescriber if hyperglycemia develops.
•Be aware that some patients use nandrolone to improve athletic performance and that long-term use may lead to abuse and addiction. Expect nandrolone abuse to cause such adverse reactions as antisocial behavior, cardiovascular complications, hepatotoxicity, and libido changes.
•If no improvement occurs after 6 months, expect prescriber to discontinue nandrolone.
PATIENT TEACHING
•Review signs of virilism with patient, and urge her to notify prescriber if such signs develop. Inform her that some signs may be permanent.
•To prevent vaginitis, advise female patient to wash after intercourse and to wear only cotton underwear.
•Instruct patient to notify prescriber immediately about menstrual changes.
•Advise patient to notify prescriber about sudden weight gain—a sign of edema, which may cause significant problems in patients with cardiac or renal disorders.
•Inform adolescent males that they may need to undergo semen evaluation every 3 to 4 months.
•Instruct diabetic patient to monitor blood glucose level frequently and to watch for signs of hyperglycemia; urge her to notify prescriber of significant changes.

naproxen

Apo-Naproxen (CAN), EC-Naprosyn, Naprosyn, Naprosyn-E (CAN), Naxen (CAN), Novo-Naprox (CAN), Nu-Naprox (CAN)

naproxen sodium

Aleve, Anaprox, Anaprox DS, Apo-Napro-Na (CAN), Naprelan, Naprosyn-SR (CAN), Novo-Naprox Sodium (CAN)

Class and Category
Chemical: Propionic acid derivative
Therapeutic: Analgesic, anti-inflammatory, antipyretic
Pregnancy category: B (first trimester), Not rated (later trimesters)

Indications and Dosages
➤ *To relieve mild to moderate musculoskeletal inflammation, including ankylosing spondylitis, osteoarthritis, and rheumatoid arthritis*
DELAYED-RELEASE TABLETS, ORAL SUSPENSION, TABLETS (NAPROXEN)
Adults. 250 to 500 mg b.i.d. *Maximum:* 1,500 mg/day for limited periods, as prescribed.
E.R. TABLETS (NAPROXEN SODIUM)
Adults. 750 to 1,000 mg q.d. *Maximum:* 1,500 mg/day.
TABLETS (NAPROXEN SODIUM)
Adults. 275 to 550 mg b.i.d. *Maximum:* 1,650 mg/day for limited periods, as prescribed.
SUPPOSITORIES (NAPROXEN SODIUM)
Adults. 500 mg h.s. in addition to daytime P.O. administration. *Maximum:* 1,500 mg/day (P.O. and suppository combined).
➤ *To relieve symptoms of juvenile rheumatoid arthritis and other inflammatory conditions in children*
ORAL SUSPENSION, TABLETS (NAPROXEN)
Children. 10 mg/kg/day in divided doses b.i.d.
➤ *To relieve symptoms of acute gouty arthritis*
DELAYED-RELEASE TABLETS, ORAL SUSPENSION, TABLETS (NAPROXEN)
Adults. *Initial:* 750 mg, then 250 mg q 8 hr until symptoms subside.
E.R. TABLETS (NAPROXEN SODIUM)
Adults. *Initial:* 1,000 to 1,500 mg on day 1, then 1,000 mg q.d. until symptoms subside. *Maximum:* 1,500 mg/day.
TABLETS (NAPROXEN SODIUM)
Adults. *Initial:* 825 mg, then 275 mg q 8 hr until symptoms subside.
➤ *To relieve mild to moderate pain, including acute tendinitis and bursitis, arthralgia, dysmenorrhea, and myalgia*
DELAYED-RELEASE TABLETS (NAPROXEN)
Adults. *Initial:* 1,000 mg q.d. *Maximum:* 1,500 mg/day.
E.R. TABLETS (NAPROXEN SODIUM)
Adults. *Initial:* 1,100 mg q.d., increased as prescribed. *Maximum:* 1,500 mg/day.

ORAL SUSPENSION, TABLETS (NAPROXEN)
Adults. *Initial:* 500 mg, then 250 mg q 6 to 8 hr, p.r.n. *Maximum:* 1,250 mg/day.
TABLETS (NAPROXEN SODIUM)
Adults. *Initial:* 550 mg, then 275 mg q 6 to 8 hr, p.r.n. *Maximum:* 1,375 mg/day.
➤ *To relieve fever, mild to moderate musculoskeletal inflammation, mild to moderate pain*
TABLETS (OTC NAPROXEN SODIUM)
Adults. 220 mg q 8 to 12 hr, or 440 mg followed by 220 mg 12 hr later. *Maximum:* 660 mg/day for 10 days unless prescriber directs otherwise.
DOSAGE ADJUSTMENT For patients over age 65, dosage reduced to 220 mg q 12 hr. *Maximum:* 440 mg for 10 days unless prescriber directs otherwise.

Route	Onset	Peak	Duration
P.O. (naproxen)*	1 hr†	2 to 4 hr†‡	7 to 12 hr†
P.O. (naproxen sodium)*	30 min†	1 hr†‡	7 to 12 hr†

Mechanism of Action
Blocks the activity of cyclooxygenase, the enzyme needed to synthesize prostaglandins, which mediate the inflammatory response and cause local vasodilation, swelling, and pain. By blocking cyclooxygenase and inhibiting prostaglandins, this NSAID reduces symptoms of inflammation and relieves pain. Naproxen's antipyretic action probably stems from its effect on the hypothalamus, which increases peripheral blood flow, causing vasodilation and heat dissipation.

Contraindications
Angioedema, asthma, bronchospasm, nasal polyps, rhinitis, or urticaria induced by aspirin, iodides, or other NSAIDs

Interactions
DRUGS
acetaminophen: Increased risk of adverse

---

* For antirheumatism, onset is in 14 days, peak is unknown, and duration is 2 to 4 wk.
† For analgesia.
‡ For gout, 1 to 2 days.

renal effects with long-term use of acetaminophen and naproxen
anticoagulants, thrombolytics: Prolonged PT, increased risk of bleeding
antihypertensives: Decreased effectiveness of antihypertensive
beta blockers: Decreased antihypertensive effects of these drugs
bone marrow depressants, such as aldesleukin and cisplatin: Increased risk of leukopenia and thrombocytopenia
cefamandole, cefoperazone, cefotetan, plicamycin, valproic acid: Increased risk of hypoprothrombinemia and bleeding
cimetidine: Altered blood naproxen level
colchicine, glucocorticoids, other NSAIDs, potassium supplements, salicylates: Increased GI irritability and bleeding
cyclosporine, gold compounds, nephrotoxic drugs: Increased risk of nephrotoxicity
digoxin: Increased blood digoxin level and risk of digitalis toxicity
diuretics: Decreased diuretic effectiveness
insulin, oral antidiabetic drugs: Increased effectiveness of these drugs; risk of hypoglycemia
lithium: Increased risk of lithium toxicity
methotrexate: Increased risk of methotrexate toxicity
phenytoin: Increased blood phenytoin level
probenecid: Increased risk of naproxen toxicity
ACTIVITIES
alcohol use, smoking: Increased risk of naproxen-induced GI ulceration

Adverse Reactions
CNS: Aseptic meningitis, depression, dizziness, dream disturbances, drowsiness, fever, headache, inability to concentrate, insomnia, light-headedness, malaise, vertigo
CV: Edema, heart failure, hypertension, palpitations, vasculitis
EENT: Stomatitis, tinnitus, vision changes
ENDO: Hyperglycemia, hypoglycemia
GI: Abdominal pain, anorexia, constipation, diarrhea, elevated liver function test results, flatulence, GI bleeding and perforation, heartburn, hematemesis, indigestion, melena, nausea, pancreatitis, thirst, vomiting
GU: Glomerulonephritis, hematuria, interstitial nephritis, menstrual irregularities, nephrotic syndrome, renal failure, renal papillary necrosis
HEME: Agranulocytosis, aplastic anemia, eosinophilia, granulocytopenia, hemolytic anemia, leukopenia, thrombocytopenia

MS: Muscle weakness, myalgia
RESP: Dyspnea, eosinophilic pneumonitis
SKIN: Alopecia, diaphoresis, ecchymosis, jaundice, photosensitivity, pruritus, purpura, rash, Stevens-Johnson syndrome, urticaria
Other: Anaphylaxis, angioedema, hyperkalemia

Nursing Considerations

•Because of naproxen's sodium content, monitor for hypertension and fluid retention.
•WARNING Anticipate increased risk of serious adverse GI reactions, such as bleeding, perforation, and ulceration, during long-term naproxen therapy. These reactions may occur at any time and without warning.
•Assess for signs of drug effectiveness in patients with ankylosing spondylitis: decreased night pain, morning stiffness, and pain at rest in affected joints.
•Assess for signs of drug effectiveness in patients with osteoarthritis: decreased joint pain or tenderness and increased mobility, range of motion, and ability to perform activities of daily living.
•Assess for signs of drug effectiveness in patients with rheumatoid arthritis: increased mobility and decreased joint swelling and morning stiffness.
•Assess for signs of drug effectiveness in patients with acute gouty arthritis: decreased heat, pain, swelling, and tenderness in affected joints.

PATIENT TEACHING

•Instruct patient to swallow delayed-release naproxen tablets whole and not to break, crush, or chew them.
•Advise patient to take drug with food to reduce GI distress.
•Instruct patient to take drug with a full glass of water and to remain upright for 15 to 30 minutes afterward to prevent drug from lodging in esophagus and causing irritation.
•Caution patient to avoid potentially hazardous activities until drug's CNS effects are known.
•Advise patient to notify prescriber immediately about dark stools, persistent abdominal pain, rash, or worsening symptoms.
•Encourage patient to keep scheduled appointments with prescriber to monitor progress.

naratriptan hydrochloride

Amerge

Class and Category

Chemical: Selective serotonin 5-HT receptor agonist
Therapeutic: Antimigraine
Pregnancy category: C

Indications and Dosages

➤ *To relieve acute migraine with or without aura*

TABLETS

Adults. 1 to 2.5 mg as a single dose, repeated in 4 hr p.r.n. if only partial relief obtained. *Maximum:* 5 mg/day.
DOSAGE ADJUSTMENT For patients with mild to moderate renal or hepatic impairment, maximum dosage reduced to 2.5 mg/day.

> ### Mechanism of Action
>
> Binds to receptors on intracranial blood vessels and sensory nerves in the trigeminal-vascular system to stimulate negative feedback, which halts the release of serotonin. In this way, naratriptan selectively constricts inflamed and dilated cranial vessels in the carotid circulation and inhibits the production of proinflammatory neuropeptides.

Contraindications

Basilar or hemiplegic migraine; cerebrovascular, peripheral vascular, or coronary artery disease (ischemic or vasospastic); hypersensitivity to naratriptan or its components; hypertension (uncontrolled); severe hepatic or renal dysfunction; use within 24 hours of another 5-HT agonist or an ergotamine-containing or ergot-type drug, such as dihydroergotamine or methysergide

Interactions

DRUGS

ergot-containing drugs: Possibly prolonged or additive vasospastic reactions
fluoxetine, fluvoxamine, paroxetine, sertraline: Possibly weakness, hyperreflexia, and incoordination
oral contraceptives: Possibly reduced clearance and increased blood level of naratriptan
other selective serotonin 5-HT receptor ago-

nists (including rizatriptan, sumatriptan, and zolmitriptan): Possibly additive effects

Adverse Reactions
CNS: Dizziness, drowsiness, fatigue, malaise, paresthesia
CV: Chest pain, pressure, or heaviness
EENT: Decreased salivation, otitis media, pharyngitis, photophobia, rhinitis, throat tightness
GI: Nausea, vomiting

Nursing Considerations
•**WARNING** Because naratriptan therapy can cause coronary artery vasospasm, monitor patient with coronary artery disease for signs or symptoms of angina while taking drug. Because naratriptan may also cause peripheral vasospastic reactions, such as ischemic bowel disease, monitor patient for abdominal pain and bloody diarrhea.
•Monitor patient for hypertension during naratriptan therapy. Drug may increase systolic blood pressure by as much as 32 mm Hg.
•Be prepared to perform a complete neurovascular assessment in any patient who reports an unusual headache or who fails to respond to first dose of naratriptan.
PATIENT TEACHING
•Inform patient that naratriptan is used to treat acute migraine attacks and that it won't prevent or reduce the number of migraines.
•Advise patient not to take more than maximum prescribed dosage during any 24-hour period.
•If patient experiences no relief from initial dose of naratriptan, instruct her to notify prescriber rather than taking another dose in 4 hours because she may need a different drug.
•Advise patient to seek reevaluation by prescriber if she experiences more than four headaches during any 30-day period while taking naratriptan.

nateglinide

Starlix

Class and Category
Chemical: Amino acid derivative
Therapeutic: Antidiabetic
Pregnancy category: C

Indications and Dosages
➤ *To control blood glucose level in type 2 diabetes mellitus as monotherapy or in combination with metformin*
TABLETS
Adults. 120 mg t.i.d. 1 to 30 min a.c.
DOSAGE ADJUSTMENT Dosage reduced to 60 mg t.i.d. in patients with near-goal glycosylated hemoglobin (HbA$_{1c}$) level.

Route	Onset	Peak	Duration
P.O.	20 min	1 hr	4 hr

Contraindications
Diabetic ketoacidosis, hypersensitivity to nateglinide or its components, type 1 diabetes mellitus

Interactions
DRUGS
corticosteroids, sympathomimetics, thiazide diuretics, thyroid products: Possibly reduced hypoglycemic effects of nateglinide
MAO inhibitors, nonselective beta-adrenergic blockers, NSAIDs, salicylates: Possibly additive hypoglycemic effects of nateglinide

Adverse Reactions
CNS: Dizziness
ENDO: Hypoglycemia
GI: Diarrhea
MS: Accidental trauma, arthropathy, back pain
RESP: Bronchitis, cough, upper respiratory tract infection
Other: Flulike symptoms

Nursing Considerations
•Administer nateglinide 1 to 30 minutes before meals to reduce the risk of hypoglycemia.
•Monitor fasting glucose and HbA$_{1c}$ levels periodically, as ordered, to evaluate treatment effectiveness.
•Monitor patient frequently in event of fever, infection, trauma, or surgery because transient loss of glucose control may occur, requiring an alteration in therapy.
PATIENT TEACHING
•Instruct patient to take nateglinide 1 to 30 minutes before meals. Advise her to skip scheduled dose if she skips a meal to reduce the risk of hypoglycemia.
•Teach patient how to measure blood glucose level and recognize signs of hyperglycemia

N
O

Mechanism of Action

Nateglinide stimulates the release of insulin from functioning beta cells of the pancreas. In patients with type 2 diabetes mellitus, a lack of functioning beta cells diminishes blood levels of insulin and causes glucose intolerance. By interacting with the adenosine triphosphatase (ATP)–potassium channel on the beta cell membrane, nateglinide prevents potassium (K^+) from leaving the cell. This causes the beta cell to depolarize and the cell membrane's calcium channel to open. Consequently, calcium (Ca^{++}) moves into the cell and insulin moves out of it. The extent of insulin release is glucose dependent; the lower the glucose level, the less insulin is secreted from the cell.

By promoting insulin secretion in patients with type 2 diabetes mellitus, nateglinide improves glucose tolerance.

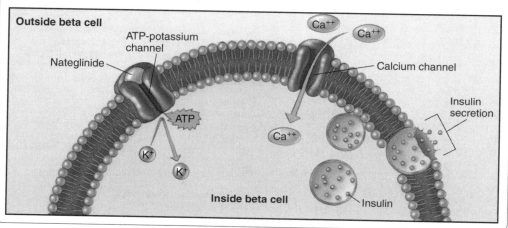

and hypoglycemia. Advise her to notify prescriber if blood glucose level is abnormal.
•Inform patient that strenuous physical exercise, insufficient caloric intake, and use of alcoholic beverages may increase the risk of hypoglycemia.
•Advise patient to monitor blood glucose levels as prescribed and to maintain follow-up appointments to monitor HbA_{1c} level because drug may become less effective over time.

nedocromil sodium

Tilade

Class and Category

Chemical: Pyranoquinoline dicarboxylic acid derivative
Therapeutic: Antiasthmatic, anti-inflammatory
Pregnancy category: B

Indications and Dosages

➤ *To control mild to moderate chronic asthma*

ORAL INHALATION

Adults and children age 6 and older. 2 inhalations (3.5 mg) q.i.d. Dosage frequency possibly reduced to b.i.d. or t.i.d. once desired response occurs.

Route	Onset	Peak	Duration
Inhalation	2 to 4 wk	Unknown	6 to 12 hr

Contraindications

Hypersensitivity to nedocromil or its components

Adverse Reactions

CNS: Dizziness, fatigue, headache (possibly severe), tremor
CV: Chest pain
EENT: Dry mouth, hoarseness, pharyngitis, rhinitis, taste perversion

GI: Abdominal pain, diarrhea, elevated liver function test results, indigestion, nausea, vomiting
HEME: Leukopenia, neutropenia
MS: Arthritis
RESP: Bronchospasm, cough, upper respiratory tract infection
SKIN: Rash, sensation of warmth

Mechanism of Action

Inhibits the activation and release of inflammatory mediators—such as histamine, leukotrienes, and prostaglandins—in the lumen and mucosa of the bronchi and bronchioles. As a result, nedocromil inhibits allergen-induced early and late asthmatic reactions when administered directly to the bronchial mucosa. The drug also may inhibit axon reflexes and release sensory neuropeptides in the lungs. This action:
• suppresses bradykinin-induced bronchoconstriction
• decreases localized tissue edema and mucus secretion
• mobilizes anti-inflammatory cells.

Nursing Considerations

• Be aware that nedocromil may be used alone or with other drugs, such as bronchodilators and corticosteroids.
• Avoid using nedocromil to reverse acute bronchospasm because drug doesn't have bronchodilator effects.
• Continue nedocromil therapy during acute exacerbations unless patient becomes intolerant of inhaled form. Intolerance is characterized by bronchospasm, cough, and wheezing.
• **WARNING** Monitor for life-threatening bronchospasm immediately after administration. If it occurs, notify prescriber and expect to discontinue nedocromil therapy and start a different drug.

PATIENT TEACHING
• Advise patient to store nedocromil at room temperature and to shake it before use.
• Instruct patient to prime drug canister with three sprays before first use and after more than 7 days of disuse.
• If patient has trouble coordinating inhalation with each spray, suggest using a spacer.
• Urge patient to take drug regularly, even when she has no symptoms.

• Inform patient that drug's full effect may not occur for 1 or more weeks after therapy starts.
• If patient uses other inhalers, instruct her to use bronchodilator first and wait 5 minutes before using nedocromil.
• Caution patient not to spray nedocromil into eyes.
• Instruct patient to wash mouthpiece after each use and not to use nedocromil mouthpiece with other aerosol drugs.
• Advise patient to gargle or rinse mouth after inhalation to relieve dry mouth, hoarseness, throat irritation, and unpleasant taste.
• Instruct patient to discard canister after 104 metered sprays.
• Urge patient to notify prescriber if symptoms worsen or fail to improve; caution against increasing the number of inhalations without consulting prescriber.

nefazodone hydrochloride

Serzone

Class and Category

Chemical: Phenylpiperazine derivative
Therapeutic: Antidepressant
Pregnancy category: C

Indications and Dosages

➤ *To treat major depression*

TABLETS
Adults. *Initial:* 100 mg b.i.d., increased by 100 to 200 mg/day q wk, as prescribed. *Maintenance:* 150 to 300 mg b.i.d. *Maximum:* 600 mg/day.
DOSAGE ADJUSTMENT Initial dosage possibly reduced to 50 mg b.i.d. for elderly or debilitated patients; then dosage adjusted as ordered, based on patient response.

Route	Onset	Peak	Duration
P.O.	Several wk	Unknown	Unknown

Mechanism of Action

Believed to inhibit serotonin reuptake at presynaptic neurons, which may increase the neuronal level of serotonin, an inhibitory neurotransmitter that is thought to regulate mood. Nefazodone also may act as a postsynaptic serotonin receptor antagonist, further increasing the amount of synaptic serotonin that's available.

Contraindications

Concurrent use of astemizole, cisapride, or terfenadine; hypersensitivity to nefazodone, other phenylpiperazine antidepressants, or their components; restarting nefazodone therapy that was discontinued because of liver injury; use within 14 days of MAO inhibitor therapy

Interactions

DRUGS

alprazolam, buspirone, carbamazepine, cyclosporine, modafinil, triazolam: Increased blood levels of these drugs

antihypertensives: Increased risk of hypotension

astemizole, cisapride, terfenadine: Increased blood levels of these drugs, prolonged QT interval, and, possibly, serious cardiovascular effects, including death from ventricular tachycardia

cilostazol: Decreased cilostazol clearance, increased adverse effects of cilostazol, such as headache

dextromethorphan, sibutramine, tramadol, trazodone: Increased risk of serotonin syndrome

digoxin: Increased blood digoxin level, increased risk of digitalis toxicity

haloperidol: Decreased haloperidol clearance

indinavir: Inhibited indinavir metabolism

levobupivacaine: Increased blood levobupivacaine level, possibly toxicity

lovastatin, simvastatin: Increased risk of rhabdomyolysis and myositis

MAO inhibitors: Possibly fatal reactions, including autonomic instability (with rapidly fluctuating vital signs), hyperthermia, mental status changes (such as severe agitation progressing to delirium and coma), muscle rigidity, and myoclonus

methadone: Increased blood level and adverse effects of methadone, additive CNS effects

nevirapine: Increased nefazodone metabolism, inhibited nevirapine metabolism

ritonavir: Inhibited nefazodone and ritonavir metabolism

sildenafil: Decreased sildenafil clearance

tacrolimus: Decreased tacrolimus clearance and increased adverse effects, including delirium and renal failure

ACTIVITIES

alcohol use: Increased risk of CNS depression

Adverse Reactions

CNS: Abnormal gait, apathy, asthenia, ataxia, chills, confusion, decreased concentration, delusions, depersonalization, dizziness, dream disturbances, euphoria, fever, hallucinations, headache, hostility, hypotonia, insomnia, light-headedness, malaise, memory loss, myoclonic jerks, neuralgia, paranoia, paresthesia, somnolence, suicidal ideation, syncope, tremor, vertigo

CV: Angina, hypertension, hypotension, peripheral edema, orthostatic hypotension, tachycardia, vasodilation, ventricular arrhythmias

EENT: Abnormal vision, blurred vision, conjunctivitis, diplopia, dry eyes and mouth, earache, epistaxis, eye pain, gingivitis, halitosis, hyperacusis, laryngitis, mydriasis, neck rigidity, periodontal abscess, pharyngitis, photophobia, stomatitis, taste perversion, tinnitus, visual field defects

ENDO: Breast pain, gynecomastia, lymphadenopathy

GI: Abdominal distention, colitis, constipation, diarrhea, elevated liver function test results, eructation, esophagitis, gastritis, gastroenteritis, hernia, hepatotoxicity, hiccups, increased appetite, indigestion, life-threatening hepatic failure, nausea, peptic ulcer, rectal bleeding, thirst, vomiting

GU: Abnormal ejaculation; amenorrhea; cystitis; hematuria; hypermenorrhea; impotence; libido changes; nocturia; pelvic pain; polyuria; renal calculi; urinary frequency, incontinence, or urgency; urine retention; UTI; vaginal bleeding; vaginitis

HEME: Anemia, leukopenia

MS: Arthralgia, arthritis, bursitis, dysarthria, gout, muscle stiffness, tenosynovitis

RESP: Asthma, bronchitis, cough, dyspnea, pneumonia

SKIN: Acne, alopecia, dry skin, ecchymosis, eczema, maculopapular rash, photosensitivity, pruritus, rash, urticaria

Other: Allergic reaction, dehydration, infection, serotonin syndrome, weight loss

Nursing Considerations

•WARNING Be aware that nefazodone should not be given with astemizole, cisapride, MAO inhibitors, or terfenadine; serious, even fatal, reactions may occur.

•WARNING Be aware that life-threatening hepatic failure has occurred during nefazodone therapy, resulting in need for transplant or even death. Monitor patient for signs of hepatic failure, such as jaundice, malaise, and elevated liver function test results.

• Follow facility policy during initial nefazodone therapy if patient is at high risk for suicide.
• Assess for signs of serotonin syndrome, such as abdominal cramps, aggressive behavior, agitation, chills, diarrhea, headache, insomnia, lack of coordination, nausea, palpitations, paresthesia, poor concentration, and worsening of obsessive thoughts.

PATIENT TEACHING
• Instruct patient to take nefazodone exactly as prescribed and not to alter dosage.
• Urge patient to immediately report signs of hepatic failure, such as jaundice, darkened urine, lack of appetite, nausea, or abdominal pain.
• Inform patient that antidepressant effects may not occur for several weeks and that treatment may last 6 months or longer.
• Caution patient to avoid alcohol during nefazodone therapy.
• Advise patient to avoid potentially hazardous activities until drug's CNS effects are known.
• Suggest that patient try sugarless gum or hard candy for dry mouth. Urge her to notify prescriber if dry mouth persists.

neomycin sulfate

Mycifradin, Neo-Fradin

Class and Category
Chemical: Aminoglycoside
Therapeutic: Antibiotic
Pregnancy category: D

Indications and Dosages
➤ *To suppress intestinal bacterial growth in preoperative bowel preparation*

TABLETS (24-HR REGIMEN)
Adults. 1 g q hr for 4 doses and then 1 g q 4 hr for remainder of 24 hr before surgery. Alternatively, for 8 a.m. surgery, 1 g of neomycin with erythromycin at 1 p.m., 2 p.m., and 11 p.m. the day before surgery.
Children. 25 mg/kg at 1 p.m., 2 p.m., and 11 p.m. the day before surgery.

TABLETS (2- TO 3-DAY REGIMEN)
Adults and children. 88 mg/kg q 4 hr in 6 equally divided doses for 2 to 3 days before surgery.

➤ *As adjunct to treat hepatic encephalopathy*

TABLETS
Adults. 4 to 12 g/day in divided doses q 6 hr for 5 to 6 days.
Children. 50 to 100 mg/kg/day in divided doses q 6 hr for 5 to 6 days.

➤ *To treat infectious diarrhea caused by enteropathic* Escherichia coli

TABLETS
Adults and children. 50 mg/kg/day in divided doses q.i.d. for 2 to 3 days.

Mechanism of Action
Is transported into bacterial cells, where it competes with messenger RNA to bind with a specific receptor protein on the 30S ribosomal subunit of DNA. This action causes abnormal, nonfunctioning proteins to form. A lack of functional proteins causes bacterial cell death.

Contraindications
Hypersensitivity or serious reaction to neomycin, other aminoglycosides, or their components; inflammatory or ulcerative GI disease; intestinal obstruction

Interactions
DRUGS
digoxin, spironolactone: Possibly reduced absorption rate of these drugs
dimenhydrinate: Possibly masked symptoms of neomycin-induced ototoxicity
methotrexate: Possibly decreased absorption and bioavailability of methotrexate
neuromuscular blockers: Potentiated neuromuscular blockade, increased risk of prolonged respiratory depression
oral anticoagulants: Possibly potentiated anticoagulant effects

Adverse Reactions
EENT: Ototoxicity
GI: Diarrhea, malabsorption syndrome (decreased serum carotene level and xylose absorption, increased fecal fat and flatulence), nausea, pseudomembranous colitis, vomiting
GU: Nephrotoxicity

Nursing Considerations
• Monitor BUN and serum creatinine levels to assess renal function before and during neomycin therapy. Expect to decrease dosage or discontinue drug, as ordered, if nephrotoxicity develops.
• Monitor blood neomycin level, as directed, to assess for therapeutic range of 5 to 10 mcg/ml.

•**WARNING** Be aware that neomycin is highly ototoxic and may cause hearing loss and tinnitus.
•Monitor for signs of pseudomembranous colitis, such as severe abdominal cramps and severe, watery diarrhea.
•Anticipate that neomycin's curare-like effect may worsen muscle weakness in patients with neuromuscular disorders, such as myasthenia gravis and parkinsonism.

PATIENT TEACHING
•Urge patient to complete the full course of neomycin therapy.
•Unless contraindicated, encourage patient to drink plenty of fluids to help prevent nephrotoxicity.
•Urge patient undergoing bowel preparation to comply with recommended regimen, including low-residue diet, bisacodyl enema administration, and neomycin use.
•Advise patient to notify prescriber about hearing loss or ringing in ears.

neostigmine bromide

Prostigmin

neostigmine methylsulfate

Prostigmin

Class and Category

Chemical: Quaternary ammonium compound
Therapeutic: Anticholinesterase, curare antidote
Pregnancy category: C

Indications and Dosages

➤ *To treat symptoms of myasthenia gravis*
TABLETS (NEOSTIGMINE BROMIDE)
Adults. *Initial:* 15 mg q 3 to 4 hr. Dosage adjusted based on clinical response. *Maintenance:* 150 mg/day in divided doses based on clinical response.
Children. 2 mg/kg/day in 6 to 8 divided doses.
I.M. OR S.C. INJECTION (NEOSTIGMINE METHYLSULFATE)
Adults. *Initial:* 0.5 mg. Dosage adjusted based on clinical response.
Children. 0.01 to 0.04 mg/kg q 2 to 3 hr.

➤ *To reverse nondepolarizing neuromuscular blockade*
I.V. INJECTION (NEOSTIGMINE METHYLSULFATE)
Adults. 0.5 to 2 mg by slow push, repeated as needed up to 5 mg; 0.6 to 1.2 mg of atropine or

0.2 to 0.6 mg of glycopyrrolate is given with or a few minutes before neostigmine, as ordered.
Children. 0.04 mg/kg by slow push; 0.02 mg of atropine/kg is given I.M. or S.C. with each dose or alternate doses.

➤ *To prevent postoperative, nonobstructive urine retention and abdominal distention (adynamic ileus)*
I.M. OR S.C. INJECTION (NEOSTIGMINE METHYLSULFATE)
Adults. 0.25 mg immediately after surgery and repeated q 4 to 6 hr for 2 to 3 days.

➤ *To treat postoperative, nonobstructive urine retention and abdominal distention (adynamic ileus)*
I.M. OR S.C. INJECTION (NEOSTIGMINE METHYLSULFATE)
Adults. 0.5 mg; injections repeated q 3 hr for at least 5 doses if patient has voided or bladder has emptied within 1 hr.

Route	Onset	Peak	Duration
P.O.	45 to 75 min*	Unknown	3 to 6 hr
I.V.	4 to 8 min†	30 min	2 to 4 hr
I.M.	20 to 30 min†	30 min	2 to 4 hr

Mechanism of Action

Inhibits the action of cholinesterase, an enzyme that destroys acetylcholine at myoneuronal junctions, thereby increasing acetylcholine accumulation at myoneuronal junctions and facilitating nerve impulse transmission across the junctions. This action:
•helps prevent or relieve urine retention by increasing detrusor muscle tone in the bladder and causing bladder contractions strong enough to induce urination
•prevents or treats postoperative abdominal distention by increasing gastric motility and tone
•improves muscle strength and increases muscle response to repetitive nerve stimulation in myasthenia gravis.

Contraindications

Hypersensitivity to neostigmine, other anticholinesterases, bromides, or their components; mechanical obstruction of intestinal or urinary tract; peritonitis

---

* For adynamic ileus, 2 to 4 hr.
† For adynamic ileus, 10 to 30 min.

Interactions

DRUGS

aminoglycosides, anesthetics, capreomycin, colistimethate, colistin, lidocaine, lincomycins, polymyxin B, quinine: Increased risk of neuromuscular blockade

anticholinergics: Possibly masked signs of cholinergic crisis

guanadrel, guanethidine, mecamylamine, trimethaphan: Possibly antagonized effects of neostigmine, possibly decreased antihypertensive effects

neuromuscular blockers: Possibly prolonged action of depolarizing—and antagonized action of nondepolarizing—neuromuscular blockers

procainamide, quinidine: Possibly antagonized effects of neostigmine

quinine: Decreased neostigmine effectiveness

Adverse Reactions

CNS: Dizziness, drowsiness, headache, seizures, syncope, weakness

CV: Arrhythmias (AV block, bradycardia, nodal rhythm, tachycardia), cardiac arrest, ECG changes, hypotension

EENT: Increased salivation, lacrimation, miosis, vision changes

GI: Abdominal cramps, diarrhea, flatulence, increased peristalsis, nausea, vomiting

GU: Urinary frequency

MS: Arthralgia, dysarthria, muscle spasms

RESP: Bronchospasm, dyspnea, increased bronchial secretions, respiratory arrest or depression

SKIN: Flushing, diaphoresis, rash, urticaria

Nursing Considerations

•Be aware that 15 mg of oral neostigmine bromide is equivalent to 0.5 mg of parenteral neostigmine methylsulfate.

•If also giving atropine, be sure to administer it before neostigmine, as prescribed.

•When giving neostigmine I.V., make sure patient is well ventilated and airway remains patent until normal respiration is assured.

•If patient has myasthenia gravis, give drug night and day, as ordered, with larger portions of daily dose during periods of increased fatigue. If patient's condition becomes refractory to neostigmine, expect to reduce dosage or discontinue drug, as prescribed, for a few days.

•**WARNING** Monitor for signs of neostigmine overdose, which can cause possibly fatal cholinergic crisis (increased muscle weakness,

including respiratory muscles). Expect to stop neostigmine and atropine, as ordered.

PATIENT TEACHING

•Instruct patient to take neostigmine exactly as prescribed.

•Advise patient to take drug with food or milk to reduce adverse GI reactions.

•Suggest that patient with myasthenia gravis keep a daily record of doses and adverse reactions during therapy.

•Instruct patient to schedule activities to minimize fatigue.

nesiritide

Natrecor

Class and Category

Chemical: Human B-type natriuretic peptide
Therapeutic: Arterial and venous smooth muscle cell relaxant
Pregnancy category: C

Indications and Dosages

➤ *To reduce dyspnea at rest or with minimal activity in patients with acute decompensated congestive heart failure*

I.V. INFUSION, I.V. INJECTION

Adults. 2-mcg/kg bolus followed by continuous infusion of 0.01 mcg/kg/min for up to 48 hr.

Route	Onset	Peak	Duration
I.V.	In 15 min	1 hr	3 hr

N
O

Mechanism of Action

Binds to the guanylate cyclase receptor of vascular smooth muscle and endothelial cells. This action increases intracellular levels of cyclic guanosine monophosphate, which leads to arterial and venous smooth muscle cell relaxation. Ultimately, nesiritide reduces pulmonary capillary wedge pressure and systemic arterial pressure in patients with congestive heart failure, which decreases the heart's workload and subsequently relieves dyspnea.

Incompatibilities

Don't infuse nesiritide through same I.V. line as bumetanide, enalaprilat, ethacrynate sodium, furosemide, heparin, hydralazine, or insulin because these drugs are chemically and physically incompatible with nesiritide. Don't infuse drugs that contain the preservative sodium metabisulfite through same I.V. line as nesiritide.

Contraindications

Hypersensitivity to nesiritide or its components; primary therapy for cardiogenic shock; systolic blood pressure less of than 90 mm Hg

Interactions
DRUGS
ACE inhibitors: Increased risk of symptomatic hypotension

Adverse Reactions

CNS: Anxiety, dizziness, headache, insomnia
CV: Angina, bradycardia, hypotension, PVCs, ventricular tachycardia
GI: Abdominal pain, nausea, vomiting
GU: Elevated serum creatinine level
MS: Back pain

Nursing Considerations

•**WARNING** Be aware that nesiritide isn't recommended for patients suspected to have low cardiac filling pressures or patients for whom vasodilating drugs aren't appropriate, such as those with constrictive pericarditis, pericardial tamponade, restrictive or obstructive cardiomyopathy, significant valvular stenosis, or other conditions in which cardiac output depends on venous return.
•Reconstitute 1.5-mg vial by adding 5 ml of diluent removed from a 250-ml plastic I.V. bag containing preservative-free D_5W, NS, $D_5.45NS$, or $D_5.2NS$.
•Don't shake vial. Rock it gently so that all surfaces, including the stopper, are in contact with the diluent to ensure complete reconstitution. Inspect drug for particulate matter and discoloration; if present, discard drug.
•Withdraw entire contents of the reconstituted solution and add it to the same 250-ml plastic I.V. bag used to withdraw the diluent to yield a solution of about 6 mcg/ml. Invert the I.V. bag several times to ensure complete mixing.
•After preparing the infusion bag, withdraw the bolus volume from the infusion bag and administer it over about 60 seconds. Immediately after the bolus, infuse drug at 0.1 ml/kg/hr, which will deliver 0.01 mcg/kg/min.

•Prime I.V. tubing with 25 ml of solution before connecting to the I.V. line and before administering the bolus dose or starting the infusion.
•Flush the I.V. line between doses of nesiritide and incompatible drugs.
•Because nesiritide binds to heparin and therefore could bind to the heparin lining of a heparin-coated catheter, don't give it through a central heparin-coated catheter.
•Store reconstituted vials at room temperature (20° to 25° C [68° to 77° F]) or refrigerate (2° to 8° C [36° to 46° F]) for up to 24 hours.
•Because nesiritide contains no antimicrobial preservatives, discard the reconstituted solution after 24 hours.
•Monitor blood pressure and heart rate and rhythm frequently during therapy.
•If hypotension occurs, notify prescriber and expect to reduce dosage or discontinued the drug. Implement measures to support blood pressure as prescribed.
•Assess patient's breath sounds and respiratory rate, rhythm, depth, and quality frequently during drug therapy.
•Monitor serum creatinine level during drug therapy and notify prescriber of abnormal results.
•Store unopened drug at controlled room temperature or refrigerate. Keep in carton until time of use.
PATIENT TEACHING
•Instruct patient to notify you or another nurse if she becomes dizzy because this may indicate hypotension.
•Reassure patient that her blood pressure, heart rate, and breathing will be monitored frequently.

netilmicin sulfate

Netromycin

Class and Category
Chemical: Aminoglycoside
Therapeutic: Antibiotic
Pregnancy category: D

Indications and Dosages

➤ *To treat serious systemic infections, such as intra-abdominal infections, lower respiratory tract infections, septicemia, and skin and soft-tissue infections, caused by* Enterobacter aerogenes, Escherichia coli, Klebsiella pneumoniae, Proteus mirabilis, Pseudomonas aeruginosa, Serratia *sp., and* Staphylococcus aureus

I.V. INFUSION, I.M. INJECTION
Adults and children age 12 and older. 1.3 to 2.2 mg/kg q 8 hr or 2 to 3.25 mg/kg q 12 hr for 7 to 14 days. *Maximum:* 7.5 mg/kg/day.
Children ages 6 weeks to 12 years. 1.8 to 2.7 mg/kg q 8 hr or 2.7 to 4 mg/kg q 12 hr for 7 to 14 days.
Infants up to age 6 weeks. 2 to 3.25 mg/kg q 12 hr for 7 to 14 days.

➤ *To treat complicated UTIs caused by* Citrobacter *sp.,* Enterobacter *sp.,* E. coli, K. pneumoniae, P. mirabilis, P. aeruginosa, Serratia *sp., and* Staphylococcus *sp.*

I.V. INFUSION, I.M. INJECTION
Adults and adolescents. 1.5 to 2 mg/kg q 12 hr for 7 to 14 days. *Maximum:* 7.5 mg/kg/day.

> ### Mechanism of Action
> Is transported into bacterial cells, where it competes with messenger RNA to bind with a specific receptor protein on the 30S ribosomal subunit of DNA. This action causes abnormal, nonfunctioning proteins to form. A lack of functional proteins causes bacterial cell death.

Incompatibilities
Don't mix netilmicin with beta-lactam antibiotics (penicillins and cephalosporins) because substantial mutual inactivation may result. If prescribed concurrently, administer these drugs at separate sites.

Contraindications
Hypersensitivity to netilmicin, other aminoglycosides, or their components

Interactions
DRUGS
capreomycin, other aminoglycosides: Increased risk of nephrotoxicity, neuromuscular blockade, and ototoxicity
cephalosporins, nephrotoxic drugs: Increased risk of nephrotoxicity
loop diuretics, ototoxic drugs: Increased risk of ototoxicity
methoxyflurane, polymyxins (parenteral): Increased risk of nephrotoxicity and neuromuscular blockade
neuromuscular blockers: Increased neuromuscular blockade

Adverse Reactions
CNS: Disorientation, dizziness, encephalopathy, headache, myasthenia gravis-like syndrome, neuromuscular blockade (acute muscle paralysis and apnea), paresthesia, peripheral neuropathy, seizures, vertigo, weakness
CV: Hypotension, palpitations
EENT: Blurred vision, hearing loss, nystagmus, tinnitus
GI: Diarrhea, elevated liver function tests results, nausea, vomiting
GU: Elevated BUN and serum creatinine levels, nephrotoxicity, oliguria, proteinuria
HEME: Anemia, eosinophilia, leukopenia, prolonged PT, thrombocytopenia, thrombocytosis
MS: Muscle twitching
RESP: Apnea
SKIN: Allergic dermatitis, erythema, pruritus, rash
Other: Angioedema; hyperkalemia; injection site hematoma, induration, and pain

Nursing Considerations
•To prepare netilmicin for I.V. use, dilute each dose in 50 to 200 ml of suitable diluent, such as NS, D_5W, or LR solution, and administer slowly over 30 to 60 minutes.
•Ensure adequate hydration during therapy to maintain adequate renal function.
•Monitor blood netilmicin level; optimum peak level is 6 to 10 mcg/ml and trough level is 0.5 to 2 mcg/ml.
•Check BUN and serum creatinine levels, urine specific gravity, and creatinine clearance during netilmicin therapy, as ordered.
•Anticipate higher risk of nephrotoxicity in elderly patients, those with impaired renal function, and those who receive high doses or prolonged netilmicin therapy.
•Reduce dosage or discontinue drug, as ordered, if signs of drug-induced auditory or vestibular toxicity develop; the damage may be permanent.

PATIENT TEACHING
•Encourage patient to drink plenty of fluids during netilmicin therapy.
•Instruct patient to notify prescriber immediately about dizziness, hearing loss, muscle twitching, nausea, numbness and tingling, ringing or buzzing in ears, seizures, significant changes in amount of urine or frequency of urination, and vomiting.
•Urge patient to keep follow-up appointments to monitor progress.

N O

nicardipine hydrochloride
Cardene, Cardene SR

Class and Category
Chemical: Dihydropyridine derivative
Therapeutic: Antianginal, antihypertensive
Pregnancy category: C

Indications and Dosages
➤ *To manage angina pectoris and Prinz-metal's angina, to manage hypertension*
CAPSULES
Adults and adolescents. 20 to 40 mg t.i.d., increased q 3 days, as prescribed.
E.R. CAPSULES
Adults. 30 mg b.i.d.
I.V. INFUSION
Adults. 0.5 to 2.2 mg/hr by continuous infusion.
➤ *To control acute hypertension*
I.V. INFUSION
Adults. *Initial:* 5 mg/hr by continuous infusion; increased by 2.5 mg/hr q 5 to 15 min, as prescribed. *Maximum:* 15 mg/hr.

Route	Onset	Peak	Duration
P.O.	20 min	1 to 2 hr	Unknown
P.O. (E.R.)	20 min	1 to 2 hr	12 hr
I.V.	Immediate	Unknown	Unknown

Mechanism of Action
May slow extracellular calcium movement into myocardial and vascular smooth-muscle cells by deforming calcium channels in cell membranes, inhibiting ion-controlled gating mechanisms, and interfering with calcium release from the sarcoplasmic reticulum. By decreasing the intracellular calcium level, nicardipine inhibits smooth-muscle cell contraction and dilates coronary and systemic arteries. As with other calcium channel blockers, these actions lead to decreased myocardial oxygen requirements and reduced peripheral resistance, blood pressure, and afterload.

Incompatibilities
Don't mix nicardipine with sodium bicarbonate or LR solution, and don't administer through same I.V. line.

Contraindications
Advanced aortic stenosis, hypersensitivity to any calcium channel blocker, second- or third-degree AV block in patient without artificial pacemaker

Interactions
DRUGS
anesthetics (hydrocarbon inhalation): Possibly hypotension
beta blockers, other antihypertensives, prazocin: Increased risk of hypotension
calcium supplements: Possibly impaired action of nicardipine
cimetidine: Increased nicardipine bioavailability
digoxin: Transiently increased blood digoxin level, increased risk of digitalis toxicity
disopyramide, flecainide: Increased risk of bradycardia, conduction defects, and heart failure
estrogens: Possibly increased fluid retention and decreased therapeutic effects of nicardipine
lithium: Increased risk of neurotoxicity
NSAIDs, sympathomimetics: Possibly decreased therapeutic effects of nicardipine
procainamide, quinidine: Possibly prolonged QT interval
FOODS
grapefruit, grapefruit juice: Possibly increased bioavailability of nicardipine
high-fat meals: Decreased blood nicardipine level
ACTIVITIES
alcohol use: Increased hypotensive effect

Adverse Reactions
CNS: Anxiety, asthenia, ataxia, confusion, dizziness, drowsiness, headache, nervousness, paresthesia, psychiatric disturbance, syncope, tremor, weakness
CV: Arrhythmias (bradycardia, tachycardia), chest pain, heart failure, hypotension, orthostatic hypotension, palpitations, peripheral edema
EENT: Altered taste, blurred vision, dry mouth, epistaxis, gingival hyperplasia, pharyngitis, rhinitis, tinnitus
ENDO: Gynecomastia, hyperglycemia
GI: Anorexia, constipation, diarrhea, elevated liver function test results, indigestion, nausea, thirst, vomiting

GU: Dysuria, nocturia, polyuria, sexual dysfunction, urinary frequency
HEME: Anemia, leukopenia, thrombocytopenia
MS: Joint stiffness, muscle spasms
RESP: Bronchitis, cough, upper respiratory tract infection
SKIN: Dermatitis, diaphoresis, erythema multiforme, flushing, photosensitivity, pruritus, rash, Stevens-Johnson syndrome, urticaria
Other: Hypokalemia, weight gain

Nursing Considerations
• Check blood pressure and pulse rate before nicardipine therapy begins, during dosage changes, and periodically throughout therapy. During prolonged therapy, periodically assess ECG tracings for arrhythmias and other changes.
• Dilute each 25-mg ampule of nicardipine with 240 ml of solution to yield 0.1 mg/ml. Mixture is stable at room temperature for 24 hours.
• Administer continuous infusion by I.V. pump or controller, and adjust according to patient's blood pressure, as prescribed.
• Change peripheral I.V. site every 12 hours, if feasible.
• Give first dose of oral nicardipine 1 hour before stopping I.V. infusion, as prescribed.
• Monitor fluid intake and output and daily weight for signs of fluid retention, which may precipitate heart failure. Also assess for signs of heart failure, such as crackles, dyspnea, jugular vein distention, peripheral edema, and weight gain.
• During prolonged therapy, periodically monitor liver and renal function test results. Expect elevated liver function test results to return to normal after drug is discontinued.
• Monitor serum potassium level during prolonged therapy. Hypokalemia increases the risk of arrhythmias.
• Because of drug's negative inotropic effect on some patients, closely monitor patients who take a beta blocker or have heart failure or significant left ventricular dysfunction.
• **WARNING** Expect to taper dosage gradually before discontinuing drug. Otherwise, angina or dangerously high blood pressure could result.
PATIENT TEACHING
• Urge patient to take nicardipine as prescribed, even if she feels well.
• Instruct patient to swallow E.R. capsules whole, not to chew, crush, cut, or open them.

• Advise patient not to take drug within 1 hour of eating a high-fat meal or grapefruit product. Urge her not to alter the amount of grapefruit products in her diet without consulting prescriber.
• **WARNING** Caution patient against stopping nicardipine abruptly because angina or dangerously high blood pressure could result.
• Teach patient how to take her pulse, and urge her to notify prescriber immediately if it falls below 50 beats/minute.
• Teach patient how to measure her blood pressure, and advise her to do so weekly if nicardipine was prescribed for hypertension. Suggest that she keep a log of blood pressure readings to take to follow-up visits.
• Advise patient to change position slowly to minimize effects of orthostatic hypotension.
• Urge patient to avoid potentially hazardous activities until drug's CNS effects are known.
• Advise patient to notify prescriber immediately about chest pain that's not relieved by rest or nitroglycerin, constipation, irregular heartbeats, nausea, pronounced dizziness, severe or persistent headache, and swelling of hands or feet.
• Encourage patient to comply with suggested lifestyle changes, such as alcohol moderation, low-sodium or low-fat diet, regular exercise, smoking cessation, stress management, and weight reduction.
• Inform patient that saunas, hot tubs, and prolonged hot showers may cause dizziness or fainting.
• Instruct patient to avoid prolonged sun exposure and to use sunscreen when going outdoors.

niclosamide
Niclocide

Class and Category
Chemical: Salicylanilide derivative
Therapeutic: Anthelmintic
Pregnancy category: B

Indications and Dosages
➤ *To treat beef* (Taenia saginata), *fish* (Diphyllobothrium latum), *or pork* (Taenia solium) *tapeworm infestations*

CHEWABLE TABLETS

Adults. 2 g as a single dose; repeated in 7 days, if needed. *Maximum:* 2 g/day.
Children who weigh more than 34 kg (75 lb). 1.5 g as a single dose; repeated in 7 days, if needed. *Maximum:* 2 g/day.
Children who weigh 11 (24 lb) to 34 kg. 1 g as a single dose; repeated in 7 days, if needed. *Maximum:* 2 g/day.
➤ To treat dwarf tapeworm (Hymenolepsis nana) *infestations*
CHEWABLE TABLETS
Adults. 2 g/day for 7 days; repeated in 7 to 14 days, if needed.
Children who weigh more than 34 kg. 1.5 g on day 1 and then 1 g/day for the next 6 days; repeated in 7 to 14 days, if needed. *Maximum:* 2 g/day.
Children who weigh 11 to 34 kg. 1 g on day 1 and then 500 mg/day for the next 6 days; repeated in 7 to 14 days, if needed. *Maximum:* 2 g/day.

Mechanism of Action

May alter anaerobic energy production in tapeworms by inhibiting oxidative phosphorylation in their mitochondria, which decreases the synthesis of ATP. Niclosamide causes the scolex (headlike segment) and proximal segment of the tapeworm to detach from the intestinal wall, which leads to parasite evacuation from the intestines through normal peristalsis.

Contraindications

Age under 2 years; hypersensitivity to niclosamide, other anthelmintics, or their components

Interactions
ACTIVITIES
alcohol use: Decreased niclosamide effects

Adverse Reactions
CNS: Dizziness, drowsiness, headache, lightheadedness
EENT: Taste perversion
GI: Abdominal distress, anorexia, constipation, diarrhea, nausea, vomiting
SKIN: Anal pruritus, rash

Nursing Considerations
•To determine type of infestation, collect several stool specimens before starting

niclosamide therapy, as ordered, because eggs and parasite segments are released irregularly.
•If patient can't chew tablets thoroughly, crush them and give with small amount of water.
•For young child, crush tablets to fine powder and mix with small amount of water to make paste.
•Be aware that treatment isn't considered successful until stools have shown no eggs or parasites for at least 3 months.
PATIENT TEACHING
•Instruct patient to take niclosamide after a light meal.
•For young child, instruct parent to crush tablets to fine powder and mix with small amount of water to make paste.
•Urge patient to complete entire course of niclosamide therapy.
•Advise patient to avoid potentially hazardous activities until drug's CNS effects are known.
•Advise patient to store niclosamide in a cool, dry, dark place. Caution against storing in bathroom, near kitchen sink, or in other damp places because heat and moisture break down drug.
•Inform patient that stool may need to be examined on day 7 of treatment and again 1 and 3 months after treatment.
•Instruct patient to wash her hands thoroughly, to wash all bedding, and to use meticulous personal and environmental hygiene to decrease the risk of autoinfection.
•Caution patient against eating undercooked fish, pork, or beef.

nicotine for inhalation
Nicotrol Inhaler
nicotine nasal solution
Nicotrol NS
nicotine polacrilex
Nicorette, Nicorette Plus (CAN)
nicotine transdermal system
Habitrol, Nicoderm, NicoDerm CQ, Nicotrol, ProStep

Class and Category
Chemical: Pyridine alkaloid
Therapeutic: Smoking cessation adjunct

Pregnancy category: C (nicotine polacrilex), D (other forms of nicotine)

Indications and Dosages

➤ *To relieve nicotine withdrawal symptoms, including craving*

CHEWING GUM

Adults. *Initial:* 2 or 4 mg p.r.n. or q 1 to 2 hr, adjusted to complete withdrawal by 4 to 6 mo. *Maximum:* 30 pieces of 2-mg gum/day or 20 pieces of 4-mg gum/day.

NASAL SOLUTION

Adults. 1 to 2 sprays (1 to 2 mg) in each nostril/hr. *Maximum:* 5 mg/hr or 40 mg/day for up to 3 mo.

ORAL INHALATION

Adults and adolescents. 6 to 16 cartridges (24 to 64 mg)/day for up to 12 wk; then dosage gradually reduced over 12 wk or less. *Maximum:* 16 cartridges (64 mg)/day for 6 mo.

TRANSDERMAL SYSTEM

Adults. *Initial:* 14 to 22 mg q.d., adjusted to lower-dose systems over 2 to 5 mo.

DOSAGE ADJUSTMENT For adolescents and for adults who weigh less than 45 kg (100 lb) and who smoke less than 10 cigarettes daily or have heart disease, initial dosage reduced to 11 to 14 mg q.d. and adjusted to lower-dose systems over 2 to 5 mo.

Mechanism of Action

Binds selectively to nicotinic-cholinergic receptors at autonomic ganglia, in the adrenal medulla, at neuromuscular junctions, and in the brain. By providing a lower dose of nicotine than cigarettes, this drug reduces nicotine craving and withdrawal symptoms.

Contraindications

Hypersensitivity to nicotine, its components, or components of transdermal system; life-threatening arrhythmias; nonsmokers; recovery from acute MI; severe angina pectoris; skin disorders (transdermal); temporomandibular joint disease (chewing gum)

Interactions

DRUGS

acetaminophen, beta blockers, imipramine, insulin, oxazepam, pentazocine, theophylline: Possibly increased therapeutic effects of these drugs (chewing gum, nasal spray, transdermal system)

alpha blockers, bronchodilators: Possibly increased therapeutic effects of these drugs (chewing gum, transdermal system)

bupropion: Potentiated therapeutic effects of nicotine, possibly increased risk of hypertension

sympathomimetics: Possibly decreased therapeutic effects of these drugs (chewing gum, transdermal system)

theophylline, tricyclic antidepressants: Possibly altered pharmacologic actions of these drugs (oral inhalation)

FOODS

acidic beverages (citrus juices, coffee, soft drinks, tea, wine): Decreased nicotine absorption from gum if beverages consumed within 15 minutes before or while chewing gum

caffeine: Increased effects of caffeine (chewing gum, nasal spray, transdermal system)

Adverse Reactions

CNS: Dizziness, dream disturbances, drowsiness, headache, irritability, light-headedness, nervousness (chewing gum, transdermal system); amnesia, confusion, difficulty speaking, headache, migraine headache, paresthesia (nasal spray); chills, fever, headache, paresthesia (oral inhalation)

CV: Arrhythmias (all forms); hypertension (chewing gum, transdermal system); peripheral edema (nasal spray)

EENT: Increased salivation, injury to teeth or dental work, mouth injury, pharyngitis, stomatitis (chewing gum); altered taste, dry mouth (chewing gum, transdermal system); altered smell and taste, burning eyes, dry mouth, earache, epistaxis, gum disorders, hoarseness, lacrimation, mouth and tongue swelling, nasal blisters, nasal irritation or ulceration, pharyngitis, rhinitis, sinus problems, sneezing, vision changes (nasal spray); altered taste, lacrimation, pharyngitis, rhinitis, sinusitis, stomatitis (oral inhalation)

GI: Eructation (chewing gum); abdominal pain, constipation, diarrhea, flatulence, increased appetite, indigestion, nausea, vomiting (chewing gum, transdermal system); abdominal pain, constipation, diarrhea, flatulence, hiccups, indigestion, nausea (nasal spray); diarrhea, flatulence, hiccups, indigestion, nausea, vomiting (oral inhalation)

GU: Dysmenorrhea (chewing gum, transdermal system); menstrual irregularities (nasal spray)

MS: Jaw and neck pain (chewing gum); arthralgia, myalgia (chewing gum, transdermal system); arthralgia, back pain, myalgia (nasal spray); back pain (oral inhalation)

RESP: Cough (chewing gum, transdermal system); bronchitis, bronchospasm, chest tightness, cough, dyspnea, increased sputum production (nasal spray); chest tightness, cough, dyspnea, wheezing (oral inhalation)

SKIN: Diaphoresis, erythema, pruritus, rash, urticaria (chewing gum, transdermal system); acne, flushing of face, pruritus, purpura, rash (nasal spray); pruritus, rash, urticaria (oral inhalation)

Other: Allergic reaction (chewing gum, transdermal system); physical dependence (nasal spray); flulike symptoms, generalized pain, withdrawal symptoms (oral inhalation)

Nursing Considerations

•When administering nicotine by oral inhalation, expect optimal effect to result from continuous puffing for 20 minutes.

PATIENT TEACHING

•Instruct patient to read and follow package instructions to obtain best results with nicotine product.

•Advise patient to notify prescriber about other drugs she takes.

•Stress that patient must stop smoking as soon as treatment starts to avoid toxicity.

•For chewing gum therapy, instruct patient to wait at least 15 minutes after drinking coffee, juice, soft drink, tea, or wine. Advise her to chew gum until she detects a tingling sensation or peppery taste and then to place the gum between her cheek and gum until tingling or peppery taste subsides. Then direct her to move the gum to a different site until tingling or taste subsides, repeating until she no longer feels the sensation—usually about 30 minutes. Caution against swallowing the gum.

•For nasal spray therapy, instruct patient to tilt her head back and spray into a nostril. Caution against sniffing, swallowing, or inhaling spray because nicotine is absorbed through nasal mucosa.

•Warn patient that prolonged use of nasal form may cause dependence.

•For oral inhalation therapy, instruct patient to use 6 to 16 cartridges per day to prevent or relieve withdrawal symptoms and craving. Starting with 1 or 2 cartridges per day yields poor success. Direct patient to inhale through device just like a cigarette, puffing frequently for 20 minutes for best results.

•For transdermal system therapy, instruct patient not to open package until immediately before use because nicotine will be lost in the air. Advise her to apply system to clean, hairless, dry site on the upper outer arm or upper body. Instruct her to change systems and rotate sites every 24 hours and not to use the same site within 7 days.

•WARNING Urge patient to keep all unused nicotine forms safely away from children and pets and to discard used forms carefully. (Enough nicotine may remain in used systems to poison children and pets.) Instruct her to contact a poison control center immediately if she suspects that a child has ingested nicotine.

•Explain to patient with asthma or COPD that nicotine may cause bronchospasm.

•Inform patient that it may take several attempts to successfully stop smoking. Urge her to join a smoking cessation program.

nifedipine

Adalat, Adalat CC, Adalat PA (CAN), Adalat XL (CAN), Apo-Nifed (CAN), Novo-Nifedin (CAN), Nu-Nifed (CAN), Procardia, Procardia XL

Class and Category

Chemical: Dihydropyridine derivative
Therapeutic: Antianginal, antihypertensive
Pregnancy category: C

Indications and Dosages

➤ *To manage angina*

CAPSULES (ADALAT, APO-NIFED, NOVO-NIFEDIN, NU-NIFED, PROCARDIA)

Adults. *Initial:* 10 mg t.i.d., increased over 1 to 2 wk as needed. *Maintenance:* 10 to 20 mg t.i.d. *Maximum:* 180 mg/day, 30 mg/dose.

E.R. TABLETS (ADALAT XL, PROCARDIA XL)

Adults. *Initial:* 30 to 60 mg q.d., increased or decreased over 7 to 14 days based on patient response. *Maximum:* 90 mg/day.

➤ *To manage hypertension*

E.R. TABLETS (ADALAT CC)

Adults. *Initial:* 30 mg q.d. *Maintenance:* 30 to 60 mg q.d., increased or decreased over 7 to 14 days based on patient response. *Maximum:* 90 mg/day.

E.R. TABLETS (ADALAT PA)
Adults. *Initial:* 10 to 20 mg b.i.d., increased q 3 wk based on patient response. *Maintenance:* 20 mg b.i.d. *Maximum:* 80 mg/day.
E.R. TABLETS (ADALAT XL)
Adults. *Initial:* 30 to 60 mg q.d., increased or decreased over 7 to 14 days based on patient response. *Maintenance:* 60 to 90 mg q.d. *Maximum:* 120 mg/day.
E.R. TABLETS (PROCARDIA XL)
Adults. 30 to 60 mg q.d., increased or decreased over 7 to 14 days based on patient response. *Maximum:* 120 mg/day.
DOSAGE ADJUSTMENT Dosage possibly reduced for elderly patients and those with heart failure or impaired hepatic or renal function.

Route	Onset	Peak	Duration
P.O. (cap)	20 min	Unknown	Unknown

Mechanism of Action
May slow extracellular calcium movement into myocardial and vascular smooth-muscle cells by deforming calcium channels in cell membranes, inhibiting ion-controlled gating mechanisms, and interfering with calcium release from the sarcoplasmic reticulum. By decreasing the intracellular calcium level, nifedipine inhibits smooth-muscle cell contraction and dilates coronary and systemic arteries. As with other calcium channel blockers, these actions lead to decreased myocardial oxygen requirements and reduced peripheral resistance, blood pressure, and afterload.

Contraindications
Hypersensitivity to any calcium channel blocker, second- or third-degree AV block without artificial pacemaker, sick sinus syndrome

Interactions
DRUGS
anesthetics (hydrocarbon inhalation): Possibly hypotension
beta blockers: Increased risk of hypotension
calcium supplements: Possibly interference with action of nifedipine
cimetidine: Increased nifedipine bioavailability
digoxin: Transiently increased blood digoxin level, increased risk of digitalis toxicity
disopyramide, flecainide: Increased risk of bradycardia, conduction defects, and heart failure

estrogens: Possibly increased fluid retention and decreased therapeutic effects of nifedipine
lithium: Increased risk of neurotoxicity
NSAIDs, sympathomimetics: Possibly decreased therapeutic effects of nifedipine
other antihypertensives, prazocin: Increased risk of hypotension
procainamide, quinidine: Possibly prolonged QT interval
FOODS
grapefruit, grapefruit juice: Possibly increased bioavailability of nifedipine
high-fat meals: Possibly delayed nifedipine absorption
ACTIVITIES
alcohol use: Additive hypotensive effect

Adverse Reactions
CNS: Anxiety, ataxia, confusion, dizziness, drowsiness, headache, nervousness (possibly extreme), nightmares, paresthesia, psychiatric disturbance, syncope, tremor, weakness
CV: Arrhythmias (bradycardia, tachycardia), chest pain, heart failure, hypotension, palpitations, peripheral edema
EENT: Altered taste, blurred vision, dry mouth, epistaxis, gingival hyperplasia, nasal congestion, pharyngitis, sinusitis, tinnitus
ENDO: Gynecomastia, hyperglycemia
GI: Anorexia, constipation, diarrhea, dyspepsia, elevated liver function test results, hepatitis, nausea, vomiting
GU: Dysuria, nocturia, polyuria, sexual dysfunction, urinary frequency
HEME: Anemia, leukopenia, positive Coombs' test, thrombocytopenia
MS: Joint stiffness, muscle cramps
RESP: Chest congestion, cough, dyspnea, respiratory tract infection, wheezing
SKIN: Dermatitis, diaphoresis, erythema multiforme, flushing, photosensitivity, pruritus, rash, urticaria

Nursing Considerations
•When starting and stopping nifedipine therapy, taper dosage, as prescribed, over 7 to 14 days.
•For closely monitored hospitalized patient with angina, plan to increase usual dosage by 10 mg every 4 to 6 hours, as ordered, to control chest pain.
•Because of drug's negative inotropic effect on some patients, frequently monitor heart rate and rhythm and blood pressure in patients who take a beta blocker or have heart failure or significant left ventricular dysfunction.

• Monitor fluid intake and output and daily weight to assess for signs of fluid retention, which may lead to heart failure. Also assess for signs of heart failure, such as crackles, dyspnea, jugular vein distention, peripheral edema, and weight gain.

PATIENT TEACHING

• Instruct patient to swallow E.R. tablets whole, not to crush, chew, or break them. Inform her that their empty shells may appear in stool.

• Urge patient to take nifedipine exactly as prescribed, even when she's feeling well. Advise her to notify prescriber if she misses two or more doses.

• Advise patient not to take drug within 1 hour of eating a high-fat meal or grapefruit product. Urge her not to alter the amount of grapefruit products in her diet without consulting prescriber.

• **WARNING** Caution patient against stopping nifedipine abruptly because angina or dangerously high blood pressure could result.

• Teach patient how to measure her pulse rate and blood pressure, and advise her to call prescriber if they drop below accepted levels. Suggest that she keep a log of weekly measurements and take it to follow-up visits.

• Instruct patient to notify prescriber immediately about chest pain, difficulty breathing, ringing in ears, and swollen gums.

• Advise patient to avoid potentially hazardous activities until drug's CNS effects are known.

• Urge patient to avoid alcoholic beverages because they may worsen dizziness, drowsiness, and hypotension.

• Teach patient to minimize constipation by increasing her intake of fluids, if allowed, and dietary fiber.

• Emphasize the need to comply with prescribed lifestyle changes, such as alcohol moderation, low-fat or low-sodium diet, regular exercise, smoking cessation, stress reduction, and weight reduction.

• Stress the need for good oral hygiene and regular dental visits.

• Caution patient that hot tubs, saunas, and prolonged hot showers may cause dizziness and fainting.

• Advise patient to avoid prolonged sun exposure and to wear sunscreen when outdoors.

nimodipine

Nimotop

Class and Category

Chemical: Dihydropyridine derivative
Therapeutic: Cerebral vasodilator
Pregnancy category: C

Indications and Dosages

➤ *To treat neurologic deficits associated with subarachnoid hemorrhage*

CAPSULES

Adults. 60 mg q 4 hr within 96 hr of hemorrhage and continued for 21 days.

DOSAGE ADJUSTMENT Dosage reduced to 30 mg q 4 hr for patients with hepatic impairment.

Mechanism of Action

Inhibits calcium ion transfer into smooth muscle cells, thereby inhibiting contraction of vascular smooth muscle. By relieving or preventing reactive vasodilation, nimodipine may prevent cerebral arterial spasms after hemorrhage.

Contraindications

Cardiogenic shock, hepatic function impairment, hypersensitivity to nimodipine or its components

Interactions

DRUGS

anesthetics (hydrocarbon inhalation): Possibly hypotension

antihypertensives, prazocin: Increased risk of hypotension

beta blockers: Increased adverse effects of beta blockers

cimetidine: Increased nimodipine bioavailability

digoxin: Transiently increased blood digoxin level and risk of digitalis toxicity

estrogens: Possibly increased fluid retention and decreased therapeutic effect of nimodipine

lithium: Increased risk of neurotoxicity

NSAIDs, sympathomimetics: Possibly decreased therapeutic effect of nimodipine

procainamide, quinidine: Increased risk of prolonged QT interval

Adverse Reactions

CNS: Dizziness, headache
CV: Hypotension, edema
GI: Diarrhea, nausea
SKIN: Rash

Nursing Considerations

•For patients who can't take oral nimodipine, be prepared to extract drug from capsule using an 18G needle and syringe, to administer drug through a nasogastric or percutaneous esophagogastrostomy tube, and then to flush tube with 30 ml of NS.

•**WARNING** Assess patients with cardiac history for progressive hemodynamic instability and cardiac arrhythmias because of nimodipine's potential effects on heart rate and conduction.

•Monitor blood pressure throughout drug therapy for possible hypotension.

•Monitor fluid intake and output and assess for signs of edema, which may indicate fluid retention, because drug promotes peripheral vasodilation. Notify prescriber if edema persists or if patient develops a negative fluid balance.

PATIENT TEACHING

•Instruct patient to swallow nimodipine capsules whole and not to crush or chew them.

•Teach patient how to monitor pulse and blood pressure. Suggest that she keep a log of weekly measurements and take it to follow-up office appointment.

•Advise patient to notify prescriber immediately if she experiences pronounced dizziness or headache or swelling of hands or feet.

nisoldipine

Sular

Class and Category

Chemical: Dihydropyridine derivative
Therapeutic: Antihypertensive
Pregnancy category: C

Indications and Dosages

➤ *To manage hypertension*

E.R. TABLETS

Adults. 20 mg q.d., increased by 10 mg q 7 days, as prescribed. *Maintenance:* 20 to 40 mg/day. *Maximum:* 60 mg/day.

DOSAGE ADJUSTMENT For patients over age 65 and patients with hepatic impairment, initial dosage reduced to 10 mg q.d.

Contraindications

Hypersensitivity to any calcium channel blocker, second- or third-degree AV block without artificial pacemaker, sick sinus syndrome

Mechanism of Action

May slow extracellular calcium movement into myocardial and vascular smooth-muscle cells by deforming calcium channels in cell membranes, inhibiting ion-controlled gating mechanisms, and interfering with calcium release from the sarcoplasmic reticulum. By decreasing the intracellular calcium level, nisoldipine inhibits smooth-muscle cell contraction and dilates coronary and systemic arteries. As with other calcium channel blockers, these actions lead to decreased myocardial oxygen requirements and reduced peripheral resistance, blood pressure, and afterload.

Interactions

DRUGS

beta blockers: Possibly increased risk of hypotension
cimetidine, ranitidine: Increased blood nisoldipine level
NSAIDs: Decreased antihypertensive effect of nisoldipine
quinidine: Possibly decreased blood nisoldipine level

FOODS

grapefruit, grapefruit juice: Possibly increased bioavailability of nisoldipine
high-fat meals: Possibly delayed nisoldipine absorption

ACTIVITIES

alcohol use: Additive hypotensive effect

Adverse Reactions

CNS: Dizziness, headache
CV: Angina, hypotension, palpitations, peripheral edema
EENT: Pharyngitis, sinusitis
GI: Constipation, nausea
RESP: Dyspnea
SKIN: Rash

Nursing Considerations

•Monitor pulse rate and rhythm and blood pressure before starting nisoldipine therapy, during dosage adjustments, and periodically throughout therapy.

•Don't break or crush E.R. tablets.

•For optimal absorption, give drug 30 minutes before or 2 hours after meals.

•Monitor fluid intake and output and daily weight to assess for signs of fluid retention, which may lead to heart failure. Also assess for signs of heart failure, such as crackles, dyspnea, jugular vein distention, peripheral edema, and weight gain.

PATIENT TEACHING

•Instruct patient to swallow E.R. nisoldipine tablets whole, not to break, crush, or chew them.

•Advise patient not to take drug within 1 hour of eating a high-fat meal or grapefruit product. Urge her not to alter the amount of grapefruit products in her diet without consulting prescriber.

•Urge patient to continue taking drug as prescribed, even if she feels well.

•**WARNING** Caution patient against stopping drug abruptly because blood pressure could rise dangerously high.

•Instruct patient to notify prescriber about constipation, difficulty breathing, dizziness, irregular heartbeat, nausea, severe headache, and swelling of hands or feet.

•Teach patient and family how to measure blood pressure, and instruct them to notify prescriber if systolic blood pressure falls below 90 mm Hg. Suggest that patient keep a log of weekly measurements and take it to follow-up visits.

•Advise patient to change position slowly to minimize effects of orthostatic hypotension. Inform her that hot tubs, saunas, and prolonged hot showers may worsen this adverse reaction.

•Caution patient to avoid potentially hazardous activities until drug's CNS effects are known.

•Urge patient to avoid alcohol and OTC alcohol-containing drugs without consulting prescriber. Many OTC preparations can raise blood pressure.

•Emphasize the need to adhere to prescribed lifestyle changes, such as alcohol moderation, low-fat and low-sodium diet, regular exercise, smoking cessation, stress reduction, and weight reduction.

nitrofurantoin

Apo-Nitrofurantoin (CAN), Furadantin, Macrobid, Macrodantin, Novo-Furantoin (CAN)

Class and Category

Chemical: Nitrofuran derivative
Therapeutic: Antibiotic
Pregnancy category: B (except near term)

Indications and Dosages

➤ *To treat acute cystitis*
CAPSULES, ORAL SUSPENSION, TABLETS
Adults. 50 to 100 mg q 6 hr. *Maximum:* 600 mg/day or 10 mg/kg/day.
Children over age 1 month. 0.75 to 1.75 mg/kg q 6 hr.
E.R. CAPSULES
Adults and children age 12 and older. 100 mg q 12 hr for 7 days.
➤ *To suppress chronic cystitis*
CAPSULES, ORAL SUSPENSION, TABLETS
Adults. 50 to 100 mg h.s. *Maximum:* 600 mg/day or 10 mg/kg/day.
Children over age 1 month. 1 mg/kg/day h.s.

Mechanism of Action

Inactivates or alters bacterial ribosomal proteins and other macromolecules. This inhibits bacterial protein synthesis, aerobic energy metabolism, DNA synthesis, RNA synthesis, and cell wall synthesis. Nitrofurantoin is bacteriostatic at low doses and bactericidal at higher doses.

Contraindications

Age under 1 month, anuria, creatinine clearance of less than 60 ml/min/1.73 m², hypersensitivity to nitrofurantoin or parabens, oliguria, pregnancy near term

Interactions

DRUGS

hepatotoxic drugs: Increased risk of hepatotoxicity
magnesium trisilicate: Decreased nitrofurantoin absorption
methyldopa, procainamide, hemolytics: Increased risk of toxic effects from nitrofurantoin
nalidixic acid: Possibly impaired therapeutic effects of this drug
neurotoxic drugs: Increased risk of neurotoxicity
probenecid, sulfinpyrazone: Increased blood nitrofurantoin level and risk of toxicity

Adverse Reactions

CNS: Chills, confusion, depression, headache, neurotoxicity, peripheral neuropathy
EENT: Optic neuritis, parotitis, tooth discoloration

GI: Abdominal pain, anorexia, diarrhea, hepatitis, nausea, pancreatitis, pseudomembranous colitis, vomiting
GU: Rust-colored to brown urine
HEME: Aplastic anemia, granulocytopenia, hemolyic anemia, leukopenia, megaloblastic anemia, methemoglobinemia, thrombocytopenia
MS: Arthralgia, myalgia
RESP: Asthma (in asthmatic patients), cyanosis, pneumonitis (acute)
SKIN: Alopecia, erythema multiforme, exfoliative dermatitis, jaundice, pruritus, rash, urticaria
Other: Anaphylaxis, angioedema, drug-induced fever

Nursing Considerations
•Obtain urine specimen for culture and sensitivity tests, as ordered; review test results if possible before giving nitrofurantoin.
•Give drug with food or milk to avoid staining teeth.
•Don't crush or break capsules.
•Shake oral suspension before pouring dose, and mix with food or milk, as needed.
•Monitor for signs of superinfection, such as abdominal pain, diarrhea, and fever.

PATIENT TEACHING
•Instruct patient to shake nitrofurantoin oral suspension before measuring dose and to take drug with food or milk.
•Caution patient against taking any preparations that contain magnesium trisilicate during therapy.
•Inform patient that urine may become brown, orange, or rust-colored during therapy.

nitroglycerin
(glyceryl trinitrate)

Deponit, Minitran, Nitro-Bid, Nitrocot, Nitro-Dur, Nitrogard, Nitroglyn E-R, Nitroject, Nitrol, Nitrolingual, Nitrong SR, Nitro-par, Nitrostat, Nitro-time, Transderm-Nitro, Tridil

Class and Category
Chemical: Nitrate
Therapeutic: Antianginal, antihypertensive, vasodilator
Pregnancy category: C

Indications and Dosages
➤ *To prevent or treat angina*

E.R. BUCCAL TABLETS
Adults. 1 mg q 5 hr while awake.

E.R. CAPSULES
Adults. 2.5, 6.5, or 9 mg q 12 hr. Frequency increased to q 8 hr based on patient's response.

E.R. TABLETS
Adults. 2.6 or 6.5 mg q 12 hr. Frequency increased to q 8 hr based on patient's response.

S.L. TABLETS
Adults. 0.3 to 0.6 mg, repeated q 5 min. *Maximum:* 3 tabs in 15 min or 10 mg/day.

TRANSDERMAL OINTMENT
Adults. 1″ to 2″ (15 to 30 mg) q 8 hr. Frequency increased to q 6 hr if angina occurs between doses. *Maximum:* 5″ (75 mg)/application.

TRANSDERMAL PATCH
Adults. 0.1 to 0.8 mg/hr, worn 12 to 14 hr.

TRANSLINGUAL SPRAY
Adults. 1 or 2 metered doses (0.4 or 0.8 mg) onto or under tongue, repeated q 5 min as needed. *Maximum:* 3 metered doses in 15 min or 1.2 mg/day.

➤ *To prevent or treat angina, to manage hypertension or heart failure*

I.V. INFUSION
Adults. 5 mcg/min, increased by 5 mcg/min q 3 to 5 min to 20 mcg/min, as prescribed, and then by 10 to 20 mcg/min q 3 to 5 min until desired effect occurs.

Route	Onset	Peak	Duration
P.O. (buccal)	3 min	Unknown	5 hr
P.O. (E.R.)	20 to 45 min	Unknown	8 to 12 hr
I.V.	1 to 2 min	Unknown	3 to 5 min
S.L.	1 to 3 min	Unknown	30 to 60 min
Trans-dermal (ointment)	In 30 min	Unknown	4 to 8 hr
Trans-dermal (patch)	In 30 min	Unknown	8 to 24 hr
Trans-lingual	2 to 4 min	Unknown	30 to 60 min

Incompatibilities
Don't administer I.V. nitroglycerin through I.V. bags or tubing made of polyvinyl chloride. Don't mix drug with other solutions.

Mechanism of Action

May interact with nitrate receptors in vascular smooth-muscle cell membranes. This interaction reduces nitroglycerin to nitric oxide, which activates the enzyme guanylate cyclase, increasing intracellular formation of cGMP. The increased cGMP level may relax vascular smooth muscle by forcing calcium out of muscle cells, causing vasodilation. Venous dilation decreases venous return to the heart, reducing left ventricular end-diastolic pressure and pulmonary artery wedge pressure. Arterial dilation decreases systemic vascular resistance, systolic arterial pressure, and mean arterial pressure. Thus, nitroglycerin reduces preload and afterload, decreasing myocardial workload and oxygen demand. Nitroglycerin also dilates coronary arteries, increasing blood flow to ischemic myocardial tissue.

Contraindications

Acute MI (S.L.), angle-closure glaucoma, cerebral hemorrhage, constrictive pericarditis (I.V.), head trauma, hypersensitivity to adhesive in transdermal form, hypersensitivity to nitrates, hypotension (I.V.), hypovolemia (I.V.), inadequate cerebral circulation (I.V.), increased intracranial pressure, orthostatic hypotension, pericardial tamponade, severe anemia

Interactions

DRUGS

acetylcholine, norepinephrine: Possibly decreased therapeutic effects of these drugs
heparin: Possibly decreased anticoagulant effect of heparin (I.V. nitroglycerin)
opioid analgesics, other antihypertensives, vasodilators: Possibly increased orthostatic hypotension
sildenafil: Possibly potentiated hypotensive effect of nitroglycerin
sympathomimetics: Possibly decreased antianginal effect of nitroglycerin and increased risk of hypotension

ACTIVITIES

alcohol use: Possibly increased orthostatic hypotension

Adverse Reactions

CNS: Agitation, anxiety, dizziness, headache, insomnia, restlessness, syncope, weakness

CV: Arrhythmias (including tachycardia), edema, hypotension, orthostatic hypotension, palpitations
EENT: Blurred vision, burning or tingling in mouth (buccal, S.L. forms), dry mouth
GI: Abdominal pain, diarrhea, indigestion, nausea, vomiting
GU: Dysuria, impotence, urinary frequency
HEME: Methemoglobinemia
MS: Arthralgia
RESP: Bronchitis, pneumonia
SKIN: Contact dermatitis (transdermal forms), flushing of face and neck, rash

Nursing Considerations

• Plan to give patient a nitroglycerin-free period of about 10 hours each day, as prescribed to maintain therapeutic effects and avoid tolerance.
• Place E.R. buccal tablets in buccal pouch with patient in sitting or lying position.
• Don't break or crush E.R. tablets or capsules. Have patient swallow them whole with a full glass of water.
• Place S.L. tablet under patient's tongue and ensure that it remains in place and completely dissolves.
• Be sure to remove cotton from S.L. tablet container to allow quick access to the drug.
• When applying transdermal ointment, apply correct amount on dose-measuring paper. Then place paper on hairless area of body and spread in a thin even layer over an area at least 2″ by 3″. Don't place on cuts or irritated areas. Wash your hands after application. Rotate sites. Store at room temperature.
• Open transdermal patch package immediately before use. Apply patch to hairless area, and press edges to seal. Rotate sites. Store at room temperature. If patient needs cardioversion or defibrillation, remove transdermal patch.
• Don't shake translingual spray container before administering. Have patient inhale and hold her breath, and then spray drug under or on her tongue.
• Be aware that I.V. nitroglycerin should be diluted only in D_5W or NS and shouldn't be mixed with other infusions. The pharmacist should add drug to a glass bottle, not a container made of polyvinyl chloride. Don't use a filter because plastic absorbs drug. Administer with infusion pump.
• Check vital signs before every dosage adjustment and frequently during therapy.

•Frequently monitor heart and breath sounds, level of consciousness, fluid intake and output, and pulmonary artery wedge pressure, if possible.

•Store premixed containers in the dark; don't freeze them.

•**WARNING** Assess for signs of overdose, such as confusion, diaphoresis, dyspnea, flushing, headache, hypotension, nausea, palpitations, tachycardia, vertigo, vision changes, and vomiting. Treat as prescribed by removing nitroglycerin source, if possible; elevating the legs above heart level; and administering an alpha-adrenergic agonist, such as phenylephrine, as prescribed, to treat severe hypotension.

PATIENT TEACHING

•Teach patient to recognize signs and symptoms of angina pectoris, including chest fullness, pain, and pressure, which may be accompanied by sweating and nausea. Pain may radiate down left arm or into neck or jaw. Inform female patients and those with diabetes mellitus or hypertension that they may experience only fatigue and shortness of breath.

•Instruct patient to read and follow package instructions to obtain full benefits of nitroglycerin.

•To prevent drug tolerance, inform patient that prescriber may order a 10- to 12-hour drug-free period at night (or at another time if she has chest pain at night or in the morning).

•Instruct patient to swallow E.R. tablets or capsules whole—not to break, crush, or chew them—with a full glass of water.

•For sublingual or buccal use, advise patient to place a tablet under her tongue or in her buccal pouch when angina starts and then to sit or lie down. Instruct her not to swallow drug, but to let it dissolve. Explain that moisture in her mouth helps drug absorption. If angina doesn't subside, instruct patient to place another tablet under her tongue or in her buccal pouch after 5 minutes and to repeat, if needed, for three doses total. If pain doesn't subside after 20 minutes, urge patient to call 911 or another emergency service.

•Advise patient to carry S.L. tablets in their original brown bottle in a purse or jacket pocket, but not one that will be affected by body heat. Instruct her to store drug in a dry place at room temperature and to discard cotton from container. Advise her to discard and replace S.L. tablets after 6 months.

•Advise patient using transdermal ointment or patch to rotate sites to avoid skin sensitization.

•Inform patient that swimming or bathing doesn't affect transdermal forms but that hot tubs, saunas, prolonged hot showers, electric blankets, and magnetic therapy over site may increase drug absorption and cause dizziness and hypotension.

•Instruct patient not to inhale translingual spray.

•Inform patient that drug commonly causes headache, which typically resolves after a few days of continuous therapy. Suggest that patient take acetaminophen, as needed.

•Advise patient to notify prescriber immediately about blurred vision, dizziness, and severe headache.

•Suggest that patient change position slowly to minimize effects of orthostatic hypotension.

•Advise patient to avoid potentially hazardous activities until drug's CNS effects are known.

•Urge patient to avoid alcohol during therapy.

nitroprusside sodium

Nipride, Nitropress

Class and Category

Chemical: Cyanonitrosylferrate
Therapeutic: Antihypertensive, vasodilator
Pregnancy category: C

Indications and Dosages

➤ *To treat hypertensive crisis and manage severe heart failure*

I.V. INFUSION

Adults and children. *Initial:* 0.25 to 0.3 mcg/kg/min, increased gradually q few minutes until blood pressure reaches desired level. *Maintenance:* 3 mcg/kg/min (range, 0.25 to 10 mcg/kg/min). *Maximum:* 10 mcg/kg/min for 10 min.

Route	Onset	Peak	Duration
I.V.	1 to 2 min	Immediate	1 to 10 min

Incompatibilities

Don't mix nitroprusside with any other drug.

Contraindications

Acute heart failure with decreased peripheral vascular resistance, congenital optic atrophy, decreased cerebral perfusion, hypersensitivity to nitroprusside or its components, hypertension from aortic coarctation or AV shunting, tobacco-induced amblyopia

Mechanism of Action
May interact with nitrate receptors in vascular smooth-muscle cell membranes. This action reduces nitroprusside to nitric oxide and then activates intracellular guanylate cyclase, which increases the cGMP level. The increased cGMP level may relax vascular smooth muscle by forcing calcium out of muscle cells. Smooth-muscle relaxation causes arteries and veins to dilate, which reduces peripheral vascular resistance and blood pressure.

Interactions
DRUGS
dobutamine: Increased cardiac output, decreased pulmonary artery wedge pressure
ganglionic blockers, general anesthetics, hypotension-producing drugs: Increased hypotensive effect
sympathomimetics: Decreased antihypertensive effect of nitroprusside

Adverse Reactions
CNS: Anxiety, dizziness, headache, increased intracranial pressure, nervousness, restlessness
CV: Hypotension, tachycardia
ENDO: Hypothyroidism
GI: Abdominal pain, ileus, nausea, vomiting
HEME: Methemoglobinemia
MS: Muscle twitching
SKIN: Diaphoresis, flushing, rash
Other: Infusion site phlebitis

Nursing Considerations
• Obtain baseline vital signs before administering nitroprusside.
• **WARNING** Don't give drug undiluted. Reconstitute with 2 ml of D_5W, and add solution to 250 to 500 ml of D_5W to produce 200 mcg/ml or 100 mcg/ml, respectively.
• Be aware that solution is stable at room temperature for 24 hours when protected from light. Don't use reconstituted solution if it contains particles or is blue, green, red, or darker than faint brown.
• Use an infusion pump. Place opaque covering over infusion container because drug is metabolized by light. I.V. tubing doesn't need to be covered.
• Keep patient supine when starting drug or titrating dose up or down.

• Monitor blood pressure continuously with intra-arterial pressure monitor. Record blood pressure every 5 minutes at start of infusion and every 15 minutes thereafter.
• If patient has severe heart failure, expect to administer an inotropic drug, such as dopamine or dobutamine, as prescribed.
• **WARNING** For patient who receives prolonged nitroprusside therapy or short-term high-dose therapy, monitor for signs of thiocyanate toxicity (ataxia, blurred vision, delirium, dizziness, dyspnea, headache, hyperreflexia, loss of consciousness, nausea, tinnitus, vomiting). Toxicity can cause arrhythmias, metabolic acidosis, severe hypotension, and death.
• Monitor serum thiocyanate level at least every 72 hours; levels above 100 mcg/ml are associated with toxicity.
• **WARNING** Assess for signs of cyanide toxicity (absence of reflexes, coma, distant heart sounds, hypotension, metabolic acidosis, mydriasis, pink skin, shallow respirations, and weak pulse). If you detect such signs, discontinue nitroprusside, as ordered, and give 4 to 6 mg/kg of sodium nitrite over 2 to 4 minutes to convert hemoglobin to methemoglobin. Follow with 150 to 200 mg/kg of sodium thiosulfate. Repeat this regimen at one-half the original doses after 2 hours, as ordered.
PATIENT TEACHING
• Advise patient to change position slowly to minimize dizziness from sudden, severe hypotension.

nizatidine
Apo-Nizatidine (CAN), Axid, Axid AR

Class and Category
Chemical: Ethenediamine derivative
Therapeutic: Antiulcer
Pregnancy category: B

Indications and Dosages
➤ *To manage active duodenal ulcer*
CAPSULES
Adults and adolescents. 300 mg h.s. or 150 mg b.i.d. for 8 wk.
DOSAGE ADJUSTMENT Dosage reduced to 150 mg/day for patients with creatinine clearance of 20 to 50 ml/min/1.73 m²; to 150 mg q.o.d. for those with creatinine clearance of less than 20 ml/min/1.73 m².
➤ *To prevent recurrence of duodenal ulcer*
CAPSULES
Adults and adolescents. 150 mg h.s.

DOSAGE ADJUSTMENT Dosage reduced to 150 mg q.o.d. for patients with creatinine clearance of 20 to 50 ml/min/1.73 m^2; to 150 mg q 3 days for those with creatinine clearance of less than 20 ml/min/1.73 m^2.

➤ *To manage acute benign gastric ulcer*
CAPSULES
Adults and adolescents. 300 mg h.s. or 150 mg b.i.d.

➤ *To manage gastroesophageal reflux disease*
CAPSULES
Adults and adolescents. 150 mg b.i.d.

➤ *To prevent or relieve acid indigestion or heartburn*
TABLETS
Adults and adolescents. 75 mg 30 min to 1 hr before meals.

Route	Onset	Peak	Duration
P.O.	Unknown	Unknown	10 to 12 hr*

Mechanism of Action
Inhibits basal and nocturnal secretion of gastric acid by reversibly and competitively blocking H$_2$ receptors, especially those in gastric parietal cells. Nizatidine also inhibits gastric acid secretion in response to stimuli, including food and caffeine.

Contraindications
Hypersensitivity to nizatidine or other H$_2$-receptor antagonists

Interactions
DRUGS
antacids: Decreased nizatidine bioavailability
itraconazole, ketoconazole: Decreased absorption of these drugs
salicylates: Increased blood level of these drugs
sucralfate: Possibly decreased nizatidine absorption

Adverse Reactions
CNS: Agitation, anxiety, confusion, depression, dizziness, fatigue, fever, hallucinations, headache, insomnia, somnolence
CV: Arrhythmias, chest pain, vasculitis
EENT: Amblyopia, dry mouth, laryngeal edema, pharyngitis, rhinitis, sinusitis

* For nocturnal acid secretion; up to 4 hr for food-stimulated acid secretion.

ENDO: Gynecomastia
GI: Abdominal pain, constipation, diarrhea, hepatitis, nausea, vomiting
GU: Decreased libido, hyperuricemia not associated with gout or nephrolithiasis, impotence
HEME: Anemia, aplastic anemia, eosinophilia, hemolytic anemia, leukopenia, neutropenia, pancytopenia, thrombocytopenia
MS: Back pain, myalgia
RESP: Bronchospasm, cough
SKIN: Alopecia, diaphoresis, erythema multiforme, exfoliative dermatitis, jaundice, pruritus, rash, Stevens-Johnson syndrome, toxic epidermal necrolysis, urticaria
Other: Anaphylaxis, angioedema, serum sickness–like reaction

Nursing Considerations
• Monitor CBC, BUN and serum creatinine levels, and liver function test results before and periodically during nizatidine therapy.
• Don't administer drug within 1 hour of an antacid.
PATIENT TEACHING
• Instruct patient not to take nizatidine within 1 hour of an antacid.
• Urge patient to take drug exactly as prescribed, even if she feels better. Inform her that ulcer may take up to 8 weeks to heal.
• If patient smokes, encourage her to stop because smoking increases gastric acid production. Suggest that she join a smoking cessation program.
• Teach patient to minimize constipation by drinking plenty of fluids (if allowed), eating high-fiber foods, and exercising regularly.
• Instruct patient to notify prescriber immediately about abdominal pain, easy bruising, extreme fatigue, and yellow skin or sclera.

norepinephrine bitartrate
(levarterenol bitartrate)
Levophed

Class and Category
Chemical: Catecholamine
Therapeutic: Cardiac stimulant, vasopressor
Pregnancy category: C

Indications and Dosages
➤ *To treat acute hypotension, cardiogenic shock, and septic shock*
I.V. INFUSION
Adults. *Initial:* 0.5 to 1 mcg/min. Increased, as ordered, until systolic blood pressure

reaches desired level. *Maintenance:* 2 to 12 mcg/min.
Children. 0.1 mcg/kg/min. *Maximum:* 1 mcg/kg/min.

➤ *To treat refractory shock*
I.V. INFUSION
Adults. Up to 30 mcg/min.

Route	Onset	Peak	Duration
I.V.	Rapid	Unknown	1 to 2 min

Mechanism of Action
At high doses (more than 4 mcg/min), directly stimulates alpha-adrenergic receptors and inhibits activity of the intracellular enzyme adenyl cyclase, which then inhibits cyclic adenosine monophosphate (cAMP) production. Inhibition of cAMP causes arterial and venous constriction and increases peripheral vascular resistance and systolic blood pressure. At low doses (less than 2 mcg/min), norepinephrine directly stimulates beta-adrenergic receptors in the myocardium and increases adenyl cyclase activity, producing positive inotropic and chronotropic effects.

Contraindications
Concurrent use of hydrocarbon inhalation anesthetics, hypersensitivity to norepinephrine or its components, hypovolemia, mesenteric or peripheral vascular thrombosis

Interactions
DRUGS
alpha blockers: Decreased vasopressor effects of norepinephrine
beta blockers: Decreased cardiac-stimulating effect of norepinephrine, possibly decreased therapeutic effects of both drugs
digoxin: Increased risk of arrhythmias, possibly potentiated inotropic effect
doxapram: Possibly increased vasopressor effects of both drugs
ergonovine, ergotamine, methylergonovine, methysergide, oxytocin: Possibly increased vasoconstriction
general anesthetics: Increased risk of arrhythmias
guanadrel, guanethidine: Increased vasopressor response to norepinephrine, possibly severe hypertension
MAO inhibitors: Possibly life-threatening adverse effects, including arrhythmias, hyperpyrexia, severe headache, severe hypertension, and vomiting
maprotiline, tricyclic antidepressants: Possibly potentiated cardiovascular and pressor effects of norepinephrine, including arrhythmias, severe hypertension, and hyperpyrexia
methylphenidate: Possibly potentiated vasopressor effect of norepinephrine
nitrates: Possibly decreased therapeutic effects of both drugs
phenoxybenzamine: Possibly arrhythmias or hypotension
sympathomimetics: Increased risk of adverse cardiovascular effects
thyroid hormones: Increased risk of coronary insufficiency

Adverse Reactions
CNS: Anxiety, dizziness, headache, insomnia, nervousness, tremor, weakness
CV: Angina, bradycardia, ECG changes, edema, hypertension, hypotension, palpitations, peripheral vascular insufficiency (including gangrene), PVCs, sinus tachycardia
GI: Nausea, vomiting
GU: Decreased renal perfusion
RESP: Apnea, dyspnea
SKIN: Pallor
Other: Infusion site sloughing and tissue necrosis, metabolic acidosis

Nursing Considerations
•Dilute norepinephrine concentrate for infusion in D₅W, D₅NS, or NS before administering. Dilutions typically range from 16 to 32 mcg/ml.
•Make sure solution contains no particles and isn't discolored before administering.
•Administer drug with infusion pump or other flow-control device.
•Check blood pressure every 2 to 3 minutes, preferably by direct intra-arterial monitoring, until stabilized and then every 5 minutes.
•**WARNING** Because extravasation can cause severe tissue damage and necrosis, expect prescriber to give multiple S.C. injections of phentolamine (5 to 10 mg diluted in 10 to 15 ml of NS) around extravasated infusion site.
•If blanching occurs along vein, change infusion site and notify prescriber at once.
•Monitor ECG tracing continuously during drug administration.
PATIENT TEACHING
•Urge patient to notify you at once about burning, leaking, or tingling around I.V. site.

norfloxacin

Noroxin

Class and Category

Chemical: Fluoroquinolone
Therapeutic: Antibiotic
Pregnancy category: C

Indications and Dosages

➤ *To treat uncomplicated UTIs caused by* Escherichia coli, Klebsiella pneumoniae, *or* Proteus mirabilis

TABLETS

Adults. 400 mg q 12 hr for 3 days.

➤ *To treat uncomplicated UTIs caused by* Citrobacter freundii, Enterobacter aerogenes, Enterobacter cloacae, Enterococcus faecalis, Proteus *sp.,* Pseudomonas aeruginosa, Staphylococcus aureus, Staphylococcus epidermidis, Staphylococcus saprophyticus, *or* Streptococcus agalactiae

TABLETS

Adults. 400 mg q 12 hr for 7 to 10 days.

➤ *To treat complicated UTIs caused by* E. coli, E. faecalis, K. pneumoniae, P. aeruginosa, P. mirabilis, *or* Serratia marcescens

TABLETS

Adults. 400 mg q 12 hr for 10 to 21 days. *Maximum:* 800 mg/day.

➤ *To treat uncomplicated gonorrhea*

TABLETS

Adults. 800 mg as a single dose.

➤ *To treat prostatitis caused by* E. coli

TABLETS

Adults. 400 mg q 12 hr for 28 days.

DOSAGE ADJUSTMENT Dosage reduced to 400 mg q.d. for patients with creatinine clearance of 30 ml/min/1.73 m^2 or less.

Mechanism of Action

Inhibits the enzyme DNA gyrase, which is responsible for unwinding and supercoiling bacterial DNA before it replicates. By inhibiting this enzyme, norfloxacin interferes with bacterial cell replication and causes cell death.

Contraindications

Hypersensitivity to norfloxacin, other fluoroquinolones, or their components

Interactions

DRUGS

aluminum-, calcium-, or magnesium-containing antacids; ferrous sulfate; magnesium-containing laxatives; sucralfate; zinc: Possibly decreased absorption and blood level of norfloxacin

cyclosporine: Possibly increased serum creatinine and blood cyclosporine levels

didanosine: Possibly decreased norfloxacin absorption

probenecid: Decreased norfloxacin excretion and risk of toxicity

warfarin: Possibly increased anticoagulant effect and risk of bleeding

Adverse Reactions

CNS: Dizziness, drowsiness, headache, insomnia, seizures, tremors

EENT: Impaired taste

GI: Abdominal cramps or pain, diarrhea, elevated liver function test results, nausea, pseudomembranous colitis, vomiting

GU: Vaginal candidiasis

MS: Tendinitis; tendon inflammation, pain, or rupture

SKIN: Blisters, diaphoresis, erythema, erythema multiforme, exfoliative dermatitis, photosensitivity, pruritus, rash, Stevens-Johnson syndrome, toxic epidermal necrolysis, urticaria

Nursing Considerations

•Obtain urine specimen for culture and sensitivity testing. Review test results, if possible, before starting norfloxacin.

•Determine if patient has a history of a CNS disorder, such as cerebral arteriosclerosis or epilepsy, because drug may lower the seizure threshold. Notify prescriber about such a history before starting therapy, and institute seizure precautions according to facility policy.

•Give drug on an empty stomach. Administer it 2 hours before or after giving antacids, didanosine, sucralfate, or vitamins that contain iron or zinc.

•Keep emergency resuscitation equipment readily available, and observe for signs of hypersensitivity, such as angioedema, dyspnea, and urticaria. If you suspect anaphylaxis, prepare to give epinephrine, corticosteroids, and diphenhydramine, as prescribed.

•If patient has myasthenia gravis, assess her frequently for a change in respiratory status because norfloxacin may worsen this condi-

N
O

tion and lead to life-threatening weakness of respiratory muscles.

PATIENT TEACHING
•Instruct patient to take norfloxacin on an empty stomach with a large glass of water to prevent crystalluria. Urge her to drink several glasses of water every day during therapy.
•Instruct patient to take drug at least 2 hours before or after eating, drinking milk, or taking antacids, didanosine, sucralfate, or vitamins that contain iron or zinc.
•Advise patient to avoid hazardous activities until drug's CNS effects are known.

nortriptyline hydrochloride

Aventyl, Pamelor

Class and Category

Chemical: Dibenzocycloheptene derivative
Therapeutic: Antidepressant
Pregnancy category: D

Indications and Dosages

➤ *To treat depression*
CAPSULES, ORAL SOLUTION
Adults. *Initial:* 25 mg t.i.d. or q.i.d. *Maximum:* 150 mg/day.
Adolescents. 25 to 50 mg/day or 1 to 3 mg/kg/day in divided doses.
Children ages 6 to 12. 10 to 20 mg/day or 1 to 3 mg/kg/day in divided doses.
DOSAGE ADJUSTMENT Dosage possibly reduced to 30 to 50 mg/day (in divided doses or h.s.) for elderly patients.

Route	Onset	Peak	Duration
P.O.	2 to 3 wk	Unknown	Unknown

Mechanism of Action
May interfere with reuptake of serotonin (and possibly other neurotransmitters) at presynaptic neurons, thus enhancing serotonin's effects at postsynaptic receptors. By restoring normal neurotransmitter levels at nerve synapses, this tricyclic antidepressant may elevate mood.

Contraindications
Acute recovery phase of CVA or MI; hypersensitivity to nortriptyline, other tricyclic antidepressants, or their components; use within 14 days of MAO inhibitor therapy

Interactions
DRUGS
amantadine, anticholinergics, antidyskinetics, antihistamines: Possibly increased anticholinergic effects, confusion, hallucinations, nightmares; increased CNS depression
anticonvulsants: Possibly increased CNS depression and risk of seizures, possibly decreased anticonvulsant effectiveness
antithyroid drugs: Possibly agranulocytosis
barbiturates, carbamazepine: Possibly decreased blood level and effectiveness of nortriptyline
bupropion, clozapine, cyclobenzaprine, haloperidol, loxapine, maprotiline, molindone, phenothiazines, thioxanthenes: Possibly increased sedative and anticholinergic effects of these drugs, possibly increased risk of seizures
cimetidine, fluoxetine: Possibly increased blood nortriptyline level and risk of toxicity
clonidine: Possibly decreased antihypertensive effect of clonidine, increased CNS depression
disulfiram: Possibly delirium
ethchlorvynol: Possibly delirium, increased CNS depression
guanadrel, guanethidine: Possibly decreased antihypertensive effect of these drugs
MAO inhibitors: Increased risk of hypertensive crisis, severe seizures, and death
oral anticoagulants: Possibly increased anticoagulant activity
pimozide, probucol: Possibly arrhythmias
sympathomimetics, including ophthalmic epinephrine and vasoconstrictive local anesthetics: Increased risk of arrhythmias, hyperpyrexia, hypertension, and tachycardia
thyroid hormones: Possibly increased therapeutic and toxic effects of both drugs
ACTIVITIES
alcohol use: Increased CNS and respiratory depression, hypertension, and alcohol effects

Adverse Reactions
CNS: Ataxia, confusion, CVA, delirium, dizziness, drowsiness, excitation, hallucinations, headache, insomnia, nervousness, nightmares, parkinsonism, tremor
CV: Arrhythmias, orthostatic hypotension
EENT: Blurred vision, dry mouth, increased intraocular pressure, taste perversion
GI: Constipation, diarrhea, heartburn, ileus, increased appetite, nausea, vomiting

GU: Sexual dysfunction, urine retention
HEME: Bone marrow depression
RESP: Wheezing
SKIN: Diaphoresis, urticaria
Other: Weight gain

Nursing Considerations
•Expect to discontinue MAO inhibitor therapy 10 to 14 days before starting nortriptyline therapy.
•Be aware that nortriptyline oral solution (10 mg/5 ml) contains 4% alcohol.
•Give drug with food to reduce adverse GI reactions.
•Monitor blood nortriptyline level; therapeutic range is 50 to 150 ng/ml.
•Monitor ECG tracing as appropriate to detect arrhythmias.

PATIENT TEACHING
•Inform patient that nortriptyline oral solution contains alcohol in case patient has a history of alcohol abuse.
•Discourage patient from drinking alcohol during nortriptyline therapy.
•Inform patient that improvement may not occur for several weeks.
•Advise patient to avoid potentially hazardous activities until drug's CNS effects are known.
•Instruct patient to change position slowly to minimize effects of orthostatic hypotension.
•Suggest that patient minimize constipation by drinking plenty of fluids (if allowed), eating high-fiber foods, and exercising regularly.

nystatin
Mycostatin, Nadostine (CAN), Nilstat, Nystex, Nystop, Pedi-Dri

Class and Category
Chemical: Amphoteric polyene macrolide
Therapeutic: Antifungal
Pregnancy category: Not rated (lozenges, oral suspension, tablets, topical forms), A (vaginal form)

Indications and Dosages
➤ *To treat oropharyngeal candidiasis (thrush)*
LOZENGES (PASTILLES)
Adults and children over age 5. 200,000 to 400,000 U dissolved in mouth 4 or 5 times/day for up to 14 days.
ORAL SUSPENSION
Adults and children. 400,000 to 600,000 U swished and swallowed q.i.d. until at least 48 hr after symptoms subside.

Infants. 200,000 U applied to each side of mouth q.i.d. until at least 48 hr after symptoms subside.
Neonates. 100,000 U applied to each side of mouth q.i.d. until at least 48 hr after symptoms subside.
TABLETS
Adults and adolescents. 500,000 to 1,000,000 U t.i.d. until at least 48 hr after symptoms subside.
Children age 5 and older. 500,000 U q.i.d. until at least 48 hr after symptoms subside.
➤ *To treat cutaneous and mucocutaneous candidiasis*
CREAM, OINTMENT, POWDER
Adults and children. 100,000 U (1 g) applied to affected area b.i.d. or t.i.d. for at least 2 wk.
➤ *To treat vulvovaginal candidiasis*
VAGINAL TABLETS
Adults and adolescents. 100,000 U (1 tab) q.d. or b.i.d. for 14 days.

Mechanism of Action
Binds to sterols in fungal cell membranes, thereby impairing membrane integrity. As a result, fungal cells lose intracellular potassium and other cellular contents and, eventually, die.

Contraindications
Hypersensitivity to nystatin or its components

Adverse Reactions
ENDO: Hyperglycemia (lozenge, oral suspension)
GI: Abdominal pain, diarrhea, nausea, vomiting (oral forms)
GU: Vaginal burning or itching (vaginal form)
SKIN: Irritation (topical forms)

Nursing Considerations
•Prepare nystatin powder for oral suspension individually for each dose because it contains no preservatives.
•Gently rub nystatin cream or ointment into skin at affected area. Keep area dry and avoid occlusive dressings.
•Don't let topical form come in contact with patient's eyes.
•When treating candidal infection of feet, dust patient's shoes and socks as well as her feet with drug.
•For vaginal form, use applicator supplied by manufacturer.

N O

PATIENT TEACHING

•Instruct patient to let nystatin lozenges dissolve slowly in her mouth, not to chew or swallow them.

•Instruct patient to swish oral suspension in her mouth for as long as possible before swallowing.

•Advise patient to gently rub ointment or cream into skin at affected area, to keep area dry, and to avoid occlusive dressings.

•Caution patient to keep topical form away from her eyes.

•Advise patient with candidal infection of feet to dust her shoes, socks, and feet with nystatin.

•Instruct patient who uses vaginal form to insert it with applicator supplied by manufacturer.

octreotide acetate

Sandostatin, Sandostatin LAR Depot

Class and Category

Chemical: Cyclic octapeptide, somatostatin analogue

Therapeutic: Antidiarrheal, hormone suppressant

Pregnancy category: B

Indications and Dosages

➤ *To control symptoms associated with vasoactive intestinal peptide tumors (watery diarrhea) and metastatic carcinoid tumors (diarrhea and flushing)*

I.M. INJECTION

Adults currently receiving S.C. injections. 20 mg q 4 wk for 2 mo, with S.C. doses continued for 2 to 4 wk after I.M. injections start. If patient has positive response to initial 2-mo regimen, dosage reduced to 10 mg q 4 wk. If symptoms persist or increase after initial 2-mo regimen, dosage increased to 30 mg q 4 wk, as prescribed.

S.C. INJECTION

Adults. *Initial:* 200 to 300 mcg/day in divided doses b.i.d. to q.i.d. for first 2 wk. *Maintenance:* Individualized. *Maximum:* 450 mcg/day.

➤ *To treat symptoms of acromegaly, to suppress the release of growth hormone from pituitary tumors*

I.V. OR S.C. INJECTION

Adults. *Initial:* 50 mcg t.i.d. *Usual:* 100 mcg t.i.d. *Maximum:* 1,500 mcg/day.

I.M. INJECTION

Adults currently receiving S.C. injections. 20 mg q 4 wk for 3 mo, then adjusted as prescribed in response to serum growth hormone level. *Maximum:* 40 mg q 4 wk.

Route	Onset	Peak	Duration
S.C.	Unknown	Unknown	Up to 12 hr

Mechanism of Action

Controls many types of secretory diarrhea by inhibiting secretion of serotonin and pituitary and GI hormones (including insulin, glucagon, growth hormone, thyrotropin, and, possibly, thyroid-stimulating hormone) as well as vasoactive intestinal peptides and pancreatic polypeptides (including gastrin, secretin, and motilin). Inhibition of serotonin and peptides increases intestinal absorption of water and electrolytes, decreases pancreatic and gastric acid secretions, and increases intestinal transit time by slowing gastric motility.

By inhibiting hormones involved in vasodilation, octreotide increases splanchnic arterial resistance and decreases GI blood flow, hepatic vein wedge pressure, hepatic blood flow, portal vein pressure, and intravariceal pressure, thus raising seated and standing blood pressures. By inhibiting serotonin secretion, the drug decreases symptoms of acromegaly, including diarrhea, flushing, wheezing, and urinary excretion of 5-hydroxyindoleacetic acid.

Incompatibilities

Don't mix octreotide in same syringe with fat emulsions or total parenteral nutrition solutions.

Contraindications

Hypersensitivity to octreotide or its components

Interactions

DRUGS

beta blockers, calcium channel blockers: Additive cardiovascular effects of these drugs

cisapride: Decreased effectiveness of both drugs

cyclosporine: Decreased blood cyclosporine level

diuretics: Increased risk of fluid and electrolyte imbalances

insulin, oral antidiabetic drugs: Increased risk of hypoglycemia
vitamin B$_{12}$: Decreased blood levels of vitamin B$_{12}$

Adverse Reactions
CNS: Dizziness, drowsiness, fatigue, headache
CV: Arrhythmias (including conduction abnormalities), edema, hypotension, orthostatic hypotension
EENT: Vision changes
ENDO: Hyperglycemia, hypoglycemia
GI: Abdominal pain, acute cholecystitis, ascending cholangitis, biliary obstruction, cholelithiasis, cholestatic hepatitis, constipation, flatulence, nausea, pancreatitis, vomiting
GU: Increased urine output
Other: Dehydration, electrolyte imbalances, injection site irritation

Nursing Considerations
•Give octreotide by I.V. injection only in an emergency, as prescribed.
•To prepare depot injection (long-acting suspension form), let powder and diluent warm to room temperature and then reconstitute according to manufacturer's instructions. Gently inject 2 ml of supplied diluent down side of vial without disturbing depot powder. Let diluent saturate powder. After 2 to 5 minutes, check sides and bottom of vial without inverting it. Once powder is completely saturated, swirl—don't shake—vial for 30 to 60 seconds to form suspension. Use immediately after reconstituting.
•Don't give depot injection by S.C. route; give only by I.M. route and only to patients who respond to and tolerate S.C. drug, as prescribed.
•To minimize pain, use smallest injection volume to deliver desired dose and rotate injection sites.
•Avoid using deltoid site for I.M. injection because injection site reactions and pain may result. Intragluteal injection is recommended.
•WARNING To avoid worsening of symptoms, expect to continue S.C. injections when switching to I.M. injections, as prescribed.
•Be aware that octreotide increases risk of acute cholecystitis, ascending cholangitis, biliary obstruction, cholestatic hepatitis, and pancreatitis.
•Monitor vital signs, bowels sounds, and stool consistency. Assess for abdominal pain

and signs of gallbladder disease.
•Monitor serum liver enzyme levels, as appropriate.
•Monitor for signs of electrolyte imbalances and dehydration.
•Carefully monitor diabetic patient for altered glucose control.
•If patient has periodic flare-ups of symptoms, expect to give additional S.C. octreotide temporarily, as prescribed.
PATIENT TEACHING
•Advise patient to change position slowly to minimize effects of orthostatic hypotension.
•Instruct patient to notify prescriber about adverse reactions, especially abdominal pain, which may indicate pancreatitis.
•Urge diabetic patient to monitor blood glucose level frequently.

ofloxacin
Floxin

Class and Category
Chemical: Fluoroquinolone
Therapeutic: Antibiotic
Pregnancy category: C

Indications and Dosages
➤ *To treat acute, uncomplicated cystitis caused by* Escherichia coli *or* Klebsiella pneumoniae
TABLETS, I.V. INFUSION
Adults. 200 mg q 12 hr for 3 days.
➤ *To treat uncomplicated cystitis caused by* Citrobacter diversus, Enterobacter aerogenes, Proteus mirabilis, *or* Pseudomonas aeruginosa
TABLETS, I.V. INFUSION
Adults. 200 mg q 12 hr for 7 days.
➤ *To treat complicated UTIs caused by* C. diversus, E. coli, K. pneumoniae, P. mirabilis, *or* P. aeruginosa
TABLETS, I.V. INFUSION
Adults. 200 mg q 12 hr for 10 days.
➤ *To treat uncomplicated gonorrhea*
TABLETS, I.V. INFUSION
Adults and adolescents. 400 mg as a single dose.
➤ *To treat urethritis or cervicitis caused by* Chlamydia trachomatis *or* Neisseria gonorrhoeae

TABLETS, I.V. INFUSION
Adults and adolescents. 300 mg b.i.d. for 7 days as an alternative to doxycycline or azithromycin.
➤ *To treat pelvic inflammatory disease caused by susceptible organisms*
TABLETS
Adults and adolescents. 400 mg b.i.d. with metronidazole P.O. for 10 to 14 days.
I.V. INFUSION
Adults and adolescents. 400 mg q 12 hr with metronidazole I.V. and then switched to oral therapy, as prescribed, after 24 hr. Complete course of therapy lasts 14 days.
➤ *To treat prostatitis caused by* E. coli
TABLETS, I.V. INFUSION
Adults. 300 mg q 12 hr for 6 wk.
➤ *To treat lower respiratory tract infections caused by* Haemophilus influenzae *or* Streptococcus pneumoniae *and skin and soft-tissue infections caused by* Staphylococcus aureus *or* Streptococcus pyogenes
TABLETS, I.V. INFUSION
Adults. 400 mg q 12 hr for 10 days.
DOSAGE ADJUSTMENT For patients with creatinine clearance of 20 to 50 ml/min/1.73 m^2, dosing frequency possibly reduced to q 24 hr; for creatinine clearance of less than 10 ml/min/1.73 m^2, dosage possibly reduced by 50% and given q 24 hr.

Mechanism of Action
Inhibits synthesis of the bacterial enzyme DNA gyrase by counteracting the excessive supercoiling of DNA during replication or transcription. Inhibition of DNA gyrase causes rapid- and slow-growing bacterial cells to die.

Incompatibilities
Don't mix ofloxacin with other I.V. drugs or additives.

Contraindications
Hypersensitivity to ofloxacin, other fluoroquinolones, or their components

Interactions
DRUGS
aluminum-, calcium-, or magnesium-containing antacids; didanosine; ferrous sulfate; magnesium-containing laxatives; multivitamins; sevelamer; sucralfate; zinc: Decreased absorption of oral ofloxacin

probenecid: Decreased ofloxacin excretion, increased risk of toxicity
procainamide: Decreased renal clearance of procainamide
warfarin: Possibly increased anticoagulant activity and risk of bleeding

Adverse Reactions
CNS: Dizziness, drowsiness, headache, insomnia
GI: Abdominal cramps or pain, diarrhea, nausea, pseudomembranous colitis, vomiting
GU: Vaginal candidiasis
MS: Tendinitis; tendon inflammation, pain, or rupture
SKIN: Blisters, diaphoresis, erythema, erythema multiforme, exfoliative dermatitis, photosensitivity, pruritus, rash, Stevens-Johnson syndrome, toxic epidermal necrolysis, urticaria
Other: Infusion site phlebitis

Nursing Considerations
•For I.V. infusion, dilute drug in NS or D$_5$W to at least 4 mg/ml, and infuse over 60 minutes to minimize the risk of hypotension. Discard unused portion.
•Stop drug and notify prescriber immediately if patient has severe (toxic) photosensitivity reaction or tendon pain.
•Maintain adequate hydration to prevent highly concentrated urine and crystalluria.
•Expect an increased risk of drug toxicity in patients with severe hepatic disease, including cirrhosis.
•Be aware that ofloxacin may stimulate the CNS and aggravate seizure disorders.
•If diarrhea develops, consider the possibility of pseudomembranous colitis, a complication of long-term use.
•Be alert for signs and symptoms of secondary fungal infection.
PATIENT TEACHING
•Encourage patient to take each oral dose with a full glass of water.
•Instruct patient not to take antacids or iron or zinc preparations within 2 hours of ofloxacin to prevent decreased or delayed drug absorption.
•Caution patient to avoid excessive exposure to sun and other forms of ultraviolet light to prevent phototoxicity.
•Advise patient to notify prescriber immediately about burning skin, hives, itching, rapid heart rate, rash, and tendon pain.
•Urge patient to seek medical attention imme-

diately for trouble breathing or swallowing, which may be signs of an allergic reaction.

olanzapine
Zydis, Zyprexa

Class and Category
Chemical: Thienobenzodiazepine derivative
Therapeutic: Antipsychotic
Pregnancy category: C

Indications and Dosages
➤ *To treat psychosis*
ORALLY DISINTEGRATING TABLETS, TABLETS
Adults. *Initial:* 5 to 10 mg q.d. *Usual:* 10 mg/day. *Maximum:* 20 mg/day
➤ *To treat manic phase of acute bipolar disorder*
ORALLY DISINTEGRATING TABLETS, TABLETS
Adults. *Initial:* 10 to 15 mg q.d.; may be increased or decreased by 5 mg q 24 hr as needed and prescribed. *Usual:* 5 to 20 mg q.d. for 3 to 4 wk. *Maximum:* 20 mg/day.
DOSAGE ADJUSTMENT Initial dosage possibly reduced to 5 mg for debilitated patients, those prone to hypotension, and nonsmoking women over age 65.

Route	Onset	Peak	Duration
P.O.	1 wk	Unknown	Unknown

Mechanism of Action
May achieve its antipsychotic effects by antagonizing dopamine and serotonin receptors. Anticholinergic effects may result from competitive binding to and antagonism of muscarinic receptors M_1 through M_5.

Contraindications
Blood dyscrasias, bone marrow depression, cerebral arteriosclerosis, coma, coronary artery disease, hepatic dysfunction, high-dose therapy with CNS depressants, hypersensitivity to olanzapine or its components, hypertension, hypotension, myeloproliferative disorders, severe CNS depression, subcortical brain damage

Interactions
DRUGS
anticholinergics: Increased anticholinergic effects, altered thermoregulation
antihypertensives: Increased effects of both drugs, increased risk of hypotension

carbamazepine, omeprazole, rifampin: Increased olanzapine clearance
CNS depressants: Additive CNS depression, potentiated orthostatic hypotension
diazepam: Increased CNS depressant effects
fluvoxamine: Decreased olanzapine clearance
levodopa: Decreased levodopa efficacy
ACTIVITIES
alcohol use: Additive CNS depression, potentiated orthostatic hypotension
smoking: Decreased blood olanzapine level

Adverse Reactions
CNS: Agitation, altered thermoregulation, amnesia, anxiety, dizziness, euphoria, fever, headache, nervousness, neuroleptic malignant syndrome, restlessness, somnolence, stuttering, tardive dyskinesia, tremor
CV: Chest pain, hypotension, orthostatic hypotension, peripheral edema, tachycardia
EENT: Amblyopia, dry mouth, increased salivation, pharyngitis, rhinitis
GI: Abdominal pain, constipation, dysphagia, increased appetite, nausea, thirst, vomiting
GU: Urinary incontinence
MS: Arthralgia, muscle spasms and twitching
RESP: Cough
SKIN: Photosensitivity
Other: Flulike symptoms, weight gain

Nursing Considerations
• Be aware that olanzapine may worsen such conditions as angle-closure glaucoma, benign prostatic hyperplasia, and seizures.
• Assess daily weight to detect fluid retention.
• Notify prescriber if patient develops tardive dyskinesia or urinary incontinence.
• Be alert for and immediately report to prescriber signs of neuroleptic malignant syndrome.
• Monitor patient for suicidal tendencies. Notify prescriber and implement suicide precautions according to facility policy.
PATIENT TEACHING
• Advise patient to avoid alcohol and smoking during olanzapine therapy.
• Teach patient to open the orally disintegrating tablet sachet by peeling back the foil on the blister and not to push tablet through the foil. Immediately after opening the blister, tell him to use dry hands to remove tablet and place it in his mouth. Explain that tablet will disintegrate rapidly in his saliva so that he can easily swallow it without liquid.

•Caution patient with phenylketonuria that disintegrating tablets contain phenylalanine.
•Urge patient to avoid potentially hazardous activities until drug's CNS effects are known.
•Instruct patient to change position slowly to minimize effects of orthostatic hypotension.

olmesartan medoxomil

Benicar

Class and Category

Chemical: Angiotensin II receptor antagonist
Therapeutic: Antihypertensive
Pregnancy category: C (first trimester), D (later trimesters)

Indications and Dosages

➤ *To manage or as adjunct to manage hypertension*

TABLETS

Adults. *Initial:* 20 mg q.d., increased in 2 wk to 40 mg q.d., if needed.

DOSAGE ADJUSTMENT Lower starting dosage is recommended for patients with possible depletion of intravascular volume, such as those treated with diuretics, especially if impaired renal function is present.

Contraindications

Hypersensitivity to olmesartan medoxomil or its components

Interactions

None known

Adverse Reactions

CNS: Dizziness, fatigue, headache, vertigo
CV: Chest pain, hypercholesterolemia, hyperlipemia, hypertriglyceridemia, insomnia, peripheral edema, tachycardia
EENT: Pharyngitis, rhinitis, sinusitis
ENDO: Hyperglycemia, hyperuricemia
GI: Abdominal pain, diarrhea, dyspepsia, gastroenteritis, nausea
GU: Elevated BUN and serum creatinine levels, hematuria, urinary tract infection
MS: Arthralgia, arthritis, back pain, myalgia, skeletal pain
RESP: Bronchitis, cough, upper respiratory infection
SKIN: Rash
Other: Facial angioedema, increased creatine phosphokinase level, flulike symptoms, pain

Nursing Considerations

•Expect to provide treatment such as NS solution I.V., as prescribed, to correct known or suspected hypovolemia before beginning olmesartan therapy.
•Monitor patient for increased BUN and serum creatinine levels, especially in a patient with impaired renal function, because drug may cause acute renal failure. If increased levels are significant or persistent, notify prescriber immediately.

Mechanism of Action

Olmesartan medoxomil blocks angiotensin II from binding to receptor sites in many tissues, including vascular smooth muscle and adrenal glands. Angiotensin II, a potent vasoconstrictor, is then free to stimulate the adrenal cortex to secrete aldosterone, and the inhibiting effects of angiotensin II reduce blood pressure.

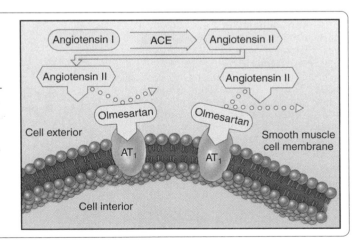

•Monitor blood pressure frequently to assess effectiveness of therapy. If blood pressure isn't controlled with olmesartan alone, expect to administer a diuretic, such as hydrochlorothiazide, as prescribed.

•**WARNING** Monitor patient's blood pressure frequently if she receives a diuretic or other antihypertensive during olmesartan therapy because of an increased risk of hypotension.

•Expect to discontinue drug temporarily if patient experiences hypotension. If hypotension occurs, place patient in supine position immediately and prepare to administer NS solution I.V., as prescribed. Expect to resume drug therapy after blood pressure stabilizes.

•If patient also receives a diuretic, provide adequate hydration, as appropriate, to help prevent hypovolemia. Monitor her for signs and symptoms of hypovolemia, such as hypotension with dizziness and fainting.

PATIENT TEACHING

•Advise patient to avoid exercise in hot weather and excessive alcohol use to reduce the risk of dehydration and hypotension. Also instruct her to notify prescriber if she experiences prolonged diarrhea, nausea, or vomiting.

•Caution patient to avoid potentially hazardous activities until drug's CNS effects are known.

•Explain the importance of regular exercise, proper diet, and other lifestyle changes in controlling hypertension.

•Advise female patient to notify prescriber immediately about known or suspected pregnancy. Explain that if she becomes pregnant, prescriber may replace olmesartan with another antihypertensive that is safe to use during pregnancy.

olsalazine sodium

Dipentum

Class and Category

Chemical: Salicylate derivative
Therapeutic: Bowel disease suppressant
Pregnancy category: C

Indications and Dosages

➤ *To maintain remission of ulcerative colitis*
TABLETS
Adults and adolescents. 500 mg b.i.d.

Mechanism of Action

Exerts an anti-inflammatory action in the GI tract after being converted by colonic bacteria to mesalamine (5-aminosalicylic acid), which inhibits cyclooxygenase. Inhibition of cyclooxygenase reduces prostaglandin production in the intestinal mucosa. This in turn reduces production of arachidonic acid metabolites, which may be increased in patients with inflammatory bowel disease. Olsalazine also exerts an anti-inflammatory effect by indirectly inhibiting leukotriene synthesis, which normally catalyzes the production of arachidonic acid.

Contraindications

Hypersensitivity to olsalazine, salicylates, or their components

Interactions

DRUGS
oral anticoagulants: Possibly prolonged PT

Adverse Reactions

CNS: Anxiety, depression, dizziness, headache, insomnia
CV: Hot flashes, pericarditis, second-degree AV block
EENT: Dry eyes and mouth, lacrimation, tinnitus
GI: Abdominal pain, anorexia, diarrhea, nausea, vomiting
GU: Dysuria, hematuria, nephrotic syndrome, urinary frequency
HEME: Hemolytic anemia, lymphopenia, neutropenia
MS: Muscle spasms, myalgia
SKIN: Acne, alopecia, erythema nodosum, photosensitivity
Other: Dehydration

Nursing Considerations

•Assess for aspirin allergy before giving olsalazine.

•Assess quantity and consistency of stools and frequency of bowel movements before, during, and after therapy.

•Give drug with food to decrease adverse GI reactions.

•Monitor skin turgor for signs of adequate hydration.

•Assess for abdominal pain and hyperactive bowel sounds.

•Monitor renal function studies, as appropriate.

N
O

PATIENT TEACHING
•Instruct patient to take olsalazine with food.
•Urge patient to continue taking drug as prescribed, even if symptoms improve.
•Advise patient to watch for signs of dehydration.

omeprazole

Losec (CAN), Prilosec

Class and Category

Chemical: Substituted benzimidazole
Therapeutic: Antiulcer
Pregnancy category: C

Indications and Dosages

➤ *To treat gastroesophageal reflux disease without esophageal lesions, to prevent erosive esophagitis*

DELAYED-RELEASE CAPSULES, DELAYED-RELEASE TABLETS

Adults. 20 mg q.d. for 4 wk.

➤ *To treat gastroesophageal reflux disease with erosive esophagitis*

DELAYED-RELEASE CAPSULES, DELAYED-RELEASE TABLETS

Adults. 20 mg q.d. for 4 to 8 wk.

➤ *To provide short-term treatment of active benign gastric ulcer*

DELAYED-RELEASE CAPSULES

Adults. 40 mg q.d. for 4 to 8 wk.

DELAYED-RELEASE TABLETS

Adults. 20 mg q.d. for 4 to 8 wk, increased to 40 mg q.d., p.r.n.

➤ *To treat duodenal or gastric ulcer associated with* Helicobacter pylori

DELAYED-RELEASE CAPSULES

Adults. 40 mg q.d. with clarithromycin for 14 days, followed by 20 mg q.d. alone for another 14 days; or 20 mg b.i.d. with amoxicillin for 14 days; or 20 mg b.i.d. with amoxicillin and clarithromycin for 10 days.

DELAYED-RELEASE TABLETS

Adults. 20 mg b.i.d. with clarithromycin and amoxicillin or metronidazole for 7 days, followed by 20 mg q.d. for up to 3 wk (for duodenal ulcer) or 20 to 40 mg q.d. for up to 12 wk (for gastric ulcer).

➤ *To provide long-term treatment of gastric hypersecretory conditions, such as multiple endocrine adenoma syndrome, systemic mastocytosis, and Zollinger-Ellison syndrome*

DELAYED-RELEASE CAPSULES, DELAYED-RELEASE TABLETS

Adults. 60 mg q.d. or in divided doses, as prescribed. *Maximum:* 120 mg t.i.d.

Route	Onset	Peak	Duration
P.O.	1 hr	In 2 hr	72 to 96 hr

Contraindications

Hypersensitivity to omeprazole, other proton pump inhibitors, or their components

Interactions

DRUGS

alprazolam, astemizole, carbamazepine, cisapride, cyclosporine, diazepam, diltiazem, erythromycin, felodipine, lidocaine, lovastatin, midazolam, quinidine, simvastatin, terfenadine, triazolam, verapamil: Decreased clearance and increased blood levels of these drugs

ampicillin, iron salts, itraconazole, ketoconazole, vitamin B_{12}: Impaired absorption of these drugs

cilostazol: Increased blood cilostazol level

digoxin: Increased digoxin bioavailability, possibly digitalis toxicity

levobupivacaine: Increased risk of levobupivacaine toxicity

methotrexate: Possibly delayed methotrexate elimination

nifedipine: Decreased nifedipine clearance, increased risk of hypotension

phenytoin: Decreased phenytoin clearance, increased risk of phenytoin toxicity

sucralfate: Decreased omeprazole absorption

Adverse Reactions

CNS: Dizziness, drowsiness, fatigue, headache, somnolence

GI: Abdominal pain, constipation, diarrhea, elevated liver function test results, flatulence, indigestion, nausea, vomiting

HEME: Anemia

SKIN: Pruritus, rash

Nursing Considerations

•Give omeprazole before meals, preferably in the morning for once-daily dosing. If necessary, also give an antacid, as prescribed.

•If necessary, open capsule and sprinkle enteric-coated granules on applesauce or yogurt or mix granules with water or an acidic fruit juice, such as apple or cranberry juice. Administer immediately.

•To give drug through an NG tube, mix granules in an acidic juice because enteric coating dissolves in alkaline pH.

•Because drug can interfere with absorption of vitamin B_{12}, monitor for macrocytic anemia.

•Be aware that long-term use of omeprazole may increase the risk of gastric carcinoma.

Mechanism of Action

Omeprazole interferes with gastric acid secretion by inhibiting the hydrogen-potassium-adenosine triphosphatase (H^+K^+-ATPase) enzyme system, or proton pump, in gastric parietal cells. Normally, the proton pump uses energy from the hydrolysis of adenosine triphosphate to drive hydrogen (H^+) and chloride (Cl^-) out of parietal cells and into the stomach lumen in exchange for potassium (K^+), which leaves the stomach lumen and enters the parietal cells. After this exchange, H^+ and Cl^- combine in the stomach to form hydrochloric acid (HCl), as shown below left. Omeprazole irreversibly blocks the exchange of intracellular H^+ and extracellular K^+, as shown below right. By preventing H^+ from entering the stomach lumen, omeprazole prevents additional HCl from forming.

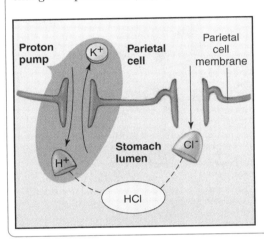

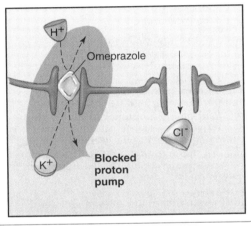

- Instruct patient to take omeprazole before eating—usually before breakfast—and to swallow delayed-release capsules or tablets whole, not chew or crush them.
- Stress the need to take drug exactly as prescribed to prevent recurrence of symptoms.
- Encourage patient to avoid alcohol, aspirin products, ibuprofen, and foods that may increase gastric secretions during therapy.
- Advise patient to notify prescriber immediately about abdominal pain or diarrhea.
- Urge female patient of childbearing age to use effective contraceptive method during therapy and to inform prescriber immediately if she becomes or suspects she may be pregnant.

ondansetron hydrochloride

Zofran, Zofran ODT

Class and Category

Chemical: Carbazole
Therapeutic: Antiemetic
Pregnancy category: B

Indications and Dosages

➤ *To prevent chemotherapy-induced nausea and vomiting*

DISINTEGRATING TABLETS, ORAL SOLUTION, TABLETS
Adults and children age 12 and older. *Initial:* 8 mg given 30 min before chemotherapy. *Postchemotherapy:* 8 mg given 8 hr after initial dose, then 8 mg q 12 hr for 1 to 2 days.
Children ages 4 to 12. *Initial:* 4 mg given 30 min before chemotherapy. *Postchemotherapy:* 4 mg given 4 and 8 hr after initial dose, then 4 mg q 8 hr for 1 to 2 days.

I.V. INFUSION
Adults. 32 mg infused over 15 min, starting 30 min before chemotherapy; or 8 mg infused over 15 min, starting 30 min before chemotherapy, followed by continuous infusion of 1 mg/hr for 24 hr.

N O

Children ages 4 to 18. 3 to 5 mg/m^2 infused over 15 min immediately before chemotherapy, followed by 4 mg P.O. q 8 hr for 5 days or less.

I.V. INFUSION (3-DOSE REGIMEN)
Adults and children ages 4 to 18. 150 mcg/kg infused over 15 min, starting 30 min before chemotherapy; then 150 mcg/kg 4 and 8 hr after first dose.

➤ *To prevent postoperative nausea and vomiting*

DISINTEGRATING TABLETS, ORAL SOLUTION, TABLETS
Adults. 16 mg as a single dose 1 hr before anesthesia induction.

I.V. INFUSION
Adults and children age 12 and older. 4 mg as a single dose just before anesthesia induction or if nausea or vomiting develops shortly after surgery.
Children ages 2 to 12 who weigh more than 40 kg (88 lb). 4 mg as a single dose just before anesthesia induction or if nausea or vomiting develops shortly after surgery.
Children ages 2 to 12 who weigh less than 40 kg. 0.1 mg/kg as a single dose just before anesthesia induction or if nausea or vomiting develops shortly after surgery.

I.M. INJECTION
Adults and children age 12 and older. 4 mg as a single dose just before anesthesia induction or if nausea or vomiting develops shortly after surgery.

➤ *To prevent nausea and vomiting after radiation therapy*

DISINTEGRATING TABLETS, ORAL SOLUTION, TABLETS
Adults and children age 12 and older. *Initial:* 8 mg as a single dose given 1 to 2 hr before radiation therapy. *Posttherapy:* 8 mg q 8 hr, as needed and tolerated.
DOSAGE ADJUSTMENT For patients with hepatic impairment, maximum dosage limited to 8 mg/day I.V. or P.O.

Incompatibilities

Don't administer ondansetron through same I.V. line as acyclovir, allopurinol, aminophylline, amphotericin B, ampicillin, ampicillin and sulbactam, amsacrine, cefepime, cefoperazone, furosemide, ganciclovir, lorazepam, methylprednisolone, mezlocillin, piperacillin, or sargramostim. Alkaline solutions and highly concentrated solutions of fluorouracil are also physically incompatible.

Mechanism of Action

Blocks serotonin receptors centrally in the chemoreceptor trigger zone and peripherally at vagal nerve terminals in the intestine. This action reduces nausea and vomiting by preventing serotonin release in the small intestine (the probable cause of chemotherapy- and radiation therapy-induced nausea and vomiting) and by blocking signals to the CNS. Ondansetron may also bind to other serotonin receptors and to mu-opioid receptors.

Contraindications

Hypersensitivity to ondansetron or its components

Interactions
DRUGS
cisplatin, cyclophosphamide: Possibly altered blood levels of these drugs
ACTIVITIES
alcohol use: Increased stimulant and sedative effects, including mood and physical sensations

Adverse Reactions

CNS: Akathisia, ataxia, dizziness, fever, headache, restlessness, seizures, weakness
CV: Chest pain, hypotension, pulmonary embolism, tachycardia
EENT: Accommodation disturbances, altered taste, blurred vision, dry mouth
GI: Abdominal pain, anorexia, constipation, diarrhea, elevated liver function test results, flatulence, indigestion, intestinal obstruction, thirst
SKIN: Flushing, hyperpigmentation, maculopapular rash, pruritus
Other: Injection site burning, pain, and redness

Nursing Considerations

•**WARNING** Be aware that oral disintegrating tablets may contain aspartame, which is metabolized to phenylalanine and must be used cautiously in patients with phenylketonuria.
•Place disintegrating tablet on patient's tongue immediately after opening package. It dissolves in seconds.
•Use calibrated container or oral syringe to measure dose of oral solution.
•Give up to 4 mg I.V. diluted in 50 ml of D$_5$W or NS.
•**WARNING** Be aware that ondansetron may mask symptoms of adynamic ileus or gastric distention after abdominal surgery.

• Advise patient to use calibrated container or oral syringe to measure dose for oral solution.
• Instruct patient to place ondansetron disintegrating tablet on his tongue immediately after opening package and to let it dissolve on his tongue before swallowing.
• Advise patient to notify prescriber immediately about signs of hypersensitivity reaction, such as rash.

orlistat

Xenical

Class and Category
Chemical: Lipase inhibitor
Therapeutic: Antiobesity
Pregnancy category: B

Indications and Dosages
➤ *To promote weight loss in patients with a body mass index above 30 kg (66 lb)/m² (27 kg [59.4 lb]/m² in patients with diabetes mellitus, hyperlipidemia, or hypertension)*

GELCAPS
Adults. 120 mg t.i.d. with fat-containing meals.

Contraindications
Cholestasis, chronic malabsorption syndrome, hypersensitivity to orlistat or its components

Interactions
DRUGS
cyclosporine: Altered cyclosporine absorption
fat-soluble vitamins: Decreased vitamin absorption, especially vitamin E and beta-carotene
pravastatin: Potentiated lipid-lowering effect

Adverse Reactions
CNS: Anxiety, depression, dizziness, fatigue, headache, sleep disturbance
CV: Pedal edema
EENT: Gingival or tooth disorder
GI: Abdominal discomfort or pain, diarrhea (infectious), fatty or oily stool, fecal incontinence or urgency, flatulence with discharge, increased frequency of bowel movements, nausea, rectal pain, vomiting
GU: Menstrual irregularities, UTI, vaginitis
MS: Arthralgia, arthritis, back pain, leg pain, myalgia, tendinitis

Mechanism of Action
In the GI tract, orlistat binds with and inactivates gastric and pancreatic enzymes known as lipases, as shown. Normally, lipase enzymes convert ingested triglycerides into absorbable free fatty acids and monoglycerides. By inactivating lipase, orlistat allows undigested triglycerides to pass through the GI tract and exit the body in feces. Blocking the absorption of some of these fats lowers the number of calories the person receives from food, which promotes weight loss.

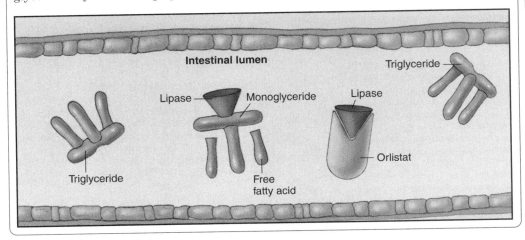

N
O

RESP: Respiratory tract infection
SKIN: Dry skin, rash
Other: Flulike symptoms

Nursing Considerations
•Give orlistat with or up to 1 hour after meals that contain fat.
•Consult prescriber if you think that patient has an eating disorder, such as anorexia nervosa or bulimia.

PATIENT TEACHING
•Instruct patient to take orlistat with or shortly after meals that contain fat.
•Advise patient to take a multivitamin that contains fat-soluble vitamins and beta-carotene at least 2 hours before or after taking drug, if indicated.
•Inform patient about drug's adverse GI effects, but explain that reducing dietary fat may decrease them. Instruct him to notify prescriber if they become too unpleasant.
•Help patient plan a reduced-fat diet (less than 30% of daily calories) and an exercise program to promote weight loss.
•Advise patient to weigh himself daily, at the same time and wearing similar clothes, to check his progress in losing weight.

orphenadrine citrate

Aniflex, Banflex, Flexoject, Miolin, Mio-Rel, Myotrol, Norflex, Orfro, Orphenate

orphenadrine hydrochloride

Disipal (CAN)

Class and Category
Chemical: Tertiary amine
Therapeutic: Skeletal muscle relaxant
Pregnancy category: C

Indications and Dosages
➤ *To relieve muscle spasms in painful musculoskeletal conditions*

E.R. TABLETS (ORPHENADRINE CITRATE)
Adults and adolescents. 100 mg b.i.d. in the morning and evening.

TABLETS (ORPHENADRINE HYDROCHLORIDE)
Adults and adolescents. 50 mg t.i.d. *Maximum:* 250 mg/day.

I.V. OR I.M. INJECTION (ORPHENADRINE CITRATE)
Adults and adolescents. 60 mg q 12 hr, p.r.n.

DOSAGE ADJUSTMENT Dosage reduced to 25 to 50 mg t.i.d. or q.i.d. if patient also receives aspirin and caffeine.

Route	Onset	Peak	Duration
P.O.	In 1 hr	Unknown	4 to 6 hr*
I.V.	Immediate	Unknown	4 to 6 hr
I.M.	30 min	Unknown	4 to 6 hr

Mechanism of Action
May reduce muscle spasms by acting on the cerebral motor centers or the medulla. Postganglionic anticholinergic effects and some antihistaminic and local anesthetic action contribute to skeletal muscle relaxation.

Contraindications
Angle-closure glaucoma; hypersensitivity to orphenadrine or its components; myasthenia gravis; obstruction of bladder neck, duodenum, or pylorus; prostatic hypertrophy; stenosing peptic ulcers

Interactions
DRUGS
amantadine, amitriptyline, amoxapine, antimuscarinics, atropine, bupropion, carbinoxamine, chlorpromazine, clemastine, clomipramine, clozapine, cyclobenzaprine, diphenhydramine, disopyramide, doxepin, imipramine, maprotiline, mesoridazine, methdilazine, nortriptyline, phenothiazines, procainamide, promazine, promethazine, protriptyline, thioridazine, triflupromazine, trimeprazine, trimipramine: Possibly additive anticholinergic effects
CNS depressants: Increased CNS depression
haloperidol: Increased schizophrenic symptoms, possibly tardive dyskinesia
propoxyphene: Increased risk of anxiety, confusion, and tremor
ACTIVITIES
alcohol use: Increased CNS depression

Adverse Reactions
CNS: Agitation, confusion, dizziness, drowsiness, light-headedness, syncope, tremor
CV: Palpitations, tachycardia
EENT: Blurred vision, dry eyes and mouth, increased contact lens awareness
GI: Abdominal distention, constipation, nausea, vomiting
GU: Urine retention

---

* 12 hr for extended-release.

Nursing Considerations

• Be aware that orphenadrine shouldn't be given to patients with tachycardia or cardiac insufficiency.
• Administer I.V. form over 5 minutes with patient in supine position. Have patient remain in this position for 5 to 10 minutes to minimize adverse reactions. Then assist him to sitting position.
• Be aware that drug can aggravate myasthenia gravis and cause tachycardia.
• Anticipate that drug's anticholinergic effects may cause blurred vision, dry eyes, and increased contact lens awareness.

PATIENT TEACHING

• Advise patient to avoid potentially hazardous activities until orphenadrine's CNS effects are known.
• Inform patient that dry mouth may occur but can be relieved with such measures as increased intake of fluid, ice chips, and sugarless candy or gum.
• Suggest that patient (especially one who wears contact lenses) use artificial tears during therapy to avoid discomfort from dry eyes.

oxacillin sodium

Bactocill, Prostaphlin

Class and Category

Chemical: Penicillin
Therapeutic class: Antibiotic
Pregnancy category: B

Indications and Dosages

➤ *To treat bacteremia, bone and joint infections (such as osteomyelitis and infectious arthritis), CNS infections (such as ventriculitis and meningitis), endocarditis, septicemia, skin and soft-tissue infections, upper and lower respiratory tract infections, and UTIs caused by penicillinase-producing strains of* Staphylococcus *or other susceptible organisms*

CAPSULES, ORAL SOLUTION

Adults and children who weigh 40 kg (88 lb) or more. 500 to 1,000 mg q 4 to 6 hr. *Maximum:* 6 g/day.
Children who weigh less than 40 kg. 50 to 100 mg/kg/day in divided doses q 4 to 6 hr.

➤ *To treat mild to moderate infections caused by penicillinase-producing strains of* Staphylococcus *or other susceptible organisms*

I.V. INFUSION, I.M. INJECTION

Adults and children who weigh 40 kg or more. 250 to 500 mg q 4 to 6 hr.
Infants and children who weigh less than 40 kg. 50 mg/kg/day in divided doses q 4 to 6 hr.
Neonates over age 7 days who weigh more than 2,000 g. 25 to 50 mg/kg q 6 hr.
Neonates over age 7 days who weigh less than 2,000 g. 25 to 50 mg/kg q 8 hr.
Neonates age 7 days and younger who weigh more than 2,000 g. 25 to 50 mg/kg q 8 hr.
Neonates age 7 days and younger who weigh 2,000 g or less. 25 to 50 mg/kg q 12 hr.

➤ *To treat severe infections caused by penicillinase-producing strains of* Staphylococcus *or other susceptible organisms*

I.V. INFUSION, I.M. INJECTION

Adults and children who weigh 40 kg or more. 1,000 mg q 4 to 6 hr.
Infants and children who weigh less than 40 kg. 100 to 200 mg/kg/day in divided doses q 4 to 6 hr.
Neonates over age 7 days who weigh more than 2,000 g. 25 to 50 mg/kg q 6 hr.
Neonates over age 7 days who weigh less than 2,000 g. 25 to 50 mg/kg q 8 hr.
Neonates age 7 days and younger who weigh more than 2,000 g. 25 to 50 mg/kg q 8 hr.
Neonates age 7 days and younger who weigh 2,000 g or less. 25 to 50 mg/kg q 12 hr.

➤ *To treat endocarditis caused by methicillin-susceptible* Staphylococcus aureus *in patients without a prosthetic valve*

I.V. INFUSION

Adults. 2 g q 4 hr for 4 to 6 wk.

➤ *To treat endocarditis caused by methicillin-susceptible* S. aureus *in patients with a prosthetic valve*

I.V. INFUSION

Adults. 2 g q 4 hr for at least 6 wk.

Incompatibilities

Don't give oxacillin at same time or in same admixture as aminoglycosides because they are chemically and physically incompatible and will inactivate each other.

Mechanism of Action
Inhibits bacterial cell wall synthesis. In susceptible bacteria, the rigid, cross-linked cell wall is assembled in several steps. Oxacillin exerts its effects in the final stage of the cross-linking process by binding with and inactivating penicillin-binding proteins (enzymes responsible for linking the cell wall strands). This action causes bacterial cell lysis and death.

Contraindications
Hypersensitivity to oxacillin, penicillins, or their components

Interactions
DRUGS
aminoglycosides: Inactivation of both drugs
chloramphenicol, erythromycins, sulfonamides, tetracyclines: Decreased therapeutic effects of oxacillin
oral contraceptives: Decreased contraceptive efficacy
probenecid: Increased blood oxacillin level
FOODS
all foods: Altered absorption of oxacillin

Adverse Reactions
CNS: Anxiety, depression, fatigue, hallucinations, headache, seizures
EENT: Oral candidiasis
GI: Diarrhea, nausea, pseudomembranous colitis, vomiting
GU: Interstitial nephritis, vaginal candidiasis
HEME: Agranulocytosis, anemia, granulocytopenia, neutropenia
SKIN: Exfoliative dermatitis, pruritus, rash, urticaria
Other: Anaphylaxis

Nursing Considerations
•Administer oxacillin at least 1 hour before other antibiotics.
•Give oral forms on an empty stomach, preferably 1 hour before or 2 hours after a meal, to prevent impaired absorption.
•Before reconstituting drug, loosen powder by tapping bottle several times. Reconstitute powder for I.M. injection with sterile water for injection, 0.45NS, or NS. Shake vial until solution is clear.
•For I.V. infusion, reconstitute only with NS or D$_5$W.

PATIENT TEACHING
•Advise patient to take oxacillin on an empty stomach.
•Instruct patient to notify prescriber immediately about a rash.
•Advise female patient who uses an oral contraceptive to use an additional contraceptive method during oxacillin therapy.

oxandrolone
Oxandrin

Class, Category, and Schedule
Chemical: Testosterone derivative
Therapeutic: Appetite stimulant
Pregnancy category: X
Controlled susbstance: Schedule III

Indications and Dosages
➤ *To promote weight gain after chronic infection, extensive surgery, failure to maintain weight despite no evidence of pathology, or severe trauma; to offset protein catabolism from prolonged use of corticosteroids*
TABLETS
Adults. 2.5 mg b.i.d. to q.i.d. for 2 to 4 wk; intermittent therapy repeated as prescribed. *Maximum:* 20 mg/day.
Children. 250 mcg/kg q.d.; intermittent therapy repeated as prescribed.

Mechanism of Action
Promotes tissue-building processes and reverses catabolic or tissue-depleting processes by promoting protein anabolism.

Contraindications
Breast cancer (males); breast cancer with hypercalcemia (females); hypersensitivity to oxandrolone, anabolic steroids, or their components; nephrosis; pregnancy; prostate cancer

Interactions
DRUGS
corticosteroids: Increased risk of edema and severe acne
hepatotoxic drugs: Increased risk of hepatotoxicity
insulin, oral antidiabetic drugs: Possibly hypoglycemia

NSAIDs, oral anticoagulants, salicylates: Increased anticoagulant effects
sodium-containing drugs: Increased risk of edema
somatrem, somatropin: Possibly accelerated epiphyseal closure

FOODS
high-sodium foods: Increased risk of edema

Adverse Reactions

CNS: Depression, excitement, insomnia
CV: Decreased serum HDL level, edema, hyperlipidemia, hypertension
ENDO: Feminization in postpubertal males (epididymitis, gynecomastia, impotence, oligospermia, priapism, testicular atrophy); glucose intolerance; virilism in females (acne, clitoral enlargement, decreased breast size, deepened voice, diaphoresis, emotional lability, flushing, hirsutism, hoarseness, libido changes, male-pattern baldness, menstrual irregularities, nervousness, oily skin or hair, vaginal bleeding, vaginitis, weight gain), virilism in prepubertal males (acne, decreased ejaculatory volume, penis enlargement, prepubertal closure of epiphyseal plates, unnatural growth of body and facial hair)
GI: Diarrhea, elevated liver function test results, hepatocellular carcinoma, nausea, vomiting
GU: Benign prostatic hyperplasia, prostate cancer, urinary frequency, urine retention (elderly males)
HEME: Iron deficiency anemia, leukemia, prolonged bleeding time
SKIN: Jaundice
Other: Fluid retention, hypercalcemia (females), physical and psychological dependence, sodium retention

Nursing Considerations

•Use oxandrolone cautiously in patients with heart disease because drug has hypercholesterolemic effects.
•Provide adequate calories and protein, as ordered, to maintain a positive nitrogen balance during oxandrolone therapy.
•Anticipate an increased risk of fluid and sodium retention in patients with cardiac, hepatic, or renal dysfunction.
•Weigh patient daily to detect fluid retention. Expect to place patient with fluid retention on sodium-restricted diet or diuretics, as prescribed.

•**WARNING** Be aware that oxandrolone may suppress spermatogenesis in males and cause permanent virilization in females.
•Monitor blood glucose level frequently in patient with diabetes mellitus.

PATIENT TEACHING
•Advise patient to consume a diet high in protein and calories to achieve maximum therapeutic effect of oxandrolone.
•Direct patient to check his weight daily during oxandrolone therapy and to notify prescriber immediately about swelling or unexplained weight gain.
•Inform patient that drug may cause libido changes.
•Inform female patient that drug may cause permanent physical changes, such as clitoral enlargement, deepened voice, and unnatural hair growth.
•Advise female patient of childbearing age to use contraception during therapy and to notify prescriber immediately about suspected or known pregnancy.
•Instruct diabetic patient to monitor blood glucose level frequently.

oxaprozin

Daypro

Class and Category

Chemical: Proprionic acid derivative
Therapeutic: Anti-inflammatory, antirheumatic
Pregnancy category: C (first trimester), Not rated (later trimesters)

Indications and Dosages

➤ *To treat rheumatoid arthritis*
TABLETS
Adults. 1,200 mg q.d. Dosage adjusted based on patient response. *Maximum:* 1,800 mg/day or 26 mg/kg/day (whichever is less) in divided doses b.i.d. or t.i.d.

➤ *To treat osteoarthritis*
TABLETS
Adults. 600 to 1,200 mg q.d. *Maximum:* 1,800 mg/day or 26 mg/kg (whichever is less) in divided doses b.i.d. or t.i.d.
DOSAGE ADJUSTMENT Initial loading dose of 1,200 to 1,800 mg possibly given to speed onset of action. Initial dose limited to 600 mg q.d. for patients with renal impairment.

Route	Onset	Peak	Duration
P.O.	In 7 days	Unknown	Unknown

Mechanism of Action

Blocks the activity of cyclooxygenase, the enzyme needed to synthesize prostaglandins, which mediate the inflammatory response and cause local vasodilation, swelling, and pain. By blocking cyclooxygenase and prostaglandins, the NSAID oxaprozin relieves pain.

Contraindications

Angioedema, asthma, bronchospasm, nasal polyps, rhinitis, or urticaria induced by aspirin, iodides, or other NSAIDs

Interactions

DRUGS

ACE inhibitors, antihypertensives: Decreased antihypertensive response, possibly impaired renal function
acetaminophen: Increased risk of adverse renal effects with long-term use of both drugs
anticoagulants, thrombolytics: Prolonged PT, increased risk of bleeding
beta blockers: Decreased antihypertensive effect
bone marrow depressants: Increased risk of leukopenia and thrombocytopenia
cefamandole, cefoperazone, cefotetan, plicamycin, valproic acid: Increased risk of hypoprothrombinemia and bleeding
cimetidine: Decreased oxaprozin clearance
corticosteroids, potassium supplements: Increased risk of adverse GI effects
digoxin: Increased blood digoxin level and risk of digitalis toxicity
diuretics: Possibly decreased diuretic effect
insulin, oral antidiabetic drugs: Increased effectiveness of these drugs; risk of hypoglycemia
lithium: Increased blood lithium level
methotrexate: Increased blood methotrexate level and risk of methotrexate toxicity
other NSAIDs, salicylates: Increased GI irritability and bleeding
probenecid: Increased risk of oxaprozin toxicity

ACTIVITIES

alcohol use, smoking: Increased risk of adverse GI effects

Adverse Reactions

CNS: Confusion, dizziness, drowsiness, fatigue, headache, insomnia, nervousness, sedation, vertigo, weakness
CV: Hypotension
EENT: Tinnitus
GI: Abdominal pain, constipation, diarrhea, dyspepsia, elevated liver function test results, nausea, vomiting
GU: Dysuria, urinary frequency
HEME: Anemia, thrombocytopenia
SKIN: Alopecia, maculopapular rash, photosensitivity

Nursing Considerations

• Monitor fluid intake and output in elderly patients, patients with hepatic or renal disease or heart failure, and patients who take diuretics or nephrotoxic drugs during oxaprozin therapy.
• Expect drug to increase fluid retention.
• Monitor liver function test results.
• Expect to monitor coagulation status for possible alterations in APTT, PT, and INR.
• Be aware that oxaprozin may mask signs of infection in patients with bone marrow suppression.

PATIENT TEACHING

• Instruct patient to take oxaprozin exactly as prescribed.
• Advise patient to take drug with a full glass of water and to remain upright for 15 to 30 minutes afterward to prevent it from lodging in esophagus and causing irritation.
• Urge patient to avoid alcohol as well as aspirin and other NSAIDs during oxaprozin therapy to avoid bleeding complications.
• Advise patient to avoid excessive sun exposure to reduce the risk of photosensitivity.
• Caution patient to avoid potentially hazardous activities until drug's CNS effects are known.
• Inform patient that risk of bleeding may continue for up to 2 weeks after stopping drug.

oxazepam

Apo-Oxazepam (CAN), Novoxapam (CAN), Serax

Class, Category, and Schedule

Chemical: Benzodiazepine
Therapeutic: Antianxiety, sedative-hypnotic
Pregnancy category: Not rated
Controlled substance: Schedule IV

Indications and Dosages

➤ *To treat anxiety*

CAPSULES, TABLETS

Adults. 10 to 15 mg t.i.d. or q.i.d. for mild to

moderate anxiety; up to 30 mg t.i.d. or q.i.d. for severe anxiety.

➤ *To help manage acute alcohol withdrawal symptoms*

CAPSULES, TABLETS

Adults. 15 to 30 mg t.i.d. or q.i.d.
DOSAGE ADJUSTMENT For elderly or debilitated patients, initial dose of 10 mg t.i.d. increased cautiously to 15 mg t.i.d. or q.i.d.

Mechanism of Action

May potentiate the effects of gamma-aminobutyric acid (GABA) and other inhibitory neurotransmitters by binding to specific benzodiazepine receptors in the limbic and cortical areas of the CNS. GABA inhibits excitatory stimulation, which helps control emotional behavior. The limbic system contains highly dense areas of benzodiazepine receptors, which may explain oxazepam's antianxiety effects.

Contraindications

Acute angle-closure glaucoma; concurrent use of itraconazole or ketoconazole; hypersensitivity to oxazepam, benzodiazepines, or their components; psychoses

Interactions

DRUGS

cimetidine, oral contraceptives: Impaired metabolism and elimination of oxazepam
clozapine: Increased risk of respiratory depression and arrest
CNS depressants: Increased risk of apnea and CNS depression
levodopa: Decreased therapeutic effects of levodopa
probenecid: Increased therapeutic effects of oxazepam and risk of oversedation

ACTIVITIES

alcohol use: Increased risk of apnea and CNS depression

Adverse Reactions

CNS: Anxiety (in daytime), ataxia, confusion, depression, dizziness, drowsiness, fatigue, headache, insomnia, nightmares, sleep disturbance, slurred speech, syncope, talkativeness, tremor, vertigo
GI: Nausea
Other: Drug tolerance, physical and psychological dependence, withdrawal symptoms

Nursing Considerations

•WARNING Be aware that oxazepam may cause physical and psychological dependence.
•Be aware that drug shouldn't be stopped abruptly after prolonged use; doing so may cause seizures or withdrawal symptoms, such as insomnia, irritability, and nervousness.
•Be aware that withdrawal symptoms can occur when therapy is discontinued after only 1 or 2 weeks.
•WARNING Monitor respiratory status in patients with pulmonary disease (such as severe COPD), respiratory depression, or sleep apnea because drug may worsen ventilatory failure.
•Expect an increased risk of falls among elderly patients from impaired cognition and motor function. Take safety precautions according to facility policy.
•Be aware that drug may worsen acute intermittent porphyria, myasthenia gravis, and severe renal impairment, possibly resulting in nephrotoxicity.
•Expect patient with late-stage Parkinson's disease to experience decreased cognition or coordination and, possibly, increased psychosis when given oxazepam.

PATIENT TEACHING

•Instruct patient to take oxazepam exactly as prescribed and not to stop taking it without consulting prescriber.
•Caution patient about possible drowsiness and reduced coordination, and advise him to avoid potentially hazardous activities until drug's CNS effects are known.
•Urge patient to avoid alcohol, which increases oxazepam's sedative effects.
•Instruct patient to notify prescriber about excessive drowsiness or nausea.

oxcarbazepine

Trileptal

Class and Category

Chemical: Tricyclic iminostilbene derivative
Therapeutic: Anticonvulsant
Pregnancy category: C

Indications and Dosages

➤ *As adjunct to treat partial seizures*

ORAL SUSPENSION, TABLETS

Adults and adolescents over age 16. *Initial:* 300 mg b.i.d. Dosage increased by 600 mg/

day q wk. *Usual:* 1,200 mg/day. *Maximum:* 2,400 mg/day.

Children ages 4 to 16. *Initial:* 4 to 5 mg/kg b.i.d. up to maximum initial dose of 600 mg/day. *Usual:* For children who weigh 20 to 29 kg (44 to 64 lb), 900 mg/day; for 29.1 to 39 kg (65 to 86 lb), 1,200 mg/day; for more than 39 kg, 1,800 mg/day. *Maximum:* 1,800 mg/day. ᴅ ᴏ ѕ ᴀ ɢ ᴇ   ᴀ ᴅ ᴊ ᴜ ѕ ᴛ ᴍ ᴇ ɴ ᴛ For patients with creatinine clearance of less than 30 ml/min/1.73 m², usual initial dosage reduced by 50%.

➤ *As monotherapy to treat partial seizures*

ᴏʀᴀʟ ѕᴜѕᴘᴇɴѕɪᴏɴ, ᴛᴀʙʟᴇᴛѕ

Adults and adolescents over age 16. *Initial:* 300 mg b.i.d. Dosage increased by 300 mg/day q 3 days as needed. *Usual:* 1,200 mg/day. *Maximum:* 2,400 mg/day.

➤ *To convert to monotherapy in the treatment of partial seizures*

ᴏʀᴀʟ ѕᴜѕᴘᴇɴѕɪᴏɴ, ᴛᴀʙʟᴇᴛѕ

Adults and adolescents over age 16. *Initial:* 300 mg b.i.d. Dosage increased by 600 mg/day q wk over 2 to 4 wk, as needed, while dosage of other anticonvulsant is reduced. *Usual:* 1,200 mg/day. *Maximum:* 2,400 mg/day.

Mechanism of Action

May prevent or halt seizures by closing or blocking sodium channels in the neuronal cell membrane. By preventing sodium from entering the cell, oxcarbazepine may slow nerve impulse transmission, thus decreasing the rate at which neurons fire.

Contraindications

Hypersensitivity to carbamazepine, oxcarbazepine, or their components

Interactions

Dʀᴜɢѕ

carbamazepine, phenobarbital, phenytoin, valproic acid: Decreased blood oxcarbazepine level, possibly increased blood levels of phenobarbital and phenytoin

felodipine, verapamil: Decreased blood levels of these drugs

oral contraceptives: Decreased effectiveness of oral contraceptives

Aᴄᴛɪᴠɪᴛɪᴇѕ

alcohol use: Possibly additive CNS depressant effects

Adverse Reactions

CNS: Abnormal gait, ataxia, dizziness, fatigue, fever, headache, somnolence, tremor

EENT: Abnormal vision, diplopia, nystagmus, rhinitis

GI: Abdominal pain, indigestion, nausea, vomiting

SKIN: Rash

Other: Hyponatremia

Nursing Considerations

•Before beginning oxcarbazepine therapy, ask patient if he has had an allergic reaction to carbamazepine; such a reaction indicates an increased risk of hypersensitivity to oxcarbazepine.

•Monitor serum sodium level for signs of hyponatremia, especially during first 3 months of therapy.

•Be prepared to monitor therapeutic oxcarbazepine levels during initiation and titration of drug therapy, and expect to adjust dosage accordingly.

•Implement seizure precautions as appropriate and according to facility policy.

Pᴀᴛɪᴇɴᴛ Tᴇᴀᴄʜɪɴɢ

•Teach patient to shake suspension well and prepare the dose immediately afterwards. Tell him to then withdraw the prescribed amount using the supplied oral dosing syringe. Instruct him to mix the dose in a small glass of water just before taking it, or tell him that he can swallow drug directly from the syringe. Instruct him to close the bottle and to rinse the syringe with warm water and allow it to dry thoroughly after each use.

•Inform patient that he may experience dizziness, double vision, and unsteady gait while taking oxcarbazepine.

•Advise patient to avoid driving and other activities that require a high level of alertness until drug's full CNS effects are known.

•Instruct patient not to drink alcohol while taking oxcarbazepine.

oxtriphylline

Apo-Oxtriphylline (ᴄᴀɴ), Choledyl, Choledyl SA

oxtriphylline and guaifenesin

Brondelate, Choledyl Expectorant (ᴄᴀɴ)

Class and Category

Chemical: Xanthine derivative
Therapeutic: Bronchodilator
Pregnancy category: C

Indications and Dosages

➤ To treat acute asthma, bronchospasm due to chronic bronchitis or COPD

DELAYED-RELEASE TABLETS (OXTRIPHYLLINE), ELIXIR (OXTRIPHYLLINE AND GUAIFENESIN)

Adults and children age 6 and older. 300 mg q.d. for 3 days and then increased to 400 mg q.d. for 3 days. *Maintenance:* 600 mg/day in divided doses q 6 to 8 hr.

E.R. TABLETS (OXTRIPHYLLINE)

Adults and children age 6 and older. 300 mg q.d. for 3 days and then increased to 400 mg q.d. for 3 days. *Maintenance:* 600 mg/day in divided doses q 12 hr.

Mechanism of Action

Inhibits phosphodiesterase enzymes, causing bronchodilation. Normally, these enzymes inactivate cAMP and cGMP, which are responsible for bronchial smooth-muscle relaxation. Other mechanisms of action may include calcium translocation, prostaglandin antagonism, catecholamine stimulation, inhibition of cGMP metabolism, and adenosine receptor antagonism. Guaifenesin eases expectoration by thinning and loosening sputum and bronchial secretions.

Contraindications

Hypersensitivity to oxtriphylline, guaifenesin, xanthines, or their components; peptic ulcer; seizure disorder unless controlled by an anticonvulsant

Interactions

DRUGS

activated charcoal, aminoglutethimide, barbiturates, ketoconazole, rifampin, sulfinpyrazone, sympathomimetics: Decreased blood theophylline level

allopurinol, beta blockers (nonselective), calcium channel blockers, cimetidine, corticosteroids, disulfiram, ephedrine, influenza virus vaccine, interferon, macrolides, mexiletine, oral contraceptives, quinolones, thiabendazole: Increased blood theophylline level

benzodiazepines, propofol: Possibly antagonized sedative effects of these drugs

carbamazepine, isoniazid, loop diuretics: Possibly increased or decreased blood theophylline level

halothane anesthetics: Increased risk of cardiotoxicity

hydantoins: Possibly decreased blood hydantoin level

ketamine: Increased risk of seizures

lithium: Decreased blood lithium level

neuromuscular blockers: Possibly reversal of neuromuscular blockade

tetracyclines: Possibly increased adverse effects of theophylline

FOODS

all foods: Altered bioavailability and absorption of E.R. oxtriphylline

charcoal broiled beef; low-carbohydrate, high-protein diet: Increased theophylline elimination

high-carbohydrate, low-protein diet: Decreased elimination and prolonged half-life of theophylline

ACTIVITIES

alcohol use: Increased CNS effects, especially with elixir

smoking (1 or more packs/day): Decreased effects of oxtriphylline

Adverse Reactions

CNS: Anxiety, dizziness, headache, insomnia, restlessness, seizures

CV: Hypotension, palpitations, sinus tachycardia

EENT: Unpleasant taste

GI: Anorexia, diarrhea, nausea, vomiting

RESP: Tachypnea

SKIN: Alopecia, flushing, rash

Nursing Considerations

• Be aware that oxtriphylline contains 64% anhydrous theophylline, so dosage is based on equivalent of 5 to 6 mg of anhydrous theophylline/kg.

• WARNING Be aware that elixir form contains 20% alcohol and shouldn't be used in children or in patients with a history of alcohol abuse.

• Be aware that food delays absorption of delayed-release and E.R. forms and that large volumes of fluid may increase absorption.

• Know that elixir is absorbed more rapidly and that delayed-release and E.R. preparations vary in their absorption rate.

• Monitor blood theophylline level because toxicity may develop at a level only slightly above therapeutic.

PATIENT TEACHING

• Advise patient to take elixir on an empty stomach with a full glass of water to enhance absorption.

• If patient complains of GI discomfort, suggest that he take drug with or just after meals.

• Urge patient to stop smoking and to notify prescriber about changes in smoking habits.

N
O

Also instruct him to avoid alcohol during oxtriphylline therapy.
•Encourage patient to keep follow-up appointments for laboratory studies.

oxybutynin chloride

Ditropan, Ditropan XL

Class and Category
Chemical: Tertiary amine
Therapeutic: Antispasmodic
Pregnancy category: B

Indications and Dosages
➤ *To treat overactive bladder, including neurogenic bladder, with urinary frequency, urgency, or incontinence from involuntary contraction of detrusor muscle*
E.R. TABLETS
Adults. *Initial:* 5 mg q.d., adjusted by 5 mg/wk, as prescribed. *Maximum:* 30 mg/day.
SYRUP, TABLETS
Adults. 5 mg b.i.d. or t.i.d. *Maximum:* 5 mg q.i.d. or 20 mg/day.
Children age 5 and older. 5 mg b.i.d. *Maximum:* 15 mg t.i.d.
DOSAGE ADJUSTMENT For elderly patients, possibly 2.5 mg b.i.d. initially, increased to maximum of 5 mg t.i.d., as prescribed.

Route	Onset	Peak	Duration
P.O.	30 to 60 min	3 to 6 hr	6 to 10 hr

Mechanism of Action
Exerts antimuscarinic (atropine-like) and potent direct antispasmodic (papaverine-like) actions on smooth muscle in the bladder and decreases detrusor muscle contractions. The result is increased bladder capacity, which decreases the urge to void.

Contraindications
Acute hemorrhage, angle-closure glaucoma, GI obstruction, hypersensitivity to oxybutynin or its components, ileus, intestinal atony in elderly or debilitated patients, myasthenia gravis, obstructive uropathy, toxic megacolon with ulcerative colitis

Interactions
DRUGS
amantadine, amitriptyline, amoxapine, antimuscarinics, brompheniramine, bupropion, *carbinoxamine, chlorpheniramine, chlorpromazine, clemastine, clomipramine, clozapine, cyclobenzaprine, dimenhydrinate, diphenhydramine, disopyramide, doxepin, doxylamine, imipramine, maprotiline, mesoridazine, methdilazine, nortriptyline, procainamide, promazine, promethazine, protriptyline, thioridazine, triflupromazine, trimeprazine, trimipramine:* Increased anticholinergic effects
CNS depressants: Increased sedation
ketoconazole: Possibly altered total absorption rate and blood level of ketoconazole
opioid agonists: Increased depressive effects of opioid agonists on GI motility and bladder function
parasympathomimetics: Decreased antimuscarinic action of oxybutynin
ACTIVITIES
alcohol use: Increased sedation

Adverse Reactions
CNS: Asthenia, dizziness, drowsiness, hallucinations, insomnia, restlessness, somnolence
CV: Palpitations, tachycardia, vasodilation
EENT: Dry mouth, nose, and throat
GI: Constipation, esophagitis, nausea
GU: Impotence, urinary hesitancy, urine retention
SKIN: Decreased sweating, flushing, urticaria
Other: Heatstroke

Nursing Considerations
•Use oxybutynin cautiously in patients with diarrhea because diarrhea may signal incomplete GI obstruction, especially in patients with colostomy or ileostomy.
•Assess urinary symptoms before and after treatment.
•Administer drug on an empty stomach or, to prevent GI irritation, with food or milk.
•Make sure patient swallows E.R. tablets whole and doesn't crush, chew, or divide them. Expect to see portions of drug in stool.
•WARNING Monitor for adverse cardiovascular reactions in patients with arrhythmias, coronary artery disease, heart failure, or hypertension because drug's antimuscarinic effects may increase their risk.
•Because decreased GI motility can precipitate adynamic ileus, assess for abdominal pain and ileus.
•Be aware that drug may aggravate benign prostatic hyperplasia, gastroesophageal reflux disease, and hyperthyroidism.

PATIENT TEACHING
•Instruct patient to take oxybutynin on an empty stomach. If adverse GI reactions develop, suggest that he take drug with food or milk.
•Advise patient not to chew, crush, or break E.R. tablets.
•Inform patient about the risk of decreased mental alertness and physical coordination. Advise him to avoid potentially hazardous activities until drug's CNS effects are known.
•Caution patient to avoid strenuous exercise and excessive sun exposure because of increased risk of heatstroke.
•Urge patient to avoid alcohol during therapy.

oxycodone and acetaminophen

Endocet, Oxycocet (CAN), Percocet, Percocet-Demi (CAN), Roxicet, Roxilox, Tylox

Class, Category, and Schedule
Chemical: Phenanthrene derivative (oxycodone), aminophenyl derivative (acetaminophen)
Therapeutic: Analgesic
Pregnancy category: Not rated
Controlled substance: Schedule II

Indications and Dosages
➤ *To control moderate to moderately severe pain*
CAPSULES, TABLETS
Adults. 5 mg of oxycodone and 325 to 500 mg of acetaminophen (1 tab or capsule) q 4 to 6 hr, p.r.n. *Maximum:* 4,000 mg/day of acetaminophen.
ORAL SOLUTION
Adults. 5 mg (5 ml) of oxycodone and 325 mg of acetaminophen q 4 to 6 hr, p.r.n. *Maximum:* 4,000 mg/day of acetaminophen.

Route	Onset	Peak	Duration
P.O.	30 min	90 min	3 to 4 hr

Contraindications
Hypercapnia; hypersensitivity to oxycodone, acetaminophen, or their components; ileus; use within 14 days of MAO inhibitor therapy

Interactions
DRUGS
antacids: Decreased and delayed acetaminophen absorption

Mechanism of Action
Produces a synergistic analgesic effect through two mechanisms of action. Oxycodone, a mu receptor agonist, alters the perception of and emotional response to pain at the spinal cord and higher levels of the CNS by blocking the release of inhibitory neurotransmitters, such as gamma-aminobutyric acid and acetylcholine.
Acetaminophen blocks the activity of cyclooxygenase, an enzyme necessary for prostaglandin synthesis. Prostaglandins, important mediators in the inflammatory response, cause local vasodilation with swelling and pain.

antianxiety drugs, benzodiazepines, brompheniramine, carbinoxamine, chlorpheniramine, clemastine, dimenhydrinate, diphenhydramine, doxylamine, general anesthetics, hypnotics, methdilazine, opioid antagonists, phenothiazines, promethazine, sedatives, skeletal muscle relaxants, tramadol, tricyclic antidepressants, trimeprazine: Potentiated respiratory depression from these drugs and oxycodone
anticholinergics: Possibly severe constipation and paralytic ileus
antidiarrheals: Possibly severe constipation and additive CNS depression
antihypertensives: Possibly exaggerated antihypertensive effects and risk of orthostatic hypotension
antineoplastics, immunosuppressants: Risk of masking signs of infection, such as fever and pain
barbiturates: Additive CNS depression
butorphanol, pentazocine: Possibly acute withdrawal symptoms in opioid-dependent patients, decreased analgesic effect
carbamazepine, phenobarbital, phenytoin, primidone, rifampin: Possibly need for increased oxycodone dosage to achieve analgesia and prevent withdrawal symptoms in opioid-dependent patients, possibly increased risk of acetaminophen-induced hepatotoxicity
cimetidine, ritonavir: Possibly apnea, confusion, disorientation, and seizures from respiratory depression and impaired CNS function, increased risk of acetaminophen-induced hepatotoxicity (ritonavir)

MAO inhibitors: Possibly fatal reactions, including cardiac arrest, coma, respiratory depression, seizures, and severe hypertension
nalbuphine, nalmefene, naloxone, naltrexone: Blocked oxycodone effects, withdrawal symptoms in opioid-dependent patients
verapamil: Increased constipation
warfarin: Increased INR and risk of bleeding
FOODS
all foods: Decreased and delayed acetaminophen absorption
ACTIVITIES
alcohol use: Additive CNS depression, increased risk of acetaminophen-induced hepatotoxicity

Adverse Reactions

CNS: Confusion, dizziness, drowsiness, euphoria, excitation, hallucinations, headache, restlessness, sedation, somnolence
CV: Bradycardia, hypotension, orthostatic hypotension, palpitations
EENT: Blurred vision, dry eyes, lens opacities, miosis
GI: Abdominal pain, constipation, elevated liver function test results, hepatotoxicity, nausea, vomiting
GU: Amenorrhea, decreased libido, erectile dysfunction, oliguria, renal tubular necrosis, urinary hesitancy, urine retention
RESP: Respiratory depression
SKIN: Erythema, flushing, pruritus, urticaria
Other: Drug tolerance, hypoprothrombinemia, physical and psychological dependence, withdrawal symptoms

Nursing Considerations

• **WARNING** Be aware that oxycodone has a high potential for abuse.
• Use drug cautiously in patients with head injury because drug may alter neurologic findings.
• Assess pain level regularly, and give drug as prescribed before pain becomes severe.
• Administer drug with a full glass of water or, to minimize GI distress, with food or milk.
• Adjust dosage to relieve pain as prescribed, keeping in mind the maximum daily dose of acetaminophen. Be prepared to adjust dosage for patient who hasn't previously received opioids until he can tolerate drug's effects.
• Avoid giving drug within 1 to 2 hours of antacids or food because of risk of decreased drug effectiveness.

• Assess for possible respiratory depression or paradoxical excitation during dosage titration.
• Assess for abdominal pain because oxycodone may mask signs and symptoms of underlying GI disorders.
• Increase patient's dietary fiber intake if needed to prevent constipation.
• Anticipate an increased risk of falling during therapy. Institute safety precautions according to facility policy.
PATIENT TEACHING
• Instruct patient not to take oxycodone and acetaminophen more often than prescribed and not to stop taking drug abruptly after long-term use.
• Encourage patient to take drug with a full glass of water and with food, if possible.
• Suggest that patient change position slowly to minimize effects of orthostatic hypotension.
• Instruct patient to avoid alcohol and potentially hazardous activities during therapy.
• Advise patient to notify prescriber about possible signs of toxicity or hypersensitivity, such as excessive light-headedness, extreme dizziness, itching, swelling, and trouble breathing.

oxycodone hydrochloride

OxyContin, Roxicodone, Supeudol (CAN)

Class, Category, and Schedule
Chemical: Phenanthrene derivative
Therapeutic: Analgesic
Pregnancy category: Not rated
Controlled substance: Schedule II

Indications and Dosages
➤ *To relieve moderate to severe pain*
ORAL SOLUTION
Adults. 5 mg q 3 to 6 hr, p.r.n., and increased as needed.
TABLETS
Adults. 5 mg q 3 to 6 hr or 10 mg q 6 to 8 hr, p.r.n.

➤ *To manage pain for more than a few days*
CONTROLLED-RELEASE TABLETS
Adults who haven't received opioids before.
Initial: 10 to 20 mg q 12 hr, adjusted q 1 to 2 days, as prescribed, based on total amount of oxycodone needed daily to control pain.
Adults who currently receive an opioid agonist or fixed-ratio combination drugs (opioid

agonist plus acetaminophen, aspirin, or NSAID). Half the 24-hr oxycodone dose q 12 hr, as prescribed. Be prepared to manage breakthrough pain with immediate-release tablets, p.r.n., and adjust q 1 to 2 days, as prescribed.

Adults who use fentanyl transdermal patch. 10 mg oxycodone for each 25 mcg/hr of fentanyl patch dosage q 12 hr, beginning 12 to 18 hr after removing patch.

DOSAGE ADJUSTMENT To provide supplemental analgesia for adults receiving controlled-release oxycodone, one-fourth to one-third the 12-hr controlled-release dose given as tablet q 3 to 6 hr, p.r.n.

Route	Onset	Peak	Duration
P.O.	10 to 15 min	1 hr	3 to 4 hr

Mechanism of Action

Alters the perception of and emotional response to pain at the spinal cord and higher levels of the CNS by blocking the release of inhibitory neurotransmitters, such as gamma-aminobutyric acid and acetylcholine.

Contraindications

Hypercapnia, hypersensitivity to oxycodone or its components, ileus, use within 14 days of MAO inhibitor therapy

Interactions

DRUGS

anticholinergics: Possibly severe constipation and ileus
antidiarrheals: Possibly severe constipation and additive CNS depression
antihypertensives: Possibly exaggerated antihypertensive effects and risk of orthostatic hypotension
butorphanol, pentazocine: Possibly acute withdrawal symptoms in opioid-dependent patients, decreased analgesic effects
carbamazepine, phenytoin, primidone, rifampin: Possibly need for increased oxycodone dosage to achieve analgesia and prevent withdrawal symptoms in opioid-dependent patients
cimetidine: Possibly apnea, confusion, disorientation, and seizures from respiratory depression and impaired CNS function
CNS depressants: Possibly increased CNS and respiratory depression and orthostatic hypotension

MAO inhibitors: Possibly fatal reactions, including cardiac arrest, coma, respiratory depression, seizures, and severe hypertension
nalbuphine, nalmefene, naloxone, naltrexone: Blocked oxycodone effects, withdrawal symptoms in opioid-dependent patients

ACTIVITIES

alcohol use: Additive CNS effects

Adverse Reactions

CNS: Dizziness, drowsiness, euphoria, excitation, headache, sedation, somnolence
CV: Bradycardia, hypotension, orthostatic hypotension, palpitations
EENT: Blurred vision, dry eyes, lens opacities, miosis
GI: Constipation, elevated liver function test results, nausea, vomiting
GU: Amenorrhea, decreased libido, erectile dysfunction, oliguria, urinary hesitancy, urine retention
RESP: Respiratory depression
SKIN: Pruritus
Other: Drug tolerance, physical and psychological dependence, withdrawal symptoms

Nursing Considerations

• WARNING Be aware that oxycodone has a high potential for abuse.
• WARNING Be aware that abuse of crushed controlled-release tablets poses a hazard of overdose and death. If you suspect abuse and determine that patient also is abusing alcohol or illicit substances, notify prescriber immediately because the risk of overdose and death is increased. If you suspect parenteral abuse, be aware that tablet excipients, especially talc, may result in local tissue necrosis, infection, pulmonary granulomas, endocarditis, and valvular heart injury.
• Assess baseline neurologic status before each dose in patient with head injury because drug may obscure progression of his condition.
• Assess pain level regularly, and give drug as prescribed before pain becomes severe.
• Be prepared to adjust dosage for patient who hasn't previously received opioids until he can tolerate drug's effects.
• Expect to give controlled-release tablets only to opioid-tolerant patients who need at least 160 mg/day.
• Assess patient for possible respiratory depression or paradoxical excitation during dosage titration.

•Assess patient for abdominal pain because oxycodone may mask signs and symptoms of underlying GI disorders.

PATIENT TEACHING

•**WARNING** Strongly warn patient to swallow tablets whole and not to break, chew, or crush them. Explain that taking broken, chewed, or crushed tablets leads to rapid release and absorption of a potentially fatal dose.

•Instruct patient not to take oxycodone more often than prescribed and not to stop taking drug abruptly after long-term use.

•Instruct patient to avoid alcohol and potentially hazardous activities during oxycodone therapy.

•Advise patient to notify prescriber about possible signs of toxicity or hypersensitivity, such as excessive light-headedness, extreme dizziness, itching, swelling, and trouble breathing.

oxymetholone

Anadrol-50, Anapolon-50 (CAN)

Class, Category, and Schedule

Chemical: Testosterone derivative
Therapeutic: Antianemic, antiangioedema (hereditary)
Pregnancy category: X
Controlled substance: Schedule III

Indications and Dosages

➤ *To treat acquired and congenital aplastic anemias, anemias caused by deficient RBC production, bone marrow failure anemias, hypoplastic anemias caused by myelotoxic drugs, and myelofibrosis; to prevent or treat hereditary angioedema*

TABLETS

Adults and children. 1 to 2 mg/kg/day for 3 to 6 mo. *Maximum:* 5 mg/kg/day.

Mechanism of Action

Combats anemia by increasing production of erythropoietin, a precursor of RBCs. Oxymetholone also increases the hemoglobin level and RBC volume.

Contraindications

Breast or prostate cancer in males patients, hypercalcemia in female patients with breast cancer, hypersensitivity to oxymetholone or anabolic steroids, nephrosis, nephrotic phase of nephritis, pregnancy, severe hepatic dysfunction

Interactions

DRUGS

corticosteroids: Increased risk of edema and severe acne
hepatotoxic drugs: Increased risk of hepatotoxicity
insulin, oral antidiabetic drugs: Possibly hypoglycemia
NSAIDs, oral anticoagulants, salicylates: Increased anticoagulant effects
sodium-containing drugs: Increased risk of edema
somatrem, somatropin: Possibly accelerated epiphyseal maturation

FOODS

high-sodium foods: Increased risk of edema

Adverse Reactions

CNS: Depression, excitement, insomnia
CV: Decreased serum HDL level, edema, hyperlipidemia, hypertension
ENDO: Feminization in postpubertal males (epididymitis, gynecomastia, impotence, oligospermia, priapism, testicular atrophy), glucose intolerance, virilism in females (acne, clitoral enlargement, decreased breast size, deepened voice, diaphoresis, emotional lability, flushing, hirsutism, hoarseness, libido changes, male-pattern baldness, menstrual irregularities, nervousness, oily hair or skin, vaginal bleeding, vaginitis, weight gain), virilism in prepubertal males (acne, decreased ejaculatory volume, penis enlargement, prepubertal closure of epiphyseal plates, unnatural growth of body and facial hair)
GI: Diarrhea, elevated liver function test results, hepatocellular carcinoma, nausea, vomiting
GU: Benign prostatic hyperplasia, prostate cancer, urinary frequency, urine retention (elderly males)
HEME: Iron deficiency anemia, leukemia, prolonged bleeding time
SKIN: Jaundice
Other: Fluid retention, hypercalcemia (females), physical and psychological dependence, sodium retention

Nursing Considerations

•Be aware that oxymetholone shouldn't be used in patients with a history of hypercal-

cemia because drug may exacerbate this condition or in patients with prostate problems because drug may promote benign or cancerous tumor growth.
•Anticipate increased risk of fluid and sodium retention in patients with cardiac, hepatic, or renal dysfunction. Monitor for signs and symptoms of fluid retention.
•Monitor daily weight. Expect to place patient with fluid retention on sodium-restricted diet or diuretics, as prescribed
•WARNING Be aware that oxymetholone may suppress spermatogenesis in males and cause permanent virilization in females.

PATIENT TEACHING
•Advise patient to consume a diet high in protein and calories to achieve maximum therapeutic effect of oxymetholone.
•Instruct patient to check his weight daily during oxymetholone therapy and to notify prescriber immediately about swelling or unexplained weight gain.
•Inform patient that drug may cause libido changes.
•Advise diabetic patient to monitor blood glucose levels frequently because drug may increase hypoglycemic effect of antidiabetic drugs.
•Inform female patient that drug may cause permanent physical changes, such as clitoral enlargement, deepened voice, and unnatural hair growth.
•Advise female patient of childbearing age to use contraception during therapy and to notify prescriber immediately about suspected or known pregnancy.

oxymorphone hydrochloride

Numorphan

Class, Category, and Schedule
Chemical: Phenanthrene derivative
Therapeutic: Analgesic
Pregnancy category: Not rated
Controlled substance: Schedule II

Indications and Dosages
➤ *To relieve moderate to severe pain, to relieve anxiety in patients with dyspnea from pulmonary edema caused by acute left ventricular dysfunction*

I.V. INJECTION
Adults. *Initial:* 0.5 mg, repeated q 3 to 6 hr, p.r.n.
I.M. OR S.C. INJECTION
Adults. *Initial:* 1 to 1.5 mg, repeated q 3 to 6 hr, p.r.n.
SUPPOSITORIES
Adults. 5 mg q 4 to 6 hr, p.r.n.
➤ *To relieve obstetric pain during labor*
I.M. INJECTION
Adults. 0.5 to 1 mg as a single dose.

Route	Onset	Peak	Duration
I.V.	5 to 10 min	15 to 30 min	3 to 4 hr
I.M.	10 to 15 min	30 to 90 min	3 to 6 hr
S.C.	10 to 20 min	30 to 90 min	3 to 6 hr
P.R.	15 to 30 min	2 hr	3 to 6 hr

Mechanism of Action
Alters the perception of and emotional response to pain at the spinal cord and higher levels of the CNS by blocking the release of inhibitory neurotransmitters, such as gamma-aminobutyric acid and acetylcholine.

Contraindications
Acute or severe asthma; hypersensitivity to oxymorphone, other morphine analogues, or their components; ileus; pulmonary edema from a chemical respiratory irritant; severe respiratory depression; upper airway obstruction

Interactions
DRUGS
anticholingerics: Increased risk of urine retention, severe constipation
antidiarrheals, antiperistaltics: Increased risk of severe constipation, CNS depression
antihypertensives, diuretics, hypotension-producing drugs: Increased hypotensive effects
buprenorphine: Reduced oxymorphone effectiveness if buprenorphine is given first, possibly withdrawal symptoms in oxymorphone-dependent patients
CNS depressants: Additive CNS depressant effects, increased risk of habituation

hydroxyzine, other opioid analgesics: Increased analgesia, CNS depression, and hypotensive effects
MAO inhibitors: Increased risk of unpredictable, severe, sometimes fatal adverse reactions
metoclopramide: Antagonized effects of metoclopramide on GI motility
naloxone: Antagonized analgesic, CNS, and respiratory depressant effects of oxymorphone
naltrexone: Withdrawal symptoms in oxymorphone-dependent patients
neuromuscular blockers: Additive respiratory depression
ACTIVITIES
alcohol use: Additive CNS depressant effects, increased risk of habituation

Adverse Reactions

CNS: Confusion, delusions, depersonalization, dizziness, drowsiness, euphoria, headache, light-headedness, nervousness, nightmares, restlessness, seizures, tiredness, tremor, weakness
CV: Bradycardia, hypertension, hypotension, palpitations, tachycardia
EENT: Blurred vision, diplopia, dry mouth, laryngeal edema, laryngospasm, tinnitus
GI: Abdominal cramps or pain, constipation, hepatotoxicity, nausea, vomiting
GU: Decreased urine output, dysuria, urinary frequency
MS: Muscle rigidity (with large doses), uncontrolled muscle movements
RESP: Atelectasis, bradypnea, bronchospasm, dyspnea, irregular breathing, respiratory depression, wheezing
SKIN: Diaphoresis, erythema, flushing of face
Other: Injection site burning, pain, redness, and swelling

Nursing Considerations

• Monitor vital signs during oxymorphone therapy to detect respiratory depression and hypotension.
• Monitor urinary and bowel status; constipation may become so severe that it causes ileus.
• Offer fluids to relieve dry mouth.
PATIENT TEACHING
• Instruct patient to take oxymorphone exactly as prescribed and not to stop taking drug abruptly; warn him that drug can cause physical dependence.
• Stress the importance of taking drug before pain becomes severe.

• Instruct patient to store suppositories in refrigerator.
• Encourage patient to increase fluid and fiber intake to prevent constipation.
• Urge patient not to drink alcohol or use CNS depressants during therapy without first consulting prescriber.
• Caution patient to avoid potentially hazardous activities until drug's CNS effects are known.
• Advise female patient to stop drug and notify prescriber about known or suspected pregnancy.

oxytetracycline

Terramycin I.M.

oxytetracycline hydrochloride

Terramycin

Class and Category

Chemical: Tetracycline derived from *Streptomyces rimosus*
Therapeutic: Antibiotic, antiprotozoal
Pregnancy category: D

Indications and Dosages

➤ *To treat systemic bacterial and protozoal infections, such as bronchitis, chlamydial infection, Lyme disease, nongonococcal urethritis, rickettsial infection, traveler's diarrhea, and UTIs*

CAPSULES (OXYTETRACYCLINE HYDROCHLORIDE)
Adults and adolescents. 250 to 500 mg q 6 hr. *Maximum:* 4,000 mg/day.
Children ages 8 to 12. 6.25 to 12.5 mg/kg q 6 hr.
I.M. INJECTION (OXYTETRACYCLINE)
Adults and adolescents. 100 mg q 8 hr, 150 mg q 12 hr, or 250 mg q.d. *Maximum:* 500 mg/day.
Children ages 8 to 12. 5 to 8.3 mg/kg q 8 hr or 7.5 to 12.5 mg/kg q 12 hr. *Maximum:* 250 mg/day.
DOSAGE ADJUSTMENT Dosage possibly reduced for patients with renal impairment.

➤ *To treat brucellosis*
CAPSULES (OXYTETRACYCLINE HYDROCHLORIDE)
Adults and adolescents. 500 mg q 6 hr for 3 wk with 1,000 mg of streptomycin I.M. q 12 hr in wk 1 and q.d. in wk 2. *Maximum:* 4,000 mg/day.

➤ *To treat uncomplicated gonorrhea*
CAPSULES (OXYTETRACYCLINE HYDROCHLORIDE)
Adults and adolescents. *Initial:* 1,500 mg, then 500 mg q 6 hr to total of 9,000 mg for full course of treatment.

➤ *To treat syphilis*
CAPSULES (OXYTETRACYCLINE HYDROCHLORIDE)
Adults and adolescents. 500 to 1,000 mg q 6 hr for 10 to 15 days to total of 30 to 40 g for full course of treatment.

Mechanism of Action
Binds with ribosomal subunits of susceptible bacteria and alters the cytoplasmic membrane, inhibiting bacterial protein synthesis and rendering the organism ineffective.

Contraindications
Hypersensitivity to tetracyclines or their components

Interactions
DRUGS
antacids, calcium supplements, cholestyramine, choline salicylates, colestipol, iron supplements, magnesium salicylates: Possibly decreased absorption of oxytetracycline
digoxin: Increased blood digoxin level
lithium: Altered blood lithium level
methoxyflurane: Increased risk of nephrotoxicity
oral anticoagulants: Increased anticoagulant effects
oral contraceptives: Decreased contraceptive effectiveness, increased risk of breakthrough bleeding and pregnancy
penicillins: Decreased bactericidal effects of penicillins
sodium bicarbonate: Possibly decreased absorption of oral oxytetracycline
vitamin A: Increased risk of benign intracranial hypertension
FOODS
all foods, especially dairy products: Possibly interference with oxytetracycline absorption

Adverse Reactions
CNS: Dizziness, light-headedness, tiredness, unsteadiness, weakness
EENT: Darkened, discolored, or sore tongue; stomatitis, tooth discoloration (in infants and children under age 8)
GI: Abdominal cramps, diarrhea, indigestion, nausea, thirst, vomiting
GU: Urinary frequency
SKIN: Photosensitivity
Other: Superinfection

Nursing Considerations
•**WARNING** Be aware that oxytetracycline shouldn't be given to premature infants because it may impair skeletal growth or to children under age 8 because it may permanently discolor teeth and cause enamel hypoplasia.
•Be aware that patient should be switched from parenteral to oral form as soon as possible.
PATIENT TEACHING
•Instruct patient to take oxytetracycline capsules 1 hour before meals and 3 hours before or after other drugs and dairy products.
•Advise patient to take drug with a full glass of water and in an upright position to minimize adverse GI reactions.
•Urge patient to complete entire course of oxytetracycline therapy, even if he feels better beforehand.
•Caution patient to avoid potentially hazardous activities until drug's CNS effects are known.
•Advise patient to avoid excessive sun exposure and to protect skin when outdoors.
•Urge female patient who uses oral contraceptives to use an additional form of birth control during oxytetracycline therapy.
•Advise patient to discard outdated capsules because drug may become toxic.

P

pamidronate disodium

Aredia

Class and Category

Chemical: Bisphosphonate
Therapeutic: Antihypercalcemic, bone resorption inhibitor
Pregnancy category: C

Indications and Dosages

➤ *To treat cancer-induced hypercalcemia that's inadequately managed by oral hydration alone*

I.V. INFUSION
Adults. 60 to 90 mg over 2 to 24 hr as a single dose when corrected serum calcium level is 12 to 13.5 mg/dl; 90 mg over 2 to 24 hr when corrected serum calcium level is greater than 13.5 mg/dl. May be repeated as prescribed after 7 days if hypercalcemia recurs.

DOSAGE ADJUSTMENT For patients with renal failure, dosage limited to 30 mg over 4 to 24 hr, as prescribed. For patients with cardiac or renal failure, drug is given in a smaller volume of fluid or at a slower rate, as prescribed.

➤ *To treat moderate to severe Paget's disease of bone*

I.V. INFUSION
Adults. 30 mg/day over 4 hr on 3 consecutive days for a total dose of 90 mg. Repeated as needed and tolerated.

➤ *To treat osteolytic bone metastases of breast cancer*

I.V. INFUSION
Adults. 90 mg over 2 hr q 3 to 4 wk.

➤ *To treat osteolytic bone metastases of multiple myeloma*

I.V. INFUSION
Adults. 90 mg over 4 hr q mo.

Incompatibilities

Don't mix pamidronate with calcium-containing infusion solutions, such as Ringer's solution.

Mechanism of Action

Inhibits bone resorption, possibly by impairing attachment of osteoclast precursors to mineralized bone matrix, thus reducing the rate of bone turnover in Paget's disease and osteolytic metastases. Pamidronate also reduces the flow of calcium from resorbing bone into the blood.

Contraindications

Hypersensitivity to pamidronate, other bisphosphonates, or their components

Interactions

DRUGS
calcium-containing preparations; vitamin D preparations, such as calcifediol and calcitriol: Antagonized pamidronate effects when used to treat hypercalcemia

Adverse Reactions

CNS: Confusion, fever, psychosis
GI: Abdominal cramps, anorexia, GI bleeding, indigestion, nausea, vomiting
GU: Azotemia
HEME: Leukopenia, lymphopenia
MS: Bone pain, muscle spasms or stiffness
Other: Hypocalcemia, hypokalemia, hypomagnesemia, hypophosphatemia, injection site pain and swelling

Nursing Considerations

•Be alert for fever during first 3 days of pamidronate therapy, especially in patients receiving high doses. If fever develops, obtain CBC with differential, as ordered.
•Assess patient with anemia, leukopenia, or thrombocytopenia for worsening of the condition during first 2 weeks of therapy.

PATIENT TEACHING
•Stress the importance of complying with prescribed administration schedule for pamidronate.
•Advise patient to avoid calcium and vitamin D supplements during therapy.

pancreatin

Donnazyme (contains 500 mg of pancreatin, 1,000 U of lipase, 12,500 U of protease, 12,500 U of amylase), Hi-Vegi-Lip (contains 2,400 mg of pancreatin, 4,800 U of lipase, 60,000 U of protease, 60,000 U of amylase), Pancrezyme 4X (contains 2,400 mg of pancreatin, 12,000 U of lipase, 60,000 U of protease, 60,000 U of amylase), 4X Pancreatin (contains 2,400 mg of pancreatin, 12,000 U of lipase, 60,000 U of protease, 60,000 U of amylase), 8X Pancreatin (contains 7,200 mg of pancreatin, 22,500 U of lipase, 180,000 U of protease, 180,000 U of amylase)

Class and Category
Chemical: Pancreatic enzyme
Therapeutic: Digestant, pancreatic enzyme replacement
Pregnancy category: C

Indications and Dosages
➤ *To treat pancreatic insufficiency, including steatorrhea*
CAPSULES, TABLETS
Adults. 8,000 to 24,000 U of lipase with meals or snacks, adjusted as prescribed, according to need for steatorrhea control. For severe insufficiency, up to 36,000 U of lipase with meals or snacks.

Mechanism of Action
Releases the enzymes pancreatin, lipase, amylase, and protease, mainly in the duodenum and upper jejunum. These enzymes facilitate the hydrolysis of fats into glycerol and fatty acids, starches into dextrins and sugars, and proteins into peptides. Pancreatin acts locally in the GI tract but is quickly inactivated by gastric acid.

Contraindications
Acute exacerbation of chronic pancreatic disease; acute pancreatitis; hypersensitivity to pancreatin, pancrelipase, or pork

Interactions
DRUGS
acarbose, miglitol: Decreased effectiveness of these drugs
aluminum hydroxide, H$_2$-receptor antagonists, omeprazole, sodium bicarbonate: Increased gastric pH, prolonged enzymatic action of pancreatin
calcium carbonate– and magnesium hydroxide–containing antacids: Decreased pancreatin effectiveness
iron supplements: Decreased iron absorption

Adverse Reactions
EENT: Stomatitis
GI: Abdominal cramps or pain, diarrhea, intestinal obstruction, nausea

SKIN: Rash, urticaria
Other: Hyperuricemia

Nursing Considerations
•**WARNING** Don't administer pancreatin to patient who is allergic to pork.
•Assess for GI disturbances and hyperuricemia in patients who are receiving high doses of pancreatin.
•If patient opens capsules and sprinkles contents on food, assess for signs of sensitization (chest tightness, dyspnea, nasal congestion, wheezing), which may result from repeated inadvertent inhalation of powder.
•Be aware that brands of pancreatin aren't interchangeable because the same doses don't contain equivalent amounts of drug.
PATIENT TEACHING
•Instruct patient to take pancreatin before or with meals or snacks to maximize effectiveness.
•To prevent capsule or tablet from lodging in esophagus, advise patient to take drug with a beverage while sitting upright, to swallow it quickly, and to follow with 1 or 2 mouthfuls of solid food.
•Caution patient not to chew tablets; doing so may irritate mouth, lips, and tongue.
•If patient has trouble swallowing capsules, advise her to open the capsule and sprinkle its contents on food without inhaling them.
•Caution patient not to take antacids that contain calcium carbonate or magnesium hydroxide during therapy.

pancrelipase

Cotazym (contains 8,000 U of lipase, 30,000 U of protease, 30,000 U of amylase), Cotazym-S (contains 5,000 U of lipase, 20,000 U of protease, 20,000 U of amylase), Ilozyme (contains 11,000 U of lipase, 30,000 U of protease, 30,000 U of amylase), Ku-Zyme HP (contains 8,000 U of lipase, 30,000 U of protease, 30,000 U of amylase), Pancrease (contains 4,500 U of lipase, 25,000 U of protease, 20,000 U of amylase), Pancrease MT 4 (contains 4,000 U of lipase, 12,000 U of protease, 12,000 U of amylase), Pancrease MT 10 (contains 10,000 U of lipase, 30,000 U of protease, 30,000 U of amylase), Pancrease MT 16 (contains 16,000 U of lipase, 48,000 U of protease, 48,000 U of amylase), Pancrease MT 20 (contains 20,000 U of lipase, 44,000 U of protease, 56,000 U of amylase), Protilase (contains 4,000 U of lipase, 25,000 U of protease, 20,000 U of amylase), Ultrase MT 12 (contains 12,000 U of lipase, 39,000 U of protease, 39,000 U of amylase), Ultrase MT 20 (contains 20,000 U of lipase, 65,000 U of protease, 65,000 U of amylase), Viokase Tablets (contains 8,000 U of lipase, 30,000 U of protease, 30,000 U of amylase), Viokase Powder (contains 16,800 U of lipase, 70,000 U of protease, 70,000 U of amylase), Zymase (contains 12,000 U of lipase, 24,000 U of protease, 24,000 U of amylase)

Class and Category
Chemical: Porcine pancreatic enzyme
Therapeutic: Pancreatic enzyme replacement
Pregnancy category: C

Indications and Dosages
➤ *To treat pancreatic insufficiency, including steatorrhea*
CAPSULES, DELAYED-RELEASE CAPSULES, POWDER, TABLETS
Adults and adolescents. 33,000 to 44,000 U of lipase before or with meals or snacks; adjusted as prescribed. For patients with severe deficiency, possibly up to 88,000 U of lipase with meals or snacks or dosing frequency increased to q hr.
Children ages 7 to 12. 4,000 to 12,000 U of lipase with meals and snacks; adjusted as needed and tolerated.
Children ages 1 to 6. 4,000 to 8,000 U of lipase with meals and 4,000 U of lipase given with each snack; adjusted as needed and tolerated.
Infants ages 6 to 11 months. 2,000 U of lipase with meals; adjusted as needed and tolerated.

Mechanism of Action
Releases high levels of the enzymes lipase, amylase, and protease, mainly in the duodenum and upper jejunum. These enzymes facilitate the hydrolysis of fats into glycerol and fatty acids, starches into dextrins and sugars, and proteins into peptides.

Contraindications
Acute exacerbation of chronic pancreatic disease; acute pancreatitis; hypersensitivity to pancreatin, pancrelipase, or pork

Interactions
DRUGS
acarbose, miglitol: Decreased effectiveness of these drugs
aluminum hydroxide, H₂-receptor antagonists, omeprazole, sodium bicarbonate: Increased gastric pH, prolonged enzymatic action of pancrelipase
calcium carbonate– and magnesium hydroxide–containing antacids: Decreased pancrelipase effectiveness
iron supplements: Decreased iron absorption

Adverse Reactions
EENT: Stomatitis
GI: Abdominal cramps or pain, diarrhea, intestinal obstruction, nausea
HEME: Anemia
SKIN: Rash, urticaria
Other: Hyperuricemia

Nursing Considerations
• WARNING Don't administer pancrelipase to patient who is allergic to pork.
• Be aware that brands of pancrelipase aren't interchangeable because the same doses don't contain equivalent amounts of drug.
• Mix powder with fluid or soft, nondairy food.
• If necessary, open delayed-release capsules and mix contents (enteric-coated spheres, microspheres, or microtablets) with liquids or soft food that requires no chewing. Administer immediately because enteric coating will dissolve after prolonged contact with foods that have a pH greater than 6.
• If patient opens capsules and sprinkles contents on food, assess for signs of sensitization (chest tightness, dyspnea, nasal congestion, wheezing), which may result from repeated inadvertent inhalation of powder.
• Give drug before or with meals and snacks, and follow with a glass of water or juice.
• Expect drug to cause stomatitis if held in mouth.
• Monitor stool for fecal fat content, as ordered.
• Monitor for iron deficiency anemia because serum iron level may decline during pancrelipase therapy.
PATIENT TEACHING
• Instruct patient to take pancrelipase before or with meals and snacks and to follow with a glass of water or juice.
• Instruct patient not to chew capsules (or capsule contents) or crush tablets and to swallow immediately because drug may cause irritation if held in mouth.

- If patient opens delayed-release capsules, urge her to avoid inhaling powder because doing so may cause chest tightness, shortness of breath, stuffy nose, trouble breathing, and wheezing.
- Inform patient that sneezing and tearing also may result from contact with powder.
- Caution patient not to use antacids because they may decrease drug effectiveness.
- Inform patient that her stool may smell foul.

pantoprazole sodium

Pantoloc (CAN), Protonix

Class and Category
Chemical: Substituted benzimidazole
Therapeutic: Antiulcer, gastric acid proton pump inhibitor
Pregnancy category: B

Indications and Dosages
➤ *To treat gastroesophageal reflux disease (GERD)*
DELAYED-RELEASE TABLETS
Adults. 40 mg q.d. for up to 8 wk. Dosage repeated for another 4 to 8 wk if healing isn't achieved.
I.V. INFUSION
Adults. 40 mg q.d. infused over 15 min for 7 to 10 days, followed by oral doses.
➤ *To maintain healing of erosive esophagitis and reduce relapse of daytime and nighttime symptoms in patients with GERD*
DELAYED-RELEASE TABLETS
Adults. 40 mg q.d. for up to 12 mo.
➤ *To treat pathological hypersecretion associated with Zollinger-Ellison syndrome or other neoplastic conditions*
I.V. INFUSION
Adults. 80 mg q 12 hr, adjusted based on patient's acid output measurements up to 80 mg q 8 hr.

Route	Onset	Peak	Duration
P.O.	1 day	1 wk	1 wk
I.V.	1 day	Unknown	1 wk

Contraindications
Hypersensitivity to pantoprazole, other substituted benzimidazoles (omeprazole, lansoprazole, rabeprazole sodium), or their components

Interactions
DRUGS
ampicillin, cyanocobalamin, digoxin, iron

salts, ketoconazole: Possibly impaired absorption of these drugs

Mechanism of Action
Interferes with gastric acid secretion by inhibiting the hydrogen-potassium-adenosine triphosphatase (H^+K^+–ATPase) enzyme system, or proton pump, in gastric parietal cells. Normally, the proton pump uses energy from the hydrolysis of ATPase to drive H^+ and chloride (Cl^-) out of parietal cells and into the stomach lumen in exchange for potassium (K^+), which leaves the stomach lumen and enters parietal cells. After this exchange, H^+ and Cl^- combine in the stomach to form hydrochloric acid (HCl). Pantoprazole irreversibly inhibits the final step in gastric acid production by blocking the exchange of intracellular H^+ and extracellular K^+, thus preventing H^+ from entering the stomach and additional HCl from forming.

Adverse Reactions
CNS: Headache, malaise
GI: Diarrhea

Nursing Considerations
- Be aware that patient may need follow-up assessment for gastric cancer, which isn't precluded by a favorable response to pantoprazole therapy.
- Ensure the continuity of gastric acid suppression during transition from oral to I.V. form (or vice versa) because even a brief interruption of effective suppression can lead to serious complications.
- Don't administer pantoprazole, as prescribed, within 4 weeks before testing for *Helicobacter pylori* because antibiotics, proton pump inhibitors, and bismuth preparations suppress *H. pylori* and may lead to false-negative results.
PATIENT TEACHING
- Instruct patient to swallow pantoprazole tablets whole and not to chew or crush them.
- Advise patient to expect relief of symptoms within 2 weeks of starting therapy.

paricalcitol

Zemplar

Class and Category
Chemical: Sterol derivative, vitamin D analogue

Therapeutic: Antihyperparathyroid
Pregnancy category: Not rated

Indications and Dosages

➤ *To prevent and treat secondary hyperparathyroidism in patients with chronic renal failure*

I.V. INJECTION

Adults. *Initial:* 0.04 to 0.1 mcg/kg (2.8 to 7 mcg) no more than q.o.d. at any time during dialysis. *Maintenance:* If initial dosage doesn't produce a satisfactory response, 2 to 4 mcg given q 2 to 4 wk. *Maximum:* 0.24 mcg/kg/dose or up to 16.8 mcg/dose.

DOSAGE ADJUSTMENT If serum parathyroid hormone (PTH) level remains the same or increases, dosage increased. If serum PTH level decreases by less than 30%, dosage increased. If serum PTH level decreases by 30% to 60%, dosage maintained. If serum PTH level decreases by more than 60%, dosage decreased. If serum PTH level is 1.5 to 3 times the upper normal limit, dosage maintained.

DOSAGE ADJUSTMENT Dosage immediately reduced or stopped if the serum calcium level is elevated or if the serum calcium-phosphorus product is greater than 75. Dosage restarted at a lower dose when these levels return to normal.

Route	Onset	Peak	Duration
I.V.	Unknown	Unknown	15 hr

Mechanism of Action

Reduces serum PTH level by an unknown mechanism. In chronic renal failure, decreased renal synthesis of vitamin D leads to chronic hypocalcemia. In an attempt to stimulate vitamin D synthesis and normalize the serum calcium levels, the parathyroid glands secrete excessive amounts of PTH, which can't produce normal serum calcium levels because of renal failure.

Contraindications

Evidence of vitamin D toxicity, hypercalcemia, hypersensitivity to paricalcitol or its components

Interactions

None known.

Adverse Reactions

CNS: Chills, fever, light-headedness, malaise
CV: Palpitations
EENT: Dry mouth
GI: GI bleeding, nausea, vomiting
RESP: Pneumonia
Other: Generalized edema, influenza, sepsis

Nursing Considerations

- Before administration, inspect drug for particulate matter and discoloration; if present, discard drug.
- Administer drug as an I.V. bolus and discard unused portion.
- Monitor serum calcium and phosphorus levels, as ordered, twice weekly early in therapy to guide dosage adjustments and then monthly.
- WARNING Be aware that paricalcitol may lead to vitamin D toxicity and hypercalcemia. Assess patient for early signs and symptoms of these conditions, including arthralgia, constipation, dry mouth, headache, metallic taste, myalgia, nausea, somnolence, vomiting, and weakness. Also assess patient for late signs and symptoms, including albuminuria, anorexia, arrhythmias, azotemia, conjunctivitis (calcific), decreased libido, elevated BUN and serum ALT and AST levels, generalized vascular calcification, hypercholesterolemia, hypertension, hyperthermia, irritability, mild acidosis, nephrocalcinosis, nocturia, pancreatitis, photophobia, polydipsia, polyuria, pruritus, rhinorrhea, and weight loss.
- If toxicity occurs, notify prescriber immediately and expect to decrease dosage or discontinue drug. Place patient on bed rest and administer fluids, a low calcium diet, and a laxative, as prescribed. If patient has a hypercalcemic crisis and dehydration, infuse NS and a loop diuretic, such as furosemide or ethacrynic acid, to increase renal calcium excretion, as prescribed.
- Expect to monitor serum PTH level every 3 months.
- If patient also takes digoxin, monitor her for signs and symptoms of digitalis glycoside toxicity, which is potentiated by hypercalcemia.
- Store drug at 25° C (77° F).

PATIENT TEACHING

- Advise patient to follow a diet high in calcium and low in phosphorus.
- Explain that patient may need phosphate binders to control serum phosphorus level.
- Teach patient the early signs and symptoms of hypercalcemia and vitamin D toxicity. Ad-

vise patient to contact prescriber immediately if they develop.
•Advise patient to avoid activities that require alertness until drug's adverse CNS effects are known.
•If patient takes digoxin, teach her the signs and symptoms of digitalis glycoside toxicity. Advise her to contact prescriber immediately if she suspects toxicity.

paroxetine hydrochloride

Paxil, Paxil CR

Class and Category

Chemical: Phenylpiperidine derivative
Therapeutic: Antidepressant, antiobsessional, antipanic
Pregnancy category: C

Indications and Dosages

➤ *To treat major depression*
C.R. TABLETS
Adults. *Initial:* 25 mg q.d., increased as prescribed and tolerated by 12.5 mg/day q wk. *Maximum:* 62.5 mg/day.
ORAL SUSPENSION, TABLETS
Adults. *Initial:* 20 mg q.d., increased as prescribed and tolerated by 10 mg/day q wk. *Maximum:* 50 mg/day.
➤ *To treat obsessive-compulsive disorder*
ORAL SUSPENSION, TABLETS
Adults. *Initial:* 20 mg q.d., increased as prescribed and tolerated by 10 mg/day q wk. *Usual:* 20 to 60 mg q.d. *Maximum:* 60 mg/day.
➤ *To treat panic disorder*
ORAL SUSPENSION, TABLETS
Adults. *Initial:* 10 mg q.d., increased as prescribed and tolerated by 10 mg/day q wk. *Usual:* 10 to 60 mg q.d. *Maximum:* 60 mg/day.
➤ *To treat social anxiety disorder*
ORAL SUSPENSION, TABLETS
Adults. *Initial:* 20 mg q.d., increased as prescribed and tolerated by 10 mg/day q wk. *Usual:* 20 to 60 mg q.d. *Maximum:* 60 mg/day.
➤ *To treat generalized anxiety disorder*
ORAL SUSPENSION, TABLETS
Adults. *Initial:* 20 mg q.d., increased as prescribed and tolerated by 10 mg/day q wk. *Usual:* 20 to 50 mg q.d. *Maximum:* 60 mg/day.

➤ *To treat posttraumatic stress disorder*
ORAL SUSPENSION, TABLETS
Adults. *Initial:* 20 mg q.d., increased as prescribed and tolerated by 10 mg/day q wk. *Usual:* 20 to 50 mg q.d. *Maximum:* 50 mg/day.
DOSAGE ADJUSTMENT For elderly or debilitated patients and those with a creatinine clearance of less than 30 ml/min/1.73 m², initial dosage reduced to 10 mg/day and maximum limited to 40 mg/day; C.R. form not recommended. For patients using C.R. tablets who have a creatinine clearance of less than 30 ml/min/1.73 m², initial dosage reduced to 12.5 mg/day and maximum limited to 50 mg/day.

Route	Onset	Peak	Duration
P.O.	1 to 4 wk	Unknown	Unknown

Mechanism of Action

Achieves its antidepressant, antiobsessional, and antipanic effects by potentiating serotonin activity in the CNS and inhibiting serotonin reuptake at the presynaptic neuronal membrane. Blocked serotonin reuptake at the neuronal membrane results in increased concentrations and prolonged activity of serotonin at synaptic receptor sites.

Contraindications

Hypersensitivity to paroxetine or its components, use within 14 days of MAO inhibitor therapy

Interactions

DRUGS
antacids: Hastened release of C.R. paroxetine
astemizole: Increased risk of arrhythmias
barbiturates, primidone: Decreased blood paroxetine level
cimetidine: Possibly increased blood paroxetine level
cisapride, isoniazid, MAO inhibitors, procarbazine: Possibly serotonin syndrome
codeine, haloperidol, metoprolol, perphenazine, propranolol, risperidone, thioridazine: Decreased metabolism and increased effects of these drugs
cyproheptadine: Decreased effects of paroxetine
dextromethorphan: Decreased dextromethorphan metabolism and increased risk of toxicity

digoxin: Possibly decreased digoxin effects
encainide, flecainide, propafenone, quinidine: Potentiated toxicity of these drugs
lithium: Possibly increased blood paroxetine level, increased risk of serotonin syndrome
methadone: Decreased methadone metabolism, increased risk of adverse effects
phenytoin: Possibly phenytoin toxicity
procyclidine: Increased blood procyclidine level and anticholinergic effects
theophylline: Possibly increased blood theophylline level and risk of toxicity
tramadol: Increased risk of serotonin syndrome and seizures
tricyclic antidepressants: Increased metabolism and blood antidepressant levels; increased risk of toxicity, including seizures
tryptophan: Increased risk of serotonin syndrome
tryptophan: Possibly serotonin syndrome
warfarin: Potentiated anticoagulant activity, increased risk of bleeding

Adverse Reactions

CNS: Agitation, confusion, dizziness, drowsiness, emotional lability, headache, insomnia, mania, restlessness, tremor
CV: Palpitations, tachycardia
EENT: Blurred vision, dry mouth, rhinitis, taste perversion
GI: Abdominal cramps or pain, constipation, diarrhea, flatulence, nausea, vomiting
GU: Decreased libido, difficult ejaculation, impotence, sexual dysfunction, urine retention
MS: Back pain, myalgia, myasthenia, myopathy
SKIN: Diaphoresis, rash
Other: Weight gain or loss

Nursing Considerations

• Shake paroxetine oral suspension well before using. Measure with an oral syringe or calibrated measuring device.
• Ensure that patient swallows C.R. tablets whole. Don't let her cut, crush, or chew them.
• Avoid giving enteric-coated tablets with antacids.
• Assess patient for worsening depression or suicidal ideation.
• Observe patient for sudden mania; all antidepressants can precipitate mania in predisposed patients.
• Be aware that paroxetine may precipitate serotonin syndrome, which may cause ar-

rhythmias, coma, disseminated intravascular coagulation, renal and respiratory failure, seizures, and severe hypertension, along with such milder symptoms as abdominal cramps, aggressive behavior, confusion, headache, nausea, palpitations, paresthesia, and increased obsessive thoughts.

PATIENT TEACHING
• Advise patient to take paroxetine in the morning to minimize insomnia and to take drug with food if adverse GI reactions develop.
• Instruct patient to avoid taking C.R. paroxetine within 2 hours of an antacid.
• Suggest that patient avoid hazardous activities until drug's CNS effects are known.
• Inform patient that drug may not achieve full effects for 4 weeks.
• Urge patient to avoid alcohol during paroxetine therapy because its effects on drug are unknown.
• Inform patient that episodes of acute depression may persist for months or longer and that they require continued follow-up.
• Instruct patient not to discontinue drug abruptly. Tell her to taper dosage as instructed to help prevent adverse reactions, such as dizziness, tingling, agitation, nausea, and sweating, as drug is discontinued.

pegfilgrastim

Neulasta

Class and Category

Chemical: Recombinant granulocyte colony-stimulating factor conjugate
Therapeutic: Antineutropenic, hematopoietic stimulator
Pregnancy category: C

Indications and Dosages

➤ *To reduce the risk of infection, as manifested by febrile neutropenia, after myelosuppressive chemotherapy*
S.C. INJECTION
Adults. 6 mg with each chemotherapy cycle.

Contraindications

Hypersensitivity to filgrastim, pegfilgrastim, or their components or to proteins derived from *Escherichia coli*

Interactions
DRUGS
lithium: Increased neutrophil production

Mechanism of Action
Is pharmacologically identical to human granulocyte colony-stimulating factor, an endogenous hormone synthesized by monocytes, endothelial cells, and fibroblasts. Pegfilgrastim induces the formation of neutrophil progenitor cells by binding directly to receptors on the surface of granulocytes, which then divide and differentiate. It also potentiates the effects of mature neutrophils, thus reducing fever and the risk of infection posed by severe neutropenia.

Adverse Reactions
CNS: Fever
GI: Elevated liver function test results, splenomegaly
GU: Elevated uric acid level
HEME: Leukocytosis, sickle cell crisis
MS: Bone pain
RESP: Dyspnea, hypoxia, pulmonary infiltrates
SKIN: Rash, urticaria
Other: Anaphylaxis

Nursing Considerations
• Be aware that pegfilgrastim should not be administered for 14 days before and 24 hours after cytotoxic chemotherapy.
• Monitor CBC, hematocrit, and platelet count before starting therapy and periodically thereafter, as ordered.
• Let pegfilgrastim warm to room temperature before injection. Discard drug if stored at room temperature for longer than 48 hours.
• Don't shake the solution.
• Discard solution if it contains particles or is discolored. Use prefilled syringe and needles to administer drug.
• **WARNING** Monitor patient for signs of an allergic reaction, such as difficulty breathing or a rash. If such a reaction occurs, discontinue infusion and notify prescriber at once. If anaphylaxis occurs, administer an antihistamine, epinephrine, a corticosteroid, and a bronchodilator, as prescribed.
• **WARNING** Be aware that patients receiving filgrastim, the parent drug of pegfilgrastim, have experienced splenic rupture and acute respiratory distress syndrome. Assess patient for signs of these conditions, such as fever, respiratory distress, and upper abdominal or shoulder tip pain.
• Assess patients with sickle cell disease for signs of sickle cell crisis, and encourage adequate hydration. Sickle cell crisis has been reported by patients using the parent drug, filgrastim.
• Administer nonnarcotic and narcotic analgesics, as ordered, if patient experiences bone pain.
• Before using drug, store it at 2° to 8° C (36° to 46° F), and protect from freezing and light.
PATIENT TEACHING
• Advise patient to immediately report potentially serious adverse reactions, such as difficulty breathing, rash, or chest tightness, during pegfilgrastim therapy. Also instruct her to report signs of a possible infection, such as fever or chills.
• If patient will be self-administering drug, teach her how to prepare, administer, and store it.
• Instruct patient to rotate injection sites among thigh, stomach (except for 2″ around the navel), buttocks, and outer, upper arms. Caution her to avoid areas that are tender, hard, red, or bruised.
• Urge patient to discard used needles and syringes in a puncture-resistant container and not to reuse them. Instruct her to return container to prescriber for proper disposal.
• Stress the importance of returning for follow-up laboratory tests.
• Advise patient to store drug in refrigerator and not to freeze it. Tell her to discard drug if left unrefrigerated for more than 48 hours.

pemoline
Cylert, Cylert Chewable

Class, Category, and Schedule
Chemical: Oxazolidine
Therapeutic: CNS stimulant
Pregnancy category: B
Controlled substance: Schedule IV

Indications and Dosages
➤ *To treat attention deficit hyperactivity disorder (ADHD)*
CHEWABLE TABLETS, TABLETS
Children age 6 and older. *Initial:* 37.5 mg q.d. in the morning. Dosage increased by 18.75 mg/day q wk until desired response

achieved. *Usual:* 56.25 to 75 mg/day. *Maximum:* 112.5 mg/day.

DOSAGE ADJUSTMENT When ADHD symptoms are controlled in children, dosage may be reduced or therapy interrupted during summer months and other periods of decreased stress; for example, drug may be given only on weekdays, with weekends and holidays drug free.

Route	Onset	Peak	Duration
P.O.	Unknown	3 to 4 wk	Unknown

Mechanism of Action

May act in the cerebral cortex and the subcortical structures to block the reuptake mechanism present in dopaminergic neurons. This action decreases hyperactivity and prolongs the attention span.

Contraindications

Hypersensitivity or abnormal susceptibility to pemoline or its components, impaired hepatic function, use within 14 days of MAO inhibitor therapy

Interactions

DRUGS

anticonvulsants: Possibly decreased seizure threshold

CNS stimulants: Possibly excessive CNS stimulation

Adverse Reactions

CNS: Depression, dizziness, drowsiness, headache, insomnia, irritability

GI: Abdominal pain, elevated liver function test results, hepatic failure, nausea

Other: Weight loss

Nursing Considerations

•Monitor for compliance in patients with emotional instability or patients who may be inclined to increase pemoline dosage without consulting prescriber.

•WARNING Expect to monitor patient's liver function test results, as ordered, before and every 2 weeks during pemoline therapy because drug may precipitate hepatic failure, especially during first 4 weeks. Assess patient for signs of acute hepatic failure, such as jaundice, dark urine, GI disturbances, and malaise.

•WARNING Monitor patients on prolonged therapy and those with a previous history of substance abuse for physical and psychologi-

cal dependence. Assess for possible withdrawal symptoms, such as abdominal pain, depression, headache, nausea or vomiting, seizures, unusual behavior, and unusual tiredness or weakness.

•Assess patients with a history of Tourette syndrome or motor or vocal tics for exacerbation of these symptoms during pemoline therapy.

•Monitor growth and development in children because drug use may adversely affect growth.

•Expect drug to be discontinued gradually during adolescence if significant clinical improvement has been achieved.

PATIENT TEACHING

•Advise patient to take pemoline in the morning with food or after a meal to reduce anorexia.

•Instruct patient to chew chewable tablet thoroughly before swallowing.

•Urge patient to avoid potentially hazardous activities until drug's CNS effects are known.

•Advise patient to notify prescriber immediately in the event her skin or eyes begin to turn yellow or she notices her urine color darkening.

•Encourage patient to comply with routinely scheduled laboratory blood tests to help detect early signs of liver dysfunction.

•Instruct parents to keep regularly scheduled follow-up appointments for child to prevent growth suppression during pemoline therapy.

•Inform parents that child may be placed on drug-free weekend and holiday schedule, as prescribed, if symptoms of ADHD are controlled.

penbutolol sulfate

Levatol

Class and Category

Chemical: Nonselective beta-adrenergic blocker

Therapeutic: Antihypertensive

Pregnancy category: Not rated

Indications and Dosages

➤ *To manage hypertension*

TABLETS

Adults. 20 mg q.d.

DOSAGE ADJUSTMENT For elderly patients, dosage individualized according to sensitivity to drug.

Route	Onset	Peak	Duration
P.O.	Unknown	1.5 to 3 hr	Unknown

Mechanism of Action
May reduce blood pressure by competing with beta-adrenergic receptor agonists, which helps reduce cardiac output, decrease sympathetic outflow to peripheral blood vessels, and inhibit renin release by the kidneys.

Contraindications
Asthma, bradycardia (fewer than 45 beats/min), cardiogenic shock, heart failure, hypersensitivity to penbutolol or its components, second- or third-degree AV block

Interactions
DRUGS

allergen immunotherapy, allergenic extracts for skin testing: Increased risk of serious systemic reaction or anaphylaxis

amiodarone: Additive depressant effect on cardiac conduction, negative inotropic effects

anesthetics (hydrocarbon inhalation): Increased risk of myocardial depression and hypotension

calcium channel blockers, clonidine, diazoxide, guanabenz, other hypotension-producing drugs, reserpine: Additive hypotension and possibly other beta blocker effects

cimetidine: Possibly increased blood penbutolol level

estrogens: Decreased antihypertensive effect of penbutolol

fentanyl and its derivatives: Possibly increased risk of initial bradycardia after induction doses of fentanyl derivative (with long-term penbutolol use)

insulin, oral antidiabetic drugs: Possibly impaired glucose control and masking of hypoglycemia symptoms such as tachycardia

lidocaine: Decreased lidocaine clearance, increased risk of lidocaine toxicity

MAO inhibitors: Increased risk of significant hypertension

neuromuscular blockers: Possibly potentiated and prolonged action of these drugs

NSAIDs: Possibly decreased hypotensive effect of penbutolol

other beta blockers: Additive beta blocker effects

phenothiazines: Increased blood levels of both drugs

phenytoin (parenteral): Additive cardiac depressant effects

sympathomimetics, xanthines: Possibly inhibited effects of penbutolol and these drugs

Adverse Reactions
CNS: Anxiety, depression, dizziness, drowsiness, fatigue, insomnia, light-headedness, nervousness, syncope, weakness
CV: Bradycardia, chest pain, edema, peripheral vascular insufficiency
EENT: Nasal congestion
GI: Constipation, diarrhea, epigastric pain, nausea, vomiting
GU: Impotence
RESP: Bronchospasm, dyspnea

Nursing Considerations
•Expect varied drug effectiveness in elderly patients, who may be more sensitive to penbutolol's antihypertensive effects because of reduced drug clearance by kidneys.
•**WARNING** Avoid discontinuing penbutolol therapy abruptly because doing so may precipitate myocardial infarction, myocardial ischemia, severe hypertension, or ventricular arrhythmias, particularly in patients with known cardiovascular disease. Monitor for tachycardia because drug may also mask certain signs of hyperthyroidism. Be aware that abrupt withdrawal of drug in patients with hyperthyroidism or thyrotoxicosis can precipitate thyroid storm.
•Monitor blood pressure and cardiac output, as appropriate, in patients with a history of systolic heart failure or left ventricular dysfunction because drug's negative inotropic effect can depress cardiac output.
•Monitor patients with diabetes mellitus who are taking antidiabetic drugs because penbutolol can prolong hypoglycemia or promote hyperglycemia. Be aware that penbutolol can also mask signs of hypoglycemia, especially tachycardia, palpitations, and tremor.
•Monitor for impaired circulation in elderly patients with age-related peripheral vascular disease or patients with Raynaud's phenomenon. Keep in mind that elderly patients are also at increased risk for beta blocker–induced hypothermia.
•Monitor drug refill frequency to help determine patient compliance.

PATIENT TEACHING
• Instruct patient to take penbutolol at the same time every day and not to change dosage without consulting prescriber.
• Advise patient not to stop taking drug abruptly, but to taper dosage gradually under prescriber's supervision.
• Instruct patient with diabetes mellitus to regularly monitor blood glucose level and test urine for ketones.
• Advise patient to consult prescriber before taking over-the-counter drugs, especially cold remedies.
• Urge patient to avoid potentially hazardous activities until drug's CNS effects are known.
• Instruct patient to inform prescriber of chest pain, fainting, light-headedness, or shortness of breath, any of which may indicate the need for a dosage change.
• Inform patient that penbutolol doesn't cure hypertension. Encourage her to follow recommended diet and lifestyle changes.

penicillamine

Cuprimine, Depen

Class and Category
Chemical: Degradation product of penicillin
Therapeutic: Antirheumatic, antiurolithic, chelating agent
Pregnancy category: Not rated

Indications and Dosages
➤ *To treat cystinuria*
CAPSULES, TABLETS
Adults and adolescents. 500 mg q.i.d.
Children. 7.5 mg/kg q.i.d.
➤ *To treat rheumatoid arthritis*
CAPSULES, TABLETS
Adults and adolescents. *Initial:* 125 or 250 mg q.d. Dosage increased by 125 or 250 mg/day q 2 to 3 mo. *Maximum:* 1,500 mg/day.
➤ *To treat Wilson's disease*
CAPSULES, TABLETS
Adults and adolescents. Dosage individualized up to 2 g/day in divided doses q.i.d., as determined by measurement of urinary copper excretion.
DOSAGE ADJUSTMENT For elderly patients, 125 mg q.d. initially, then increased by 125 mg/day q 2 to 3 mo, up to maximum of 750 mg/day; for pregnant women, maximum dose of 1 g/day; for women undergoing

planned cesarean section, dosage limited to 250 mg/day during last 6 wk of pregnancy and until wound healing completed.

Route	Onset	Peak	Duration
P.O.	2 to 3 mo*	Unknown	Unknown

Mechanism of Action
Combines with copper to form a ring-shaped complex that is excreted in urine, thereby reducing copper levels in the body. Penicillamine also lowers urine cystine levels by binding with cystine to form penicillamine-cysteine disulfide, which is more soluble than cystine and more easily excreted in urine. The decrease in urine cystine levels also helps prevent the formation of cystine calculi and may help existing cystine calculi dissolve over time. In addition, penicillamine improves lymphocyte function by reducing IgM rheumatoid factor and immune complexes in serum and synovial fluid, which may play a role in the treatment of rheumatoid arthritis.

Contraindications
Hypersensitivity to penicillin, penicillamine, or their components; penicillamine-related aplastic anemia or agranulocytosis; renal insufficiency (for patients with rheumatoid arthritis)

Interactions
DRUGS
4-aminoquinolines, bone marrow depressants, gold compounds, immunosuppressants (excluding glucocorticoids), phenylbutazone: Possibly increased risk of serious hematologic or renal adverse reactions
iron supplements: Possibly decreased effectiveness of penicillamine
pyridoxine: Decreased effectiveness of pyridoxine, possibly increased risk of anemia or peripheral neuritis reaction

Adverse Reactions
CNS: Fever
EENT: Loss of taste, stomatitis
GI: Anorexia, diarrhea, mild epigastric pain, nausea, vomiting
GU: Glomerulonephropathy

---

* For rheumatoid arthritis; 1 to 3 mo for Wilson's disease.

HEME: Agranulocytosis, aplastic anemia, hemolytic anemia, leukopenia, thrombocytopenia
MS: Arthralgia
SKIN: Pemphigus, pruritus, rash, urticaria

Nursing Considerations

•Administer penicillamine 1 hour before or 2 hours after meals and at least 1 hour before or after any other drug, food, or milk. Give last dose of day at least 3 hours after evening meal to ensure maximum absorption.
•For patient who has difficulty swallowing capsules or tablets, open capsule and mix contents in 15 to 30 ml of pureed fruit or fruit juice to mask drug's sulfur odor. Alternatively, request pharmacist to prepare an elixir for oral administration.
•Expect to administer 25 mg of pyridoxine, as prescribed, to patients being treated with penicillamine because penicillamine increases intake requirements for this vitamin.
•Monitor for febrile reactions in patients who developed a fever during previous penicillamine administration. Expect drug to be discontinued if patient develops drug-induced fever.
•Assess skin and mucous membranes for possible sensitivity reactions, such as skin lesions and mouth ulcers. Be prepared to discontinue drug as prescribed.
•Expect to monitor urine laboratory test results, as ordered, for proteinuria or hematuria, which may precipitate nephrotic syndrome, especially in patients with renal disease or history of renal insufficiency. Also, weigh patient daily, observe for signs of edema, and monitor intake and output because penicillamine may exacerbate underlying renal disease.
•Because of the potential for cross-sensitivity between penicillamine and penicillin, monitor for symptoms of an allergic reaction in patients with a history of penicillin allergy.
•Notify prescriber if patient complains of decreased sense of taste, especially for salty and sweet foods. Expect normal taste sensation to be restored (except in patients with Wilson's disease) with administration of 5 to 10 mg of copper a day, as prescribed.
•Monitor patients with diabetes mellitus for reduced insulin requirements to prevent the risk of nighttime hypoglycemia because penicillamine may promote the formation of anti-insulin antibodies.

PATIENT TEACHING
•Advise patient to take penicillamine on an empty stomach.
•Instruct adult males and nonpregnant females with cystinuria to increase fluid intake and follow prescribed low-methionine diet to minimize cystine production and enhance drug's effectiveness. Encourage patient to drink about 1 pint of fluid at bedtime and again during the night because this is when urine is more concentrated.
•Instruct patient being treated for Wilson's disease to follow a diet low in copper, avoiding such foods as broccoli, chocolate, copper-enriched cereals, liver, molasses, mushrooms, nuts, and shellfish. Inform her that improvement in her condition may require 1 to 3 months of therapy.
•Advise patient to consult prescriber before having dental work done during penicillamine therapy because drug can promote mouth ulcers.
•Instruct patient to avoid iron-containing preparations during penicillamine therapy because iron can decrease drug's effectiveness.
•Inform patient that her sense of taste may decrease during penicillamine therapy. Advise her to notify prescriber if decreased taste becomes intolerable.
•Inform patient with rheumatoid arthritis that improvement in condition may require 2 to 3 months of therapy.
•Caution female patient to notify prescriber immediately if she becomes or may be pregnant because dosage may need to be reduced to prevent serious birth defects.

penicillin G benzathine

Bicillin L-A, Megacillin (CAN), Permapen

penicillin G potassium

Megacillin (CAN), Pentids, Pfizerpen

penicillin G procaine

Ayercillin (CAN), Crysticillin 300 AS, Pfizerpen-AS, Wycillin

penicillin G sodium

penicillin V potassium

Apo-Pen-VK (CAN), Beepen-VK, Betapen-VK, Ledercillin VK, Nadopen-V 200 (CAN), Nadopen-V 400 (CAN), Novo-Pen-VK (CAN), Nu-Pen

VK (CAN), Pen Vee (CAN), Pen Vee K, V-Cillin K (CAN), Veetids

Class and Category

Chemical: Penicillin
Therapeutic: Antibiotic
Pregnancy category: B

Indications and Dosages

➤ *To treat systemic infections caused by gram-positive organisms (including* Bacillus anthracis, Corynebacterium diphtheriae, *enterococci,* Listeria monocytogenes, Staphylococcus aureus, *and* Staphylococcus epidermidis)*, gram-negative organisms (including* Neisseria gonorrhoeae, Neisseria meningitidis, Pasteurella multocida, *and* Streptobacillus moniliformis *[rat-bite fever]), and gram-positive anaerobes (including* Actinomyces israelii *[actinomycosis],* Clostridium perfringens, Clostridium tetani, Pasteurella multocida, Peptococcus *sp.,* Peptostreptococcus *sp., and spirochetes, especially* Treponema carateum *[pinta],* Treponema pallidum, *and* Treponema pertenue *[yaws])*

ORAL SOLUTION, TABLETS (PENICILLIN G POTASSIUM)
Adults and adolescents. 200,000 to 500,000 U (125 to 312 mg) q 4 to 6 hr. *Maximum:* 2 million U/day.
Children. 4,167 to 15,000 U/kg q 4 hr, 6,250 to 22,500 U/kg q 6 hr, or 8,333 to 30,000 U/kg q 8 hr.

TABLETS (PENICILLIN V POTASSIUM)
Adults and adolescents. 200,000 to 800,000 U (125 to 500 mg) q 6 to 8 hr. *Maximum:* 11,520,000 U (7,200 mg)/day
Children. 4,167 to 13,280 U (2.5 to 8.3 mg)/kg q 4 hr, 6,250 to 20,000 U (3.75 to 12.5 mg)/kg q 6 hr, or 8,333 to 26,720 U (5 to 16.7 mg)/kg q 8 hr.

I.V. INFUSION, I.M. INJECTION (PENICILLIN G POTASSIUM, PENICILLIN G SODIUM)
Adults and adolescents. 1 to 5 million U q 4 to 6 hr. *Maximum:* 80 million U/day.
Children. 8,333 to 16,667 U/kg q 4 hr or 12,500 to 25,000 U/kg q 6 hr.
Premature and full-term neonates. 30,000 U/kg q 12 hr.

I.M. INJECTION (PENICILLIN G PROCAINE)
Adults and adolescents. 600,000 to 1,200,000 U/day in divided doses q 12 to 24 hr.

➤ *To treat moderately severe to severe streptococcal infections*
I.M. INJECTION (PENICILLIN G BENZATHINE)
Adults and children weighing more than 45 kg (100 lb). 1.2 million U as a single injection.
Children weighing 27 to 45 kg (59 to 100 lb). 900,000 U as a single injection.
Children weighing less than 27 kg. 300,000 to 600,000 U as a single injection.

➤ *To treat congenital syphilis*
I.M. INJECTION (PENICILLIN G BENZATHINE)
Children under age 2. 50,000 U/kg as a single injection.

➤ *To treat syphilis of less than 1 year's duration*
I.M. INJECTION (PENICILLIN G BENZATHINE)
Adults and adolescents. 2.4 million U as a single injection.
Children. 50,000 U/kg up to adult dosage as a single injection. *Maximum:* 2.4 million U/dose.

➤ *To treat syphilis of more than 1 year's duration*
I.M. INJECTION (PENICILLIN G BENZATHINE)
Adults and adolescents. 2.4 million U q wk for 3 wk.
Children. 50,000 U/kg q wk for 3 wk.

➤ *To treat bacterial meningitis*
I.V. INFUSION, I.M. INJECTION (PENICILLIN G POTASSIUM)
Adults. 50,000 U/kg q 4 hr or 24 million U/day in divided doses q 2 to 4 hr.

Mechanism of Action

Inhibits final stage of bacterial cell wall synthesis by competitively binding to penicillin-binding proteins inside the cell wall. Penicillin-binding proteins are responsible for various steps in bacterial cell wall synthesis. By binding to these proteins, penicillin leads to cell wall lysis.

Contraindications

Hypersensitivity to penicillin or its components

Incompatibilities

Don't mix any penicillin in the same syringe or container with aminoglycosides because aminoglycosides will be inactivated. Don't mix penicillin G with drugs that may result in a pH below 5.5 or above 8.

Interactions

DRUGS
ACE inhibitors, potassium-containing drugs, potassium-sparing diuretics: Increased risk

of hyperkalemia (with penicillin G potassium)

chloramphenicol, erythromycin, sulfonamides, tetracycline, thrombolytics: Possibly interference with penicillin's bactericidal effect
cholestyramine, colestipol: Possibly impaired absorption of oral penicillin G
methotrexate: Decreased methotrexate clearance, increased risk of toxicity
oral contraceptives: Decreased contraceptive effectiveness (with penicillin V)
probenecid: Increased blood penicillin level
FOODS
acidic beverages, such as fruit juices: Possibly altered effects of oral penicillin G

Adverse Reactions
CNS: Confusion, dizziness, dysphasia, hallucinations, headache, lethargy, sciatic nerve irritation, seizures
CV: Labile blood pressure, palpitations
EENT: Black "hairy" tongue, oral candidiasis, stomatitis, taste perversion
GI: Abdominal pain, diarrhea, elevated liver function test results (transient), indigestion, nausea, pseudomembranous colitis
GU: Interstitial nephritis (acute), vaginal candidiasis
MS: Muscle twitching
SKIN: Rash
Other: Electrolyte imbalances; injection site necrosis, pain, or redness

Nursing Considerations
•Obtain body tissue and fluid samples for culture and sensitivity tests as ordered before giving first dose. Expect to begin drug therapy before test results are known.
•Reconstitute vials of penicillin for injection with sterile water for injection, D_5W, or sodium chloride for injection.
•Administer penicillin at least 1 hour before other antibiotics.
•Inject I.M. form deep into large muscle mass. Apply ice to relieve pain.
•**WARNING** Give penicillin G procaine only by deep I.M. injection; I.V. injection may be fatal, and intra-arterial injection may cause extensive tissue and organ necrosis.
•Be aware that I.M. drug is absorbed slowly, which may make allergic reactions difficult to treat.
•Assess for signs of secondary infection, such as profuse, watery diarrhea.

•Monitor serum sodium level and assess for early signs of heart failure in patients receiving high doses of penicillin G sodium.
PATIENT TEACHING
•Instruct patient to report previous allergies to penicillins and to notify prescriber immediately about adverse reactions, including fever.
•Advise patient who uses oral contraceptives to use an additional form of contraception during penicillin V therapy.

pentamidine isethionate
NebuPent, Pentacarinat (CAN), Pentam 300, Pneumopent (CAN)

Class and Category
Chemical: Diamidine derivative
Therapeutic: Antiprotozoal
Pregnancy category: C

Indications and Dosages
➤ *To prevent* Pneumocystis carinii *pneumonia*
ORAL INHALATION (NEBUPENT, PENTACARINAT)
Adults and adolescents. 300 mg q 4 wk or 150 mg q 2 wk, using nebulizer and continuing until nebulizer chamber is empty (30 to 45 min).
ORAL INHALATION (PNEUMOPENT)
Adults and adolescents. *Initial:* 60 mg q 24 to 72 hr for 5 doses over 2 wk, using ultrasonic nebulizer and continuing until nebulizer chamber is empty (about 15 min). *Maintenance:* 60 mg q 2 wk, using ultrasonic nebulizer and continuing until nebulizer chamber is empty.

➤ *To treat* P. carinii *pneumonia*
I.V. INFUSION, I.M. INJECTION
Adults and children. 4 mg/kg q.d. for 14 to 21 days, given deep I.M. or by I.V. infusion over 1 to 2 hr.
DOSAGE ADJUSTMENT Dosage possibly reduced or I.V. infusion time or dosing interval extended for patients with renal failure.

Incompatibilities
Don't mix pentamidine with other drugs or with saline solutions because precipitation may occur.

Contraindications
History of anaphylactic reaction to pentamidine or its components (inhalation form)

Mechanism of Action

May bind to DNA and inhibit DNA replication in *Pneumocystis carinii*. Pentamidine also may inhibit dihydrofolate reductase, an enzyme needed to convert dihydrofolic acid to tetrahydrofolic acid in this organism. This action inhibits the formation of coenzymes that are essential to the growth and replication of *P. carinii*.

Interactions

DRUGS

bone marrow depressants, drugs that cause blood dyscrasias: Increased risk of adverse hematologic effects

didanosine: Increased risk of pancreatitis

erythromycin (I.V.): Increased risk of torsades de pointes

foscarnet: Increased risk of severe but reversible hypocalcemia, hypomagnesemia, and nephrotoxicity

nephrotoxic drugs: Increased risk of nephrotoxicity

Adverse Reactions

CNS: Chills, confusion, dizziness, fatigue, fever, hallucinations, headache (I.V., I.M. forms)

CV: Arrhythmias, edema, hypotension, prolonged QT interval, torsades de pointes, ventricular tachycardia (I.V., I.M. forms)

EENT: Bitter or metallic taste (all forms), pharyngitis (inhalation form)

ENDO: Diabetes mellitus, hyperglycemia (I.V., I.M. forms); hypoglycemia (all forms)

GI: Abdominal pain, anorexia, diarrhea, elevated liver function test results, nausea, vomiting (I.V., I.M. forms); pancreatitis (all forms)

GU: Elevated serum creatinine level (I.V., I.M. forms); renal insufficiency (inhalation form)

HEME: Anemia, leukopenia, thrombocytopenia, unusual bleeding or bruising (I.V., I.M. forms)

MS: Myalgia (I.V., I.M. forms)

RESP: Bronchospasm, chest pain or congestion, cough, dyspnea, extrapulmonary pneumocystosis, pneumothorax (inhalation form)

SKIN: Night sweats (I.V., I.M. forms); rash (all forms)

Other: Hyperchloremic acidosis; hyperkalemia; hypocalcemia; hypomagnesemia; infusion site sterile abscess (I.V. form); injection site induration, pain, and phlebitis (I.M. form)

Nursing Considerations

• Store pentamidine at room temperature, protected from light. Use within 24 hours after reconstitution.

• For I.V. use, dissolve contents of 300-mg vial with 3 to 5 ml of sterile water for injection or D_5W. Further dilute in 50 to 250 ml of D_5W and infuse over 1 to 2 hours.

• For I.M. use, dissolve contents of vial in 3 ml of sterile water for injection and inject deep into large muscle mass. Be aware that I.M. administration increases the risk of sterile abscess formation at injection site.

• When giving drug I.V. or I.M., keep patient supine and monitor blood pressure frequently during and after administration. Keep emergency resuscitation equipment readily available.

• Assess for hypoglycemia and arrhythmias in patient receiving I.V. or I.M. pentamidine. Although uncommon, these adverse reactions can be severe.

• For inhalation, reconstitute contents of vial with 6 ml of sterile water for injection (if using NebuPent or Pentacarinat) or 3 to 5 ml of sterile water for injection or inhalation (if using Pneumopent). Reconstitute immediately before use. Don't use NS because it causes precipitation. Place reconstituted drug into Respirgard II nebulizer, and set flow rate at 5 to 7 L/min for use with NebuPent or Pentacarinat. Don't mix with any other drugs. For Pneumopent administration, place reconstituted drug in Fisoneb ultrasonic nebulizer and set flow rate at the mid-flow mark.

• Administer aerosolized pentamidine with patient in supine or recumbent position for best distribution of drug.

• If patient who uses inhalation form has a history of asthma or smoking, notify prescriber if bronchospasm or a cough develops. She may need an aerosolized bronchodilator before each dose of pentamidine.

• Monitor CBC; platelet count; liver function test results; BUN, serum creatinine and calcium, and blood glucose levels; and ECG tracing throughout therapy, as ordered.

• Monitor blood glucose level because pentamidine use can induce insulin release from pancreas, causing severe hypoglycemia that can last from 1 day to several weeks.

• Be aware that hyperglycemia and diabetes mellitus can occur up to several months after discontinuation of parenteral therapy.

P

PATIENT TEACHING
• Stress the importance of complying with
the prescribed administration schedule when
pentamidine is used to prevent *P. carinii*
pneumonia.
• Advise patient to avoid potentially hazardous activities until drug's CNS effects are
known.
• Instruct patient to notify prescriber about
unusual bleeding or bruising and to take
precautions to avoid bleeding, such as using
a soft-bristled toothbrush and an electric
shaver.
• Caution patient about possible hypoglycemic effects of pentamidine therapy.
• Advise patient to have follow-up laboratory
studies to test for diabetes mellitus, which
can occur up to several months after stopping pentamidine therapy.

pentazocine lactate

Talwin, Talwin-Nx

Class, Category, and Schedule
Chemical: Synthetic opioid
Therapeutic: Analgesic
Pregnancy category: C
Controlled substance: Schedule IV

Indications and Dosages
➤ *To relieve moderate to severe pain*
I.V., I.M., OR S.C. INJECTION
Adults. *Initial:* 30 mg q 3 to 4 hr, p.r.n. *Maxi-
mum:* 30 mg/single dose I.V., 60 mg/single
dose I.M. or S.C., or 360 mg/24 hr for all
parenteral forms.
➤ *To relieve obstetric pain*
I.V. INJECTION
Adults. 20 mg when contractions become
regular; repeated 2 or 3 times q 2 to 3 hr, as
prescribed.
I.M. INJECTION
Adults. 30 mg as a single dose.

Route	Onset	Peak	Duration
I.V.	2 to 3 min	15 to 30 min	2 to 3 hr
I.M., S.C.	15 to 20 min	30 to 60 min	2 to 3 hr

Incompatibilities
Don't mix pentazocine in same syringe with
a soluble barbiturate because precipitation
will occur.

Mechanism of Action
Binds with opioid receptors, primarily
kappa and sigma receptors, at many CNS
sites to alter the perception of and emotional response to pain.

Contraindications
Hypersensitivity to pentazocine or its components

Interactions
DRUGS
anticholinergics: Increased risk of urine retention and severe constipation
antidiarrheals, antiperistaltics: Increased risk
of severe constipation and CNS depression
*antihypertensives, diuretics, other hypotension-
producing drugs:* Additive hypotensive effects
buprenorphine: Decreased pentazocine effectiveness, increased respiratory depression
CNS depressants: Increased CNS depression,
increased risk of habituation
hydroxyzine, other opioid analgesics: Increased analgesia, CNS depression, and hypotensive effects
MAO inhibitors: Increased risk of unpredictable, severe, and sometimes fatal adverse reactions
metoclopramide: Antagonized metoclopramide effects on GI motility
naloxone: Antagonized analgesic, CNS, and
respiratory depressant effects of pentazocine
naltrexone: Withdrawal symptoms in patients
who are physically dependent on pentazocine
neuromuscular blockers: Increased respiratory depression
ACTIVITIES
alcohol use: Additive CNS depression and
increased risk of habituation

Adverse Reactions
CNS: Dizziness, drowsiness, euphoria, fa-
tigue, headache, light-headedness, nervous-
ness, nightmares, restlessness, weakness
CV: Hypotension, tachycardia
EENT: Blurred vision, diplopia, dry mouth,
laryngeal edema, laryngospasm
GI: Constipation, hepatotoxicity, nausea,
vomiting
GU: Decreased urine output, dysuria, urinary
frequency
MS: Muscle rigidity (with large doses)
RESP: Atelectasis, bronchospasm, dyspnea,
hypoventilation, wheezing

SKIN: Diaphoresis, facial flushing, pruritus, rash, urticaria
Other: Facial edema; injection site burning, pain, redness, or swelling; physical and psychological dependence

Nursing Considerations
• Use pentazocine with extreme caution in patients who have a head injury, an intracranial lesion, or increased intracranial pressure because drug may mask neurologic signs and symptoms.
• Use drug cautiously in patients who are physically dependent on opioid agonists because drug may prompt withdrawal symptoms; in patients with acute MI because drug's cardiovascular effects can increase cardiac workload; in patients with renal or hepatic dysfunction because drug is metabolized in the liver and excreted in urine; and in patients with respiratory conditions because drug depresses the respiratory system.
• When giving repeated parenteral doses, use I.M. or I.V. route when possible and as prescribed because S.C. route may cause severe tissue damage at injection site. Rotate I.M. sites to avoid tissue damage.
• After giving parenteral form, expect to taper dosage gradually, as prescribed, to reduce the risk of withdrawal symptoms.
PATIENT TEACHING
• Caution patient that prolonged use of pentazocine may result in drug dependence.
• Inform patient about possible dizziness, drowsiness, and other adverse CNS effects. Advise her to avoid potentially hazardous activities until drug's CNS effects are known.
• Caution patient not to use alcohol or OTC drugs without consulting prescriber.
• Advise patient to notify prescriber if she notices signs of an allergic reaction, such as a rash or itching.

pentobarbital sodium

Nembutal, Nova Rectal (CAN), Novopentobarb (CAN)

Class, Category, and Schedule
Chemical: Barbiturate
Therapeutic: Anticonvulsant, sedative-hypnotic
Pregnancy category: D
Controlled substance: Schedule II (oral, parenteral), III (rectal)

Indications and Dosages
➤ *To provide daytime sedation*
ELIXIR
Adults. 20 mg t.i.d. or q.i.d.
Children. 2 to 6 mg/kg q.d.
SUPPOSITORIES
Adults. 30 mg b.i.d. to q.i.d.
Children. 2 mg/kg t.i.d.
➤ *To provide short-term treatment of insomnia*
CAPSULES, ELIXIR
Adults. 100 mg h.s.
I.V. INJECTION
Adults. *Initial:* 100 mg, with additional small doses at 1-min intervals, as prescribed. *Maximum:* 500 mg.
I.M. INJECTION
Adults. 150 to 200 mg h.s.
SUPPOSITORIES
Adults and adolescents over age 14. 120 to 200 mg h.s.
Children ages 12 to 14. 60 to 120 mg h.s.
Children ages 5 to 12. 60 mg h.s.
Children ages 1 to 4. 30 to 60 mg h.s.
Infants ages 2 months to 1 year. 30 mg h.s.
➤ *To provide preoperative sedation*
CAPSULES, ELIXIR
Adults. 100 mg before surgery.
Children. 2 to 6 mg/kg before surgery. *Maximum:* 100 mg/dose.
I.M. INJECTION
Adults. 150 to 200 mg before surgery.
Children. 2 to 6 mg/kg before surgery. *Maximum:* 100 mg/dose.
SUPPOSITORIES
Children ages 12 to 14. 60 to 120 mg before surgery.
Children ages 5 to 12. 60 mg before surgery.
Children ages 1 to 4. 30 to 60 mg before surgery.
Infants ages 2 months to 1 year. 30 mg before surgery.
➤ *To provide emergency treatment of seizures associated with eclampsia, meningitis, status epilepticus, tetanus, or toxic reactions to local anesthetics or strychnine*
I.V. INJECTION
Adults. 100 mg, with additional small doses at 1-min intervals, as prescribed. *Maximum:* 500 mg.
Children. 50 mg, with additional small doses at 1-min intervals, as prescribed, until desired effect occurs.

I.M. INJECTION
Children. 50 mg, with additional small doses at 1-min intervals, as prescribed, until desired effect occurs.

DOSAGE ADJUSTMENT Dosage possibly reduced for elderly or debilitated patients and those with hepatic dysfunction.

Route	Onset	Peak	Duration
P.O., P.R.	15 to 60 min	1 to 4 hr	3 to 4 hr
I.V.	In 1 min	Unknown	15 min
I.M.	10 to 25 min	Unknown	3 to 4 hr

Mechanism of Action
Inhibits ascending conduction in the reticular formation, which controls CNS arousal to produce drowsiness, hypnosis, and sedation. Pentobarbital also decreases the spread of seizure activity in the cortex, thalamus, and limbic system. It promotes an increased threshold for electrical stimulation in the motor cortex, which may contribute to its anticonvulsant properties.

Contraindications
Hepatic disease; history of addiction to hypnotics or sedatives; hypersensitivity to pentobarbital, barbiturates, or their components; nephritis; porphyria; severe respiratory disease with airway obstruction or dyspnea

Interactions
DRUGS
acetaminophen: Possibly decreased effects of acetaminophen (with long-term pentobarbital use)
carbamazepine, chloramphenicol, corticosteroids, cyclosporine, dacarbazine, digoxin, disopyramide, doxycycline, griseofulvin, metronidazole, oral contraceptives, phenylbutazone, quinidine, theophyllines, vitamin D: Decreased effectiveness of these drugs
CNS depressants: Increased CNS depression and risk of habituation
divalproex sodium, valproic acid: Increased risk of CNS toxicity and neurotoxicity
guanadrel, guanethidine: Possibly increased risk of orthostatic hypotension
halogenated hydrocarbon anesthetic: Increased risk of hepatotoxicity (with long-term pentobarbital use)

haloperidol: Possibly decreased blood haloperidol level, possibly altered seizure pattern or frequency
hydantoins: Possibly interference with hydantoin metabolism
leucovorin: Possibly decreased anticonvulsant effect of pentobarbital
maprotiline: Possibly enhanced CNS depression and decreased therapeutic effects of pentobarbital
mexiletine: Possibly decreased blood mexiletine level
oral anticoagulants: Possibly decreased therapeutic effects of these drugs, possibly increased risk of bleeding when pentobarbital is discontinued
tricyclic antidepressants: Possibly decreased therapeutic effects of these drugs
ACTIVITIES
alcohol use: Increased CNS depression

Adverse Reactions
CNS: Agitation, anxiety, ataxia, confusion, delusions, depression, dizziness, drowsiness, fever, hallucinations, headache, insomnia, irritability, nervousness, nightmares, paradoxical stimulation, seizures, syncope, tremor
CV: Orthostatic hypotension
EENT: Vision changes
GI: Anorexia, constipation, hepatic dysfunction, nausea, vomiting
HEME: Agranulocytosis
MS: Arthralgia, bone pain, muscle twitching or weakness
RESP: Respiratory depression
SKIN: Exfoliative dermatitis, rash, Stevens-Johnson syndrome
Other: Physical and psychological dependence, weight loss

Nursing Considerations
•Use pentobarbital with extreme caution in patients with depression, a history of drug abuse, or suicidal tendencies.
•Use drug cautiously in elderly or debilitated patients and those with acute or chronic pain because it may induce paradoxical stimulation.
•When using I.V. route, inject drug at 50 mg/min or less to avoid adverse respiratory and circulatory reactions.
•If patient shows premonitory signs of hepatic coma, withhold drug and notify prescriber immediately.

•Monitor I.V. site closely and be careful to avoid extravasation. Drug is highly alkaline and may cause local tissue damage and necrosis.

PATIENT TEACHING

•Inform patient that pentobarbital is habit-forming, and stress the importance of taking it exactly as prescribed.

•Instruct patient who takes elixir form to use a calibrated measuring device and to close container tightly after use.

•Instruct patient who uses suppositories to refrigerate them.

•Advise patient to avoid potentially hazardous activities until drug's CNS effects are known.

•Urge patient to avoid alcohol and other CNS depressants because they may increase drug's adverse CNS effects.

pentosan polysulfate sodium

Elmiron

Class and Category

Chemical: Low-molecular-weight heparin-like compound
Therapeutic: Local anti-inflammatory (bladder-specific)
Pregnancy category: B

Indications and Dosages

➤ *To relieve bladder discomfort or pain caused by interstitial cystitis*

CAPSULES

Adults. 100 mg t.i.d. for up to 3 mo, possibly followed by another 3 mo if no improvement and no adverse reactions occur.

Mechanism of Action

Adheres to the mucosal membrane of the bladder wall and may block irritating solutes from reaching the cells, thereby decreasing local pain and discomfort.

Contraindications

Hypersensitivity to pentosan, other structurally related compounds, or their components

Interactions

DRUGS

alteplase (recombinant), aspirin (high doses), heparin, oral anticoagulants, streptokinase: Increased risk of hemorrhage

Adverse Reactions

CNS: Depression, dizziness, emotional lability, headache
GI: Abdominal pain, diarrhea, hepatic dysfunction, indigestion, nausea
HEME: Unusual bleeding or bruising
SKIN: Alopecia, rash

Nursing Considerations

•Use pentosan with extreme caution in patients with conditions that increase the risk of bleeding, such as aneurysm, diverticula, GI ulceration, hemophilia, polyps, and thrombocytopenia (especially heparin-induced).

•Use drug cautiously in patients with hepatic dysfunction because drug is desulfated in the liver and spleen.

•Monitor for abnormal bleeding, such as unexplained bruises and epistaxis, because drug is a weak anticoagulant.

PATIENT TEACHING

•Instruct patient to take pentosan with a full glass of water at least 1 hour before or 2 hours after meals.

•Explain the pattern of exacerbations and remissions associated with interstitial cystitis. Reassure patient that symptoms should improve within 3 months after starting therapy.

•Advise patient to take bleeding precautions during therapy, such as using an electric shaver and a soft-bristled toothbrush.

•If alopecia develops, explain that it's usually confined to a single area.

pentoxifylline

Trental

Class and Category

Chemical: Xanthine derivative
Therapeutic: Blood viscosity reducer
Pregnancy category: C

Indications and Dosages

➤ *To treat peripheral vascular disease*

E.R. TABLETS

Adults. 400 mg t.i.d. with meals.

DOSAGE ADJUSTMENT Dosage possibly reduced to 400 mg b.i.d. for patients who experience adverse GI or CNS reactions.

Route	Onset	Peak	Duration
P.O.	2 to 4 wk	Unknown	Unknown

P

Mechanism of Action

Relieves symptoms of peripheral vascular disease through several actions. Pentoxifylline:
• reduces blood viscosity by decreasing the plasma fibrinogen level and inhibiting RBC and platelet aggregation
• improves erythrocyte flexibility by inhibiting phosphodiesterase and increasing the amount of cAMP in RBCs
• decreases peripheral vascular resistance and improves microcirculatory blood flow and tissue oxygenation.

Contraindications

Hypersensitivity to pentoxifylline, methylxanthines (such as caffeine, theophylline, and theobromine), or their components; recent cerebral or retinal hemorrhage

Interactions
DRUGS

antihypertensives: Potentiated antihypertensive effects
cefamandole, cefoperazone, cefotetan, heparin, oral anticoagulants, other platelet aggregation inhibitors, plicamycin, thrombolytics, valproic acid: Increased risk of bleeding
cimetidine: Increased blood pentoxifylline level, increased risk of adverse effects
sympathomimetics, xanthines: Enhanced CNS stimulation
ACTIVITIES
smoking: Possibly decreased therapeutic effects of pentoxifylline

Adverse Reactions

CNS: Dizziness, headache
GI: Indigestion, nausea, vomiting

Nursing Considerations

• Use pentoxifylline cautiously in elderly patients and those with hepatic or renal dysfunction.
• Administer drug with meals and, if needed, an antacid to reduce adverse GI reactions.
PATIENT TEACHING
• Instruct patient to swallow pentoxifylline E.R. tablets whole and not to crush, break, or chew them.
• Advise patient to take drug with meals to reduce GI irritation. If adverse GI reactions occur anyway, advise her to also take an antacid with meals.

• Although symptoms may not improve for several weeks, urge patient to continue taking drug as prescribed to achieve maximum therapeutic effect.
• Instruct patient not to smoke during therapy because smoking constricts blood vessels and may reduce drug effectiveness.
• Advise patient to notify prescriber about adverse reactions; dosage may need to be reduced.

pergolide mesylate

Permax

Class and Category

Chemical: Semisynthetic ergot alkaloid derivative
Therapeutic: Antidyskinetic
Pregnancy category: B

Indications and Dosages

➤ *As adjunct to relieve symptoms of Parkinson's disease*
TABLETS
Adults. *Initial:* 0.05 mg q.d on days 1 and 2. Dosage increased by 0.1 or 0.15 mg q 3 days over next 12 days, then increased by 0.25 mg q 3 days until therapeutic effect is achieved. *Maximum:* 5 mg/day.

Mechanism of Action

Directly stimulates postsynaptic dopamine receptors to inhibit the firing of striatal neurons (such as cholinergic neurons), which helps control alterations in voluntary muscle movement—such as tremors and rigidity—associated with Parkinson's disease.

Contraindications

Hypersensitivity to pergolide mesylate, other ergot alkaloid derivatives, or their components

Interactions
DRUGS

antihypertensives, other hypotension-producing drugs: Possibly additive hypotensive effects
droperidol, haloperidol, loxapine, methyldopa, metoclopramide, molindone, papaverine, phenothiazines, reserpine, thioxanthenes: Possibly decreased effectiveness of pergolide

Adverse Reactions

CNS: Anxiety, confusion, dizziness, drowsiness, dyskinesia, fatigue, hallucinations, insomnia, weakness
CV: Hypertension, hypotension, orthostatic hypotension, peripheral edema
EENT: Dry mouth, facial swelling, rhinitis, vision changes
GI: Anorexia, constipation, diarrhea, indigestion, nausea, vomiting
GU: UTI
HEME: Anemia
MS: Low back pain, muscle weakness
Other: Flulike symptoms

Nursing Considerations

• Monitor heart rate and rhythm of patients at risk for cardiac arrhythmias because they're more likely to develop premature atrial contractions and sinus tachycardia during pergolide therapy.
• Monitor blood pressure for symptomatic orthostatic hypotension or sustained hypertension, especially during early stages of treatment. Be aware that tolerance usually develops with gradual titration.
• **WARNING** Be aware that drug should not be discontinued or dosage changed abruptly because doing so may precipitate neuroleptic malignant syndrome (NMS). During drug discontinuation or dosage change, assess patient for signs and symptoms of NMS, such as difficulty breathing, rapid heartbeat, high fever, labile blood pressure, diaphoresis, loss of bladder control, muscle stiffness, and seizures. Be prepared to institute appropriate supportive measures and notify prescriber immediately.
• Assess patient for mouth discomfort and oral candidiasis, especially if she complains of dry mouth. Notify prescriber immediately if symptoms persist or infection develops.
• Monitor patient with a psychiatric disorder for confusion and hallucinations, which may be exacerbated by pergolide therapy.

PATIENT TEACHING
• Stress the importance of taking pergolide regularly and in exact dosage prescribed. Caution patient that altering dose or dosing interval may increase the risk of adverse reactions and decrease drug's effectiveness.
• Instruct patient or caregiver to avoid abrupt drug discontinuation because this may precipitate neuroleptic malignant syndrome.

• Inform patient that several weeks or months may pass before drug's therapeutic effects are achieved.
• Inform patient or caregiver that patient may experience orthostatic hypotension early during pergolide treatment but that she'll probably develop a tolerance to it over time.
• Advise patient to rise slowly from a seated or lying position during initial therapy to reduce the risk of dizziness or fainting.
• Advise patient not to drive or participate in activities requiring high level of mental alertness until drug's full CNS effects are known.
• Urge patient to avoid alcoholic beverages, especially if she experiences adverse CNS reactions from drug.
• Advise patient with a history of psychiatric disorders (or caregiver) to notify prescriber immediately if confusion or hallucinations worsen during pergolide therapy.
• Suggest that patient chew sugarless gum or suck on hard candy to prevent dry mouth.
• Advise her to have regular dental checkups to decrease the risk of gingival disorders due to dry mouth.

perindopril erbumine

Aceon

Class and Category

Chemical: Perindoprilat prodrug
Therapeutic: Antihypertensive
Pregnancy category: C (first trimester), D (later trimesters)

Indications and Dosages

➤ *To manage hypertension*
TABLETS
Adults. *Initial:* 4 mg/day as a single dose or in divided doses b.i.d., increased as prescribed until blood pressure is controlled or maximum dosage is reached. *Maintenance:* 4 to 8 mg/day. *Maximum:* 8 mg/day.
DOSAGE ADJUSTMENT For patients who already take a diuretic, initial dosage possibly reduced to 2 to 4 mg/day; for patients with renal failure, initial dosage possibly reduced to 2 mg/day.

Contraindications

History of angioedema from previous ACE inhibitor treatment; hypersensitivity to perindopril, other ACE inhibitors, or their components

P

Mechanism of Action
Is converted to the active metabolite perindoprilat, which competes with angiotensin I binding sites, blocking the conversion of angiotensin I to angiotensin II, a potent vasoconstrictor. As a result, this ACE inhibitor reduces vasoconstriction and blood pressure. A decrease in the plasma angiotensin II level also reduces aldosterone secretion, leading to increased excretion of water and sodium by the kidneys.

Interactions
DRUGS
diuretics: Increased risk of hypotension
lithium: Increased blood lithium level and risk of toxicity
potassium-sparing diuretics, potassium supplements: Increased risk of hyperkalemia

Adverse Reactions
CNS: Amnesia, anxiety, dizziness, fatigue, fever, headache, hypertonia, migraine, syncope, vertigo
CV: Chest pain, ECG changes, heart murmur, hypotension, orthostatic hypotension, palpitations, PVCs
EENT: Conjunctivitis, earache, epistaxis, hoarseness, pharyngitis, rhinitis, sinusitis, sneezing, tinnitus
GI: Abdominal pain, diarrhea, elevated liver function test results, flatulence, increased appetite, indigestion
GU: Flank pain, renal calculi, urinary frequency and urgency, vaginitis
HEME: Hematoma, leukopenia, neutropenia
MS: Arthritis, back pain, gout, limb pain, myalgia, neck pain
RESP: Cough
SKIN: Canker sores, diaphoresis, dry skin, ecchymosis, erythema, pruritus, rash
Other: Angioedema, facial edema

Nursing Considerations
•Use perindopril cautiously in patients with heart failure, renal artery stenosis, or renal dysfunction.
•Monitor patients with hepatic dysfunction for enhanced therapeutic drug effects because drug's bioavailability is increased.
•Monitor serum potassium level to detect hyperkalemia, especially in patients with renal insufficiency or diabetes mellitus and those who use a potassium-containing salt substitute or take a potassium-sparing diuretic or potassium supplement.

PATIENT TEACHING
•Instruct patient to take perindopril exactly as prescribed, even if she feels well.
•**WARNING** Urge patient to stop taking drug and notify prescriber immediately if she experiences signs of angioedema, including swelling of the face, extremities, eyes, lips, and tongue and trouble breathing or swallowing.
•Advise patient to notify prescriber at once about fever, sore throat, or other signs that may indicate neutropenia.
•Urge patient to avoid taking potassium supplements and using potassium-containing salt substitutes unless prescriber approves.
•Instruct patient to avoid potentially hazardous activities until drug's CNS effects are known.
•Advise female patients to notify prescriber promptly about suspected, known, or intended pregnancy because drug could harm fetus during second and third trimesters.

perphenazine
Apo-Perphenazine (CAN), PMS Perphenazine (CAN), Trilafon, Trilafon Concentrate

Class and Category
Chemical: Piperazine phenothiazine
Therapeutic: Antiemetic, antipyschotic
Pregnancy category: Not rated

Indications and Dosages
➤ *To treat psychotic disorders*
ORAL SOLUTION
Hospitalized adults and adolescents. 8 to 16 mg b.i.d. to q.i.d., adjusted as prescribed and tolerated. *Maximum:* 64 mg/day.
TABLETS
Adults and adolescents. 4 to 16 mg b.i.d. to q.i.d., adjusted as prescribed and tolerated. *Maximum:* 64 mg/day.
I.M. INJECTION
Adults and adolescents. 5 to 10 mg q 6 hr, adjusted as prescribed and tolerated. *Maximum:* 15 mg/day for outpatients, 30 mg/day for hospitalized patients.
➤ *To treat severe nausea and vomiting*
TABLETS
Adults and adolescents. 8 to 16 mg/day in divided doses, decreased as appropriate. *Maximum:* 24 mg/day.

I.V. INFUSION OR INJECTION
Adults and adolescents. 1 mg q 1 to 2 min, up to 5 mg total.
I.M. INJECTION
Adults and adolescents. 5 mg, increased to 10 mg as prescribed and tolerated for rapid control of severe vomiting. *Maximum:* 15 mg/day for outpatients, 30 mg/day for hospitalized patients.
DOSAGE ADJUSTMENT Initial dose possibly reduced and gradually increased for elderly, emaciated, or debilitated patients. Lower end of adult dosage range possibly needed for adolescents.

Route	Onset	Peak	Duration
P.O.	Several wk	4 to 7 days	Unknown
I.M.	Unknown	1 to 2 hr	6 hr

Mechanism of Action
Depresses areas of the brain that control activity and aggression, including the cerebral cortex, hypothalamus, and limbic system, by an unknown mechanism. Perphenazine also prevents nausea and vomiting by inhibiting or blocking dopamine receptors in the medullary chemoreceptor trigger zone and peripherally by blocking the vagus nerve in the GI tract.

Incompatibilities
Don't mix perphenazine oral solution with beverages that contain caffeine or tannins (such as coffee, colas, and teas) or pectinates (such as apple juice) because they're physically incompatible.

Contraindications
Blood dyscrasias; bone marrow depression; cerebral arteriosclerosis; coma; concurrent use of CNS depressants (large doses); coronary artery disease; hepatic impairment; hypersensitivity to perphenazine, other phenothiazines, or their components; myeloproliferative disorders; severe CNS depression; severe hypertension or hypotension; subcortical brain damage

Interactions
DRUGS
aluminum- and magnesium-containing antacids, antidiarrheals (adsorbent): Decreased absorption of oral perphenazine

amantadine, anticholinergics, antidyskinetics, antihistamines: Increased adverse anticholinergic effects
amphetamines: Decreased therapeutic effects of both drugs
anticonvulsants: Decreased seizure threshold, inhibited metabolism and toxicity of anticonvulsant
antithyroid drugs: Increased risk of agranulocytosis
apomorphine: Additive CNS depression, decreased emetic response to apomorphine if perphenazine is given first
appetite suppressants (except phenmetrazine): Antagonized anorectic effect of appetite suppressants
beta blockers: Increased blood levels of both drugs and risk of arrhythmias, hypotension, irreversible retinopathy, and tardive dyskinesia
bromocriptine: Possibly interference with bromocriptine's effects
CNS depressants: Increased CNS and respiratory depression and hypotensive effects
dopamine: Antagonized peripheral vasoconstriction with high doses of dopamine
ephedrine: Decreased vasopressor response to ephedrine
epinephrine: Blocked alpha-adrenergic effects of epinephrine, possibly causing severe hypotension and tachycardia
hepatotoxic drugs: Increased risk of hepatotoxicity
hypotension-causing drugs: Increased risk of severe orthostatic hypotension
levodopa: Inhibited antidyskinetic effects of levodopa
lithium: Possibly neurotoxicity (disorientation, extrapyramidal symptoms, unconsciousness)
maprotiline, selective serotonin reuptake inhibitors, tricyclic antidepressants: Prolonged and intensified sedative and anticholinergic effects of these drugs or perphenazine
metrizamide: Decreased seizure threshold
opioid analgesics: Increased CNS and respiratory depression, increased risk of orthostatic hypotension and severe constipation
ototoxic drugs, especially antibiotics: Possibly masking of some symptoms of ototoxicity, such as dizziness, tinnitus, and vertigo
probucol, other drugs that prolong QT interval: Prolonged QT interval, which may increase risk of ventricular tachycardia

thiazide diuretics: Possibly hyponatremia and water intoxication

ACTIVITIES

alcohol use: Increased CNS and respiratory depression, hypotensive effects, and risk of heatstroke

Adverse Reactions

CNS: Behavioral changes, cerebral edema, dizziness, drowsiness, extrapyramidal reactions (such as akathisia, dystonia, pseudoparkinsonism), fever, headache, neuroleptic malignant syndrome, seizures, syncope, tardive dyskinesia (persistent)

CV: Bradycardia, cardiac arrest, hypertension, hypotension, orthostatic hypotension, tachycardia

EENT: Blurred vision, dry mouth, glaucoma, laryngeal edema, miosis, mydriasis, nasal congestion, ocular changes (corneal opacification, retinopathy)

ENDO: Decreased libido, galactorrhea, gynecomastia, syndrome of inappropriate ADH secretion

GI: Anorexia, constipation, diarrhea, fecal impaction, nausea, vomiting

GU: Bladder paralysis, ejaculation failure, menstrual irregularities, polyuria, urinary frequency, urinary incontinence, urine retention

HEME: Agranulocytosis, eosinophilia, hemolytic anemia, leukopenia, pancytopenia, thrombocytopenic purpura

RESP: Asthma

SKIN: Diaphoresis, eczema, erythema, exfoliative dermatitis, hyperpigmentation, jaundice, pallor, photosensitivity, pruritus, urticaria

Other: Anaphylaxis, angioedema

Nursing Considerations

• Use perphenazine cautiously in patients with depression or hepatic, pulmonary, or renal dysfunction and in elderly patients, who are at increased risk for increased plasma concentrations and tardive dyskinesia.

• When using I.V. route, dilute drug to 0.5 mg/ml with sodium chloride for injection. Protect solution from light. Slight yellowing is acceptable, but discard solution if it's markedly discolored or contains precipitate.

• Obtain blood samples for CBC and liver and renal function tests, as ordered, to detect adverse reactions.

• Monitor temperature frequently, and notify prescriber if it rises; a significant increase suggests drug intolerance.

• Monitor blood pressure of patient who takes large doses of perphenazine, especially if surgery is indicated, because of the increased risk of hypotension.

PATIENT TEACHING

• Instruct patient to take perphenazine exactly as prescribed to ensure optimal effectiveness and minimize adverse reactions.

• Remind patient who takes oral solution to use a calibrated measuring device.

• Instruct patient taking oral solution to dilute every 5 ml (teaspoon) of drug in 2 fluid oz of water, milk, tomato juice, fruit juice (except apple), soup, or carbonated beverage. Caution her not to mix drug in beverages that contain caffeine or tannins, such as cola, coffee, and tea.

• Caution patient not to spill oral solution on skin or clothing because it can cause contact dermatitis and damage clothing.

• Urge patient to avoid alcohol and other CNS depressants during perphenazine therapy and to avoid potentially hazardous activities until drug's CNS effects are known.

• Advise patient to avoid excessive sun exposure and to protect skin when outdoors.

• Instruct patient to notify prescriber about persistent or severe adverse reactions.

• Urge patient to comply with long-term follow-up to detect adverse reactions and determine possible need for dosage adjustments.

phenazopyridine hydrochloride

Azo-Standard, Baridium, Eridium, Geridium, Phenazo (CAN), Phenazodine, Pyridiate, Pyridium, Urodine, Urogesic, Viridium

Class and Category

Chemical: Azo dye
Therapeutic: Urinary analgesic
Pregnancy category: B

Indications and Dosages

➤ *To relieve burning and pain on urination, and urinary frequency and urgency*

TABLETS

Adults and adolescents. 200 mg t.i.d. with or without food for no longer than 2 days.
Children. 4 mg/kg t.i.d. with food for no longer than 2 days.

Contraindications

Hypersensitivity to phenazopyridine or its components, renal insufficiency

Mechanism of Action
Exerts a topical or local anesthetic effect on the mucosa of the urinary tract as drug is excreted in urine. Phenazopyridine's exact mechanism is unknown.

Adverse Reactions
CNS: Headache
GI: Indigestion, nausea, vomiting
GU: Reddish orange urine
SKIN: Pruritus, rash
Other: Discoloration of body fluids

Nursing Considerations
•Notify prescriber if yellowish skin or sclerae develop in patient taking phenazopyridine because this may indicate drug accumulation from impaired renal excretion. Expect prescriber to discontinue drug.
•Be aware that phenazopyridine treatment should be limited to 2 days in patients with UTIs.

PATIENT TEACHING
•Instruct patient not to take phenazopyridine for longer than 2 days and to notify prescriber if symptoms persist beyond that time.
•If GI distress develops, advise patient to take drug with meals.
•Inform patient that drug turns urine orange to red and may discolor other body fluids, such as tears.
•Advise patient not to wear contact lenses during therapy because they may become stained.

phenelzine sulfate
Nardil

Class and Category
Chemical: Hydrazine derivative
Therapeutic: Antidepressant
Pregnancy category: C

Indications and Dosages
➤ *To treat depression*

TABLETS
Adults. *Initial:* 1 mg/kg/day, increased gradually as prescribed and tolerated. *Maintenance:* 45 mg/day. *Maximum:* 90 mg/day.
DOSAGE ADJUSTMENT For elderly patients, initial dosage possibly reduced to 0.8 to 1 mg/kg/day in divided doses and increased as prescribed and tolerated to maximum of 60 mg/day.

Route	Onset	Peak	Duration
P.O.	7 to 10 days	4 to 8 wk	10 days

Contraindications
Cardiovascular disease; cerebrovascular disease; heart failure; hepatic disease; history of headaches; hypersensitivity to phenelzine or its components; hypertension; pheochromocytoma; severe renal impairment; use of anesthetics, antihypertensives, bupropion, buspirone, carbamazepine, CNS depressants, cyclobenzaprine, dextromethorphan, meperidine, selective serotonin-reuptake inhibitors, sympathomimetics, or tricyclic antidepressants; use within 14 days of other MAO inhibitor

Interactions
DRUGS
anticholinergics, antidyskinetics, antihistamines: Increased anticholinergic effect, prolonged CNS depression (antihistamines)
anticonvulsants: Increased CNS depression, possibly altered pattern of seizures
beta blockers: Increased risk of bradycardia
bromocriptine: Possibly interference with bromocriptine effects
bupropion: Increased risk of bupropion toxicity
buspirone: Increased risk of hypertension
caffeine-containing drugs: Increased risk of dangerous arrhythmias and severe hypertension
carbamazepine, cyclobenzaprine, maprotiline, other MAO inhibitors: Increased risk of hyperpyretic crisis, hypertensive crisis, severe seizures, and death; altered pattern of seizures (with carbamazepine)
CNS depressants: Increased CNS depression
dextromethorphan: Increased risk of excitation, hypertension, and hyperpyrexia
diuretics: Increased hypotensive effect
doxapram: Increased vasopressor effects of either drug
fluoxetine: Increased risk of agitation, confusion, GI symptoms, hyperpyretic episodes, hypertensive crisis, potentially fatal serotonin syndrome, restlessness, and severe seizures.
guanadrel, guanethidine: Increased risk of hypertension
haloperidol, loxapine, molindone, phenothiazines, pimozide, thioxanthenes: Prolonged and intensified anticholinergic, hypotensive, and sedative effects of these drugs or phenelzine

P

Mechanism of Action

Phenelzine relieves symptoms of unipolar depressive disorders by inhibiting the enzyme monoamine oxidase (MAO). Normally, MAO breaks down monoamine neurotransmitters, such as serotonin, as shown below left. By inhibiting this enzyme, phenelzine increases the concentration of serotonin in the vesicles of monoamine nerve endings, allowing more serotonin to be released and engage with receptors on postsynaptic cells, as shown below right. A serotonin deficiency may be responsible in part for endogenous depression.

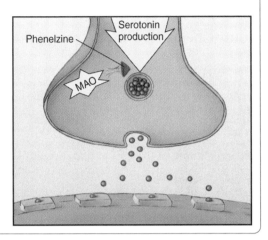

insulin, oral antidiabetic drugs: Increased hypoglycemic effects

levodopa: Increased risk of sudden, moderate to severe hypertension

local anesthetics (with epinephrine or levonordefrin): Possibly severe hypertension

meperidine, other opioid analgesics: Increased risk of coma, hyperpyrexia, hypotension, immediate excitation, rigidity, seizures, severe hypertension, severe respiratory depression, sweating, vascular collapse, and death

methyldopa: Increased risk of hallucinations, headache, hyperexcitability, and severe hypertension

methylphenidate: Increased CNS stimulant effect of methylphenidate

metrizamide: Decreased seizure threshold, increased risk of seizures

oral anticoagulants: Increased anticoagulant activity

paroxetine, sertraline, trazodone, tricyclic antidepressants: Increased risk of potentially fatal serotonin syndrome

phenylephrine (nasal or ophthalmic): Potentiated vasopressor effect of phenylephrine

rauwolfia alkaloids: Increased risk of moderate to severe hypertension, CNS depression (when phenelzine is added to rauwolfia alkaloid therapy), CNS excitation and hypertension (when rauwolfia alkaloid is added to phenelzine therapy)

spinal anesthetics: Increased risk of hypotension

succinylcholine: Possibly increased neuromuscular blockade of succinylcholine

sympathomimetics: Prolonged and intensified cardiac stimulant and vasopressor effects

tryptophan: Increased risk of confusion, disorientation, hyperreflexia, hyperthermia, hyperventilation, mania or hypomania, and shivering

FOODS

foods and beverages high in tyramine or other pressor amines, such as aged cheese; beer; fava beans or other broad beans; cured meat or sausage; liqueurs; overripe fruit; red and white wine; reduced-alcohol and alcohol-free beer and wine; sauerkraut; sherry; smoked or pickled fish, meats, and poultry; yeast or protein extracts: Increased risk of sudden, severe hypertension

ACTIVITIES
alcohol use: Increased CNS depressant effects and hypertensive crisis

Adverse Reactions
CNS: Agitation, dizziness, drowsiness, headache, overstimulation, restlessness, sedation, sleep disturbance, weakness
CV: Bradycardia, edema, hypertensive crisis, orthostatic hypotension, palpitations, tachycardia
EENT: Blurred vision, dry mouth, photophobia
GI: Abdominal pain, constipation, diarrhea, elevated liver function test results, increased appetite, nausea
GU: Impotence, priapism, sexual dysfunction, urinary frequency, urine retention
MS: Muscle twitching
SKIN: Diaphoresis, rash
Other: Hypernatremia, weight gain

Nursing Considerations
• Use phenelzine cautiously in patients with epilepsy because drug may alter seizure threshold.
• Expect to observe some therapeutic effect within 7 to 10 days, but keep in mind that full effect may not occur for 4 to 8 weeks.
• Monitor cardiovascular status closely for changes in heart rate (especially if patient receives more than 30 mg/day) and signs of life-threatening hypertensive crisis. Question patient frequently about headaches and palpitations. If either occurs, notify prescriber and expect to discontinue drug.
• Keep phentolamine readily available to treat hypertensive crisis. Give 5 mg by slow I.V., as prescribed, to reduce blood pressure without causing excessive hypotension. Use external cooling measures, as prescribed, to manage fever.
• To avoid hypertensive crisis, expect to wait 10 to 14 days, as prescribed, when switching patient from one MAO inhibitor to another or when switching from a dibenzazepine-related drug, such as amitriptyline or perphenazine.

PATIENT TEACHING
• Inform patient and family members that therapeutic effects of phenelzine may take several weeks to appear and that she should continue taking drug as prescribed.
• Caution patient to rise slowly from a lying or sitting position to minimize effects of orthostatic hypotension.

• **WARNING** Instruct patient to avoid the following foods, beverages, and drugs during phenelzine therapy and for 2 weeks afterward: alcohol-free and reduced-alcohol beer and wine; appetite suppressants; beer; broad beans; cheese (except cottage and cream cheese); chocolate and caffeine in large quantities; dry sausage (including Genoa salami, hard salami, pepperoni, and Lebanon bologna); hay fever drugs; inhaled asthma drugs; liver; meat extract; OTC cold and cough preparations (including those containing dextromethorphan), nasal decongestants (tablets, drops, or spray); pickled herring; products that contain tryptophan; protein-rich foods that may have undergone protein changes by aging, pickling, fermenting, or smoking; sauerkraut; sinus drugs; weight-loss preparations; yeast extracts (including brewer's yeast in large quantities); yogurt; and wine.
• Advise patient to inform all health care providers (including dentists) that she takes an MAO inhibitor because certain drugs are contraindicated within 2 weeks of therapy.
• Urge patient to avoid potentially hazardous activities until drug's CNS effects are known.
• Stress the importance of reporting headaches and other unusual, persistent, or severe symptoms.
• Urge patient with diabetes mellitus who's taking insulin or oral antidiabetic drug to monitor blood glucose level frequently during therapy because phenelzine may affect glucose control.

phenobarbital
Ancalixir (CAN), Barbita, Solfoton

phenobarbital sodium
Luminal

Class, Category, and Schedule
Chemical: Barbiturate
Therapeutic: Anticonvulsant, sedative-hypnotic
Pregnancy category: D
Controlled substance: Schedule IV

Indications and Dosages
➤ *To treat seizures*
CAPSULES, ELIXIR, TABLETS
Adults. 60 to 250 mg/day as a single dose or in divided doses.

Children. 1 to 6 mg/kg/day as a single dose or in divided doses.

I.V. INJECTION
Adults. 100 to 320 mg, repeated as needed and as prescribed. *Maximum:* 600 mg/day.
Children. *Initial:* 10 to 20 mg/kg as a single dose. *Maintenance:* 1 to 6 mg/kg/day.

➤ *To treat status epilepticus*
I.V. INFUSION OR INJECTION
Adults. 10 to 20 mg/kg given slowly and repeated as needed and as prescribed.
Children. 15 to 20 mg/kg over 10 to 15 min.

➤ *To provide short-term treatment of insomnia*
CAPSULES, ELIXIR, TABLETS
Adults. 100 to 320 mg h.s.
I.V., I.M., OR S.C. INJECTION
Adults. 100 to 325 mg h.s.

➤ *To provide daytime sedation*
CAPSULES, ELIXIR, TABLETS
Adults. 30 to 120 mg/day in divided doses b.i.d. or t.i.d.
Children. 2 mg/kg t.i.d.

I.V., I.M., OR S.C. INJECTION
Adults. 30 to 120 mg/day in divided doses b.i.d. or t.i.d.

➤ *To provide preoperative sedation*
CAPSULES, ELIXIR, TABLETS
Children. 1 to 3 mg/kg before surgery.
I.M. INJECTION
Adults. 130 to 200 mg 60 to 90 min before surgery.
I.V. OR I.M. INJECTION
Children. 1 to 3 mg/kg 60 to 90 min before surgery.

DOSAGE ADJUSTMENT Dosage possibly reduced for elderly or debilitated patients to minimize confusion, depression, and excitement.

Route	Onset	Peak	Duration
P.O.	20 to 60 min	Unknown	Unknown
I.V.	5 min	30 min	4 to 6 hr
I.M., S.C.	5 to 20 min	Unknown	4 to 6 hr

Contraindications
Hepatic disease; history of addiction to hypnotics or sedatives; hypersensitivity to phenobarbital, other barbiturates, or their components; nephritis; porphyria; severe respiratory disease with airway obstruction or dyspnea

Mechanism of Action
Inhibits ascending conduction of impulses in the reticular formation, which controls CNS arousal to produce drowsiness, hypnosis, and sedation. Phenobarbital also decreases the spread of seizure activity in the cortex, thalamus, and limbic system. It promotes an increased threshold for electrical stimulation in the motor cortex, which may contribute to its anticonvulsant properties.

Interactions
DRUGS
acetaminophen: Decreased acetaminophen effectiveness with long-term phenobarbital therapy
amphetamines: Delayed intestinal absorption of phenobarbital
anesthetics (halogenated hydrocarbon): Possibly hepatotoxicity
anticonvulsants (hydantoin): Unpredictable effects on metabolism of anticonvulsant
anticonvulsants (succinimide), including carbamazepine: Decreased blood levels and elimination half-lives of these drugs
calcium channel blockers: Possibly excessive hypotension
carbonic anhydrase inhibitors: Enhanced osteopenia induced by phenobarbital
chloramphenicol, corticosteroids, cyclosporine, dacarbazine, digoxin, metronidazole, quinidine: Decreased effectiveness of these drugs from enhanced metabolism
CNS depressants: Additive CNS depression
cyclophosphamide: Possibly reduced half-life and increased leukopenic activity of cyclophosphamide
disopyramide: Possibly ineffectiveness of disopyramide
doxycycline, fenoprofen: Shortened half-life of these drugs
griseofulvin: Possibly decreased absorption and effectiveness of griseofulvin
guanadrel, guanethidine: Possibly increased orthostatic hypotension
haloperidol: Decreased seizure threshold, decreased blood haloperidol level
ketamine (high doses): Increased risk of hypotension and respiratory depression
leucovorin: Interference with phenobarbital's anticonvulsant effect

levothyroxine, oral contraceptives, phenylbutazone, tricyclic antidepressants: Decreased effectiveness of these drugs
loxapine, phenothiazines, thioxanthenes: Decreased seizure threshold
MAO inhibitors: Prolonged phenobarbital effects, possibly altered pattern of seizure activity
maprotiline: Increased CNS depression, decreased seizure threshold at high doses, decreased phenobarbital effectiveness
methoxyflurane: Possibly hepatotoxicity and nephrotoxicity
methylphenidate: Increased risk of phenobarbital toxicity
mexiletine: Decreased blood mexiletine level
oral anticoagulants: Decreased anticoagulant activity, increased risk of bleeding when phenobarbital is discontinued
pituitary hormones (posterior): Increased risk of arrhythmias and coronary insufficiency
primidone: Altered pattern of seizures, increased CNS effects of both drugs
valproate, valproic acid: Decreased phenobarbital metabolism, increased risk of barbiturate toxicity
vitamin D: Decreased phenobarbital effectiveness
xanthines: Increased xanthine metabolism, antagonized hypnotic effect of phenobarbital
ACTIVITIES
alcohol use: Additive CNS depression

Adverse Reactions
CNS: Anxiety, depression, dizziness, drowsiness, headache, irritability, lethargy, mood changes, paradoxical stimulation, sedation, vertigo
CV: Hypotension, sinus bradycardia
EENT: Miosis, ptosis
GI: Constipation, diarrhea, nausea, vomiting
GU: Decreased libido, impotence, sexual dysfunction
MS: Arthralgia, bone tenderness
RESP: Bronchospasm, respiratory depression
SKIN: Dermatitis, photosensitivity, rash, urticaria
Other: Injection site phlebitis (I.V.), physical and psychological dependence

Nursing Considerations
•Be aware that phenobarbital shouldn't be given during third trimester of pregnancy because repeated use can cause dependence in neonate. It also shouldn't be given to breast-feeding women because it may cause CNS depression in infants.
•Use I.V. route cautiously in patients with cardiovascular disease, hypotension, pulmonary disease, or shock because drug may cause adverse hemodynamic or respiratory effects.
•Because drug can cause respiratory depression, assess respiratory rate and depth before use, especially in patient with bronchopneumonia, pulmonary disease, respiratory tract infection, or status asthmaticus.
•Give elixir undiluted or mix with water, milk, or fruit juice. Use a calibrated device to measure doses.
•If necessary, crush tablets and mix with food or fluids.
•Reconstitute sterile powder with at least 10 ml of sterile water for injection. Don't use reconstituted solution if it fails to clear within 5 minutes. Further dilute prescribed dose with NS or D_5W and infuse over 30 to 60 minutes.
•Don't administer more rapidly than 60 mg/min by I.V. injection.
•During I.V. administration, monitor blood pressure, respiratory rate, and heart rate and rhythm. Anticipate increased risk of hypotension, even when giving drug at recommended rate. Keep resuscitation equipment readily available.
•During I.M. use, don't inject more than 5 ml into any one I.M. site to prevent sterile abscess formation.
•Be aware that drug may cause physical and psychological dependence.
•Anticipate that phenobarbital's CNS effects may exacerbate major depression, suicidal tendencies, or other mental disorders.
•Take safety precautions for elderly patients, as appropriate, because they're more likely to experience confusion, depression, and excitement as adverse CNS reactions.
•Anticipate that phenobarbital may cause paradoxical stimulation in children.
•Be aware that drug may trigger signs and symptoms in patients with acute intermittent porphyria.
PATIENT TEACHING
•Instruct patient to take phenobarbital elixir undiluted or to mix it with water, milk, or fruit juice. Advise her to use a calibrated device to measure doses.
•If patient has trouble swallowing tablets, suggest that she crush them and mix with food or fluid.

P

•Caution patient about possible drowsiness and reduced alertness. Advise her to avoid potentially hazardous activities until drug's CNS effects are known.

•Urge patient to avoid alcohol during therapy.

•Inform parents that a child may react with paradoxical excitement. Tell them to notify prescriber if this occurs.

•Instruct female patient to notify prescriber about suspected, known, or intended pregnancy. Advise against breast-feeding during therapy.

phentolamine mesylate

Regitine

Class and Category

Chemical: Imidazoline
Therapeutic: Antihypertensive, diagnostic aid, vasodilator
Pregnancy category: Not rated

Indications and Dosages

➤ *To diagnose pheochromocytoma*

I.V. INJECTION

Adults. 2.5 mg as a single dose. After negative result, repeat test with 5-mg dose, as prescribed.

Children. 1 mg as a single dose. After negative result, repeat test with 0.1-mg/kg dose, as prescribed.

➤ *To manage hypertension before or during pheochromocytomectomy*

I.V. OR I.M. INJECTION

Adults. 5 mg 1 to 2 hr before surgery, repeated as needed and as prescribed. During surgery, 5 mg I.V., as ordered.

Children. 1 mg 1 to 2 hr before surgery, repeated as needed and as prescribed. During surgery, 1 mg I.V., as ordered.

➤ *To prevent dermal necrosis or sloughing after extravasation of I.V. norepinephrine*

I.V. INJECTION

Adults, children, and infants. 10 mg/L of I.V. fluid that contains norepinephrine at rate determined by patient response.

➤ *To treat dermal necrosis or sloughing after extravasation of I.V. norepinephrine*

INTRADERMAL INJECTION

Adults. 5 to 10 mg in 10 ml of NS infiltrated in affected area within 12 hr of extravasation.

Children. 0.1 to 0.2 mg/kg. *Maximum:* 10 mg.

Mechanism of Action

Blocks the actions of circulating epinephrine and norepinephrine by antagonizing $alpha_1$ and $alpha_2$ receptors. Phentolamine causes peripheral vasodilation through direct relaxation of vascular smooth muscle and alpha blockade. Positive inotropic and chronotropic effects increase cardiac output. A positive inotropic effect primarily raises blood pressure, but in larger doses, phentolamine causes peripheral vasodilation and can reduce blood pressure.

In patients with pheochromocytoma, phentolamine causes systolic and diastolic blood pressures to fall dramatically. In those without pheochromocytoma, it causes blood pressure to fall or rise slightly or remain the same.

Contraindications

Angina, hypersensitivity to phentolamine or its components, MI

Interactions

DRUGS

antihypertensives: Additive hypotensive effect
dopamine: Antagonized vasopressor activity of dopamine
epinephrine, methoxamine, norepinephrine, phenylephrine: Inhibited alpha adrenergic effects of these drugs
metaraminol: Possibly decreased vasopressor effect of metaraminol

ACTIVITIES

alcohol use: Additive vasodilation, increased risk of hypotension and tachycardia

Adverse Reactions

CNS: Dizziness
CV: Angina; arrhythmias, including tachycardia; hypotension
EENT: Nasal congestion
GI: Diarrhea, nausea, vomiting
GU: Ejaculation disorders, priapism
MS: Muscle weakness
SKIN: Flushing

Nursing Considerations

•Reconstitute each 5-mg vial of phentolamine with 1 ml of sterile water for injection.

•Use reconstituted solution immediately; don't store unused portion.

•Dilute 5 to 10 mg of reconstituted solution in 500 ml of D_5W.

• Inspect drug for particles and discoloration before administering.

• When using drug to diagnose pheochromocytoma, withhold all nonessential drugs, as ordered, for at least 24 hours (preferably 48 to 72 hours) before test.

• Before giving I.V. test dose for pheochromocytoma, place patient in supine position and determine baseline blood pressure by taking readings every 10 minutes for at least 30 minutes.

• Expect patient with pheochromocytoma to have excessive hypotension after receiving drug.

• Take safety precautions according to facility policy if patient experiences dizziness.

PATIENT TEACHING

• Instruct patient to move slowly after phentolamine administration to minimize dizziness and avoid falls.

phenylephrine hydrochloride

Alconefrin Nasal Drops 12, Alconefrin Nasal Drops 25, Alconefrin Nasal Drops 50, Alconefrin Nasal Spray 25, Doktors, Duration, Neo-Synephrine, Neo-Synephrine Nasal Drops, Neo-Synephrine Nasal Jelly, Neo-Synephrine Nasal Spray, Neo-Synephrine Pediatric Nasal Drops, Nostril Spray Pump, Nostril Spray Pump Mild, Rhinall, Rhinall-10 Children's Flavored Nose Drops, Vicks Sinex

Class and Category

Chemical: Sympathomimetic amine
Therapeutic: Antiarrhythmic, decongestant, vasoconstrictor, vasopressor
Pregnancy category: C (parenteral), Not rated (nasal)

Indications and Dosages

➤ *To manage mild to moderate hypotension*
I.V. INJECTION
Adults. *Initial:* 0.1 to 0.5 mg. *Usual:* 0.2 mg, repeated no more than q 10 to 15 min, as prescribed.
I.M. OR S.C. INJECTION
Adults. *Initial:* 1 to 5 mg. *Usual:* 2 to 5 mg (range, 1 to 10 mg), repeated no more than q 10 to 15 min, as prescribed.
➤ *To treat severe hypotension or shock*
I.V. INFUSION
Adults. *Initial:* 100 to 180 mcg/min (0.1 to 0.18 mg/min) until blood pressure is stable.

Maintenance: 40 to 60 mcg/min (0.04 to 0.06 mg/min). Infusion concentration and flow rate adjusted as prescribed, based on patient response.
➤ *To prevent hypotension during spinal anesthesia*
I.M. OR S.C. INJECTION
Adults. 2 to 3 mg 3 or 4 min before injection of spinal anesthetic.
Children. 0.5 to 1 mg for each 11.3 kg (25 lb).
➤ *To treat hypotension during spinal anesthesia*
I.V. INJECTION
Adults. *Initial:* 0.2 mg, increased by no more than 0.2 mg, as prescribed. *Maximum:* 0.5 mg/dose.
Children. 0.5 to 1 mg for each 11.3 kg (25 lb).
➤ *To treat paroxysmal supraventricular tachycardia*
I.V. INJECTION
Adults. *Initial:* Up to 0.5 mg by rapid injection; later doses increased 0.1 to 0.2 mg higher than preceding dose, as prescribed. *Maximum:* 1 mg/dose.
➤ *To treat sinus, nasal, and eustachian tube congestion*
NASAL JELLY OR SOLUTION
Adults and children age 12 and older. 2 or 3 drops or sprays of 0.25% or 0.5% solution q 4 hr, p.r.n., or small quantity of 0.5% nasal jelly in each nostril q 3 to 4 hr, p.r.n. A 1% solution may be used for severe congestion.
Children ages 6 to 12. 2 or 3 drops or sprays of 0.25% solution in each nostril q 4 hr, p.r.n.
Children ages 2 to 6. 2 or 3 drops or sprays of 0.125% or 0.16% solution in each nostril q 4 hr, p.r.n.

Route	Onset	Peak	Duration
I.V.	Immediately	Unknown	15 to 20 min
I.M.	10 to 15 min	Unknown	30 min to 2 hr
S.C.	10 to 15 min	Unknown	50 min to 1 hr
Nasal	Unknown	Unknown	30 min to 4 hr

Incompatibilities

Don't combine nasal form with alkalies, butacaine, ferrous salts, metals, or oxidizing agents.

Mechanism of Action

Directly stimulates alpha-adrenergic receptors and inhibits activity of the intracellular enzyme adenyl cyclase, which then inhibits production of cAMP. The inhibition of cAMP causes arterial and venous constriction and increases peripheral vascular resistance and systolic blood pressure. With greater-than-therapeutic doses, phenylephrine directly stimulates beta-adrenergic receptors in the myocardium, which increases the activity of adenyl cyclase and produces a positive inotropic and chronotropic effect. Intranasal administration directly stimulates alpha-adrenergic receptors on the nasal mucosa, constricting local vessels and decreasing blood flow and mucosal edema.

Contraindications

Hypersensitivity to bisulfites, phenylephrine, or their components; severe coronary artery disease or hypertension; use within 14 days of MAO inhibitor therapy; ventricular tachycardia

Interactions

DRUGS

alpha blockers, haloperidol, loxapine, phenothiazines, thioxanthenes: Possibly decreased vasoconstrictor effect of phenylephrine; decreased decongestant effect of nasal phenylephrine (with phenothiazines)
antihypertensives, diuretics: Possibly decreased antihypertensive effects
atropine: Possibly enhanced vasopressor effect of phenylephrine
beta blockers: Decreased therapeutic effects of both drugs
bretylium: Possibly potentiated vasopressor effect and arrhythmias
doxapram: Increased vasopressor effect of both drugs
ergot alkaloids: Possibly cerebral blood vessel rupture, increased vasopressor effect, peripheral vascular ischemia, and gangrene (with ergotamine)
guanadrel, guanethidine: Increased vasopressor effect of phenylephrine, increased risk of severe hypertension and arrhythmias
hydrocarbon inhalation anesthetics: Increased risk of serious arrhythmias
MAO inhibitors: Increased and prolonged cardiac stimulation, increased vasopressor effect, increased risk of severe cardiovascular and cerebrovascular effects, hyperpyrexia, vomiting
maprotiline, tricyclic antidepressants: Increased risk of severe cardiovascular effects (including arrhythmias, hyperpyrexia, severe hypertension); possibly increased or decreased sensitivity to I.V. phenylephrine
mecamylamine, methyldopa: Decreased hypotensive effects of these drugs, increased vasopressor effect of phenylephrine
nitrates: Possibly decreased vasopressor effect of phenylephrine and decreased antianginal effect of nitrates
oxytocin: Possibly severe, persistent hypertension
phenoxybenzamine: Decreased vasoconstrictor effect of phenylephrine, possibly hypotension and tachycardia
theophylline: Possibly enhanced toxicity (including cardiotoxicity); decreased blood theophylline level (with nasal phenylephrine)
thyroid hormones: Increased cardiovascular effects of both drugs
urinary acidifiers: Possibly increased elimination and decreased therapeutic effects (with nasal phenylephrine)
urinary alkalizers: Possibly decreased elimination and toxic effects (with nasal phenylephrine)

Adverse Reactions

CNS: Dizziness, headache, insomnia, nervousness, paresthesia, restlessness, sleep disturbance (nasal), tremor, weakness
CV: Angina, bradycardia, hypertension, hypotension, palpitations, peripheral vasoconstriction that may lead to necrosis or gangrene, tachycardia, ventricular arrhythmias
EENT: Burning, dry, or stinging nasal mucosa; rebound congestion; and rhinitis (nasal forms)
GI: Nausea, vomiting
RESP: Dyspnea
SKIN: Extravasation with tissue necrosis and sloughing, pallor
Other: Allergic reaction

Nursing Considerations

• Don't dilute phenylephrine for I.M. or S.C. use.
• To reduce the risk of tissue extravasation, don't inject S.C. drug intradermally.
• For I.V. use, dilute with D_5W or sodium chloride for injection and prepare as prescribed—usually 10 mg/500 ml.

• After nasal application, rinse spray bottle tip or nasal dropper with hot water and dry with clean tissue. Wipe tip of nasal jelly tube with clean tissue.
• To prevent transmission of infection, don't use nasal form on more than one patient.
• Assess for signs and symptoms of angina, arrhythmias, and hypertension because phenylephrine may increase myocardial oxygen demand and the risk of proarrhythmias and blood pressure changes.
• WARNING Monitor patient with thyroid disease for increased sensitivity to catecholamines and, possibly, thyrotoxicity or cardiotoxicity.
• WARNING Be aware that extravasation may cause tissue necrosis, gangrene, and other reactions around injection site. Expect to use phentolamine if extravasation occurs.

PATIENT TEACHING
• Inform patient who uses nasal form of phenylephrine that excessive use may cause rebound congestion. Urge her not to exceed recommended dosage and to use for only 3 to 5 days.
• Teach patient who uses nasal form how to care for spray bottle, dropper, or tube.
• Advise patient to avoid potentially hazardous activities until drug's CNS effects are known.

phenytoin

Dilantin-30 (CAN), Dilantin-125, Dilantin Infatabs

phenytoin sodium

Dilantin, Dilantin Kapseals, Phenytex

Class and Category
Chemical: Hydantoin derivative
Therapeutic: Anticonvulsant
Pregnancy category: C

Indications and Dosages
➤ *To treat tonic-clonic, simple, or complex partial seizures in patients who have had no prior treatment*
CHEWABLE TABLETS, ORAL SUSPENSION (PHENYTOIN)
Adults and adolescents. *Initial:* 125 mg suspension or 100 to 125 mg tablet t.i.d., adjusted q 7 to 10 days as needed and tolerated.
Children. *Initial:* 5 mg/kg/day in divided doses b.i.d. or t.i.d., adjusted as needed and

tolerated. *Maintenance:* 4 to 8 mg/kg/day in divided doses b.i.d. or t.i.d. *Maximum:* 300 mg/day.
EXTENDED CAPSULES (PHENYTOIN SODIUM)
Adults and adolescents. *Initial:* 100 mg t.i.d., adjusted q 7 to 10 days as needed and tolerated. *Maintenance:* Once seizures are controlled, adjusted dosage given q.d. if needed and tolerated.
DOSAGE ADJUSTMENT For hospitalized patients without hepatic or renal disease, oral loading dose of 400 mg followed in 2 hr by 300 mg and then in 2 more hr by another 300 mg for a total of 1 g.
Children. *Initial:* 5 mg/kg/day in divided doses b.i.d. or t.i.d., adjusted as needed and tolerated. *Maintenance:* 4 to 8 mg/kg/day in divided doses b.i.d. or t.i.d. *Maximum:* 300 mg/day.
PROMPT CAPSULES (PHENYTOIN SODIUM)
Adults and adolescents. 100 mg t.i.d., adjusted q 7 to 10 days as needed and tolerated.
Children. *Initial:* 5 mg/kg/day in divided doses b.i.d. or t.i.d., adjusted as needed and tolerated. *Maintenance:* 4 to 8 mg/kg/day in divided doses b.i.d. or t.i.d. *Maximum:* 300 mg/day.

➤ *To treat status epilepticus*
I.V. INJECTION (PHENYTOIN SODIUM)
Adults and adolescents. *Initial:* 15 to 20 mg/kg by slow push in 50 ml of sodium chloride for injection at no more than 50 mg/min. *Maintenance:* Beginning within 12 to 24 hr of initial dose, 5 mg/kg/day P.O. in divided doses b.i.d. to q.i.d., or 100 mg I.V. q 6 to 8 hr.
Children. 15 to 20 mg/kg at no more than 1 mg/kg/min. *Maximum:* 50 mg/min.
DOSAGE ADJUSTMENT For elderly or very ill patients and those with CV or hepatic disease, dosage reduced to 25 mg/min, as prescribed, or possibly as low as 5 to 10 mg/min to reduce the risk of adverse reactions.

➤ *To prevent or treat seizures during neurosurgery*
I.V. INJECTION (PHENYTOIN SODIUM)
Adults. 100 to 200 mg q 4 hr at no more than 50 mg/min during or immediately after neurosurgery.

Incompatibilities
Don't mix phenytoin in same syringe with any other drugs or with any I.V. solutions other than sodium chloride for injection because precipitate will form.

P

Mechanism of Action

Limits the spread of seizure activity and the start of new seizures by regulating voltage-dependent sodium and calcium channels in neurons, inhibiting calcium movement across neuronal membranes, and enhancing sodium-potassium ATP activity in neurons and glial cells. These actions all help stabilize the neurons.

Contraindications

Adams-Stokes syndrome, hypersensitivity to phenytoin or its components, SA block, second- or third-degree heart block, sinus bradycardia

Interactions

DRUGS

acetaminophen: Possibly hepatotoxicity, decreased acetaminophen effects

activated charcoal, antacids, calcium salts, enteral feedings, sucralfate: Decreased absorption of oral phenytoin

allopurinol, benzodiazepines, chloramphenicol, cimetidine, disulfiram, fluconazole, isoniazid, itraconazole, methylphenidate, metronidazole, miconazole, omeprazole, phenacemide, ranitidine, sulfonamides, trazodone, trimethoprim: Decreased metabolism and increased effects of phenytoin

amiodarone, ticlopidine: Possibly increased blood phenytoin level

antifungals (azole): Increased blood phenytoin level, decreased blood antifungal level

antineoplastics, nitrofurantoin, pyridoxine: Decreased phenytoin effects

barbiturates: Variable effects on blood phenytoin level

bupropion, clozapine, loxapine, MAO inhibitors, maprotiline, molindone, phenothiazines, pimozide, thioxanthenes, tricyclic antidepressants: Decreased seizure threshold, decreased anticonvulsant effect of phenytoin

calcium channel blockers: Increased metabolism and decreased effects of these drugs, possibly increased blood phenytoin level

carbamazepine: Decreased blood level and effects of carbamazepine, possibly phenytoin toxicity

carbonic anhydrase inhibitors: Increased risk of osteopenia from phenytoin

chlordiazepoxide, diazepam: Possibly increased blood phenytoin level, decreased effects of these drugs

clonazepam: Possibly decreased blood level and effects of clonazepam, possibly phenytoin toxicity

corticosteroids, cyclosporine, dicumarol, digoxin, disopyramide, doxycycline, estrogens, furosemide, lamotrigine, levodopa, methadone, metyrapone, mexiletine, oral contraceptives, quinidine, sirolimus, tacrolimus, theophylline: Increased metabolism and decreased effects of these drugs

dopamine: Increased risk of severe hypotension and bradycardia (with I.V. phenytoin)

fluoxetine: Increased blood phenytoin level and risk of phenytoin toxicity

folic acid, leucovorin: Decreased blood phenytoin level, increased risk of seizures

haloperidol: Decreased effects of haloperidol, decreased anticonvulsant effect of phenytoin

halothane anesthetics: Increased risk of hepatotoxicity and phenytoin toxicity

ifosfamide: Decreased phenytoin effects, possibly increased toxicity

influenza virus vaccine: Possibly decreased phenytoin effects

insulin, oral antidiabetic drugs: Possibly hyperglycemia, increased blood phenytoin level (with tolbutamide)

levonorgestrel, mebendazole, streptozocin, sulfonylureas: Decreased effects of these drugs

lidocaine, propranolol (possibly other beta blockers): Increased cardiac depressant effects (with I.V. phenytoin), possibly decreased blood level and increased adverse effects of phenytoin

lithium: Increased risk of lithium toxicity, increased risk of neurologic symptoms with normal blood lithium level

meperidine: Increased metabolism and decreased effects of meperidine, possibly meperidine toxicity

methadone: Possibly increased metabolism of methadone and withdrawal symptoms

neuromuscular blockers: Shorter duration of action and decreased effects of neuromuscular blockers

oral anticoagulants: Decreased metabolism and increased effects of phenytoin; early increase in anticoagulant effect followed by decrease

paroxetine: Decreased bioavailability of both drugs

phenylbutazone, salicylates: Increased phenytoin effects, possibly phenytoin toxicity *primidone:* Increased primidone effects, possibly primidone toxicity

rifampin: Increased hepatic metabolism of phenytoin

valproic acid: Possibly decreased phenytoin metabolism, resulting in increased phenytoin effects; possibly decreased blood valproic acid level

vitamin D: Possibly decreased vitamin D effects, resulting in rickets or osteomalacia (with long-term use of phenytoin)

ACTIVITIES
alcohol use: Additive CNS depression, increased phenytoin clearance

Adverse Reactions

CNS: Ataxia, confusion, depression, dizziness, drowsiness, excitement, fever, headache, involuntary motor activity, lethargy, nervousness, peripheral neuropathy, restlessness, slurred speech, tremor, weakness
CV: Cardiac arrest, hypotension, vasculitis
EENT: Amblyopia, conjunctivitis, diplopia, earache, epistaxis, eye pain, gingival hyperplasia, hearing loss, loss of taste, nystagmus, pharyngitis, photophobia, rhinitis, sinusitis, taste perversion, tinnitus
ENDO: Gynecomastia, hyperglycemia
GI: Abdominal pain, anorexia, constipation, diarrhea, epigastric pain, hepatic dysfunction, hepatic necrosis, hepatitis, nausea, vomiting
GU: Glycosuria, priapism, renal failure
HEME: Acute intermittent porphyria (exacerbation), agranulocytosis, anemia, eosinophilia, leukopenia, pancytopenia, thrombocytopenia
MS: Arthralgia, arthropathy, bone fractures, muscle twitching, osteomalacia, polymyositis
RESP: Apnea, asthma, bronchitis, cough, dyspnea, hypoxia, increased sputum production, pneumonia, pneumothorax, pulmonary fibrosis
SKIN: Exfoliative dermatitis, jaundice, maculopapular or morbilliform rash, purpuric dermatitis, Stevens-Johnson syndrome, toxic epidermal necrolysis, unusual hair growth, urticaria
Other: Facial feature enlargement, injection site pain, lupus-like symptoms, lymphadenopathy, polyarteritis, weight gain or loss

Nursing Considerations

•Be aware that preferred administration routes for phenytoin are oral and I.V. injection. With I.M. administration, phenytoin has a variable absorption rate.

•If patient has difficulty swallowing, open prompt (rapid-release) capsules and mix contents with food or fluid.

•Shake oral suspension before measuring dose, and use a calibrated measuring device.

•To minimize GI distress, give phenytoin with or just after meals.

•Inspect I.V. form for particles and discoloration before administering.

•**WARNING** Avoid rapid I.V. injection because it may cause cardiac arrest, CNS depression, or severe hypotension.

•To decrease vein irritation, follow I.V. injection with flush of sodium chloride for injection through same I.V. catheter.

•Continuously monitor ECG tracings and blood pressure when administering I.V. phenytoin.

•Frequently assess I.V. site for signs of extravasation because drug can cause tissue necrosis.

•If patient has an NG tube in place, minimize drug absorption by polyvinyl chloride tubing by diluting suspension threefold with sodium chloride for injection, D_5W, or sterile water. After administration, flush tube with at least 20 ml of diluent.

•Separate oral phenytoin administration by at least 2 hours from antacids and calcium salts.

•Expect continuous enteral feedings to disrupt phenytoin absorption and, possibly, reduce blood phenytoin level. Discontinue tube feedings 1 to 2 hours before and after phenytoin administration, as prescribed. Anticipate giving increased phenytoin doses to compensate for reduced bioavailability during continuous tube feedings.

•Monitor blood phenytoin level. Therapeutic level ranges from 10 to 20 mcg/L.

•**WARNING** Monitor hematologic status during therapy because phenytoin can cause blood dyscrasias. A patient with a history of agranulocytosis, leukopenia, or pancytopenia may have an increased risk of infection because phenytoin can cause myelosuppression.

•Anticipate that drug may worsen intermittent porphyria.

•Frequently monitor blood glucose level of patient with diabetes mellitus because drug can stimulate glucagon secretion and impair insulin secretion, either of which can raise blood glucose level.

P

• Monitor blood thyroid hormone levels as appropriate in patient receiving thyroid replacement therapy because phenytoin may decrease circulating thyroid hormone levels and increase thyroid-stimulating hormone level.

• Be aware that long-term phenytoin therapy may increase patient's requirements for folic acid or vitamin D supplements. However, keep in mind that a diet high in folic acid may decrease seizure control.

PATIENT TEACHING

• Instruct patient to crush or thoroughly chew phenytoin chewable tablets before swallowing or to shake oral solution well before using.

• Advise patient to take drug exactly as prescribed and not to change brands or dosage or stop taking drug unless instructed by prescriber.

• Instruct patient to avoid taking antacids or calcium products within 2 hours of phenytoin.

• Urge patient to avoid alcohol during therapy.

• Caution patient to avoid potentially hazardous activities until drug's CNS effects are known.

• Inform patient with diabetes mellitus about the increased risk of hyperglycemia and the possible need for increased antidiabetic drug dosage during therapy. Advise her to monitor her blood glucose level frequently.

• Stress the importance of good oral hygiene, and encourage patient to inform her dentist that she's taking phenytoin.

• Encourage patient to obtain medical identification that indicates her diagnosis and drug therapy.

physostigmine salicylate

Antilirium

Class and Category

Chemical: Salicylic acid derivative
Therapeutic: Anticholinergic antidote, cholinesterase inhibitor
Pregnancy category: Not rated

Indications and Dosages

➤ *To counteract toxic anticholinergic effects (anticholinergic syndrome)*

I.V. OR I.M. INJECTION

Adults and adolescents. 0.5 to 2 mg at no more than 1 mg/min; then 1 to 4 mg, repeated q 20 to 30 min as needed and as prescribed.

Children. 0.02 mg/kg I.V. at a rate not to exceed 0.5 mg/min, repeated q 5 to 10 min as needed and as prescribed. *Maximum:* 2 mg/dose.

Route	Onset	Peak	Duration
I.V.	3 to 8 min	5 min	30 to 60 min
I.M.	3 to 8 min	20 to 30 min	30 to 60 min

Mechanism of Action

Inhibits the destruction of acetylcholine by acetylcholinesterase. This action increases the concentration of acetylcholine at cholinergic transmission sites and prolongs and exaggerates the effects of acetylcholine that are blocked by toxic doses of anticholinergics.

Contraindications

Asthma; cardiovascular disease; diabetes mellitus; gangrene; GI or GU obstruction; hypersensitivity to physostigmine, sulfites, or their components

Interactions

DRUGS

choline esters: Enhanced effects of carbachol and bethanechol with concurrent use of physostigmine, enhanced effects of acetylcholine and methacholine with prior use of physostigmine
succinylcholine: Prolonged neuromuscular paralysis

Adverse Reactions

CNS: CNS stimulation, fatigue, hallucinations, restlessness, seizures (with too-rapid I.V. administration), weakness
CV: Bradycardia (with too-rapid I.V. administration), irregular heartbeat, palpitations
EENT: Increased salivation, lacrimation, miosis
GI: Abdominal pain, diarrhea, nausea, vomiting
GU: Urinary urgency
MS: Muscle twitching
RESP: Bronchospasm, chest tightness, dyspnea (with too-rapid I.V. administration), increased bronchial secretions, wheezing
SKIN: Diaphoresis

Nursing Considerations

• Use physostigmine cautiously in patients with bradycardia, epilepsy, or Parkinson's disease.

- Avoid rapid I.V. administration because it may lead to bradycardia, respiratory distress, or seizures.
- Frequently monitor pulse and respiratory rates, blood pressure, and neurologic status during therapy.
- Monitor ECG tracing during I.V. administration.
- Closely monitor patient with asthma for asthma attack because drug may precipitate attack by causing bronchoconstriction.
- Monitor for seizures in patient with a history of seizures because drug can induce seizures by causing CNS stimulation.
- **WARNING** Be alert for signs of a life-threatening cholinergic crisis, which may indicate a physostigmine overdose: confusion, diaphoresis, hypotension, miosis, muscle weakness, nausea, paralysis (including respiratory paralysis), salivation, seizures, sinus bradycardia, and vomiting. If you detect such signs, prepare to give atropine (the antidote) and use resuscitation equipment. Keep in mind that atropine counteracts only muscarinic cholinergic effects; paralytic effects may continue.

PATIENT TEACHING
- Reassure patient that her vital signs will be monitored frequently to help prevent or detect adverse reactions.
- Instruct patient to notify prescriber immediately about signs of cholinergic crisis.

pindolol

NovoPindol (CAN), SynPindol (CAN), Visken

Class and Category
Chemical: Nonselective beta blocker
Therapeutic: Antihypertensive
Pregnancy category: B

Indications and Dosages
➤ *To manage hypertension*
TABLETS
Adults. *Initial:* 5 mg b.i.d., increased by 10 mg/day q 3 to 4 wk, as prescribed. *Maintenance:* 10 to 30 mg/day. *Maximum:* 60 mg/day (U.S.), 45 mg/day (Canadian).

Route	Onset	Peak	Duration
P.O.	Unknown	1 to 2 hr	Up to 24 hr

Contraindications
Advanced AV block; asthma; bronchospasm; cardiogenic shock; heart failure; hepatic disease; hypersensitivity to pindolol, other beta blockers, or their components; hypotension (with systolic pressure less than 100 mm Hg); sinus bradycardia

Mechanism of Action
Blocks sympathetic stimulation of beta$_1$ receptors in the heart and beta$_2$ receptors in vascular and bronchial smooth muscle by competing with adrenergic neurotransmitters, such as catecholamines. Pindolol's negative chronotropic effects slow the resting heart rate and reduce exercise-induced tachycardia. Its negative inotropic effects reduce cardiac output, myocardial contractility, systolic and diastolic blood pressure, and myocardial oxygen consumption during stress or exercise. Among beta blockers, pindolol has the most intrinsic sympathomimetic activity and nonselective antagonism.

Interactions
DRUGS
allergy extracts or immunotherapy, iodinated contrast media: Increased risk of systemic reaction or anaphylaxis
aluminum salts, barbiturates, calcium salts, certain penicillins, cholestyramine, colestipol, NSAIDs, rifampin, salicylates, sulfinpyrazone: Decreased blood level and effects of pindolol
antihypertensives: Additive hypotensive effect
calcium channel blockers, quinidine: Possibly increased effects of both drugs, symptomatic bradycardia (with diltiazem or verapamil), excessive hypertension or heart failure (with nifedipine)
cimetidine: Increased blood pindolol level
epinephrine: Possibly hypertension followed by bradycardia
ergotamine: Possibly severe peripheral vasoconstriction with pain and cyanosis
estrogens: Decreased antihypertensive effect
fentanyl, fentanyl derivatives: Risk of bradycardia after anesthesia induction
insulin, oral antidiabetic drugs: Masked symptoms of hypoglycemia, increased risk of hyperglycemia
lidocaine: Increased risk of lidocaine toxicity
MAO inhibitors: Possibly hypertension
neuromuscular blockers: Possibly increased or prolonged neuromuscular blockade

phenothiazines: Increased blood levels of both drugs

phenytoin: Possibly increased cardiac depressant effects

prazosin, reserpine: Increased risk of orthostatic hypotension, bradycardia (with reserpine)

quinolones: Possibly increased bioavailability of pindolol

xanthines: Possibly decreased effects of both drugs, decreased xanthine clearance

Adverse Reactions

CNS: Anxiety, confusion, CVA, depression, dizziness, fatigue, fever, hallucinations, hypothermia, insomnia, memory loss, paresthesia, peripheral neuropathy, syncope, weakness
CV: Arrhythmias (including AV block and bradycardia), chest pain, decreased peripheral circulation, heart failure, hyperlipidemia, hypotension, MI, orthostatic hypotension, peripheral edema and ischemia, thrombosis of renal or mesenteric artery
EENT: Pharyngitis
ENDO: Hyperglycemia, hypoglycemia
GI: Colitis (ischemic), constipation, diarrhea, elevated liver function test results, gastritis, nausea, pancreatitis, vomiting
GU: Cystitis, decreased libido, renal colic, renal failure, urinary frequency, urine retention, UTI
HEME: Agranulocytosis, bleeding, eosinophilia, leukopenia, nonthrombocytopenic purpura, thrombocytopenia, thrombocytopenic purpura, unusual bleeding or bruising
MS: Arthralgia, back pain
RESP: Bronchospasm, pulmonary edema, pulmonary emboli
SKIN: Acne; alopecia; crusted, red, or scaly skin; diaphoresis; eczema; exfoliative dermatitis; hyperpigmentation; pruritus; purpura; rash
Other: Angioedema, positive ANA titer

Nursing Considerations

• Monitor blood pressure and pulse rate frequently, especially at start of pindolol therapy. Also monitor fluid intake and output and daily weight, and assess for signs of heart failure, such as dyspnea, edema, fatigue, and jugular vein distention.
• Be aware that drug shouldn't be stopped abruptly because MI, myocardial ischemia, severe hypertension, or ventricular arrhythmias may result.
• Expect to discontinue drug up to 2 days before surgery, as prescribed, to reduce the risk of heart failure.

• Assess distal circulation and peripheral pulses in patient with Raynaud's phenomenon or other peripheral vascular disorder because drug can worsen these conditions.
• Be aware that pindolol can mask tachycardia from hyperthyroidism and that abrupt withdrawal can cause thyroid storm. Drug also may potentiate diplopia and muscle weakness in patient with myasthenia gravis; decrease blood glucose level, prolong or mask symptoms of hypoglycemia, and promote hyperglycemia in patient with diabetes mellitus; and worsen psoriasis.
PATIENT TEACHING
• Instruct patient to weigh herself daily during pindolol therapy and to notify prescriber if she gains more than 2 lb (0.9 kg) in 1 day or 5 lb (2.3 kg) in 1 week.
• Caution patient not to stop taking drug abruptly.
• Advise patient to rise slowly from a seated or lying position to minimize effects of orthostatic hypotension.
• Advise patient to avoid potentially hazardous activities until drug's CNS effects are known.
• Instruct patient to contact prescriber about bleeding or bruising, cough at night, depression, dizziness, edema, rash, shortness of breath, slow pulse rate, or sore throat.
• Advise diabetic patient to monitor her blood glucose level more often during pindolol therapy because drug may mask symptoms of hypoglycemia.
• Inform patient with psoriasis that drug may aggravate this condition.

pioglitazone hydrochloride

Actos

Class and Category

Chemical: Thiazolidinedione
Therapeutic: Antidiabetic
Pregnancy category: C

Indications and Dosages

➤ *To achieve glucose control in type 2 diabetes mellitus as monotherapy or in combination with insulin, metformin, or a sulfonylurea*
TABLETS
Adults. *Initial:* 15 or 30 mg q.d. *Maximum:* 45 mg/day.

DOSAGE ADJUSTMENT For patients taking insulin, insulin dosage decreased by 10% to 25%, as prescribed, once glucose level reaches 100 mg/dl or less. If hypoglycemia occurs, dosage of any concurrent antidiabetic is reduced, as prescribed.

Mechanism of Action
Decreases insulin resistance by enhancing the sensitivity of insulin-dependent tissues, such as adipose tissue, skeletal muscle, and the liver, and reduces glucose output from the liver. Pioglitazone is a potent and highly selective agonist for peroxisome proliferator-activated receptor-gamma (PPARγ). In adipose tissue, skeletal muscle, and the liver, activation of PPARγ receptors by pioglitazone modulates the transcription of a number of insulin-responsive genes involved in glucose control and lipid metabolism. In this way, pioglitazone reduces hyperglycemia, hyperinsulinemia, and hypertriglyceridemia in patients with type 2 diabetes mellitus and insulin resistance. However, to work effectively, pioglitazone depends on the presence of endogenous insulin. Unlike sulfonylureas, the drug does not increase pancreatic insulin secretion.

Contraindications
Diabetic ketoacidosis, hypersensitivity to pioglitazone or its components, severe hepatic dysfunction, type 1 diabetes mellitus

Interactions
DRUGS
ketoconazole: Possibly decreased metabolism of pioglitazone
oral contraceptives: Possibly decreased effectiveness of oral contraceptives

Adverse Reactions
CNS: Headache
CV: Congestive heart failure, edema
EENT: Pharyngitis, sinusitis, tooth disorders
MS: Myalgia
RESP: Upper respiratory tract infection
Other: Weight gain

Nursing Considerations
•Be aware that pioglitazone isn't recommended for patients classified by the New York Heart Association with a cardiac status of Class III or IV.
•Be prepared to monitor liver function test results before therapy begins, then every 2 months

during first year of therapy and annually thereafter, as ordered, because drug is extensively metabolized in the liver. Be prepared to discontinue drug if patient develops jaundice or if ALT values are greater than 2½ times normal.
•**WARNING** Monitor patient for signs and symptoms of congestive heart failure—such as shortness of breath, rapid weight gain, or edema—because pioglitazone can cause fluid retention that may lead to or worsen heart failure. Notify prescriber immediately of any deterioration in the patient's cardiac status, and expect to discontinue the drug, as ordered.
•Assess for signs and symptoms of hypoglycemia, especially if patient is also taking another antidiabetic drug.
•Monitor fasting glucose level, as ordered, to evaluate effectiveness of therapy.
•Monitor glycosylated hemoglobin level to assess long-term effectiveness of drug therapy.
PATIENT TEACHING
•Stress the need for patient to continue exercise program, diet control, and weight management during pioglitazone therapy.
•Advise patient to notify prescriber immediately if he experiences shortness of breath, fluid retention, or sudden weight gain because drug may need to be discontinued.
•Instruct patient to keep appointments for liver function tests, as ordered, typically every 2 months during first year of therapy and annually thereafter.
•Inform female patient who uses oral contraceptives that drug decreases their effectiveness; suggest that she use another method of contraception while taking pioglitazone.

piperacillin sodium
Pipracil

Class and Category
Chemical: Piperazine derivative of ampicillin, acylureidopenicillin
Therapeutic: Antibiotic
Pregnancy category: B

Indications and Dosages
➤ *To treat moderate to severe bacterial infections, including bone and joint infections, gynecologic infections, intra-abdominal infections, lower respiratory tract infections, septicemia, and skin and soft-tissue infections, caused by susceptible strains of* Acinetobacter *sp.,* anaerobic cocci, Bacteroides *sp.,* Enterobacter *sp.,*

Escherichia coli, Haemophilus influenzae, Klebsiella *sp.*, Proteus *sp.*, Pseudomonas aeruginosa, *and* Serratia *sp.*

I.V. INFUSION

Adults and adolescents. 12 to 18 g/day or 200 to 300 mg/kg/day in divided doses q 4 to 6 hr. *Maximum:* 24 g/day.

➤ *To treat bacterial meningitis*

I.V. INFUSION

Adults and adolescents. 4 g q 4 hr or 75 mg/kg q 6 hr. *Maximum:* 24 g/day.

➤ *To treat uncomplicated UTIs and community-acquired pneumonia caused by susceptible organisms, including* E. coli, Klebsiella *sp., and* Serratia *sp.*

I.V. INFUSION, I.M. INJECTION

Adults. 6 to 8 g/day or 100 to 125 mg/kg/day in divided doses q 6 to 12 hr.

➤ *To treat complicated UTIs caused by susceptible organisms, including* Acinetobacter *sp.,* Klebsiella *sp., and* Serratia *sp.*

I.V. INFUSION

Adults. 8 to 16 g/day or 125 to 200 mg/kg/day in divided doses q 6 to 8 hr.

➤ *To treat uncomplicated gonorrhea caused by susceptible strains of* Neisseria gonorrhoeae

I.M. INJECTION

Adults. 2 g as a single dose 30 min after 1-g dose of probenecid P.O.

➤ *To provide surgical prophylaxis in intraabdominal procedures, including GI and biliary surgery*

I.V. INFUSION

Adults. 2 g 20 to 30 min before anesthesia, 2 g during surgery, and 2 g q 6 hr for 24 hr after surgery.

➤ *To provide surgical prophylaxis in abdominal hysterectomy*

I.V. INFUSION

Adults. 2 g 20 to 30 min before anesthesia, 2 g just after surgery, and 2 g 6 hr later.

➤ *To provide surgical prophylaxis in vaginal hysterectomy*

I.V. INFUSION

Adults. 2 g 20 to 30 min before anesthesia, then 2 g 6 and 12 hr after initial dose.

➤ *To provide surgical prophylaxis in cesarean section*

I.V. INFUSION

Adults. 2 g after cord is clamped, then 2 g 4 and 8 hr after initial dose.

Mechanism of Action

Binds to specific penicillin-binding proteins and inhibits the third and final stage of bacterial cell wall synthesis by interfering with an autolysin inhibitor. Uninhibited autolytic enzymes destroy the cell wall and result in cell lysis.

Incompatibilities

Don't mix piperacillin sodium in same container with aminoglycosides because of chemical incompatibility (depending on concentrations, diluents, pH, and temperature). Don't mix with solutions that contain only sodium bicarbonate because of chemical instability.

Contraindications

Hypersensitivity to cephalosporins, penicillins, or their components

Interactions

DRUGS

aminoglycosides: Additive or synergistic effects against some bacteria, possibly mutual inactivation

anti-inflammatory drugs (including aspirin and NSAIDs), heparin, oral anticoagulants, platelet aggregation inhibitors, sulfinpyrazone, thrombolytics: Increased risk of bleeding

hepatotoxic drugs (including labetalol and rifampin): Increased risk of hepatotoxicity

methotrexate: Increased blood methotrexate level and risk of toxicity

probenecid: Increased blood piperacillin level and risk of toxicity

Adverse Reactions

CNS: CVA, dizziness, fever, hallucinations, headache, lethargy, seizures

CV: Cardiac arrest, hypotension, palpitations, tachycardia, vasodilation, vasovagal reactions

EENT: Oral candidiasis, pharyngitis

GI: Diarrhea, epigastric distress, intestinal necrosis, nausea, pseudomembranous colitis, vomiting

GU: Hematuria, impotence, nephritis, neurogenic bladder, priapism, proteinuria, renal failure, vaginal candidiasis

HEME: Eosinophilia, leukopenia, neutropenia, thrombocytopenia

MS: Arthralgia

RESP: Dyspnea, pulmonary embolism, pulmonary hypertension

SKIN: Exfoliative dermatitis, mottling, rash

Other: Anaphylaxis; facial edema; hypokalemia; hyponatremia; injection site pain, phlebitis, and skin ulcer; superinfection

Nursing Considerations
•Obtain blood, sputum, or other samples for culture and sensitivity testing, as ordered, before giving piperacillin. Expect to begin piperacillin therapy before results are available.
•Be aware that sunlight may darken powder for dilution but won't alter drug potency.
•For initial dilution for I.V. infusion, reconstitute each gram of piperacillin with at least 5 ml of sterile water for injection, sodium chloride for injection, D_5W, D_5NS, or bacteriostatic water that contains parabens or benzyl alcohol. Shake solution vigorously after adding diluent to help drug dissolve, and inspect for particles and discoloration before administering.
•For further dilution, use sodium chloride for injection, D_5W, D_5NS, LR solution, or dextran 6% in NS. Be aware that solutions diluted with LR solution should be given within 2 hours.
•For intermittent infusion, infuse appropriate dose over 20 to 30 minutes.
•For I.M. injection, reconstitute each gram of piperacillin with at least 2 ml of an appropriate diluent listed above.
•Don't administer more than 2 g I.M. at any one site. Use the deltoid area cautiously and only if well developed to avoid injuring the radial nerve.
•Assess for bleeding or excessive bruising because drug can decrease platelet aggregation.
•Monitor serum potassium level to detect hypokalemia, which may result from urinary potassium loss.
•Monitor for diarrhea during or shortly after drug therapy; diarrhea may signal pseudomembranous colitis.
•Administer aminoglycosides 1 hour before or after piperacillin, using separate site, I.V. bag, and tubing.

PATIENT TEACHING
•Advise patient to consult prescriber before using OTC drugs during piperacillin therapy because of the risk of interactions.
•Inform patient that increased bruising may occur if she takes anti-inflammatory drugs, such as aspirin and NSAIDs, during therapy.
•Advise patient to notify prescriber if she experiences signs of superinfection, such as severe diarrhea or white patches on tongue or in mouth.

piperacillin sodium and tazobactam sodium
Tazocin (CAN), Zosyn

Class and Category
Chemical: Piperazine derivative of ampicillin, acylureidopenicillin (piperacillin); penicillinate sulfone (tazobactam)
Therapeutic: Antibiotic
Pregnancy category: B

Indications and Dosages
➤ *To treat moderate to severe gram-negative or anaerobic infections, such as appendicitis, community-acquired pneumonia, diabetic foot ulcers, intra-abdominal infections, pelvic inflammatory disease, peritonitis, postpartum endometritis, and uncomplicated or complicated skin or soft-tissue infections caused by susceptible organisms, such as* Bacteroides *sp. (including many strains of* Bacteroides fragilis*),* Clostridium *sp.,* Enterobacter *sp.,* Enterococcus faecalis, Escherichia coli, Haemophilus influenzae, Klebsiella pneumoniae, Morganella morganii, Neisseria gonorrhoeae, Proteus mirabilis, Proteus vulgaris, Pseudomonas aeruginosa, and* Serratia *sp.*

I.V. INFUSION
Adults and adolescents. 3.375 g q 6 hr. *Maximum:* 4.5 g q 6 to 8 hr.

➤ *To treat nosocomial pneumonia caused by susceptible organisms*
I.V. INFUSION
Adults and adolescents. 3.375 g q 4 hr in addition to aminoglycoside therapy for 7 to 14 days.

DOSAGE ADJUSTMENT Dosage possibly decreased to 2.25 g q 6 hr for patients with creatinine clearance of 20 to 40 ml/min/1.73 m^2; to 2.25 g q 8 hr for those with creatinine clearance of less than 20 ml/min/1.73 m^2.

Incompatibilities
Don't mix piperacillin and tazobactam in same container with aminoglycosides because of chemical incompatibility (depending on concentrations, diluents, pH, and temperature).

P

Mechanism of Action
Binds to specific penicillin-binding proteins and inhibits the third and final stage of bacterial cell wall synthesis. Piperacillin does this by interfering with an autolysin inhibitor. Uninhibited autolytic enzymes destroy the cell wall and result in cell lysis.

Tazobactam doesn't change piperacillin's action, but it protects piperacillin against Richmond and Sykes types II, III, IV, and V beta-lactamases; staphylococcal beta-lactamases; and extended-spectrum beta-lactamases.

Contraindications
Hypersensitivity to beta-lactamase inhibitors, cephalosporins, penicillins, piperacillin, tazobactam, or their components

Interactions
DRUGS
aminoglycosides: Additive or synergistic effects against some bacteria, possibly mutual inactivation
anti-inflammatory drugs (including aspirin and NSAIDs), heparin, oral anticoagulants, platelet aggregation inhibitors, sulfinpyrazone, thrombolytics: Increased risk of bleeding
hepatotoxic drugs (including labetalol and rifampin): Increased risk of hepatotoxicity
methotrexate: Increased blood methotrexate level and risk of toxicity
probenecid: Increased blood piperacillin level and risk of toxicity

Adverse Reactions
CNS: Chills, CVA, dizziness, fever, hallucinations, headache, lethargy, seizures
CV: Cardiac arrest, hypotension, palpitations, tachycardia, vasodilation, vasovagal reactions
EENT: Epistaxis, oral candidiasis, pharyngitis
GI: Diarrhea, elevated liver function test results, epigastric distress, intestinal necrosis, nausea, pseudomembranous colitis, vomiting
GU: Hematuria, impotence, nephritis, neurogenic bladder, priapism, proteinuria, renal failure, vaginal candidiasis
HEME: Eosinophilia, leukopenia, neutropenia, thrombocytopenia
MS: Arthralgia, prolonged muscle relaxation

RESP: Dyspnea, pulmonary embolism, pulmonary hypertension
SKIN: Erythema multiforme, exfoliative dermatitis, mottling, rash, Stevens-Johnson syndrome
Other: Anaphylaxis, facial edema, hypokalemia, hyponatremia

Nursing Considerations
• Obtain blood, sputum, or other samples for culture and sensitivity testing, as ordered, before giving piperacillin and tazobactam. Expect to begin therapy before results are available.
• Be aware that sunlight may darken powder for dilution but won't alter drug potency.
• Reconstitute with sterile water for injection, sodium chloride for injection, D_5W, or bacteriostatic water or NS that contains parabens or benzyl alcohol.
• For additional dilution (50 to 150 ml except as noted), use appropriate solution, such as sodium chloride for injection, sterile water for injection (no more than 50 ml), D_5W, or dextran 6% in NS.
• Shake solution vigorously after adding diluent to help drug dissolve, and inspect for particles and discoloration before administering.
• Administer over at least 30 minutes.
• Assess for bleeding or excessive bruising because drug can decrease platelet aggregation.
• Monitor serum potassium level to detect hypokalemia, which may result from urinary potassium loss.
• Monitor for diarrhea during or shortly after drug therapy; diarrhea may signal pseudomembranous colitis.
• Administer aminoglycosides 1 hour before or after piperacillin and tazobactam, using separate site, I.V. bag, and tubing.
PATIENT TEACHING
• Advise patient to consult prescriber before using OTC drugs during treatment with piperacillin and tazobactam because of the risk of interactions.
• Inform patient that increased bruising may occur if she takes anti-inflammatory drugs, such as aspirin and NSAIDs, during piperacillin and tazobactam therapy.
• Advise patient to notify prescriber if she experiences signs of superinfection, such as severe diarrhea or white patches on tongue or in mouth.

pirbuterol acetate

Maxair, Maxair Autohaler

Class and Category

Chemical: Sympathomimetic amine
Therapeutic: Bronchodilator
Pregnancy category: C

Indications and Dosages

➤ *To prevent or treat bronchospasm caused by COPD, to treat bronchospasm caused by asthma*

ORAL INHALATION

Adults and adolescents. 1 or 2 inhalations (200 to 400 mcg) q 4 to 6 hr. *Maximum:* 12 inhalations (2.4 mg)/day.

Route	Onset	Peak	Duration
Oral in-halation	In 5 min	In 30 to 90 min	3 to 6 hr

Mechanism of Action

Attaches to beta$_2$ receptors on bronchial cell membranes, which stimulates the intracellular enzyme adenyl cyclase to convert adenosine triphosphate (ATP) to cAMP. The increased intracellular level of cAMP relaxes bronchial smooth-muscle cells and inhibits histamine release. Pirbuterol also stabilizes mast cells and inhibits the release of histamine.

Contraindications

Hypersensitivity to pirbuterol or its components, tachycardia

Interactions

DRUGS

beta-adrenergic bronchodilators: Additive effects
beta blockers (ophthalmic): Possibly decreased pirbuterol effects, increased risk of bronchospasm
beta blockers (systemic): Decreased effects of both drugs, increased risk of bronchospasm
MAO inhibitors, tricyclic antidepressants: Potentiated cardiovascular effects

Adverse Reactions

CNS: Anxiety, confusion, depression, dizziness, headache, nervousness, tiredness, tremor
CV: Arrhythmias (including PVCs and tachycardia), chest pain, ECG changes (including flattening of T waves, prolonged QT interval, and ST-segment depression), hypotension, palpitations
EENT: Dry mouth
GI: Abdominal cramps, diarrhea, nausea, vomiting
RESP: Bronchospasm, cough
SKIN: Alopecia, rash, urticaria
Other: Facial edema, hypokalemia

Nursing Considerations

•For patient with a cardiovascular disorder, such as arrhythmias, hypertension, or ischemic cardiac disease, monitor blood pressure and heart rate and rhythm to detect significant changes after pirbuterol use.
•Be aware that elderly patients have a greater risk of adverse reactions than younger adults.
•WARNING Discontinue drug and notify prescriber immediately if patient experiences paradoxical bronchospasm, a life-threatening adverse reaction.

PATIENT TEACHING

•Teach patient how to use an inhaler and spacer correctly, and urge her to keep the inhaler readily available at all times.
•Recommend the use of an autohaler if patient has trouble coordinating inhalations with a regular inhaler.
•Advise patient to clean the inhaler's mouthpiece at least once daily.
•Caution patient against overusing drug because doing so may increase adverse reactions.
•Teach patient how to use a peak flow meter and how to determine her personal best reading.
•WARNING Advise patient to notify prescriber if symptoms worsen, if bronchospasm occurs more frequently, if she needs to use the inhaler more often, or if the inhaler becomes less effective.

piroxicam

Apo-Piroxicam (CAN), Feldene, Novo-Pirocam (CAN), Nu-Pirox (CAN), PMS-Piroxicam (CAN)

Class and Category

Chemical: Oxicam derivative
Therapeutic: Anti-inflammatory, antirheumatic
Pregnancy category: Not rated

Indications and Dosages

➤ *To treat acute and chronic osteoarthritis and rheumatoid arthritis*

CAPSULES

Adults. *Initial:* 20 mg q.d. or 10 mg b.i.d.

Route	Onset	Peak	Duration
P.O.	Unknown	Several days to 1 wk*	Unknown

Mechanism of Action

Blocks the activity of cyclooxygenase, the enzyme needed for prostaglandin synthesis. Prostaglandins, important mediators of the inflammatory response, cause local vasodilation with swelling and pain. By blocking cyclooxygenase activity and inhibiting prostaglandins, this NSAID reduces inflammatory symptoms and pain.

Contraindications

Angioedema, asthma, bronchospasm, nasal polyps, rhinitis, or urticaria induced by aspirin, iodides, or other NSAIDs; hypersensitivity to piroxicam or its components

Interactions

DRUGS

acetaminophen: Possibly increased adverse renal effects with long-term use of both drugs
antihypertensives: Possibly decreased or reversed effects of antihypertensives
aspirin, other NSAIDs: Increased risk of bleeding and adverse GI effects, possibly increased blood piroxicam level
cefamandole, cefoperazone, cefotetan: Increased risk of hypoprothrombinemia and bleeding
colchicine: Increased risk of GI bleeding, hemorrhage, and ulcers
corticosteroids, potassium supplements: Increased risk of adverse GI effects
cyclosporine: Increased risk of nephrotoxicity from both drugs, increased blood cyclosporine level
diuretics: Decreased antihypertensive, diuretic, and natriuretic effects of diuretics
gold compounds, nephrotoxic drugs: Increased risk of adverse renal effects

heparin, oral anticoagulants, thrombolytics: Increased anticoagulant effects, increased risk of hemorrhage
insulin, oral antidiabetic drugs: Possibly increased hypoglycemic effect of these drugs
lithium: Possibly increased blood lithium level and toxicity
methotrexate: Decreased methotrexate clearance, increased risk of methotrexate toxicity
platelet aggregation inhibitors: Increased risk of bleeding and GI ulceration or hemorrhage
plicamycin, valproic acid: Increased risk of hypoprothrombinemia and GI bleeding, hemorrhage, and ulceration
probenecid: Possibly increased blood level, effectiveness, and risk of toxicity of piroxicam

ACTIVITIES

alcohol use: Increased risk of adverse GI effects

Adverse Reactions

CNS: Anxiety, asthenia, confusion, depression, dizziness, dream disturbances, drowsiness, fever, headache, insomnia, malaise, nervousness, paresthesia, somnolence, syncope, tremor, vertigo
CV: Edema, heart failure, hypertension, tachycardia
EENT: Blurred vision, dry mouth, epistaxis, glossitis, stomatitis, tinnitus
GI: Abdominal pain; anorexia; constipation; diarrhea; elevated liver function test results; esophagitis; flatulence; gastritis; GI bleeding, perforation, or ulceration; heartburn; hematemesis; hepatitis; indigestion; melena; nausea; vomiting
GU: Cystitis, dysuria, elevated serum creatinine level, hematuria, interstitial nephritis, nephrotic syndrome, oliguria, polyuria, proteinuria, renal failure or insufficiency
HEME: Anemia, coagulation abnormalities, eosinophilia, leukopenia, thrombocytopenia
RESP: Asthma, dyspnea
SKIN: Alopecia, diaphoresis, ecchymosis, erythema, jaundice, photosensitivity, pruritus, purpura, rash, urticaria
Other: Flulike symptoms, hyperkalemia, infection, sepsis, weight loss or gain

Nursing Considerations

• Administer piroxicam with food to decrease GI upset.
• Monitor patient's fluid intake and output as well as BUN and serum creatinine levels, as ordered, for evidence of adverse renal effects.

---

* With severe inflammation, 2 wk or more.

•Monitor hepatic function periodically, as ordered, during long-term therapy.

•Assess for signs of GI bleeding and ulceration, which can occur without warning during long-term piroxicam therapy.

•Be aware that drug's anti-inflammatory actions may mask signs and symptoms of infection.

•**WARNING** Be aware that drug may cause premature closure of ductus arteriosus in growing fetus during third trimester of pregnancy. Be prepared to suggest referral for high-risk pregnancy.

PATIENT TEACHING

•Advise patient to take piroxicam with meals to minimize GI distress. Also direct her to take drug with a full glass of water and to remain upright for 30 minutes afterward to decrease the risk of drug lodging in esophagus and causing irritation.

•Instruct patient to swallow capsules whole and not to crush, break, chew, or open them.

•Advise patient to avoid alcohol, aspirin, and other NSAIDs, unless prescribed, while taking piroxicam.

•Caution patient to avoid potentially hazardous activities until drug's CNS effects are known.

•If patient also takes an anticoagulant, advise her to watch for and immediately report bleeding problems, such as bloody or tarry stools and bloody vomitus.

•If patient also takes insulin or an oral antidiabetic drug, advise her to closely monitor her blood glucose level to prevent hypoglycemia. Encourage her to carry candy or other simple sugars to treat mild hypoglycemia. Advise her to notify prescriber if hypoglycemic episodes are frequent or severe.

•Instruct female patient to consult prescriber if she becomes pregnant because drug may cause premature closure of ductus arteriosus in growing fetus during third trimester of pregnancy.

polymyxin B sulfate

Aerosporin

Class and Category

Chemical: Bacillus polymyxa derivative
Therapeutic: Antibiotic
Pregnancy category: Not rated

Indications and Dosages

➤ *To treat infections that are resistant to less toxic drugs, such as bacteremia, septicemia, and UTIs caused by susceptible organisms, including* Enterobacter aerogenes, Escherichia coli, Haemophilus influenzae, *and* Klebsiella pneumoniae

I.V. INFUSION

Adults and children age 2 and older. 15,000 to 25,000 U/kg/day in divided doses q 12 hr or as a continuous infusion. *Maximum:* 2 million U/day.

Infants and children under age 2. Up to 40,000 U/kg/day in divided doses q 12 hr or as a continuous infusion.

I.M. INJECTION

Adults and children age 2 and older. 25,000 to 30,000 U/kg/day in divided doses q 4 to 6 hr. *Maximum:* 2 million U/day.

Infants and children under age 2. Up to 40,000 U/kg/day in divided doses q 4 to 6 hr.

DOSAGE ADJUSTMENT Dosage reduced by 50% for patients with creatinine clearance of 5 to 20 ml/min/1.73 m^2; by 85% for patients with creatinine clearance of less than 5 ml/min/1.73 m^2.

➤ *To prevent bacteriuria and bacteremia in patients with an indwelling catheter*

BLADDER IRRIGATION

Adults and children age 2 and older. Combination of 200,000 U (20 mg) of polymyxin B sulfate and 57 mg of neomycin sulfate added to 1,000 ml of NS daily as a continuous bladder irrigation for up to 10 days; rate adjusted as prescribed, based on patient's urine output.

➤ *To treat meningitis caused by susceptible strains of* Pseudomonas aeruginosa *or* H. influenzae

INTRATHECAL INJECTION

Adults and children age 2 and older. 50,000 U q.d. for 3 to 4 days, then 50,000 U q.o.d. for at least 2 wk after CSF cultures are negative and glucose content is normal.

Infants and children under age 2. 20,000 U q.d. for 3 to 4 days, then 25,000 U q.o.d. for at least 2 wk after CSF cultures are negative and glucose content is normal.

Incompatibilities

Don't mix polymyxin B sulfate with amphotericin B, calcium salts, chloramphenicol, chlorothiazide, heparin sodium, magnesium salts, nitrofurantoin, penicillins, prednisolone, and tetracyclines. They're incompatible.

Mechanism of Action

Binds to cell membrane phospholipids in gram-negative bacteria, increasing the permeability of the cell membrane. Polymyxin B also acts as a cationic detergent, altering the osmotic barrier of the membrane and causing essential intracellular metabolites to leak out. Both actions lead to cell death.

Contraindications

Hypersensitivity to polymyxin B or its components

Interactions

DRUGS

general anesthetics, neuromuscular blockers, skeletal muscle relaxants: Increased or prolonged skeletal muscle relaxation, possibly respiratory paralysis

nephrotoxic and neurotoxic drugs (such as aminoglycosides, amphotericin B, colistin, sodium citrate, streptomycin, tobramycin, and vancomycin): Increased risk of nephrotoxicity and neurotoxicity

Adverse Reactions

CNS: Ataxia, confusion, dizziness, drowsiness, fever, giddiness, headache, increased leukocyte and protein levels in CSF, neurotoxicity, paresthesia (circumoral or peripheral), slurred speech
CV: Thrombophlebitis
EENT: Blurred vision, nystagmus
GU: Albuminuria, azotemia, cylindruria, decreased urine output, hematuria, nephrotoxicity
HEME: Eosinophilia
RESP: Respiratory muscle paralysis
SKIN: Rash, urticaria
Other: Anaphylaxis, drug-induced fever, facial flushing, injection site pain, stiff neck (with intrathecal injection), superinfection

Nursing Considerations

•Be aware that patients receiving polymyxin B sulfate are hospitalized to allow appropriate supervision.
•Obtain blood, urine, or other samples for culture and sensitivity tests, as ordered, before giving drug. Expect to begin polymyxin B therapy before results are known. Keep in mind that baseline renal function tests should have been performed before adminis-

tration. Check these test results, if available, and notify prescriber of abnormalities.
•For I.M. injection, reconstitute sterile powder with 2 ml of sterile water for injection or sodium chloride for injection.
•Be aware that I.M. route isn't usually recommended (especially for infants and children) because it can cause severe pain at injection site.
•For I.V. infusion, dissolve polymyxin B in 300 to 500 ml of D_5W and infuse over 60 to 90 minutes.
•For intrathecal route, add 10 ml of sodium chloride for injection to vial of polymyxin B.
•Inspect for particles and discoloration before giving drug.
•During therapy, monitor renal function, including BUN and serum creatinine levels, especially in patients with a history of renal insufficiency.
•WARNING Be aware that declining urine output and rising BUN level suggest nephrotoxicity, which also is characterized by albuminuria, azotemia, cylindruria, excessive excretion of electrolytes, hematuria, leukocyturia, and rising blood drug level. Notify prescriber immediately if you detect any of these signs.
•WARNING Notify prescriber immediately if patient experiences blurred vision, circumoral or peripheral paresthesia, confusion, dizziness, drowsiness, facial flushing, giddiness, myasthenia, nystagmus, or slurred speech. These may be signs of neurotoxicity, a serious adverse reaction that may lead to respiratory arrest or paralysis if untreated.
•Assess for signs of superinfection, such as mouth sores, severe diarrhea, and white patches on tongue or in mouth, especially in debilitated or elderly patients.
•Monitor fluid intake and output and provide adequate fluids to reduce the risk of nephrotoxicity.

PATIENT TEACHING

•Encourage patient to maintain adequate fluid intake during polymyxin B therapy.
•Instruct patient to notify prescriber immediately about diarrhea, mouth sores, or vaginitis, which may be early signs of superinfection.

potassium acetate

(contains 2 or 4 mEq of elemental potassium per 1 ml of injection)

potassium bicarbonate

(contains 6.5 mEq of elemental potassium per tablet, 20 or 25 mEq of elemental potassium per effervescent tablet for oral solution)

K+Care ET, K-Electrolyte, K-Ide, Klor-Con/EF, K-Lyte, K-Vescent

potassium bicarbonate and potassium chloride

(contains 20 mEq of elemental potassium per 2.8-g granule packet; 20, 25, or 50 mEq of elemental potassium per effervescent tablet for oral solution)

Klorvess Effervescent Granules, K-Lyte/Cl, K-Lyte/Cl 50, Neo-K (CAN), Potassium Sandoz (CAN)

potassium bicarbonate and potassium citrate

(contains 25 or 50 mEq of elemental potassium per effervescent tablet for oral solution)

Effer-K, K-Lyte DS

potassium chloride

(contains 8 or 10 mEq of elemental potassium per E.R. capsule; 6.7, 8, 10, 12, or 20 mEq of elemental potassium per E.R. tablet; 10, 20, 30, or 40 mEq of elemental potassium per 15 ml of oral solution; 10, 15, 20, or 25 mEq of elemental potassium per packet for oral solution; 20 mEq of elemental potassium per packet for oral suspension; 0.1, 0.2, 0.3, 0.4, 1.5, 2, 3, or 10 mEq of elemental potassium per 1 ml of injection)

Apo-K (CAN), Cena-K, Gen-K, K-8, K-10 (CAN), K+ 10, Kalium Durules (CAN), Kaochlor 10%, Kaochlor S-F 10%, Kaon-Cl, Kato, Kay Ciel, K+ Care, KCL 5% (CAN), K-Dur, K-Ide, K-Lease, K-Long (CAN), K-Lor, Klor-Con 10, Klor-Con Powder, Klor-Con/25 Powder, Klorvess 10% Liquid, Klotrix, K-Lyte/Cl Powder, K-Med 900 (CAN), K-Norm, K-Sol, K-Tab, Micro-K, Micro-K 10, Potasalan, Roychlor 10% (CAN), Rum-K, Slow-K, Ten-K

potassium gluconate

(contains 20 mEq of elemental potassium per 15 ml of elixir; 2, 2.3, or 2.5 mEq of elemental potassium per tablet)

Glu-K, Kaon, Kaylixir, K-G Elixir, Potassium-Rougier (CAN)

potassium gluconate and potassium chloride

(contains 20 mEq of elemental potassium per 15 ml of oral solution; 20 mEq of elemental potassium per 5-g packet for oral solution)

Kolyum

potassium gluconate and potassium citrate

(contains 20 mEq of elemental potassium per 15 ml of oral solution)

Twin-K

trikates

(contains 15 mEq of elemental potassium per 5 ml of oral solution)

Tri-K

Class and Category
Chemical: Electrolyte cation
Therapeutic: Electrolyte replacement
Pregnancy category: C

Indications and Dosages
➤ *To prevent or treat hypokalemia in patients who can't ingest sufficient dietary potassium or who are losing potassium because of certain conditions (such as hepatic cirrhosis and prolonged vomiting) or drugs (such as potassium-wasting diuretics and certain antibiotics)*

EFFERVESCENT TABLETS (POTASSIUM BICARBONATE)
Adults and adolescents. 25 to 50 mEq/g q.d. or b.i.d., as needed and tolerated. *Maximum:* 100 mEq/day.

EFFERVESCENT TABLETS (POTASSIUM BICARBONATE AND POTASSIUM CHLORIDE)
Adults and adolescents. 20, 25, or 50 mEq q.d. or b.i.d., as needed and tolerated. *Maximum:* 100 mEq/day.

EFFERVESCENT TABLETS (POTASSIUM BICARBONATE AND POTASSIUM CITRATE)
Adults and adolescents. 25 or 50 mEq q.d. or b.i.d., as needed and tolerated. *Maximum:* 100 mEq/day.

ELIXIR (POTASSIUM GLUCONATE)
Adults and adolescents. 20 mEq b.i.d. to q.i.d., as needed and tolerated. *Maximum:* 100 mEq/day.
Children. 2 to 3 mEq/kg/day in divided doses.

E.R. CAPSULES (POTASSIUM CHLORIDE)
Adults and adolescents. 40 to 100 mEq/day in divided doses b.i.d. or t.i.d. for treatment; 16

to 24 mEq/day in divided doses b.i.d. or. t.i.d. for prevention. *Maximum*: 100 mEq/day.
E.R. TABLETS (POTASSIUM CHLORIDE)
Adults and adolescents. 6.7 to 20 mEq t.i.d. *Maximum:* 100 mEq/day.
GRANULE PACKETS (POTASSIUM BICARBONATE AND POTAS-SIUM CHLORIDE)
Adults and adolescents. 20 mEq q.d. or b.i.d., as needed and tolerated. *Maximum:* 100 mEq/day.
GRANULES FOR ORAL SUSPENSION (POTASSIUM CHLORIDE)
Adults and adolescents. 20 mEq 1 to 5 times/day, as needed. *Maximum:* 100 mEq/day.
ORAL SOLUTION (POTASSIUM CHLORIDE)
Adults and adolescents. 20 mEq q.d. to q.i.d., as needed and tolerated. *Maximum:* 100 mEq/day.
Children. 1 to 3 mEq/kg/day in divided doses.
ORAL SOLUTION (POTASSIUM GLUCONATE AND POTASSIUM CHLORIDE, POTASSIUM GLUCONATE AND POTASSIUM CITRATE)
Adults and adolescents. 20 mEq b.i.d. to q.i.d., as needed and tolerated. *Maximum:* 100 mEq/day.
Children. 2 to 3 mEq/kg/day in divided doses.
POWDER PACKET FOR ORAL SOLUTION (POTASSIUM CHLORIDE)
Adults. 15 to 25 mEq b.i.d. to q.i.d., as needed and tolerated. *Maximum:* 100 mEq/day.
Children. 1 to 3 mEq/kg/day in divided doses, as needed and tolerated.
POWDER PACKET FOR ORAL SOLUTION (POTASSIUM GLU-CONATE AND POTASSIUM CHLORIDE)
Adults and adolescents. 20 mEq b.i.d. to q.i.d., as needed and tolerated. *Maximum:* 100 mEq/day.
Children. 2 to 3 mEq/kg/day in divided doses.
ORAL TRIKATES SOLUTION (POTASSIUM ACETATE, POTAS-SIUM BICARBONATE, AND POTASSIUM CITRATE)
Adults and adolescents. 15 mEq t.i.d. to q.i.d., as needed and tolerated. *Maximum:* 100 mEq/day.
Children. 2 to 3 mEq/kg/day in divided doses.
TABLETS (POTASSIUM GLUCONATE)
Adults and adolescents. 5 to 10 mEq b.i.d. to q.i.d., as needed and tolerated. *Maximum:* 100 mEq/day.
I.V. INFUSION (POTASSIUM ACETATE AND POTASSIUM CHLORIDE)
Adults and adolescents with serum potassium level above 2.5 mEq/L. Up to 10 mEq/hr. *Maximum:* 200 mEq/day.
Adults and adolescents with serum potassium level below 2 mEq/L, ECG changes, or paralysis. Up to 20 mEq/hr. *Maximum:* 400 mEq/day.
Children. 3 mEq/kg/day.

DOSAGE ADJUSTMENT Dosage adjusted as prescribed based on patient's ECG patterns and serum potassium level.

Mechanism of Action
Acts as the major cation in intracellular fluid, activating many enzymatic reactions that are essential for physiologic processes, including nerve impulse transmission and cardiac and skeletal muscle contraction. Potassium also helps maintain electroneutrality in cells by controlling the exchange of intracellular and extracellular ions. It also helps maintain normal renal function and acid-base balance.

Incompatibilities
Don't mix potassium chloride for injection in same syringe with amino acid solutions, lipid solutions, or mannitol because these drugs may precipitate from solution. Administration with blood or blood products can cause lysis of infused RBCs.

Contraindications
Acute dehydration, Addison's disease (untreated), concurrent use of potassium-sparing diuretics, crush syndrome, heat cramps, hyperkalemia, hypersensitivity to potassium salts or their components, renal impairment with azotemia or oliguria, severe hemolytic anemia

Interactions
DRUGS
ACE inhibitors, beta blockers, blood products, cyclosporine, heparin, NSAIDs, potassium-containing drugs, potassium-sparing diuretics: Increased risk of hyperkalemia
amphotericin B, corticosteroids (glucocorticoids or mineralocorticoids), gentamicin, penicillins, polymyxin B: Possibly hypokalemia
anticholinergics, drugs with anticholinergic activity: Increased risk of GI ulceration, stricture, and perforation
calcium salts (parenteral): Possibly arrhythmias
digoxin: Increased risk of digitalis toxicity
insulin, laxatives, sodium bicarbonate: Decreased serum potassium level
sodium polystyrene sulfonate: Possibly decreased serum potassium level and fluid retention

thiazide diuretics: Possibly hyperkalemia when diuretic is discontinued
FOODS
low-salt milk, salt substitutes: Increased risk of hyperkalemia

Adverse Reactions
CNS: Confusion, paralysis, paresthesia, weakness
CV: Arrhythmias, ECG changes
EENT: Throat pain when swallowing
GI: Abdominal pain; bloody stools; diarrhea; flatulence; GI bleeding, perforation, or ulceration; intestinal obstruction; nausea; vomiting
RESP: Dyspnea
SKIN: Rash
Other: Hyperkalemia

Nursing Considerations
•Administer oral potassium with or immediately after meals.
•Mix potassium chloride for oral solution or potassium gluconate elixir in cold water, orange juice, tomato juice (if patient isn't sodium restricted), or apple juice, and stir for 1 full minute before administering.
•Mix potassium bicarbonate, potassium bicarbonate and potassium chloride, and potassium bicarbonate and potassium citrate effervescent tablets with cold water and allow to dissolve completely.
•Be aware that liquid form of oral potassium is prescribed for patients with delayed gastric emptying, esophageal compression, or intestinal obstruction or stricture to decrease the risk of tissue damage.
•**WARNING** Be aware that direct injection of a potassium concentrate may be immediately fatal. Dilute potassium concentrate for injection with an adequate volume of solution before I.V. use. Maximum concentration suggested is 40 mEq/L, although stronger concentrations (up to 80 mEq/L) may be used for severe hypokalemia. Inappropriate solutions or improper technique may cause extravasation, fever, hyperkalemia, hypervolemia, I.V. site infection, phlebitis, venospasm, and venous thrombosis.
•Infuse potassium slowly to avoid phlebitis and decrease the risk of adverse cardiac reactions. Keep in mind that different forms of potassium salts contain different amounts of elemental potassium per gram and that not all forms are dosage equivalent.

•Monitor serum potassium level before and regularly during administration of I.V. potassium.
•**WARNING** Be aware that some forms of potassium contain tartrazine, which may cause an allergic reaction, such as asthma.
•Regularly assess patient for signs of hypokalemia, such as arrhythmias, fatigue, and weakness, and for signs of hyperkalemia, such as arrhythmias, confusion, dyspnea, and paresthesia.
•Because adequate renal function is needed for potassium supplementation, monitor serum creatinine level and urine output during administration. Notify prescriber about signs of decreased renal function.
PATIENT TEACHING
•Inform patient that potassium is a normal part of a regular diet and that most meats, seafoods, fruits, and vegetables contain sufficient potassium to meet the recommended daily intake. Also advise her not to exceed the recommended daily amount of potassium.
•Teach patient the correct way to take the prescribed potassium. This can vary from swallowing a tablet with a full glass of water to mixing certain preparations with one-half to a full glass of cold water or juice.
•Caution patient not to crush or chew E.R. forms unless instructed otherwise.
•Instruct patient to take drug with or right after food.
•Teach patient how to take her radial pulse, and advise her to notify prescriber about significant changes in heart rate or rhythm.
•Advise patient to watch stools for changes in color and consistency and to notify prescriber if they become black or tarry or bright red from blood.
•Inform patient that although she may see waxy form of E.R. tablet in stools, she has received all of the potassium.
•Urge patient to keep follow-up laboratory appointments as directed by prescriber to determine serum potassium level.

potassium iodide
(KI, SSKI)
Pima, Thyro-Block

Class and Category
Chemical: Iodine

Therapeutic: Antithyroid, radiation protectant
Pregnancy category: D

Indications and Dosages

➤ *To prepare for thyroidectomy*
ORAL SOLUTION

Adults and children. 50 to 250 mg t.i.d. for 10 to 14 days before surgery.
➤ *To manage thyrotoxic crisis*
ORAL SOLUTION

Adults. 50 to 250 mg t.i.d. or 500 mg q 4 hr.
➤ *To protect thyroid gland during radiation exposure*
ORAL SOLUTION, SYRUP, TABLETS

Adults and adolescents. 100 to 150 mg 24 hr before administration of or exposure to radioactive isotopes of iodine and q.d. for 3 to 10 days afterward. *Maximum:* 12 g/day.
Children age 1 and older. 130 mg q.d. for 10 days after administration of or exposure to radioactive isotopes of iodine.
Children under age 1. 65 mg q.d. for 10 days after administration of or exposure to radioactive isotopes of iodine.

Route	Onset	Peak	Duration
P.O.*	24 hr	10 to 15 days	Up to 6 wk

Mechanism of Action
Inhibits the release of thyroid hormone into the circulation, thus alleviating symptoms caused by excessive thyroid hormone stimulation. Potassium iodide also blocks thyroidal uptake of radioactive iodine isotopes that are released as a result of radiation exposure.

Contraindications
Acute bronchitis, Addison's disease, dehydration, heat cramps, hyperkalemia, hypersensitivity to iodides or their components, hyperthyroidism, iodism, renal impairment, tuberculosis

Interactions
DRUGS

antithyroid drugs, lithium: Increased risk of hypothyroidism and goiter
captopril, enalapril, lisinopril, potassium-sparing diuretics: Increased risk of hyperkalemia

Adverse Reactions
CNS: Confusion, fatigue, headache, heaviness or weakness in legs, paresthesia

CV: Irregular heartbeat
EENT: Burning in mouth or throat, increased salivation, metallic taste, sore teeth or gums
GI: Diarrhea, epigastric pain, indigestion, nausea, vomiting
HEME: Eosinophilia
MS: Arthralgia
SKIN: Acneiform lesions, urticaria
Other: Angioedema, lymphadenopathy

Nursing Considerations
• Be aware that potassium iodide shouldn't be given to patients with tuberculosis because drug may cause pulmonary irritation and increased secretions.
• **WARNING** Monitor serum potassium level regularly in patients with renal impairment because of the risk of hyperkalemia.
• Monitor thyroid function test results periodically to assess drug's effectiveness.
PATIENT TEACHING

• Advise patient taking potassium iodide oral solution or syrup to use a calibrated liquid-measuring device to ensure accurate doses.
• Urge patient to mix solution or syrup in a full glass (8 oz) of water, fruit juice, milk, or broth to improve taste and lessen GI reactions. Advise patient taking tablet form to dissolve each tablet in half a glass (4 oz) of water or milk before ingestion.
• If crystals form in solution, advise patient to place the closed container in warm water and gently shake to dissolve.
• Instruct patient to discard bottle and obtain a new one if solution turns brownish yellow.

potassium phosphates

K-Phos Original, Neutra-Phos-K

potassium and sodium phosphates

K-Phos M.F., K-Phos-Neutral, K-Phos No. 2, Neutra-Phos

sodium phosphates

Class and Category
Chemical: Anion, soluble salts
Therapeutic: Antiurolithic, electrolyte replenisher, urinary acidifier
Pregnancy category: C

Indications and Dosages
➤ *As adjunct to treat UTIs, to prevent renal calculus formation*

MONOBASIC TABLETS (POTASSIUM PHOSPHATES)
Adults and adolescents. 1 g in 180 to 240 ml of water q.i.d., after meals and h.s.
MONOBASIC TABLETS (POTASSIUM AND SODIUM PHOSPHATES)
Adults and adolescents. 250 mg in 240 ml of water q.i.d., after meals and h.s. Dosage interval may be increased to q 2 hr if urine is difficult to acidify. *Maximum:* 2 g/24 hr.

➤ *To prevent or treat hypophosphatemia*
CAPSULES (POTASSIUM PHOSPHATES)
Adults and children age 4 and older. 1.45 g in 75 ml of water or juice q.i.d., after meals and h.s.
Children up to age 4. 200 mg in 60 ml of water or juice q.i.d., after meals and h.s.
CAPSULES (POTASSIUM AND SODIUM PHOSPHATES)
Adults and children age 4 and older. 1.25 g in 75 ml of water or juice q.i.d., after meals and h.s.
Children up to age 4. 200 mg in 60 ml of water or fruit juice q.i.d., after meals and h.s.
MONOBASIC TABLETS (POTASSIUM PHOSPHATES)
Adults and children age 4 and older. 1 g in 180 to 240 ml of water q.i.d., after meals and h.s.
Children up to age 4. 200 mg in 60 ml of water q.i.d., after meals and h.s.
MONOBASIC TABLETS (POTASSIUM AND SODIUM PHOSPHATES)
Adults and children age 4 and older. 250 mg in 240 ml of water q.i.d., after meals and h.s.
Children up to age 4. 200 mg in 60 ml of water q.i.d., after meals and h.s.
ORAL SOLUTION (POTASSIUM PHOSPHATES, POTASSIUM AND SODIUM PHOSPHATES)
Adults and children age 4 and older. 250 mg q.i.d., after meals and h.s.
Children up to age 4. 200 mg q.i.d., after meals and h.s.
TABLETS (POTASSIUM AND SODIUM PHOSPHATES)
Adults and children age 4 and older. 250 mg in a full glass of water q.i.d., after meals and h.s.
Children up to age 4. 200 mg in 60 ml of water q.i.d., after meals and h.s.
I.V. INFUSION (SODIUM PHOSPHATES)
Adults and adolescents. 10 to 15 mmol (310 to 465 mg)/day.
Children. 1.5 to 2 mmol (46.5 to 62 mg)/kg/day.

Incompatibilities
Don't add phosphates to calcium- or magnesium-containing solutions because precipitate may form.

Mechanism of Action
Reverses symptoms of hypophosphatemia by replenishing the body's supply of phosphate; acidifies urine by causing hydrogen to be exchanged for sodium in the renal distal tubule; and inhibits formation of calcium renal calculi by preventing solidification of calcium oxalate.

Contraindications
Hyperkalemia (potassium formulations only), hypernatremia (sodium formulations only), hyperphosphatemia, magnesium ammonium phosphate urolithiasis accompanied by infection, severe renal insufficiency, UTIs caused by urea-splitting organisms

Interactions
DRUGS
ACE inhibitors, cyclosporine, heparin (long-term use), NSAIDs, potassium-containing drugs, potassium-sparing diuretics: Increased risk of hyperkalemia (potassium formulations only)
aluminum- or magnesium-containing antacids: Possibly impaired phosphate absorption
anabolic steroids, androgens, corticosteroids, estrogens: Increased risk of edema (sodium formulations only)
calcium-containing drugs: Increased risk of calcium deposition in soft tissues
iron supplements: Decreased absorption of oral iron
phosphate-containing drugs, vitamin D: Increased risk of hyperphosphatemia
salicylates: Increased blood salicylate level
zinc supplements: Reduced zinc absorption
FOODS
low-salt milk, salt substitutes: Increased risk of hyperkalemia
oxalates (in spinach and rhubarb), phyates (in bran and whole grains): Decreased absorption of phosphate

Adverse Reactions
CNS: Anxiety, confusion, dizziness, fatigue, headache, paresthesia, seizures, tremor, weakness
CV: Arrhythmias, edema of legs, tachycardia
GI: Diarrhea, epigastric pain, nausea, thirst, vomiting
GU: Decreased urine output
MS: Muscle cramps or weakness

P

RESP: Dyspnea
Other: Hyperkalemia, hypernatremia, hyperphosphatemia, hypocalcemia, weight gain

Nursing Considerations
•Monitor serum phosphorus level, as appropriate, in patient who receives phosphates and has a condition that may be associated with an elevated phosphorus level, such as chronic renal disease, hypoparathyroidism, and rhabdomyolysis; phosphates may further increase serum phosphorus level.
•Monitor serum calcium level, as appropriate, in patient who receives phosphates and has a condition that may be associated with a low calcium level, such as acute pancreatitis, chronic renal disease, hypoparathyroidism, osteomalacia, rhabdomyolysis, and rickets; phosphates may further decrease serum calcium level.
•Monitor serum potassium level, as appropriate, in patient who receives potassium phosphate and has a condition that may be associated with an elevated potassium level, such as acute dehydration, adrenal insufficiency, extensive tissue breakdown (as in severe burns), myotonia congenita, pancreatitis, rhabdomyolysis, and severe renal insufficiency; she may have an increased risk of hyperkalemia.
•Monitor serum sodium level in patient who receives sodium phosphates and has a condition that may be exacerbated by sodium excess, such as heart failure, hypernatremia, hypertension, peripheral or pulmonary edema, preeclampsia, renal impairment, and severe hepatic disease.
•Monitor urine pH, as ordered, to assess drug effectiveness when it's used to acidify urine.
•When administering sodium phosphates, monitor ECG tracing frequently during I.V. infusion to detect arrhythmias.

PATIENT TEACHING
•Instruct patient to take phosphates after meals to avoid GI upset and decrease laxative effect.
•Stress the importance of not swallowing capsules or tablets whole; instead, advise patient to soak tablets in water or fruit juice for 2 to 3 minutes to dissolve them.
•Suggest chilling the diluted drug to improve the flavor, but caution against freezing.
•Encourage increased intake of fluids (8 oz/hour, if not contraindicated) to prevent kidney stones.

•Urge patient to notify prescriber immediately about muscle weakness or cramps, unexplained weight gain, or shortness of breath.
•Instruct patient who needs an iron supplement to take it 1 to 2 hours after taking phosphates.

pralidoxime chloride

(2-PAM chloride, 2-pyridine aldoxime methochloride)

Protopam Chloride

Class and Category
Chemical: Quaternary ammonium oxime
Therapeutic: Anticholinesterase antidote
Pregnancy category: C

Indications and Dosages
➤ *As adjunct to reverse organophosphate pesticide toxicity*
I.V. INFUSION, I.M. OR S.C. INJECTION
Adults. *Initial:* 1 to 2 g in 100 ml of NS infused over 15 to 30 min, given concurrently with atropine 2 to 6 mg q 5 to 60 min until muscarinic signs and symptoms disappear; may be repeated in 1 hr and then q 3 to 8 hr if muscle weakness persists. If I.V. route isn't feasible, administer I.M. or S.C.
Children. *Initial:* 20 mg/kg in 100 ml of NS infused over 15 to 30 min, given concurrently with atropine (dosage individualized); may be repeated in 1 hr and then q 3 to 8 hr if muscle weakness persists. If I.V. route isn't feasible, administer I.M. or S.C.

➤ *To treat anticholinesterase overdose secondary to myasthenic drugs (including ambenonium, neostigmine, and pyridostigmine)*
I.V. INJECTION
Adults. *Initial:* 1 to 2 g, followed by 250 mg q 5 min.

➤ *To treat exposure to nerve agents*
I.V. INJECTION
Adults. *Initial:* 1 atropine-containing autoinjector followed by 1 pralidoxime-containing autoinjector as soon as atropine's effects are evident; both injections repeated q 15 min for 2 additional doses if nerve agent symptoms persist.

DOSAGE ADJUSTMENT Dosage reduced for patients with renal insufficiency.

Mechanism of Action

Reverses muscle paralysis by removing the phosphoryl group from inhibited cholinesterase molecules at the neuromuscular junction of skeletal and respiratory muscles. Reactivation of cholinesterase restores the body's ability to metabolize acetylcholine, which is inhibited by the effects of organophosphate pesticides, anticholinesterase overdose, or nerve agent poisoning.

Contraindications

Hypersensitivity to pralidoxime chloride or its components

Interactions

DRUGS

aminophylline, morphine, phenothiazines, reserpine, succinylcholine, theophylline: Increased symptoms of organophosphate poisoning

barbiturates: Potentiated barbiturate effects

Adverse Reactions

CNS: Dizziness, drowsiness, headache
CV: Increased systolic and diastolic blood pressure, tachycardia
EENT: Accommodation disturbances, blurred vision, diplopia
GI: Nausea, vomiting
MS: Muscle weakness
RESP: Hyperventilation
Other: Injection site pain

Nursing Considerations

• Be aware that pralidoxime must be administered within 36 hours of toxicity to be effective.
• Use drug with extreme caution in patients with myasthenia gravis who are being treated for organophosphate poisoning because pralidoxime may precipitate myasthenic crisis.
• Reconstitute drug according to manufacturer's guidelines and administration route.
• For intermittent infusion, further dilute with NS to a volume of 100 ml and infuse over 15 to 30 minutes.
• Avoid too-rapid administration, which may cause hypertension, laryngospasm, muscle spasms, neuromuscular blockade, and tachycardia. Also be sure to avoid intradermal injection.
• Closely monitor neuromuscular status during therapy.

• Monitor BUN and serum creatinine levels, as appropriate, in patients with renal insufficiency because drug is excreted in urine.
• When pralidoxime is administered with atropine, expect signs of atropination, such as dry mouth and nose, flushing, mydriasis, and tachycardia, to occur earlier than might be expected when atropine is given alone.

PATIENT TEACHING

• Inform patient receiving I.M. pralidoxime that she'll experience pain at the injection site for 40 to 60 minutes afterward.
• Reassure patient that she'll be closely monitored throughout therapy.

pramipexole dihydrochloride

Mirapex

Class and Category

Chemical: Benzothiazolamine derivative
Therapeutic: Antidyskinetic
Pregnancy category: C

Indications and Dosages

➤ *To treat Parkinson's disease, with or without concurrent levodopa therapy*

TABLETS

Adults. *Initial:* 0.125 mg t.i.d. for 1 wk, increased weekly thereafter as follows: for week 2, 0.25 mg t.i.d.; for week 3, 0.5 mg t.i.d.; for week 4, 0.75 mg t.i.d.; for week 5, 1 mg t.i.d.; for week 6, 1.25 mg t.i.d.; and for week 7, 1.5 mg t.i.d. *Maintenance:* 1.5 to 4.5 mg/day in divided doses t.i.d. *Maximum:* 4.5 mg/day.

DOSAGE ADJUSTMENT For patients with renal impairment, dosage reduced as follows: for creatinine clearance of 35 to 59 ml/min/ 1.73 m^2, initial dose of 0.125 mg b.i.d., maximum of 3 mg/day; for creatinine clearance of 15 to 34 ml/min/1.73 m^2, initial dose of 0.125 mg q.d., maximum of 1.5 mg/day. Drug should not be given to patients with creatinine clearance of less than 15 ml/min/ 1.73 m^2.

Mechanism of Action

May stimulate dopamine receptors in the brain, thereby easing symptoms of Parkinson's disease, which is thought to be caused by a dopamine deficiency.

P

Contraindications

Hypersensitivity to pramipexole or its components

Interactions

DRUGS

carbidopa, levodopa: Possibly increased peak blood levodopa level and potentiation of levodopa's dopaminergic adverse effects
diltiazem, quinidine, quinine, ranitidine, triamterene, verapamil: Decreased pramipexole clearance
haloperidol, metoclopramide, phenothiazines, thioxanthenes: Decreased pramipexole effectiveness

Adverse Reactions

CNS: Amnesia, anxiety, asthenia, confusion, dream disturbances, drowsiness, dyskinesia, dystonia, fever, hallucinations, insomnia, malaise, paranoia, restlessness
CV: Edema, orthostatic hypotension
EENT: Diplopia, dry mouth, rhinitis, vision changes
GI: Anorexia, constipation, dysphagia, nausea
GU: Decreased libido, impotence, urinary frequency, urinary incontinence
MS: Arthralgia, myalgia, myasthenia
RESP: Pneumonia
SKIN: Diaphoresis, rash
Other: Weight loss

Nursing Considerations

•Use pramipexole cautiously in patients with hallucinations, hypotension, or retinal problems (such as macular degeneration) because drug may exacerbate these conditions.
•Also use cautiously in patients with renal impairment because pramipexole elimination may be decreased.
•Take safety precautions according to facility policy until drug's CNS effects are known.
•Don't discontinue pramipexole therapy abruptly. Sudden withdrawal may cause a symptom complex resembling neuroleptic malignant syndrome, consisting of hyperpyrexia, muscle rigidity, altered level of consciousness, and autonomic instability.

PATIENT TEACHING

•Advise patient to take pramipexole with meals if nausea occurs.
•Caution patient about possible dizziness, drowsiness, or light-headedness, which may result from orthostatic hypotension. Advise her not to rise quickly from a lying or sitting position to minimize these effects.
•Instruct patient to notify prescriber immediately about vision problems or urinary frequency or incontinence.
•Inform patient that improvement in motor performance and activities of daily living may take 2 to 3 weeks.

pravastatin sodium

Pravachol

Class and Category

Chemical: Mevinic acid derivative
Therapeutic: Antihyperlipidemic
Pregnancy category: X

Indications and Dosages

➤ *To prevent coronary and cardiovascular events in patients at risk, to treat hyperlipidemia*

TABLETS

Adults. *Initial:* 10 to 40 mg q.d. h.s., increased q 4 wk, as needed. *Maintenance:* 10 to 80 mg h.s.
DOSAGE ADJUSTMENT For patients with significant renal or hepatic impairment, those taking immunosuppressants, and elderly patients, initial dosage reduced to 10 mg q.d. h.s. For elderly patients and those taking immunosuppressants, maintenance dosage usually limited to 20 mg/day.

Mechanism of Action

Inhibits cholesterol synthesis in the liver by blocking the enzyme needed to convert hydroxymethylglutaryl-CoA (HMG-CoA) to mevalonate, an early precursor of cholesterol. When cholesterol synthesis is blocked, the liver also increases the breakdown of LDL cholesterol.

Contraindications

Active hepatic disease or unexplained, persistent elevated liver function test results; breast-feeding; hypersensitivity to pravastatin or its components; pregnancy

Interactions

DRUGS

cholestyramine, colestipol: Decreased pravastatin bioavailability
cyclosporine, erythromycin, gemfibrozil, immunosuppressants, niacin: Increased risk of rhabdomyolysis and acute renal failure

oral anticoagulants: Increased bleeding or prolonged PT

Adverse Reactions
CNS: Dizziness, fatigue, headache
CV: Chest pain
EENT: Rhinitis
GI: Abdominal pain, constipation, diarrhea, flatulence, heartburn, nausea, pancreatitis, vomiting
MS: Myalgia, myopathy, rhabdomyolysis
RESP: Cough
SKIN: Rash

Nursing Considerations
•Use pravastatin cautiously in patients with renal or hepatic impairment and in elderly patients.
•Give drug 1 hour before or 4 hours after giving cholestyramine or colestipol.
•Monitor BUN and serum creatinine levels and liver function test results periodically for abnormal elevations.
•Monitor blood lipoprotein level, as indicated, to evaluate response to therapy.

PATIENT TEACHING
•Instruct patient to take drug at bedtime, without regard to meals.
•Advise patient to notify prescriber immediately about muscle pain, tenderness, and weakness and other symptoms of myopathy.
•Urge female patient of childbearing age to use a reliable method of contraception during therapy and to notify prescriber at once if she becomes or might be pregnant.
•Instruct patient not to discontinue drug without consulting prescriber, even when cholesterol level returns to normal.
•Encourage at-risk patients, especially those with previous cardiac history, to continue following low-fat, low-cholesterol diet to reduce the risk of heart attack or stroke.

prazosin hydrochloride

Minipress

Class and Category
Chemical: Quinazoline derivative
Therapeutic: Antihypertensive
Pregnancy category: C

Indications and Dosages
➤ *To manage hypertension*

CAPSULES
Adults. *Initial:* 1 mg b.i.d. or t.i.d. *Maintenance:* 6 to 15 mg/day in divided doses b.i.d. or t.i.d. *Maximum:* 40 mg/day.

Children. *Initial:* 50 to 400 mcg/kg/day in divided doses b.i.d. or t.i.d. *Maximum:* 7 mg/dose, 15 mg/day.

TABLETS
Adults. *Initial:* 0.5 mg b.i.d. or t.i.d. for at least 3 days, then increased to 1 mg b.i.d. or t.t.i.d., if tolerated, for an additional 3 days. Subsequent dosages adjusted gradually, as needed and tolerated. *Maintenance:* 6 to 15 mg/day in divided doses b.i.d. or t.i.d. *Maximum:* 40 mg/day.
Children. *Initial:* 50 to 400 mcg/kg/day in divided doses b.i.d. or t.i.d. *Maximum:* 7 mg/dose, 15 mg/day.
DOSAGE ADJUSTMENT For elderly patients and those with renal impairment, initial dosage possibly reduced to 1 mg q.d. to b.i.d.

Route	Onset	Peak	Duration
P.O.	0.5 to 1.5 hr	2 to 4 hr*	7 to 10 hr

Mechanism of Action
Selectively and competitively inhibits alpha$_1$-adrenergic receptors. This action promotes peripheral arterial and venous dilation and reduces peripheral vascular resistance, thereby lowering blood pressure.

Contraindications
Hypersensitivity to prazosin, other quinazolines, or their components

Interactions
DRUGS
beta blockers, diuretics, other antihypertensives: Increased risk of hypotension and syncope
dopamine: Antagonized peripheral vasoconstrictive effect of dopamine (with high doses)
ephedrine: Decreased vasopressor response to ephedrine
epinephrine: Possibly severe hypotension and tachycardia
metaraminol: Decreased vasopressor effect of metaraminol
methoxamine, phenylephrine: Possibly decreased vasopressor effect and shortened duration of action of these drugs
NSAIDs, sympathomimetics: Decreased effectiveness of prazosin

P

* For a single dose; 3 to 4 wk for multiple doses.

Adverse Reactions

CNS: Dizziness, drowsiness, fatigue, headache, malaise, nervousness, syncope
CV: Edema, orthostatic hypotension, palpitations
EENT: Dry mouth
GI: Nausea
GU: Urinary frequency, urinary incontinence

Nursing Considerations

•Use prazosin cautiously in patients with renal impairment because of increased sensitivity to prazosin's effects; in those with angina pectoris because drug may induce or aggravate angina; in those with narcolepsy because prazosin may exacerbate cataplexy; and in elderly patients because they're at increased risk for drug-induced hypotension.
•Monitor blood pressure regularly to evaluate effectiveness of therapy.

PATIENT TEACHING

•Instruct patient who is beginning prazosin therapy to take drug at bedtime to minimize effects of first-dose hypotension.
•Stress the importance of taking drug even when feeling well.
•Advise patient to avoid drinking alcohol, standing for long periods, and exercising in hot weather because these activities increase the risk of orthostatic hypotension.
•Suggest rising slowly from a lying or sitting position to minimize the effects of orthostatic hypotension.
•Urge patient to avoid potentially hazardous activities until drug's CNS effects are known.
•Advise patient to notify prescriber immediately about adverse reactions, especially dizziness and fainting.
•Instruct patient not to take any drugs, including OTC preparations, without first consulting prescriber to avoid serious interactions.

prednisolone

Cotolone, Delta-Cortef, Prelone

prednisolone acetate

Articulose-50, Key-Pred, Predacort 50, Predalone 50, Predate 50, Predcor-25, Predcor-50, Pred-Ject 50

prednisolone sodium phosphate

Pediapred

prednisolone tebutate

Nor-Pred T.B.A., Predalone T.B.A., Predate TBA, Predcor-TBA

Class and Category

Chemical: Glucocorticoid
Therapeutic: Anti-inflammatory, immunosuppressant
Pregnancy category: C

Indications and Dosages

➤ *To treat adrenal insufficiency and acute and chronic inflammatory and immunosuppressive disorders*

SYRUP, TABLETS (PREDNISOLONE); ORAL SOLUTION (PREDNISOLONE SODIUM PHOSPHATE)
Adults and adolescents. 5 to 60 mg q.d. or in divided doses. *Maximum:* 250 mg/day.

I.M. INJECTION (PREDNISOLONE ACETATE)
Adults and adolescents. 4 to 60 mg/day.

INTRA-ARTICULAR, INTRALESIONAL, OR SOFT-TISSUE INJECTION (PREDNISOLONE ACETATE, PREDNISOLONE TEBUTATE)
Adults and adolescents. 4 to 100 mg of prednisolone acetate, repeated as needed, or 4 to 40 mg of prednisolone tebutate, repeated q 1 to 3 wk, as needed.

➤ *To treat adrenocortical insufficiency in children*

SYRUP, TABLETS (PREDNISOLONE); ORAL SOLUTION (PREDNISOLONE SODIUM PHOSPHATE)
Children. 0.14 mg/kg/day in divided doses t.i.d.

I.M. INJECTION (PREDNISOLONE ACETATE)
Children. 0.14 mg/kg over a 24-hr period in divided doses t.i.d. q third day.

➤ *To treat acute exacerbations of multiple sclerosis*

SYRUP, TABLETS (PREDNISOLONE); ORAL SOLUTION (PREDNISOLONE SODIUM PHOSPHATE)
Adults. 200 mg/day for 1 wk, followed by 80 mg q.o.d. for 1 mo.

Contraindications

Hypersensitivity to prednisolone or its components, idiopathic thrombocytopenic purpura (I.M. form), systemic fungal infection

Interactions

DRUGS

acetaminophen: Possibly hepatotoxicity (with long-term use or high doses of acetaminophen)

acetazolamide: Possibly hypernatremia or edema
amphotericin B (parenteral): Possibly severe hypokalemia
anabolic steroids, androgens: Possibly edema and severe acne
anticholinergics: Increased intraocular pressure
asparaginase: Increased hyperglycemic effect of asparaginase, possibly neuropathy and disturbances in erythropoiesis
carbonic anhydrase inhibitors: Possibly hypocalcemia, hypokalemia, and osteoporosis
digoxin: Possibly arrhythmias and digitalis toxicity from hypokalemia
diuretics: Possibly decreased natriuretic and diuretic effects of diuretics, severe hypokalemia (with potassium-depleting diuretics)
ephedrine: Increased metabolic clearance of prednisolone
estrogens, oral contraceptives: Decreased clearance, increased elimination half-life, and increased therapeutic and toxic effects of prednisolone
folic acid: Increased folic acid requirements (with long-term prednisolone use)
heparin, oral anticoagulants, streptokinase, urokinase: Possibly decreased anticoagulant effect and increased risk of GI ulceration and bleeding
immunosuppressants: Increased risk of infection, lymphomas, and other lymphoproliferative disorders
isoniazid: Decreased blood isoniazid level
mexiletine: Possibly accelerated metabolism and decreased blood level of mexiletine
neuromuscular blockers: Increased neuromuscular blockade
NSAIDs: Increased risk of GI ulceration and bleeding, possibly added therapeutic effect when NSAIDs are used to treat arthritis
potassium supplements: Decreased effectiveness of both drugs
rifampin, other hepatic enzyme inducers: Decreased prednisolone effect
ritodrine: Increased risk of pulmonary edema in pregnant women
salicylates: Possibly decreased blood salicylate level, increased risk of GI ulceration and bleeding
sodium-containing drugs: Possibly edema and hypertension
somatrem, somatropin: Inhibited growth response to somatrem or somatropin

streptozocin: Increased risk of hyperglycemia
toxoids, vaccines: Possibly loss of antibody response, increased risk of neurologic complications
tricyclic antidepressants: Possibly exacerbated adverse psychiatric effects of prednisolone
troleandomycin: Increased therapeutic and toxic effects of prednisolone

FOODS
sodium-containing foods: Increased risk of edema and hypertension

ACTIVITIES
alcohol use: Increased risk of GI ulceration and bleeding

Route	Onset	Peak	Duration
P.O. (prednisolone)	Unknown	1 to 2 hr	1.25 to 1.5 days
I.M. (prednisolone acetate)	Slow	Unknown	Unknown
Intra-articular, intralesional, soft-tissue injection (prednisolone tebutate)	1 to 2 days	Unknown	1 to 3 wk

Mechanism of Action

Binds to intracellular glucocorticoid receptors and suppresses inflammatory and immune responses by:
•inhibiting neutrophil and monocyte accumulation at inflammation site and suppressing their phagocytic and bactericidal activity
•stabilizing lysosomal membranes
•suppressing antigen response of macrophages and helper T cells
•inhibiting synthesis of inflammatory response mediators, such as cytokines, interleukins, and prostaglandins.

Adverse Reactions

CNS: Euphoria, headache, insomnia, nervousness, psychosis, restlessness, seizures, vertigo
CV: Edema, heart failure, hypertension
EENT: Cataracts, exophthalmos, glaucoma, increased ocular pressure

P

ENDO: Adrenal insufficiency, Cushing's syndrome, growth suppression in children, hyperglycemia
GI: Anorexia, GI bleeding and ulceration, increased appetite, indigestion, intestinal perforation, nausea, pancreatitis, vomiting
GU: Menstrual irregularities
MS: Avascular necrosis of joints, bone fractures, muscle atrophy or weakness, myalgia, osteoporosis, tendon rupture (local injection only)
SKIN: Acne; cutaneous or subcutaneous atrophy (with frequent repository injections); diaphoresis; ecchymosis; flushing; petechiae; striae; thin, fragile skin
Other: Delayed wound healing, hypernatremia, hypokalemia, injection site scarring, negative nitrogen balance

Nursing Considerations

•**WARNING** Avoid using prednisolone in patients with a history of active tuberculosis because drug can reactivate the disease.
•Administer once-daily doses in the morning to match the body's normal cortisol secretion schedule.
•Inspect injectable form for particulates and discoloration before administering.
•For I.M. injection, shake suspension well before withdrawing. Notify prescriber if patient has idiopathic thrombocytopenic purpura because I.M. injections are contraindicated.
•For intra-articular injection, attach a 20G to 24G needle to an empty syringe, using aseptic technique, so prescriber can remove a few drops of synovial fluid to confirm that needle is in the joint. The aspirating syringe is then exchanged with a prenisolone-filled syringe to inject drug into joint.
•Because prednisolone can produce many adverse reactions, assess patient regularly for signs and symptoms of such reactions, including heart failure and hypertension. Also monitor patient's intake, output, and daily weight.
•Monitor growth pattern in children because prednisolone may retard bone growth.
•Be aware that prolonged use may cause hypothalamic-pituitary-adrenal suppression.
•**WARNING** Withdraw drug gradually, as ordered, if therapy lasts longer than 2 weeks. Abrupt discontinuation may cause acute adrenal insufficiency or, possibly, death.
•Be aware that patient may be at risk for

emotional instability or psychic disturbance while taking prednisolone, especially if she is predisposed to these conditions or is taking high doses.

PATIENT TEACHING
•Instruct patient to take oral prednisolone with food to decrease stomach upset and to take once-daily dose in the morning.
•Stress the importance of taking drug exactly as prescribed; taking too much increases the risk of serious adverse reactions.
•Caution patient not to discontinue drug abruptly.
•Urge patient to avoid alcohol during therapy because of increased risk of GI ulcers and bleeding.
•Encourage patient to avoid potentially hazardous activities until drug's CNS effects are known.
•Advise patient to avoid people with contagious infections because drug has an immunosuppressant effect. Urge her to notify prescriber immediately about exposure to measles or chickenpox.
•Caution against receiving vaccinations or other immunizations and coming in contact with people who have recently received the oral poliovirus vaccine.
•Teach patient about potential side effects of prednisolone therapy, including restlessness, mood swings, nervousness, and delayed wound healing.
•Instruct patient to notify prescriber immediately about joint pain, swelling, tarry stools, and visual disturbances. Also instruct her to report signs of infection or injury for up to 12 months after therapy.
•Advise patient to restrict joint use after intra-articular injection and to obtain activity guidelines from prescriber.
•Instruct diabetic patient to monitor her blood glucose level frequently because prednisolone may cause hyperglycemia.
•Advise patient to comply with follow-up visits to assess drug's effectiveness and detect adverse reactions.
•Encourage patient to carry or wear medical identification notifying others of prednisolone therapy.

prednisone

Apo-Prednisone (CAN), Deltasone Liquid
Pred, Meticorten, Orasone 1, Orasone 5,

Orasone 10, Prednicen-M, Prednicot, Prednisone Intensol, Sterapred, Sterapred DS, Winpred (CAN)

Class and Category
Chemical: Glucocorticoid
Therapeutic: Anti-inflammatory, immunosuppressant
Pregnancy category: Not rated

Indications and Dosages
➤ *To treat adrenal insufficiency and acute and chronic inflammatory and immunosuppressive disorders*
ORAL SOLUTION, SYRUP, TABLETS
Adults and adolescents. 5 to 60 mg/day as a single dose or in divided doses. *Maximum:* 250 mg/day.
➤ *To treat adrenogenital syndrome*
ORAL SOLUTION, SYRUP, TABLETS
Adults and adolescents. 5 to 10 mg q.d.
Children. 5 mg/m^2/day in divided doses b.i.d.
➤ *To treat acute exacerbations of multiple sclerosis*
ORAL SOLUTION, SYRUP, TABLETS
Adults. 200 mg q.d. for 1 wk, then 80 mg q.o.d. for 1 mo. *Maximum:* 250 mg/day.
➤ *To treat nephrosis in children*
ORAL SOLUTION, SYRUP, TABLETS
Children age 10 and older. 20 mg q.i.d.
Children ages 4 to 10. 15 mg q.i.d.
Children ages 18 months to 4 years. 7.5 to 10 mg q.i.d.
➤ *To treat rheumatic carditis, leukemia, and tumors in children*
ORAL SOLUTION, SYRUP, TABLETS
Children. 0.5 mg/kg q.i.d. for 2 to 3 wk, then 0.375 mg/kg q.i.d. for 4 to 6 wk.
➤ *As adjunct to treat tuberculosis in children (with concurrent antitubercular therapy)*
ORAL SOLUTION, SYRUP, TABLETS
Children. 0.5 mg/kg q.i.d. for 2 mo.

Route	Onset	Peak	Duration
P.O.	Rapid	1 to 2 hr	1.25 to 1.5 days

Contraindications
Hypersensitivity to prednisone or its components, systemic fungal infection

Mechanism of Action
Binds to intracellular glucocorticoid receptors and suppresses inflammatory and immune responses by:
• inhibiting neutrophil and monocyte accumulation at inflammation site and suppressing their phagocytic and bactericidal activity
• stabilizing lysosomal membranes
• suppressing antigen response of macrophages and helper T cells
• inhibiting synthesis of inflammatory response mediators, such as cytokines, interleukins, and prostaglandins.

Interactions
DRUGS
acetaminophen: Possibly hepatotoxicity (with long-term use or high doses of acetaminophen)
acetazolamide sodium: Possibly hypernatremia or edema
amphotericin B (parenteral): Possibly severe hypokalemia
anabolic steroids, androgens: Possibly edema and severe acne
antacids: Decreased absorption of prednisone (with long-term use)
anticholinergics: Increased intraocular pressure
asparaginase: Increased hyperglycemic effect of asparaginase, possibly neuropathy and disturbances in erythropoiesis
carbonic anhydrase inhibitors: Possibly hypocalcemia, hypokalemia, and osteoporosis
digoxin: Possibly arrhythmias and digitalis toxicity from hypokalemia
diuretics: Possibly decreased natriuretic and diuretic effects of diuretics, severe hypokalemia (with potassium-depleting diuretics)
ephedrine: Increased metabolic clearance of prednisone
estrogens, oral contraceptives: Decreased clearance, increased elimination half-life, and increased therapeutic and toxic effects of prednisone
folic acid: Increased folic acid requirements (with long-term prednisone use)
heparin, oral anticoagulants, streptokinase, urokinase: Possibly decreased anticoagulant effect and increased risk of GI ulceration and bleeding
immunosuppressants: Increased risk of infection, lymphomas, and other lymphoproliferative disorders

isoniazid: Decreased blood isoniazid level
mexiletine: Possibly accelerated metabolism and decreased blood level of mexiletine
neuromuscular blockers: Increased neuromuscular blockade
NSAIDs: Increased risk of GI ulceration and bleeding, possibly added therapeutic effect when NSAIDs are used to treat arthritis
potassium supplements: Decreased effectiveness of both drugs
ritodrine: Increased risk of pulmonary edema in pregnant women
salicylates: Possibly decreased blood salicylate level, increased risk of GI ulceration and bleeding
sodium-containing drugs: Possibly edema and hypertension
somatrem, somatropin: Inhibited growth response to somatrem or somatropin
streptozocin: Increased risk of hyperglycemia
toxoids, vaccines: Possibly loss of antibody response, increased risk of neurologic complications
tricyclic antidepressants: Possibly exacerbated adverse psychiatric effects of prednisone
troleandomycin: Increased therapeutic and toxic effects of prednisone

FOODS
sodium-containing foods: Increased risk of edema and hypertension

ACTIVITIES
alcohol use: Increased risk of GI ulceration and bleeding

Adverse Reactions

CNS: Euphoria, headache, insomnia, nervousness, psychosis, restlessness, seizures, vertigo
CV: Edema, heart failure, hypertension
EENT: Cataracts, exophthalmos, glaucoma, increased ocular pressure
ENDO: Adrenal insufficiency, Cushing's syndrome, growth suppression in children, hyperglycemia
GI: Anorexia, GI bleeding and ulceration, increased appetite, indigestion, intestinal perforation, nausea, pancreatitis, vomiting
GU: Menstrual irregularities
MS: Avascular necrosis of joints, bone fractures, muscle atrophy or weakness, myalgia, osteoporosis
SKIN: Acne; diaphoresis; ecchymosis; flushing; petechiae; striae; thin, fragile skin
Other: Delayed wound healing, hypernatremia, hypokalemia, negative nitrogen balance

Nursing Considerations

•Administer once-daily doses of prednisone in the morning to match the body's normal cortisol secretion schedule.
•Because prednisone can produce many adverse reactions, assess regularly for signs and symptoms of such reactions as heart failure and hypertension. Also monitor fluid intake and output and daily weight.
•Monitor growth pattern in children because prednisone may retard bone growth.
•Be aware that prolonged use may cause hypothalamic-pituitary-adrenal suppression.
•**WARNING** Withdraw drug gradually, as ordered, if therapy lasts longer than 2 weeks. Abrupt discontinuation may cause acute adrenal insufficiency and, possibly, death.

PATIENT TEACHING
•Instruct patient to take prednisone with food to decrease GI distress and to take once-daily dose in the morning.
•Stress the importance of taking drug exactly as prescribed; taking more than prescribed dosage increases the risk of serious adverse reactions.
•Caution patient not to discontinue drug abruptly.
•Urge patient to avoid alcohol during therapy because of the increased risk of GI ulcers and bleeding.
•Encourage patient to avoid potentially hazardous activities until drug's CNS effects are known.
•Advise patient to avoid people with contagious infections because drug has an immunosuppressant effect. Urge her to notify prescriber immediately about possible exposure to measles or chickenpox.
•Caution against receiving vaccinations or other immunizations and coming in contact with people who have recently received the oral poliovirus vaccine.
•Instruct patient to notify prescriber immediately about joint pain, swelling, tarry stools, and visual disturbances. Also instruct her to report signs of infection or injury for up to 12 months after therapy.
•Instruct diabetic patient to monitor her blood glucose level frequently because prednisone may cause hyperglycemia.
•Advise patient to comply with follow-up visits to assess drug effectiveness and detect adverse reactions.
•Encourage patient to carry or wear medical

identification to notify others of prednisone therapy.

primidone

Apo-Primidone (CAN), Myidone, Mysoline, PMS Primidone (CAN), Sertan (CAN)

Class and Category

Chemical: Prodrug of phenobarbital
Therapeutic: Anticonvulsant
Pregnancy category: Not rated

Indications and Dosages

➤ *To manage generalized tonic-clonic seizures, nocturnal myoclonic seizures, complex partial seizures, and simple partial seizures caused by epilepsy*

CHEWABLE TABLETS, ORAL SUSPENSION, TABLETS

Adults and children age 8 and older. *Initial:* 100 or 125 mg h.s. for first 3 days, then increased to 100 or 125 mg b.i.d. for next 3 days, followed by 100 or 125 mg t.i.d. for next 3 days. On 10th day, begin maintenance dosage as prescribed. *Maintenance:* 250 mg t.i.d. or q.i.d., adjusted as needed. *Maximum:* 2 g/day.

Children up to age 8. *Initial:* 50 mg h.s. for first 3 days, then increased to 50 mg b.i.d. for next 3 days, followed by increase to 100 mg b.i.d. for next 3 days. On 10th day, begin maintenance dosage. *Maintenance:* 125 to 250 mg t.i.d., adjusted as needed.

Mechanism of Action

Prevents seizures by decreasing the excitability of neurons and increasing the motor cortex's threshold of electrical stimulation.

Contraindications

Hypersensitivity to primidone, phenobarbital, or their components; porphyria

Interactions

DRUGS

acetaminophen: Decreased acetaminophen effectiveness, increased risk of hepatotoxicity
adrenocorticoids, chloramphenicol, cyclosporine, dacarbazine, disopyramide, doxycycline, levothyroxine, metronidazole, mexiletine, oral anticoagulants, oral contraceptives (estrogen-containing), quinidine, tricyclic antidepressants: Decreased effectiveness of these drugs
amphetamines: Possibly delayed absorption of primidone
anticonvulsants: Possibly altered pattern of seizures
carbamazepine: Decreased effectiveness of primidone
carbonic anhydrase inhibitors: Increased risk of osteopenia
CNS depressants: Possibly enhanced CNS and respiratory depressant effects of both drugs
cyclophosphamide: Reduced half-life and increased leukopenic activity of cyclophosphamide
enflurane, halothane, methoxyflurane: Increased risk of hepatotoxicity; increased risk of nephrotoxicity (with methoxyflurane)
fenoprofen: Decreased elimination half-life of fenoprofen
folic acid: Increased folic acid requirements
griseofulvin: Decreased antifungal effects of griseofulvin
guanadrel, guanethidine: Possibly aggravated orthostatic hypotension
haloperidol, loxapine, maprotiline, molindone, phenothiazines, thioxanthenes: Possibly lowered seizure threshold and increased CNS depression
leucovorin: Possibly decreased anticonvulsant effects of primidone (with large doses)
MAO inhibitors: Possibly prolonged effects of primidone and altered pattern of seizures
methylphenidate: Possibly increased blood primidone level, resulting in toxicity
phenobarbital: Increased sedative effects of either drug, possibly altered pattern of seizures
phenylbutazone: Decreased primidone effectiveness, increased metabolism and decreased half-life of phenylbutazone
rifampin: Decreased blood primidone level
valproic acid: Increased blood primidone level, leading to increased CNS depression and neurotoxicity; decreased half-life of valproic acid and enhanced risk of hepatotoxicity
vitamin D: Decreased effects of vitamin D
xanthines: Increased metabolism and clearance of xanthines (except dyphylline)

ACTIVITIES

alcohol use: Possibly increased CNS and respiratory depressant effects of primidone

Adverse Reactions

CNS: Ataxia, confusion, dizziness, drowsiness, excitement, mental changes, mood changes, restlessness
EENT: Diplopia, nystagmus
GI: Anorexia, nausea, vomiting
GU: Impotence
RESP: Dyspnea
Other: Folic acid deficiency

Nursing Considerations

• Monitor blood levels of primidone and phenobarbital (its active metabolite), as ordered, to determine therapeutic level or detect toxic levels.
• Anticipate that drug may cause confusion, excitement, or mood changes in elderly patients and children.
• Assess for signs of folic acid deficiency: mental dysfunction, neuropathy, tiredness, and weakness.

PATIENT TEACHING

• Instruct patient to crush primidone tablets and mix with foods or fluids, as needed.
• Advise patient taking oral suspension to shake the bottle well and measure doses with a calibrated device.
• Suggest that patient take drug with meals to minimize adverse GI reactions.
• Urge patient not to stop taking primidone abruptly because doing so can precipitate seizures.
• Caution patient about possible decreased alertness.
• Advise her to avoid potentially hazardous activities until drug's CNS effects are known.
• Urge patient to avoid alcohol and other CNS depressants during primidone therapy.

probenecid

Benemid, Benuryl (CAN), Probalan

Class and Category

Chemical: Sulfonamide derivative
Therapeutic: Antibiotic adjunct, antigout, uricosuric
Pregnancy category: Not rated

Indications and Dosages

➤ *To treat chronic gouty arthritis and hyperuricemia due to chronic gout*
TABLETS

Adults and adolescents. *Initial:* 250 mg b.i.d. for 1 wk, then increased to maintenance dos-

age. *Maintenance:* 500 mg b.i.d.; if not effective or 24-hr uric acid excretion isn't greater than 700 mg, dosage increased by 500 mg/day q 4 wk, as needed and prescribed, up to a maximum of 3 g/day. If no acute attacks of gout occur over next 6 mo and serum uric acid level is within normal limits, dosage decreased, as prescribed, by 500 mg q 6 mo until lowest effective maintenance dose is reached. *Maximum:* 3 g/day.

DOSAGE ADJUSTMENT Dosage possibly increased for patients with mild renal dysfunction, except for elderly patients, who require a dosage reduction.

➤ *As adjunct to antibiotic therapy with penicillins and some cephalosporins*
TABLETS

Adults, adolescents age 14 and older, and children weighing more than 50 kg (110 lb). 500 mg q.i.d.; if given with I.V. or I.M. antibiotic, administer at least 30 min before antibiotic.

Children ages 2 to 14 weighing up to 50 kg. 25 mg/kg as a single dose, followed by 10 mg/kg q.i.d.; if given with I.V. or I.M. antibiotic, administer at least 30 min before antibiotic.

➤ *As adjunct to treat sexually transmitted diseases*
TABLETS

Adults and adolescents. 1 g as a single dose administered together with appropriate antibiotic.

➤ *As adjunct to treat pediatric gonorrhea*
TABLETS

Postpubertal children and children weighing more than 45 kg (99 lb). 1 g as a single dose administered together with appropriate antibiotic.

➤ *As adjunct to treat neurosyphilis*
TABLETS

Adults and adolescents. 500 mg q.i.d. concurrently with 1 daily dose (2.4 million U) of penicillin G procaine for 10 to 14 days.

Route	Onset	Peak	Duration
P.O.	Unknown	30 min*	8 hr†

---

* For renal clearance of uric acid; 2 hr for effect on blood antibiotic level.
† For effect on blood antibiotic level; unknown for renal clearance of uric acid.

Mechanism of Action

Increases urinary excretion of uric acid and lowers serum uric acid level, which may prevent or resolve urate deposits, tophus formation, and joint changes. Eventually, the incidence of acute gout attacks decreases. Probenecid also inhibits renal excretion of penicillins and some cephalosporin antibiotics, thereby increasing their serum concentration and prolonging their duration of action.

Contraindications

Age less than 2 years, blood dyscrasias, hypersensitivity to probenecid or its components, renal calculi (urate)

Interactions

DRUGS

acyclovir: Decreased renal tubular secretion of acyclovir
allopurinol: Additive antihyperuricemic effects
aminosalicylate sodium, cephalosporins, ciprofloxacin, clofibrate, dapsone, ganciclovir, imipenem, methotrexate, nitrofurantoin, norfloxacin, penicillins: Increased and possibly prolonged blood levels of these drugs, increased risk of toxicity
antineoplastics (rapidly cytolytic): Possibly uric acid nephropathy
diazoxide, mecamylamine, pyrazinamide: Increased risk of hyperuricemia, decreased probenecid effectiveness
dyphylline: Increased half-life of dyphylline
furosemide: Increased blood furosemide level
heparin: Increased and prolonged anticoagulant effect
indomethacin, ketoprofen, other NSAIDs: Possibly increased adverse effects
lorazepam, oxazepam, temazepam: Increased effects of these drugs and, possibly, excessive sedation
riboflavin: Decreased GI absorption of riboflavin
rifampin, sulfonamides: Increased blood levels of these drugs and, possibly, toxicity
salicylates: Decreased uricosuric effects of probenecid
sodium benzoate and sodium phenylacetate: Decreased renal elimination of these drugs
sulfonylureas: Increased sulfonylurea half-life

thiopental: Prolonged thiopental effect
zidovudine: Increased risk of zidovudine toxicity

ACTIVITIES

alcohol use: Increased risk of hyperuricemia, decreased probenecid effectiveness

Adverse Reactions

CNS: Dizziness, headache
EENT: Sore gums
GI: Anorexia, nausea, vomiting
GU: Hematuria, renal calculi (urate), renal colic, urinary frequency
MS: Costovertebral pain; joint pain, redness, and swelling
SKIN: Facial flushing, pruritus, rash, urticaria

Nursing Considerations

• Be aware that probenecid therapy shouldn't be started until acute gout attack has subsided. If acute gout attack begins during therapy, continue drug therapy as prescribed.
• Use drug cautiously in patients with peptic ulcer disease.
• Expect to give sodium bicarbonate (3 to 7.5 g/day) or potassium citrate (7.5 g/day), as prescribed, to keep urine alkaline and prevent renal calculus formation.
• Monitor CBC, serum uric acid level, and liver and renal function test results during therapy.
• Closely monitor patients receiving intermittent therapy because they're more likely to develop allergic reactions.
• Monitor blood glucose level frequently in diabetic patient who takes a sulfonylurea because of the risk of drug interactions.

PATIENT TEACHING

• Advise patient to take probenecid with meals to minimize GI distress.
• Encourage patient to increase fluid intake (up to 3 L/day, if not contraindicated) to help prevent renal calculus formation.
• Instruct patient to notify prescriber immediately if she experiences signs of an acute gout attack (joint pain, swelling, and redness) or of kidney stones (flank pain and blood in urine).
• Caution patient against taking salicylates while taking probenecid. Instead, advise her to use acetaminophen to treat mild pain or fever.

probenecid and colchicine

ColBenemid, Col-Probenecid, Proben-C

P

Class and Category

Chemical: Sulfonamide derivative (probenecid), colchicium alkaloid derivative (colchicine)
Therapeutic: Antigout
Pregnancy category: Not rated

Indications and Dosages

➤ *To treat chronic gouty arthritis in patients who experience frequent attacks*

TABLETS

Adults. *Initial:* 1 tablet (500 mg of probenecid/0.5 mg of colchicine) q.d. for 1 wk, then increased to maintenance dosage. *Maintenance:* 1 tablet b.i.d.; if not effective or 24-hr uric acid excretion isn't greater than 700 mg, dosage increased by 1 tablet/day q 4 wk, as needed and prescribed, up to a maximum of 4 tablets/day. If no acute attacks of gout occur over next 6 mo and serum uric acid level is within normal limits, dosage decreased, as prescribed, by 1 tablet q 6 mo until lowest effective maintenance dose is reached.

DOSAGE ADJUSTMENT Dosage possibly increased for patients with mild renal dysfunction.

Mechanism of Action

Reduces the frequency of gout attacks through several mechanisms. Probenecid increases urinary excretion of uric acid and reduces the serum level of uric acid, which may prevent or resolve urate deposits, tophus formation, and joint changes. Eventually, the incidence of acute gout attacks may decrease.

Colchicine helps to stop inflammation, probably by disrupting microtubules in leukocytes. Microtubules contribute to cell structure and movement. When colchicine binds to tubulin (the protein from which microtubules are made), it causes microtubules to fall apart. This, in turn, disrupts cell function and prevents leukocytes from continuing to invade joints and produce inflammation.

Contraindications

Age less than 2 years; blood dyscrasias; hypersensitivity to colchicine, probenecid, or their components; renal calculi (urate)

Interactions

DRUGS

acyclovir: Decreased renal tubular secretion of acyclovir

allopurinol: Additive antihyperuricemic effects
aminosalicylate sodium, cephalosporins, ciprofloxacin, clofibrate, dapsone, ganciclovir, imipenem, methotrexate, nitrofurantoin, norfloxacin, penicillins: Increased and possibly prolonged blood levels of these drugs, increased risk of toxicity
antineoplastics (rapidly cytolytic): Possibly uric acid nephropathy
cyclosporine: Possibly impaired renal function and risk of nephrotoxicity
diazoxide, mecamylamine, pyrazinamide: Increased risk of hyperuricemia, decreased probenecid effectiveness
dyphylline: Increased half-life of dyphylline
erythromycin: Impaired metabolism of colchicine
furosemide: Increased blood furosemide level
heparin: Increased and prolonged anticoagulant effect
indomethacin, ketoprofen, other NSAIDs: Possibly increased adverse effects
lorazepam, oxazepam, temazepam: Increased effects of these drugs and, possibly, excessive sedation
riboflavin: Decreased GI absorption of riboflavin
rifampin, sulfonamides: Increased blood levels of these drugs and, possibly, toxicity
salicylates: Decreased uricosuric effects of probenecid and colchicine
sodium benzoate and sodium phenylacetate: Decreased renal elimination of these drugs
sulfonylureas: Increased sulfonylurea half-life
thiopental: Prolonged thiopental effect
vitamin B_{12} (cyanocobalamin): Reversible decrease in blood vitamin B_{12} level
zidovudine: Increased risk of zidovudine toxicity

ACTIVITIES

alcohol use: Increased risk of hyperuricemia, decreased antigout effects

Adverse Reactions

CNS: Dizziness, fever, headache, peripheral neuritis
EENT: Sore gums
GI: Abdominal pain, anorexia, diarrhea, hepatic necrosis, nausea, vomiting
GU: Hematuria, nephropathy (urate), nephrotic syndrome, renal calculi (urate), renal colic, urinary frequency
HEME: Agranulocytosis, anemia, aplastic anemia, hemolytic anemia, leukopenia

MS: Back or rib pain, gout attacks, muscle weakness
SKIN: Alopecia, dermatitis, flushing, purpura
Other: Anaphylaxis

Nursing Considerations

• Be aware that probenecid and colchicine therapy shouldn't be started until acute gout attack has subsided. If acute gout attack begins during therapy, expect to continue drug therapy.
• Use drug cautiously in patients with peptic ulcer disease.
• Expect to give sodium bicarbonate (3 to 7.5 g/day) or potassium citrate (7.5 g/day), as prescribed, to keep urine alkaline and prevent renal calculus formation.
• Monitor CBC, serum uric acid level, and liver and renal function test results during therapy.
• Closely monitor patients receiving intermittent therapy because they are more prone to allergic reactions.
• Frequently monitor blood glucose level of diabetic patient who takes a sulfonylurea because of the risk of drug interactions.

PATIENT TEACHING

• Advise patient to take probenecid and colchicine with meals to minimize stomach upset.
• Encourage increased fluid intake (up to 3 L/day, if not contraindicated) to help prevent renal calculus formation.
• Instruct patient to notify prescriber immediately if she experiences a gouty arthritis flare-up (joint pain, swelling, and redness) or signs of kidney stones, such as flank pain and blood in urine.
• Caution patient against taking salicylates while taking drug. Instead, advise her to use acetaminophen to treat mild pain or fever.

procainamide hydrochloride

Procanbid, Procan SR, Promine, Pronestyl, Pronestyl-SR

Class and Category

Chemical: Ethyl benzamide monohydrochloride
Therapeutic: Antiarrhythmic
Pregnancy category: C

Indications and Dosages

➤ *To treat life-threatening ventricular arrhythmias*

CAPSULES, TABLETS

Adults. 50 mg/kg/day in 8 divided doses (q 3 hr), adjusted as needed and tolerated. *Maximum:* 6 g/day (maintenance).
Children. 12.5 mg/kg q.i.d.

E.R. TABLETS

Adults. *Maintenance:* 50 mg/kg/day in divided doses q.i.d. (q 6 hr), adjusted as needed and tolerated. *Maximum:* 6 g/day (maintenance).

I.V. INFUSION OR INJECTION

Adults. *Initial:* 100 mg diluted in D_5W and administered at a rate not to exceed 50 mg/min. Dosage repeated q 5 min until arrhythmia is controlled or maximum total dose of 1 g is reached. Alternatively, 10 to 15 mg/kg I.V. bolus administered at a rate of 25 to 50 mg/min. *Maintenance:* 1 to 4 mg/min by continuous infusion.

I.M. INJECTION

Adults. 50 mg/kg/day in divided doses q 3 to 6 hr.

➤ *To treat ventricular extrasystoles and arrhythmias associated with anesthesia and surgery*

I.V. INFUSION OR INJECTION

Adults. *Initial:* 100 mg diluted in D_5W and administered at a rate not to exceed 50 mg/min. Dosage repeated q 5 min until arrhythmia is controlled or maximum total dose of 1 g is reached. Alternatively, 10 to 15 mg/kg I.V. bolus administered at a rate of 25 to 50 mg/min. *Maintenance:* 1 to 4 mg/min by continuous infusion.

I.M. INJECTION

Adults. 100 to 500 mg q 3 to 6 hr.
DOSAGE ADJUSTMENT For elderly patients or those with cardiac or hepatic insufficiency, dosage possibly reduced or dosing intervals increased. For patients with creatinine clearance less than 50 ml/min/1.73 m^2, initial dosage reduced to 1 to 2 mg/min.

Route	Onset	Peak	Duration
P.O.	Unknown	Unknown	60 to 90 min
P.O. (E.R.)	Unknown	60 to 90 min	Unknown
I.V.	Unknown	Immediate	Unknown
I.M.	10 to 30 min	15 to 60 min	Unknown

Mechanism of Action
Prolongs the recovery period after myocardial repolarization by inhibiting sodium influx through myocardial cell membranes. This action prolongs the refractory period, causing myocardial automaticity, excitability, and conduction velocity to decline.

Contraindications
Complete heart block, hypersensitivity to procainamide or its components, systemic lupus erythematosus, torsades de pointes

Interactions
DRUGS
antiarrhythmics: Additive cardiac effects
anticholinergics, antidyskinetics, antihistamines: Possibly intensified atropine-like adverse effects, increased risk of ileus
antihypertensives: Additive hypotensive effects
antimyasthenics: Possibly antagonized effect of antimyasthenic on skeletal muscle
bethanechol: Possibly antagonized cholinergic effect of bethanechol
bone marrow depressants: Possibly increased leukopenic or thrombocytopenic effects
bretylium: Possibly decreased inotropic effect of bretylium and enhanced hypotension
neuromuscular blockers: Possibly increased or prolonged neuromuscular blockade
pimozide: Possibly prolonged QT interval, leading to life-threatening arrhythmias

Adverse Reactions
CNS: Chills, disorientation, dizziness, lightheadedness
CV: Heart block (second-degree), hypotension, pericarditis, prolonged QT interval, tachycardia
EENT: Bitter taste
GI: Abdominal distress, anorexia, diarrhea, nausea, vomiting
HEME: Agranulocytosis, neutropenia, thrombocytopenia
MS: Arthralgia, myalgia
RESP: Pleural effusion
SKIN: Pruritus, rash
Other: Drug-induced fever

Nursing Considerations
•Place patient in a supine position before administering procainamide I.M. or I.V. to minimize hypotensive effects. Monitor blood pressure frequently and ECG tracings continuously during administration and for 30 minutes afterward.
•Inspect parenteral solution for particles and discoloration before giving drug; discard if particles are present or solution is darker than light amber.
•When possible, give drug by I.V. infusion or injection, as prescribed, rather than by I.M. injection.
•If drug is to be administered I.M. and patient's platelet count is below 50,000/mm^3, notify prescriber immediately because patient may develop bleeding, bruising, or hematomas from procainamide-induced bone marrow suppression and thrombocytopenia. Expect to administer procainamide I.V.
•For I.V. injection, dilute procainamide with D_5W according to manufacturer's instructions before administration.
•For I.V. infusion, dilute 200 to 1,000 mg of procainamide to a concentration of 2 or 4 mg/ml using 50 to 500 ml of D_5W.
•Administer I.V. infusion with an infusion pump or other controlled-delivery device.
•Don't exceed 500 mg in 30 minutes by I.V. infusion or 50 mg/min by I.V. injection because heart block or cardiac arrest may occur.
•Anticipate that patient has reached maximum clinical response when ventricular tachycardia resolves, hypotension develops, or QRS complex is 50% wider than original width.
•Expect to administer first oral dose 3 to 4 hours after last I.V. dose.

PATIENT TEACHING
•Instruct patient to swallow E.R. procainamide tablets whole, without breaking, crushing, or chewing them.
•If patient has trouble swallowing, advise her to crush regular-release tablets or open capsules and mix contents with food or fluid.
•Instruct patient to take drug 1 hour before or 2 hours after meals with a full glass of water. Inform her that she may take procainamide with food if GI irritation develops.
•Urge patient to obtain needed dental work before therapy starts or after blood count returns to normal because drug can cause myelosuppression and increased risk of bleeding and infection. Stress the need for good oral hygiene during therapy, and urge patient to consult prescriber before scheduling dental procedures.
•Advise patient to notify prescriber immediately about bruising, chills, diarrhea, fever, or rash.

prochlorperazine

Compazine, Stemetil (CAN)

prochlorperazine edisylate

Compazine

prochlorperazine maleate

Compazine Spansule, Nu-Prochlor (CAN), Stemetil (CAN)

Class and Category

Chemical: Phenothiazine, piperazine
Therapeutic: Antianxiety, antiemetic, antipsychotic
Pregnancy category: Not rated

Indications and Dosages

➤ *To control nausea and vomiting related to surgery*

I.V. INFUSION OR INJECTION (PROCHLORPERAZINE EDISYLATE)

Adults and adolescents. 5 to 10 mg at a rate not to exceed 5 mg/ml 15 to 30 min before anesthesia or during or after surgery, as needed. Dosage repeated once, if necessary. *Maximum:* 10 mg/dose, 40 mg/day.

I.M. INJECTION (PROCHLORPERAZINE EDISYLATE)

Adults and adolescents. 5 to 10 mg 1 to 2 hr before anesthesia or during or after surgery, as needed. Dosage repeated once in 30 min, if necessary. *Maximum:* 10 mg/dose, 40 mg/day.

➤ *To control severe nausea and vomiting*

E.R. CAPSULES (PROCHLORPERAZINE MALEATE)

Adults and adolescents. 15 to 30 mg q.d. in the morning, or 10 mg q 12 hr. *Maximum:* 40 mg/day.

ORAL SOLUTION (PROCHLORPERAZINE EDISYLATE)

Adults and adolescents. 5 to 10 mg t.i.d. or q.i.d. *Maximum:* 40 mg/day.
Children weighing 18 to 39 kg (40 to 86 lb). 2.5 mg t.i.d. or 5 mg b.i.d. *Maximum:* 15 mg/day.
Children weighing 14 to 18 kg (31 to 40 lb). 2.5 mg b.i.d. or t.i.d. *Maximum:* 10 mg/day.
Children weighing 9 to 14 kg (20 to 31 lb). 2.5 mg q.d. or b.i.d. *Maximum:* 7.5 mg/day.

TABLETS (PROCHLORPERAZINE MALEATE)

Adults and adolescents. 5 to 10 mg t.i.d. or q.i.d. *Maximum:* 40 mg/day.

I.V. INFUSION OR INJECTION (PROCHLORPERAZINE EDISYLATE)

Adults and adolescents. 2.5 to 10 mg at a rate not to exceed 5 mg/min. *Maximum:* 40 mg/day.

I.M. INJECTION (PROCHLORPERAZINE EDISYLATE)

Adults and adolescents. 5 to 10 mg q 3 to 4 hr, p.r.n. *Maximum:* 40 mg/day.
Children ages 2 to 12. 132 mcg/kg/dose to maximum of 10 mg on day 1, then increased as needed. *Maximum:* On day 1, 10 mg for all children; thereafter, 25 mg/day for children ages 6 to 12, 20 mg/day for children ages 2 to 6.

SUPPOSITORIES (PROCHLORPERAZINE)

Adults and adolescents. 25 mg b.i.d.
Children weighing 18 to 39 kg. 2.5 mg t.i.d. or 5 mg b.i.d. *Maximum:* 15 mg/day.
Children weighing 14 to 18 kg. 2.5 mg b.i.d. or t.i.d. *Maximum:* 10 mg/day.
Children weighing 9 to 14 kg. 2.5 mg q.d. or b.i.d. *Maximum:* 7.5 mg/day.

➤ *To manage psychotic disorders, such as schizophrenia*

ORAL SOLUTION (PROCHLORPERAZINE EDISYLATE)

Adults and adolescents. 5 to 10 mg t.i.d. or q.i.d., increased gradually q 2 to 3 days, as needed and tolerated. *Maximum:* 150 mg/day.
Children ages 2 to 12. 2.5 mg b.i.d. or t.i.d. *Maximum:* On day 1, 10 mg for all children; thereafter, 25 mg/day for children ages 6 to 12, 20 mg/day for children ages 2 to 6.

TABLETS (PROCHLORPERAZINE MALEATE)

Adults and adolescents. 5 to 10 mg t.i.d. or q.i.d., increased gradually q 2 to 3 days, as needed and tolerated. *Maximum:* 150 mg/day.

I.M. INJECTION (PROCHLORPERAZINE EDISYLATE)

Adults and adolescents. *Initial:* 10 to 20 mg, repeated q 2 to 4 hr, as prescribed, to bring symptoms under control (usually 3 to 4 doses). *Maintenance:* 10 to 20 mg q 4 to 6 hr. *Maximum:* 200 mg/day.
Children ages 2 to 12. 132 mcg/kg/dose on day 1, then increased as needed. *Maximum:* On day 1, 10 mg for all children; thereafter, 25 mg/day for children ages 6 to 12, 20 mg/day for children ages 2 to 6.

➤ *To provide short-term treatment of anxiety*

E.R. CAPSULES (PROCHLORPERAZINE MALEATE)

Adults and adolescents. 15 mg q.d. in the morning, or 10 mg q 12 hr. *Maximum:* 20 mg/day for no longer than 12 wk.

ORAL SOLUTION, TABLETS (PROCHLORPERAZINE EDISYLATE)

Adults and adolescents. 5 mg t.i.d. or q.i.d. *Maximum:* 20 mg/day for no longer than 12 wk.

P

I.V. INFUSION OR INJECTION (PROCHLORPERAZINE EDISYLATE)

Adults and adolescents. 2.5 to 10 mg at a rate not to exceed 5 mg/min. *Maximum:* 40 mg/day.

I.M. INJECTION (PROCHLORPERAZINE EDISYLATE)

Adults and adolescents. 5 to 10 mg q 3 to 4 hr, p.r.n.

DOSAGE ADJUSTMENT Initial dose usually reduced and subsequent dosage increased more gradually for elderly, emaciated, and debilitated patients.

Route	Onset	Peak	Duration
P.O., I.V., I.M., P.R.	Up to several wk*	Up to 6 mo	Unknown

Mechanism of Action

Alleviates psychotic symptoms by blocking dopamine receptors, depressing the release of selected hormones, and producing an alpha-adrenergic blocking effect in the brain.

Prochlorperazine also alleviates nausea and vomiting by centrally blocking dopamine receptors in the medullary chemoreceptor trigger zone and by peripherally blocking the vagus nerve in the GI tract.

Anticholinergic effects and alpha-adrenergic blockade reduce anxiety by decreasing arousal and filtering internal stimuli to the brain stem reticular activating system.

Incompatibilities

Don't mix prochlorperazine in same syringe with other drugs. A precipitate may form when prochlorperazine edisylate is mixed in same syringe with morphine sulfate.

Contraindications

Age less than 2 years, blood dyscrasias, bone marrow depression, cerebral arteriosclerosis, coma, coronary artery disease, hepatic dysfunction, hypersensitivity to phenothiazines, myeloproliferative disorders, pediatric surgery, severe CNS depression, severe hypertension or hypotension, subcortical brain damage, use of large quantities of CNS depressants, weight less than 9 kg (20 lb)

---

* For antipsychotic effects; unknown for other indications.

Interactions

DRUGS

aluminum- or magnesium-containing antacids, antidiarrheals (adsorbent): Possibly inhibited absorption of oral prochlorperazine
amantadine, anticholinergics, antidyskinetics, antihistamines: Possibly intensified anticholinergic adverse effects, increased risk of prochlorperazine-induced hyperpyretic effect
amphetamines: Decreased stimulant effect of amphetamines, decreased antipsychotic effect of prochlorperazine
anticonvulsants: Lowered seizure threshold
antithyroid drugs: Increased risk of agranulocytosis
apomorphine: Possibly decreased emetic response to apomorphine, additive CNS depression
appetite suppressants: Possibly antagonized anorectic effect of appetite suppressants (except for phenmetrazine)
astemizole, cisapride, disopyramide, erythromycin, pimozide, probucol, procainamide: Additive QT interval prolongation, increased risk of ventricular tachycardia
beta blockers: Increased risk of additive hypotensive effects, irreversible retinopathy, arrhythmias, and tardive dyskinesia
bromocriptine: Decreased effectiveness of bromocriptine
CNS depressants: Additive CNS depression
dopamine: Possibly antagonized peripheral vasoconstriction (with high doses of dopamine)
ephedrine, epinephrine: Decreased vasopressor effects of these drugs
hepatotoxic drugs: Increased incidence of hepatotoxicity
hypotension-producing drugs: Possibly severe hypotension with syncope
levodopa: Inhibited antidyskinetic effect of levodopa
lithium: Reduced absorption of oral prochlorperazine, increased excretion of lithium, increased extrapyramidal effects, possibly masking of early symptoms of lithium toxicity
MAO inhibitors, maprotiline, tricyclic antidepressants: Possibly prolonged and intensified anticholinergic and sedative effects, increased blood antidepressant levels, inhibited prochlorperazine metabolism, and increased risk of neuroleptic malignant syndrome

mephentermine: Possibly antagonized antipsychotic effect of prochlorperazine and vasopressor effect of mephentermine
metrizamide: Increased risk of seizures
opioid analgesics: Increased risk of CNS and respiratory depression, orthostatic hypotension, severe constipation, and urine retention
ototoxic drugs: Possibly masking of some symptoms of ototoxicity, such as dizziness, tinnitus, and vertigo
phenytoin: Possibly inhibited phenytoin metabolism and increased risk of phenytoin toxicity
thiazide diuretics: Possibly potentiated hyponatremia and water intoxication
ACTIVITIES
alcohol use: Additive CNS depression

Adverse Reactions

CNS: Akathisia, altered temperature regulation, dizziness, drowsiness, extrapyramidal reactions (such as dystonia, pseudoparkinsonism, tardive dyskinesia)
CV: Hypotension, orthostatic hypotension, tachycardia
EENT: Blurred vision, dry mouth, nasal congestion, ocular changes, pigmentary retinopathy
ENDO: Galactorrhea, gynecomastia
GI: Constipation, epigastric pain, nausea, vomiting
GU: Dysuria, ejaculation disorders, menstrual irregularities, urine retention
SKIN: Decreased sweating, photosensitivity, pruritus, rash
Other: Weight gain

Nursing Considerations

•Avoid contact between skin and solution forms of prochlorperazine because contact dermatitis could result.
•Inject I.M. form slowly and deeply into upper outer quadrant of buttocks. Keep patient lying down for 30 minutes after injection to minimize hypotensive effects.
•Rotate I.M. injection sites to prevent irritation and sterile abscesses.
•Be aware that I.V. form may be administered undiluted as injection or diluted in isotonic solution as infusion (mesylate form requires dilution in at least 1 L). Both forms should be administered at a rate not to exceed 5 mg/min.
•Protect prochlorperazine from light.

•Be aware that parenteral solution may develop a slight yellowing that won't affect potency. Don't use if discoloration is pronounced or precipitate is present.
•Expect antipsychotic effects to occur in 2 to 3 weeks, although the range is days to months.
•**WARNING** Monitor closely for numerous adverse reactions that may be serious.
•Be aware that adverse reactions may occur for up to 12 weeks after discontinuation of E.R. capsules.
PATIENT TEACHING
•Instruct patient to take prochlorperazine with food or a full glass of milk or water to minimize GI distress.
•Advise patient to swallow E.R. capsules whole, not to crush or chew them.
•Instruct patient using a suppository to refrigerate it for 30 minutes or hold it under running cold water before removing the wrapper if it softens during storage.
•Teach patient the correct administration technique for suppository.
•Caution patient receiving long-term therapy not to stop taking prochlorperazine abruptly because doing so may lead to such adverse reactions as nausea, vomiting, and trembling.
•Urge patient to avoid alcohol and OTC drugs that may contain CNS depressants.
•Advise patient to rise slowly from lying and sitting positions to minimize effects of orthostatic hypotension.
•Urge patient to avoid potentially hazardous activities because of the risk of drowsiness and impaired judgment and coordination.
•Instruct patient to avoid excessive sun exposure and to wear sunscreen when outdoors.
•Urge patient to notify prescriber about involuntary movements and restlessness.
•Inform patient that adverse reactions may occur for up to 12 weeks after discontinuing E.R. capsules.

procyclidine hydrochloride

Kemadrin, PMS-Procyclidine (CAN), Procyclid (CAN)

Class and Category

Chemical: Synthetic tertiary amine

Therapeutic: Antidyskinetic
Pregnancy category: C

Indications and Dosages

➤ *To treat parkinsonism*

ELIXIR, TABLETS

Adults and adolescents. *Initial:* 2.5 mg t.i.d. after meals; may be increased gradually to 5 mg t.i.d., as needed. If necessary, a 4th dose of 5 mg may be given h.s.

➤ *To treat drug-induced extrapyramidal symptoms*

ELIXIR, TABLETS

Adults and adolescents. *Initial:* 2.5 mg t.i.d.; dosage increased in daily increments of 2.5 mg, as needed and tolerated.

Route	Onset	Peak	Duration
P.O.	Unknown	Unknown	4 hr

Mechanism of Action

Competes with acetylcholine to block muscarinic cholinergic receptors in the CNS, which may decrease salivation and relax smooth muscle. Procyclidine also may block dopamine reuptake and storage in CNS cells, thus prolonging dopamine's effects.

Contraindications

Achalasia, angle-closure glaucoma, bladder neck obstructions, hypersensitivity to procyclidine or its components, megacolon, myasthenia gravis, prostatic hypertrophy, pyloric or duodenal obstruction, stenosing peptic ulcers

Interactions

DRUGS

amantadine, other anticholinergics, MAO inhibitors: Additive anticholinergic effects
antidiarrheals (adsorbent): Decreased therapeutic effect of procyclidine
carbidopa-levodopa, levodopa: Potentiated dopaminergic effects of levodopa
chlorpromazine: Decreased blood chlorpromazine level
CNS depressants: Increased sedative effects
digoxin: Increased risk of digitalis toxicity
haloperidol: Possibly worsening of schizophrenic symptoms, decreased blood haloperidol level, tardive dyskinesia

ACTIVITIES

alcohol use: Increased sedative effects

Adverse Reactions

CNS: Drowsiness, euphoria, headache, memory loss, nervousness, paresthesia, unusual excitement
CV: Orthostatic hypotension, tachycardia
EENT: Blurred vision; dry mouth, nose, or throat
GI: Constipation, indigestion, nausea, vomiting
GU: Dysuria
MS: Muscle cramps
SKIN: Decreased sweating, photosensitivity

Nursing Considerations

• Use procyclidine cautiously in patients with cardiac disorders because of drug's anticholinergic effects. Frequently monitor blood pressure and heart rate and rhythm.
• Monitor for drug abuse because procyclidine provides a false sense of well-being that may tempt patient to abuse it.

PATIENT TEACHING

• Instruct patient to take procyclidine after meals to minimize GI distress.
• Advise patient to avoid alcohol and OTC drugs that may contain CNS depressants because of potential for drug interactions.
• Urge patient to avoid potentially hazardous activities because of risk of drowsiness and reduced alertness.
• Caution patient not to stop taking procyclidine abruptly because doing so may cause sudden adverse reactions.
• If patient reports dry mouth, suggest sugarless hard candy or gum and increased fluid intake.
• Inform patient that exercise and increased fluid intake can help prevent constipation.
• Encourage patient to avoid extreme temperatures because procyclidine may cause decreased sweating, thereby increasing the risk of heatstroke. Also advise patient to wear sunscreen when outdoors.
• Explain to contact lens wearer that drug may increase lens awareness or blur vision. Suggest using artificial tears for relief.
• Instruct patient to notify prescriber about adverse reactions.

promethazine hydrochloride

Anergan 25, Anergan 50, Antinaus 50, Histantil (CAN), Pentazine, Phenazine 25, Phenazine 50, Phencen-50, Phenergan, Phenergan

Fortis, Phenergan Plain, Phenerzine, Pheno-ject-50, Pro-50, Promacot, Pro-Med 50, Promet, Prorex-25, Prorex-50, Prothazine, Shogan, V-Gan-25, V-Gan-50

Class and Category

Chemical: Phenothiazine derivative
Therapeutic: Antiemetic, antihistamine, anti-vertigo, sedative-hypnotic
Pregnancy category: C

Indications and Dosages

➤ *To prevent or treat motion sickness*

SYRUP, TABLETS

Adults and adolescents. 25 mg 30 to 60 min before travel and repeated 8 to 12 hr later, if needed. *Maximum:* 150 mg/day.

➤ *To treat vertigo*

SYRUP, TABLETS

Adults and adolescents. 25 mg b.i.d., p.r.n. *Maximum:* 150 mg/day.
Children age 2 and older. 0.5 mg/kg or 10 to 25 mg q 12 hr, p.r.n.

SUPPOSITORIES

Adults and adolescents. 25 mg b.i.d., p.r.n. *Maximum:* 150 mg/day.
Children age 2 and older. 0.5 mg/kg or 12.5 to 25 mg q 12 hr.

➤ *To prevent or treat nausea and vomiting associated with certain types of anesthesia and surgery*

SYRUP, TABLETS

Adults and adolescents. *Initial:* 25 mg, then 10 to 25 mg q 4 to 6 hr, p.r.n. *Maximum:* 150 mg/day.
Children age 2 and older. 0.25 to 0.5 mg/kg or 10 to 25 mg q 4 to 6 hr, p.r.n.

I.V. OR I.M. INJECTION

Adults and adolescents. 12.5 to 25 mg q 4 hr, p.r.n. *Maximum:* 150 mg/day.

I.M. INJECTION

Children age 2 and older. 0.25 to 0.5 mg/kg or 12.5 to 25 mg q 4 to 6 hr, p.r.n.

SUPPOSITORIES

Adults and adolescents. *Initial:* 25 mg, then 12.5 to 25 mg q 4 to 6 hr, p.r.n. *Maximum:* 150 mg/day.
Children age 2 and older. 0.25 to 0.5 mg/kg or 12.5 to 25 mg q 4 to 6 hr.

➤ *To treat signs and symptoms of allergic response*

SYRUP, TABLETS

Adults and adolescents. 10 to 12.5 mg q.i.d. before meals and h.s., p.r.n. Alternatively, 25 mg h.s., p.r.n. *Maximum:* 150 mg/day.

Children age 2 and older. 0.125 mg/kg q 4 to 6 hr or 5 to 12.5 mg t.i.d., p.r.n. Alternatively, 0.5 mg/kg or 25 mg h.s., p.r.n.

I.V. INJECTION

Adults and adolescents. 25 mg, repeated within 2 hr, if needed.

I.M. INJECTION, SUPPOSITORIES

Adults and adolescents. 25 mg, repeated in 2 hr, p.r.n. *Maximum:* 150 mg/day.
Children age 2 and older. 0.125 mg/kg q 4 to 6 hr or 6.25 to 12.5 mg t.i.d., p.r.n. Alternatively, 0.5 mg/kg or 25 mg h.s., p.r.n.

➤ *To provide nighttime, preoperative, or postoperative sedation*

SYRUP, TABLETS

Adults and adolescents. 25 to 50 mg as a single dose. *Maximum:* 150 mg/day.
Children age 2 and older. 0.5 to 1 mg/kg or 10 to 25 mg as a single dose. Alternatively, for preoperative sedation, 1.1 mg/kg along with 1.1 mg/kg of meperidine and appropriate dose of an atropine-like drug.

I.V. INJECTION

Adults and adolescents. 25 to 50 mg as a single dose. Alternatively, for preoperative and postoperative sedation, 25 to 50 mg combined with appropriately reduced dosages of analgesics and anticholinergics.

I.M. INJECTION, SUPPOSITORIES

Adults and adolescents. 25 to 50 mg as a single dose. Alternatively, for preoperative and postoperative sedation, 25 to 50 mg combined with appropriately reduced dosages of analgesics and anticholinergics.
Children age 2 and older. 0.5 to 1 mg/kg or 12.5 to 25 mg as a single dose. Alternatively, for preoperative sedation, 1.1 mg/kg along with 1.1 mg/kg of meperidine and an appropriate dose of an atropine-like drug.

➤ *To relieve apprehension and promote sleep the night before surgery*

SYRUP, TABLETS, SUPPOSITORIES

Adults and adolescents. 50 mg along with 50 mg of meperidine and an appropriate dose of an atropine-like drug h.s. on the night before surgery.

DOSAGE ADJUSTMENT Dosage usually decreased for elderly patients.

➤ *To provide obstetric sedation*

I.V. OR I.M. INJECTION

Adults and adolescents. 50 mg for early stages of labor, followed by 1 or 2 doses of 25 to 75 mg after labor is definitely established and repeated q 4 hr during course of normal labor.

Route	Onset	Peak	Duration
P.O.	15 to 60 min	Unknown	4 to 6 hr
I.V.	3 to 5 min	Unknown	4 to 6 hr
I.M., P.R.	20 min	Unknown	4 to 6 hr

Mechanism of Action

Competes with histamine for H$_1$-receptor sites, thereby antagonizing many histamine effects and reducing allergy signs and symptoms. Promethazine also prevents motion sickness, nausea, and vertigo by acting centrally on the medullary chemoreceptive trigger zone and by decreasing vestibular stimulation and labyrinthine function in the inner ear. In addition, it promotes sedation and relieves anxiety by blocking receptor sites within the CNS, directly reducing stimuli to the brain.

Contraindications

Angle-closure glaucoma, benign prostatic hyperplasia, bladder neck obstruction, bone marrow depression, breast-feeding, coma, hypersensitivity to promethazine or its components, hypertensive crisis, pyloroduodenal obstruction, stenosing peptic ulcer, use of large quantities of CNS depressants

Interactions

DRUGS
amphetamines: Decreased stimulant effect of amphetamines
anticholinergics: Possibly intensified anticholinergic adverse effects
anticonvulsants: Lowered seizure threshold
appetite suppressants: Possibly antagonized anorectic effect of appetite suppressants
beta blockers: Increased risk of additive hypotensive effects, irreversible retinopathy, arrhythmias, and tardive dyskinesia
bromocriptine: Decreased effectiveness of bromocriptine
CNS depressants: Additive CNS depression
dopamine: Possibly antagonized peripheral vasoconstriction (with high doses of dopamine)
ephedrine, metaraminol, methoxamine: Decreased vasopressor response to these drugs
epinephrine: Blocked alpha-adrenergic effects of epinephrine, increased risk of hypotension

guanadrel, guanethidine: Decreased antihypertensive effects of these drugs
hepatotoxic drugs: Increased risk of hepatotoxicity
hypotension-producing drugs: Possibly severe hypotension with syncope
levodopa: Inhibited antidyskinetic effects of levodopa
MAO inhibitors: Possibly prolonged and intensified anticholinergic and CNS depressant effects of promethazine
metrizamide: Increased risk of seizures
ototoxic drugs: Possibly masking of some symptoms of ototoxicity, such as dizziness, tinnitus, and vertigo
quinidine: Additive cardiac effects
riboflavin: Increased riboflavin requirements
ACTIVITIES
alcohol use: Additive CNS depression

Adverse Reactions

CNS: Akathisia, CNS stimulation, confusion, dizziness, drowsiness, dystonia, insomnia, irritability, paradoxical stimulation, pseudoparkinsonism, restlessness, tardive dyskinesia
CV: Hypotension, tachycardia
EENT: Blurred vision; dry mouth, nose, and throat; tinnitus; vision changes
GI: Anorexia, ileus, rectal burning or stinging (suppository form)
GU: Dysuria
RESP: Tenacious bronchial secretions
SKIN: Diaphoresis, photosensitivity, rash

Nursing Considerations

•Use promethazine cautiously in children and elderly patients because they may be more sensitive to drug's effects.
•Also use drug cautiously in patients with asthma because of its anticholinergic effects.
•Inject I.M. form deep into large muscle mass and rotate sites.
•**WARNING** Avoid inadvertent intra-arterial injection of promethazine because it can cause arteriospasm; gangrene may develop from impaired circulation.
•Administer I.V. injection at a rate not to exceed 25 mg/min; rapid I.V. administration may produce a transient fall in blood pressure.
•Monitor respiratory function because drug may suppress cough reflex and cause thickening of bronchial secretions, aggravating such conditions as asthma and COPD.
•Be aware that patient shouldn't undergo intradermal allergen tests within 72 hours of

receiving promethazine because drug may cause significant alterations of flare response.
PATIENT TEACHING
•Instruct patient to use a calibrated measuring device when using promethazine syrup to ensure accurate dose.
•Teach patient correct administration technique for suppository, if necessary.
•Advise patient to avoid OTC drugs unless approved by prescriber.
•Instruct patient to notify prescriber immediately if she experiences involuntary movements and restlessness.
•Urge patient to avoid alcohol and other CNS depressants while taking promethazine.
•Instruct patient to avoid potentially hazardous activities until drug's CNS effects are known.
•Suggest that patient relieve dry mouth with frequent rinsing and use of sugarless gum or hard candy.
•Advise patient to avoid excessive sun exposure and to use sunscreen when outdoors.

propafenone hydrochloride

Rythmol

Class and Category
Chemical: 3-Phenylpropriophenone
Therapeutic: Class IC antiarrhythmic
Pregnancy category: C

Indications and Dosages
➤ *To treat life-threatening ventricular arrhythmias*
TABLETS
Adults. *Initial:* 150 mg q 8 hr; after 3 or 4 days, increased to 225 mg q 8 hr (in the U.S.) or 300 mg q 12 hr (in Canada), if needed; after an additional 3 or 4 days, further increased to 300 mg q 8 hr, if needed. *Maximum:* 900 mg/day.

Mechanism of Action
Prolongs the recovery period after myocardial repolarization by inhibiting sodium influx through myocardial cell membranes. This action prolongs the refractory period, causing myocardial automaticity, excitability, and conduction velocity to decline.

Contraindications
Bronchospastic disorders, such as asthma; cardiogenic shock; electrolyte imbalances; heart failure (uncontrolled); hypersensitivity to propafenone or its components; severe hypotension; sinus bradycardia or AV conduction disturbances (in patient without artificial pacemaker)

Interactions
DRUGS
anesthetics (local): Increased risk of adverse CNS effects
antiarrhythmics: Increased therapeutic benefit, risk of additive adverse CV effects
digoxin: Increased risk of digitalis toxicity
metoprolol, propranolol: Increased blood level and half-life of these drugs
quinidine: Inhibited propafenone metabolism
warfarin: Increased blood warfarin level and risk of bleeding

Adverse Reactions
CNS: Dizziness, fatigue, headache
CV: Angina, bradycardia, heart failure, irregular heartbeat, tachycardia
EENT: Altered taste, blurred vision, dry mouth
GI: Constipation, diarrhea, nausea, vomiting
SKIN: Rash

Nursing Considerations
•Assess for electrolyte imbalances, such as hyperkalemia, before beginning therapy with propafenone or any antiarrhythmic to reduce the risk of adverse cardiac reactions.
•Use propafenone cautiously in patients with heart failure or myocardial dysfunction because drug's beta-blocking activity may further depress myocardial contractility.
•Monitor ECG tracings, blood pressure, and pulse rate, particularly at the start of therapy.
•Institute continuous cardiac monitoring, as ordered, at the start of therapy and with dosage increases.
PATIENT TEACHING
•Instruct patient to take a missed dose of propafenone if she remembers within 4 hours; otherwise, she should skip the missed dose and resume the regular dosing schedule.
•Advise patient not to discontinue drug or change dosage without consulting prescriber.
•Urge patient to carry or wear medical identification indicating her use of propafenone.
•Advise patient to avoid potentially hazardous activities until drug's CNS effects are known.

•Encourage patient to increase fluid intake and add fiber to diet if she becomes constipated.
•Inform patient that drug may cause an unusual taste in her mouth. Advise her to notify prescriber if taste interferes with compliance.

propantheline bromide

Pro-Banthine, Propanthel (CAN)

Class and Category

Chemical: Quaternary amine
Therapeutic: Anticholinergic
Pregnancy category: C

Indications and Dosages

➤ *As adjunct to treat peptic ulcer disease*
TABLETS
Adults. 15 mg t.i.d. before meals and 30 mg h.s., adjusted as needed and tolerated. *Maximum:* 120 mg/day.
Children. 0.375 mg/kg q.i.d., adjusted as needed and tolerated.
DOSAGE ADJUSTMENT For elderly patients with mild symptoms or patients of below-average weight, dosage possibly reduced to 7.5 mg t.i.d. or q.i.d.

Route	Onset	Peak	Duration
P.O.	Unknown	Unknown	6 hr

Mechanism of Action

Prevents the neurotransmitter acetylcholine from combining with receptors on the postganglionic parasympathetic nerve terminal, thereby reducing smooth-muscle spasms in the GI system, slowing GI motility, and inhibiting gastric acid secretion. All these effects help heal peptic ulcers.

Contraindications

Adhesions between iris and lens, angle-closure glaucoma, hemorrhage accompanied by hemodynamic instability, hepatic dysfunction, hypersensitivity to propantheline or its components, ileus, myasthenia gravis, myocardial ischemia, obstructive GI or urinary disease, renal dysfunction, severe ulcerative colitis, tachycardia

Interactions

DRUGS
amantadine, other anticholinergics, tricyclic antidepressants: Additive anticholinergic effects
antacids, antidiarrheals (adsorbent): Possibly reduced absorption of propantheline
antimyasthenics: Possibly further reduction in intestinal motility
atenolol: Increased effects of atenolol
cyclopropane: Possibly ventricular arrhythmias
digoxin: Possibly digitalis toxicity
haloperidol: Decreased antipsychotic effect of haloperidol in schizophrenic patients
ketoconazole: Decreased ketoconazole absorption
metoclopramide: Possibly decreased metoclopramide effect on GI motility
opioid analgesics: Increased risk of severe constipation and urine retention
phenothiazines: Possibly decreased antipsychotic effects
potassium chloride: Possibly increased severity of potassium chloride–induced GI ulceration, stricture, or perforation
urinary alkalizers: Delayed urinary excretion of propantheline

Adverse Reactions

CNS: Dizziness, excitement, insomnia, nervousness, paradoxical CNS stimulation
CV: Palpitations, tachycardia
EENT: Blurred vision; dry mouth, nose, and throat
GI: Constipation, dysphagia, heartburn, ileus, nausea, vomiting
GU: Impotence, urinary hesitancy, urine retention
SKIN: Decreased sweating, dry skin, flushing

Nursing Considerations

•Don't administer propantheline within 1 hour of antacids or antidiarrheals.
•Monitor elderly patients closely because they may respond to usual drug dose with agitation, confusion, drowsiness, or excitement.
•**WARNING** Be aware that drug can interfere with sweating reflex, thereby increasing the risk of heatstroke.
PATIENT TEACHING
•Instruct patient to take propantheline 30 to 60 minutes before meals and at bedtime, as prescribed.
•Inform patient that drug may cause dizziness. Advise her not to perform hazardous activities until drug's CNS effects are known.

•Encourage patient to increase her fluid and fiber intake to decrease constipation. Instruct her to report persistent constipation and urine retention.

•Advise patient to avoid excessive exposure to heat to reduce the risk of heat prostration and heatstroke, because propantheline decreases sweating.

•Suggest that patient relieve dry mouth with frequent rinsing and sugar-free hard candy or gum.

propofol

(disoprofol)

Diprivan

Class and Category

Chemical: 2,6-diisopropylphenol derivative
Therapeutic: Sedative-hypnotic
Pregnancy category: B

Indications and Dosages

➤ *To provide sedation for critically ill patients in intensive care*

I.V. INFUSION
Adults. 2.8 to 130 mcg/kg/min. *Usual:* 27 mcg/kg/min.

Route	Onset	Peak	Duration
I.V.	Within 40 sec	Unknown	3 to 5 min

Mechanism of Action

Decreases cerebral blood flow, cerebral metabolic oxygen consumption, and intracranial pressure and increases cerebrovascular resistance, which may play a role in propofol's hypnotic effects.

Incompatibilities

Don't mix propofol with other drugs before administration. Don't administer propofol through same I.V. line as blood or plasma products because globular component of emulsion will aggregate.

Contraindications

Hypersensitivity to propofol or its components

Interactions

DRUGS
CNS depressants: Additive CNS depressant, respiratory depressant, and hypotensive ef-

fects; possibly decreased emetic effects of opioids
droperidol: Possibly decreased control of nausea and vomiting

ACTIVITIES
alcohol use: Additive CNS depressant, respiratory depressant, and hypotensive effects

Adverse Reactions

CV: Bradycardia, hypotension
GI: Nausea, vomiting
MS: Involuntary muscle movements (transient)
RESP: Apnea
Other: Injection site burning, pain, or stinging

Nursing Considerations

•Use propofol cautiously in patients with cardiac disease, peripheral vascular disease, impaired cerebral circulation, or increased intracranial pressure because drug may aggravate these disorders.

•If ordered to dilute drug before administration, use only D_5W to yield a final concentration of 2 mg/ml or more.

•Consult prescriber about pretreating injection site with 1 ml of 1% lidocaine to minimize pain, burning, or stinging that may occur with propofol administration. Administering drug through a larger vein in the forearm or antecubital fossa may also minimize injection site discomfort.

•Shake container well before using and administer drug promptly after opening.

•Use a drop counter, syringe pump, or volumetric pump to safely control infusion rate. Don't infuse drug through filter with a pore size of less than 5 microns because doing so could cause emulsion to break down.

•Discard all unused portions of propofol solution as well as reservoirs, I.V. tubing, and solutions immediately after or within 12 hours of administration (6 hours if propofol was transferred from original container) to prevent bacterial growth in stagnant solution. Also, protect solution from light.

•Expect patient to recover from sedation within 8 minutes.

PATIENT TEACHING
•Encourage patient and family to voice concerns and ask questions before propofol administration.

•Reassure patient that she'll be closely monitored throughout drug administration and that her vital functions, including breathing, will be supported as needed.

propoxyphene hydrochloride

Cotanol-65, Darvon, PP-Cap

propoxyphene hydrochloride and acetaminophen

E-Lor, Wygesic

propoxyphene hydrochloride, aspirin, and caffeine

Darvon Compound-65, PC-Cap, Propoxyphene Compound-65

propoxyphene napsylate

Darvon-N

propoxyphene napsylate and acetaminophen

Darvocet-N 50, Darvocet-N 100, Propacet 100

propoxyphene napsylate and aspirin

Darvon-N with A.S.A. (CAN)

propoxyphene napsylate, aspirin, and caffeine

Darvon-N Compound (CAN)

Class, Category, and Schedule

Chemical: Synthetic opioid
Therapeutic: Analgesic
Pregnancy category: Not rated
Controlled substance: Schedule IV

Indications and Dosages

➤ *To relieve mild to moderate pain*

CAPSULES (PROPOXYPHENE HYDROCHLORIDE, ASPIRIN, AND CAFFEINE)

Adults. 1 capsule (65 mg of propoxyphene/ 389 mg of aspirin/32.4 mg of caffeine) q 4 hr, p.r.n. *Maximum:* 390 mg of propoxyphene hydrochloride/day.

CAPSULES (PROPOXYPHENE NAPSYLATE AND ASPIRIN)

Adults. 1 capsule (100 mg of propoxyphene/ 325 mg of aspirin) q 4 hr, p.r.n. *Maximum:* 600 mg of propoxyphene napsylate/day.

CAPSULES (PROPOXYPHENE NAPSYLATE, ASPIRIN, AND CAFFEINE)

Adults. 1 capsule (100 mg of propoxyphene/ 375 mg of aspirin/30 mg of caffeine) q 4 hr, p.r.n. *Maximum:* 600 mg of propoxyphene napsylate/day.

CAPSULES, ORAL SUSPENSION, TABLETS (PROPOXYPHENE NAPYSLATE)

Adults. 100 mg q 4 hr, p.r.n. *Maximum:* 600 mg/day.

CAPSULES, TABLETS (PROPOXYPHENE HYDROCHLORIDE)

Adults. 65 mg q 4 hr, p.r.n. *Maximum:* 390 mg/day.

TABLETS (PROPOXYPHENE HYDROCHLORIDE AND ACETAMINOPHEN)

Adults. 1 tablet (65 mg of propoxyphene/ 650 mg of acetaminophen) q 4 hr, p.r.n.

TABLETS (PROPOXYPHENE HYDROCHLORIDE, ASPIRIN, AND CAFFEINE)

Adults. 1 tablet (65 mg of propoxyphene/ 375 mg of aspirin/30 mg of caffeine) q 4 hr, p.r.n. *Maximum:* 390 mg of propoxyphene hydrochloride/day.

TABLETS (PROPOXYPHENE NAPSYLATE AND ACETAMINOPHEN)

Adults. 1 tablet (100 mg of propoxyphene/ 650 mg of acetaminophen) or 2 tablets (each containing 50 mg of propoxyphene/325 mg of acetaminophen) q 4 hr, p.r.n.

Route	Onset	Peak	Duration
P.O.	15 to 60 min	2 hr	4 to 6 hr

Contraindications

Hypersensitivity to propoxyphene or its components (including acetaminophen and aspirin), respiratory depression, severe asthma, upper airway obstruction, use within 14 days of MAO inhibitor therapy

Interactions

DRUGS

amphetamines: Possibly fatal seizures (with propoxyphene overdose)
anticholinergics: Increased risk of severe constipation and urine retention
antidiarrheals: Severe constipation, possibly increased CNS depression
antihypertensives: Possibly exaggerated antihypertensive response
buprenorphine: Possibly decreased propoxyphene effectiveness, increased respiratory depression
carbamazepine: Possibly carbamazepine toxicity
CNS depressants: Increased CNS and respiratory depression, hypotensive effects, and risk of habituation
hydroxyzine: Increased analgesic, CNS depressant, and hypotensive effects of propoxyphene
MAO inhibitors: Severe, possibly fatal reactions, including hypertensive crisis

metoclopramide: Possibly antagonized effects of metoclopramide on GI motility
naloxone: Antagonized analgesic and CNS and respiratory depressant effects of propoxyphene
naltrexone: Risk of withdrawal symptoms in patients who are dependent on propoxyphene, possibly decreased analgesic effect of propoxyphene
neuromuscular blockers: Additive respiratory depressant effects
opioid analgesics: Additive CNS and respiratory depressant and hypotensive effects
warfarin: Increased anticoagulation effects

ACTIVITIES
alcohol use: Increased CNS and respiratory depression, hypotensive effects, and risk of habituation
nicotine chewing gum, other smoking deterrents, smoking cessation: Decreased effectiveness of propoxyphene

Mechanism of Action

Produces analgesia through a synergistic analgesic effect.

Propoxyphene strongly agonizes mu receptors, blocking the release of such inhibitory neurotransmitters as gamma-aminobutyric acid (GABA) and acetylcholine. It also mediates analgesia by changing pain perception at the spinal cord and higher CNS levels and by altering the emotional response to pain.

Acetaminophen acts centrally to increase the pain threshold by inhibiting cyclooxygenase, an enzyme involved in prostaglandin synthesis.

Aspirin possesses analgesic, anti-inflammatory, antiplatelet, and antipyretic properties. It interferes with arachidonate metabolism as it acetylates proteins and inhibits prostaglandin synthesis by irreversibly inhibiting cyclooxygenase-2, one of two major enzymes that act on arachidonic acid. Aspirin also decreases the perception of pain.

Caffeine exhibits a direct stimulant effect at all levels of the CNS and cardiovascular system. It stimulates the medullary respiratory center, relaxes bronchial smooth muscle, stimulates gastric acid secretion, increases renal blood flow, and acts as a mild diuretic.

Adverse Reactions

CNS: Dizziness, drowsiness, fatigue, insomnia, light-headedness, malaise, nervousness, sedation, tremor
CV: Orthostatic hypotension, tachycardia
EENT: Blurred vision, diplopia, dry mouth, tinnitus
GI: Abdominal cramps, anorexia, constipation, nausea, vomiting
GU: Decreased urine output
MS: Muscle weakness
RESP: Dyspnea, respiratory depression, wheezing
SKIN: Flushing of face, pruritus, rash, urticaria
Other: Psychological dependence

Nursing Considerations

• Use propoxyphene cautiously in patients with hepatic or renal dysfunction because delayed elimination may occur. Monitor hepatic and renal function test results.
• WARNING Be aware that long-term, high-dose propoxyphene therapy may lead to psychological dependence in some patients. Assess for opioid and alcohol use, which increase the risk of drug abuse or dependence.
• Be aware that abruptly discontinuing drug can result in withdrawal symptoms.

PATIENT TEACHING
• Inform patient that she may take propoxyphene with food if she experiences GI distress.
• Instruct patient not to take more than the prescribed amount because drug may be addictive.
• Inform patient that drug may cause blurred vision, drowsiness, dizziness, and impaired judgment and coordination. Urge her to avoid potentially hazardous activities until drug's CNS effects are known.
• Instruct patient to avoid alcohol and other sedatives while taking drug.
• Advise smokers to inform prescriber if they attempt to stop smoking during propoxyphene therapy because increased drug dosage may be required for effective analgesia.
• Urge patient to notify prescriber immediately if pain isn't relieved or worsens.

propranolol hydrochloride

Apo-Propranolol (CAN), Detensol (CAN), Inderal, Inderal LA, Novopranol (CAN), pms Propranolol (CAN)

Class and Category

Chemical: Beta-adrenergic blocker
Therapeutic: Antianginal, antiarrhythmic, antihypertensive, anti-MI, antimigraine, anti-tremor, hypertrophic cardiomyopathy and pheochromocytoma therapy adjunct
Pregnancy category: C

Indications and Dosages

➤ *To manage hypertension*

E.R. TABLETS

Adults. *Initial:* 80 mg q.d., increased gradually up to 160 mg q.d. *Maximum:* 640 mg/day.

ORAL SOLUTION, TABLETS

Adults. *Initial:* 40 mg b.i.d., increased gradually to 120 to 240 mg/day, as needed. *Maximum:* 640 mg/day.

Children. *Initial:* 0.5 to 1 mg/kg/day in divided doses b.i.d. to q.i.d., adjusted as needed. *Maintenance:* 2 to 4 mg/kg/day in divided doses b.i.d.

➤ *To treat chronic angina*

E.R. TABLETS

Adults. *Initial:* 80 mg q.d., increased q 3 to 7 days, as prescribed. *Maximum:* 320 mg/day.

ORAL SOLUTION, TABLETS

Adults. 80 to 320 mg/day in divided doses b.i.d., t.i.d., or q.i.d.

➤ *To treat supraventricular arrhythmias and ventricular tachycardia*

ORAL SOLUTION, TABLETS

Adults. 10 to 30 mg t.i.d. or q.i.d., adjusted as needed.

I.V. INJECTION

Adults. 1 to 3 mg at a rate not to exceed 1 mg/min; repeated after 2 min and again after 4 hr, if needed.

Children. 0.01 to 0.1 mg/kg at a rate not to exceed 1 mg/min; repeated q 6 to 8 hr, as needed. *Maximum:* 1 mg/dose.

➤ *To control tremor*

ORAL SOLUTION, TABLETS

Adults. *Initial:* 40 mg b.i.d., adjusted as needed and prescribed. *Maximum:* 320 mg/day.

➤ *To prevent vascular migraine headaches*

E.R. TABLETS

Adults. *Initial:* 80 mg q.d., increased gradually, as needed. *Maximum:* 240 mg/day.

ORAL SOLUTION, TABLETS

Adults. *Initial:* 20 mg q.i.d., increased gradually, as needed. *Maximum:* 240 mg/day.

➤ *As adjunct to treat hypertrophic cardiomyopathy*

ORAL SOLUTION, TABLETS

Adults. 20 to 40 mg t.i.d. or q.i.d., adjusted as needed.

➤ *As adjunct to manage pheochromocytoma*

ORAL SOLUTION, TABLETS

Adults. For operable tumors, 20 mg t.i.d. to 40 mg t.i.d. or q.i.d. for 3 days before surgery, concomitantly with an alpha blocker. For inoperable tumors, 30 to 160 mg/day in divided doses.

➤ *To prevent MI*

ORAL SOLUTION, TABLETS

Adults. 180 to 240 mg/day in divided doses.

DOSAGE ADJUSTMENT Dosage increased or decreased for elderly patients, depending on sensitivity to propranolol.

Route	Onset	Peak	Duration
P.O.	Unknown	1 to 1.5 hr*	Unknown

Mechanism of Action

Exerts the following effects through its beta-blocking actions:

• prevents arterial dilation and inhibits renin secretion, resulting in decreased blood pressure (in hypertension and pheochromocytoma) and relief of migraine headaches

• decreases the heart rate, which helps resolve tachyarrhythmias

• improves myocardial contractility, which helps ease the symptoms of hypertrophic cardiomyopathy

• decreases myocardial oxygen demand, which helps prevent angina pain and death of myocardial tissue

In addition, peripheral beta-adrenergic blockade may play a role in propranolol's ability to alleviate tremor.

Contraindications

Asthma, cardiogenic shock, greater than first-degree AV block, heart failure (unless secondary to tachyarrhythmia that's responsive to propranolol), hypersensitivity to propranolol or its components, sinus bradycardia

---

* For regular-release form; unknown for E.R. form.

Interactions

DRUGS

allergen immunotherapy, allergenic extracts for skin testing: Increased risk of serious systemic adverse reactions or anaphylaxis

amiodarone: Additive depressant effects on conduction, negative inotropic effects

anesthetics (hydrocarbon inhalation): Increased risk of myocardial depression and hypotension

beta blockers: Additive beta blockade effects

calcium channel blockers, clonidine, diazoxide, guanabenz, resperpine, other hypotension-producing drugs: Additive hypotensive effect and, possibly, other beta blockade effects

cimetidine: Possibly interference with propranolol clearance

estrogens: Decreased antihypertensive effect of propranolol

fentanyl, fentanyl derivatives: Possibly increased risk of initial bradycardia after induction doses of fentanyl or a derivative (with long-term propranolol use)

glucagon: Possibly blunted hyperglycemic response

insulin, oral antidiabetic drugs: Possibly impaired glucose control, masking of tachycardia in response to hypoglycemia

lidocaine: Decreased lidocaine clearance, increased risk of lidocaine toxicity

MAO inhibitors: Increased risk of significant hypertension

neuromuscular blockers: Possibly potentiated and prolonged action of these drugs

NSAIDs: Possibly decreased hypotensive effects

phenothiazines: Increased blood levels of both drugs

phenytoin: Additive cardiac depressant effects (with parenteral phenytoin)

propafenone: Increased blood level and half-life of propranolol

sympathomimetics, xanthines: Possibly mutual inhibition of therapeutic effects

ACTIVITIES

nicotine chewing gum, smoking cessation, smoking deterrents: Increased therapeutic effects of propranolol

Adverse Reactions

CNS: Anxiety, depression, dizziness, drowsiness, fatigue, insomnia, lethargy, nervousness, weakness

CV: AV conduction disorders, cold extremities, heart failure, hypotension, sinus bradycardia

EENT: Nasal congestion

GI: Abdominal pain, constipation, diarrhea, nausea, vomiting

GU: Sexual dysfunction

MS: Muscle weakness

RESP: Bronchospasm, dyspnea, wheezing

Nursing Considerations

• Monitor blood pressure, apical and radial pulses, fluid intake and output, daily weight, respiration, and circulation in extremities before and during propranolol therapy.

• Administer I.V. injection at a rate not to exceed 1 mg/minute.

• **WARNING** Institute continuous ECG monitoring, as ordered, when administering I.V. injection. Have emergency drugs and equipment available to intervene in case hypotension or cardiac arrest occurs.

• Protect injection solution from light.

• Because drug's negative inotropic effect can depress cardiac output, monitor cardiac output in patients with heart failure, particularly those with severely compromised left ventricular dysfunction.

• Be aware that propranolol can mask tachycardia that occurs in hyperthyroidism and that abrupt withdrawal of drug in patients with hyperthyroidism or thyrotoxicosis can precipitate thyroid storm.

• Monitor diabetic patient who is receiving antidiabetic drugs because propranolol can prolong hypoglycemia or promote hyperglycemia. Propranolol also can mask signs of hypoglycemia, especially tachycardia, palpitations, and tremor, but it doesn't suppress diaphoresis or hypertensive response to hypoglycemia.

• **WARNING** Be aware that abrupt discontinuation may cause myocardial ischemia, MI, ventricular arrhythmias, or severe hypertension, particularly in patients with preexisting cardiac disease.

PATIENT TEACHING

• Instruct patient to take propranolol at the same time every day.

• Caution patient not to change dosage without consulting prescriber and not to stop taking drug abruptly.

• Advise patient to notify prescriber immediately if she experiences shortness of breath.

• Instruct diabetic patient to regularly monitor blood glucose level and test urine for ketones.

P

- Advise patient to consult prescriber before taking OTC drugs, especially cold remedies.
- Urge patient to avoid potentially hazardous activities until drug's CNS effects are known.
- Advise smoker to notify prescriber immediately if she stops smoking because smoking cessation may decrease drug metabolism, calling for dosage adjustments.

propylthiouracil
(PTU)
Propyl-Thyracil (CAN)

Class and Category
Chemical: Thiourea derivative
Therapeutic: Antithyroid
Pregnancy category: D

Indications and Dosages
➤ *To treat hyperthyroidism*
TABLETS
Adults and adolescents. *Initial:* For mild to moderate hyperthyroidism, 300 to 900 mg/day in 1 to 4 divided doses until patient becomes euthyroid; for severe hyperthyroidism, 300 to 1,200 mg/day in 1 to 4 divided doses until patient becomes euthyroid. *Maintenance:* 50 to 600 mg/day in 1 to 4 divided doses.
Children age 10 and older. *Initial:* 50 to 300 mg/day in 1 to 4 divided doses. *Maintenance:* Dosage adjusted based on response to initial dosage.
Children ages 6 to 10. *Initial:* 50 to 150 mg/day in 1 to 4 divided doses. *Maintenance:* Dosage adjusted based on response to initial dosage.
Neonates. 10 mg/kg/day in divided doses.
➤ *As adjunct to treat thyrotoxic crisis*
TABLETS
Adults and adolescents. 200 to 400 mg q 4 hr on day 1 along with other measures. Dosage gradually decreased as crisis subsides.
DOSAGE ADJUSTMENT For patients with creatinine clearance of 10 to 50 ml/min/1.73 m², recommended dosage reduced by 25%; for creatinine clearance of less than 10 ml/min/1.73 m², recommended dosage reduced by 50%.

Route	Onset	Peak	Duration
P.O.	Unknown	17 wk	Unknown

Mechanism of Action
Inhibits the conversion of peripheral thyroxine to triiodothyronine by interfering with the incorporation of iodide into thyroglobulin; the drug remains iodinated and degraded within the thyroid gland. The diversion of oxidized iodine away from thyroglobulin diminishes thyroid hormone synthesis, thereby reducing levels of circulating thyroid hormone.

Contraindications
Breast-feeding, hypersensitivity to propylthiouracil or its components

Interactions
DRUGS
amiodarone, iodinated glycerol, iodine, potassium iodide: Decreased efficacy of propylthiouracil
digoxin: Risk of digitalis toxicity
oral anticoagulants: Possibly enhanced anticoagulant effect
sodium iodide 131 (radioactive iodine, ^{131}I): Decreased thyroid uptake of ^{131}I

Adverse Reactions
CNS: Dizziness, paresthesia, peripheral neuropathy
CV: Vasculitis
ENDO: Hypothyroidism
GI: Abdominal pain, nausea, vomiting
HEME: Agranulocytosis, leukopenia
MS: Arthralgia, joint redness or swelling
SKIN: Pruritus, rash, urticaria
Other: Lupus-like symptoms

Nursing Considerations
- Monitor CBC, PT, and liver and thyroid function test results in patients taking propylthiouracil. Elevated serum triiodothyronine (T_3) level may be the sole indicator of inadequate treatment.
- Be aware that propylthiouracil should be stopped 3 to 4 days before ^{131}I treatment to prevent decreased thyroid uptake of ^{131}I; therapy may be resumed 3 to 5 days after radiation, if needed.
- Be aware that serum T_3 and thyroxine levels should decrease after about 3 weeks of therapy.
- Expect prescriber to decrease beta blocker or theophylline dosage once patient is euthyroid.
PATIENT TEACHING
- Instruct patient to take propylthiouracil with meals to decrease adverse GI reactions.

• Advise patient to avoid dietary sources of iodine, such as iodized salt and shellfish.
• Instruct patient to monitor pulse rate and weight daily and to report increased heart rate and excessive weight loss to prescriber.
• Urge patient to report signs of infection, such as fever and sore throat, or possible signs of hepatic dysfunction, such as anorexia and right-upper-quadrant pain.
• Instruct patient to notify prescriber immediately if she becomes pregnant.
• Advise patient to report signs and symptoms of hypothyroidism, such as cold intolerance, depression, and increased fatigue.
• Instruct patient to consult prescriber before using OTC cold remedies because some of them contain iodides.

protamine sulfate

Class and Category
Chemical: Simple low-molecular-weight protein
Therapeutic: Heparin antagonist
Pregnancy category: C

Indications and Dosages
➤ *To treat heparin toxicity or hemorrhage associated with heparin therapy*

I.V. INJECTION
Adults and children. 1 mg for each 100 U of heparin to be neutralized, or as indicated by coagulation test results. *Maximum:* 100 mg (within 2-hr period).

Route	Onset	Peak	Duration
I.V.	5 min	Unknown	2 hr

Mechanism of Action
Neutralizes anticoagulant activity. A strong basic polypeptide, protamine combines with strongly acidic heparin complex to form an inactive stable salt, thereby neutralizing the anticoagulant activity of both drugs.

Incompatibilities
Don't mix protamine sulfate in same syringe with other drugs unless they're known to be compatible. Several cephalosporins, penicillins, and other antibiotics are incompatible.

Contraindications
Allergy to fish, hypersensitivity to protamine or its components

Interactions
DRUGS
heparin: Neutralized anticoagulant effect of both drugs

Adverse Reactions
CNS: Weakness
CV: Bradycardia, hypertension, hypotension, shock
GI: Nausea, vomiting
HEME: Unusual bleeding or bruising
RESP: Dyspnea, pulmonary edema (noncardiogenic), pulmonary hypertension
SKIN: Flushing, sensation of warmth
Other: Anaphylaxis

Nursing Considerations
• Expect to administer I.V. protamine undiluted. However, dilute drug if needed (for patients other than neonates) with 5 ml of bacteriostatic water for injection containing 0.9% benzyl alcohol. For neonates, reconstitute with preservative-free sterile water for injection.
• Inject drug slowly at a rate of 5 mg/minute; administer no more than 50 mg in 10 minutes or 100 mg in 2 hours.
• **WARNING** Be aware that rapid administration may cause severe hypotension and anaphylaxis.
• Be prepared to obtain coagulation studies (APTT, activated clotting time) 5 to 15 minutes after administering drug and to repeat studies in 2 to 8 hours to assess for heparin-rebound hypotension, shock, and bleeding.
• Monitor vital signs, hemodynamic parameters, and fluid intake and output, and assess for flushing sensation.
• Have fluids—epinephrine 1:1,000, dobutamine, or dopamine—available for allergic or hypotensive reactions.
• Be aware that vasectomized males have an increased risk of hypersensitivity reaction because of possible accumulation of antiprotamine antibodies.
PATIENT TEACHING
• Instruct patient to report adverse reactions immediately.

protriptyline hydrochloride

Triptil (CAN), Vivactil

Class and Category
Chemical: Dibenzocycloheptene derivative

P

Therapeutic: Antidepressant
Pregnancy category: Not rated

Indications and Dosages

➤ *To treat depression*

TABLETS

Adults. *Initial:* 5 to 10 mg t.i.d. or q.i.d., increased q wk by 10 mg/day, as needed. *Maximum:* 60 mg/day.

Children age 12 and older. *Initial:* 5 mg t.i.d., increased as needed.

DOSAGE ADJUSTMENT For elderly patients, initial dosage limited to 5 mg t.i.d., then adjusted as needed.

Route	Onset	Peak	Duration
P.O.	2 to 3 wk	Unknown	Unknown

Mechanism of Action

May block the reuptake of norepinephrine and serotonin (and possibly other neurotransmitters) at neuronal membranes, thus enhancing their effects at postsynaptic receptors. These neurotransmitters may play a role in relieving symptoms of depression.

Contraindications

Acute recovery phase after MI, hypersensitivity to protriptyline or its components, use within 14 days of MAO inhibitor therapy

Interactions

DRUGS

amantadine, anticholinergics, antidyskinetics, antihistamines: Additive anticholinergic effects, potentiated effects of antihistamines or protriptyline, possibly impaired detoxification of atropine and related drugs

anticonvulsants: Possibly lowered seizure threshold and decreased anticonvulsant effectiveness; enhanced CNS depression

antithyroid drugs: Possibly agranulocytosis

barbiturates, carbamazepine: Decreased therapeutic effects of protriptyline

bupropion, clozapine, cyclobenzaprine, haloperidol, loxapine, maprotiline, molindone, phenothiazines, thioxanthenes: Prolonged and intensified anticholinergic and sedative effects, lowered seizure threshold, increased risk of neuroleptic malignant syndrome; increased blood protriptyline level and inhibited phenothiazine metabolism (with phenothiazine use)

cimetidine: Increased risk of protriptyline toxicity

clonidine, guanadrel, guanethidine: Decreased hypotensive effects of these drugs; increased CNS depression (with clonidine use)

CNS depressants: Possibly serious potentiation of CNS and respiratory depression and hypotensive effect

disulfiram, etchlorvynol: Possibly transient delirium; increased CNS depression (with ethchlorvynol use)

fluoxetine: Increased blood protriptyline level

MAO inhibitors: Increased risk of hyperpyretic crisis, severe seizures, and death

methylphenidate: Possibly antagonized effects of methylphenidate and increased blood protriptyline level

metrizamide: Increased risk of seizures

naphazoline, oxymetazoline, phenylephrine, xylometazoline: Possibly increased vasopressor effects of these drugs

oral anticoagulants: Possibly increased anticoagulant activity

pimozide, probucol: Possibly prolonged QT interval and ventricular tachycardia

sympathomimetics: Possibly potentiated cardiovascular effects, decreased vasopressor effects of ephedrine and mephentermine

thyroid hormones: Increased therapeutic and toxic effects of both drugs

ACTIVITIES

alcohol use: Possibly increased response to alcohol

Adverse Reactions

CNS: Agitation, ataxia, confusion, dizziness, drowsiness, exacerbation of psychosis, extrapyramidal reactions, fatigue, lack of coordination, paresthesia, peripheral neuropathy, tremor, weakness

CV: Arrhythmias, including heart block and tachycardia; CVA; hypertension; hypotension; MI; orthostatic hypotension; palpitations

EENT: Black tongue, blurred vision, dry mouth, increased intraocular pressure, lacrimation, stomatitis, tongue swelling

ENDO: Hyperglycemia, hypoglycemia

GI: Abdominal cramps, anorexia, constipation, diarrhea, epigastric discomfort, hepatic dysfunction, nausea, vomiting

GU: Impotence, libido changes, nocturia, urinary frequency and hesitancy, urine retention

SKIN: Diaphoresis, petechiae, photosensitivity, rash, urticaria

Other: Facial edema, weight gain or loss

Nursing Considerations
•Use protriptyline cautiously in patients with a history of seizures because drug can lower seizure threshold.
•Use drug cautiously in patients with a history of urine retention or increased intraocular pressure because of drug's autonomic activity.
•WARNING Avoid administering protriptyline with an MAO inhibitor. If patient is being switched from an MAO inhibitor to protriptyline, ensure that MAO inhibitor has been discontinued for 14 days before starting protriptyline.

PATIENT TEACHING
•Inform patient that protriptyline therapy may take several weeks to reach full effect.
•Instruct patient to avoid potentially hazardous activities until drug's CNS effects are known.
•Advise patient to change position slowly to minimize effects of orthostatic hypotension.
•Urge patient to avoid alcohol while taking drug.
•Suggest that patient drink water and use sugarless gum or hard candy to relieve dry mouth.
•Advise patient to avoid sunlight and tanning booths and to wear protective clothing, a hat, and sunscreen when outdoors.
•Instruct diabetic patient to check blood glucose level frequently during first few weeks of protriptyline therapy.

pyrazinamide
pms-Pyrazinamide (CAN), Tebrazid (CAN)

Class and Category
Chemical: Pyrazine analogue of nicotinamide
Therapeutic: Antitubercular
Pregnancy category: C

Indications and Dosages
➤ *As adjunct to treat tuberculosis, along with other antitubercular drugs*

TABLETS
Adults and children. 15 to 30 mg/kg q.d.; alternatively, 50 to 70 mg/kg 2 or 3 times/wk. *Maximum:* 2 g/day for daily regimen, 4 g/day for 2 times/wk regimen, and 3 g/day for 3 times/wk regimen.
DOSAGE ADJUSTMENT For patients with HIV infection, 20 to 30 mg/kg/day for first 2 mo of therapy.

Mechanism of Action
Inhibits the growth of *Mycobacterium tuberculosis* organisms by decreasing the pH level; exhibits bactericidal or bacteriostatic action, depending on blood pyrazinamide level.

Contraindications
Acute gout, hypersensitivity to pyrazinamide or its components, severe hepatic damage

Interactions
DRUGS
allopurinol, colchicine, probenecid, sulfinpyrazone: Possibly increased blood uric acid level and decreased efficacy of antigout therapy
cyclosporine: Possibly decreased blood level and therapeutic effects of cyclosporine

Adverse Reactions
CNS: Fever
GI: Anorexia, hepatotoxicity, nausea, vomiting
GU: Dysuria
HEME: Porphyria
MS: Arthralgia, gout, myalgia
SKIN: Acne, photosensitivity, pruritus, rash, urticaria

Nursing Considerations
•Review liver function test results before and every 2 to 4 weeks during pyrazinamide therapy.
•Be aware that drug can affect the accuracy of certain urine ketone strip test results.
•Because drug is metabolized by liver, monitor for signs of hepatotoxicity, such as darkened urine, fever, jaundice, malaise, nausea, severe pain in feet or toes, and vomiting.

PATIENT TEACHING
•Explain the importance of complying with long-term pyrazinamide therapy.
•Advise diabetic patient to use alternative methods of ketone determination while taking drug.
•Instruct patient to report darkened urine, fever, malaise, nausea, severe pain in feet or toes, vomiting, and yellowing of skin or eyes.
•Inform patient of need for regular blood tests and follow-up visits with prescriber.
•Urge patient to minimize exposure to sun and to wear protective clothing, hat, sunglasses, and sunscreen when outdoors.

pyridostigmine bromide

Mestinon, Mestinon-SR (CAN), Mestinon Timespans, Regonol (CAN)

Class and Category
Chemical: Bromide dimethylcarbamate
Therapeutic: Antimyasthenic
Pregnancy category: Not rated

Indications and Dosages
➤ *To treat symptoms of myasthenia gravis*
E.R. TABLETS
Adults and adolescents. 180 to 540 mg q.d. or b.i.d. (with at least 6 hr between doses).
SYRUP, TABLETS
Adults and adolescents. *Initial:* 30 to 60 mg q 3 to 4 hr, adjusted as needed. *Maintenance:* 60 mg to 1.5 g/day.
Children. 7 mg/kg/day in 5 or 6 divided doses.
I.V. OR I.M. INJECTION
Adults and adolescents. 2 mg q 2 to 3 hr.
I.M. INJECTION
Neonates of myasthenic mothers. 0.05 to 0.15 mg/kg q 4 to 6 hr.
➤ *To reverse the effects of neuromuscular blockers*
I.V. INJECTION
Adults and adolescents. 10 to 20 mg after 0.6 to 1.2 mg of I.V. atropine has been given.
DOSAGE ADJUSTMENT Dosage possibly reduced for patients with renal impairment.

Route	Onset	Peak	Duration
P.O.	30 to 45 min	1 to 2 hr	3 to 6 hr
P.O. (E.R.)	30 to 60 min	1 to 2 hr	6 to 12 hr
I.V.	2 to 5 min	Unknown	2 to 4 hr
I.M.	15 min	Unknown	2 to 4 hr

Mechanism of Action
Improves muscle strength compromised by myasthenia gravis or neuromuscular blockade by competing with acetylcholine for its binding site on acetylcholinesterase. This action potentiates the effects of acetylcholine on skeletal muscle and the GI tract. Inhibited destruction of acetylcholine allows freer transmission of nerve impulses across the neuromuscular junction.

Contraindications
Hypersensitivity to pyridostigmine or its components, mechanical obstruction of GI or urinary tract

Interactions
DRUGS
aminoglycosides (systemic), anesthetics (hydrocarbon inhalation), capreomycin, lidocaine (I.V.), lincomycins, polymyxins, quinine: Possibly antagonized effect of pyridostigmine on skeletal muscle; possibly decreased neuromuscular blocking activity of these drugs (with large doses of pyridostigmine)
anesthetics (local): Inhibited neuronal transmission, increased anesthesia effects
anticholinergics: Possibly masking of signs of pyridostigmine overdose and reduced intestinal motility
cholinesterase inhibitors: Increased risk of additive toxicity
edrophonium: Possibly worsening of patient's condition
guanadrel, guanethidine, mecamylamine, neuromuscular blockers, procainamide: Possibly prolonged phase I blocking effect or reversal of nondepolarization blockade
quinidine, trimethaphan: Possibly antagonized effects of pyridostigmine

Adverse Reactions
EENT: Increased salivation, lacrimation, miosis
GI: Abdominal cramps, diarrhea, increased peristalsis, nausea, vomiting
GU: Urinary frequency, incontinence, or urgency
MS: Fasciculations, muscle spasms or weakness
RESP: Increased tracheobronchial secretions
SKIN: Diaphoresis

Nursing Considerations
• Use pyridostigmine cautiously in patients with renal disease because drug is mainly excreted unchanged by kidneys. Monitor BUN and serum creatinine levels as appropriate.
• WARNING Maintain a rigid dosing schedule because a missed or late dose can precipitate myasthenic crisis.
• Observe for cholinergic reactions when administering drug I.V. or I.M.
• WARNING Be aware that pyridostigmine overdose may obscure the diagnosis of myasthenic crisis because the primary symptom in both is muscle weakness. Respiratory muscle involvement can lead to death. Be prepared to treat cholinergic crisis by immediately stopping anticholinesterase therapy, adminis-

tering atropine as prescribed, and assisting with endotracheal intubation and mechanical ventilation, if needed.

• Be aware that reversal of neuromuscular blockade usually occurs in 15 to 30 minutes. Be prepared to maintain patent airway and ventilation until normal voluntary respiration returns completely. Assess respiratory measurements and muscle tone with peripheral nerve stimulator device, as indicated.

PATIENT TEACHING

• Instruct patient to take pyridostigmine as directed and on schedule. Explain that a late or missed dose can precipitate a crisis. Suggest the use of a battery-operated alarm clock as a reminder.

• Advise patient to take the oral form with a full glass of water or with food or milk if GI distress occurs.

• Instruct patient not to crush or chew E.R. tablets.

• Ask patient to record pyridostigmine dosage, times taken, and effects to help determine optimal dosage and schedule for her needs.

• Urge patient to carry medical identification describing her condition and drug regimen.

P

Q·R·S

quazepam

Doral

Class, Category, and Schedule

Chemical: Benzodiazepine
Therapeutic: Sedative-hypnotic
Pregnancy category: X
Controlled substance: Schedule IV

Indications and Dosages

➤ *To treat insomnia*

TABLETS

Adults. 15 mg h.s.

DOSAGE ADJUSTMENT In elderly and debilitated patients, dosage possibly reduced to 7.5 mg h.s. after 1 or 2 nights of therapy.

Mechanism of Action

Believed to agonize mu receptors at limbic, thalamic, and hypothalamic regions of the brain, blocking release of such inhibitory neurotransmitters as gamma-aminobutyric acid (GABA) and acetylcholine. Central receptors interact with GABA receptors, allowing for greater influx of chloride into the neuron, thereby suppressing neuronal excitability. GABA effects may inhibit spinal afferent pathways and block the cortical and limbic arousal that normally occurs when reticular pathways are stimulated. These effects result in various levels of CNS depression, including sleep.

Contraindications

Hypersensitivity to quazepam or its components, pregnancy, sleep apnea (known or suspected)

Interactions

DRUGS

addictive drugs: Possibly habituation
carbamazepine: Decreased blood quazepam level, possibly increased blood carbamazepine level
cimetidine, diltiazem, disulfiram, erythromycin, fluoxetine, fluvoxamine, isoniazid, itraconazole, ketoconazole, nefazodone, oral con-traceptives, propoxyphene, ranitidine, verapamil: Possibly potentiated effects of quazepam
clozapine: Possibly syncope, with respiratory depression or arrest
CNS depressants, tricyclic antidepressants: Increased CNS depression
digoxin: Possibly increased blood digoxin level and risk of digitalis toxicity
levodopa: Possibly decreased therapeutic effects of levodopa
phenytoin: Increased risk of phenytoin toxicity
theophyllines: Possibly antagonized effects of quazepam
zidovudine: Increased risk of zidovudine toxicity

FOODS

grapefruit juice: Increased blood quazepam level

ACTIVITIES

alcohol use: Additive CNS depression
smoking: Possibly decreased effectiveness of quazepam

Adverse Reactions

CNS: Amnesia (anterograde), anxiety, ataxia, confusion, depression, dizziness, drowsiness, euphoria, fatigue, headache, light-headedness, paresthesia, slurred speech, tremor, weakness
CV: Chest pain, palpitations, tachycardia
EENT: Blurred vision, dry mouth, hyperacusis, photophobia, worsening of glaucoma
GI: Abdominal cramps, constipation, diarrhea, heartburn, nausea, thirst, vomiting
GU: Renal dysfunction, urinary incontinence, urine retention
MS: Muscle spasms
RESP: Increased tracheobronchial secretions

Nursing Considerations

•Use quazepam cautiously in patients with angle-closure glaucoma because of drug's anticholinergic effects; in patients with hepatic dysfunction because this condition may prolong quazepam's half-life; in patients with myasthenia gravis because drug may worsen condition; in patients with severe COPD because adverse effects of quazepam may compromise respiratory function; and in patients with renal dysfunction because accumulation of metabolites may result in toxicity.
•WARNING Notify prescriber immediately if eye pain develops in patient with angle-closure glaucoma.
•WARNING Be aware that quazepam may intensify signs and symptoms of depression.

Q
R
S

Monitor closely for suicidal ideation. Institute suicide precautions, as appropriate, according to facility policy.

PATIENT TEACHING
• Urge patient to avoid alcohol during quazepam therapy because it may increase drug's sedative effects.
• Instruct patient not to discontinue drug abruptly after prolonged use (6 weeks or longer).
• Instruct female patient of childbearing age to use effective contraception during therapy and to notify prescriber immediately of known or suspected pregnancy.

quetiapine fumarate

Seroquel

Class and Category

Chemical: Dibenzothiazepine derivative
Therapeutic: Antipsychotic
Pregnancy category: C

Indications and Dosages

➤ *To manage psychotic disorders, including schizophrenia*

TABLETS
Adults. *Initial:* 25 mg b.i.d. on day 1. Dosage increased by 25 to 50 mg b.i.d. or t.i.d. on days 2 and 3. *Usual:* 300 to 400 mg/day by day 4, in divided doses b.i.d. or t.i.d. Dosage increased q 2 days in increments of 25 to 50 mg b.i.d., as needed. *Maximum:* 800 mg/day.

Mechanism of Action

May produce antipsychotic effects by interfering with dopamine binding to dopamine type 2 (D_2)-receptor sites in the brain and by antagonizing serotonin 5-HT_2, dopamine type 1 (D_1), histamine H_1, and adrenergic alpha$_1$ and alpha$_2$ receptors.

Contraindications

Hypersensitivity to quetiapine or its components

Interactions

DRUGS
antihypertensives: Possibly enhanced antihypertensive effects of these drugs
cimetidine, erythromycin, fluconazole, itraconazole, ketoconazole: Decreased clearance and possibly increased effects of quetiapine

CNS depressants: Possibly increased CNS depression
lorazepam: Possibly increased effects of lorazepam
phenytoin, thioridazine: Increased clearance and possibly decreased effectiveness of quetiapine

ACTIVITIES
alcohol use: Possibly enhanced CNS depression

Adverse Reactions

CNS: Dizziness, drowsiness, extrapyramidal reactions, hypertonia, tardive dyskinesia
CV: Orthostatic hypotension, palpitations
EENT: Dry mouth, pharyngitis, rhinitis
GI: Anorexia, constipation, indigestion
HEME: Leukopenia
MS: Dysarthria, muscle weakness
RESP: Cough, dyspnea
SKIN: Diaphoresis
Other: Flulike symptoms, weight gain

Nursing Considerations

• **WARNING** Monitor patient taking quetiapine fumarate for predisposing factors that may contribute to development of neuroleptic malignant syndrome; these include heat stress, physical exhaustion, dehydration, and organic brain disease. The syndrome is characterized by hyperpyrexia, muscle rigidity, altered mental status, and autonomic instability (which may include irregular pulse or blood pressure, tachycardia, diaphoresis, and arrhythmias).
• Monitor patient for signs of tardive dyskinesia, a potentially irreversible complication characterized by involuntary, dyskinetic movements of the tongue, mouth, jaw, eyelids, or face. Notify prescriber if such signs develop because quetiapine therapy may need to be discontinued.
• Monitor for orthostatic hypotension, especially during initial dosage titration period. Be prepared to correct underlying conditions, such as hypovolemia and dehydration, before starting therapy, as prescribed.
• Monitor patient during treatment for signs and symptoms of hypothyroidism because drug can cause dose-dependent decreases in total and free thyroxine (T_4) levels.
• Monitor laboratory results during first 3 weeks of therapy for transient elevations in hepatic enzyme levels. Notify prescriber if elevations persist or become progressively worse.

- Instruct patient to take quetiapine with food to reduce stomach upset.
- Advise patient not to stop taking quetiapine suddenly because doing so may exacerbate his symptoms.
- Inform patient that drug may cause dizziness or drowsiness. Advise him not to drive or perform other activities that require alertness until drug's full CNS effects are known.
- Instruct patient to rise slowly from a seated or lying position to reduce the risk of dizziness or fainting.
- Urge patient to avoid consuming alcoholic beverages because they can increase dizziness and drowsiness.
- Encourage patient on long-term therapy to have regular eye examinations so that cataracts can be detected.

quinapril hydrochloride

Accupril

Class and Catgeory
Chemical: Ethylester of quinaprilat
Therapeutic: Antihypertensive
Pregnancy category: C (first trimester), D (later trimesters)

Indications and Dosages
➤ *To treat hypertension*
TABLETS
Adults. *Initial:* 10 or 20 mg q.d., adjusted q 2 wk based on clinical response. *Maintenance:* 20 to 80 mg q.d. or in divided doses b.i.d.
DOSAGE ADJUSTMENT Initial dosage reduced to 5 mg q.d. for patients who are dehydrated from previous diuretic therapy, those who are still receiving diuretic therapy, and those with creatinine clearance of 30 to 60 ml/min/1.73 m². Dosage reduced to 2.5 mg q.d. for patients with creatinine clearance of 10 to 30 ml/min/1.73 m².

Route	Onset	Peak	Duration
P.O.	In 1 hr	2 to 4 hr	Up to 24 hr

Contraindications
History of angioedema related to previous treatment with ACE inhibitor, hypersensitivity to quinapril or its components

Mechanism of Action
Blocks conversion of angiotensin I to angiotensin II, leading to vasodilation, and reduces aldosterone secretion, which prevents water retention. Quinapril also reduces peripheral arterial resistance. These combined actions lead to a reduction in blood pressure.

Interactions
DRUGS
allopurinol, bone marrow depressants, corticosteroids (systemic), procainamide: Increased risk of fatal neutropenia or agranulocytosis
CNS depressants, other hypotension-producing drugs: Additive hypotensive effects
cyclosporine, potassium preparations, potassium-sparing diuretics: Possibly hyperkalemia
lithium: Possibly increased blood lithium level and risk of toxicity
NSAIDs, sympathomimetics: Decreased antihypertensive effect of quinapril
tetracyclines: Reduced tetracycline absorption
FOODS
low-salt milk, salt substitutes: Increased risk of hyperkalemia
ACTIVITIES
alcohol use: Additive hypotensive effects

Adverse Reactions
CNS: Depression, dizziness, drowsiness, fatigue, fever, headache, insomnia, light-headedness, malaise, paresthesia, sleep disturbance, syncope, vertigo
CV: Chest pain, hypotension, orthostatic hypotension, palpitations, tachycardia
EENT: Amblyopia, dry mouth, loss of taste, pharyngitis
GI: Abdominal pain, constipation, diarrhea, nausea, vomiting
GU: Impotence
MS: Arthralgia, back pain, myalgia
RESP: Cough, dyspnea
SKIN: Alopecia, diaphoresis, flushing, photosensitivity, pruritus, rash, urticaria
Other: Angioedema

Nursing Considerations
- Use quinapril cautiously in patients with renal impairment.
- WARNING Be aware that patients with heart failure, hyponatremia, or severe volume or salt depletion; those who've recently received

intensive diuresis or an increase in diuretic dosage; and those undergoing dialysis may be at risk for excessive hypotension. Monitor blood pressure frequently for first 2 weeks of therapy and whenever quinapril or diuretic dosage increases. If excessive hypotension occurs, notify prescriber immediately, place patient in a supine position, and, if prescribed, infuse NS.

•WARNING Because of the risk of angioedema, be prepared to discontinue drug and administer emergency measures, including S.C. epinephrine 1:1,000 (0.3 to 0.5 ml), if swelling of tongue, glottis, or larynx causes airway obstruction.

•Monitor blood pressure frequently to assess drug's effectiveness.

PATIENT TEACHING

•Instruct patient to notify prescriber immediately and stop taking quinapril if he experiences swelling of the face, eyes, lips, or tongue or difficulty breathing.

•Explain that drug may cause dizziness and light-headedness, especially during first few days of therapy. Advise patient to avoid potentially hazardous activities until drug's CNS effects are known and to notify prescriber immediately if he faints.

•Inform female patient of childbearing age of risks of taking quinapril during pregnancy, especially during the second and third trimesters. Caution her to use effective contraception and to notify prescriber immediately of known or suspected pregnancy.

•Advise patient planning to undergo surgery or anesthesia to inform specialist that he's taking quinapril.

•Instruct patient to consult prescriber before using potassium supplements or salt substitutes that contain potassium.

quinidine gluconate

Quinaglute Dura-tabs, Quinate (CAN), Quin-Release

quinidine polygalacturonate

Cardioquin

quinidine sulfate

Apo-Quinidine (CAN), Novoquinidin (CAN), Quinidex Extentabs

Class and Category

Chemical: Dextrorotatory isomer of quinine
Therapeutic: Class IA antiarrhythmic
Pregnancy category: C

Indications and Dosages

➤ *To prevent or treat cardiac arrhythmias, including established atrial fibrillation, atrial flutter, paroxysmal atrial fibrillation, paroxysmal atrial tachycardia, paroxysmal atrioventricular junctional rhythm, paroxysmal ventricular tachycardia not associated with complete heart block, and premature atrial and ventricular contractions*

E.R. TABLETS (QUINIDINE GLUCONATE)
Adults. 324 to 660 mg q 8 to 12 hr. *Maximum:* 1,944 mg/day.

E.R. TABLETS (QUINIDINE SULFATE)
Adults. 300 to 600 mg q 8 to 12 hr.

TABLETS (QUINIDINE GLUCONATE)
Adults. *Initial:* 325 mg q 2 to 3 hr for 5 to 8 doses, gradually increasing dosage as needed and prescribed. *Maintenance:* 325 to 488 mg t.i.d. or q.i.d.

TABLETS (QUINIDINE POLYGALACTURONATE)
Adults. *Initial:* 275 to 825 mg q 3 to 4 hr for 3 or 4 doses, then increased by 137.5 to 275 mg q 3rd or 4th dose until rhythm is restored or toxic effects occur. *Maintenance:* 275 mg b.i.d. or t.i.d.

TABLETS (QUINIDINE SULFATE)
Adults. *Initial:* For premature atrial and ventricular contractions, 200 to 300 mg t.i.d. or q.i.d.; for paroxysmal supraventricular tachycardia, 400 to 600 mg q 2 to 3 hr until terminated; for atrial flutter, individual titration after digitalization; for conversion of atrial fibrillation, 200 mg q 2 to 3 hr for 5 to 8 doses, followed by subsequent daily increases, as needed. *Maintenance:* 200 to 400 mg t.i.d. or q.i.d.
Children. 6 mg/kg 5 times/day.

I.V. INFUSION (QUINIDINE GLUCONATE)
Adults. 800 mg in 40 ml of D_5W at a rate of up to 0.25 mg/kg/min.

I.M. INJECTION (QUINIDINE SULFATE)
Adults. 190 to 380 mg q 2 to 4 hr. *Maximum:* 3 g/day.

Route	Onset	Peak	Duration
P.O.	Unknown	Unknown	6 to 8 hr
P.O. (E.R.)	Unknown	Unknown	12 hr

Mechanism of Action

Depresses excitability, conduction velocity, and contractility of the myocardium and increases the effective refractory period to suppress arrhythmic activity in the atria, ventricles, and His-Purkinje system.

Contraindications

Digitalis toxicity; history of quinidine-induced thrombocytopenic purpura or torsades de pointes; hypersensitivity to quinidine, other cinchona derivatives, or their components; long-QT syndrome; myasthenia gravis; pacemaker-dependent conduction disturbances

Interactions

DRUGS

antiarrhythmics, phenothiazines, rauwolfia alkaloids: Additive cardiac effects
anticholinergics: Possibly intensified atropine-like adverse effects
antimyasthenics: Antagonized antimyasthenic effects on skeletal muscle
barbiturates, rifampin: Possibly accelerated elimination and decreased effectiveness of quinidine
cimetidine: Increased elimination half-life, possibly leading to quinidine toxicity
digoxin: Possibly digitalis toxicity
hepatic enzyme inducers: Possibly decreased blood quinidine level
neuromuscular blockers: Possibly potentiated neuromuscular blockade
oral anticoagulants: Additive hypoprothrombinemia, increased risk of bleeding
pimozide: Risk of arrhythmias
quinine: Increased risk of quinidine toxicity
urinary alkalizers (such as antacids, carbonic anhydrase inhibitors, citrates, sodium bicarbonate, thiazide diuretics): Increased renal tubular reabsorption of quinidine, possibly leading to quinidine toxicity
verapamil: Possibly AV block, bradycardia, pulmonary edema, significant hypotension, and ventricular tachycardia

Adverse Reactions

CNS: Anxiety, asthenia, ataxia, confusion, delirium, difficulty speaking, dizziness, drowsiness, extrapyramidal reactions, fever, headache, hypertonia, syncope, vertigo
CV: Complete heart block, orthostatic hypotension, palpitations, peripheral edema, prolonged QT interval, torsades de pointes, vasculitis, ventricular arrhythmias, widening QRS complex
EENT: Blurred vision, change in color perception, diplopia, dry mouth, hearing loss (high-frequency), pharyngitis, photophobia, rhinitis, tinnitus
GI: Abdominal pain, anorexia, constipation, diarrhea, indigestion, nausea, vomiting
HEME: Agranulocytosis, hemolytic anemia, leukopenia, neutropenia, thrombocytopenia, thrombocytopenic purpura
MS: Arthralgia, myalgia
RESP: Dyspnea
SKIN: Diaphoresis, eczema, exfoliative dermatitis, flushing, hyperpigmentation, photosensitivity, pruritus, psoriasis, purpura, rash, urticaria
Other: Angioedema, flulike symptoms, weight gain

Nursing Considerations

• Administer I.M. form of quinidine undiluted.
• For intermittent I.V. infusion, dilute drug in 40 ml of D_5W and administer using an infusion pump at a rate of 0.25 mg/kg/min or less. Rapid administration may cause hypotension. Monitor ECG tracings and blood pressure throughout administration.
• Monitor therapeutic blood level of quinidine, as ordered, in all patients receiving drug.
• Monitor heart rate and rhythm closely because quinidine may cause serious adverse reactions and can be cardiotoxic, especially at dosages exceeding 2.4 g/day. Implement continuous cardiac monitoring, as ordered.
• Assess for early signs and symptoms of cinchonism, including blurred vision, change in color perception, confusion, diplopia, headache, and tinnitus, which may indicate quinidine toxicity.

PATIENT TEACHING

• Advise patient to take quinidine at the same times every day and at evenly spaced intervals.
• Instruct patient to swallow E.R. tablets whole, with a full glass of water, preferably while sitting upright.
• Advise patient to take drug with food if GI upset occurs.
• Urge patient to inform prescriber immediately of blurred or double vision, change in color perception, confusion, diarrhea, fever, headache, loss of hearing, or tinnitus.

Q
R
S

quinine sulfate

Class and Category
Chemical: Cinchona alkaloid
Therapeutic: Antimalarial
Pregnancy category: X

Indications and Dosages
➤ *As adjunct to treat chloroquine-resistant malaria caused by* Plasmodium falciparum
CAPSULES, TABLETS
Adults. 600 to 650 mg q 8 hr for at least 3 days with one of the following: 250 mg of tetracycline q 6 hr for 7 days; 1.5 g of sulfadoxine and 75 mg of pyrimethamine combined as a single dose; 900 mg of clindamycin q 8 hr for 3 days; or 100 mg of doxycycline q 12 hr for 7 days.
Children over age 8. 8.3 mg/kg q 8 hr for at least 3 days with one of the following: 5 mg/kg of tetracycline q 6 hr for 7 days; 6.7 to 13.3 mg/kg of clindamycin q 8 hr for 3 days; or 1.25 mg/kg of pyrimethamine and 25 mg/kg of sulfadoxine combined as a single dose.

Mechanism of Action
May disrupt function in malarial parasite by elevating intracellular pH in parasitic acid vesicles.

Contraindications
G6PD deficiency, history of quinine-induced blackwater fever or thrombocytopenic purpura, hypersensitivity to quinine or its components, optic neuritis, pregnancy, tinnitus

Interactions
DRUGS
acetazolamide, sodium bicarbonate: Increased risk of quinine toxicity
aluminum-containing antacids: Possibly delayed or decreased quinine absorption
antimyasthenics: Possibly antagonized antimyasthenic effect on skeletal muscle
cimetidine: Possibly reduced clearance of quinine
digoxin: Increased blood digoxin level
hemolytics, neurotoxic drugs, ototoxic drugs: Increased risk of toxicity of these drugs
hepatic enzyme inducers: Possibly decreased blood quinine level
mefloquine: Increased risk of seizures
neuromuscular blockers: Potentiated neuromuscular blockade
oral anticoagulants: Possibly increased anticoagulant effects and risk of bleeding
quinidine: Increased risk of prolonged QT interval

Adverse Reactions
CNS: Headache
EENT: Blurred vision, hearing loss, tinnitus, vision changes
ENDO: Hypoglycemia
GI: Abdominal or epigastric pain, diarrhea, nausea, vomiting
HEME: Thrombocytopenia

Nursing Considerations
• Be aware that quinine shouldn't be used in patients with blackwater fever, which can follow chronic malaria, because they're at increased risk for anemia and hemolysis with renal failure.
• Be aware that quinine shouldn't be given I.M. Doing so may cause bleeding, bruising, or hematomas because of quinine's effect on platelets.
• Monitor patient with type 2 diabetes mellitus for alterations in blood glucose level because quinine stimulates release of insulin and may promote hypoglycemia.
• Be aware that quinine can exacerbate optic neuritis or tinnitus. It may also exacerbate muscle weakness and cause dysphagia and respiratory distress in myasthenic patients.
• Assess for early signs and symptoms of cinchonism, including blurred vision, confusion, diplopia, fever, headache, loss of hearing, and tinnitus, which may indicate quinine toxicity.
PATIENT TEACHING
• Instruct patient not to crush or chew quinine tablets; they taste bitter and can irritate the mouth and throat.
• Advise patient to take drug with food or after meals to minimize GI irritation.
• Urge patient to notify prescriber immediately if he experiences blurred or double vision, confusion, fever, headache, loss of hearing, or tinnitus, which are indicators of quinine toxicity.
• Advise patient to avoid potentially hazardous activities until he knows how quinine will affect his vision.

quinupristin and dalfopristin

Synercid

Class and Category
Chemical: Pristinamycin I and IIa derivative, streptogramin
Therapeutic: Antibiotic
Pregnancy category: B

Indications and Dosages
➤ To treat serious or life-threatening infections, such as bacteremia caused by vancomycin-resistant Enterococcus faecium

I.V. INFUSION
Adults and adolescents age 16 and older.
7.5 mg/kg q 8 hr.

➤ To treat complicated skin and soft-tissue infections caused by methicillin-susceptible strains of Staphylococcus aureus or Streptococcus pyogenes

I.V. INFUSION
Adults and adolescents age 16 and older.
7.5 mg/kg q 12 hr for at least 7 days.

Mechanism of Action
Inhibits bacterial protein synthesis by irreversibly blocking ribosome functioning.
   Quinupristin inhibits the late phase of protein synthesis by binding to the 50S ribosomal subunit. Dalfopristin inhibits the early phase of protein synthesis by binding to the 70S or 50S ribosomal subunit. Additionally, this combined activity inhibits transfer RNA (tRNA) synthetase activity, which decreases the amount of free tRNA within the cell. Without tRNA, the bacterial cell cannot incorporate amino acids into peptide chains, resulting in bacterial cell death.

Incompatibilities
Don't mix quinupristin and dalfopristin in saline solutions, including NS, .45NS, 3% sodium chloride, and 5% sodium chloride, because drug is physically incompatible with these solutions.

Contraindications
Hypersensitivity to quinupristin or dalfopristin, other streptogramin antibiotics, or their components

Interactions
DRUGS
alfentanil, alprazolam, carbamazepine, delavirdine, diazepam, diltiazem, disopyramide, dofetilide, donepezil, erythromycin, ethinyl estradiol, felodipine, fexofenadine, indinavir, lidocaine, lovastatin, methylprednisolone, nevirapine, norethindrone, quinidine, ritonavir, saquinavir, simvastatin, tacrolimus, triazolam, trimetrexate, verapamil, vinblastine: Decreased elimination of these drugs, possibly resulting in toxicity
astemizole, cisapride, terfenadine: Decreased elimination of these drugs, possibly prolonged QT interval
cyclosporine, midazolam, nifedipine, terfenadine: Possibly increased blood levels of these drugs

Adverse Reactions
CNS: Anxiety, confusion, dizziness, fever, headache, hypertonia, insomnia, paresthesia
CV: Chest pain, palpitations, peripheral edema, thrombophlebitis, vasodilation
EENT: Oral candidiasis, stomatitis
GI: Abdominal pain, constipation, diarrhea, elevated liver function test results, indigestion, nausea, pancreatitis, pseudomembranous colitis, vomiting
GU: Hematuria, vaginitis
MS: Arthralgia, gout, muscle spasms, myalgia, myasthenia
RESP: Dyspnea, pleural effusion
SKIN: Diaphoresis, pruritus, rash, urticaria
Other: Injection site edema, inflammation, pain, or thrombophlebitis

Nursing Considerations
• Store unopened vials of quinupristin and dalfopristin in refrigerator.
• **WARNING** Reconstitute and further dilute drug with dextrose in water or sterile water for injection only. Don't use saline solutions because drug is physically incompatible with them.
• Dilute prescribed dose in 250 ml dextrose 5% in water (D_5W), and infuse over 1 hour through a peripheral I.V. line. If administered by central venous catheter, dilute prescribed dose in 100 ml of D_5W. Central venous administration may decrease incidence of infusion site reaction. Use an infusion pump or device to control rate of infusion.
• Further dilute reconstituted solution within

30 minutes. Vials are for single use only. Discard any unused portion.
•Don't flush I.V. catheter with saline or heparin flush solution because of possible incompatibility. Flush I.V. catheter only with D$_5$W before and after drug administration.
•Monitor patient for diarrhea, a possible indication of overgrowth of normal intestinal flora, such as *Clostridium difficile*. Be aware that pseudomembranous colitis may result from a toxin produced by *C. difficile*.
•If you suspect that patient has pseudomembranous colitis, notify prescriber and expect to stop drug immediately.
•If patient develops pseudomembranous colitis, be aware that drugs that inhibit peristalsis are contraindicated because of the risk of toxic megacolon.

PATIENT TEACHING
•Instruct patient to complete the full course of quinupristin and dalfopristin therapy, as prescribed.
•Advise patient to notify prescriber at once if he develops diarrhea or abdominal pains.
•Inform patient that if he requires long-term therapy, drug will be given in hospital or clinic or by a home health care nurse.

rabeprazole sodium

AcipHex

Class and Category
Chemical: Substituted benzimidazole
Therapeutic: Antiulcer
Pregnancy category: B

Indications and Dosages
➤ *To provide short-term treatment of erosive esophagitis or ulcerative gastroesophageal reflux disease (GERD)*
DELAYED-RELEASE TABLETS
Adults. For mild to moderate disease, 20 mg q.d. for 4 to 8 wk; course may be repeated if healing has not occurred at the end of 8 wk. For severe reflux with ulceration or stricture formation, 40 mg q.d. for 4 to 8 wk.
➤ *To treat symptomatic GERD*
DELAYED-RELEASE TABLETS
Adults. 20 mg q.d. for 4 wk. Course may be repeated if symptoms aren't completely resolved.

➤ *To provide maintenance treatment of erosive esophagitis or GERD*
DELAYED-RELEASE TABLETS
Adults. 20 mg q.d.
➤ *To promote healing of duodenal ulcer, as adjunct to treat* Helicobacter pylori–*positive duodenal ulcer*
DELAYED-RELEASE TABLETS
Adults. 20 mg q.d. after breakfast for up to 4 wk for ulcer healing and for 2 wk when used in combination with antibiotic therapy to eradicate *H. pylori*.
➤ *To treat hypersecretory conditions, such as Zollinger-Ellison syndrome*
DELAYED-RELEASE TABLETS
Adults. *Initial:* 60 mg q.d.; may be increased, if needed, to 100 mg q.d. or 60 mg b.i.d.
DOSAGE ADJUSTMENT Dosage reduction may be necessary for patients with severe hepatic dysfunction.

Mechanism of Action
Decreases gastric acid secretion by suppressing its release at the secretory surface of gastric parietal cells. Rabeprazole also increases gastric pH and decreases basal acid output, which helps to heal ulcerated areas. In gastric parietal cells, it's transformed to an active sulfonamide, which increases the clearance rate of *Helicobacter pylori*, the underlying cause of some duodenal ulcers.

Contraindications
Hypersensitivity to rabeprazole, other substituted benzimidazoles (omeprazole, lansoprazole), or their components

Interactions
DRUGS
cyclosporine: Possibly inhibited cyclosporine metabolism
digoxin: Increased risk of digitalis toxicity

Adverse Reactions
CNS: Dizziness, headache, malaise
GI: Diarrhea, nausea, vomiting
SKIN: Rash

Nursing Considerations
•Use rabeprazole cautiously in patients with hepatic dysfunction.
•Monitor serum gastrin level during long-term therapy, as ordered, to detect elevations.
•Closely monitor Japanese men receiving rabeprazole for adverse reactions because

they're more likely than other patients to have increased blood drug levels.

PATIENT TEACHING
• Instruct patient to swallow delayed-release rabeprazole tablets whole.
• Inform patients with hypersecretory conditions, such as Zollinger-Ellison syndrome, that treatment can last as long as 1 year.
• Advise patient to avoid potentially hazardous activities until drug's CNS effects are known.

raloxifene hydrochloride

(keoxifene hydrochloride)

Evista

Class and Category

Chemical: Benzothiophene derivative
Therapeutic: Osteoporosis prophylactic
Pregnancy category: X

Indications and Dosages

➤ *To prevent osteoporosis in postmenopausal women*

TABLETS
Adults. 60 mg q.d.

Mechanism of Action

Prevents osteoporosis by binding to estrogen receptors, which decreases bone resorption and increases bone mineral density in postmenopausal women.

Contraindications

History of thromboembolic disease, hypersensitivity to raloxifene or its components, pregnancy

Interactions

DRUGS
ampicillin, cholestyramine: Decreased raloxifene absorption
warfarin: Possibly decreased PT

Adverse Reactions

CNS: Depression, fever, insomnia, migraine
CV: Chest pain, hot flashes, peripheral edema, thromboembolism
EENT: Laryngitis, pharyngitis, sinusitis
GI: Abdominal pain, flatulence, indigestion, nausea, vomiting

GU: Cystitis, infertility, leukorrhea, UTI, vaginitis
MS: Arthralgia, arthritis, leg cramps, myalgia
RESP: Cough, pneumonia
SKIN: Diaphoresis, rash
Other: Flulike symptoms, weight gain

Nursing Considerations

• **WARNING** Monitor distal extremities for impaired circulation and pain, which may indicate thromboembolism, during raloxifene therapy.
• Expect prescriber to discontinue drug at least 72 hours before and during periods of prolonged immobilization, such as after surgery and during bed rest. Resume drug as prescribed after patient is fully ambulatory.

PATIENT TEACHING
• Advise patient to avoid lengthy immobilization during travel while taking raloxifene because of the increased risk of thromboembolism.
• Instruct patient to report adverse reactions she experiences to prescriber.
• Stress the importance of compliance with long-term raloxifene therapy.

ramipril

Altace

Class and Category

Chemical: Ethylester of ramiprilat
Therapeutic: Antihypertensive
Pregnancy category: C (first trimester), D (later trimesters)

Indications and Dosages

➤ *To treat heart failure after MI*

CAPSULES
Adults. *Initial:* 1.25 to 2.5 mg b.i.d. *Maintenance:* 5 mg b.i.d.

➤ *To treat hypertension*

CAPSULES
Adults. *Initial:* 2.5 mg q.d. *Maintenance:* 2.5 to 20 mg q.d. or in divided doses b.i.d.
DOSAGE ADJUSTMENT Initial dosage reduced to 1.25 mg q.d. for patients who are dehydrated from prior diuretic therapy, those receiving diuretic therapy, and those with creatinine clearance of less than 40 ml/min/ 1.73 m^2; dosage then slowly increased until blood pressure is under control or maximum daily dose of 5 mg is reached.

Q
R
S

Route	Onset	Peak	Duration
P.O.	1 to 2 hr	4 to 6.5 hr	24 hr

Mechanism of Action
Blocks conversion of angiotensin I to angiotensin II, leading to vasodilation, and reduces aldosterone secretion, which prevents water retention. Ramipril also reduces peripheral arterial resistance. These combined actions lead to a reduction in blood pressure.

Contraindications
History of angioedema from earlier treatment with ACE inhibitor, hypersensitivity to ramipril or its components

Interactions
DRUGS
allopurinol, bone marrow depressants, corticosteroids (systemic), procainamide: Increased risk of fatal neutropenia or agranulocytosis
CNS depressants, other hypotension-producing drugs: Additive hypotensive effect
cyclosporine, potassium preparations, potassium-sparing diuretics: Possibly hyperkalemia
lithium: Increased risk of lithium toxicity
NSAIDs, sympathomimetics: Decreased antihypertensive effect of ramipril
tetracyclines: Reduced tetracycline absorption
FOODS
low-salt milk, salt substitutes: Increased risk of hyperkalemia
ACTIVITIES
alcohol use: Additive hypotensive effects

Adverse Reactions
CNS: Depression, dizziness, drowsiness, fatigue, fever, headache, insomnia, light-headedness, malaise, paresthesia, sleep disturbance, syncope, vertigo
CV: Chest pain, hypotension, orthostatic hypotension, palpitations, tachycardia
EENT: Amblyopia, dry mouth, loss of taste, pharyngitis
GI: Abdominal pain, constipation, diarrhea, nausea, vomiting
GU: Impotence
MS: Arthralgia, back pain, myalgia
RESP: Cough, dyspnea
SKIN: Alopecia, diaphoresis, flushing, photosensitivity, pruritus, rash, urticaria
Other: Angioedema

Nursing Considerations
• Use ramipril cautiously in patients with renal impairment.
• **WARNING** Be aware that patients with dehydration, heart failure, or hyponatremia; those who've recently received intensive diuresis or an increase in diuretic dosage; and those undergoing dialysis may be at risk for excessive hypotension. Maintain close supervision for the first 2 weeks of therapy and whenever ramipril or diuretic dosage increases. If excessive hypotension occurs, notify prescriber immediately, place patient in a supine position, and, if prescribed, infuse NS.
• **WARNING** Because of the risk of angioedema, be prepared to discontinue drug and administer emergency measures, including S.C. epinephrine 1:1,000 (0.3 to 0.5 ml), if swelling of tongue, glottis, or larynx causes airway obstruction.
• Monitor blood pressure frequently during therapy to assess drug's effectiveness.
PATIENT TEACHING
• Advise patient to stop taking ramipril and inform prescriber immediately if she experiences swelling of the face, eyes, lips, or tongue or has difficulty breathing.
• Explain that drug may cause dizziness and light-headedness, especially during first few days of therapy. Advise patient to avoid potentially hazardous activities until drug's CNS effects are known. Instruct her and a family member to use safety precautions and to notify prescriber immediately if patient faints.
• Inform female patient of childbearing age of the risks of taking ramipril during pregnancy, especially during the second and third trimesters. Caution patient to use effective contraception and to report known or suspected pregnancy immediately.
• Advise patient planning to undergo surgery or anesthesia to inform specialist that she's taking ramipril.
• Instruct patient to consult prescriber before using potassium supplements or salt substitutes containing potassium.

ranitidine hydrochloride
Apo-Ranitidine (CAN), Gen-Ranitidine (CAN), Novo-Ranitidine (CAN), Nu-Ranit (CAN), Zantac, Zantac EFFERdose Tablets, Zantac 150 GELdose, Zantac 300 GELdose

Class and Category

Chemical: Aminoalkyl-substituted puran derivative
Therapeutic: Antiulcer agent, gastric acid secretion inhibitor
Pregnancy category: B

Indications and Dosages

➤ *To prevent duodenal and gastric ulcers*
CAPSULES, EFFERVESCENT GRANULES, EFFERVESCENT TABLETS, SYRUP, TABLETS
Adults and adolescents. 150 mg h.s.
➤ *To provide short-term treatment of active duodenal and benign gastric ulcers*
CAPSULES, EFFERVESCENT GRANULES, EFFERVESCENT TABLETS, SYRUP, TABLETS
Adults and adolescents. 150 mg b.i.d. for gastric ulcers; 150 mg b.i.d. or 300 mg h.s. for duodenal ulcers.
Children. 2 to 4 mg/kg b.i.d. *Maximum:* 300 mg/day.
CONTINUOUS I.V. INFUSION
Adults and adolescents. 6.25 mg/hr. *Maximum:* 400 mg/day.
INTERMITTENT I.V. INFUSION
Adults and adolescents. 50 mg diluted to total volume of 100 ml and infused over 15 to 20 min q 6 to 8 hr. *Maximum:* 400 mg/day.
Children. 2 to 4 mg/kg/day diluted to a suitable volume and infused over 15 to 20 min.
I.V. INJECTION
Adults and adolescents. 50 mg diluted to total volume of 20 ml and injected slowly over no less than 5 min q 6 to 8 hr. *Maximum:* 400 mg/day.
I.M. INJECTION
Adults and adolescents. 50 mg q 6 to 8 hr. *Maximum:* 400 mg/day.
➤ *To treat acute gastroesophageal reflux disease*
CAPSULES, EFFERVESCENT GRANULES, EFFERVESCENT TABLETS, SYRUP, TABLETS
Adults and adolescents. 150 mg b.i.d.
Children. 2 to 8 mg/kg t.i.d.
INTERMITTENT I.V. INFUSION
Children. 2 to 8 mg/kg diluted to suitable volume and infused over 15 to 20 min t.i.d.
➤ *To treat erosive esophagitis*
CAPSULES, EFFERVESCENT GRANULES, EFFERVESCENT TABLETS, SYRUP, TABLETS
Adults and adolescents. 150 mg q.i.d.
➤ *To treat hypersecretory GI conditions, such as Zollinger-Ellison syndrome, systemic mastocytosis, and multiple endocrine adenoma syndrome*
CAPSULES, EFFERVESCENT GRANULES, EFFERVESCENT TABLETS, SYRUP, TABLETS
Adults and adolescents. *Initial:* 150 mg b.i.d., adjusted as needed. *Maximum:* 6 g/day in divided doses.
CONTINUOUS I.V. INFUSION
Adults and adolescents. *Initial:* 1 mg/kg/hr, increased by 0.5 mg/kg/hr up to 2.5 mg/kg/hr. *Maximum:* 400 mg/day.
INTERMITTENT I.V. INFUSION
Adults. 50 mg diluted to total volume of 100 ml and infused over 15 to 20 min q 6 to 8 hr. *Maximum:* 400 mg/day.
I.V. INJECTION
Adults and adolescents. 50 mg diluted to total volume of 20 ml and injected slowly over no less than 5 min q 6 to 8 hr. *Maximum:* 400 mg/day.
I.M. INJECTION
Adults. 50 mg q 6 to 8 hr.
➤ *To prevent acid indigestion, heartburn, and sour stomach*
TABLETS
Adults and adolescents. 75 mg 30 to 60 min before consuming food or beverages expected to cause symptoms. *Maximum:* 150 mg/day over no more than 2 continuous wk.
➤ *To treat acid indigestion, heartburn, and sour stomach*
TABLETS
Adults and adolescents. 75 mg at onset of symptoms; dosage repeated once within 24 hr, if needed.
DOSAGE ADJUSTMENT For patients with creatinine clearance of less than 50 ml/min/1.73 m^2, 150 mg P.O. q 24 hr with dosage interval increased thereafter to q 12 hr, as needed; or 50 mg I.V. q 18 to 24 hr with dosage interval increased thereafter to q 12 hr, as needed. Dosage reduction may also be necessary for patients with hepatic dysfunction.

Route	Onset	Peak	Duration
P.O., I.V., I.M.	Unknown	1 to 3 hr	13 hr

Contraindications

Acute porphyria, hypersensitivity to ranitidine or its components

Interactions

DRUGS
antacids: Decreased ranitidine absorption

bone marrow depressants: Increased risk of neutropenia or other blood dyscrasias
diazepam, itraconazole, ketoconazole, sucralfate: Decreased absorption of these drugs
glipizide, glyburide, metoprolol, midazolam, nifedipine, phenytoin, theophylline, warfarin: Increased effects of these drugs, possibly leading to toxic reactions

ACTIVITIES
alcohol use: Increased blood alcohol level (with oral ranitidine)

Mechanism of Action
Inhibits basal and nocturnal secretion of gastric acid and pepsin by competitively inhibiting the action of histamine at H_2 receptors on gastric parietal cells. This action reduces total volume of gastric juices and, thus, irritation of GI mucosa.

Adverse Reactions
CNS: Dizziness, drowsiness, headache, insomnia
CV: Vasculitis
GI: Abdominal distress, constipation, diarrhea, nausea, vomiting
GU: Impotence
MS: Arthralgia, myalgia
SKIN: Alopecia, erythema multiforme, rash

Nursing Considerations
•Be aware that ranitidine must be diluted for I.V. administration if premixed solution is not being used. For I.V. injection, dilute to total volume of 20 ml with NS, D_5W or $D_{10}W$, LR, or 5% sodium bicarbonate. For I.V. infusion, dilute to total volume of 100 ml of same solutions.
•Administer I.V. injection at no more than 4 ml/min, intermittent I.V. infusion at 5 to 7 ml/min, and continuous I.V. infusion at 6.25 mg/hr (except in patients with hypersecretory conditions, for whom initial infusion rate is 1 mg/kg/hr and then gradually increased after 4 hours, as needed, in increments of 0.5 mg/kg/hr).
•Don't add additives to premixed solution.
•Stop primary I.V. solution infusion during piggyback administration.

PATIENT TEACHING
•Instruct patient to dissolve ranitidine effervescent tablets or granules in 6 to 8 oz of water.
•Alert patient with phenylketonuria that effervescent tablets and granules contain phenylalanine.

•Inform patient that she may take drug with food.
•Advise patient to take antacids, if needed, 2 hours before or after taking ranitidine.
•Inform patient that healing of an ulcer may require 4 to 8 weeks of therapy.

rasburicase
Elitek

Class and Category
Chemical: Tetrameric protein
Therapeutic: Uric acid reducer
Pregnancy category: C

Indications and Dosages
➤ *To manage plasma uric acid levels initially in pediatric patients with leukemia, lymphoma, or solid tumor malignancies who receive anticancer therapy that elevates plasma uric acid*

I.V. INFUSION
Children. 0.15 or 0.20 mg/kg infused over 30 min q.d. for 5 days.

Mechanism of Action
Converts uric acid into an inactive and soluble metabolite at the end of the purine catabolic pathway. This prevents plasma uric acid levels from rising due to tumor lysis from anticancer therapy.

Contraindications
Glucose-6-phosphatase dehydrogenase (G6PD) deficiency; history of anaphylaxis or hypersensitivity reactions, hemolytic reactions, or methemoglobinemia reactions; hypersensitivity to rasburicase or its components

Interactions
None known

Adverse Reactions
CNS: Anxiety, fever, headache, paresthesia, rigors, seizures
CV: Arrhythmia, cardiac failure or arrest, cerebrovascular disorder, chest pain, hemorrhage, hypotension, myocardial infarction, pulmonary edema, thrombophlebitis, thrombosis
EENT: Mucositis, retinal hemorrhage
ENDO: Hot flashes

GI: Abdominal pain, constipation, diarrhea, ileus, intestinal obstruction, nausea, vomiting
GU: Acute renal failure
HEME: Anemia, hemolysis, methemoglobinemia, neutropenia, pancytopenia
RESP: Cyanosis, dyspnea, pneumonia, pulmonary hypertension, respiratory distress
SKIN: Cellulitis, rash
Other: Anaphylaxis, dehydration, infection, sepsis

Nursing Considerations
• Be aware that children at high risk for G6PD, such as patients of African or Mediterranean ancestry, should be screened before administering rasburicase because severe hemolysis can occur.
• Expect to administer only one course of therapy because of the high risk for severe allergic reactions.
• Reconstitute rasburicase using only the diluent provided. Add 1 ml of the diluent to each vial needed, and mix by swirling very gently. Don't shake vial or mix by turning it from top to bottom
• Inject reconstituted solution into an infusion bag containing the appropriate volume of 0.9% NaCl to obtain a final volume of 50 ml. Infuse over 30 minutes using a different line than for the infusion of other drugs. If a separate line isn't possible, flush the line with at least 15 ml of NS solution before and after rasburicase infusion. Don't use filters for the infusion.
• Store reconstituted solution at 2° to 8° C (36° to 46° F) for no longer than 24 hours. Protect drug from light.
• **WARNING** Monitor patient closely for severe hypersensitivity reactions including anaphylaxis (chest pain, dyspnea, hypotension, urticaria), hemolysis (severe anxiety, pain, dyspnea), and methemoglobinemia (anxiety, hypoxemia, shortness of breath). If any occur, discontinue rasburicase immediately, notify prescriber, and institute emergency treatment. Rasburicase shouldn't be reinstituted at any time after such a reaction occurs.
• Ensure that blood samples to measure uric acid levels are collected in pre-chilled tubes containing heparin anticoagulant and are immediately immersed and maintained in ice water until analysis is done (within 4 hours); blood samples left at room temperature will

result in low uric acid levels because of enzyme degradation of uric acid at room temperature.
PATIENT TEACHING
• Inform child and parents that chemotherapy will be started 4 to 24 hours after rasburicase administration.
• Stress the importance of reporting any adverse reaction immediately.

remifentanil hydrochloride
Ultiva

Class, Category, and Schedule
Chemical: Fentanyl analogue
Therapeutic: Anesthesia adjunct
Pregnancy category: C
Controlled substance: Schedule II

Indications and Dosages
➤ *As adjunct to induce general anesthesia*
INTERMITTENT I.V. INFUSION
Adults and children age 2 and older. 0.5 to 1 mcg/kg in addition to inhalation or I.V. anesthetic.
➤ *To maintain general anesthesia*
INTERMITTENT I.V. INFUSION
Adults and children age 2 and older. 0.05 to 0.2 mcg/kg, followed by 0.5 to 1 mcg/kg q 2 to 5 min, as needed.
➤ *To continue analgesic effect in immediate postoperative period*
CONTINUOUS I.V. INFUSION
Adults and children age 2 and older. *Initial:* 0.1 mcg/kg/min, adjusted by 0.025 mcg/kg/min q 5 min, as prescribed, to balance level of analgesia and respiratory rate. *Maximum:* 0.2 mcg/kg/min.
➤ *To supplement local or regional anesthesia in a monitored anesthetic setting*
I.V. INFUSION
Adults and children age 2 and older. *With a benzodiazepine:* 0.05 mcg/kg/min, beginning 5 min before placement of local or regional block; after placement of block, decreased to 0.025 mcg/kg/min and then further adjusted q 5 min in increments of 0.025 mcg/kg/min, as needed. *Without a benzodiazepine:* 0.1 mcg/kg/min, beginning 5 min before placement of local or regional block; after placement of block, decreased to 0.05 mcg/kg/min and then

further adjusted q 5 min in increments of 0.025 mcg/kg/min, as needed.

I.V. INJECTION

Adults and children age 2 and older. *With a benzodiazepine:* 0.5 mcg/kg administered over 30 to 60 sec as a single dose 60 to 90 sec before local anesthetic is administered. *Without a benzodiazepine:* 1 mcg/kg administered over 30 to 60 sec as a single dose 60 to 90 sec before local anesthetic is administered.

DOSAGE ADJUSTMENT For elderly patients, starting dose possibly reduced by one-half. For patients who weigh more than 30% over ideal body weight, starting dose based on ideal body weight.

Route	Onset	Peak	Duration
I.V.	1 min	1 to 2 min	5 to 10 min

Incompatibilities

Don't administer remifentanil through same I.V. line as blood because nonspecific esterases in blood products may inactivate drug.

Contraindications

Epidural or intrathecal administration, hypersensitivity to fentanyl analogues

Interactions

DRUGS

anesthetics (barbiturate, inhalation), benzodiazepines, propofol: Possibly synergistic effects, increasing risk of hypotension and respiratory depression

atropine, glycopyrrolate: Possibly reversal of remifentanil-induced bradycardia

ephedrine, epinephrine, norepinephrine: Possibly reversal of remifentanil-induced hypotension

neuromuscular blockers: Prolonged remifentanil-induced skeletal muscle rigidity

opioid antagonists: Possibly reversal of remifentanil's effects

Adverse Reactions

CNS: Headache
CV: Bradycardia, hypotension
GI: Nausea, vomiting
MS: Skeletal muscle rigidity
RESP: Apnea, dyspnea, respiratory depression

Nursing Considerations

•Inject remifentanil into I.V. tubing at or as close as possible to venous cannula.
•Use an infusion device to administer continuous infusion.

Mechanism of Action

Remifentanil decreases the transmission and perception of pain by stimulating mu-opioid receptors in neurons. This action decreases the activity of adenyl cyclase in neurons, which in turn decreases cAMP production. With less cAMP available, potassium (K^+) is forced out of neurons, and calcium (Ca^{++}) is prevented from entering neurons. As a result, neuron excitability declines, and fewer neurotransmitters (such as substance P) leave the neurons, thereby decreasing pain transmission.

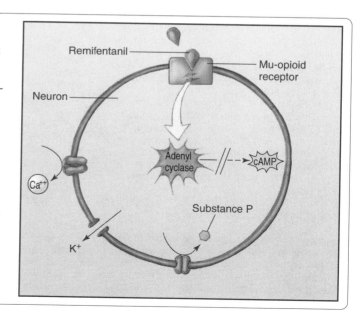

• Monitor vital signs and oxygenation continuously during administration.
• Expect analgesic effects to dissipate rapidly when drug is discontinued. Expect to start adequate postoperative analgesia, as prescribed, before stopping drug.
• WARNING After stopping drug, clear I.V. tubing to prevent inadvertent later administration.
• Monitor respiratory status continuously because of risk of respiratory depression from residual effects of other anesthetics for up to 30 minutes after infusion stops.

PATIENT TEACHING
• Explain expected drug effects to patient, and reassure her that she'll be monitored continuously during drug administration.

repaglinide

Prandin

Class and Category

Chemical: Meglitinide
Therapeutic: Antidiabetic drug
Pregnancy category: C

Indications and Dosages

➤ *To achieve glucose control in type 2 diabetes mellitus as monotherapy or in combination with metformin*

TABLETS
Adults. *Initial:* 0.5 mg 15 to 30 min before each meal. Dosage increased up to 4 mg according to glucose response. *Maximum:* 16 mg/day.
DOSAGE ADJUSTMENT For patients previously treated with a glucose-lowering drug, initial dosage increased to 1 to 2 mg. For patients with moderate to severe hepatic or renal impairment, interval between dosage adjustments increased.

Contraindications

Diabetic ketoacidosis, hypersensitivity to repaglinide or its components, severe hepatic or renal impairment, type 1 diabetes mellitus

Interactions

DRUGS
barbiturates, carbamazepine, rifampin, troglitazone: Possibly increased repaglinide metabolism
beta blockers, chloramphenicol, MAO inhibitors, NSAIDs, oral anticoagulants, probenecid, salicylates, sulfonamides: Enhanced hypoglycemic effects of repaglinide

calcium channel blockers, corticosteroids, diuretics, estrogens, isoniazid, niacin, oral contraceptives, phenothiazines, phenytoin, sympathomimetics, thyroid hormones: Possibly loss of glucose control
erythromycin, ketoconazole, miconazole: Possibly inhibited repaglinide metabolism

Mechanism of Action

Stimulates the release of insulin from functioning pancreatic beta cells. In patients with type 2 diabetes mellitus, a shortage of functioning beta cells diminishes blood levels of insulin and causes glucose intolerance. By interacting with the adenosine triphosphatase (ATP)-potassium channel on the beta cell membrane, repaglinide prevents potassium (K^+) from leaving the cell. This causes the beta cell to depolarize and the cell membrane's calcium channel to open. As a result, calcium (Ca^{++}) moves into the cell and insulin moves out of it. The extent of insulin release is glucose dependent; the lower the glucose level, the less insulin is secreted from the cell.

Adverse Reactions

CNS: Headache
EENT: Rhinitis, sinusitis
ENDO: Hypoglycemia
GI: Diarrhea, nausea
MS: Arthralgia, back pain
RESP: Bronchitis, upper respiratory tract infection

Nursing Considerations

• Administer repaglinide 15 to 30 minutes before each meal.
• Be aware that some patients with type 2 diabetes mellitus may also receive metformin as an adjunct to repaglinide therapy.
• Expect to check glycosylated hemoglobin (HbA_{1c}) level every 3 months, as ordered, until patient's blood glucose level is controlled to assess long-term glucose control.
• During periods of increased stress, such as infection, surgery, and trauma, monitor blood glucose level frequently to detect hyperglycemia and assess the need for supplemental insulin.

PATIENT TEACHING
• Instruct patient to take repaglinide 15 to 30 minutes before meals and to skip dose whenever she skips a meal.

Q
R
S

•Explain that repaglinide is an adjunct to diet in managing type 2 diabetes mellitus.
•Emphasize the continued need for exercise, diet, hygiene, foot care, and avoiding infection.
•Teach patient how to monitor her blood glucose level and when to notify prescriber.
•Review signs and symptoms of hyperglycemia and hypoglycemia with patient and family. Instruct patient to notify prescriber immediately if she experiences anxiety, confusion, dizziness, excessive sweating, headache, increased thirst, increased urination, or nausea.
•Advise patient to carry identification indicating that she has diabetes. Encourage her to carry candy or other simple carbohydrates with her to treat mild episodes of hypoglycemia.
•Inform patient that her HbA$_{1c}$ level will be tested every 3 to 6 months until her blood glucose level is controlled.

reserpine

Novoreserpine (CAN), Reserfia (CAN), Serpalan, Serpasil (CAN)

Class and Category
Chemical: Rauwolfia alkaloid
Therapeutic: Antihypertensive
Pregnancy category: C

Indications and Dosages
➤ *To treat hypertension*
TABLETS
Adults. 0.1 to 0.25 mg q.d.
Children. 0.005 to 0.02 mg/kg/day q.d. or in divided doses b.i.d.
DOSAGE ADJUSTMENT Lower dosage possibly required for elderly or severely debilitated patients.

Route	Onset	Peak	Duration
P.O.	Days to 3 wk	3 to 6 wk	1 to 6 wk

Mechanism of Action

Reserpine reduces blood pressure by decreasing norepinephrine stores in presynaptic sympathetic neurons.

Normally, when a nerve impulse activates a sympathetic neuron, the nerve ending releases norepinephrine, which stimulates alpha or beta receptors on target cell membranes, as shown below left. Stimulation of alpha receptors may produce vasoconstriction; stimulation of beta receptors may increase the heart rate and force of myocardial contraction, which raises cardiac output. Through a reuptake mechanism, some norepinephrine returns to the neuron and is stored in vesicles for reuse.

Reserpine displaces norepinephrine from vesicles in the nerve fiber, and MAO degrades the displaced norepinephrine, as shown below right. These actions reduce the amount of norepinephrine available to stimulate postsynaptic alpha and beta receptors, leading to a reduction in vasoconstriction, cardiac output, and blood pressure.

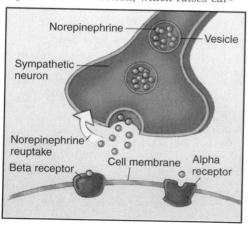

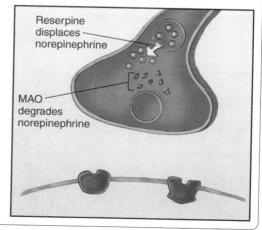

Contraindications

Active peptic ulcer, electroconvulsive therapy, hypersensitivity to reserpine or its components, mental depression (current or history of), ulcerative colitis

Interactions

DRUGS

anticholinergics: Decreased effectiveness of anticholinergics
barbiturates: Increased CNS depression
beta blockers: Additive and, possibly, excessive beta-adrenergic blockade
bromocriptine: Possibly interference with bromocriptine's effects
digoxin, procainamide, quinidine: Increased risk of arrhythmias
hypotension-producing drugs: Increased antihypertensive effect; increased risk of orthostatic hypotension or bradycardia (with guanadrel or guanethidine)
levodopa: Decreased levodopa effectiveness
MAO inhibitors: Increased risk of severe hypertension and hyperpyrexia, additive CNS depression
NSAIDs: Decreased antihypertensive effect
sympathomimetics: Increased vasopressor effects, decreased antihypertensive effect

ACTIVITIES

alcohol use: Increased CNS depression

Adverse Reactions

CNS: Anxiety, depression, dizziness, drowsiness, headache, nervousness, nightmares, sleep disturbance, syncope, weakness
CV: Arrhythmias, such as bradycardia; chest pain; peripheral edema
EENT: Conjunctival injection, dry mouth, epistaxis, glaucoma, hearing loss, nasal congestion, optic atrophy, uveitis
ENDO: Breast engorgement
GI: Abdominal cramps or pain, anorexia, diarrhea, increased gastric secretions, melena, nausea, vomiting
GU: Decreased libido, galactorrhea, gynecomastia, impotence
MS: Myalgia
RESP: Dyspnea
SKIN: Purpura
Other: Weight gain

Nursing Considerations

• Use reserpine cautiously in patients with a history of depression because drug may cause depression that is masked as somatic complaints.
• Monitor blood pressure frequently during drug therapy.
• Alert anesthesiologist if patient is scheduled for surgery. Drug may cause circulatory instability even if withheld before procedure.

PATIENT TEACHING

• Instruct patient to take reserpine with food or milk to minimize stomach upset.
• Caution patient about possible drowsiness, and advise her to avoid potentially hazardous activities until drug's CNS effects are known.
• Explain the need for frequent appointments to monitor blood pressure and adjust dosage at start of therapy.

reteplase

Retavase

Class and Category

Chemical: Recombinant plasminogen activator (r-PA)
Therapeutic: Thrombolytic
Pregnancy category: C

Indications and Dosages

➤ *To improve ventricular function, prevent heart failure, and reduce mortality after acute MI*

I.V. INJECTION

Adults. 10 U over 2 min; repeated after 30 min.

Mechanism of Action

Converts plasminogen to plasmin, which works to break up fibrin clots that have formed in the coronary arteries. Elimination of the clots improves cardiac blood and oxygen flow to the area, thus improving ventricular function.

Incompatibilities

Don't add other drugs to reteplase injection solution or administer them through same I.V. line as reteplase.

Contraindications

Active internal bleeding, aneurysm, arteriovenous malformation, bleeding diathesis, brain tumor, history of CVA or other cerebrovascular disease, hypersensitivity to reteplase or its components, intracranial or intraspinal surgery

Q
R
S

or trauma during previous 2 months, severe uncontrolled hypertension (systolic 200 mm Hg or higher, diastolic 110 mm Hg or higher)

Interactions
DRUGS
antifibrinolytics (including aminocaproic acid, aprotinin, and tranexamic acid): Decreased effectiveness of reteplase
antineoplastics, antithymocyte globulin, certain cephalosporins (such as cefamandole, cefoperazone, and cefotetan), heparin, oral anticoagulants, platelet aggregation inhibitors (such as abciximab, aspirin, and dipyridamole), strontium-89 chloride, sulfinpyrazone, valproic acid: Increased risk of bleeding

Adverse Reactions
CNS: Intracranial hemorrhage
GI: GI bleeding, nausea, vomiting
HEME: Thrombocytopenia
RESP: Hemoptysis
SKIN: Bleeding from wounds, ecchymosis, hematoma, purpura
Other: Allergic reaction, injection site bleeding

Nursing Considerations
•Expect to begin reteplase therapy, as prescribed, as soon as possible after MI symptoms begin.
•Closely monitor patient with atrial fibrillation, severe hypertension, or other cardiac disease for signs and symptoms of cerebral embolism.
•To reconstitute, use diluent, syringe, needle, and dispensing pin provided. Withdraw 10 ml of preservative-free sterile water for injection. Remove and discard needle from syringe, and connect dispensing pin to syringe. Remove protective cap from spike end of dispensing pin, and insert spike into reteplase vial. Inject 10 ml of sterile water into the vial. With the spike still in the vial, swirl gently to dissolve the powder. Don't shake. Expect to see slight foaming. Let the vial stand for several minutes. When the bubbles dissipate, withdraw 10 ml of reconstituted solution into the syringe (about 0.7 ml may remain in the vial). Now detach the syringe from the dispensing pin and attach the 20G needle.
•Use the solution within 4 hours. Discard if it's discolored or contains particulates.
•Don't administer heparin and reteplase in the same solution. Instead, flush the heparin line with NS or D$_5$W before and after reteplase injection.

•Because fibrin is lysed during therapy, closely monitor all possible bleeding sites (catheter insertions, arterial and venous punctures, cutdowns, and needle punctures).
•Avoid I.M. injections, venipunctures, and nonessential handling of patient during therapy.
•If arterial puncture is necessary, use an arm vessel that can be compressed, if possible. After sample is obtained, apply pressure for at least 30 minutes, and then apply a pressure dressing. Check site frequently for bleeding.
•If bleeding occurs and can't be controlled by local pressure, notify prescriber immediately. Be prepared to stop concurrent anticoagulant therapy immediately and to discontinue second reteplase bolus, as prescribed.
•Anticipate that reperfusion arrhythmias—premature ventricular contractions, ventricular tachycardia—may follow coronary thrombolysis.
PATIENT TEACHING
•Advise patient to report adverse reactions immediately.

rifabutin

Mycobutin

Class and Category
Chemical: Spiropiperidyl derivative
Therapeutic: Antimycobacterial antibiotic
Pregnancy category: B

Indications and Dosages
➤ *To prevent disseminated* Mycobacterium avium *complex in patients with advanced HIV infection*
CAPSULES
Adults. 300 mg q.d. or 150 mg b.i.d.

> ### Mechanism of Action
> Suppresses RNA synthesis by inhibiting DNA-dependent RNA polymerase in a wide variety of bacteria, including *Mycobacterium avium*. Exhibits dose-dependent bactericidal or bacteriostatic action.

Contraindications
Hypersensitivity to rifabutin or rifamycins

Interactions
DRUGS
aminophylline, barbiturates, beta blockers, chloramphenicol, clofibrate, corticosteroids, cyclosporine, dapsone, diazepam, digoxin,

disopyramide, estramustine, estrogens, keto-conazole, mexiletine, oral anticoagulants, oral antidiabetic drugs, oral contraceptives (containing estrogen), oxtriphylline, pheny-toin, quinidine, theophylline, tocainide, ve-rapamil (oral): Reduced therapeutic effects of these drugs
fluconazole: Increased blood rifabutin level
methadone: Possibly withdrawal symptoms
zidovudine: Decreased blood zidovudine level

Adverse Reactions

CNS: Asthenia, fever, headache, insomnia
CV: Chest pain
EENT: Discolored saliva, tears, and sputum
GI: Abdominal pain, anorexia, diarrhea, dis-colored feces, elevated liver function test re-sults, eructation, flatulence, indigestion, nau-sea, vomiting
GU: Discolored urine
HEME: Neutropenia, thrombocytopenia
MS: Myalgia
SKIN: Discolored skin and sweat, rash

Nursing Considerations

• Monitor laboratory values during rifabutin therapy to detect neutropenia and thrombo-cytopenia.
• Expect drug to cause reddish orange to red-dish brown discoloration of skin and body fluids.
• Be aware that drug may cause myelosup-pression and increased risk of infection. No-tify prescriber immediately if signs of infec-tion, such as fever, develop.

PATIENT TEACHING
• Advise patient to take rifabutin with food if GI distress develops.
• Encourage patient to have any necessary den-tal work done before rifabutin therapy starts to reduce the risk of bleeding or infection.
• Explain that drug may turn urine, feces, saliva, sputum, sweat, tears, and skin red-dish orange to reddish brown.
• Caution patient against wearing soft con-tact lenses during therapy because drug may permanently stain them.
• Advise patient to notify prescriber about signs of Mycobacterium avium complex (chills, fever, night sweats, weight loss), tu-berculosis, myositis, or uveitis.
• Advise woman of childbearing age who is using an oral contraceptive to change to a nonhormonal method of birth control be-cause rifabutin may decrease contraceptive's effectiveness.

rifampin

(rifampicin)

Rifadin, Rifadin IV, Rimactane, Rofact (CAN)

Class and Category

Chemical: Semisynthetic antibiotic derivative of rifamycin
Therapeutic: Antimycobacterial antitubercular
Pregnancy category: C

Indications and Dosages

➤ *As adjunct to treat tuberculosis caused by all strains of* Mycobacterium tuberculosis

CAPSULES, ORAL SUSPENSION, I.V. INFUSION
Adults. 10 mg/kg q.d. in combination with other antitubercular drugs for 2 mo. *Maxi-mum:* 600 mg/day.
Infants and children. 10 to 20 mg/kg q.d. in combination with other antitubercular drugs for 2 mo. *Maximum:* 600 mg/day.

➤ *To eliminate meningococci from naso-pharynx of asymptomatic carriers of* Neisseria meningitidis

CAPSULES, ORAL SUSPENSION, I.V. INFUSION
Adults. 600 mg q 12 hr for 2 days (total of 4 doses).
Infants age 1 month and older and children. 10 mg/kg q 12 hr for 2 days (total of 4 doses). *Maximum:* 600 mg/day.
Infants under age 1 month. 5 mg/kg q 12 hr for 2 days (total of 4 doses). *Maximum:* 600 mg/day.

DOSAGE ADJUSTMENT For patients with he-patic impairment, maximum dosage of 8 mg/kg/day. For patients with creatinine clear-ance of 10 ml/min/1.73 m² or less, recom-mended dosage usually decreased by 50%.

Mechanism of Action

Inhibits bacterial and mycobacterial RNA synthesis by binding to DNA-dependent RNA polymerase, thereby blocking RNA transcription. Exhibits dose-dependent bac-tericidal or bacteriostatic action. Rifampin is highly effective against rapidly dividing bacilli in extracellular cavitary lesions, such as those found in the nasopharynx.

Incompatibilities

Don't administer rifampin in the same I.V. line as diltiazem.

Q
R
S

Contraindications

Concurrent use of nonnucleoside reverse transcriptase inhibitors or protease inhibitors (by patients with HIV), hypersensitivity to rifamycins

Interactions

DRUGS

aminophylline, oxtriphylline, theophylline: Increased metabolism and clearance of these theophylline preparations

anesthetics (hydrocarbon inhalation, except isoflurane), hepatotoxic drugs, isoniazid: Increased risk of hepatotoxicity

beta blockers, chloramphenicol, clofibrate, corticosteroids, cyclosporine, dapsone, digitalis glycosides, disopyramide, hexobarbital, itraconazole, ketoconazole, mexiletine, oral anticoagulants, oral antidiabetic drugs, phenytoin, propafenone, quinidine, tocainide, verapamil (oral): Increased metabolism, resulting in lower blood levels of these drugs

bone marrow depressants: Increased leukopenic or thrombocytopenic effects

clofazimine: Reduced absorption of rifampin, delaying its peak concentration and increasing its half-life

diazepam: Enhanced elimination of diazepam, resulting in decreased drug effectiveness

estramustine, estrogens, oral contraceptives: Decreased estrogenic effects

methadone: Possibly impaired absorption of methadone, leading to withdrawal symptoms

probenecid: Increased blood level or prolonged duration of rifampin, increasing risk of toxicity

nonnucleoside reverse transcriptase inhibitors, protease inhibitors (indinavir, nelfinavir, ritonavir, saquinavir): Accelerated metabolism of these drugs (by patients with HIV), resulting in subtherapeutic levels; delayed metabolism of rifampin, increasing risk of toxicity

trimethoprim: Increased elimination and shortened elimination half-life of trimethoprim

ACTIVITIES

alcohol use: Increased risk of hepatotoxicity

Adverse Reactions

CNS: Chills, dizziness, drowsiness, fatigue, headache, paresthesia

EENT: Discolored saliva, tears, and sputum; mouth or tongue soreness; periorbital edema

GI: Abdominal cramps, anorexia, diarrhea, discolored feces, elevated liver function test results, epigastric discomfort, flatulence, heartburn, hepatitis, nausea, pseudomembranous colitis, vomiting

GU: Discolored urine

MS: Arthralgia, myalgia

SKIN: Discolored skin and sweat

Other: Facial edema, flulike symptoms

Nursing Considerations

- Obtain blood samples or other specimens for culture and sensitivity testing, as ordered, before giving rifampin and throughout therapy to monitor response to drug.
- Expect to monitor liver function test results before therapy and every 2 to 4 weeks during therapy. Notify prescriber immediately of abnormalities.
- For I.V. infusion, reconstitute by adding 10 ml of sterile water for injection to 600-mg vial of rifampin. Swirl gently to dissolve. Withdraw appropriate dose and add to 500 ml of D_5W (preferred solution) or NS and infuse over 3 hours. Alternatively, withdraw appropriate dose and add to 100 ml of D_5W (preferred solution) or NS and infuse over 30 minutes. Use reconstituted drug promptly because rifampin may precipitate out of D_5W solution after 4 hours. NS solution is stable for up to 24 hours at room temperature.
- Be aware that patient receiving intermittent therapy (once or twice weekly) is at increased risk for adverse reactions.
- Expect drug to cause reddish orange to reddish brown discoloration of skin and body fluids.
- Be aware that rifampin can cause myelosuppression and increase risk of infection. Notify prescriber immediately if signs of infection, such as fever, develop.

PATIENT TEACHING

- Instruct patient to take rifampin 1 hour before or 2 hours after a meal with a full glass of water.
- Stress the need to take drug exactly as prescribed. Explain that interruptions can lead to increased adverse reactions.
- Explain that drug may turn urine, feces, saliva, sputum, sweat, tears, and skin reddish orange to reddish brown.
- Caution patient against wearing soft contact lenses during therapy because drug may permanently stain them.
- Advise patient who takes an oral contraceptive to use an additional form of birth control during rifampin therapy.

• Urge patient to notify prescriber about flu-like symptoms, anorexia, darkened urine, fever, joint pain or swelling, malaise, nausea, vomiting, and yellowish skin or eyes, which may indicate hepatitis.
• Advise patient to avoid alcohol during rifampin therapy.
• Instruct patient to notify prescriber if no improvement occurs within 2 to 3 weeks.

riluzole

Rilutek

Class and Category

Chemical: Benzothiazole
Therapeutic: Amyotrophic lateral sclerosis treatment agent
Pregnancy category: C

Indications and Dosages

➤ *To treat amyotrophic lateral sclerosis*
TABLETS
Adults. 50 mg q 12 hr.

Mechanism of Action

Inhibits release of glutamate (glutamic acid), an excitatory amino acid neurotransmitter, in the CNS, thus reducing glutamate's effects on target cells. Glutamic acid is believed to play a role in the degeneration of neurons that occurs in amyotrophic lateral sclerosis; thus, reducing the glutamate level may help to slow the disease.

Contraindications

Hypersensitivity to riluzole or its components

Interactions

DRUGS
allopurinol, hepatotoxic drugs, methyldopa, sulfasalazine: Increased risk of hepatotoxicity
amitriptyline, phenacetin, quinolones, tacrine, theophylline: Delayed elimination of riluzole
omeprazole, rifampin: Increased riluzole clearance
FOODS
charbroiled foods: Increased riluzole elimination
ACTIVITIES
alcohol use: Increased risk of hepatotoxicity
smoking: Increased riluzole elimination

Adverse Reactions

CNS: Asthenia, dizziness, headache, insomnia, paresthesia (circumoral), somnolence, spasticity, vertigo

CV: Peripheral edema
EENT: Dry mouth, rhinitis, stomatitis
GI: Abdominal pain, anorexia, constipation, diarrhea, elevated liver function test results, flatulence, indigestion, nausea, vomiting
HEME: Neutropenia
MS: Back or muscle pain or stiffness
RESP: Dyspnea, increased cough, pneumonia
SKIN: Alopecia, eczema, pruritus

Nursing Considerations

• Use riluzole cautiously in patients with impaired hepatic or renal function.
• Also use cautiously in elderly patients, women, and Japanese patients because of increased risk of toxicity from decreased drug clearance.
• Monitor liver function test results before and during riluzole therapy.
PATIENT TEACHING
• Instruct patient to take riluzole regularly, every 12 hours, 1 hour before or 2 hours after a meal, and at the same time each day.
• Instruct patient to store riluzole at room temperature, protected from bright light.
• Encourage patient to avoid excessive alcohol, smoking, and charboiled foods because they cause drug to be excreted faster.
• Advise patient to notify prescriber if he develops a fever.

risedronate sodium

Actonel

Class and Category

Chemical: Pyridinyl bisphosphonate
Therapeutic: Bone resorption inhibitor
Pregnancy category: C

Indications and Dosages

➤ *To treat Paget's disease of bone when serum alkaline phosphatase level is at least twice normal and patient is symptomatic or at risk for complications*
TABLETS
Adults. 30 mg q.d. for 2 mo. Repeated after 2-mo observation period if relapse occurs or if serum alkaline phosphatase level fails to normalize.

➤ *To prevent or treat postmenopausal or glucocorticoid-induced osteoporosis*
TABLETS
Adults. 5 mg q.d. Alternatively, for postmenopausal osteoporosis, 35 mg once/wk.

Q
R
S

Route	Onset	Peak	Duration
P.O.	Unknown	3 mo	16 mo

Mechanism of Action
Hinders excessive bone remodeling characteristic of Paget's disease by binding to bone and reducing the rate at which osteoclasts are resorbed by bone.

Contraindications
Hypersensitivity to risedronate or its components, hypocalcemia

Interactions
DRUGS
aspirin, NSAIDs: Increased risk of GI irritation
calcium-containing preparations, including antacids: Impaired absorption of risedronate
FOODS
all foods: Decreased risedronate bioavailability

Adverse Reactions
CNS: Dizziness, headache, weakness
CV: Chest pain, peripheral edema
EENT: Amblyopia, dry eyes, sinusitis, tinnitus
GI: Abdominal pain, colitis, constipation, diarrhea, eructation, nausea
MS: Arthralgia, leg cramps, myasthenia
RESP: Bronchitis
SKIN: Rash
Other: Flulike symptoms

Nursing Considerations
•Administer supplemental calcium and vitamin D, as prescribed, during risedronate therapy if patient's dietary intake of these nutrients is inadequate.
•Give calcium supplements and antacids at different time of day than risedronate administration to avoid impaired drug absorption and altered effectiveness.
PATIENT TEACHING
•Instruct patient to take risedronate at least 1 hour before first food or drink of day (except water) while in an upright position and with 6 to 8 oz of water. Caution against lying down for at least 30 minutes after taking drug to prevent it from lodging in esophagus and causing irritation.
•Advise patient to take calcium supplements or antacids at different time of day than risedronate.

risperidone
Risperdal

Class and Category
Chemical: Benzisoxazole derivative
Therapeutic: Antipsychotic
Pregnancy category: C

Indications and Dosages
➤ *To manage psychotic disorders*
ORAL SOLUTION, TABLETS
Adults. 1 mg b.i.d. on day 1; 2 mg b.i.d. on day 2; 3 mg b.i.d. on day 3. Alternatively, 0.5 to 1 mg b.i.d., increased as needed q 3 to 5 days until total daily dose of 4 to 8 mg is reached. Daily dosage then increased by 1 to 2 mg at 1- to 2-wk intervals, as needed. *Maximum:* 16 mg/day.
DOSAGE ADJUSTMENT Initial dose limited to 0.5 mg b.i.d. for elderly or debilitated patients, those with renal or hepatic impairment, and those at increased risk for hypotension, then increased by 0.5 mg b.i.d. q wk, as needed. Dosage given q.d. after target dosage has been maintained for 2 or 3 days. Maximum for patients with severe hepatic dysfunction, 4 mg/day; for elderly patients, 3 mg/day.

Mechanism of Action
Selectively blocks serotonin and dopamine receptors in the mesocortical tract of the CNS to suppress psychotic symptoms.

Incompatibilities
Don't mix risperidone oral solution with cola or tea.

Contraindications
Hypersensitivity to risperidone or its components

Interactions
DRUGS
antihypertensives: Increased antihypertensive effects
bromocriptine, levodopa, pergolide: Possibly antagonized effects of these drugs
carbamazepine: Increased risperidone clearance with long-term concurrent use
clozapine: Decreased risperidone clearance with long-term concurrent use
CNS depressants: Additive CNS depression

ACTIVITIES
alcohol use: Additive CNS depression

Adverse Reactions
CNS: Aggressiveness, agitation, anxiety, asthenia, decreased concentration, dizziness, dream disturbances, drowsiness, dystonia, fatigue, headache, lassitude, memory loss, nervousness, neuroleptic malignant syndrome, parkinsonism, restlessness, somnolence
CV: Chest pain, orthostatic hypotension, palpitations, tachycardia
EENT: Decreased or increased salivation, dry mouth, pharyngitis, rhinitis, sinusitis, vision changes
ENDO: Galactorrhea
GI: Abdominal pain, constipation, diarrhea, indigestion, nausea, vomiting
GU: Amenorrhea, decreased libido, dysmenorrhea, dysuria, hypermenorrhea, polyuria, sexual dysfunction
MS: Arthralgia, back pain
RESP: Cough, dyspnea
SKIN: Diaphoresis, dry skin, hyperpigmentation, photosensitivity, pruritus, rash, seborrhea
Other: Weight gain or loss

Nursing Considerations
•Use risperidone cautiously in patients with hepatic or renal dysfunction or hypotension and in debilitated or elderly patients because of their increased sensitivity to drug.
•Monitor for orthostatic hypotension, especially in patients with cardiac or cerebrovascular disease.
•**WARNING** Immediately notify prescriber and be prepared to stop drug if patient shows signs of neuroleptic malignant syndrome (altered mental status, autonomic instability, hyperpyrexia, muscle rigidity), which can be fatal.

PATIENT TEACHING
•Instruct patient to dilute risperidone oral solution with water, coffee, orange juice, or low-fat milk but not with cola or tea.
•Advise patient to avoid potentially hazardous activities until drug's CNS effects are known and to rise slowly from a lying or sitting position to minimize effects of orthostatic hypotension.
•Urge patient to avoid alcohol because of its additive CNS effects.

rivastigmine tartrate
Exelon

Class and Category
Chemical: Carbamate derivative
Therapeutic: Antidementia
Pregnancy category: B

Indications and Dosages
➤ *To treat mild to moderate Alzheimer's-type dementia*
CAPSULES
Adults. *Initial:* 1.5 mg b.i.d. Dosage increased by 3 mg/day q 2 wk, as needed. *Maximum:* 12 mg/day.
DOSAGE ADJUSTMENT If patient develops nausea or vomiting during therapy, treatment should be discontinued for several doses, as prescribed, and restarted at lowest dose and increased by 3 mg/day q 2 wk, as needed.

Mechanism of Action
May slow the decline of cognitive function in patients with Alzheimer's disease by increasing the concentration of acetylcholine at cholinergic transmission sites. This action prolongs and exaggerates the effects of acetylcholine that are otherwise blocked by toxic levels of anticholinergics. The cognitive decline in these patients is partially related to cholinergic deficits along neuronal pathways projecting from the basal forebrain to the cerebral cortex and hippocampus that are involved in memory, attention, learning, and cognition. Rivastigmine, a cholinesterase inhibitor, may inhibit the destruction of acetylcholine by cholinesterase, thereby slowing the disease process.

Contraindications
Hypersensitivity to carbamate derivatives, rivastigmine, or their components

Interactions
DRUGS
anticholinergics: Possibly decreased effectiveness of anticholinergics
bethanechol, succinylcholine: Possibly synergistic effects

Adverse Reactions
CNS: Aggression, anxiety, asthenia, confusion, depression, dizziness, fatigue, fever,

hallucinations, headache, insomnia, malaise, seizures, somnolence, tremor
CV: Hypertension
EENT: Rhinitis
GI: Abdominal pain, anorexia, constipation, diarrhea, flatulence, indigestion, nausea, vomiting
GU: UTI
SKIN: Increased sweating
Other: Flulike symptoms, weight loss

Nursing Considerations

•**WARNING** Be aware that rivastigmine should be started at lowest recommended dosage and adjusted to an effective maintenance dosage because initial therapy at high dosage can cause serious adverse GI reactions, including anorexia, nausea, and weight loss. Also, higher than recommended starting dosage may cause severe vomiting and possibly esophageal rupture. If treatment is interrupted for longer than several days, expect to restart drug at lowest recommended dosage.
•Be aware that drug shouldn't be discontinued abruptly because doing so may increase behavioral disturbances and precipitate a further decline in cognitive function.
•Monitor respiratory status of patients with pulmonary disease, including asthma, chronic bronchitis, and emphysema, because rivastigmine has a weak affinity for peripheral cholinesterase, which may increase bronchoconstriction and bronchial secretions.
•Monitor patient for adequate urine output because cholinomimetics, such as rivastigmine, may induce or exacerbate urinary tract or bladder obstruction.
•Monitor patients with Parkinson's disease for exaggerated parkinsonian symptoms, which may result from drug's increased cholinergic effects on CNS.

PATIENT TEACHING

•Explain to patient and family that rivastigmine can't cure Alzheimer's disease but may slow the progressive deterioration of memory and improve patient's ability to perform activities of daily living.
•Advise patient and family that drug should be taken with food to reduce adverse GI effects.
•Instruct a family member to supervise patient's use of rivastigmine.
•Urge caregiver to contact prescriber and to withhold drug if patient stops taking it for more than several days.

rizatriptan benzoate

Maxalt, Maxalt-MLT

Class and Category

Chemical: Selective 5-hydroxytryptamine
Therapeutic: Antimigraine
Pregnancy category: C

Indications and Dosages

➤ *To relieve acute migraine headache*
DISINTEGRATING TABLETS, TABLETS
Adults. 5 to 10 mg when migraine starts; repeated q 2 hr, p.r.n. *Maximum:* 30 mg/day.
DOSAGE ADJUSTMENT For patients taking propranolol, initial dosage reduced to 5 mg, then repeated q 2 hr, p.r.n., up to maximum of 15 mg/day.

Mechanism of Action

Binds to selective 5-hydroxytryptamine receptor sites on cerebral blood vessels, causing vessels to constrict. This may decrease the characteristic pulsing sensation and thus relieve the pain of migraines. Rizatriptan also may relieve pain by inhibiting the release of proinflammatory neuropeptides and reducing transmission of trigeminal nerve impulses from sensory nerve endings during a migraine attack.

Contraindications

Basilar or hemiplegic migraine, hypersensitivity to rizatriptan or its components, ischemic coronary artery disease, uncontrolled hypertension, use within 14 days of MAO inhibitor therapy, use within 24 hours of other serotonin-receptor agonists or ergotamine-containing or ergot-type drugs

Interactions
DRUGS

ergot-containing drugs: Prolonged vasospastic reactions
MAO inhibitors, propranolol: Increased blood rizatriptan level
selective serotonin-reuptake inhibitors: Increased risk of weakness, hyperreflexia, and lack of coordination
serotonin-receptor agonists: Additive vasospastic effects

Adverse Reactions
CNS: Altered temperature sensation, anxiety, asthenia, ataxia, chills, confusion, depres-

sion, disorientation, dizziness, dream disturbances, drowsiness, euphoria, fatigue, hangover, headache, hypoesthesia, insomnia, mental impairment, nervousness, paresthesia, somnolence, tremor, vertigo
CV: Arrhythmias, such as bradycardia and tachycardia; chest pain; hot flashes; hypertension; palpitations
EENT: Blurred vision; burning eyes; dry eyes, mouth, and throat; earache; eye pain or irritation; lacrimation; nasal congestion and irritation; pharyngeal edema; pharyngitis; tinnitus; tongue swelling
GI: Abdominal distention, constipation, diarrhea, dysphagia, flatulence, heartburn, indigestion, nausea, thirst, vomiting
GU: Menstrual irregularities, polyuria, urinary frequency
MS: Arthralgia; dysarthria; muscle spasms, stiffness, or weakness; myalgia
RESP: Dyspnea, upper respiratory tract infection, wheezing
SKIN: Diaphoresis, flushing, pruritus, rash, urticaria
Other: Angioedema, dehydration, facial edema

Nursing Considerations
• Use rizatriptan cautiously in patients with renal or hepatic dysfunction because of impaired drug metabolism or excretion. Monitor BUN and serum creatinine levels and liver function test results, as appropriate.
• Also use cautiously in patients with peripheral vascular disease because drug may cause vasospastic reactions, leading to vascular and colonic ischemia with abdominal pain and bloody diarrhea. Assess peripheral circulation and bowel sounds frequently during therapy.
• Assess cardiovascular status and institute continuous ECG monitoring, as ordered, immediately after rizatriptan administration in patients with cardiovascular risk factors because of possible asymptomatic cardiac ischemia.
• Monitor blood pressure regularly in patients with hypertension because rizatriptan may increase blood pressure.
PATIENT TEACHING
• Instruct patient taking rizatriptan disintegrating tablets to remove tablet from blister pack with dry hands just before taking, to place tablet on tongue, and to allow it to dissolve and be swallowed with saliva.
• Advise phenylketonuric patient not to use disintegrating tablet form because it contains phenylalanine.

• Instruct patient to seek emergency care immediately if cardiac symptoms, such as chest pain, occur after administration.
• Caution patient about possible adverse CNS reactions, and advise her to avoid potentially hazardous activities until drug's CNS effects are known.

rofecoxib
Vioxx
Class and Category
Chemical: Furanone derivative
Therapeutic: Anti-inflammatory
Pregnancy category: C

Indications and Dosages
➤ *To treat osteoarthritis*
ORAL SUSPENSION, TABLETS
Adults. *Initial:* 12.5 mg q.d.; may be increased, if needed, to 25 mg q.d. *Maximum:* 50 mg q.d.
➤ *To treat rheumatoid arthritis*
ORAL SUSPENSION, TABLETS
Adults. 25 mg q.d. *Maximum:* 25 mg q.d.
➤ *To manage acute pain and primary dysmenorrhea*
ORAL SUSPENSION, TABLETS
Adults. 50 mg q.d. for up to 5 days.

Mechanism of Action
Selectively inhibits the enzyme activity of cyclooxygenase-2, which is responsible for the conversion of arachidonic acid to prostaglandin. Reduced prostaglandin synthesis results in analgesic, antipyretic, and anti-inflammatory effects.

Contraindications
Angioedema, asthma, bronchospasm, nasal polyps, rhinitis, or urticaria induced by aspirin, iodides, or other NSAIDs

Interactions
DRUGS
ACE inhibitors: Decreased antihypertensive effects
aspirin: Increased risk of GI ulceration
cimetidine: Increased blood rofecoxib level
furosemide, thiazide diuretics: Decreased diuretic effectiveness, increased risk of renal failure
lithium, methotrexate: Increased blood levels of these drugs, possibly toxicity

Q R S

oral anticoagulants: Increased hyperpro-thrombinemia, increased risk of bleeding
rifampin: Decreased blood level and, possibly, effectiveness of rofecoxib

Adverse Reactions
CNS: Asthenia, dizziness, fatigue, headache, lethargy
CV: Hypertension, peripheral edema, thrombotic event
EENT: Sinusitis
GI: Abdominal pain, cholecystits, diarrhea, epigastric discomfort, GI bleeding or ulceration, heartburn, hepatotoxicity, indigestion, nausea
GU: UTI
MS: Back pain
RESP: Bronchitis
SKIN: Jaundice, pruritus, rash
Other: Flulike symptoms

Nursing Considerations
•Use rofecoxib cautiously in patients with renal or hepatic dysfunction. Monitor BUN and serum creatinine levels and liver function test results, as appropriate.
•Use drug cautiously in patients with history of ischemic heart disease because of potential CV adverse reactions.
•Monitor for evidence of GI bleeding and ulceration in elderly and debilitated patients; in patients with predisposing risk factors, such as a history of GI ulcer disease, long-term NSAID therapy, smoking, or alcoholism; and in patients who are using oral corticosteroids or anticoagulants.
PATIENT TEACHING
•Urge patient taking rofecoxib to notify prescriber immediately of rash, unexplained weight gain, swelling in arms or legs, and signs of GI ulceration or bleeding, such as black or tarry stools.
•Instruct patient to stop taking drug and immediately notify prescriber if signs of hepatotoxicity occur, such as fatigue, flulike symptoms, lethargy, nausea, pruritus, and yellow skin or eyes.
•Caution patient not to exceed 5 days of therapy when taking drug for acute pain related to primary dysmenorrhea.

ropinirole hydrochloride
Requip

Class and Category
Chemical: Non-ergot alkaloid dopamine agonist
Therapeutic: Antidyskinetic
Pregnancy category: C

Indications and Dosages
➤ *To treat signs and symptoms of Parkinson's disease*
TABLETS
Adults. *Initial:* 0.25 mg t.i.d. Dosage titrated upward q wk according to the following schedule: 0.25 mg t.i.d. in wk 1; 0.5 mg t.i.d. in wk 2; 0.75 mg t.i.d. in wk 3; 1 mg t.i.d. in wk 4. After wk 4, dosage increased by 1.5 mg/day q wk up to 9 mg/day, then by 3 mg/day up to 24 mg/day. *Maximum:* 24 mg/day.

Mechanism of Action
Directly stimulates postsynaptic dopamine type 2 (D_2) receptors within the brain and acts as an agonist at peripheral D_2 receptors. These actions inhibit the firing of striatal cholinergic neurons, thus helping to control alterations in voluntary muscle movement (such as tremors and rigidity) associated with Parkinson's disease.

Contraindications
Hypersensitivity to ropinirole or its components

Interactions
DRUGS
carbamazepine, cimetidine, ciprofloxacin, clarithromycin, diltiazem, enoxacin, erythromycin, fluvoxamine, mexiletine, norfloxacin, omeprazole, phenobarbital, phenytoin, rifampin, ritonavir, troleandomycin: Altered drug clearance and increased blood level of ropinirole
chlorprothixene, domperidone, droperidol, haloperidol, metoclopramide, phenothiazines, thiothixene: Possibly decreased effectiveness of ropinirole
ethinyl estradiol: Possibly reduced clearance of ropinirole

Adverse Reactions
CNS: Asthenia, confusion, dizziness, fatigue, hallucinations, headache, malaise, neuralgia, somnolence, syncope
CV: Orthostatic hypotension, peripheral edema
EENT: Abnormal vision, dry mouth, pharyngitis
GI: Abdominal pain, constipation, indigestion, nausea, vomiting
GU: Elevated BUN level, UTI
HEME: Anemia
MS: Arthralgia, arthritis

RESP: Bronchitis, upper respiratory tract infection
SKIN: Diaphoresis, flushing
Other: Viral infection, weight loss

Nursing Considerations
•**WARNING** Expect to reassess patient periodically during ropinirole treatment for excessive sedation. Patient may develop excessive and acute drowsiness as late as 1 year after beginning therapy.
•When ropinirole is administered as adjunct to levodopa, expect concurrent dosage of levodopa to be gradually decreased as tolerated.
•Expect to discontinue ropinirole gradually over a 7-day period, as follows: over first 4 days, dosing frequency should be reduced from t.i.d to b.i.d.; during last 3 days, frequency should be reduced to q.d., followed by complete withdrawal of drug.
•**WARNING** Monitor patient for altered mental status during drug withdrawal. Rapid dosage reduction may lead to symptom complex resembling neuroleptic malignant syndrome (fever, muscle rigidity, altered level of consciousness, and autonomic instability).
•Monitor for orthostatic hypotension, especially in patients with early Parkinson's disease. Orthostatic hypotension can occur more than 4 weeks after start of therapy or after a dosage reduction because ropinirole may impair systemic regulation of blood pressure.
•Monitor for exacerbation of preexisting dyskinesia because ropinirole may potentiate dopaminergic adverse effects of levodopa.
•Avoid using CNS depressants, sleep aids, and other CNS-interacting drugs during ropinirole therapy because they increase the risk of somnolence.

PATIENT TEACHING
•Inform patient that ropinirole helps to improve muscle control and movement but doesn't cure Parkinson's disease.
•Encourage patient to take ropinirole with food to decrease risk of adverse GI effects.
•If patient falls asleep during normal activities, advise him to notify prescriber.
•Encourage patient to avoid using alcohol during ropinirole therapy because it may enhance drug's CNS depressant effects.

rosiglitazone maleate

Avandia

Class and Category
Chemical: Thiazolidinedione

Therapeutic: Antidiabetic drug
Pregnancy category: C

Indications and Dosages
➤ *To achieve glucose control in type 2 diabetes mellitus as monotherapy or in combination with metformin*
TABLETS
Adults. *Initial:* 4 mg q.d. or 2 mg b.i.d., increased to 8 mg q.d. or 4 mg b.i.d. if glucose control is inadequate after 12 wk. *Maximum:* 8 mg q.d.

Mechanism of Action
Increases tissue sensitivity to insulin. This peroxisome proliferator-activated receptor agonist regulates the transcription of insulin-responsive genes found in key target tissues, such as adipose tissue, skeletal muscle, and the liver. Enhanced tissue sensitivity to insulin lowers blood glucose level.

Contraindications
Hypersensitivity to rosiglitazone or its components

Adverse Reactions
CNS: Fatigue, headache
CV: Congestive heart failure, edema
EENT: Sinusitis
ENDO: Hyperglycemia
GI: Diarrhea
HEME: Anemia
MS: Back pain
RESP: Upper respiratory tract infection

Nursing Considerations
•Use rosiglitazone cautiously in patients with edema, heart failure, or hepatic impairment because of potential adverse reactions.
•Be aware that drug isn't recommended for patients classified by the New York Heart Association with a cardiac status of Class III or IV.
•**WARNING** Monitor patient for signs and symptoms of congestive heart failure—such as shortness of breath, rapid weight gain, or edema—because rosiglitazone can cause fluid retention that may lead to or worsen heart failure. Notify prescriber immediately of any deterioration in the patient's cardiac status, and expect to discontinue the drug, as ordered.
•Monitor fasting glucose and glycosylated hemoglobin A_{1c} levels periodically, as ordered, to evaluate treatment effectiveness.
•Be aware that because drug is effective only in the presence of endogenous insulin.

•Stress the need to continue exercise program and diet control during rosiglitazone therapy.
•Advise patient to notify prescriber immediately if he experiences shortness of breath, fluid retention, or sudden weight gain because drug may need to be discontinued.
•Instruct patient to keep appointments for liver function tests, as prescribed, about every 2 months for first year and then annually.
•Inform premenopausal, anovulatory patient that drug may induce ovulation, increasing risk of pregnancy. Advise her to use contraception if she wishes to avoid pregnancy.

salmeterol xinafoate

Serevent, Serevent Diskus

Class and Category
Chemical: Sympathomimetic amine
Therapeutic: Bronchodilator
Pregnancy category: C

Indications and Dosages
➤ *To prevent asthma-induced bronchospasm*
ORAL INHALATION AEROSOL (SEREVENT)
Adults and children age 12 and older. 2 inhalations (42 or 50 mcg) q 12 hr.
ORAL INHALATION POWDER (SEREVENT DISKUS)
Adults and children age 4 and older. 1 inhalation (50 mcg) q 12 hr.
➤ *To prevent COPD-induced bronchospasm*
ORAL INHALATION AEROSOL
Adults. 2 inhalations (42 or 50 mcg) q 12 hr.
ORAL INHALATION POWDER
Adults. 1 inhalation (50 mcg) q 12 hr.
➤ *To prevent exercise-induced bronchospasm*
ORAL INHALATION AEROSOL
Adults and children age 12 and older. 2 inhalations (42 or 50 mcg) 30 to 60 min before exercise.
ORAL INHALATION POWDER
Adults and children age 4 and older. 1 inhalation (50 mcg) at least 30 min before exercise.

Route	Onset	Peak	Duration
Inhalation	10 to 20 min	3 to 4 hr	12 hr

Contraindications
Hypersensitivity to salmeterol or its components

Mechanism of Action
Attaches to beta$_2$ receptors on bronchial cell membranes, stimulating the intracellular enzyme adenylate cyclase to convert adenosine triphosphate to cAMP. The resulting increase in the intracellular cAMP level relaxes bronchial smooth-muscle cells, stabilizes mast cells, and inhibits histamine release.

Interactions
DRUGS
beta blockers: Mutual inhibition of therapeutic effects
loop or thiazide diuretics: Increased risk of hypokalemia and potentially life-threatening arrhythmias
MAO inhibitors, tricyclic antidepressants: Potentiated adverse vascular effects, such as hypertensive crisis

Adverse Reactions
CNS: Dizziness, fever, headache, nervousness, paresthesia, tremor
CV: Tachycardia
EENT: Dry mouth, nose, and throat; sinus problems
GI: Nausea
MS: Arthralgia
RESP: Cough, paradoxical bronchospasm
SKIN: Contact dermatitis, eczema
Other: Generalized aches and pains

Nursing Considerations
•Be aware that salmeterol shouldn't be used to relieve bronchospasm quickly because of its prolonged onset of action and that patients already taking drug twice daily shouldn't take additional doses for exercise-induced bronchospasm.
•Assess for arrhythmias and changes in blood pressure after use in patients with cardiovascular disorders, including ischemic cardiac disease, hypertension, and arrhythmias, because of drug's beta-adrenergic effects.
•Be aware that Serevent Diskus delivers full dose of salmeterol in only one inhalation.
PATIENT TEACHING
•Advise patient who is using salmeterol to prevent asthma-induced bronchospasm to take doses 12 hours apart for optimum effect. Caution against using drug more than every 12 hours.
•Teach patient how to use oral inhaler correctly. Instruct him to shake the canister,

place the mouthpiece between his teeth, close his lips firmly around the mouthpiece, and press down on the canister while taking a slow, deep inhalation. If he's using the diskus, instruct him to slide the lever only once when preparing dose to avoid wasting doses. Advise him to exhale immediately before using the diskus and then to place the mouthpiece to his lips and inhale through his mouth, not his nose. Then he should remove the mouthpiece from his mouth, hold his breath for at least 10 seconds, and exhale slowly.
• If patient requires more than one inhalation of oral inhalation *aerosol* (not diskus), instruct him to wait 1 minute, shake the inhaler again, and repeat the procedure.
• Urge patient not to let anyone else use his inhaler.
• Advise patient to rinse his mouth with water after each dose to minimize dry mouth.
• Advise patient to discard diskus 6 weeks after removing it from overwrap or when dose indicator reads zero.
• Instruct patient to notify prescriber if he needs four or more oral inhalations of rapid-acting inhaled bronchodilator a day for 2 or more consecutive days, or if he uses more than one canister of rapid-acting bronchodilator in an 8-week period.

salsalate

(salicylsalicylic acid)

Amigesic, Anaflex 750, Argesic-SA, Disalcid, Marthritic, Mono-Gesic, Salflex, Salsitab

Class and Category

Chemical: Salicylic acid ester
Therapeutic: Analgesic, anti-inflammatory
Pregnancy category: C

Indications and Dosages

➤ *To relieve symptoms of rheumatoid arthritis and related rheumatic disorders*
CAPSULES
Adults and adolescents. *Initial:* 1 g t.i.d.; dosage then titrated, as needed.
TABLETS
Adults and adolescents. *Initial:* 0.5 to 1 g b.i.d. or t.i.d.; dosage then titrated, as needed.

Route	Onset	Peak	Duration
P.O.	Unknown	2 to 3 wk	Unknown

Mechanism of Action
Exerts peripherally induced analgesic and anti-inflammatory effects by blocking pain impulses and inhibiting prostaglandin synthesis.

Contraindications
Bleeding disorders; hypersensitivity to NSAIDs, salicylates, or their components

Interactions
DRUGS
acetaminophen: Increased risk of renal dysfunction with prolonged use of both drugs
anticoagulants, thrombolytics: Increased risk and severity of GI bleeding
antiemetics: Masked symptoms of salicylate-induced ototoxicity
bismuth subsalicylate: Increased risk of salicylate toxicity with large doses of salsalate
cefamandole, cefoperazone, cefotetan, platelet aggregation inhibitors, plicamycin, valproic acid: Possibly hypoprothrombinemia
corticosteroids: Possibly decreased blood salsalate level; additive therapeutic effects when both drugs are used to treat arthritis
furosemide: Increased risk of ototoxicity and salicylate toxicity
hydantoins: Possibly decreased hydantoin metabolism, leading to toxicity
insulin, oral antidiabetic drugs: Potentiated hypoglycemic effect
laxatives (cellulose-containing): Possibly reduced salsalate effectiveness due to impaired absorption
methotrexate: Increased risk of methotrexate toxicity
NSAIDs: Increased risk of adverse GI effects
ototoxic drugs, vancomycin: Increased risk of ototoxicity
probenecid, sulfinpyrazone: Decreased uricosuric effects
topical salicylic acid, other salicylates: Increased risk of salicylate toxicity if significant quantities are absorbed
urinary acidifiers (ammonium chloride, ascorbic acid, potassium or sodium phosphates): Decreased salicylate excretion, possibly leading to salicylate toxicity
urinary alkalizers (antacids [long-term high-dose use], carbonic anhydrase inhibitors, citrates, sodium bicarbonate): Increased salicylate excretion, leading to reduced effective-

Q R S

ness and shortened half-life; increased risk of salicylate toxicity with carbonic anhydrase inhibitor–induced metabolic acidosis
vitamin K: Increased vitamin K requirements
ACTIVITIES
alcohol use: Increased risk of GI bleeding

Adverse Reactions

CNS: CNS depression, confusion, dizziness, drowsiness, fever, headache, lassitude
EENT: Hearing loss, tinnitus, vision changes
GI: Anorexia, diarrhea, epigastric discomfort, GI bleeding, heartburn, hepatotoxicity, indigestion, nausea, thirst, vomiting
HEME: Hemolytic anemia, leukopenia, prolonged bleeding time, thrombocytopenia
SKIN: Diaphoresis, purpura, rash, urticaria
Other: Angioedema, Reye's syndrome

Nursing Considerations

•Avoid using salsalate in patients with hypoprothrombinemia or vitamin K deficiency because drug's hypoprothrombinemic effect may precipitate bleeding.
•Monitor hepatic and renal function, as appropriate, during long-term salsalate therapy.
•Assess for signs and symptoms of GI bleeding, such as abdominal pain or black, tarry stools, especially in patient with peptic ulcer disease.
•Assess for symptoms of ototoxicity, such as ringing or roaring in ears.
PATIENT TEACHING
•Instruct patient to take salsalate with food or a full glass of water and to remain upright for 1 hour after administration to prevent drug from lodging in esophagus and causing irritation.
•Inform patient that therapeutic response may not occur for 2 to 3 weeks.
•Urge patient to notify prescriber immediately of abdominal pain or black, tarry stools; these symptoms may indicate GI bleeding or drug toxicity.

scopolamine hydrobromide

scopolamine transdermal system

Transderm-Scōp, Transderm-V (CAN)

Class and Category

Chemical: Belladonna alkaloid, tertiary amine
Therapeutic: Anesthesia adjunct, anticholin-
ergic, antiemetic, antispasmodic, antivertigo
Pregnancy category: C

Indications and Dosages

➤ *To treat biliary tract disorders, enuresis, nausea and vomiting, and nocturia*
I.V., I.M., OR S.C. INJECTION (HYDROBROMIDE)
Adults and adolescents. 300 to 600 mcg (0.3 to 0.6 mg) as a single dose.
Children. 6 mcg (0.006 mg)/kg as a single dose.
➤ *To prevent excessive salivation and respiratory tract secretions during anesthesia*
I.M. INJECTION (HYDROBROMIDE)
Adults and adolescents. 0.2 to 0.6 mg 30 to 60 min before induction of anesthesia.
Children ages 8 to 12. 0.3 mg 45 to 60 min before induction of anesthesia.
Children ages 3 to 8. 0.2 mg 45 to 60 min before induction of anesthesia.
Children ages 7 months to 3 years. 0.15 mg 45 to 60 min before induction of anesthesia.
Infants ages 4 to 7 months. 0.1 mg 45 to 60 min before induction of anesthesia.
➤ *As adjunct to anesthesia to induce sleep and calmness*
I.V., I.M., OR S.C. INJECTION (HYDROBROMIDE)
Adults and adolescents. 0.6 mg t.i.d. or q.i.d.
➤ *As adjunct to anesthesia to induce amnesia*
I.V., I.M., OR S.C. INJECTION (HYDROBROMIDE)
Adults and adolescents. 0.32 to 0.65 mg.
➤ *To prevent nausea, vomiting, and vertigo associated with motion sickness*
TRANSDERMAL SYSTEM
Adults and adolescents. 1 U.S. transdermal system (0.5 mg) applied behind ear for 3-day period, beginning at least 4 hr before antiemetic effect is required. Alternatively, 1 Canadian transdermal system (1 mg) applied behind ear for 3-day period, beginning at least 12 hr before antiemetic effect is required.
DOSAGE ADJUSTMENT Dosage reduction possible for elderly patients because of their increased sensitivity to scopolamine.

Contraindications

Angle-closure glaucoma; hemorrhage with hemodynamic instability; hepatic dysfunction; hypersensitivity to barbiturates, scopolamine, other belladonna alkaloids, or their components; ileus; intestinal atony; myasthenia gravis; myocardial ischemia; obstructive GI disease, such as pyloric stenosis; obstructive uropathy, as in prostatic hyperplasia;

renal impairment; tachycardia; toxic mega-colon; ulcerative colitis

Route	Onset	Peak	Duration
I.V., I.M., S.C.*	30 min	1 to 2 hr	4 to 6 hr
I.V.†	10 min	50 to 80 min	2 hr
I.M.‡	15 to 30 min	Unknown	4 hr
Trans-dermal	4 hr	Unknown	72 hr

Mechanism of Action
Competitively inhibits acetylcholine at autonomic postganglionic cholinergic receptors. Because the most sensitive receptors are in the salivary, bronchial, and sweat glands, this action reduces secretions from these glands. Scopolamine reduces GI smooth-muscle tone; decreases gastric secretions and GI motility; reduces bladder detrusor muscle tone; reduces nasal, oropharyngeal, and bronchial secretions; and decreases airway resistance by relaxing smooth muscles in the bronchi and bronchioles.

Scopolamine also blocks neural pathways in the inner ear to relieve motion sickness and depresses the cerebral cortex to produce sedation and hypnotic effects.

Interactions
DRUGS
adsorbent antidiarrheals, antacids: Decreased absorption and therapeutic effects of scopolamine
anticholinergics (other): Possibly intensified anticholinergic effects
antimyasthenics: Possibly reduced intestinal motility
CNS depressants: Possibly potentiated effects of either drug, resulting in additive sedation
cyclopropane: Increased risk of ventricular arrhythmias (with I.V. scopolamine)
haloperidol: Decreased antipsychotic effect of haloperidol

ketoconazole: Decreased ketoconazole absorption
lorazepam (parenteral): Possibly hallucinations, irrational behavior, and sedation
metoclopramide: Possibly antagonized effect of metoclopramide on GI motility
opioid analgesics: Increased risk of severe constipation and ileus
potassium chloride: Possibly increased severity of potassium chloride–induced GI lesions
urinary alkalizers (antacids, carbonic anhydrase inhibitors, citrates, sodium bicarbonate): Delayed excretion of scopolamine, possibly leading to increased therapeutic and adverse effects
ACTIVITIES
alcohol use: Additive CNS effects

Adverse Reactions
CNS: Dizziness, drowsiness, euphoria, insomnia, memory loss, paradoxical stimulation
CV: Palpitations, tachycardia
EENT: Blurred vision; dry eyes, mouth, nose, and throat; mydriasis
GI: Constipation, dysphagia
GU: Urinary hesitancy, urine retention
SKIN: Decreased sweating, dry skin, flushing
Other: Injection site irritation or redness

Nursing Considerations
•For I.V. injection, dilute scopolamine with sterile water for injection.
•Assess for bladder distention and monitor urine output because drug's antimuscarinic effects can cause urine retention.
•Monitor for pain. In presence of pain, drug may act as a stimulant and produce delirium if used without morphine or meperidine.
•Monitor heart rate for transient tachycardia, which may occur with high doses of drug. Rate should return to normal within 30 minutes.
PATIENT TEACHING
•Instruct patient to apply scopolamine transdermal patch on hairless area behind ear and to wash hands thoroughly with soap and water before and after applying.
•Advise patient to avoid potentially hazardous activities until drug's CNS effects are known.
•Instruct patient to avoid alcohol while taking oral forms of scopolamine.
•If patient complains of dry eyes, suggest lubricating drops.

Q
R
S

* For inhibition of saliva.
† For amnesia.
‡ For antiemesis.

secobarbital sodium
Novosecobarb (CAN), Seconal

Class, Category, and Schedule

Chemical: Barbiturate
Therapeutic: Sedative-hypnotic
Pregnancy category: D
Controlled substance: Schedule II

Indications and Dosages

➤ *To induce sedation before surgery*
CAPSULES
Adults. 200 to 300 mg 1 to 2 hr before surgery.
Children. 2 to 6 mg/kg 1 to 2 hr before surgery. *Maximum:* 100 mg.

➤ *To provide short-term treatment of insomnia*
CAPSULES
Adults. 100 mg h.s.

➤ *To relieve apprehension, daytime anxiety, and tension*
CAPSULES
Adults. 30 to 50 mg t.i.d. or q.i.d.
Children. 2 mg/kg t.i.d.
DOSAGE ADJUSTMENT Reduced dosage required for elderly or debilitated patients and those with renal or hepatic dysfunction.

Route	Onset	Peak	Duration
P.O.	10 to 15 min	15 to 30 min	1 to 4 hr

Mechanism of Action

Inhibits upward conduction of nerve impulses to the reticular formation of the brain, thereby disrupting impulse transmission to the cortex. This action depresses the CNS, producing drowsiness, hypnosis, and sedation.

Contraindications

History of barbiturate addiction; hypersensitivity to secobarbital, other barbiturates, or their components; nephritis; porphyria; severe hepatic or respiratory impairment

Interactions
DRUGS

acetaminophen, adrenocorticoids, beta blockers, chloramphenicol, cyclosporine, dacarbazine, digoxin, disopyramide, estrogens, metronidazole, oral anticoagulants, oral contraceptives, quinidine, thyroid hormones, tricyclic antidepressants: Decreased effectiveness of these drugs

addictive drugs: Increased risk of addiction
calcium channel blockers: Possibly excessive hypotension
carbamazepine, succinimide anticonvulsants: Decreased blood levels and increased elimination of these drugs
carbonic anhydrase inhibitors: Increased risk of osteopenia
CNS depressants: Increased CNS depressant effects
cyclophosphamide: Increased risk of leukopenic activity and reduced half-life of cyclophosphamide
divalproex sodium, valproic acid: Increased CNS depression and neurologic toxicity
doxycycline, fenoprofen: Increased elimination of these drugs
general anesthetics (enflurane, halothane, methoxyflurane): Increased risk of hepatotoxicity; increased risk of nephrotoxicity (with methoxyflurane)
griseofulvin: Decreased griseofulvin absorption
guanadrel, guanethidine: Possibly increased orthostatic hypotension
haloperidol: Possibly altered pattern or frequency of seizures, decreased blood haloperidol level
ketamine: Increased risk of hypotension or respiratory depression (when secobarbital is used as preanesthetic)
leucovorin (large doses): Decreased anticonvulsant effect of secobarbital
loxapine, phenothiazines, thioxanthenes: Possibly lowered seizure threshold
MAO inhibitors: Possibly prolonged CNS depressant effects of secobarbital
maprotiline: Increased CNS depressant effect; possibly lowered seizure threshold and decreased anticonvulsant effect with high doses of maprotiline
methylphenidate: Increased risk of barbiturate toxicity
mexiletine: Decreased blood mexiletine level
phenylbutazone: Decreased effectiveness of secobarbital
posterior pituitary hormones: Increased risk of arrhythmias and coronary insufficiency
primidone: Increased sedative effect of either drug, change in seizure pattern
vitamin D: Decreased vitamin D effects
xanthines (aminophylline, oxtriphylline, theophylline): Increased metabolism of xanthines (except dyphylline), decreased hypnotic effect of secobarbital

FOODS

caffeine: Increased caffeine metabolism, decreased hypnotic effect of secobarbital

ACTIVITIES

alcohol use: Increased CNS depression

Adverse Reactions

CNS: Anxiety, clumsiness, confusion, depression, dizziness, drowsiness, hangover, headache, insomnia, irritability, lethargy, nervousness, nightmares, paradoxical stimulation, syncope

CV: Hypotension

EENT: Laryngospasm

GI: Anorexia, constipation, nausea, vomiting

MS: Arthralgia, muscle weakness

RESP: Apnea, bronchospasm, respiratory depression

SKIN: Jaundice

Other: Drug dependence, weight loss

Nursing Considerations

• Be aware that prolonged use of secobarbital may lead to tolerance and physical and psychological dependence.

• WARNING To avoid withdrawal symptoms, expect to taper drug after long-term therapy. Withdrawal symptoms usually appear 8 to 12 hours after stopping drug and may include anxiety, insomnia, muscle twitching, nausea, orthostatic hypotension, vomiting, weakness, and weight loss. Severe symptoms may include delirium, hallucinations, and seizures. Generalized tonic-clonic seizures may occur within 16 hours or up to 5 days after last dose.

• Assess patient for signs and symptoms of barbiturate toxicity, including dyspnea, severe confusion, and severe drowsiness. Notify prescriber immediately if they appear because barbiturate toxicity may be life-threatening.

• Expect prescriber to provide patient with the least possible quantity of secobarbital to minimize the risk of acute or chronic overdosage. For patients who are depressed, suicidal, or drug-dependent or who have a history of drug abuse, institute precautions to prevent drug hoarding and overdosage.

PATIENT TEACHING

• Instruct patient to take secobarbital exactly as prescribed because of the risk of addiction.

• Inform patient that taking drug with food may reduce adverse GI effects.

• Advise patient to avoid alcohol and caffeine and potentially hazardous activities during therapy.

• Inform patient about possible hangover effect.

• If patient takes an oral contraceptive, recommend using an additional form of birth control during therapy.

• Caution patient not to stop taking drug abruptly.

• Instruct patient to notify prescriber of bone pain, muscle weakness, or unexplained weight loss during therapy.

secobarbital sodium and amobarbital sodium

Tuinal

Class, Category, and Schedule

Chemical: Barbiturate
Therapeutic: Sedative-hypnotic
Pregnancy category: D
Controlled substance: Schedule II

Indications and Dosages

➤ *To provide short-term treatment of insomnia*

CAPSULES

Adults. 100 to 200 mg (50 to 100 mg each of secobarbital sodium and amobarbital sodium) h.s.

➤ *To induce sedation before surgery*

CAPSULES

Adults. 100 to 200 mg (50 to 100 mg each of secobarbital sodium and amobarbital sodium) 1 hr before surgery.

DOSAGE ADJUSTMENT Dosage possibly reduced for elderly or debilitated patients and for those with renal or hepatic dysfunction.

Route	Onset	Peak	Duration
P.O.*	10 to 15 min	15 to 30 min	1 to 4 hr
P.O.†	45 to 60 min	Unknown	6 to 8 hr

Contraindications

History of barbiturate addiction; hypersensitivity to secobarbital, amobarbital, or their components; nephritis; porphyria; severe hepatic or respiratory dysfunction

Interactions

DRUGS

antihistamines, CNS depressants: Additive CNS depressant effects

---

* Secobarbital.
† Amobarbital.

Q
R
S

corticosteroids, oral anticoagulants: Increased metabolism of these drugs, causing decreased anticoagulant response
doxycycline: Shortened half-life and increased elimination of doxycycline
estradiol, estrone, progesterone, other steroidal hormones: Increased metabolism of these hormones, leading to decreased effectiveness
griseofulvin: Decreased absorption of griseofulvin
MAO inhibitors: Inhibited metabolism of secobarbital and amobarbital, causing prolonged CNS depressant effects
phenytoin: Possibly accelerated metabolism of phenytoin
sodium valproate, valproic acid: Decreased metabolism of secobarbital and amobarbital
vitamin D: Decreased effects of vitamin D
FOODS
caffeine: Increased metabolism of caffeine; decreased hypnotic effect of secobarbital and amobarbital
ACTIVITIES
alcohol use: Increased CNS depressant effects

Mechanism of Action
Nonselectively acts on the CNS to alter cerebral function, decrease motor activity, depress the sensory cortex, and produce drowsiness, hypnosis, and sedation. Drug appears to reduce wakefulness and alertness by acting in the thalamus, where it depresses the reticular activating system and interferes with impulse transmission from the periphery to the cortex. It produces CNS depressant effects, ranging from mild sedation and reduction of anxiety to anesthesia and coma, depending on the dosage, route, and individual patient's response. Secobarbital and amobarbital have different rates of action and dissipation. When used together, they provide a balanced sedative-hypnotic effect.

Adverse Reactions
CNS: Anxiety, clumsiness, CNS depression, confusion, dizziness, drowsiness, hallucinations, hangover, headache, insomnia, irritability, light-headedness, nervousness, nightmares, paradoxical stimulation, syncope, unsteadiness
CV: Bradycardia, hypotension

GI: Constipation, hepatic dysfunction, nausea, vomiting
HEME: Agranulocytosis, megaloblastic anemia, thrombocytopenia
MS: Osteopenia, rickets
RESP: Apnea, hypoventilation
SKIN: Exfoliative dermatitis, rash, Stevens-Johnson syndrome
Other: Angioedema, physical and psychological dependence, potentially fatal withdrawal syndrome, tolerance

Nursing Considerations
• Be aware that this combination drug is used for short-term treatment of insomnia because drug loses its effectiveness after 2 weeks.
• Monitor patient for paradoxical drug effects, such as confusion, excitement, or mental depression, especially in elderly patients.
• Be aware that drug has the potential to exaggerate depression, suicidal tendencies, and other mental disorders.
• Be aware that drug shouldn't be discontinued abruptly because withdrawal symptoms can occur.
• Assess patient for signs and symptoms of possible exfoliative dermatitis, such as fever and red, scaly, or thickened skin. If this occurs, notify prescriber and expect to discontinue drug immediately because this condition may indicate a potentially fatal hypersensitivity reaction.
• Be aware that drug may cause physical and psychological dependence.
PATIENT TEACHING
• Instruct patient to take secobarbital and amobarbital exactly as prescribed because of the risk of addiction.
• Instruct patient to report severe dizziness, persistent drowsiness, rash, or skin lesions.
• Advise patient to use caution when driving or performing tasks that require alertness.
• Instruct patient not to consume alcohol or other CNS depressants (unless prescribed) because they increase drug's effects.
• If female patient takes an oral contraceptive, recommend that she use an added form of birth control during therapy. Advise patient to notify prescriber immediately of known or suspected pregnancy. Also, caution against breast-feeding while taking drug.
• Encourage patient to use other nondrug therapies to treat insomnia. Offer suggestions for improved sleep, such as getting moderate

exercise during the day, setting regular sleep habits, and using relaxation techniques.

selegiline hydrochloride

Apo-Selegiline (CAN), Carbex, Eldepryl, Gen-Selegiline (CAN), Novo-Selegiline (CAN), Nu-Selegiline (CAN), SD Deprenyl (CAN), Selegiline-5 (CAN)

Class and Category

Chemical: Phenethylamine derivative
Therapeutic: Antidyskinetic
Pregnancy category: C

Indications and Dosages

➤ *As adjunct to carbidopa-levodopa therapy to treat Parkinson's disease*

CAPSULES, TABLETS
Adults. 10 mg q.d., or 5 mg b.i.d. with breakfast and lunch.
DOSAGE ADJUSTMENT For patient with levodopa-induced adverse effects, 2.5 mg q.i.d.

> ### Mechanism of Action
> Reduces dopamine metabolism by noncompetitively inhibiting the brain enzyme monoamine oxidase type B. This increases the amount of dopamine available to relieve symptoms associated with parkinsonism. Selegiline's metabolites may also enhance dopamine transmission by inhibiting its reuptake at synapses.

Contraindications

Hypersensitivity to selegiline or its components, use within 14 days of meperidine

Interactions

DRUGS
fluoxetine, fluvoxamine, nefazodone, paroxetine, sertraline, venlafaxine: Increased risk of adverse reactions similar to those of serotonin syndrome (confusion, hypomania, restlessness, myoclonus), autonomic instability, delirium, muscle rigidity, and severe agitation
levodopa: Increased risk of confusion, dyskinesia, hallucinations, nausea, and orthostatic hypotension
meperidine, possibly other opioid agonists: Increased risk of diaphoresis, excitation, muscle rigidity, and severe hypertension
tricyclic antidepressants: Possibly serious CNS reactions, including decreased level of

consciousness, hyperpyrexia, hypertension, muscle rigidity, seizures, and syncope
FOODS
caffeine: Increased risk of hypertension
foods that contain tyramine or other high-pressor amines: Increased risk of sudden and severe hypertension
ACTIVITIES
alcohol use: Increased risk of hypertension

Adverse Reactions

CNS: Anxiety, chills, confusion, dizziness, drowsiness, dyskinesia, euphoria, extrapyramidal reactions, fatigue, hallucinations, headache, insomnia, irritability, lethargy, memory loss, mood changes, nervousness, paresthesia, restlessness, syncope, tremor, weakness
CV: Arrhythmias, chest pain, hypertension, orthostatic hypotension, palpitations, peripheral edema
EENT: Altered taste, blepharospasm, blurred vision, burning lips or mouth, diplopia, dry mouth, tinnitus
GI: Abdominal pain, anorexia, constipation, diarrhea, GI bleeding, heartburn, nausea, vomiting
GU: Dysuria, urinary hesitancy, urinary urgency, urine retention
MS: Arthralgia, back and leg pain, muscle fatigue and spasms
RESP: Asthma
SKIN: Diaphoresis, photosensitivity, rash

Nursing Considerations

• Assess patient for mental status and mood changes because selegiline can exacerbate such conditions as dementia, severe psychosis, tardive dyskinesia, and tremor.
• Monitor patient who is also taking levodopa for levodopa-induced adverse reactions, including confusion, dyskinesia, hallucinations, nausea, and orthostatic hypotension.
• Monitor for decreased symptoms of Parkinson's disease to evaluate drug's effectiveness.
• Be aware that drug can reactivate gastric ulcers because it prevents breakdown of gastric histamine. Assess for related signs and symptoms, such as abdominal pain.
PATIENT TEACHING
• Advise patient to avoid taking selegiline in the late afternoon or evening because it may interfere with sleep.

Q
R
S

778 sertraline hydrochloride

• Caution patient to take only prescribed amount because increased dosage may cause severe adverse reactions.
• Urge patient to avoid potentially hazardous activities until drug's CNS effects are known.
• Advise patient to change position slowly to minimize effects of orthostatic hypotension.
• Suggest that patient elevate his legs when sitting to reduce ankle swelling.
• Urge patient to avoid excessive sun exposure.
• Instruct patient to notify prescriber of symptoms that could indicate overdose, including muscle twitching and eye spasms.
• Urge patient to notify prescriber if dry mouth lasts longer than 2 weeks. Advise him to have routine dental checkups.

sertraline hydrochloride

Zoloft

Class and Category

Chemical: Naphthylamine derivative
Therapeutic: Antidepressant, antiobsessant, antipanic
Pregnancy category: C

Indications and Dosages

➤ *To treat major depression*
ORAL CONCENTRATE, TABLETS
Adults. *Initial:* 50 mg/day, increased after several wk in increments of 50 mg/day q wk, as needed. *Maximum:* 200 mg/day.
➤ *To treat obsessive-compulsive disorder*
ORAL CONCENTRATE, TABLETS
Adults and adolescents. *Initial:* 50 mg/day, increased after several wk in increments of 50 mg/day q wk, as needed. *Maximum:* 200 mg/day.
Children ages 6 to 12. *Initial:* 25 mg/day, increased q wk, as needed. *Maximum:* 200 mg/day.

➤ *To treat panic disorder, with or without agoraphobia; to treat posttraumatic stress disorder*
ORAL CONCENTRATE, TABLETS
Adults. *Initial:* 25 mg q.d., increased to 50 mg q.d. after 1 wk; then increased by 50 mg/day q wk, as needed. *Maximum:* 200 mg/day.
DOSAGE ADJUSTMENT Initial dosage reduction recommended for elderly patients and those with hepatic impairment.

➤ *To treat premenstrual dysphoric disease (PMDD)*
ORAL CONCENTRATE, TABLETS
Adult women. *Initial:* 50 mg q.d., in morning or evening, throughout menstrual cycle; or 50 mg q.d., in morning or evening, during luteal phase of menstrual cycle only. Dosage increased each menstrual cycle in 50 mg increments up to 150 mg/day, or each luteal phase up to 100 mg/day, as needed. Once 100 mg/day dosage established for luteal phase, each successive cycle requires a 50 mg titration step for 3 days at the beginning of each luteal phase. *Maximum:* 150 mg/day for dosing throughout menstrual cycle, or 100 mg/day for dosing during luteal phase only.

Route	Onset	Peak	Duration
P.O.	2 to 4 wk*	Unknown	Unknown

Mechanism of Action

Inhibits reuptake of the neurotransmitter serotonin by CNS neurons, thereby increasing the amount of serotonin available in nerve synapses. An elevated serotonin level may result in elevated mood and reduced depression. This action may also relieve symptoms of other psychiatric conditions attributed to serotonin deficiency.

Contraindications

Concurrent use of disulfiram (oral concentrate) or pimozide; hypersensitivity to sertraline or its components; use within 14 days of an MAO inhibitor

Interactions
DRUGS
astemizole, terfenadine: Possibly increased blood levels of these drugs, leading to increased risk of arrhythmias
cimetidine: Increased sertraline half-life
MAO inhibitors: Possibly hyperpyretic episodes, hypertensive crisis, serotonin syndrome, and severe seizures
moclobemide, serotonergics: Increased risk of potentially fatal serotonin syndrome
tolbutamide: Possibly hypoglycemia

---

* For antidepressant and antipanic effects; for antiobsessant effect, longer than 4 wk.

tricyclic antidepressants: Possibly impaired metabolism of tricyclic antidepressants, resulting in increased risk of toxicity
warfarin: Increased anticoagulant activity and risk of bleeding

Adverse Reactions
CNS: Agitation, anxiety, dizziness, drowsiness, fatigue, headache, insomnia, nervousness, paresthesia, tremor, weakness, yawning
CV: Palpitations
EENT: Dry mouth, vision changes
ENDO: Syndrome of inappropriate ADH secretion
GI: Abdominal cramps, anorexia, constipation, diarrhea, flatulence, increased appetite, indigestion, nausea, vomiting
GU: Anorgasmia, decreased libido, ejaculation disorders, impotence
SKIN: Diaphoresis, flushing, rash
Other: Weight loss

Nursing Considerations
•Monitor liver function test results and BUN and serum creatinine levels, as appropriate, in patients with hepatic or renal dysfunction.
•Monitor patient for hypo-osmolarity of serum and urine and for hyponatremia, which may indicate sertraline-induced syndrome of inappropriate ADH secretion.
•Be aware that effective antidepressant therapy can promote mania in predisposed individuals. If manic symptoms develop, notify prescriber immediately and expect to withhold sertraline.
PATIENT TEACHING
•Teach patient to dilute oral concentrate before taking. Tell him to use supplied dropper to remove prescribed amount of oral concentrate and mix it with 4 oz (½ cup) of water, ginger ale, lemon or lime soda, lemonade, or orange juice. Warn him not to mix oral concentrate with anything other than these liquids. Explain that a slight haze may appear after mixing and that this is normal.
•Tell patient to take dose immediately after mixing it.
•If patient has latex sensitivity, advise him to use an alternate dispenser because the supplied dropper dispenser contains dry natural rubber.
•Advise patient to avoid potentially hazardous activities until drug's CNS effects are known.
•Caution patient not to stop taking drug abruptly. Explain that gradual tapering helps to avoid withdrawal symptoms.

sevelamer hydrochloride
Renagel

Class and Category
Chemical: Polyallylamine-epichlorhydrin polymer
Therapeutic: Antihyperphosphatemic
Pregnancy category: C

Indications and Dosages
➤ *To lower serum phosphate level during end-stage renal disease*
CAPSULES
Adults. 2 capsules (806 mg) t.i.d. if serum phosphorus level is 6 to 7.5 mg/dl; 3 capsules (1,209 mg) t.i.d. if serum phosphorus level is 7.6 to 8.9 mg/dl; or 4 capsules (1,612 mg) t.i.d. if serum phosphorus level is 9 mg/dl or more. Dosage increased or decreased gradually by 1 capsule (403 mg)/meal, as needed. *Maximum:* 30 capsules (12.1 g)/day.

Mechanism of Action
Inhibits absorption of phosphate in the intestine by binding dietary phosphate in the GI tract, thereby lowering the serum phosphorus level.

Contraindications
Fecal impaction, GI obstruction, hypersensitivity to sevelamer or its components, hypophosphatemia, ileus

Interactions
DRUGS
antiarrhythmics, anticonvulsants, digoxin, levothyroxine, liothyronine, quinolones, tetracyclines, theophylline, warfarin: Possibly altered absorption of these drugs
phosphate salts, phosphorus salts: Neutralized therapeutic effects of sevelamer

Adverse Reactions
CNS: Headache
CV: Hypertension, hypotension, thrombosis
GI: Constipation, diarrhea, flatulence, indigestion, nausea, vomiting
RESP: Increased cough
Other: Infection

Nursing Considerations
•Give other drugs at least 1 hour before or 3 hours after sevelamer to prevent possible interaction.

Q
R
S

•Be aware that severe hypophosphatemia may develop in patient with dysphagia, major GI tract surgery, or severe GI motility disorder because sevelamer prevents phosphates from being absorbed by the body.
•Monitor blood pressure frequently to detect hypertension or hypotension.
•Monitor serum phosphorus level to determine drug's effectiveness; monitor other serum electrolyte levels to detect imbalances.

PATIENT TEACHING
•Instruct patient to take sevelamer with meals and to swallow capsules whole with water, not to open or chew them.
•Caution patient to take other drugs 1 hour before or 3 hours after sevelamer.
•Review symptoms of thrombosis with patient, and advise him to notify prescriber immediately if they occur.

sibutramine hydrochloride monohydrate

Meridia

Class, Category, and Schedule
Chemical: Cyclobutanemethanamine
Therapeutic: Antiobesity
Pregnancy category: C
Controlled substance: Schedule IV

Indications and Dosages
➤ *As adjunct to dieting to manage obesity*
CAPSULES
Adults. *Initial:* 10 mg q.d., increased to 15 mg/day after 4 wk if weight loss is inadequate. *Maximum:* 15 mg q.d.
DOSAGE ADJUSTMENT Reduction to 5 mg/day may be needed if patient can't tolerate 10-mg dose.

Mechanism of Action
Inhibits central reuptake of dopamine, norepinephrine, and serotonin, thereby suppressing appetite and lowering food intake, leading to weight loss.

Contraindications
Anorexia nervosa, concomitant use of other centrally acting appetite suppressants, hypersensitivity to sibutramine or its components, use within 14 days of MAO inhibitor therapy

Interactions
DRUGS
certain decongestants and cough, cold, and allergy drugs; ephedrine; phenylpropanolamine; pseudoephedrine: Increased risk of elevated blood pressure or heart rate
certain opioid analgesics (dextromethorphan, fentanyl, meperidine, pentazocine), dihydroergotamine, lithium, MAO inhibitors, serotonergics, sumatriptan, tryptophan, zolmitriptan: Increased risk of potentially fatal serotonin syndrome
erythromycin, ketoconazole: Possibly decreased sibutramine clearance

Adverse Reactions
CNS: Anxiety, depression, dizziness, drowsiness, headache, insomnia, nervousness, paresthesia, somnolence
CV: Chest pain, edema, hypertension, palpitations, tachycardia
EENT: Dry mouth, earache, rhinitis, sinusitis, taste perversion
GI: Abdominal pain, anorexia, constipation, diarrhea, gastritis, increased appetite, indigestion, nausea, thirst, vomiting
GU: Dysmenorrhea, UTI, vaginal candidiasis
MS: Arthralgia, back or neck pain, myalgia, tenosynovitis
SKIN: Acne, diaphoresis, flushing
Other: Flulike symptoms

Nursing Considerations
•WARNING Use sibutramine cautiously in patients with a history of substance abuse. Observe for signs of misuse, including drug-seeking behavior, drug tolerance, and increasing dosage.
•Measure blood pressure and pulse rate before and during sibutramine therapy.
•Because serotonin release from nerve terminals has been linked to cardiac valve dysfunction, assess for development of third heart sound.
•WARNING Monitor patient taking drugs for migraine headache for signs and symptoms of serotonin syndrome: agitation, anxiety, ataxia, chills, confusion, diaphoresis, disorientation, dysarthria, emesis, excitement, hemiballismus, hyperreflexia, hyperthermia, hypomania, lack of coordination, loss of consciousness, mydriasis, myoclonus, restlessness, tachycardia, tremor, and weakness. Notify prescriber immediately if such signs occur.

•Because drug decreases salivary flow and causes dry mouth, monitor for signs and symptoms of dental caries, oral candidiasis, and periodontal disease.

PATIENT TEACHING

•Caution patient not to take sibutramine more often than prescribed.

•Teach patient how to measure his blood pressure and pulse rate during therapy.

•Emphasize that sibutramine is intended as an adjunct to a calorie-reducing diet, not a replacement for it.

•Advise patient against taking OTC products that may contain ephedrine because of the increased risk of hypertension.

•Urge patient to avoid potentially hazardous activities until drug's CNS effects are known.

•If patient reports dry mouth, suggest sugar-free hard candy or gum or a saliva substitute.

sildenafil citrate

Viagra

Class and Category

Chemical: Pyrazolopyrimidinone derivative
Therapeutic: Anti-impotence
Pregnancy category: B

Indications and Dosages

➤ *To treat erectile dysfunction*

TABLETS

Adults. 50 mg q.d., taken 1 hr before sexual activity; increased as prescribed, based on clinical response. *Maximum:* 100 mg/day.

DOSAGE ADJUSTMENT Initial dose reduced to 25 mg for elderly patients, those with hepatic cirrhosis or severe renal impairment (creatinine clearance less than 30 ml/min/1.73 m^2), and those taking potent cytochrome P-450 3A4 inhibitors or ritonavir. *Maximum:* 25 mg/48 hr.

Route	Onset	Peak	Duration
P.O.	In 30 min	Unknown	4 hr

Mechanism of Action

Enhances effect of nitric oxide (released in the penis by sexual stimulation), which increases the cGMP level, relaxes smooth muscle, and increases blood flow into the corpus cavernosum, thus producing a penile erection.

Contraindications

Concomitant continuous or intermittent nitrate therapy, hypersensitivity to sildenafil or its components

Interactions

DRUGS

cimetidine, erythromycin, itraconazole, ketoconazole, mibefradil: Prolonged sildenafil effect
nitrates: Profound hypotension
protease inhibitors: Increased sildenafil effect
rifampin: Decreased sildenafil effect

FOODS

high-fat meals: Drug absorption delayed by up to 60 minutes

Adverse Reactions

CNS: Dizziness, headache, migraine, syncope
CV: Heart failure, hypotension, myocardial ischemia, orthostatic hypotension, palpitations, tachycardia
EENT: Blurred vision, change in color perception, nasal congestion, photophobia
ENDO: Uncontrolled diabetes mellitus
GI: Diarrhea, indigestion
GU: Cystitis, dysuria, painful erection, priapism, UTI
MS: Arthralgia, back pain
RESP: Upper respiratory tract infection
SKIN: Flushing, photosensitivity

Nursing Considerations

•Use sildenafil cautiously in men with renal or hepatic dysfunction, in elderly men, and in men with penile abnormalities that may predispose them to priapism.

•Monitor blood pressure and heart rate and rhythm before and frequently during therapy.

•Monitor blood glucose level frequently in diabetic patient because sildenafil may alter glucose control.

PATIENT TEACHING

•Explain that sildenafil may be taken up to 4 hours before sexual activity but that taking it 1 hour beforehand provides most effective results.

•WARNING Instruct patient not to take sildenafil if he also takes any form of organic nitrate, either continuously or intermittently, because profound hypotension and death could result.

•Advise patient to seek sexual counseling to enhance drug's effects.

•Inform patient that drug confers no protection from sexually transmitted diseases, including HIV infection. Counsel him about protective measures, as needed.

Q
R
S

•To avoid possible penile damage and permanent loss of erectile function, urge patient to notify prescriber immediately if erection is painful or lasts longer than 4 hours.
•Instruct diabetic patient to monitor his blood glucose level frequently because drug may affect glucose control.

simvastatin
Zocor

Class and Category
Chemical: Synthetically derived fermentation product of *Aspergillus terreus*
Therapeutic: Antihyperlipidemic
Pregnancy category: X

Indications and Dosages
➤ *To treat hyperlipidemia*
TABLETS
Adults. *Initial:* 20 to 40 mg/day in the evening. Dosage adjusted at 4-wk intervals, as needed, to achieve target LDL-cholesterol level. *Maintenance:* 5 to 80 mg/day. *Maximum:* 80 mg/day.
➤ *To treat homozygous familial hypercholesterolemia*
TABLETS
Adults. 40 mg/day in the evening, or 80 mg/day in 3 divided doses (20 mg, 20 mg, and 40 mg in the evening). Dosage adjusted q 4 wk, as needed, to achieve target LDL-cholesterol level. *Maintenance:* 5 to 40 mg/day. *Maximum:* 80 mg/day.
DOSAGE ADJUSTMENT For patients who take cyclosporine, initial dosage reduced to 5 mg/day and maximum dosage reduced to 10 mg/day. For elderly patients and those with renal impairment, initial dosage reduced to 5 mg/day. For patients who take fibric-acid derivative lipid-lowering drugs, such as gemfibrozil, or lipid-lowering doses of niacin (1 g/day or more), maximum dosage reduced to 10 mg/day. For patients who take amiodarone or verapamil, maximum dosage shouldn't exceed 20 mg/day.

Route	Onset	Peak	Duration
P.O.	2 wk	4 to 6 wk	Unknown

Contraindications
Active hepatic disease, breast-feeding, hypersensitivity to simvastatin or its components, pregnancy

Mechanism of Action
Interferes with the hepatic enzyme hydroxymethylglutaryl-coenzyme A reductase. This action reduces the formation of mevalonic acid, a cholesterol precursor, thus interrupting the pathway necessary for cholesterol synthesis. When the cholesterol level declines in hepatic cells, LDLs are consumed, which in turn reduces the levels of circulating total cholesterol and serum triglycerides.

Interactions
DRUGS
amiodarone, antiretroviral protease inhibitors (amprenavir, indinavir, nelfinavir, ritonavir, saquinavir), clarithromycin, cyclosporine, gemfibrozil and other fibrates, itraconazole, ketoconazole, erythromycin, nefazodone, niacin (1 g/day or more), verapamil: Increased risk of myopathy or rhabdomyolysis
azole antifungals, cyclosporine, gemfibrozil, immunosuppressants, macrolide antibiotics (including erythromycin), niacin, verapamil: Increased risk of acute renal failure
bile acid sequestrants, cholestyramine, colestipol: Decreased bioavailability of simvastatin
digoxin: Possibly slight elevation in blood digoxin level
diltiazem, verapamil: Possibly increased blood simvastatin level, increased risk of myopathy
oral anticoagulants: Increased bleeding or prolonged PT
FOODS
grapefruit juice (1 or more quarts/day): Possibly increased blood simvastatin level

Adverse Reactions
CNS: Dizziness, fatigue, headache
CV: Chest pain
EENT: Rhinitis
GI: Abdominal pain, constipation, diarrhea, elevated liver function test results, flatulence, heartburn, nausea, pancreatitis, vomiting
MS: Myalgia, rhabdomyolysis
SKIN: Rash

Nursing Considerations
•Use simvastatin cautiously in elderly patients and those with renal or hepatic impairment.
•Give drug 1 hour before or 4 hours after giving bile acid sequestrant, cholestyramine, or colestipol.

•Expect to monitor liver function test results every 3 to 6 months for abnormal elevations.
•Monitor serum lipoprotein level, as ordered, to evaluate response to therapy.

PATIENT TEACHING

•Advise patient to take simvastatin in the evening.
•Emphasize the importance of complying with dosage instructions to ensure drug's effectiveness.
•Encourage patient to follow a low-fat, cholesterol-lowering diet.
•Urge patient to notify prescriber immediately about muscle pain, tenderness, or weakness and other symptoms of myopathy.
•Inform female patient of childbearing age of need to use reliable contraceptive method while taking drug. Instruct her to notify prescriber at once if she suspects pregnancy.
•Advise patient to avoid grapefruit juice to decrease risk of drug toxicity.

sirolimus

(rapamycin)

Rapamune

Class and Category

Chemical: Macrocyclic lactone
Therapeutic: Immunosuppressant
Pregnancy category: C

Indications and Dosages

➤ *To prevent kidney transplant rejection*

ORAL SOLUTION

Adults and adolescents over age 13 weighing 40 kg or more. *Initial:* 6-mg loading dose. *Maintenance:* 2 mg q.d.
Adolescents over age 13 weighing less than 40 kg. *Initial:* 3-mg/m² loading dose. *Maintenance:* 1 mg/m² q.d.

DOSAGE ADJUSTMENT Maintenance dosage reduced by one-third for patients with impaired hepatic function.

Route	Onset	Peak	Duration
P.O.	Unknown	Unknown	Up to 6 mo after discontinuation

Contraindications

Hypersensitivity to sirolimus or its components, malignancy

Mechanism of Action

Inhibits activation and proliferation of T lymphocytes and antibody production. Sirolimus also inhibits cell cycle progression from the G1 to the S phase, possibly by inhibiting a key regulatory kinase believed to suppress cytokine-driven T-cell proliferation.

Interactions

DRUGS

aminoglycosides, amphotericin B: Possibly impaired renal function
bromocriptine, cimetidine, cisapride, clarithromycin, clotrimazole, cyclosporine, danazol, diltiazem, erythromycin, fluconazole, indinavir, itraconazole, ketoconazole, metoclopramide, nicardipine, ritonavir, troleandomycin, verapamil: Possibly increased blood sirolimus level and toxicity
carbamazepine, phenobarbital, phenytoin, rifabutin, rifapentine: Possibly decreased blood sirolimus level
HMG-CoA reductase inhibitors: Increased risk of rhabdomyolysis when administered concurrently with sirolimus and cyclosporine
rifampin: Significantly increased sirolimus clearance
vaccines (killed virus): Possibly decreased immune response to vaccines
vaccines (live virus): Increased risk of contracting disease from live virus

FOODS

grapefruit juice: Possibly decreased metabolism of sirolimus
high-fat diet: Reduced rate of sirolimus absorption

Adverse Reactions

CNS: Asthenia, fever, headache, insomnia, tremor
CV: Atrial fibrillation, chest pain, hyperlipidemia, hypertension, peripheral edema
GI: Abdominal pain, constipation, diarrhea, nausea, vomiting
GU: UTI
HEME: Anemia, lymphoma, thrombocytopenia
MS: Arthralgia, low back or flank pain
RESP: Dyspnea on exertion
SKIN: Acne, rash
Other: Hypercholesterolemia, hypokalemia, hypophosphatemia, weight gain or loss

Q
R
S

Nursing Considerations
•Monitor patients with existing or recent (including recent exposure to) chickenpox and patients with herpes zoster for worsening symptoms because they have an increased risk of developing severe generalized disease while taking sirolimus.
•For patients with hyperlipidemia, be prepared to institute dietary changes, an exercise program, or a lipid-lowering drug regimen if blood cholesterol or triglyceride levels increase because drug may aggravate hyperlipidemia.
•Mix oral sirolimus with at least 2 oz (60 ml) of water or orange juice in a glass or plastic container. Don't dilute drug in grapefruit juice or any other liquid.
•Stir well and have patient drink solution immediately. Then rinse glass with at least 4 oz (120 ml) of additional liquid, stir well, and have patient drink that liquid to make sure that all of drug is taken.
•Give initial dose as soon after transplant as possible and daily dose 4 hours after cyclosporine, as prescribed.
•Monitor patient for signs and symptoms of infection and check CBC results, as ordered, to detect sirolimus-induced blood dyscrasias or changes in neutrophil count, which may indicate infection.

PATIENT TEACHING
•Advise patient to take sirolimus consistently either with or without food (but not food high in fat) to prevent changes in absorption rate.
•Instruct patient to take daily dose with at least 2 oz (60 ml) of water or orange juice. Caution him *not* to dilute drug in grapefruit juice or any other liquid. Advise him to stir mixture well and drink immediately, then to add at least another 4 oz (120 ml) of liquid to empty container, stir mixture again, and drink that liquid to ensure that he has swallowed all of drug.
•Urge patient to avoid people with colds, flu, or other infections because his immunosuppressed state makes him more vulnerable to infection.
•Instruct patient not to take live vaccines, such as measles, mumps, rubella, oral polio, bacille Calmette-Guérin, yellow fever, varicella, and TY21a typhoid, during sirolimus therapy.
•Advise patient to keep follow-up appointments for blood tests, as ordered.

sodium bicarbonate
Arm and Hammer Pure Baking Soda, Bell/ans, Citrocarbonate, Soda Mint

Class and Category
Chemical: Electrolyte
Therapeutic: Antacid, electrolyte replenisher, systemic and urinary alkalizer
Pregnancy category: C

Indications and Dosages
➤ *To treat hyperacidity*
EFFERVESCENT POWDER
Adults and adolescents. 3.9 to 10 g in a glass of water after meals. *Maximum:* 19.5 g/day.
Children ages 6 to 12. 1 to 1.9 g in a glass of water after meals.
ORAL POWDER
Adults and adolescents. ½ tsp in a glass of water q 2 hr, p.r.n. *Maximum:* 4 tsp/day in patients up to age 60.
TABLETS
Adults and adolescents. 325 mg to 2 g q.d. to q.i.d., p.r.n. *Maximum:* 16 g/day.
Children ages 6 to 12. 520 mg, repeated once after 30 min, p.r.n.
➤ *To provide urinary alkalization*
ORAL POWDER
Adults and adolescents. 1 tsp in a glass of water q 4 hr. *Maximum:* 4 tsp/day in patients up to age 60.
TABLETS
Adults and adolescents. *Initial:* 4 g, then 1 to 2 g q 4 hr. *Maximum:* 16 g/day.
Children. 23 to 230 mg/kg/day, adjusted p.r.n.
I.V. INFUSION
Adults and children. 2 to 5 mEq/kg over 4 to 8 hr.
➤ *To treat metabolic acidosis during cardiac arrest*
I.V. INJECTION
Adults and children. *Initial:* 1 mEq/kg, followed by 0.5 mEq/kg q 10 min while arrest continues.
➤ *To treat less urgent forms of metabolic acidosis*
I.V. INFUSION
Adults and children. 2 to 5 mEq/kg over 4 to 8 hr.
DOSAGE ADJUSTMENT Dosage reduction possible for elderly patients because of age-related renal impairment.

Mechanism of Action

Increases plasma bicarbonate level, buffers excess hydrogen ions, and raises blood pH, thereby reversing metabolic acidosis. Sodium bicarbonate also increases the excretion of free bicarbonate ions in urine, raising urine pH; increased alkalinity of urine may help to dissolve uric acid calculi. In addition, it relieves symptoms of hyperacidity by neutralizing or buffering existing stomach acid, thereby increasing the pH of stomach contents.

Incompatibilities

Don't admix I.V. form of sodium bicarbonate in same solution or administer through same I.V. line as other drugs because precipitate may form.

Contraindications

Hypocalcemia in which alkalosis may lead to tetany; hypochloremic alkalosis secondary to vomiting, diuretics, or nasogastric suction; preexisting metabolic or respiratory alkalosis

Interactions

DRUGS

amphetamines, quinidine: Decreased urinary excretion of these drugs, possibly resulting in toxicity

anticholinergics: Decreased anticholinergic absorption and effectiveness

calcium-containing products: Increased risk of milk-alkali syndrome

chlorpropamide, lithium, salicylates, tetracyclines: Increased renal excretion and decreased absorption of these drugs

ciprofloxacin, norfloxacin, ofloxacin: Decreased solubility of these drugs, leading to crystalluria and nephrotoxicity

citrates: Increased risk of systemic alkalosis; increased risk of calcium calculus formation and hypernatremia in patients with history of uric acid calculi

digoxin: Possibly elevated blood digoxin level

enteric-coated drugs: Increased risk of gastric or duodenal irritation from rapid removal of enteric coating

ephedrine: Increased ephedrine half-life and duration of action

H_2-receptor antagonists, iron supplements or preparations, ketoconazole: Decreased absorption of these drugs

mecamylamine: Decreased excretion and prolonged effect of mecamylamine

methenamine: Decreased methenamine effectiveness

mexiletine: Possibly mexiletine toxicity

potassium supplements: Decreased serum potassium level

sucralfate: Interference with binding of sucralfate to gastric mucosa

urinary acidifiers (ammonium chloride, ascorbic acid, potassium and sodium phosphates): Counteracted effects of urinary acidifiers

FOODS

dairy products: Increased risk of milk-alkali syndrome with prolonged use of sodium bicarbonate

Adverse Reactions

CNS: Mental or mood changes

CV: Irregular heartbeat, peripheral edema (with large doses), weak pulse

EENT: Dry mouth

GI: Abdominal cramps, thirst

MS: Muscle spasms, myalgia

SKIN: Extravasation with necrosis, tissue sloughing, or ulceration

Nursing Considerations

•Monitor sodium intake of patient taking sodium bicarbonate because effervescent powder contains 700.6 mg of sodium/3.9 g; oral powder contains 952 mg of sodium/tsp; and tablets contain 325 mg/3.9-mEq tablet, 520 mg/6.2-mEq tablet, and 650 mg/7.7-mEq tablet.

•For I.V. infusion, dilute drug with NS, D_5W, or other standard electrolyte solution before administration.

•Avoid rapid I.V. infusion, which can cause severe alkalosis. Be aware that during cardiac arrest, risk of death from acidosis may outweigh risks of rapid infusion.

•Monitor urine pH, as ordered, to determine drug's effectiveness as urinary alkalizer.

•If patient receiving long-term sodium bicarbonate therapy is on a diet that includes calcium or milk, monitor for milk-alkali syndrome, characterized by anorexia, confusion, headache, hypercalcemia, metabolic acidosis, nausea, renal insufficiency, and vomiting.

•Be aware that parenteral formulations are hypertonic and that increased sodium intake can produce edema and weight gain.

•Assess I.V. site frequently for signs and symptoms of extravasation. If this occurs, notify prescriber immediately and remove I.V. catheter. Elevate the extremity, apply warm com-

Q
R
S

presses, and expect prescriber to administer a local injection of hyaluronidase or lidocaine.

PATIENT TEACHING

• Advise patient not to take sodium bicarbonate with large amounts of dairy products or for longer than 2 weeks, unless directed by prescriber.

• Caution patient not to take more than the prescribed amount of drug to avoid adverse reactions.

• Direct patient not to take drug within 2 hours of other oral drugs.

• Advise patient to avoid taking OTC drugs without prescriber's approval because many drugs interact with sodium bicarbonate.

sodium ferric gluconate

(contains 62.5 mg of elemental iron per 5 ml)

Ferrlecit

Class and Category

Chemical: Iron salt, mineral
Therapeutic: Antianemic
Pregnancy category: B

Indications and Dosages

➤ *To treat iron deficiency anemia in patients receiving long-term hemodialysis and erythropoietin*

I.V. INFUSION OR INJECTION

Adults. 125 mg of elemental iron. *Usual:* Minimum cumulative dose of 1 g of elemental iron given over eight sequential dialysis treatment. Dosage repeated at lowest dosage necessary to maintain target levels of hemoglobin and hematocrit and acceptable limits of blood iron levels.

Mechanism of Action

Acts to replenish iron stores lost during hemodialysis because of increased blood loss or increased iron utilization from epoetin therapy. Iron is an essential component of hemoglobin, myoglobin, and several enzymes, including cytochromes, catalase, and peroxidase, and is needed for catecholamine metabolism and normal neutrophil function. Sodium ferric gluconate also normalizes RBC production by binding with hemoglobin or being stored as ferritin in reticuloendothelial cells of the liver, spleen, and bone marrow.

Incompatibilities

Don't mix sodium ferric gluconate with other drugs or parenteral nutrition solutions for I.V. infusion.

Contraindications

Anemia other than iron deficiency, hypersensitivity to iron salts or their components, iron overload

Interactions

DRUGS

oral iron preparations: Possibly reduced absorption of oral iron supplements

Adverse Reactions

CNS: Asthenia, dizziness, fatigue, fever, headache, hypertonia, nervousness, paresthesia, syncope
CV: Chest pain, generalized edema, hypertension, hypotension, tachycardia
EENT: Dry mouth
GI: Abdominal pain, diarrhea, nausea, vomiting
HEME: Hemorrhage
MS: Back pain, leg cramps
RESP: Cough, dyspnea, upper respiratory tract infection
SKIN: Pruritus
Other: Generalized pain, hyperkalemia, hypersensitivity, infusion or injection site reaction

Nursing Considerations

• To reconstitute sodium ferric gluconate for I.V. infusion, dilute prescribed dosage in 100 ml of NS immediately before infusion. Infuse over 1 hour. Discard any unused diluted solution.

• Inspect drug for particles and discoloration before administration and discard if present.

• Administer undiluted drug by slow I.V. injection at a rate up to 12.5 mg/min, not to exceed 125 mg per injection.

• Be aware that most patients need a minimum cumulative dose of 1 gram of elemental iron administered over eight sequential dialysis treatments.

• **WARNING** Assess patient for signs and symptoms of an allergic reaction, including chills, facial flushing, pruritus, and rash, and of a hypersensitivity reaction, including diaphoresis, dyspnea, nausea, severe lower back pain, vomiting, and wheezing. Discontinue drug and notify prescriber immediately if patient develops an allergic or hypersensitivity reaction, and be prepared to provide emergency interventions.

•**WARNING** Assess blood pressure frequently after drug administration because hypotension may occur and may be related to infusion rate or total cumulative dose. Avoid rapid infusion and be prepared to provide I.V. fluids for volume expansion.

•Expect to monitor blood hemoglobin level, hematocrit, serum ferritin level, and transferrin saturation, as ordered, before, during, and after sodium ferric gluconate therapy. Make sure that serum iron level is tested 48 hours after last dose. To prevent iron toxicity, notify prescriber and expect to discontinue therapy if blood iron level is normal or elevated.

•Assess patient for possible iron overload, characterized by bleeding in GI tract and lungs, decreased activity, pale conjunctivae, and sedation.

PATIENT TEACHING
•Warn patient not to take any oral iron preparations during sodium ferric gluconate therapy without first consulting prescriber.
•Inform patient that symptoms of iron deficiency may include decreased stamina, learning problems, shortness of breath, and fatigue.

sodium phenylbutyrate

Buphenyl

Class and Category
Chemical: Phenylacetate prodrug
Therapeutic: Antihyperammonemic
Pregnancy category: C

Indications and Dosages
➤ *As adjunct to treat urea cycle disorders in combination with low-protein diet*

POWDER, TABLETS
Adults and children who weigh more than 20 kg (44 lb). 9.9 to 13 g/m^2/day in 4 to 6 divided doses with meals.
Children who weigh up to 20 kg. 450 to 600 mg/kg/day in 4 to 6 divided doses with meals.

Contraindications
Acute hyperammonemia, hypersensitivity to sodium phenylbutyrate or its components

Mechanism of Action
Provides alternate pathway for eliminating waste nitrogen by forming phenylacetate, an active metabolite that conjugates with glutamine to produce phenylacetylglutamine, which is excreted by the kidneys.

Interactions
DRUGS
corticosteroids: Increased serum ammonia level
haloperidol, valproate: Increased risk of hyperammonemia
probenecid: Decreased excretion of conjugated product of sodium phenylbutyrate

Adverse Reactions
CNS: Depression, disorientation, fatigue, headache, light-headedness, memory loss, syncope
CV: Arrhythmias
EENT: Hypoacusis, taste perversion
GI: Abdominal pain, anorexia, constipation, elevated liver function test results, gastritis, nausea, peptic ulcer, rectal bleeding, vomiting
GU: Amenorrhea, menstrual irregularities
HEME: Anemia, aplastic anemia, leukocytosis, leukopenia, thrombocytopenia
SKIN: Rash
Other: Body odor, hyperchloremia, hypoalbuminemia, hypophosphatemia, metabolic acidosis, metabolic alkalosis, weight gain

Nursing Considerations
•Mix powder form of sodium phenylbutyrate with food or liquid, but not with acidic beverages such as coffee and tea.
•Be aware that drug shouldn't be used to treat acute hyperammonemia, which is a medical emergency.
•Monitor patient with history of heart failure or severe renal failure for fluid retention because of drug's sodium content.

PATIENT TEACHING
•Instruct patient to take sodium phenylbutyrate with meals but not to mix it with acidic beverages such as coffee and tea.
•Advise patient to comply with follow-up laboratory tests, as prescribed.
•Urge patient to notify prescriber immediately about changes in body odor because they may be early signs of metabolic imbalance.

Q
R
S

sodium phosphate monobasic monohydrate and sodium phosphate dibasic anhydrous

(contains 1.5 g of sodium phosphate per tablet)
Visicol

Class and Category

Chemical: Acid salt
Therapeutic: Hyperosmotic laxative
Pregnancy category: C

Indications and Dosages

➤ *To cleanse colon in preparation for colonoscopy*

TABLETS

Adults. A total of 40 tablets (60 g of sodium phosphate) taken as follows: the evening before scheduled colonoscopy, 3 tablets q 15 min with 2 tablets as last dose; the day of the procedure (starting 3 to 5 hr beforehand), 3 tablets q 15 min with 2 tablets as last dose.

Route	Onset	Peak	Duration
P.O.	Unknown	Unknown	1 to 3 hr

Mechanism of Action

Increases the concentration gradient and osmotic pressure within the bowel by drawing large amounts of water into the small intestine. Bowel distention and increased fluid accumulation loosen stool and stimulate peristalsis, promoting bowel evacuation. Sodium phosphate also causes the release of cholecystokinin from the intestinal mucosa, which enhances the drug's laxative effect.

Contraindications

Acute colitis; ascites; bowel perforation; disorders associated with hypomotility, such as hypothyroidism and scleroderma; gastric retention; heart failure; hypersensitivity to sodium phosphate salts or their components; ileus, acute obstruction, or pseudo-obstruction; severe chronic constipation; toxic megacolon; unstable angina pectoris

Interactions

DRUGS

all oral drugs: Possibly malabsorption of these drugs

potassium-sparing diuretics, potassium supplements: Possibly decreased blood potassium level with long-term use of sodium phosphate; possibly decreased effects of potassium-sparing diuretics

Adverse Reactions

CNS: Dizziness, headache
GI: Abdominal cramps, distention, or pain; diarrhea; nausea; rectal irritation; thirst; vomiting
Other: Hypernatremia, hyperphosphatemia, hypocalcemia, hypokalemia

Nursing Considerations

• Expect to correct electrolyte abnormalities, such as hypocalcemia, hypokalemia, hypernatremia, or hyperphosphatemia, as ordered, before beginning sodium phosphate therapy.

• Ensure that patient maintains a clear liquid diet for 12 hours before first dose, as ordered.

• Administer each dose with 8 oz of clear liquid to prevent excessive fluid loss and hypovolemia.

• Be aware that drug should not be given within 7 days of prior use.

• **WARNING** Monitor patient for hypocalcemia, hypokalemia, hypernatremia, and hyperphosphatemia during therapy. Notify prescriber at once if patient develops an electrolyte imbalance, and prepare to administer corrective therapy as prescribed. Expect electrolyte imbalances to return to baseline within 48 to 72 hours.

• During drug administration and for up to 72 hours afterward, monitor serum electrolyte levels, as ordered, of patients with impaired renal function, those with preexisting electrolyte disturbances, and those taking drugs that may affect electrolyte levels.

• Monitor patients at risk for severe electrolyte imbalance, including hypokalemia and hypocalcemia, for prolonged QT interval because serious arrhythmias may occur.

• Monitor fluid intake and output during bowel preparation to prevent or detect excessive fluid loss and hypovolemia.

• Monitor patients with a history of inflammatory bowel disease for persistent acute abdominal pain, which may indicate ulceration of colonic mucosa. Notify prescriber immediately if pain persists or intensifies.

• Be aware that undigested or partially digested tablets may be visible in watery stools or during colonoscopy.

PATIENT TEACHING

• Instruct patient to maintain a clear liquid diet for 12 hours before first dose of sodium phosphate, as ordered.

• Teach patient prescribed dosage and dosing interval. Inform him that bowel preparation will begin the evening before the scheduled procedure and will continue 3 to 5 hours beforehand. Encourage him to drink at least 8 oz of clear liquids every time he takes drug to prevent dehydration.

• Instruct patient not to use additional bowel-cleansing agents, especially those containing sodium phosphate, while he's taking this drug.

• Inform patient that stools may be watery during and immediately after drug therapy.

• Explain that he may see undigested or partially digested tablets (either of sodium phosphate or of other drugs) in stools; reassure him that this is a normal occurrence.

sodium polystyrene sulfonate

Kayexalate, K-Exit (CAN), Kionex, PMS-Sodium Polystyrene Sulfonate (CAN), SPS Suspension

Class and Category

Chemical: Sulfonated cation-exchange resin
Therapeutic: Antihyperkalemic
Pregnancy category: C

Indications and Dosages

➤ _To treat hyperkalemia_

ORAL POWDER, SUSPENSION

Adults. 15 g (4 level tsp) q.d. to q.i.d. _Maximum:_ 40 g q.i.d.

Children. 1 g/kg/dose, as needed.

RECTAL POWDER, SUSPENSION

Adults. 25 to 100 g as retention enema, as needed.

Children. 1 g/kg/dose as retention enema, as needed.

Route	Onset	Peak	Duration
P.O.	2 to 12 hr	Unknown	Unknown

Contraindications

Hypersensitivity to sodium polystyrene sulfonate or its components, hypokalemia

Mechanism of Action

Releases sodium ions in exchange for other cations in intestines. Resin enters large intestine and releases sodium ions in exchange for hydrogen ions. As the resin moves through the intestines, hydrogen ions are then exchanged for potassium ions, which are in greater concentration. Bound resin leaves the body in feces, carrying potassium and other ions with it, thereby reducing serum potassium level.

Interactions

DRUGS

antacids, laxatives: Increased risk of metabolic alkalosis
potassium-sparing diuretics, potassium supplements: Increased risk of fluid retention

Adverse Reactions

CV: Peripheral edema
GI: Abdominal cramps, anorexia, constipation, epigastric pain, fecal impaction, indigestion, nausea, vomiting
GU: Decreased urine output
Other: Hypernatremia, hypocalcemia, hypokalemia, weight gain

Nursing Considerations

• Use sodium polystyrene sulfonate cautiously in patients with heart failure, hypertension, or marked edema.

• Be aware that drug is available as powdered resin or as solution that contains sorbitol to facilitate movement of resin through intestines. As a result, patient may experience abdominal cramps, diarrhea, nausea, and vomiting.

• Because the drug doesn't take effect for several hours, be aware that it's inappropriate for acute, life-threatening hyperkalemia.

• If patient has hypokalemia or hypocalcemia, notify prescriber immediately and expect to withhold drug because it reduces total body levels of potassium and calcium. Evidence of hypokalemia includes abdominal cramps, acidic urine, anorexia, drowsiness, ECG changes, hypotension, hypoventilation, muscle weakness, and tachycardia. Evidence of hypocalcemia includes abdominal pain, agitation, anxiety, ECG changes, hypotension, muscle twitching, psychosis, seizures, and tetany.

•To administer powdered resin as oral suspension, mix in water, syrup (such as sorbitol), or food and give promptly. If necessary, administer through gastric feeding tube.
•Precede rectal administration with a cleansing enema, as ordered.
•When administering rectally, suspend powdered resin in 100 ml of aqueous solution warmed to body temperature, in bag connected to soft, large (French 28) catheter. Have patient lie on his left side with his lower leg straight and upper leg flexed or with his knees to his chest. Gently insert the tube into the rectum and well into the sigmoid colon. The solution should flow into the colon by way of gravity and be retained for 30 to 60 minutes or longer, if possible. After patient is unable to retain the solution any longer, administer a non-sodium-containing cleansing enema, as prescribed.
•After administration, assess for constipation and fecal impaction.

PATIENT TEACHING
•Instruct patient not to mix oral form of sodium polystyrene sulfonate with foods and liquids high in potassium content, such as bananas and orange juice.
•Teach patient who will self-administer the rectal solution the correct technique and body position. Remind him to allow the solution to flow into the colon by way of gravity and to retain it for 30 to 60 minutes or longer, if possible.
•Advise patient to notify prescriber immediately about abdominal cramps, nausea, and vomiting.

sodium thiosalicylate

Rexolate, Tusal

Class and Category
Chemical: Salicylic acid derivative
Therapeutic: Analgesic, anti-inflammatory
Pregnancy category: Not rated

Indications and Dosages
➤ *To relieve symptoms of acute gout*
I.V. OR I.M. INJECTION
Adults. *Initial:* 100 mg q 3 to 4 hr for 2 days, then 100 mg/day.
➤ *To relieve pain from musculoskeletal conditions*
I.V. OR I.M. INJECTION
Adults. 50 to 100 mg q.d. or q.o.d.

➤ *To relieve symptoms of osteoarthritis*
I.V. OR I.M. INJECTION
Adults. 100 mg 3 times/wk for several wk, then once/wk, usually up to a total dosage of 2.5 g. After 1 to 2 wk, another course of treatment may be given.
➤ *To treat rheumatic fever*
I.V. OR I.M. INJECTION
Adults. *Initial:* 100 to 150 mg q 4 to 8 hr for 3 days, then 100 mg b.i.d.

Mechanism of Action
Exerts peripherally induced analgesic and anti-inflammatory effects by blocking pain impulses and inhibiting prostaglandin synthesis.

Contraindications
GI bleeding; hemophilia; hemorrhage; hypersensitivity to sodium thiosalicylate, NSAIDs, or their components; Reye's syndrome

Interactions
DRUGS
ACE inhibitors, beta blockers: Decreased antihypertensive effect of these drugs
activated charcoal: Decreased sodium thiosalicylate absorption
antacids, urinary alkalizers: Increased sodium thiosalicylate excretion, leading to reduced effectiveness and shortened half-life
carbonic anhydrase inhibitors (such as acetazolamide): Increased risk of salicylate toxicity; possibly displacement of acetazolamide from protein-binding sites, resulting in toxicity
corticosteroids: Possibly increased sodium thiosalicylate excretion
insulin, oral antidiabetic drugs: Altered glucose control (with large doses of sodium thiosalicylate)
loop diuretics: Possibly decreased effectiveness of loop diuretics in patients with renal or hepatic impairment
methotrexate: Increased risk of methotrexate toxicity
nizatidine: Increased blood sodium thiosalicylate level
probenecid, sulfinpyrazone: Decreased uricosuric effects
spironolactone: Possibly inhibited diuretic effect of spironolactone
urinary acidifiers (including ammonium chloride, ascorbic acid, methionine): Decreased

sodium thiosalicylate excretion, possibly leading to salicylate toxicity

ACTIVITIES
alcohol use: Increased risk of GI ulceration

Adverse Reactions
GI: Anorexia, diarrhea, GI bleeding, heartburn, hepatotoxicity, indigestion, nausea, thirst, vomiting
HEME: Leukopenia, platelet dysfunction, prolonged bleeding time, thrombocytopenia
RESP: Bronchospasm
SKIN: Rash, urticaria
Other: Angioedema

Nursing Considerations
• Use sodium thiosalicylate cautiously in patients with asthma, chronic urticaria, or nasal polyps because they are more prone to drug hypersensitivity.
• Expect to monitor hepatic and renal function during long-term drug therapy.
• After repeated administration or large doses, assess for signs of salicylate toxicity: CNS depression, confusion, diaphoresis, diarrhea, difficulty hearing, dizziness, headache, hyperventilation, lassitude, tinnitus, and vomiting.
• Be aware that tinnitus usually means that blood sodium thiosalicylate level has reached or exceeded upper limits for therapeutic effects.

PATIENT TEACHING
• Instruct patient to report bleeding or symptoms of salicylate toxicity immediately.

somatropin
Genotropin, Humatrope, Norditropin, Nutropin, Nutropin AQ, Saizen, Serostim

Class and Category
Chemical: Recombinant DNA product
Therapeutic: Growth hormone
Pregnancy category: B (Serostim) or C (Genotropin, Humatrope, Norditropin, Nutropin, Nutropin AQ, Saizen)

Indications and Dosages
➤ *To treat growth failure caused by growth hormone deficiency*

S.C. INJECTION (NUTROPIN, NUTROPIN AQ)
Adults. 0.3 mg (0.9 IU)/kg/wk.

I.M. OR S.C. INJECTION (HUMATROPE, NUTROPIN, SAIZEN)
Children. 0.18 to 0.3 mg (0.54 to 0.9 IU)/kg/wk, divided into equal doses administered q.d. or q.o.d. over 6 to 7 days.

S.C. INJECTION (GENOTROPIN, NORDITROPIN)
Children. 0.16 to 0.24 mg (0.48 to 0.72 IU)/kg/wk, divided into equal doses administered q.d. over 6 to 7 days.

➤ *To treat growth failure caused by chronic renal insufficiency*

S.C. INJECTION (NUTROPIN, NUTROPIN AQ)
Children. Up to 0.35 mg (1.05 IU)/kg/wk, divided into equal doses administered q.d.

➤ *To treat growth failure caused by Turner's syndrome*

S.C. INJECTION (NUTROPIN, NUTROPIN AQ)
Adults and children. Up to 0.375 mg (1.125 IU)/kg/wk, divided into equal doses administered q.d. or q.o.d. over 7 days.

➤ *To provide long-term treatment of growth failure in children born small for gestational age who fail to show catch-up growth by age 2*

S.C. INJECTION (GENOTROPIN)
Children. 0.48 mg/kg/wk, divided into equal doses and administered q.d. over 6 to 7 days.

➤ *To treat AIDS-associated cachexia or weight loss*

S.C. INJECTION (SEROSTIM)
Adults who weigh more than 55 kg (121 lb). 6 mg h.s.
Adults who weigh 45 to 55 kg (99 to 121 lb). 5 mg h.s.
Adults who weigh 35 to 45 kg (77 to 99 lb). 4 mg h.s.
Adults who weigh less than 35 kg. 0.1 mg/kg h.s.

Route	Onset	Peak	Duration
I.M., S.C.	Unknown	Unknown	12 to 48 hr

Contraindications
Cancer; closed epiphyses; hypersensitivity to somatropin, its components, or benzyl alcohol

Interactions
DRUGS
anabolic steroids, androgens, estrogens, thyroid hormones: Possibly accelerated epiphyseal closure
corticosteroids, corticotropin: Inhibited growth response to somatropin

Adverse Reactions
CNS: Headache, weakness
CV: Peripheral edema

EENT: Papilledema, vision changes
ENDO: Gynecomastia, hyperglycemia, hypothyroidism
GI: Nausea, vomiting
MS: Carpal tunnel syndrome, myalgia
SKIN: Increased growth of nevi, rash
Other: Injection site inflammation

Mechanism of Action

Increases production of somatomedins (or insulin-like growth factor) in the liver and other tissues. This action mediates somatropin's anabolic and growth-promoting effects. The drug binds to specific receptors throughout the body, stimulating amino acid transport; DNA, RNA, and protein synthesis; cell proliferation; and growth of bone and soft tissue.

Somatropin also exerts the following actions:
• decreases insulin cell receptor sensitivity, thereby increasing blood glucose level
• stimulates triglyceride hydrolysis in adipose tissue and hepatic glucose output
• aids bone growth by promoting a positive calcium balance and retention of sodium and potassium.

Nursing Considerations

• Reconstitute somatropin according to package directions. (Nutropin AQ doesn't require reconstitution.) In general, swirl vial gently, rather than shaking it, to dissolve contents.
• Don't reconstitute with diluent that contains benzyl alcohol if drug will be given to neonate. Instead, use sterile water for injection.
• Store Nutropin AQ vials and cartridges refrigerated in a dark place.
• **WARNING** Anticipate increased risk of headache, nausea, papilledema, vision changes, and vomiting, especially during first 8 weeks of therapy.
• Because somatropin is a protein, monitor patient for a local or systemic allergic reaction.
• Assess patients with Turner's syndrome for otitis media and other ear and hearing disorders.
• Frequently check blood glucose level in diabetic patient who takes insulin because drug may induce insulin resistance.

PATIENT TEACHING

• Instruct diabetic patient who takes insulin to monitor blood glucose level frequently because

somatropin may induce insulin resistance.
• Inform parents of child with Turner's syndrome about increased risk of ear infections associated with treatment.
• Advise family to observe patient for limping, which may indicate a slipped epiphysis.

sotalol hydrochloride

Betapace, Betapace AF, Sotacor (CAN)

Class and Category

Chemical: Methanesulfonanilide
Therapeutic: Class III antiarrhythmic
Pregnancy category: B

Indications and Dosages

➤ *To treat life-threatening ventricular arrhythmias*

TABLETS

Adults. *Initial:* 80 mg b.i.d. *Maintenance:* 160 to 320 mg/day in divided doses b.i.d. or t.i.d. *Maximum:* 640 mg/day.

DOSAGE ADJUSTMENT For patients with creatinine clearance of 30 to 60 ml/min/1.73 m^2, dosage interval extended to q 24 hr; for creatinine clearance less than 30 ml/min/1.73 m^2, dosage interval extended to q 36 to 48 hr, according to clinical response; for creatinine clearance less than 10 ml/min/1.73 m^2, dosage individualized as prescribed.

➤ *To maintain normal sinus rhythm in patients with highly symptomatic atrial fibrillation who are currently in sinus rhythm*

TABLETS

Adults. *Initial:* 80 mg q.d. if creatinine clearance is 40 to 60 ml/min/1.73 m^2, or 80 mg b.i.d. if creatinine clearance exceeds 60 ml/min/ 1.73 m^2. *Maintenance:* After at least 3 days (five or six doses with q.d. dosing), if 80-mg dose is tolerated and QT interval remains less than 500 msec, current dosage maintained and patient discharged. Or, during hospitalization, patient monitored closely to determine maintenance dosage while dosage is increased to 120 mg b.i.d. for 3 days (five or six doses if q.d. dosing). *Maximum:* 160 mg b.i.d. if creatinine clearance exceeds 60 ml/min/1.73 m^2.

DOSAGE ADJUSTMENT If 80-mg q.d. or b.i.d dosage doesn't reduce frequency of atrial fibrillation relapses and is tolerated without excessive QT interval prolongation (greater than 520 msec), dosage increased to 120 mg q.d. or b.i.d., depending on creatinine clearance. If 120-mg dose doesn't reduce frequency of early relapse and is tolerated without excessive QT interval prolongation (greater than 520 msec), dosage increased to 160 mg q.d. or b.i.d., depending on creatinine clearance.

DOSAGE ADJUSTMENT Dosage reduced if QT interval is 520 msec or greater until QT interval returns to less than 520 msec. Drug discontinued if QT interval is greater than 520 msec with lowest maintenance dosage of 80 mg. Daily dosage reduced by half and given q.d. if renal function deteriorates.

Route	Onset	Peak	Duration
P.O.	Unknown	2 to 3 hr	Unknown

Mechanism of Action
Combines class II and class III antiarrhythmic activity to increase sinus cycle length. This beta blocker decreases AV nodal conduction and increases AV nodal refractoriness. Suppression of SA node automaticity and AV node conductivity decreases atrial and ventricular ectopy.

Contraindications
Asthma, atrial arrhythmias (if baseline QT interval exceeds 450 msec or creatinine clearance is less than 40 ml/min/1.73 m²), cardiogenic shock, congenital or acquired QT syndromes, COPD, heart failure (unless it results from tachyarrhythmia that's treatable by sotalol), hypersensitivity to sotalol or its components, second- or third-degree AV block without functioning pacemaker, sinus bradycardia

Interactions
DRUGS
allergen immunotherapy, allergenic extracts for skin testing: Increased risk of serious systemic adverse reaction or anaphylaxis
amiodarone: Additive depressant effect on conduction, negative inotropic effect
anesthetics (hydrocarbon inhalation): Increased risk of myocardial depression and hypotension
antacids: Altered sotalol effectiveness
astemizole, class I antiarrhythmics, phenothiazines, terfenadine, tricyclic antidepressants: Prolonged QT interval, life-threatening torsades de pointes

beta blockers (other): Additive beta blockade
beta₂-receptor stimulants: Decreased effectiveness of these drugs
calcium channel blockers, clonidine, diazoxide, guanabenz, reserpine and other antihypertensives: Additive antihypertensive effect and, possibly, other beta-blocking effects
cimetidine: Possibly impaired sotalol clearance
glucagon: Possibly blunted hyperglycemic response
insulin, oral antidiabetic drugs: Impaired glucose control, increased risk of hyperglycemia
lidocaine: Decreased lidocaine clearance, increased risk of lidocaine toxicity
MAO inhibitors: Increased risk of significant hypertension
neuromuscular blockers: Possibly potentiated and prolonged neuromuscular blockade
phenothiazines: Increased blood levels of both drugs
propafenone: Increased blood level and half-life of sotalol
sympathomimetics, xanthines: Possibly mutual inhibition of therapeutic effects

Adverse Reactions
CNS: Anxiety, depression, dizziness, drowsiness, fatigue, insomnia, lethargy, nervousness, weakness
CV: AV conduction disorders, bradycardia, heart failure, hypotension, peripheral vascular insufficiency
EENT: Nasal congestion
ENDO: Hyperglycemia, hypoglycemia
GI: Abdominal pain, constipation, diarrhea, nausea, vomiting
GU: Sexual dysfunction
MS: Muscle weakness
RESP: Bronchospasm, dyspnea, wheezing

Nursing Considerations
•Obtain baseline creatinine clearance and QT interval before starting sotalol therapy, as ordered.
•Monitor blood pressure, apical and radial pulse rates, fluid intake and output, daily weight, and respiratory rate, and assess circulation in extremities before and during sotalol therapy.
•If prescriber is discontinuing amiodarone, be aware that sotalol shouldn't be started until QT interval has returned to baseline because of possible adverse cardiac effects.

Q
R
S

•Be aware that sotalol shouldn't be discontinued abruptly because doing so may lead to life-threatening reactions.
•Monitor serum electrolyte levels because drug can increase risk of torsades de pointes in patients with electrolyte imbalances, especially hypokalemia or hypomagnesemia.
•Carefully evaluate assessment findings if patient has diabetes mellitus or thyrotoxicosis because these conditions may mask signs and symptoms of hypoglycemia or hyperthyroidism.

PATIENT TEACHING
•Advise patient to notify prescriber immediately if he has difficulty breathing.
•Encourage patient to consult with prescriber before taking OTC drugs, especially cold remedies, which may decrease sotalol's effectiveness.
•Urge patient to avoid potentially hazardous activities until drug's CNS effects are known.

sparfloxacin

Zagam

Class and Category
Chemical: Fluoroquinolone
Therapeutic: Antibiotic
Pregnancy category: C

Indications and Dosages
➤ *To treat community-acquired pneumonia caused by* Chlamydia pneumoniae, Haemophilus influenzae, H. parainfluenzae, Moraxella catarrhalis, Mycoplasma pneumoniae, *or* Streptococcus pneumoniae *and acute bacterial exacerbations of chronic bronchitis caused by* C. pneumoniae, Enterobacter cloacae, H. influenzae, H. parainfluenzae, Klebsiella pneumoniae, M. catarrhalis, Staphylococcus aureus, *or* S. pneumoniae

TABLETS
Adults. 400 mg on day 1, followed by 200 mg/day for 10 days.
DOSAGE ADJUSTMENT For patients with creatinine clearance less than 50 ml/min/1.73 m², 400 mg on day 1 and then dosing interval extended to 200 mg q 48 hr for 9 days.

Mechanism of Action
Causes bacterial cells to die by inhibiting the enzyme DNA gyrase, which is responsible for unwinding and supercoiling bacterial DNA before it replicates.

Contraindications
History of photosensitivity, hypersensitivity to quinolone derivatives, job or lifestyle that precludes compliance with safety measures to prevent phototoxicity, prolonged QTc interval or concurrent use of drugs that can prolong QTc interval

Interactions
DRUGS
aluminum-, calcium-, or magnesium-containing antacids; ferrous sulfate; magnesium-containing laxatives; sucralfate; zinc: Decreased bioavailability of sparfloxacin
amiodarone, astemizole, bepridil, cisapride, class IA antiarrhythmics (disopyramide, quinidine, procainamide), class III antiarrhythmics (ibutilide, sotalol), erythromycin, pentamidine, phenothiazines, terfenadine, tricyclic antidepressants, other drugs that can prolong QTc interval: Possibly prolonged QTc interval and torsades de pointes

Adverse Reactions
CNS: Asthenia, dizziness, drowsiness, headache, insomnia, light-headedness, nervousness, seizures, somnolence
CV: Prolonged QTc interval, vasodilation
EENT: Taste perversion
GI: Abdominal pain, diarrhea, nausea, pseudomembranous colitis, vomiting
GU: Vaginal candidiasis
MS: Tendinitis, tendon rupture
SKIN: Photosensitivity, pruritus, rash

Nursing Considerations
•Use sparfloxacin cautiously in patients with known or suspected CNS disorders because of risk of seizures. Institute seizure precautions according to facility policy.
•Monitor renal and liver function test results, as appropriate, during prolonged sparfloxacin therapy.
•Measure QTc interval regularly because sparfloxacin has been found to increase QTc interval, placing patient at risk for torsades de pointes.
•Monitor for severe diarrhea, which may indicate pseudomembranous colitis; be prepared to administer fluid, electrolyte, and protein replacement, as ordered.

PATIENT TEACHING
•Urge patient to avoid hazardous activities until sparfloxacin's CNS effects are known.
•Advise patient to notify prescriber immediately about aching or throbbing tendon pain.

•Instruct patient to wait 4 hours after taking sparfloxacin before taking antacids that contain aluminum, calcium, or magnesium; laxatives that contain magnesium; or vitamins that contain iron or zinc.
•Caution patient to avoid exposure to sunlight, bright natural light, and other sources of ultraviolet light during therapy and for 5 days afterward. Urge him to wear sunscreen and protective clothing when outdoors.
•Urge patient to notify prescriber at first sign of photosensitivity reaction (blistering, burning or swelling sensation, itching, rash, redness).

spectinomycin hydrochloride

Trobicin

Class and Category
Chemical: Aminocyclitol, aminoglycoside derivative
Therapeutic: Antibiotic
Pregnancy category: Not rated

Indications and Dosages
➤ *To treat acute endocervical, rectal, and urethral gonorrhea caused by susceptible strains of* Neisseria gonorrhoeae
I.M. INJECTION
Adults and children who weigh 45 kg (99 lb) or more. 2 g as a single dose, repeated as prescribed for adult if reinfection occurs or is strongly suspected. *Maximum:* 4 g for adults, 2 g for children.
Children who weigh less than 45 kg (except infants). 40 mg/kg as a single dose.

Mechanism of Action
Binds to negatively charged sites on the bacteria's outer cell membrane, disrupting cell integrity. Spectinomycin also binds to bacterial ribosomal subunits and inhibits protein synthesis. Both actions lead to bacterial cell death.

Contraindications
Hypersensitivity to spectinomycin or its components

Interactions
None known.

Adverse Reactions
CNS: Dizziness, insomnia

GI: Abdominal cramps, nausea, vomiting
Other: Injection site pain

Nursing Considerations
•To reconstitute spectinomycin, add 3.2 ml of bacteriostatic water for injection (with benzyl alcohol) to each 2-g vial or 6.2 ml of diluent to each 4-g vial. Shake vial vigorously before withdrawing dose.
•Administer I.M. injection deep into large muscle mass, preferably upper outer quadrant of gluteal muscle.
PATIENT TEACHING
•Advise patient that he'll be tested for syphilis at the start of treatment and 3 months later because spectinomycin treatment may mask or delay syphilis symptoms.
•Inform patient of risk factors for sexually transmitted diseases, and teach correct use of condoms.
•Advise patient to encourage sexual partner to be tested for gonorrhea.
•Instruct patient to notify prescriber if symptoms fail to improve within a few days.

spironolactone

Aldactone, Novospiroton (CAN)

Class and Category
Chemical: Aldosterone antagonist
Therapeutic: Aldosterone antagonist, antihypertensive, diagnostic aid for primary hyperaldosteronism, diuretic
Pregnancy category: Not rated

Indications and Dosages
➤ *To treat edema due to heart failure, hepatic cirrhosis, or nephrotic syndrome*
TABLETS
Adults. *Initial:* 25 to 200 mg/day in divided doses b.i.d. to q.i.d. for at least 5 days. *Maintenance:* 75 to 400 mg/day in divided doses b.i.d. to q.i.d. *Maximum:* 400 mg/day.
Children. *Initial:* 1 to 3 mg/kg/day as a single dose or in divided doses b.i.d. to q.i.d. for at least 2 wk; adjusted, as needed, after 5 days. *Maximum:* 3 times initial dose.

➤ *To manage hypertension*
TABLETS
Adults. *Initial:* 50 to 100 mg/day as a single dose or in divided doses b.i.d. to q.i.d. for at least 2 wk; gradually adjusted q 2 wk, as needed, to control blood pressure, up to 200 mg/day. *Maximum:* 400 mg/day.

Children. *Initial:* 1 to 3 mg/kg/day as a single dose or in divided doses b.i.d. to q.i.d. for at least 2 wk; adjusted, as needed, after 5 days. *Maximum:* 3 times initial dose.

➤ *To aid in the diagnosis of primary hyperaldosteronism*

TABLETS

Adults. For long test, 400 mg/day in divided doses b.i.d. to q.i.d. for 3 to 4 wk; for short test, 400 mg/day in divided doses b.i.d. to q.i.d. for 4 days.

➤ *To treat primary hyperaldosteronism*

TABLETS

Adults. 100 to 400 mg/day in divided doses b.i.d. to q.i.d. before surgery. *Maximum:* 400 mg/day.

DOSAGE ADJUSTMENT Long-term maintenance dosage decreased for patients at risk for complications during surgery.

➤ *To substitute as therapy for diuretic-induced hypokalemia*

TABLETS

Adults. 25 to 100 mg/day as a single dose or in divided doses b.i.d. to q.i.d. *Maximum:* 400 mg/day.

Route	Onset	Peak	Duration
P.O.*	Unknown	2 to 3 days	2 to 3 days

Contraindications

Acute renal insufficiency, anuria, hyperkalemia, hypersensitivity to spironolactone or its components

Interactions

DRUGS

ACE inhibitors, cyclosporine, other potassium-sparing diuretics, potassium-containing drugs, potassium supplements: Increased risk of hyperkalemia

digoxin: Possibly increased half-life of digoxin

exchange resins (sodium cycle), such as sodium polystyrene sulfonate: Increased risk of hypokalemia and fluid retention

heparin, oral anticoagulants: Decreased anticoagulant effect of these drugs

---

* For diuretic effect; others unknown.

Mechanism of Action

Normally, aldosterone attaches to receptors on the walls of distal convoluted tubule cells, causing sodium (Na^+) and water (H_2O) reabsorption in the blood, as shown below left.

Spironolactone competes with aldosterone for these receptors, thereby preventing sodium and water reabsorption and causing their excretion through the distal convoluted tubules, as shown below right. Increased urinary excretion of sodium and water reduces blood volume and blood pressure.

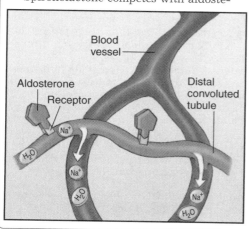

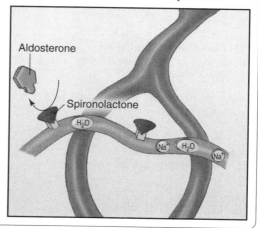

hypotension-producing drugs: Possibly potentiated antihypertensive or diuretic effect of spironolactone
lithium: Possibly lithium toxicity
NSAIDs, sympathomimetics: Decreased antihypertensive effect of spironolactone
FOODS
low-salt milk, salt substitutes: Increased risk of hyperkalemia

Adverse Reactions
CNS: Dizziness, encephalopathy, fatigue, headache
EENT: Increased intraocular pressure, nasal congestion, tinnitus, vision changes
ENDO: Gynecomastia
GI: Abdominal pain, anorexia, constipation, diarrhea, flatulence, nausea, vomiting
GU: Impotence
HEME: Aplastic anemia, neutropenia
RESP: Cough, dyspnea
MS: Arthralgia, back and leg pain, muscle weakness, myalgia
Other: Hyperkalemia

Nursing Considerations
•Be aware that for children or patients who have difficulty swallowing, pharmacist may crush spironolactone tablets, mix with a flavored syrup, and dispense as a suspension that is stable for 1 month when refrigerated.
•During diagnosis for primary aldosteronism, the test is considered positive if patient's serum potassium level rises when drug is given and falls when it's discontinued.
•Monitor serum potassium level, as appropriate. Withhold drug and notify prescriber if hyperkalemia develops.
•Evaluate spironolactone's effectiveness by monitoring blood pressure and assessing for edema.
•Stop drug for several days, as prescribed, before patient undergoes adrenal vein catheterization to measure serum aldosterone level and plasma renin activity.
PATIENT TEACHING
•Instruct patient to take spironolactone with meals or milk.
•If patient has trouble swallowing tablets, mention that pharmacist can crush them, mix them with a flavored syrup, and dispense as a suspension.
•Teach patient who takes drug for hypertension how to measure his blood pressure. Urge him to monitor it regularly and report measurements greater than 140 mm Hg systolic or 90 mm Hg diastolic to prescriber.
•Caution patient that he may experience dizziness during spironolactone therapy if fluid balance is altered.

streptokinase
Kabikinase, Streptase

Class and Category
Chemical: Purified beta-hemolytic *Streptococcus* filtrate
Therapeutic: Thrombolytic
Pregnancy category: C

Indications and Dosages
➤ *To lyse coronary artery thrombi*
I.V. INFUSION
Adults. 1,500,000 IU within 60 min of event.
INTRACORONARY INFUSION
Adults. 20,000-IU bolus, followed by 2,000 IU/min for 60 min for total dose of 140,000 IU.

➤ *To lyse acute arterial thromboembolism or thrombosis, acute pulmonary embolism, or deep vein thrombosis*
I.V. INFUSION
Adults. 250,000-IU bolus over 30 min, followed by 100,000 IU/hr for 24 to 72 hr.
➤ *To clear occluded arteriovenous cannula*
I.V. INJECTION
Adults. 100,000 to 250,000 IU instilled slowly into each occluded lumen.

Route	Onset	Peak	Duration
I.V.	Immediate	20 to 120 min	4 hr

Mechanism of Action
Binds to fibrin in thrombus and converts trapped plasminogen to plasmin. Plasmin breaks down fibrin, fibrinogen, and other clotting factors, thereby dissolving the thrombus.

Incompatibilities
Don't mix streptokinase in same syringe or administer through same I.V. line as other drugs.

Contraindications
Active internal bleeding, AV malformation or aneurysm, bleeding diathesis, history of CVA

or intracranial or intraspinal surgery within the past 2 months, hypersensitivity to streptokinase or its components, intracranial cancer, severe uncontrolled hypertension

Interactions

DRUGS

anticoagulants, enoxaparin, heparin, NSAIDs, platelet aggregation inhibitors: Increased risk of bleeding

antifibrinolytics: Antagonized effects of both drugs

antihypertensives: Increased risk of severe hypotension, especially when streptokinase is administered rapidly to treat coronary artery occlusion

cefamandole, cefoperazone, cefotetan, plicamycin, valproic acid: Possibly hypoprothrombinemia and increased risk of severe hemorrhage

corticosteroids, ethacrynic acid, salicylates: Possibly GI ulceration or bleeding

Adverse Reactions

CNS: Chills, fever
CV: Arrhythmias, hypotension
HEME: Unusual bleeding or bruising

Nursing Considerations

• Obtain hematocrit, platelet count, APTT, PT, and INR, as ordered, before giving streptokinase.
• To prevent foaming, don't shake drug during reconstitution.
• Frequently assess for bleeding at I.V. site and for blood in urine and stool. Perform neurologic assessment to detect intracranial bleeding.
• If serious spontaneous bleeding (not controlled by local pressure) occurs, stop streptokinase infusion immediately and notify prescriber.
• Monitor heart rate and rhythm by continuous ECG, as ordered.
• Treat fever with acetaminophen, as prescribed, rather than aspirin to reduce the risk of bleeding.

PATIENT TEACHING

• Explain to patient that he'll be on bed rest during streptokinase therapy.
• Inform patient that minor bleeding may occur at arterial puncture or surgical sites. Reassure him that appropriate care measures will be taken if bleeding occurs.
• Advise patient to obtain medical alert identification stating that he takes streptokinase.

• Inform patient that if he experiences chest pain within 12 months of therapy, he should notify health care providers that he has received streptokinase because repeated administration within 12 months may be ineffective.

streptomycin sulfate

Class and Category

Chemical: Aminoglycoside
Therapeutic: Antibiotic
Pregnancy category: D

Indications and Dosages

➤ *To treat gram-negative bacillary bacteremia, meningeal infections, pneumonia, systemic infections, and UTIs caused by susceptible strains of* Aerobacter aerogenes, Brucella, Calymmatobacterium granulomatis, Enterococcus faecalis, Escherichia coli, Haemophilus ducreyi, H. influenzae, Klebsiella pneumoniae, *and* Proteus

I.M. INJECTION

Adults. 1 to 2 g/day in divided doses q 6 to 12 hr. *Maximum:* 2 g/day.
Children. 20 to 40 mg/kg/day in divided doses q 6 to 12 hr.

➤ *As adjunct to treat endocarditis caused by* Streptococcus viridans *or* E. faecalis

I.M. INJECTION

Adults. 1 g b.i.d. for 1 wk *(S. viridans)* or 2 wk *(E. faecalis)* in conjunction with a penicillin. Then, 500 mg b.i.d. for 1 wk *(S. viridans)* or 4 wk *(E. faecalis)*.

➤ *As adjunct to treat tuberculosis caused by* Mycobacterium tuberculosis

I.M. INJECTION

Adults. 1 g/day in combination with other antibiotics; dosage reduced to 1 g 2 or 3 times/wk, as appropriate and prescribed. *Maximum:* 2 g/day.
Children. 20 mg/kg/day in combination with other antibiotics. *Maximum:* 1 g/day.

DOSAGE ADJUSTMENT For elderly patients, dosage decreased to 500 to 750 mg/day in combination with other antibiotics.

➤ *To treat plague caused by* Yersinia pestis

I.M. INJECTION

Adults. 2 g/day in 2 equally divided doses for at least 10 days.
Children. 30 mg/kg/day in divided doses b.i.d. or t.i.d. for 10 days.

➤ *To treat tularemia caused by* Francisella tularensis

I.M. INJECTION
Adults. 1 to 2 g/day in divided doses for 7 to 14 days.
DOSAGE ADJUSTMENT For patients with creatinine clearance of 50 to 80 ml/min/1.73 m², dosage reduced to 7.5 mg/kg I.M. q 24 hr; for creatinine clearance of 10 to 49 ml/min/1.73 m², 7.5 mg/kg I.M. q 24 to 72 hr; for creatinine clearance less than 10 ml/min/1.73 m², 7.5 mg/kg I.M. q 72 to 96 hr.

Mechanism of Action
Binds to negatively charged sites on the bacteria's outer cell membrane, disrupting cell integrity. Streptomycin also binds to bacterial ribosomal subunits and inhibits protein synthesis. Both actions lead to bacterial cell death.

Incompatibilities
Don't mix streptomycin in same solution or administer through same I.V. line as other antibiotics.

Contraindications
Hypersensitivity to streptomycin or other aminoglycosides

Interactions
DRUGS
antimyasthenics: Possibly decreased effect of antimyasthenics on skeletal muscle
beta-lactam antibiotics: Inactivation of streptomycin
capreomycin, other aminoglycosides: Increased potential for ototoxicity, nephrotoxicity, and neuromuscular blockade
indomethacin (I.V.): Decreased renal clearance of streptomycin when given to premature neonates, possibly leading to aminoglycoside toxicity
methoxyflurane, polymyxins (parenteral): Increased risk of nephrotoxicity and neuromuscular blockade
nephrotoxic and ototoxic drugs: Increased risk of nephrotoxicity and ototoxicity
neuromuscular blockers: Increased neuromuscular blockade

Adverse Reactions
CNS: Clumsiness, dizziness, neurotoxicity, paresthesia, peripheral neuropathy, seizures, unsteadiness, vertigo

EENT: Hearing loss, sensation of fullness in ears, tinnitus, vision loss
GI: Anorexia, nausea, thirst, vomiting
GU: Decreased or increased urine output, nephrotoxicity
MS: Muscle twitching
SKIN: Erythema, pruritus, rash, urticaria

Nursing Considerations
•Use streptomycin cautiously in patients with renal impairment. In severely uremic patients, single dose can produce high blood level of drug for several days; cumulative effects may produce ototoxicity.
•Expect prescriber to order baseline renal function studies and to assess cranial nerve VIII function (responsible for hearing) at start of streptomycin therapy to allow for later comparisons.
•Monitor serum peak and trough levels, as ordered, to ensure adequate but not toxic drug level.
•Be aware that streptomycin should be given only by I.M. injection.
•To reconstitute streptomycin, add 4.2 to 4.5 ml of sodium chloride for injection or sterile water for injection to each 1-g vial to provide a concentration of 200 mg/ml, or add 3.2 to 3.5 ml of diluent to each 5-g vial to provide a concentration of 250 mg/ml. Alternatively, add 6.5 ml of diluent to each 5-g vial to provide a concentration of 500 mg/ml.
•Don't give a concentration greater than 500 mg/ml.
•Rotate injection sites to prevent sterile abscess formation.
PATIENT TEACHING
•Advise patient to refrigerate streptomycin solution at 36° to 46° F (2° to 8° C).
•Inform patient that treatment for tuberculosis lasts at least 1 year.
•Urge patient to notify prescriber if he experiences fullness or ringing in ears, hearing loss, or vertigo.

sucralfate

Apo-sucralfate (CAN), Carafate, Sulcrate (CAN), Sulcrate Suspension Plus (CAN)

Class and Category
Chemical: Disulfated disaccharide, aluminum salt
Therapeutic: Antiulcer
Pregnancy category: B

Q
R
S

Indications and Dosages

➤ *To prevent duodenal ulcer*

TABLETS

Adults and adolescents. 1 g b.i.d.

➤ *To treat active duodenal ulcer*

ORAL SUSPENSION

Adults and adolescents. 1 g q.i.d. 1 hr before meals and h.s. for 4 to 8 wk or, possibly, less. Alternatively, 2 g b.i.d. on empty stomach on waking and h.s. for 4 to 8 wk or, possibly, less.

TABLETS

Adults and adolescents. 1 g q.i.d. 1 hr before meals and h.s. for 4 to 8 wk or, possibly, less.

Mechanism of Action

May react with hydrochloric acid in the stomach to form a complex that buffers acid. The complex adheres electrostatically to proteins on the ulcer's surface and creates a protective barrier at the ulcer site. Sucralfate also inhibits back-diffusion of hydrogen ions and adsorbs pepsin and bile acids, actions that promote healing of an existing duodenal ulcer and prevent ulcer formation.

Interactions

DRUGS

aluminum-containing drugs (such as antacids, antidiarrheals, buffered aspirin with aluminum, and vaginal douches): Possibly aluminum toxicity in patients with renal failure

antacids: Possibly interference with binding of sucralfate to GI mucosa

cimetidine, ciprofloxacin, digoxin, norfloxacin, ofloxacin, phenytoin, ranitidine, tetracycline, theophylline: Decreased bioavailability of these drugs

Adverse Reactions

CNS: Dizziness, drowsiness, light-headedness

EENT: Dry mouth

GI: Constipation, diarrhea, indigestion, nausea, vomiting

MS: Back pain

SKIN: Pruritus, rash, urticaria

Nursing Considerations

• Use sucralfate cautiously in patients with chronic renal failure because of increased risk of aluminum toxicity.

• Administer drug to patient when he has an empty stomach.

PATIENT TEACHING

• Instruct patient to take sucralfate on an empty stomach at least 1 hour before meals and at bedtime.

• Advise patient not to take antacids within 30 minutes of sucralfate.

• Caution patient to check with prescriber before taking another drug within 2 hours of sucralfate.

sulfadiazine

Class and Category

Chemical: Sulfonamide

Therapeutic: Antibiotic, antiprotozoal

Pregnancy category: C

Indications and Dosages

➤ *To treat asymptomatic carriers of meningitis*

TABLETS

Adults and adolescents. 1 g q 12 hr for 2 days.

Children ages 1 to 12. 500 mg q 12 hr for 2 days.

Children ages 2 to 12 months. 500 mg q.d. for 2 days.

➤ *To prevent recurrent rheumatic fever*

TABLETS

Adults and adolescents. 500 mg q.d. (for patients weighing less than 30 kg [66 lb]) to 1 g q.d. (for patients weighing 30 kg or more).

➤ *To treat inclusive nocardiosis*

TABLETS

Adults and adolescents. 4 to 8 g/day for at least 6 wk.

➤ *As adjunct to treat toxoplasmosis in patients with AIDS*

TABLETS

Adults and adolescents. 1 to 2 g q 6 hr, together with 50 to 100 mg/day of pyrimethamine and 10 to 25 mg/day of leucovorin.

Children age 2 months and older. 50 mg/kg b.i.d. for 12 mo, together with 2 mg/kg/day of pyrimethamine for 2 days, then 1 mg/kg/day of pyrimethamine for 2 to 6 mo, then 1 mg/kg/day of pyrimethamine 3 times/wk for remainder of 12 mo; in addition, 5 mg of leucovorin given 3 times/wk for 12 mo. *Maximum:* 6 g/day.

➤ *To treat toxoplasmosis in pregnant women after week 16 of gestation*

TABLETS

Adults. 1 g q 6 hr, together with 25 mg/day of pyrimethamine and 5 to 15 mg/day of leucovorin.

Mechanism of Action
Inhibits para-aminobenzoic acid, a bacterial enzyme responsible for synthesizing folic acid, which susceptible bacteria require for growth. By inactivating bacteria, sulfadiazine prevents or alleviates infection.

Contraindications
Breast-feeding; hypersensitivity to sulfadiazine, its components, or other chemically related drugs, such as sulfonamides; pregnancy at term

Interactions
DRUGS
bone marrow depressants: Increased risk of leukopenic or thrombocytopenic effects
cyclosporine: Decreased blood cyclosporine level, increased risk of nephrotoxicity
estrogen-containing oral contraceptives: Increased risk of breakthrough bleeding and pregnancy
hemolytics: Increased risk of adverse effects
hepatotoxic drugs: Increased risk of hepatotoxicity
hydantoins, oral anticoagulants, oral antidiabetic drugs: Increased or prolonged effects of these drugs, possibly toxicity
indomethacin, probenecid, salicylates: Increased blood level of free sulfadiazine caused by displacement from plasma protein-binding sites
methotrexate: Increased risk of leukopenic or thrombocytopenic effects of methotrexate
phenylbutazone, sulfinpyrazone: Increased blood sulfadiazine level
uricosuric drugs: Potentiated uricosuric action

Adverse Reactions
CNS: Dizziness, fatigue, fever, headache, lethargy, weakness
EENT: Pharyngitis
GI: Anorexia, diarrhea, dysphagia, nausea, vomiting
GU: Crystalluria
HEME: Agranulocytosis, aplastic anemia, hemolytic anemia, leukopenia, thrombocytopenia, unusual bleeding or bruising
MS: Arthralgia, myalgia
SKIN: Blisters, erythema, jaundice, pallor, photosensitivity, pruritus, rash
Other: Drug-induced fever

Nursing Considerations
• Use sulfadiazine cautiously in patients with blood dyscrasias or megaloblastic anemia from folate deficiency because drug may cause blood dyscrasias; in those with G6PD deficiency because hemolysis may occur; in those with hepatic or renal impairment because of increased risk of toxicity; and in those with porphyria because drug may precipitate an acute attack.
• Obtain blood sample for CBC and body tissue or fluid specimen for culture and sensitivity tests, as ordered, before giving drug. Expect first dose to be given before results are available.
• **WARNING** Monitor patient for drug-induced fever, which may develop 7 to 10 days after he starts taking sulfadiazine. Signs and symptoms include abdominal pain, anorexia, ataxia, depression, diarrhea, headache, insomnia, nausea, peripheral neuropathy, tinnitus, and vomiting.
• Monitor fluid intake and output during therapy. Altered fluid balance may increase risk of crystalluria.
• Frequently monitor blood glucose level and assess for signs and symptoms of hypoglycemia in patients who take an oral antidiabetic drug. Be prepared to respond if hypoglycemia develops.
PATIENT TEACHING
• Instruct patient to take sulfadiazine exactly as prescribed and to complete the full course even if he feels better.
• Advise patient to take drug with a full glass of water and to drink plenty of fluids during therapy.
• Urge patient to notify prescriber if urine turns reddish brown; this may indicate crystalluria.
• Inform patient about possible dizziness, and urge him to avoid potentially hazardous activities until drug's CNS effects are known.
• Advise patient to avoid prolonged exposure to sunlight and to wear sunscreen and protective clothing when outdoors.
• Urge patient who takes oral contraceptives to use an additional method of birth control during therapy.
• Advise patient who takes an oral antidiabetic drug to check his blood glucose level frequently because of the increased risk of hypoglycemia during therapy.

sulfamethizole

Thiosulfil Forte

Class and Category

Chemical: Sulfonamide
Therapeutic: Antibiotic
Pregnancy category: C

Indications and Dosages

➤ *To treat cystitis and other UTIs caused by* Enterobacter *sp.,* Escherichia coli, Klebsiella *sp.,* Proteus mirabilis, P. vulgaris, *or* Staphylococcus aureus

TABLETS

Adults. 0.5 to 1 g q 6 to 8 hr.
Children age 2 months and older. 7.5 to 11.25 mg/kg q 6 hr.
DOSAGE ADJUSTMENT Dosage usually reduced for patients with impaired renal function.

> ### Mechanism of Action
>
> Inhibits para-aminobenzoic acid, a bacterial enzyme responsible for synthesizing folic acid, which susceptible bacteria require for growth. By inactivating bacteria, sulfamethizole prevents or alleviates infection.

Contraindications

Breast-feeding; hypersensitivity to sulfamethizole, its components, or other chemically related drugs, such as sulfonamides; pregnancy at term

Interactions

DRUGS

bone marrow depressants: Increased risk of leukopenic or thrombocytopenic effects
cyclosporine: Decreased blood cyclosporine level, increased risk of nephrotoxicity
estrogen-containing oral contraceptives: Increased risk of breakthrough bleeding and pregnancy
hemolytics: Increased risk of adverse effects
hepatotoxic drugs: Increased risk of hepatotoxicity
hydantoins, oral anticoagulants, oral antidiabetic drugs: Increased or prolonged effects of these drugs, possibly toxicity
indomethacin, probenecid, salicylates: Increased blood level of free sulfamethizole caused by displacement from plasma protein-binding sites

methotrexate: Increased risk of leukopenic or thrombocytopenic effects of methotrexate
phenylbutazone, sulfinpyrazone: Increased blood sulfamethizole level
uricosuric drugs: Potentiated uricosuric action

Adverse Reactions

CNS: Dizziness, fatigue, fever, headache, lethargy, weakness
EENT: Pharyngitis
GI: Anorexia, diarrhea, dysphagia, nausea, vomiting
GU: Crystalluria
HEME: Agranulocytosis, aplastic anemia, hemolytic anemia, leukopenia, thrombocytopenia, unusual bleeding or bruising
MS: Arthralgia, myalgia
SKIN: Blisters, erythema, jaundice, pallor, photosensitivity, pruritus, rash
Other: Drug-induced fever

Nursing Considerations

•Use sulfamethizole cautiously in patients with blood dyscrasias or megaloblastic anemia from folate deficiency because drug may cause blood dyscrasias; in those with G6PD deficiency because hemolysis may occur; in those with hepatic or renal impairment because of increased risk of toxicity; and in those with porphyria because drug may precipitate an acute attack.
•Obtain blood sample for CBC and body tissue or fluid specimen for culture and sensitivity tests, as ordered, before giving drug. Expect first dose to be given before results are available.
•WARNING Monitor patient for drug-induced fever, which may develop 7 to 10 days after he starts taking sulfamethizole. Signs and symptoms include abdominal pain, anorexia, ataxia, depression, diarrhea, headache, insomnia, nausea, peripheral neuropathy, tinnitus, and vomiting.
•Monitor fluid intake and output during therapy. Altered fluid balance may increase risk of crystalluria.
•Frequently monitor blood glucose level and assess for signs and symptoms of hypoglycemia in patients who take an oral antidiabetic drug. Be prepared to respond if hypoglycemia develops.

PATIENT TEACHING

•Instruct patient to take sulfamethizole exactly as prescribed and to complete the full course even if he feels better.

•Advise patient to take drug with a full glass of water and to drink plenty of fluids during therapy.
•Urge patient to notify prescriber if urine turns reddish brown; this may indicate crystalluria.
•Inform patient about possible dizziness, and urge him to avoid potentially hazardous activities until drug's CNS effects are known.
•Advise patient to avoid prolonged exposure to sunlight and to wear sunscreen and protective clothing when outdoors.
•Urge patient who takes oral contraceptives to use an additional method of birth control during therapy.
•Advise patient who takes an oral antidiabetic drug to check his blood glucose level frequently because of the increased risk of hypoglycemia during therapy.

sulfamethoxazole

Apo-Sulfamethoxazole (CAN), Gantanol, Urobak

Class and Category

Chemical: Sulfonamide
Therapeutic: Antibiotic, antiprotozoal
Pregnancy category: C

Indications and Dosages

➤ *To treat chlamydial conjunctivitis; malaria (as adjunct to quinine sulfate and pyrimethamine); toxoplasmosis (as adjunct to pyrimethamine); and UTIs, including pyelonephritis and cystitis, caused by susceptible organisms*

TABLETS
Adults. *Initial:* 2 g, then 1 g q 8 to 12 hr.
Children age 2 months and older. *Initial:* 50 to 60 mg/kg, then 25 to 30 mg/kg q 12 hr. *Maximum:* 2 g for initial dose, 75 mg/kg/day for subsequent doses.
DOSAGE ADJUSTMENT Dosage reduction usually needed for patients with impaired renal function.

➤ *To treat uncomplicated urethritis, cervicitis, and proctitis caused by* Chlamydia trachomatis

TABLETS
Adults. 1 g q 12 hr for 10 days.
DOSAGE ADJUSTMENT For patients with creatinine clearance of 10 to 30 ml/min/1.73 m^2, recommended dose reduced by 50% or dosing interval extended; for creatinine clearance of less than 10 ml/min/1.73 m^2, recommended dose reduced by 75% or dosing interval extended, as prescribed.

Mechanism of Action

Inhibits para-aminobenzoic acid, a bacterial enzyme responsible for synthesizing folic acid, which susceptible bacteria require for growth. By inactivating bacteria, sulfamethoxazole prevents or alleviates infection.

Contraindications

Breast-feeding; hypersensitivity to sulfamethoxazole, its components, or other chemically related drugs, such as sulfonamides; pregnancy at term

Interactions

DRUGS
bone marrow depressants: Increased risk of leukopenic or thrombocytopenic effects
cyclosporine: Decreased blood cyclosporine level, increased risk of nephrotoxicity
estrogen-containing oral contraceptives: Increased risk of breakthrough bleeding and pregnancy
hemolytics: Increased risk of adverse effects
hepatotoxic drugs: Increased risk of hepatotoxicity
hydantoins, oral anticoagulants, oral antidiabetic drugs: Increased or prolonged effects of these drugs, possibly toxicity
indomethacin, probenecid, salicylates: Increased blood level of free sulfamethoxazole caused by displacement from plasma protein-binding sites
methotrexate: Increased risk of leukopenic or thrombocytopenic effects of methotrexate
phenylbutazone, sulfinpyrazone: Increased blood sulfamethoxazole level
uricosuric drugs: Potentiated uricosuric action

Adverse Reactions

CNS: Dizziness, fatigue, fever, headache, lethargy, weakness
EENT: Pharyngitis
GI: Anorexia, diarrhea, dysphagia, nausea, vomiting
GU: Crystalluria
HEME: Agranulocytosis, aplastic anemia, hemolytic anemia, leukopenia, thrombocytopenia, unusual bleeding or bruising

Q
R
S

MS: Arthralgia, myalgia
SKIN: Blisters, erythema, jaundice, pallor, photosensitivity, pruritus, rash
Other: Drug-induced fever

Nursing Considerations

•Use sulfamethoxazole cautiously in patients with blood dyscrasias or megaloblastic anemia from folate deficiency because drug may cause blood dyscrasias; in those with G6PD deficiency because hemolysis may occur; in those with hepatic or renal impairment because of increased risk of toxicity; and in those with porphyria because drug may precipitate an acute attack.

•Obtain blood sample for CBC and body tissue or fluid specimen for culture and sensitivity tests, as ordered, before giving drug. Expect first dose to be given before results are available.

•**WARNING** Monitor patient for drug-induced fever, which may develop 7 to 10 days after he starts taking sulfamethoxazole. Signs and symptoms include abdominal pain, anorexia, ataxia, depression, diarrhea, headache, insomnia, nausea, peripheral neuropathy, tinnitus, and vomiting.

•Monitor fluid intake and output during therapy. Altered fluid balance may increase risk of crystalluria.

•Frequently monitor blood glucose level and assess for signs and symptoms of hypoglycemia in patients who take an oral antidiabetic drug. Be prepared to respond if hypoglycemia develops.

PATIENT TEACHING

•Instruct patient to take sulfamethoxazole exactly as prescribed and to complete the full course even if he feels better.

•Advise patient to take drug with a full glass of water and to drink plenty of fluids during therapy.

•Urge patient to notify prescriber if urine turns reddish brown; this may indicate crystalluria.

•Inform patient about possible dizziness, and urge him to avoid potentially hazardous activities until drug's CNS effects are known.

•Advise patient to avoid prolonged exposure to sunlight and to wear sunscreen and protective clothing when outdoors.

•Urge patient who takes oral contraceptives to use an additional method of birth control during therapy.

•Advise patient who takes an oral antidiabetic drug to check his blood glucose level frequently because of increased risk of hypoglycemia during therapy.

sulfasalazine

Alti-Sulfasalazine (CAN), Azulfidine, Azulfidine EN-Tabs, PMS-Sulfasalazine (CAN), PMS-Sulfasalazine E.C. (CAN), Salazopyrin EN-Tabs (CAN), S.A.S.-500 (CAN), S.A.S. Enteric-500 (CAN)

Class and Category

Chemical: Salicylate, sulfonamide
Therapeutic: Anti-inflammatory, antirheumatic, immunomodulator
Pregnancy category: B

Indications and Dosages

➤ *To treat inflammatory bowel diseases, such as ulcerative colitis, and to maintain or prolong remission*
DELAYED-RELEASE TABLETS, TABLETS
Adults and adolescents. *Initial:* 500 to 1,000 mg q 6 to 8 hr. Or 500 mg q 6 to 12 hr to decrease adverse GI reactions. *Maintenance:* 500 mg q 6 hr.
Children over age 2. *Initial:* 6.7 to 10 mg/kg q 4 hr, 10 to 15 mg/kg q 6 hr, or 13.3 to 20 mg/kg q 8 hr. *Maintenance:* 7.5 mg/kg q 6 hr.

➤ *To treat rheumatoid arthritis*
DELAYED-RELEASE TABLETS, TABLETS
Adults. *Initial:* 500 to 1,000 mg q.d. during wk 1, increased by 500 mg/day q wk, as needed, up to 2,000 mg/day in divided doses. If no response after 12 wk, increased to 3,000 mg/day. *Maintenance:* 1,000 mg q 12 hr. *Maximum:* 3,000 mg/day.

➤ *To treat juvenile rheumatoid arthritis in patients who have not responded to salicylates or other NSAIDs*
DELAYED-RELEASE TABLETS
Children ages 6 to 16. 30 to 50 mg/kg/day in divided doses b.i.d. *Maximum:* 2 g/day.

Contraindications

Children under age 2; hypersensitivity to salicylates, sulfasalazine, sulfonamides, chemically related drugs, or their components; intestinal or urinary obstruction; porphyria

Mechanism of Action

Sulfasalazine is a prodrug of sulfapyridine and 5-aminosalicylic acid (mesalamine) that delivers more sulfapyridine
and mesalamine to the colon than either
metabolite could provide alone. Sulfapyridine provides antibacterial action along
the intestinal wall; mesalamine inhibits
cyclooxygenase, thereby decreasing the
production of arachidonic acid metabolites and reducing colonic inflammation.

Interactions
DRUGS
bone marrow depressants: Increased leukopenic and thrombocytopenic effects of both
drugs
digoxin: Possibly inhibited absorption and
decreased blood level of digoxin
folic acid (vitamin B_9): Decreased folic acid
absorption
hepatotoxic drugs: Increased risk of hepatotoxicity
*hydantoins, oral anticoagulants, oral antidia-
betic drugs:* Increased, prolonged, or toxic effects of these drugs
methotrexate, phenylbutazone, sulfinpyrazone:
Possibly potentiated effects of these drugs

Adverse Reactions

CNS: Ataxia, chills, depression, fatigue,
fever, Guillain-Barré syndrome, headache,
insomnia, meningitis, peripheral neuropathy,
seizures, vertigo, weakness
EENT: Hearing loss, orange-yellow tears,
pharyngitis, tinnitus
GI: Abdominal pain, anorexia, diarrhea, hepatitis, indigestion, nausea, pancreatitis, ulcerative colitis exacerbation, vomiting
GU: Crystalluria, decreased ejaculatory volume, male infertility, nephritis, nephrotic syndrome, orange-yellow urine, toxic nephrosis
HEME: Agranulocytosis, aplastic anemia,
Heinz body or hemolytic anemia, leukopenia,
neutropenia, thrombocytopenia, unusual
bleeding or bruising
MS: Arthralgia
RESP: Idiopathic pulmonary fibrosis, lymphocytic interstitial pneumonitis
SKIN: Cyanosis, jaundice, photosensitivity,
pruritus, purpura, rash, Stevens-Johnson syndrome, toxic epidermal necrolysis, urticaria

Nursing Considerations
•Monitor CBC, liver function test results, and
BUN and serum creatinine levels before and
periodically during prolonged sulfasalazine
therapy.
•Be aware that sulfasalazine doses over 4 g
or a blood level over 50 mcg/ml increases the
risk of adverse and toxic reactions.
•Monitor fluid intake and output and urine
color, pH, and consistency. Acidic urine may
require alkalization to prevent crystalluria.
PATIENT TEACHING
•Instruct patient to take sulfasalazine with
meals, milk, or an antacid to decrease GI
distress and to swallow tablets whole.
•Advise patient to prevent crystalluria by
taking drug with a full glass of water and
drinking at least 64 oz of fluid per day.
•Instruct patient and family to administer
drug around the clock.
•Inform patient that symptom relief may
take 2 to 5 days for ulcerative colitis and 4
to 12 weeks for rheumatoid arthritis.
•Alert patient that drug may turn urine and
skin orange-yellow.
•Advise contact lens wearer to consider wearing glasses during therapy because drug can
permanently stain contact lenses yellow.
•Instruct patient to avoid prolonged sun exposure and to wear protective clothing and
sunscreen when outdoors.
•Advise patient to brush with a soft-bristled
toothbrush and to use dental floss and tooth-
picks gently because leukopenic and thrombocytopenic drug effects increase the risk of
infections and gingival bleeding.
•Urge patient to return periodically for laboratory tests and follow-up visits to monitor
drug's effect.

sulfinpyrazone

Anturane, Apo-Sulfinpyrazone (CAN),
Novopyrazone (CAN)

Class and Category
Chemical: Pyrazalone derivative
Therapeutic: Antigout, uricosuric
Pregnancy category: Not rated

Indications and Dosages
➤ *To treat chronic or intermittent gouty
arthritis*

CAPSULES, TABLETS
Adults. *Initial:* 100 to 200 mg b.i.d., increased by 200 mg/day q 2 to 4 days, if needed. *Maintenance:* 100 to 200 mg b.i.d. *Maximum:* 400 mg b.i.d. during wk 1; then 200 to 400 mg b.i.d. until serum urate level is controlled.

Route	Onset	Peak	Duration
P.O.	Unknown	Unknown	4 to 10 hr

Mechanism of Action

Inhibits renal tubular reabsorption of uric acid, thereby increasing uric acid excretion and decreasing serum urate level. Decreased serum urate level prevents urate deposition, tophus formation, and chronic joint changes. It also helps resolve existing urate deposits and eventually reduces the number of gouty arthritis attacks.

Contraindications

Active peptic ulcer disease, blood dyscrasias, hypersensitivity to sulfinpyrazone or its components, symptoms of GI inflammation or ulceration

Interactions

DRUGS
acetaminophen: Increased risk of hepatotoxicity, decreased acetaminophen effects
aminosalicylate sodium: Increased blood level and prolonged duration of this drug, possibly leading to toxicity
antineoplastics: Increased risk of uric acid nephropathy
bismuth subsalicylate and other salicylates: Decreased sulfinpyrazone effects
cefamandole, cefoperazone, cefotetan, moxalactam, plicamycin, valproic acid: Possibly hypoprothrombinemia, increased risk of severe hemorrhage
diazoxide, mecamylamine, pyrazinamide: Possibly increased serum uric acid level
hydantoins: Increased blood hydantoin level, possibly leading to hydantoin toxicity
niacin: Possibly decreased uricosuric effect of sulfinpyrazone
nitrofurantoin: Decreased nitrofurantoin effectiveness, possibly nitrofurantoin toxicity
NSAIDs, oral anticoagulants, platelet aggregation inhibitors, thrombolytics: Increased risk of bleeding

oral antidiabetic drugs: Increased risk of hypoglycemia
probenecid: Increased sulfinpyrazone effects
theophylline: Possibly decreased blood theophylline level
verapamil: Increased clearance and decreased bioavailability of verapamil
ACTIVITIES
alcohol use: Possibly increased serum uric acid level

Adverse Reactions

CNS: Dizziness
EENT: Tinnitus
GI: Abdominal pain, epigastric discomfort, GI bleeding, indigestion, nausea, vomiting
GU: Dysuria, flank pain, hematuria, renal calculi, renal colic, renal failure
HEME: Agranulocytosis, anemia, aplastic anemia, leukopenia, thrombocytopenia
MS: Arthralgia, gouty arthritis (acute attack)
RESP: Bronchospasm, dyspnea, wheezing
SKIN: Erythema, rash

Nursing Considerations

• Expect to administer full maintenance dose immediately, as prescribed, for patient who is switched to sulfinpyrazone from another uricosuric.
• Monitor serum uric acid level periodically, as ordered, to evaluate drug effectiveness.
• Assess for signs of acute gouty arthritis, especially during first few months of therapy.
PATIENT TEACHING
• Instruct patient to take sulfinpyrazone with food, milk, or an antacid to prevent GI distress.
• Stress the importance of taking drug every day, even when feeling better, to prevent acute gouty arthritis attacks.
• Inform patient that acute gouty arthritis may worsen during initial therapy but should improve as treatment continues. Explain that he may not experience drug's full therapeutic effect for 6 months.
• If an acute gouty arthritis attack occurs, advise patient to seek additional treatment but to continue taking sulfinpyrazone, as prescribed, to help prevent exacerbation.
• Advise patient to drink at least 80 oz of fluids per day to decrease the risk of renal calculus formation.
• Instruct patient to consult prescriber before taking OTC products that contain aspirin or acetaminophen.

• Advise patient to avoid alcohol while taking sulfinpyrazone.
• Encourage patient to return for ordered follow-up laboratory tests to check for blood dyscrasias.

sulfisoxazole

Apo-Sulfisoxazole (CAN), Gantrisin, Novo-Soxazole (CAN), Sulfizole (CAN)

sulfisoxazole acetyl

Gantrisin

Class and Category
Chemical: Sulfonamide
Therapeutic: Antibiotic, antiprotozoal
Pregnancy category: C

Indications and Dosages
➤ *To treat nocardiosis; plague; malaria (as adjunct to quinine sulfate and pyrimethamine); and UTIs, including pyelonephritis and cystitis, caused by susceptible organisms*
ORAL SUSPENSION, ORAL SYRUP, TABLETS
Adults and adolescents. *Initial:* 2 to 4 g/day in divided doses. *Maintenance:* 4 to 8 g/day in divided doses q 4 to 6 hr. *Maximum:* 8 g/day.
Children over age 2 months. *Initial:* 75 mg/kg, followed by 120 to 150 mg/kg/day in divided doses q 4 to 6 hr. *Maximum:* 6 g/day.

➤ *To treat uncomplicated cystitis in women*
ORAL SUSPENSION, ORAL SYRUP, TABLETS
Adults. 2 g as a single dose.

➤ *To treat acute or recurrent otitis media in combination with erythromycin in penicillin-allergic patients*
ORAL SUSPENSION, ORAL SYRUP, TABLETS
Children. 150 mg of sulfisoxazole/kg/day and 50 mg of erythromycin/kg/day in divided doses q.i.d.

➤ *To treat lymphogranuloma venereum*
ORAL SUSPENSION, ORAL SYRUP, TABLETS
Adults. 500 mg q 6 hr for 21 days.

➤ *To treat uncomplicated urethritis, cervicitis, or proctitis caused by* Chlamydia trachomatis
ORAL SUSPENSION, ORAL SYRUP, TABLETS
Adults. 500 mg q 6 hr.
DOSAGE ADJUSTMENT For patients with renal impairment, dosing interval changed to q 8 to 24 hr, as prescribed.

Mechanism of Action
Inhibits para-aminobenzoic acid, a bacterial enzyme responsible for synthesizing folic acid, which susceptible bacteria require for growth. By inactivating bacteria, sulfisoxazole prevents or alleviates infection.

Contraindications
Breast-feeding; hypersensitivity to sulfisoxazole, other chemically related drugs, such as sulfonamides, or their components; pregnancy at term

Interactions
DRUGS
bone marrow depressants, methotrexate: Increased risk of leukopenia or thrombocytopenia
cyclosporine: Increased risk of nephrotoxicity
diuretics: Increased incidence of thrombocytopenic purpura
hemolytics (such as doxapram and methyldopa): Increased risk of toxic reaction
hepatotoxic drugs (such as amiodarone): Increased risk of hepatotoxicity
hydantoins, oral anticoagulants, oral antidiabetic drugs: Increased or prolonged effects of these drugs, possibly toxicity
indomethacin, probenecid, salicylates: Increased blood sulfisoxazole level
oral contraceptives: Increased risk of breakthrough bleeding with long-term sulfisoxazole use
phenylbutazone, sulfinpyrazone: Risk of increased blood sulfisoxazole level
thiopental: Increased anesthetic effect of thiopental
tolbutamide: Prolonged half-life of tolbutamide
uricosurics: Potentiated uricosuric action

Adverse Reactions
CNS: Dizziness, fatigue, fever, headache, lethargy, weakness
EENT: Pharyngitis
GI: Anorexia, diarrhea, dysphagia, nausea, vomiting
GU: Crystalluria
HEME: Agranulocytosis, aplastic anemia, hemolytic anemia, leukopenia, thrombocytopenia, unusual bleeding or bruising
MS: Arthralgia, myalgia
SKIN: Blisters, erythema, jaundice, pallor, photosensitivity, pruritus, rash
Other: Drug-induced fever

Q
R
S

Nursing Considerations

• Use sulfisoxazole cautiously in patients with blood dyscrasias or megaloblastic anemia from folate deficiency because drug may cause blood dyscrasias; in those with G6PD deficiency because hemolysis may occur; in those with hepatic or renal impairment because of increased risk of toxicity; and in those with porphyria because drug may precipitate an acute attack.

• Obtain blood sample for CBC and tissue or fluid specimen for culture and sensitivity testing, as ordered, before beginning sulfisoxazole therapy. Expect to give first dose before results are available.

• WARNING Expect prescriber to discontinue sulfisoxazole if patient exhibits signs of blood dyscrasias, including fever, jaundice, maculopapular or other rash, pallor, pharyngitis, or purpura.

• Monitor CBC frequently, as appropriate, during treatment for signs of adverse reactions.

• Closely monitor patients with AIDS, who are at increased risk for adverse reactions.

• WARNING Monitor patient for drug-induced fever, which may develop 7 to 10 days after he starts taking sulfisoxazole. Signs and symptoms include abdominal pain, anorexia, ataxia, depression, diarrhea, headache, insomnia, nausea, peripheral neuropathy, tinnitus, and vomiting.

• Monitor fluid intake and output. Unless contraindicated, provide sufficient fluids to maintain a daily urine output of at least 1,200 ml.

• For otitis media caused by *Haemophilus influenzae*, expect to give drug with erythromycin, as prescribed.

• Frequently monitor blood glucose level and assess for signs of hypoglycemia in patients who take oral antidiabetic drugs.

PATIENT TEACHING

• Instruct patient to take sulfisoxazole exactly as prescribed and to complete the full course of therapy even if he feels better.

• Advise patient to take drug with a full glass of water.

• Inform patient that tablet may be chewed or crushed and mixed with liquid to ease swallowing.

• Advise patient to shake oral suspension well before use and to measure oral suspension or syrup dose with calibrated device to ensure accuracy.

• Inform patient that oral suspension or syrup may be stored at room temperature.

• Advise patient to drink 2 to 3 L of fluid daily to maintain hydration, unless contraindicated.

• Advise patient to avoid potentially hazardous activities until drug's CNS effects are known.

• Instruct patient who takes an oral antidiabetic drug to monitor blood glucose level frequently because of the risk of hypoglycemia.

• Advise patient to avoid prolonged exposure to sunlight and to use sunscreen and wear protective clothing when outdoors.

sulindac

Apo-Sulin (CAN), Clinoril, Novo-Sundac (CAN)

Class and Category

Chemical: Pyrroleacetic acid derivative
Therapeutic: Antigout, anti-inflammatory, antirheumatic
Pregnancy category: Not rated

Indications and Dosages

➤ *To decrease pain and inflammation in ankylosing spondylitis, acute attacks of gout or pseudogout, bursitis, moderately painful arthralgia, osteoarthritis, rheumatoid arthritis, and tendinitis*

TABLETS

Adults and adolescents over age 14. *Initial:* 150 to 200 mg b.i.d., adjusted based on patient's response. *Maximum:* 200 mg b.i.d.

➤ *To relieve symptoms of acute gouty arthritis, acute subacromial bursitis, and supraspinatus tendinitis*

TABLETS

Adults and adolescents over age 14. 200 mg b.i.d. for 7 to 14 days; decreased to lowest effective dosage after satisfactory response occurs.

DOSAGE ADJUSTMENT For elderly patients, dosage reduced to 50% of usual adult dosage, if needed.

Route	Onset	Peak	Duration
P.O.	In 1 wk*	2 to 3 wk*	Unknown

Contraindications

Angioedema, asthma, bronchospasm, nasal polyps, rhinitis, or urticaria induced by aspirin, iodides, or other NSAIDs

* For antirheumatic effects; unknown for antigout or anti-inflammatory effects.

Mechanism of Action

May block the activity of cyclooxygenase, an enzyme needed to synthesize prostaglandins, which mediate the inflammatory response and cause local vasodilation, swelling, and pain. By blocking cyclooxygenase and inhibiting prostaglandins, this NSAID reduces inflammatory symptoms and pain.

Interactions

DRUGS

acetaminophen, cyclosporine, gold compounds, nephrotoxic drugs: Increased risk of adverse renal effects
antacids: Decreased blood level and effects of sulindac
antihypertensives: Risk of decreased antihypertensive effect
aspirin, salicylates: Decreased sulindac effects, increased risk of GI hemorrhage
bone marrow depressants: Increased risk of leukopenia and thrombocytopenia
cefamandole, cefoperazone, cefotetan, colchicine, oral anticoagulants, plicamycin, thrombolytics, valproic acid: Increased risk of bleeding
cimetidine, ranitidine: Increased bioavailability of both drugs
digoxin: Increased blood digoxin level and risk of digitalis toxicity
dimethyl sulfoxide (DMSO): Decreased sulindac effectiveness, possibly peripheral neuropathy with topical application of DMSO
diuretics: Possibly decreased loop diuretic effects and increased thiazide diuretic effects
glucocorticoids, other NSAIDs, potassium supplements: Increased risk of adverse GI effects
hydantoins: Increased blood hydantoin level and risk of phenytoin toxicity
insulin, oral antidiabetic drugs: Increased risk of hypoglycemia
lithium: Possibly increased blood level and toxic effects of lithium
methotrexate: Decreased methotrexate excretion, possibly leading to toxicity
platelet aggregation inhibitors: Increased risk of bleeding, additive effects of these drugs
probenecid: Increased blood level and adverse and toxic effects of sulindac

ACTIVITIES

alcohol use: Increased risk of adverse GI effects, including GI bleeding

Adverse Reactions

CNS: Chills, drowsiness, fever, headache, malaise, nervousness
CV: Edema, heart failure, hypertension, palpitations
EENT: Tinnitus
GI: Abdominal cramps or pain, anorexia, constipation, diarrhea, esophageal irritation, flatulence, gastritis, hepatic failure, hepatitis, hepatotoxicity, indigestion, nausea, vomiting
GU: Decreased urine output, nephrotic syndrome, polyuria, proteinuria
RESP: Pulmonary edema, wheezing
SKIN: Diaphoresis, exfoliative dermatitis, jaundice, maculopapular rash, pruritus, purpura
Other: Facial edema

Nursing Considerations

•WARNING Monitor for adventitious breath sounds and dyspnea; sulindac may cause fluid retention, which may precipitate heart failure in susceptible patients.
•Monitor for elevated liver function test results. Be prepared to discontinue drug, as prescribed, if elevations persist or worsen or if signs and symptoms of hepatic dysfunction develop.
•Be aware that drug's anti-inflammatory action may mask signs of infection.
•Assess for signs and symptoms of GI ulceration and bleeding, especially with prolonged drug use.
•Expect patient to undergo audiometric examinations before and periodically during prolonged therapy, as ordered.

PATIENT TEACHING

•Instruct patient to take sulindac exactly as prescribed. Explain that taking drug in higher doses doesn't increase effectiveness and may increase risk of adverse reactions.
•Advise patient to crush tablet and mix with food, if needed, to aid in swallowing.
•Instruct patient to take drug with or immediately after meals to decrease GI distress, to take with a full glass of water, and to remain upright for 20 to 30 minutes after administration to prevent drug from lodging

in esophagus and causing esophageal irritation.
•Urge patient to notify prescriber immediately of chills, fever, rash, or sweating, which may indicate hypersensitivity.
•Advise patient to consult prescriber before using acetaminophen, alcohol, aspirin, other NSAIDs, or any OTC drugs during sulindac therapy.
•Caution patient to avoid potentially hazardous activities until drug's CNS effects are known.
•Inform patient of need for periodic physical examinations and laboratory tests during prolonged therapy to monitor drug effectiveness.

sumatriptan succinate

Imitrex

Class and Category
Chemical: Serotonin 5-HT$_1$-receptor agonist
Therapeutic: Antimigraine
Pregnancy category: C

Indications and Dosages
➤ *To relieve acute migraine attacks, with or without aura, or cluster headaches*
TABLETS
Adults. 25 to 100 mg as a single dose as soon as possible after onset of symptoms, repeated q 2 hr, as needed and prescribed. *Maximum:* 300 mg/day.
DOSAGE ADJUSTMENT For patients with hepatic dysfunction, 50 mg is maximum single dose.
S.C. INJECTION
Adults. *Initial:* 6 mg, repeated after 1 or 2 hr, if needed. *Maximum:* 2 (6-mg) injections/24 hr. If migraine symptoms return after initial S.C. injection, 50 mg P.O. q 2 hr up to 200 mg/day.
NASAL SPRAY
Adults. 1 or 2 sprays (5 or 10 mg) into one nostril as a single dose or 1 spray (20 mg) into one nostril as a single dose. One additional dose may be taken if another attack occurs after at least 2 hr. *Maximum:* 40 mg q.d.

Route	Onset	Peak	Duration
P.O.	In 30 min	2 to 4 hr	Up to 24 hr
S.C.	In 10 min	1 to 2 hr	Up to 24 hr
Nasal	In 15 min	Unknown	Up to 24 hr

Mechanism of Action
May stimulate 5-HT$_1$ receptors, causing selective vasoconstriction of inflamed and dilated cranial blood vessels in carotid circulation, thus decreasing carotid arterial blood flow and relieving acute migraines.

Contraindications
Basilar or hemiplegic migraine, cardiovascular disease, concurrent use of ergotamine-containing drugs, hypersensitivity to sumatriptan or its components, ischemic heart disease, Prinzmetal's angina, use within 14 days of MAO inhibitor therapy, use within 24 hours of another serotonin 5-HT$_1$-receptor agonist

Interactions
DRUGS
antidepressants, lithium: Increased risk of serious adverse effects
ergotamine-containing drugs: Possibly additive or prolonged vasoconstrictive effects
fluoxetine, fluvoxamine, paroxetine, sertraline: Possibly incoordination, hyperreflexia, and weakness
MAO inhibitors: Risk of decreased sumatriptan clearance, increased risk of serious adverse effects

Adverse Reactions
CNS: Dizziness, drowsiness, fatigue, fever, headache, malaise, sedation, seizures, vertigo, weakness
CV: Arrhythmias; chest heaviness, pain, pressure, or tightness; coronary artery vasospasm; ECG changes; hypertension; hypotension; palpitations
EENT: Abnormal vision; nasal burning (P.O., S.C.); jaw or mouth discomfort; nasal irritation (nasal); nose or throat discomfort; photophobia (P.O., S.C.); taste perversion (nasal); tongue numbness or soreness
SKIN: Dermatitis, diaphoresis, erythema, flushing, pallor, photosensitivity (P.O., S.C.), pruritus, rash, urticaria
Other: Injection site burning, pain, and redness

Nursing Considerations
•Be aware that sumatriptan shouldn't be given to elderly patients because they're more likely to have decreased hepatic function, coronary artery disease (CAD), and more pronounced blood pressure increases.

• Assess for chest pain and monitor blood pressure in patients with CAD before and for at least 1 hour after sumatriptan administration.
• Don't administer sumatriptan within 24 hours of another 5-HT$_1$-receptor agonist, such as naratriptan, rizatriptan, or zolmitriptan.
• After nasal administration, rinse tip of bottle with hot water (don't suction water into bottle) and dry with a clean tissue. Replace cap after cleaning.
• Inspect injection solution for particles and discoloration before administering. Discard solution if you detect these changes.
• Be aware that drug shouldn't be administered I.V. because this may precipitate coronary artery vasospasm.
• Assess patients with risk factors for CAD for arrhythmias, chest pain, and other signs of heart disease.
• For patients with seizure disorder, institute seizure precautions according to facility policy because sumatriptan may lower seizure threshold.

PATIENT TEACHING
• Advise patient to use sumatriptan as soon as possible after the onset of migraine symptoms.
• Urge patient to contact prescriber and avoid taking sumatriptan if headache symptoms aren't typical.
• Remind patient not to exceed prescribed daily dosage.
• Advise patient to swallow tablets whole and drink fluids to disguise unpleasant taste.
• Show patient suitable sites for S.C. injection, and teach him how to load, administer, and discard autoinjector.
• Instruct patient to administer no more than two S.C. doses in 24 hours and not to take a second dose if first dose doesn't provide significant relief.
• Inform patient that he may experience burning, pain, and redness for 10 to 30 minutes after S.C. injection. Suggest that he apply ice to relieve pain and redness.
• Teach patient how to use nasal form correctly.
• To avoid cross-contamination, advise patient not to use the same nasal container for more than one person.
• Encourage patient to lie down in a dark, quiet room after taking drug to help relieve migraine.

• Instruct patient to seek emergency care for chest, jaw, or neck tightness after drug use because drug may cause coronary artery vasospasm; subsequent doses may require ECG monitoring.
• Urge patient to report palpitations or rash to prescriber.
• Advise patient to avoid potentially hazardous activities until drug's CNS effects are known.
• Alert patient with seizure disorder that drug may lower seizure threshold.
• Encourage yearly ophthalmologic examinations for patients who require prolonged drug therapy.

T

tacrine hydrochloride

(tetrahydroaminoacridine, THA)

Cognex

Class and Category
Chemical: Monoamine acridine
Therapeutic: Dementia treatment
Pregnancy category: C

Indications and Dosages
➤ *To treat mild to moderate Alzheimer's type dementia*

CAPSULES

Adults. *Initial:* 10 mg q.i.d. for 4 wk, increased to 20 mg q.i.d. and adjusted q 4 wk as prescribed. *Maximum:* 160 mg/day in 4 divided doses.

Contraindications
Hypersensitivity to tacrine, other acridine derivatives, or their components; jaundice from previous tacrine use; serum bilirubin level that exceeds 3 mg/dl

Interactions
DRUGS
anticholinergics: Decreased effects of both drugs
cholinergics, other cholinesterase inhibitors: Increased effects of these drugs and tacrine, possibly leading to toxicity
cimetidine: Increased blood tacrine level, possibly leading to toxicity
neuromuscular blockers: Prolonged or exaggerated muscle relaxation
NSAIDs: Increased gastric acid secretion, possibly GI irritation and bleeding
theophylline: Increased blood theophylline level, possibly leading to toxicity

Mechanism of Action
Tacrine may relieve dementia by increasing the acetylcholine level in the CNS. In Alzheimer's disease, some cholinergic neurons lose their ability to function, which decreases the acetylcholine level. The remaining functioning cholinergic neurons release acetylcholine, but it's enzymatically broken down by cholinesterases into acetic acid and choline, as shown below left. Without acetylcholine to activate muscarinic (M) and nicotinic (N) receptors on postsynaptic cell membranes, nerve transmission and excitability decrease.

Tacrine binds with and inhibits cholinesterases, making more intact acetylcholine available in cholinergic synapses, as shown below right. This prolongs and enhances acetylcholine's effects, which increases nerve transmission and reduces symptoms of dementia.

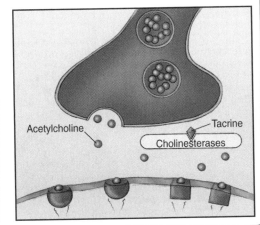

Foods
all foods: Reduced tacrine bioavailability
Activities
smoking: Possibly decreased tacrine effectiveness

Adverse Reactions

CNS: Agitation, anxiety, asthenia, ataxia, confusion, depression, dizziness, fatigue, hallucinations, headache, hostility, insomnia, seizures, somnolence, syncope, tremor
CV: Arrhythmias, chest pain, conduction disturbances, hypertension, hypotension, palpitations, peripheral edema, sick sinus syndrome
EENT: Rhinitis
GI: Abdominal pain, anorexia, constipation, diarrhea, elevated liver function test results, flatulence, indigestion, nausea, vomiting
GU: Bladder obstruction, urinary frequency and incontinence, UTI
MS: Back pain, muscle stiffness, myalgia
RESP: Asthma, cough, upper respiratory tract infection, wheezing
SKIN: Flushing, jaundice, purpura, rash
Other: Weight loss

Nursing Considerations

•Monitor patients with asthma for wheezing and increased mucus production because drug may increase bronchoconstriction and bronchial secretions.
•Expect to monitor hepatic enzyme levels (specifically ALT), as ordered, every other week from at least week 4 to week 16 of tacrine therapy.
•If patient has elevated serum ALT level, monitor for signs and symptoms of hepatitis, such as jaundice and right-upper-quadrant pain. ALT level should return to normal 4 to 6 weeks after therapy stops.
•Once ALT level returns to normal, expect to begin tacrine again (starting at 10 mg q.i.d.) as prescribed, and check hepatic enzyme levels weekly for 16 weeks, monthly for 2 months, and every 3 months thereafter, as ordered.
•Monitor patient for bradyarrhythmias, conduction disturbances, and sick sinus syndrome because tacrine may have a vagotonic effect on the heart rate.
•**WARNING** Be aware that tacrine's cholinergic effects may exacerbate seizures or parkinsonian symptoms.
•Monitor patient's urine output and assess for abdominal distention and abnormal bowel sounds because drug's cholinergic effects may exacerbate conditions involving urinary tract or GI obstruction or ileus.
•Be aware that patients with peptic ulcer disease and those receiving NSAIDs are at increased risk for developing diarrhea, nausea, and vomiting because tacrine increases gastric acid secretion.
•Asess patient for increased symptoms because drug becomes less effective as Alzheimer's disease progresses and the number of intact cholinergic neurons declines.

Patient Teaching
•Instruct patient to take tacrine on an empty stomach, and advise caregiver to make sure that drug is swallowed.
•If patient experiences GI distress, suggest taking drug with meals. Mention that drug's effects may be delayed.
•Urge patient to seek assistance when walking and changing position until drug's effects are known. Instruct her to avoid potentially hazardous activities during this period.
•Advise patient not to smoke because it decreases drug's effectiveness.
•Caution patient not to stop taking drug abruptly. Doing so may impair cognitive ability.
•Inform caregiver that drug becomes less effective as Alzheimer's disease progresses.
•Urge caregiver to make sure patient returns regularly for follow-up visits and laboratory tests to monitor drug effectiveness.

tamoxifen citrate

Apo-Tamox (CAN), Gen-Tamoxifen (CAN), Nolvadex, Novo-Tamoxifen (CAN), Tamofen (CAN), Tamone (CAN)

Class and Category

Chemical: Triphenylethylene derivative
Therapeutic: Nonsteroidal antiestrogen agent, partial estrogen agonist
Pregnancy category: D

Indications and Dosages

➤ *To treat metastatic breast cancer in men and women; to treat node-negative breast cancer in women, or node-positive breast cancer in postmenopausal women, after total or segmental mastectomy, axillary dissection, and breast irradiation*
Tablets
Adults. 20 to 40 mg q.d. Dosages greater than 20 mg administered b.i.d.

➤ *To reduce the risk of invasive breast cancer in women with ductal carcinoma in situ (DCIS) after surgery and radiation, to reduce the risk of breast cancer in women at high risk*

TABLETS

Adults. 20 mg q.d. for 5 yr.

> ## Mechanism of Action
> May block the effects of estrogen on breast tissue by competing with estrogen for estrogen-receptor binding sites. Estrogen may stimulate cancer cell growth.

Contraindications

Hypersensitivity to tamoxifen or its components; women at high risk for breast cancer and women with DCIS who have a history of deep vein thrombosis or pulmonary embolus or who require concomitant coumarin-type anticoagulant therapy

Interactions

DRUGS

bromocriptine: Possibly increased blood tamoxifen level
estrogens: Possibly altered therapeutic effect of tamoxifen
warfarin and other coumarin-type anticoagulants: Increased anticoagulant effect of these drugs

Adverse Reactions

CNS: Confusion, CVA, depression, dizziness, fatigue, headache, light-headedness, somnolence, weakness
CV: Edema, hyperlipidemia, thrombosis
EENT: Keratopathy, ocular toxicity (including cataracts), optic neuritis, retinopathy
GI: Elevated liver function test results, hepatotoxicity, nausea, vomiting
GU: Endometrial cancer, endometrial hyperplasia, endometrial polyps, genital itching, menstrual irregularities, ovarian cysts, uterine malignancies, vaginal discharge (females); impotence, decreased libido (males)
HEME: Anemia, leukopenia, thrombocytopenia
MS: Transient bone or tumor pain
RESP: Pulmonary embolism
SKIN: Bullous pemphigoid, dry skin, erythema multiforme, rash, Stevens-Johnson syndrome, thinning hair

Other: Angioedema, hot flashes, hypercalcemia, weight gain

Nursing Considerations

•**WARNING** Ensure that patient has been informed of potential for serious and life-threatening adverse effects associated with tamoxifen before therapy begins. Be aware that women with ductal carcinoma in situ or those at high risk for breast cancer are more likely to develop uterine cancer, stroke, or pulmonary emboli than others receiving tamoxifen.
•If patient is premenopausal, begin drug therapy in the middle of menstruation; if patient's menstrual cycles are irregular, verify that she has had a negative pregnancy test.
•Expect patient to undergo an ophthalmologic examination before and periodically during tamoxifen therapy to monitor for adverse ocular reactions such as cataracts.
•Assess patient for signs and symptoms of thromboembolic events, such as shortness of breath, leg pain, and change in mental status.
•Periodically monitor platelet and WBC count, cholesterol and triglyceride levels, and liver function test results, as ordered.
•Monitor blood calcium level and assess patient for signs and symptoms of hypercalcemia, such as nausea, vomiting, and thirst; tamoxifen may cause hypercalcemia in breast cancer patients with bone metastasis within a few weeks of starting treatment.
•Store tamoxifen in a closed, light-resistant container at room temperature.

PATIENT TEACHING

•Advise patient to swallow tamoxifen tablet whole with water.
•Instruct premenopausal patient to use a nonhormonal form of contraception, such as a condom or diaphragm, during tamoxifen therapy. Emphasize that she shouldn't become pregnant while taking drug and for 2 months afterward. Advise her to notify prescriber at once if she becomes pregnant during therapy.
•Inform patient of the most common side effects—hot flashes, vaginal discharge, and irregular menses.
•Urge patient to immediately notify prescriber if she notices a rash, itching, difficulty breathing, or facial swelling, which may signify a hypersensitivity reaction.
•Advise patient to notify prescriber if she experiences leg pain or calf swelling, which may indicate a blood clot.

T

• Instruct patient to report signs of hepato-toxicity, such as tiredness, nausea, yellow skin, and flulike symptoms.

• Advise patient to have regular gynecologic checkups and to report abnormal symptoms, including abdominal or pelvic pain, new breast lumps, and unusual vaginal discharge or bleeding.

• Urge patients taking tamoxifen for prophy-laxis to obtain regular mammograms because drug doesn't prevent all cancers.

• Stress the importance of taking tamoxifen regularly. Urge patient to consult prescriber if adverse reactions, such as nausea and vomiting, are interfering with dosage schedule. These symptoms may be a sign of hypercalcemia.

tamsulosin hydrochloride

Flomax

Class and Category

Chemical: Sulfamoylphenethylamine deriva-tive
Therapeutic: Benign prostatic hyperplasia (BPH) treatment
Pregnancy category: B

Indications and Dosages

➤ *To treat BPH*

CAPSULES

Adults. *Initial:* 0.4 mg q.d. 30 min p.c. for 2 to 4 wk, increased to 0.8 mg q.d. if no response to initial dosage. *Maximum:* 0.8 mg q.d.

Mechanism of Action

Blocks alpha$_1$-adrenergic receptors in the prostate. This action inhibits smooth-mus-cle contraction in the prostate, prostatic capsule, prostatic urethra, and bladder neck, which improves the rate of urine flow and reduces the symptoms of BPH.

Contraindications

Hypersensitivity to tamsulosin, quinazolines, or their components

Interactions

DRUGS

alpha blockers: Additive effects of both drugs
cimetidine: Risk of decreased tamsulosin clearance

Adverse Reactions

CNS: Asthenia, dizziness, drowsiness, head-ache, insomnia, syncope, vertigo

CV: Chest pain, orthostatic hypotension
EENT: Amblyopia, diplopia, pharyngitis, rhinitis
GI: Diarrhea, nausea
GU: Decreased libido, ejaculation disorders
MS: Back pain
SKIN: Pruritus, rash, urticaria

Nursing Considerations

• Be aware that prostate cancer should be ruled out before tamsulosin therapy begins.

• Give drug about 30 minutes after the same meal each day.

• If patient takes drug on an empty stomach, monitor his blood pressure because of the in-creased risk of orthostatic hypotension.

• If patient doesn't take drug for several days, resume therapy at 0.4 mg/dose, as pre-scribed.

PATIENT TEACHING

• Instruct patient not to open, crush, or chew tamsulosin capsules and to take drug about 30 minutes after the same meal each day.

• Instruct patient to notify prescriber if he misses several days of therapy; caution him against restarting drug at previous dosage.

• Advise patient to avoid potentially haz-ardous activities until drug's CNS effects are known. Mention the need for caution if dos-age is increased.

• Advise patient to change position slowly, especially after initial dose and each dosage increase, to minimize effects of orthostatic hypotension.

tegaserod maleate

Zelnorm

Class and Category

Chemical: 3-(5-methoxy-1H-indol-3-ylmethylene)-N-pentylcarbazimidamide hydrogen maleate
Therapeutic: Gastrointestinal 5-HT4 receptor partial agonist
Pregnancy category: B

Indications and Dosages

➤ *To treat constipation in women with ir-ritable bowel syndrome short term when it is the primary symptom*

TABLETS

Adult females. 6 mg b.i.d. before meals for 4 to 6 wk; may continue for another 4 to 6 wk, as needed, if initial response is positive.

Mechanism of Action
Activates 5-HT4 receptors in the GI tract
to stimulate peristaltic reflex and intestinal secretion and to inhibit visceral sensitivity. These actions enhance basal
motor activity and normalize impaired
motility throughout the GI tract.

Contraindications
History of abdominal adhesions, bowel obstruction, symptomatic gallbladder disease,
or suspected sphincter of Oddi dysfunction;
hypersensitivity to tegaserod maleate or its
components; moderate or severe hepatic impairment; severe renal impairment

Interactions
None known

Adverse Reactions
CNS: Dizziness, headache, migraine
GI: Abdominal pain, diarrhea, flatulence,
nausea
MS: Arthropathy, back or leg pain
Other: Accidental trauma

Nursing Considerations
•Be aware that tegaserod shouldn't be given
to women who are currently having diarrhea
or who experience frequent diarrhea.
•Give drug at least 1 hour before or 2 to
3 hours after a meal because food reduces
the drug's bioavailablity.
•WARNING Discontinue tegaserod immediately if patient develops new or sudden
worsening of abdominal pain.
PATIENT TEACHING
•Tell patient to take tegaserod at least 1 hour
before meals.
•Advise patient not to take 2 tablets to make
up for a missed dose but to skip the missed
dose and then resume her regular dosing
schedule.
•Instruct patient to notify prescriber if severe
diarrhea occurs during therapy or if diarrhea
is accompanied by severe cramping, abdominal pain, or dizziness.
•Advise patient to notify prescriber if she
develops new or worsening abdominal pain
without diarrhea.
•Inform patient about possible dizziness.
Advise her to avoid potentially hazardous
activities until drug's CNS effects are known.

telmisartan
Micardis

Class and Category
Chemical: Nonpeptide angiotensin II antago-
nist
Therapeutic: Antihypertensive
Pregnancy category: C (first trimester), D
(later trimesters)

Indications and Dosages
➤ *To manage hypertension, alone or with
other antihypertensives*
TABLETS
Adults. *Initial:* 40 mg q.d. *Maintenance:* 20 to
80 mg q.d. *Maximum:* 80 mg/day.

Route	Onset	Peak	Duration
P.O.	Unknown	In 4 wk	Unknown

Mechanism of Action
Blocks angiotensin II from binding to receptor sites in many tissues, including
vascular smooth muscle and adrenal
glands. This inhibits the vasoconstrictive
and aldosterone-secreting effects of angiotensin II, which reduces blood pressure.

Contraindications
Hypersensitivity to telmisartan or its components

Interactions
DRUGS
digoxin: Increased peak blood digoxin level
and risk of digitalis toxicity
diuretics, other antihypertensives: Enhanced
hypotensive effect

Adverse Reactions
CNS: Dizziness, fatigue, headache
CV: Chest pain, hypertension, hypotension,
orthostatic hypotension, peripheral edema
EENT: Pharyngitis, sinusitis
GI: Abdominal pain, diarrhea, indigestion,
nausea, vomiting
GU: Renal dysfunction, UTI
MS: Back pain, myalgia
RESP: ACE cough, upper respiratory tract
infection
Other: Angioedema, flulike symptoms, hypo-
volemia

Nursing Considerations
•Administer telmisartan cautiously to patients with dehydration or hyponatremia.

•Expect prescriber to add a diuretic to regimen if patient's blood pressure isn't well controlled by telmisartan.

•Be prepared to treat symptomatic hypotension by placing patient in a supine position and administering NS, as prescribed.

•Monitor BUN and serum creatinine levels and urine output in patients with impaired renal function because they're at increased risk for oliguria, progressive azotemia, and possibly acute renal failure.

•Monitor liver function test results, as appropriate, and assess for signs of drug toxicity in patients with severe hepatic disease because they're at increased risk for toxicity from increased drug accumulation.

•Avoid using telmisartan in pregnant women during second and third trimesters because drug can increase the risk of fetal harm.

PATIENT TEACHING
•Advise patient to avoid potentially hazardous activities until telmisartan's CNS effects are known.

•Instruct patient to change position slowly to minimize effects of orthostatic hypotension.

•Urge patient to notify prescriber immediately about diarrhea, dizziness, severe nausea, or vomiting.

•Instruct patient to consult prescriber before taking any new drug.

•Advise patient to drink adequate fluids during hot weather and when exercising to prevent dehydration.

•Advise female patients of childbearing age to notify presciber immediately about known or suspected pregnancy.

temazepam

Apo-Temazepam (CAN), Novo-Temazepam (CAN), Restoril

Class, Category, and Schedule
Chemical: Benzodiazepine
Therapeutic: Sedative-hypnotic
Pregnancy category: X
Controlled substance: Schedule IV

Indications and Dosages
➤ *To provide short-term management of insomnia*

CAPSULES
Adults. 7.5 to 15 mg 30 min before h.s. *Maximum:* 30 mg/day.

DOSAGE ADJUSTMENT For elderly or debilitated patients, 7.5 mg 30 min before bedtime. *Maximum:* 15 mg/day.

> ### Mechanism of Action
> May potentiate the effects of gamma-aminobutyric acid (GABA) and other inhibitory neurotransmitters by binding to specific benzodiazepine receptor sites in the limbic and cortical areas of the CNS. By binding to these receptor sites, temazepam increases GABA's inhibitory effects and blocks cortical and limbic arousal.

Contraindications
Hypersensitivity to temazepam, other benzodiazepines, or their components; pregnancy

Interactions
DRUGS
antihistamines (such as brompheniramine, carbinoxamine, chlorpheniramine, clemastine, cyproheptadine, diphenhydramine, trimeprazine), anxiolytics, barbiturates, general anesthetics, opioid analgesics, phenothiazines, promethazine, sedative-hypnotics, tramadol, tricyclic antidepressants: Increased sedation or respiratory depression
clozapine: Risk of respiratory depression or arrest
digoxin: Increased risk of elevated blood digoxin level and digitalis toxicity
flumazenil: Increased risk of withdrawal symptoms
levodopa: Possibly decreased levodopa effects
oral contraceptives: Decreased response to temazepam
phenytoin: Possibly phenytoin toxicity
probenecid: Increased response to temazepam
zidovudine: Possibly zidovudine toxicity
ACTIVITIES
alcohol use: Increased CNS depression and risk of apnea
smoking: Increased temazepam clearance

Adverse Reactions
CNS: Aggressiveness, anxiety (in daytime), ataxia, confusion, decreased concentration, depression, dizziness, drowsiness, euphoria, fatigue, headache, insomnia, nightmares, slurred speech, syncope, talkativeness, tremor, vertigo, wakefulness during last third of night
CV: Palpitations, tachycardia
EENT: Abnormal or blurred vision, increased salivation

GI: Abdominal pain, constipation, diarrhea, hepatic dysfunction, nausea, thirst, vomiting
GU: Decreased libido
HEME: Agranulocytosis, anemia, leukopenia, neutropenia, thrombocytopenia
MS: Muscle spasm or weakness
RESP: Increased bronchial secretions
SKIN: Diaphoresis, flushing, jaundice, pruritus, rash
Other: Physical and psychological dependence

Nursing Considerations
• Use temazepam cautiously in patients with a history of depression or suicidal thoughts.
• **WARNING** Monitor for signs of physical and psychological dependence during therapy.
• Implement safety precautions, according to facility policy, especially in elderly patients, because they're more sensitive to drug's CNS effects.
• Assess patients with respiratory depression, severe COPD, or sleep apnea for signs of ventilatory failure.
• Be aware that temazepam can aggravate acute intermittent porphyria, myasthenia gravis, and severe renal impairment.
• Be aware that temazepam may cause worsening psychosis or deterioration of cognition or coordination in patients with late-stage Parkinson's disease.
• Be aware that drug shouldn't be discontinued abruptly, even after only 1 to 2 weeks of therapy, because doing so may cause seizures or withdrawal symptoms, such as insomnia, irritability, and nervousness.

PATIENT TEACHING
• Instruct patient to take temazepam exactly as prescribed and not to stop taking it or change dosage without consulting prescriber.
• Explain the risks associated with abrupt cessation, including abdominal cramps, acute sense of hearing, confusion, depression, nausea, numbness, perceptual disturbances, photophobia, sweating, tachycardia, tingling, trembling, and vomiting.
• Advise patient to avoid alcohol because it increases drug's sedative effects.
• Caution patient about possible drowsiness. Advise her to avoid potentially hazardous activities until drug's CNS effects are known.
• Urge patient to notify prescriber immediately about excessive drowsiness, nausea, and known or suspected pregnancy.

tenecteplase
TNKase

Class and Category
Chemical: Purified glycoprotein
Therapeutic: Thrombolytic
Pregnancy category: C

Indications and Dosages
➤ *To reduce mortality associated with acute MI*
I.V. INJECTION
Adults. Single bolus administered over 5 sec in individualized dosage based on patient's weight, as follows: 30 mg (6 ml) for patients who weigh less than 60 kg; 35 mg (7 ml) for patients who weigh 60 to 69 kg; 40 mg (8 ml) for patients who weigh 70 to 79 kg; 45 mg (9 ml) for patients who weigh 80 to 89 kg; 50 mg (10 ml) for patients who weigh 90 kg or more. Maximum: 50 mg total dose.

Mechanism of Action
Binds to fibrin and converts plasminogen to plasmin. Plasmin breaks down fibrin, fibrinogen, and other clotting factors, resulting in dissolution of a coronary artery thrombus.

Incompatibilities
Don't administer tenecteplase through an I.V. line containing dextrose because precipitation may occur.

Contraindications
Active internal bleeding, aneurysm, arteriovenous malformation, bleeding disorders, brain tumor, history of cerebrovascular accident, hypersensitivity to tenecteplase or its components, intracranial or intraspinal surgery or trauma within past 2 months, severe uncontrolled hypertension

Interactions
DRUGS
abciximab, aspirin, clopidogrel, dipyridamole, heparin, oral anticoagulants, ticlopidine: Possibly increased risk of bleeding

Adverse Reactions
CNS: Intracranial hemorrhage
EENT: Epistaxis, gingival bleeding, pharyngeal bleeding
GI: GI and retroperitoneal bleeding

T

GU: Genitourinary bleeding, prolonged or heavy menstrual bleeding
HEME: Hematoma
RESP: Hemoptysis
SKIN: Bleeding at puncture sites, surgical incision sites, or venous cutdown sites

Nursing Considerations

•**WARNING** Reconstitute tenecteplase for injection immediately before use because drug contains no antibacterial preservatives. If reconstituted drug isn't used immediately, refrigerate vial at 36° to 46° F (2° to 8° C). Discard solution if not used within 8 hours.
•To reconstitute and administer drug, use supplied 10-ml syringe with dual cannula device. Withdraw 10 ml of supplied (preservative-free) sterile water for injection into syringe, and inject entire contents into vial containing tenecteplase dry powder, directing stream of diluent into powder. Gently swirl—don't shake—vial until contents are completely dissolved. If slight foaming occurs during reconstitution, allow drug to stand undisturbed for a few minutes to allow large bubbles to dissipate. Then withdraw prescribed dose of tenecteplase from reconstituted drug in vial, using supplied syringe. Make sure that reconstituted preparation is a colorless to pale yellow transparent solution. Discard any unused solution.
•Administer drug as a single I.V. bolus over 5 seconds. Although supplied syringe is intended for use with needleless I.V. systems, be aware that it is also compatible with a conventional needle. Follow manufacturer's directions for use with each system. Flush any dextrose-containing I.V. lines with saline solution before and after administering tenecteplase.
•**WARNING** Monitor for signs and symptoms of GI bleeding, including bloody or black, tarry stools; bloody or coffee-ground vomitus; and severe stomach pain. Notify prescriber immediately if any of these signs or symptoms develops.
•Assess tenecteplase injection site for signs and symptoms of hematoma, including deep, dark purple bruises under skin and itching, pain, redness, or swelling. Also monitor for superficial bleeding, delayed bleeding at puncture sites, and bleeding from surgical incisions.
•Assess for signs and symptoms of intracranial bleeding (such as decreased level of consciousness), retroperitoneal bleeding (such as abdominal pain or swelling and back pain), genitourinary bleeding (such as hematuria), or respiratory tract bleeding (such as hemoptysis). Notify prescriber immediately if patient develops any of these signs or symptoms.
•If serious bleeding (not controllable by local pressure) occurs, expect to discontinue concomitant heparin or oral antiplatelet therapy immediately.
•If possible, avoid I.M. injections and nonessential handling of patient for first few hours after drug administration.
•If arterial puncture becomes necessary during first few hours after tenecteplase administration, expect to use an upper extremity that's accessible to manual compression. Apply pressure for at least 30 minutes after procedure, use a pressure dressing, and frequently monitor puncture site for signs of bleeding.

PATIENT TEACHING
•Advise patient to immediately report any bleeding, including from nose or gums.
•Instruct patient to limit physical activity during tenecteplase administration to reduce the risk of injury or bleeding.

terazosin hydrochloride

Hytrin

Class and Category

Chemical: Quinazoline derivative
Therapeutic: Antihypertensive, benign prostatic hyperplasia (BPH) treatment
Pregnancy category: C

Indications and Dosages

➤ *To manage hypertension*
CAPSULES
Adults. *Initial:* 1 mg h.s. *Maintenance:* 1 to 5 mg/day as a single dose or in divided doses q 12 hr. *Maximum:* 20 mg/day.
➤ *To treat symptomatic BPH*
CAPSULES
Adults. *Initial:* 1 mg h.s., increased in increments to 2 mg, 5 mg, and then 10 mg, as prescribed, based on symptom improvement and urine flow rate. *Maintenance:* 5 to 10 mg/day as a single dose or in divided doses q 12 hr. *Maximum:* 20 mg/day.

Route	Onset	Peak	Duration
P.O.	15 min	2 to 3 hr	24 hr

Mechanism of Action

Blocks postsynaptic alpha$_1$-adrenergic receptors in many tissues, including vascular smooth muscle, the bladder neck, and the prostate. This action promotes vasodilation, which reduces blood pressure and improves urine flow.

Contraindications

Hypersensitivity to terazosin, other quinazolines, or their components

Interactions

DRUGS

clonidine: Possibly decreased clonidine effects
diuretics, other antihypertensives: Additive hypotensive effect
dopamine: Risk of decreased terazosin effects and antagonized vasoconstrictive effect of dopamine (in high doses)
epinephrine: Risk of decreased terazosin effects, possibly severe hypotension and tachycardia
indomethacin, other NSAIDS: Altered terazosin effects related to sodium and fluid retention
methoxamine, phenylephrine: Decreased vasopressor effects, and shortened duration of action of these drugs
sympathomimetics: Decreased terazosin effects

Adverse Reactions

CNS: Asthenia, dizziness, headache, lethargy, nervousness, paresthesia, somnolence, syncope, vertigo
CV: Chest pain, hypotension, orthostatic hypotension, palpitations, peripheral edema, sinus tachycardia
EENT: Blurred vision, dry mouth, nasal congestion, sinusitis
GI: Constipation, diarrhea, nausea, vomiting
MS: Arthralgia, back pain
Other: Flulike symptoms, weight gain

Nursing Considerations

• Be aware that prostate cancer should be ruled out before terazosin is used to treat BPH.
• Expect prescriber to reduce terazosin dosage if a diuretic or another antihypertensive is added to patient's regimen.
• Monitor blood pressure 2 to 3 hours after initial dose because of possible first-dose hypotension and again after 24 hours to evaluate patient's response.
• If patient requires administration by feeding tube, place capsule in 60 ml of warm tap water. Stir until capsule shell dissolves and liquid contents are released into water (5 to 10 minutes).
• Be aware that elderly patients may have exaggerated hypotension and other adverse reactions.

PATIENT TEACHING

• Instruct patient to take terazosin at the same time each night.
• Explain possible first-dose hypotension. Advise patient to change position and rise slowly to prevent syncope early in therapy. Suggest sitting or lying down if dizziness or light-headedness occurs.
• Advise patient to avoid potentially hazardous activities until drug's CNS effects are known.
• Instruct patient to notify prescriber if she misses several doses in a row; caution her against resuming therapy at previous dose.
• Inform patient that drug may take 2 to 6 weeks to improve urinary hesitancy.
• Advise patient to avoid alcohol use, prolonged standing, and excessive exercise or exposure to hot weather because these activities can worsen orthostatic hypotension.
• Stress the importance of regular follow-up visits with prescriber to evaluate patient's response to drug.

terbinafine hydrochloride

Lamisil

Class and Category

Chemical: Allylamine derivative
Therapeutic: Antifungal
Pregnancy category: B

Indications and Dosages

➤ *To treat onychomycosis of fingernails and toenails*

TABLETS

Adults and adolescents. 125 mg b.i.d. or 250 mg q.d. for 6 to 12 wk.
DOSAGE ADJUSTMENT For patients with stable chronic hepatic dysfunction or renal dysfunction (creatinine clearance less than 50 ml/min/1.73 m^2 or serum creatinine greater than 3.4 mg/dl), dosage reduced by 50%.

T

Mechanism of Action

Inhibits the conversion of squalene mono-oxygenase to squalene epoxidase, a key enzyme in fungal biosynthesis. The resulting squalene accumulation weakens cell membranes and creates a deficiency of ergosterol, the fungal membrane component necessary for normal fungal growth.

Contraindications

Hypersensitivity to terbinafine or its components

Interactions

DRUGS

cimetidine, other hepatic enzyme inhibitors: Significantly decreased terbinafine clearance, possibly increased adverse reactions
cyclosporine, other hepatic enzyme inducers, rifampin: Increased clearance and possibly decreased effectiveness of these drugs
hepatotoxic drugs: Increased risk of hepatotoxicity

FOODS

caffeine: Decreased caffeine clearance

ACTIVITIES

alcohol use: Increased risk of severe hepatitis

Adverse Reactions

CNS: Headache
EENT: Taste perversion
GI: Abdominal pain, anorexia, diarrhea, elevated liver function test results, flatulence, hepatic failure, indigestion, nausea, vomiting
SKIN: Pruritus, rash, urticaria

Nursing Considerations

• Because terbinafine has been linked to serious adverse hepatic effects, expect to send nail specimens for laboratory testing to confirm onychomycosis before beginning therapy.
• Be aware that drug shouldn't be given to patients with chronic or active hepatic disease or renal impairment.
• Monitor patient for signs and symptoms of hepatic failure, including anorexia, dark urine, fatigue, jaundice, nausea, pale stools, right upper abdominal pain, and vomiting. Expect to discontinue drug and obtain liver function tests if these signs and symptoms develop.

PATIENT TEACHING

• Instruct patient to space doses evenly if taking terbinafine more than once a day.
• Stress the importance of complying with the full course of therapy to prevent relapse of infection.
• Advise patient to avoid alcohol while taking terbinafine.
• Instruct patient to contact prescriber if she sees no improvement in onychomycosis in a few weeks.

terbutaline sulfate

Brethaire, Brethine, Bricanyl, Bricanyl Turbuhaler (CAN)

Class and Category

Chemical: Sympathomimetic amine
Therapeutic: Bronchodilator
Pregnancy category: B

Indications and Dosages

➤ *To prevent or reverse bronchospasm caused by asthma, bronchitis, or emphysema*

TABLETS (BRETHINE, BRICANYL)

Adults and adolescents age 15 and older. 2.5 to 5 mg t.i.d. at 6-hr intervals while awake. *Maximum:* 15 mg/day.
Children ages 12 to 15. 2.5 mg t.i.d. at 6-hr intervals while awake. *Maximum:* 7.5 mg/day.
Children ages 6 to 11. 50 to 75 mcg/kg t.i.d. at 6-hr intervals while awake. *Maximum:* 150 mcg/kg/dose or 5 mg/day.

S.C. INJECTION (BRICANYL)

Adults and children age 12 and older. *Initial:* 0.25 mg, repeated in 15 to 30 min as needed and as prescribed. *Maximum:* 0.5 mg/4-hr period.
Children ages 6 to 12. 5 to 10 mcg (0.005 to 0.01 mg)/kg q 15 to 20 min, up to 3 doses. *Maximum:* 400 mcg (0.4 mg)/dose.

INHALATION AEROSOL (BRETHAIRE)

Adults and children. 2 inhalations (400 mcg) q 4 to 6 hr, as needed and as prescribed.

INHALATION AEROSOL (BRICANYL TURBUHALER)

Adults and children. 1 inhalation (500 mcg), repeated after 5 min, as needed and as prescribed. *Maximum:* 6 inhalations/day.

Route	Onset	Peak	Duration
P.O.	30 to 90 min	2 to 3 hr	4 to 8 hr
S.C.	15 to 30 min	30 to 60 min	1.5 to 4 hr
Inhalation	In 5 min	30 to 90 min	3 to 6 hr

Mechanism of Action
Stimulates beta$_2$-adrenergic receptors in the lungs, which is believed to increase production of cAMP. The increased cAMP level relaxes bronchial smooth muscles, thereby increasing bronchial airflow and relieving bronchospasm.

Contraindications
Hypersensitivity to terbutaline sulfate, other sympathomimetic amines, or their components

Interactions
DRUGS
antihypertensives, diuretics: Decreased antihypertensive effect
beta blockers: Mutual inhibition of therapeutic effects, increased risk of bronchospasm
CNS stimulants: Additive CNS stimulation, possibly resulting in adverse effects
digoxin: Increased risk of arrhythmias, possibly digitalis toxicity
halogenated anesthetics: Possibly ventricular arrhythmias
MAO inhibitors: Possibly potentiated action of terbutaline; headache, hyperpyrexia, hypertension, possibly leading to hypertensive crisis
maprotiline, tricyclic antidepressants: Possibly potentiated action of terbutaline
nitrates: Decreased effectiveness of nitrates
ritodrine: Increased effects of either drug and potential for adverse effects
sympathomimetics: Increased CNS stimulation and risk of adverse cardiovascular effects, including prolonged QT interval
thyroid hormones: Increased effects of either drug, risk of coronary insufficiency in patients with coronary artery disease
xanthines (theophylline): Increased CNS stimulation and other additive toxic effects
FOODS
caffeine: Increased CNS stimulation and other additive toxic effects

Adverse Reactions
CNS: Anxiety, dizziness, drowsiness, headache, insomnia, light-headedness, nervousness, restlessness, tremor, weakness
CV: Chest pain, irregular heartbeat, palpitations, tachycardia
EENT: Dry mouth, taste perversion
ENDO: Hyperglycemia

GI: Heartburn, nausea, vomiting
MS: Muscle spasms
RESP: Dyspnea
SKIN: Diaphoresis, flushing, rash

Nursing Considerations
•Use terbutaline cautiously in patients with cardiovascular disease because drug can adversely affect cardiovascular function. Monitor patient's heart rate and rhythm and blood pressure and assess for chest pain.
•For S.C. injection, inject into lateral deltoid area.
•Reevaluate patient's respiratory rate, depth, and quality; oxygen saturation; and activity tolerance at regular intervals because continuous use of beta$_2$-agonists for 12 months or longer accelerates the decline in pulmonary function.
PATIENT TEACHING
•Teach patient how to use terbutaline aerosol inhaler or administer S.C. injection, as appropriate.
•Instruct patient not to increase dose or frequency without consulting prescriber.
•Urge patient to seek immediate medical attention if symptoms worsen.
•Inform patient that she may experience transient nervousness or tremors during terbutaline therapy.

tetracycline hydrochloride

Achromycin, Achromycin V, Apo-Tetra (CAN), Novo-Tetra (CAN), Nu-Tetra (CAN), Panmycin, Robitet, Sumycin, Tetracap, Tetracyn, Tetracyn 500

Class and Category
Chemical: Chlortetracycline derivative
Therapeutic: Antibiotic
Pregnancy category: D

Indications and Dosages
➤ *To treat actinomycosis caused by susceptible organisms*
CAPSULES, ORAL SUSPENSION, TABLETS
Adults and adolescents. 250 to 500 mg q 6 hr or 500 to 1,000 mg q 12 hr. *Maximum:* 4 g/day.
Children age 8 and older. 6.25 to 12.5 mg/kg q 6 hr or 12.5 to 25 mg/kg q 12 hr.
➤ *To treat acne vulgaris*
CAPSULES, ORAL SUSPENSION, TABLETS
Adults and adolescents. *Initial:* 500 to 2,000 mg/day in divided doses until improvement

occurs (usually in 3 wk); then dosage reduced gradually. *Maintenance:* 125 to 1,000 mg/day. *Maximum:* 4 g/day.

➤ *To treat brucellosis caused by susceptible organisms*

CAPSULES, ORAL SUSPENSION, TABLETS
Adults and adolescents. 500 mg q 6 hr for 3 wk, given concurrently with 1 g of streptomycin I.M. q 12 hr in week 1 and q.d. in week 2. *Maximum:* 4 g/day.
Children ages 8 to 12. 6.25 to 12.5 mg/kg q 6 hr, or 12.5 to 25 mg/kg q 12 hr.

➤ *To treat gonorrhea caused by* Neisseria gonorrhoeae

CAPSULES, ORAL SUSPENSION, TABLETS
Adults and adolescents. 1,500 mg, then 500 mg q 6 hr for 5 days. *Maximum:* 4 g/day.

➤ *To treat syphilis caused by* Treponema pallidum

CAPSULES, ORAL SUSPENSION, TABLETS
Adults and adolescents. 500 mg q 6 hr for 15 days (for early syphilis) or 30 days (for late syphilis). *Maximum:* 4 g/day.
Children ages 9 to 12. 6.25 to 12.5 mg/kg q 6 hr, or 12.5 to 25 mg/kg q 12 hr.

➤ *To treat uncomplicated endocervical, rectal, or urethral infections caused by* Chlamydia trachomatis

CAPSULES, ORAL SUSPENSION, TABLETS
Adults and adolescents. 500 mg q.i.d. for at least 7 days. *Maximum:* 4 g/day.
DOSAGE ADJUSTMENT For patients with renal impairment, dosage possibly reduced because of extended half-life.

Mechanism of Action
Exerts a bacteriostatic effect against a wide variety of gram-positive and gram-negative organisms by passing through the bacterial lipid bilayer, where it binds reversibly to 30S ribosomal subunits. Bound tetracycline blocks the binding of aminoacyl transfer RNA to messenger RNA, thus inhibiting bacterial protein synthesis.

Contraindications
Hypersensitivity to tetracycline or its components

Interactions
DRUGS
aluminum-, calcium-, or magnesium-containing antacids; iron supplements (oral); magne-sium-containing laxatives; magnesium salicylate; multivitamins (containing manganese or zinc salts); sodium bicarbonate: Possibly impaired absorption of oral tetracycline and formation of nonabsorbable complexes
cholestyramine, colestipol: Possibly impaired absorption of oral tetracycline
digoxin: Possibly increased blood digoxin level
methoxyflurane: Possibly nephrotoxicity
oral contraceptives (containing estrogen): Possibly reduced contraceptive reliability and increased risk of breakthrough bleeding (with long-term tetracycline use)
penicillins: Possibly decreased bactericidal effect of penicillins
vitamin A: Possibly benign intracranial hypertension
FOODS
dairy products and other foods: Possibly impaired absorption of oral tetracycline

Adverse Reactions
CNS: Dizziness, light-headedness, unsteadiness
EENT: Darkened or discolored tongue, enamel hypoplasia, oral candidiasis, tooth discoloration (in children)
GI: Abdominal pain, diarrhea, hepatotoxicity, nausea, rectal candidiasis, vomiting
GU: Vaginal candidiasis
SKIN: Photosensitivity

Nursing Considerations
• Avoid giving tetracycline to children under age 8 because drug may cause permanent brown or yellow tooth discoloration and enamel hypoplasia.
• Be aware that tooth discoloration and enamel hypoplasia may occur in breast-feeding infants, along with inhibition of linear skeletal growth, oral and vaginal candidiasis, and photosensitivity.
• To reduce the risk of esophageal irritation or ulceration, avoid bedtime dosing of tetracycline for patient with esophageal obstruction or compression.
• Assess for photosensitivity, which can develop within a few minutes or up to several hours after exposure to sunlight or other ultraviolet (UV) light. Effects may last for 1 to 2 days after discontinuation of drug.
• Be aware that citric acid in tetracycline preparations may accelerate drug deterioration and that using outdated drug may cause Fanconi's syndrome, characterized by multiple defects in renal tubular function. Symp-

toms include acidosis, bicarbonate wasting, glycosuria, hypokalemia, osteomalacia, and phosphaturia.

PATIENT TEACHING
• Instruct patient to take oral tetracycline at least 1 hour before meals or 2 hours after meals because dairy products and some foods may interfere with absorption.
• Advise patient to take each dose with a full glass of water while in an upright position to avoid esophageal or GI irritation.
• Instruct patient taking oral suspension to shake container well before measuring dose and to use a calibrated measuring device.
• Advise patient to avoid taking other drugs, including OTC antacids and other preparations, within 3 hours of taking oral tetracycline.
• Urge patient to complete the entire course of tetracycline therapy even if she feels better.
• Caution her to avoid exposure to direct sunlight or UV light and to wear sunscreen when outdoors.
• Advise women who use oral contraceptives containing estrogen to use another method of contraception while taking tetracycline because contraceptives may be less effective.
• Stress the importance of discarding outdated or decomposed tetracycline because of the risk of toxic effects.
• Encourage patient to take safety precautions if she experiences dizziness or other adverse CNS reactions.

thalidomide

Thalomid

Class and Category
Chemical: Glutamic-acid derivative
Therapeutic: Anti-inflammatory, immunomodulator
Pregnancy category: X

Indications and Dosages
➤ *To treat acute cutaneous erythema nodosum leprosum*
CAPSULES
Adults and adolescents. 100 to 400 mg q.d. h.s. or at least 1 hr after the evening meal.
Usual: 200 mg.
DOSAGE ADJUSTMENT For those weighing less than 50 kg (110 lb), dosage started at 100 mg.

➤ *To prevent or suppress recurrence of cutaneous erythema nodosum leprosum*
CAPSULES
Adults and adolescents. Minimum dosage necessary to control reaction; dosage tapered q 3 to 6 mo in increments of 50 mg q 2 to 4 wk, as prescribed.

Mechanism of Action
Suppresses the production of tumor necrosis factor-alpha, which reduces neutrophils and CD4 T cells in erythema nodosum leprosum lesions, thus preventing or controlling symptoms.

Contraindications
Hypersensitivity to thalidomide or its components, pregnancy, women of childbearing age who aren't using two reliable contraceptive methods or aren't abstaining from heterosexual intercourse

Interactions
DRUGS
antihistamines, anxiolytics, barbiturates, chlorpromazine, CNS depressants, hypnotics, opioid analgesics, reserpine, sedatives: Increased CNS depression
chloramphenicol, cisplatin, dapsone, didanosine, ethambutol, ethionamide, hydralazine, isoniazid, lithium, metronidazole, nitrofurantoin, nitrous oxide, other drugs associated with peripheral neuropathy, phenytoin, stavudine, vincristine, zalcitabine: Increased risk of peripheral neuropathy
ACTIVITIES
alcohol use: Increased CNS depression

Adverse Reactions
CNS: Agitation, asthenia, chills, dizziness, drowsiness, fever, headache, insomnia, malaise, mood changes, nervousness, paresthesia, peripheral neuropathy, somnolence, tremor, vertigo
CV: Bradycardia, hyperlipidemia, orthostatic hypotension, peripheral edema, tachycardia
EENT: Dry mouth, oral candidiasis, pharyngitis, rhinitis, sinusitis, tooth pain
GI: Abdominal pain, anorexia, constipation, diarrhea, elevated liver function test results, flatulence, hepatic dysfunction, increased appetite, nausea
GU: Albuminuria, hematuria, impotence
HEME: Anemia, leukopenia, neutropenia
MS: Back pain, neck pain or rigidity

SKIN: Acne, dermatitis, diaphoresis, photosensitivity, pruritus, rash
Other: Facial edema, lymphadenopathy, pain (generalized)

Nursing Considerations

•Be aware that all patients receiving thalidomide must complete an informed consent form and participate in a confidential monitoring registry. Thalidomide may be obtained only through physicians and pharmacies registered in the System for Thalidomide Education and Prescribing Safety (STEPS) Program, a comprehensive safety program designed to prevent fetal exposure to thalidomide. Thalidomide may be dispensed only in original packaging and in no more than a 28-day supply. Prescriptions older than 7 days may not be filled.
•Be aware that female patients of childbearing age are required to use two methods of contraception during thalidomide therapy. Pregnancy testing must be performed 24 hours before beginning thalidomide, weekly during first month of therapy, then monthly thereafter in women with regular menstrual cycles or every 2 weeks in women with irregular menstrual cycles.
•**WARNING** Be aware that thalidomide shouldn't be given to pregnant patient. A single dose during pregnancy may cause severe birth defects or fetal death.
•Assess patient's medication history for use of carbamazepine, griseofulvin, HIV-protease inhibitors, rifabutin, and rifampin. These drugs can decrease the effectiveness of hormonal contraceptives used to prevent pregnancy during thalidomide therapy.
•To minimize sedative effect, give thalidomide in divided doses t.i.d. or q.i.d., as prescribed, with larger dose in the evening.
•Assess for early signs of peripheral neuropathy (muscle cramps, numbness and tingling in toes and fingers, pain or superficial sensory loss in feet or hands) in patients receiving long-term thalidomide therapy. Early detection and drug discontinuation, as prescribed, prevents further damage and increases the chance for reversal.
•Expect to discontinue thalidomide therapy if patient's absolute neutrophil count is less than 750/mm^3. Routine monitoring of WBC count is recommended every other week during first 3 months of treatment in HIV-positive and other immunosuppressed patients, and monthly in non-immunosuppressed patients.

PATIENT TEACHING
•Instruct patient to have thalidomide prescription filled as soon as possible because prescriptions more than 7 days old may not be filled.
•Urge patient to take drug exactly as prescribed.
•Inform female patient of drug's potential harm to fetus, and stress the importance of avoiding pregnancy. Tell her that pregnancy tests will be done before and frequently during therapy.
•Instruct female patient to abstain from sexual intercourse or to use two reliable methods of birth control simultaneously, starting 4 weeks before drug therapy and continuing for up to 4 weeks after therapy has been completed. One contraceptive method must be highly effective, such as an intrauterine device, oral contraceptive, or tubal ligation; the other may be a cervical cap, diaphragm, or latex condom.
•**WARNING** Inform male patient, even one who has had a vasectomy, that he must use barrier contraception (latex condom) when having sexual intercourse with a woman of childbearing age.
•Caution patient to avoid potentially hazardous activities until drug's CNS effects are known.
•Suggest that patient change position slowly to minimize effects of orthostatic hypotension.
•Instruct patient to immediately report to prescriber early signs of peripheral neuropathy, including numbness, pain, or tingling in feet and hands.
•Inform HIV-positive patient of the need for viral-load testing after first and third months of therapy and every 3 months thereafter.
•Urge patient to avoid using alcohol and donating blood or sperm during thalidomide therapy.

theophylline

Aerolate, Aerolate III, Aerolate Jr., Aerolate Sr., Apo-Theo LA (CAN), Asmalix, Elixophyllin, Lanophyllin, PMS Theophylline (CAN), Pulmophylline (CAN), Quibron-T Dividose, Quibron-T/SR Dividose, Respbid, Slo-Bid

Gyrocaps, Slo-Phyllin, Theo-24, Theo-SR (CAN), Theobid Duracaps, Theochron, Theoclear, Theoclear LA, Theo-Dur, Theolair, Theolair-SR, Theovent Long-Acting, T-Phyl, Truxophyllin, Uni-Dur, Uniphyl

Class and Category

Chemical: Xanthine derivative
Therapeutic: Bronchodilator
Pregnancy category: C

Indications and Dosages

➤ *As loading dose to treat reversible airway obstruction in patients not currently receiving theophylline*

CAPSULES, ELIXIR, ORAL SOLUTION, SYRUP, TABLETS
Adults and children. 5 mg/kg as a single dose.

I.V. INFUSION
Adults and children. 5 mg/kg infused over 20 to 30 min.

➤ *As partial loading dose to treat reversible airway obstruction in patients currently receiving theophylline*

CAPSULES, ELIXIR, ORAL SOLUTION, SYRUP, TABLETS, I.V. INFUSION
Adults and children. Individualized dosage based on blood theophylline level, as prescribed. Loading dose based on principle that 0.5 mg/kg of theophylline will produce a 1-mcg/ml increase in blood theophylline level.

➤ *To provide maintenance treatment of reversible airway obstruction associated with asthma or COPD*

CAPSULES, TABLETS
Adults and children weighing more than 45 kg (99 lb). *Initial:* 300 mg/day in equally divided doses q 6 to 8 hr; after 3 days, if tolerated, increased to 400 mg/day in divided doses q 6 to 8 hr; after 3 more days, if tolerated, increased to 600 mg/day in divided doses q 6 to 8 hr. Dosages above 600 mg/day are based on blood theophylline level and clinical response.
Children age 1 and older weighing 45 kg or less. *Initial:* 12 to 14 mg/kg/day up to maximum of 300 mg/day in equally divided doses q 4 to 6 hr; after 3 days, if tolerated, increased to 16 mg/kg up to maximum of 400 mg/day in equally divided doses q 4 to 6 hr; after 3 more days, if tolerated, 20 mg/kg/day up to maximum of 600 mg/day in equally divided doses q 4 to 6 hr. Dosages above 600

mg/day are based on blood theophylline level and clinical response.

ELIXIR
Adults. *Initial:* 300 mg/day in equally divided doses q 6 to 8 hr; after 3 days, if tolerated, increased to 400 mg/day in divided doses q 6 to 8 hr; after 3 more days, if tolerated, increased to 600 mg/day in divided doses q 6 to 8 hr. Dosages above 600 mg/day are based on blood theophylline level and clinical response.

E.R. CAPSULES OR TABLETS
Adults and children weighing 45 kg or more. *Initial:* 300 mg/day in equally divided doses q 8 to 12 hr; after 3 days, if tolerated, increased to 400 mg/day in divided doses q 8 to 12 hr; after 3 more days, if tolerated, increased to 600 mg/day in divided doses q 8 to 12 hr. Dosages above 600 mg/day are based on blood theophylline level and clinical response.
Children age 1 and older weighing less than 45 kg. *Initial:* 12 to 14 mg/kg/day up to maximum of 300 mg/day in equally divided doses q 8 to 12 hr; after 3 days, if tolerated, increased to 16 mg/kg up to maximum of 400 mg/day in equally divided doses q 8 to 12 hr; after 3 more days, if tolerated, dosage increased to 20 mg/kg/day up to maximum of 600 mg/day in equally divided doses q 8 to 12 hr. Dosages above 600 mg/day are based on blood theophylline level and clinical response.

ORAL SOLUTION, SYRUP
Adults and children weighing more than 45 kg. *Initial:* 300 mg/day in equally divided doses q 6 to 8 hr; after 3 days, if tolerated, increased to 400 mg/day in divided doses q 6 to 8 hr; after 3 more days, if tolerated, increased to 600 mg/day in divided doses q 6 to 8 hr. Dosages above 600 mg/day are based on blood theophylline level and clinical response.
Children age 1 and older weighing 45 kg or less. *Initial:* 12 to 14 mg/kg/day up to maximum of 300 mg/day in equally divided doses q 4 to 6 hr; after 3 days, if tolerated, increased to 16 mg/kg up to a maximum of 400 mg/day in equally divided doses q 4 to 6 hr; after 3 more days, if tolerated, dosage increased to 20 mg/kg/day up to maximum of 600 mg/day in equally divided doses q 4 to 6 hr. Dosages above 600 mg/day are based on blood theophylline level and clinical response.

Full-term infants ages 26 to 52 weeks. Dosage individualized in mg/kg/day, as prescribed, and administered in equally divided doses q 6 hr.

Full-term infants up to age 26 weeks. Dosage individualized in mg/kg/day, as prescribed, and administered in equally divided doses q 8 hr.

Premature infants age 24 days and older. 1.5 mg/kg q 12 hr.

Premature infants under age 24 days. 1 mg/kg q 12 hr.

I.V. INFUSION

Adults and adolescents age 16 and older. 0.4 mg/kg/hr for nonsmokers, 0.7 mg/kg/hr for smokers.

DOSAGE ADJUSTMENT For elderly patients and adults with cardiac decompensation, cor pulmonale, or hepatic impairment, I.V. dosage reduced to 0.2 mg/kg/hr.

Children ages 9 to 16. 0.7 mg/kg/hr.

Children ages 1 to 9. 0.8 mg/kg/hr.

Full-term infants up to age 1. Dosage individualized in mg/kg/day as prescribed.

Mechanism of Action

Inhibits phosphodiesterase enzymes, causing bronchodilation. Normally, these enzymes inactivate cAMP and cGMP, which are responsible for bronchial smooth-muscle relaxation. Theophylline also may cause calcium translocation, antagonize prostaglandins and adenosine receptors, stimulate catecholamines, and inhibit cGMP metabolism.

Incompatibilities

Don't mix parenteral theophylline solution with any additives. Don't infuse theophylline through same I.V. line as Hetastarch (Hespan), a colloidal plasma volume expander, which is incompatible with theophylline.

Contraindications

Hypersensitivity to theophylline or its components, peptic ulcer disease, uncontrolled seizure disorder

Interactions

DRUGS

adenosine: Decreased adenosine effectiveness
allopurinol, cimetidine, ciprofloxacin, clarithromycin, disulfiram, enoxacin, erythromycin, fluvoxamine, interferon alpha (human recombinant), methotrexate, mexiletine, pentoxifylline, propafenone, propranolol, tacrine, thiabendazole, ticlopidine, troleandomycin, verapamil: Increased blood theophylline level and risk of toxicity
aminoglutethimide, carbamazepine, isoproterenol (I.V.), moricizine, oral contraceptives (containing estrogen), phenobarbital, phenytoin, rifampin: Decreased blood theophylline level and possibly drug effectiveness
benzodiazepines: Possibly reversal of benzodiazepine sedation
beta blockers: Possibly decreased bronchodilator effect of theophylline
ephedrine: Increased adverse effects, including insomnia, nausea, and nervousness
halothane anesthetics: Increased risk of ventricular arrhythmias
ketamine: Lowered seizure threshold
lithium: Decreased lithium effectiveness
neuromuscular blockers: Possibly antagonized neuromuscular blockade
sucralfate: Decreased absorption of oral theophylline

FOODS

high-carbohydrate, low-protein diet: Possibly decreased theophylline elimination
low-carbohydrate, high-protein diet; daily intake of charbroiled beef: Possibly increased theophylline elimination

ACTIVITIES

alcohol use: Increased blood theophylline level and risk of toxicity
smoking: Increased drug clearance, decreased drug effectiveness

Adverse Reactions

CNS: Agitation, anxiety (I.V. form), behavioral changes, confusion, disorientation, headache, insomnia, nervousness, seizures, tremor
CV: Hypotension, tachycardia, ventricular arrhythmias
ENDO: Hyperglycemia
GI: Abdominal pain, diarrhea, heartburn, nausea, vomiting
GU: Increased urine output

Nursing Considerations

• Be aware that ideal body weight is used to calculate theophylline dosages because drug doesn't bind well in body fat.
• Be aware that E.R. capsules and tablets shouldn't be used for oral loading doses.
• Infuse theophylline loading dose, bolus,

or intermittent infusion at a rate that doesn't exceed 25 mg/min.

•Administer continuous theophylline infusion with rate-controlled infusion device.

•Monitor blood theophylline level, as ordered, to gauge therapeutic level and detect toxicity.

•Frequently assess heart rate and rhythm because theophylline can exacerbate existing arrhythmias.

•Be especially alert for signs of toxicity in patient with acute pulmonary edema, hypothyroidism, influenza vaccination, prolonged fever, sepsis with multiple organ failure, shock, or viral pulmonary infection because of decreased drug clearance.

•Monitor blood theophylline level in patients with uncorrected acidemia because they have an increased risk of toxicity.

•Expect patient with cystic fibrosis or hyperthyroidism to experience increased theophylline clearance and decreased drug effectiveness. Monitor blood theophylline level, as ordered.

•Suspect toxicity if patient experiences vomiting, and be prepared to obtain blood theophylline level.

PATIENT TEACHING

•Instruct patient to swallow theophylline tablets whole and not to chew or crush them, unless scored for breaking.

•Explain that patient may open capsules and mix contents with soft food but that she shouldn't chew or crush granules.

•Instruct patient to take drug with a full glass of water on an empty stomach (30 to 60 minutes before meals or 2 hours after meals). However, suggest that she take drug with food or antacids if GI distress occurs.

•Encourage patient to take drug at the same times every day.

•Advise patient to notify prescriber if she develops a fever, makes a significant dietary change, or starts or stops smoking or taking other drugs because these factors may alter blood theophylline level.

thiethylperazine maleate

Torecan

Class and Category

Chemical: Piperazine phenothiazine

Therapeutic: Antiemetic
Pregnancy category: Not rated

Indications and Dosages

➤ *To treat nausea and vomiting*

TABLETS, I.M. INJECTION, SUPPOSITORIES

Adults and adolescents. 10 mg q.d. to t.i.d.
Maximum: 30 mg q.d.

Route	Onset	Peak	Duration
P.O.	30 to 60 min	Unknown	4 hr

Mechanism of Action

Relieves nausea and vomiting by centrally blocking dopamine receptors in the medullary chemoreceptor trigger zone.

Contraindications

Breast-feeding; coma; hypersensitivity to thiethylperazine, sulfites, tartrazine dye, or their components; jaundice; severe CNS depression

Interactions

DRUGS

aluminum- or magnesium-containing antacids, antidiarrheals (adsorbent): Decreased absorption of thiethylperazine

anticonvulsants (including barbiturates): Lowered seizure threshold

antihistamines, tricyclic antidepressants: Additive CNS and GI effects, including ileus and severe constipation

antihypertensives: Enhanced hypotensive effect of both drugs

antimuscarinics (including antiparkinsonian drugs, MAO inhibitors, meperidine, and phenothiazines): Additive GI effects, including ileus and severe constipation

appetite suppressants: Decreased anorectic effect

barbiturates, benzodiazepines, CNS depressants, general anesthetics, opioid analgesics: Additive CNS effects

beta blockers: Increased blood levels of both drugs; additive hypotensive effects; possibly arrhythmias, irreversible retinopathy, and tardive dyskinesia

bromocriptine: Possibly decreased effectiveness of bromocriptine

hepatotoxic drugs: Increased risk of hepatotoxicity

levodopa: Decreased effectiveness of levodopa

lithium: Possibly acute encephalopathy

T

methoxsalen, porfimer: Possibly increased photosensitivity
metrizamide: Increased risk of seizures
ototoxic drugs: Possibly masked symptoms of ototoxicity (dizziness, tinnitus, and vertigo)
phenytoin: Increased risk of phenytoin toxicity
quinidine: Possibly adverse cardiac effects
riboflavin: Increased requirements for riboflavin
sympathomimetics: Reduced vasopressor response and duration of action of sympathomimetics
tramadol: Additive CNS effects, increased risk of seizures

ACTIVITIES
alcohol use: Additive CNS effects

Adverse Reactions
CNS: Confusion, dizziness, EEG abnormalities, extrapyramidal reactions (dystonia, pseudoparkinsonism), sedation
CV: ECG changes, hypotension, orthostatic hypotension, tachycardia
EENT: Blurred vision, dry mouth
ENDO: Gynecomastia
GI: Constipation, increased appetite
GU: Darkened urine, ejaculation disorders, menstrual irregularities, urine retention
HEME: Agranulocytosis, leukopenia (transient)
SKIN: Contact dermatitis, photosensitivity
Other: Weight gain

Nursing Considerations
• Avoid using thiethylperazine in patients with neurologic impairment because drug can disrupt central temperature regulation.
• Avoid inadvertent I.V. administration of thiethylperazine; injection is for I.M. administration only.
• Keep patient in recumbent position for 30 to 60 minutes after I.M. injection to minimize the risk of hypotension.
• Be aware that parenteral preparations contain sulfites and that tablets contain tartrazine dye.
• Moisten suppository with water or water-soluble lubricant before insertion. If suppository has softened excessively, chill for 30 minutes or run under cold water before removing wrapper.
• Avoid skin contact with drug to prevent contact dermatitis.
• Because thiethylperazine may cause reactions from anticholinergic effects and adrenergic blockade, assess for blurred vision, constipation, dry mouth, impotence, urine reten-

tion (from cholinergic activity) and priapism (from alpha-adrenergic blockade).
• During prolonged therapy, assess for visual disturbances because drug may cause corneal keratopathy and retinal discoloration (pigmentary retinopathy).
• **WARNING** Be aware that thiethylperazine may cause neuroleptic malignant syndrome, a rare but extremely serious reaction characterized by cardiovascular instability, decreased level of consciousness, extrapyramidal effects, and hyperpyrexia.
• Monitor CBC with differential, as ordered, because drug may worsen existing blood dyscrasias, such as agranulocytosis, neutropenia, and thrombocytopenia, in patients with bone marrow suppression. Be aware that drug may worsen angle-closure glaucoma, encephalopathy, organic or traumatic brain damage, or tardive dyskinesia.
• When possible, avoid combining thiethylperazine with CNS depressants because these drugs may potentiate thiethylperazine's effects.
• Monitor patient with cardiac disease for exaggerated cardiovascular reactions.
• Implement seizure precautions and monitor for seizures in patients with known seizure disorder because drug may lower seizure threshold.
• Implement safety precautions, according to facility policy, for elderly patients. They may be especially sensitive to drug's sedative and extrapyramidal effects.
• Be prepared to discontinue drug 48 hours before myelography and to resume drug 24 to 48 hours afterward to minimize the risk of seizures.
• Be aware that photosensitivity may turn patient's skin yellow-brown, gray, or purple because of hyperpigmentation.
• Be aware that drug shouldn't be given to pregnant patient because it may cause jaundice and extrapyramidal symptoms in her neonate.

PATIENT TEACHING
• Instruct patient to stay recumbent for 1 hour after taking thiethylperazine to minimize effects of orthostatic hypotension.
• Advise patient to notify prescriber immediately about adverse CNS reactions, decreased urine output, or vision changes.
• Urge patient to avoid alcohol use and potentially hazardous activities during therapy.
• Encourage patient to avoid excessive sun exposure and to use sunscreen when she's outdoors.

•Advise patient on long-term therapy to have periodic eye examinations to detect possible eye disorders.

thiopental sodium

Pentothal

Class, Category, and Schedule
Chemical: Barbiturate
Therapeutic: Anticonvulsant, sedative-hypnotic
Pregnancy category: C
Controlled substance: Schedule III

Indications and Dosages
➤ *To control seizures from anesthesia or other causes*
I.V. INJECTION
Adults. *Initial:* 75 to 125 mg (3 to 5 ml of 2.5% solution) as soon as possible after onset of seizure. *Maximum:* 250 mg given over 10 min.
➤ *To facilitate narcoanalysis*
I.V. INFUSION OR INJECTION
Adults. Dosage individualized based on patient's age, condition, sex, and weight; injected at 100 mg/min (4 ml/min of 2.5% solution) with patient counting backwards from 100. Expect to discontinue injection once patient becomes confused with her counting but is still awake. Or, use 0.2% concentration in D_5W for injection and infuse at 50 ml/min.
➤ *To treat cerebral hypertension*
I.V. INFUSION OR INJECTION
Adults. 1.5 to 3.5 mg/kg, repeated as required, to reduce elevated intracranial pressure (ICP).

Route	Onset	Peak	Duration
I.V.	10 to 40 sec	Unknown	10 to 30 min

Mechanism of Action
Depresses the CNS and may inhibit the ascending transmission of impulses in the reticular formation. Thiopental possibly enhances or mimics the inhibitory action of gamma-aminobutyric acid, thereby having an anticonvulsant effect and producing sedation and hypnosis. Thiopental may reduce ICP by increasing cerebral vascular resistance, which decreases cerebral blood flow and volume.

Incompatibilities
Don't mix thiopental with acidic I.V. drugs or solutions, succinylcholine, or tubocurarine.

Contraindications
History of porphyria; hypersensitivity to thiopental, its components, or other barbiturates

Interactions
DRUGS
clonidine, CNS depressants, guanabenz, magnesium sulfate, methyldopa, metyrosine, pargyline, rauwolfia alkaloids: Additive CNS depressant effects
diazoxide, diuretics, guanadrel, guanethidine, mecamylamine, trimethaphan: Possibly additive hypotensive effect
ketamine: Increased risk of hypotension or respiratory depression; possibly countered hypnotic effect of thiopental
phenothiazines: Possibly increased CNS depression or excitation, increased hypotensive effect
ACTIVITIES
alcohol use: Additive CNS depressant effects

Adverse Reactions
CNS: Agitation, anxiety, seizures
CV: Bradycardia, hypotension, shock, tachycardia, thrombophlebitis
GI: Hiccups
RESP: Apnea, bronchospasm, cough, laryngospasm, respiratory depression, wheezing
SKIN: Hives, itching, rash, redness
Other: Angioedema

Nursing Considerations
•Before administering thiopental, expect to premedicate patient with an anticholinergic, such as atropine or glycopyrrolate, to minimize secretions.
•Be prepared to administer a test dose of 25 to 75 mg (1 to 3 ml of 2.5% solution) to determine tolerance or sensitivity. Expect to observe patient for at least 1 minute after administering test dose.
•Dilute drug with a compatible I.V. solution before administering, such as D_5W for injection, NS for injection, or sterile water for injection. Be aware that sterile water for injection shouldn't be used to prepare 0.2% or 0.4% solution because it would result in a hypotonic solution and cause hemolysis.
•To prepare 0.2% solution, dilute 1 g of thiopental with 500 ml of compatible diluent to produce a final concentration of 2 mg/ml.

T

•To prepare 0.4% solution, dilute 1 g of thiopental with 250 ml of compatible diluent or 2 g of thiopental with 500 ml of compatible diluent to produce a final concentration of 4 mg/ml.

•To prepare 2.5% solution, dilute 1 g of thiopental with 40 ml of compatible diluent or 5 g of thiopental with 200 ml of compatible diluent to produce a final concentration of 25 mg/ml.

•Inspect solution for particles before administration. Use solution within 24 hours of reconstitution, and discard unused portion after 24 hours.

•Monitor blood and tissue oxygenation and vital signs during I.V. administration. Keep emergency equipment and drugs nearby in case respiratory depression occurs.

•If patient has a history of CV disease or hypotension, monitor her for CV depressant effects, such as bradycardia, hypotension, or shock.

•In patient with a history of seizures, institute seizure precautions according to facility protocol.

•Monitor respiratory rate, rhythm, and quality for signs of respiratory depression in debilitated patient or one with a history of respiratory disease.

•Monitor neurologic status every hour, or as ordered, in patient with increased ICP.

PATIENT TEACHING

•Explain the need for frequent hemodynamic monitoring.

•Advise patient to use caution when driving or performing tasks that require alertness for at least 24 hours after thiopental administration.

•Instruct patient not to consume alcohol or other CNS depressants for at least 24 hours after thiopental administration (unless prescribed) because they increase the effects of thiopental.

•Instruct patient to report persistent drowsiness, rash, severe dizziness, or skin lesions to prescriber.

thioridazine

Mellaril (CAN), Mellaril-S, Novo-Ridazine (CAN)

thioridazine hydrochloride

Apo-Thioridazine (CAN), Mellaril, Mellaril Concentrate, Novo-Ridazine (CAN), PMS Thioridazine

Class and Category

Chemical: Piperidine phenothiazine
Therapeutic: Antipsychotic drug
Pregnancy category: Not rated

Indications and Dosages

➤ *To treat schizophrenia in patients unresponsive to other antipsychotic drugs*

ORAL SOLUTION, ORAL SUSPENSION, TABLETS

Adults and adolescents. *Initial:* 50 to 100 mg t.i.d., gradually increased, as needed and tolerated. *Maintenance:* 200 to 800 mg/day in two to four divided doses. *Maximum:* 800 mg/day.

Children ages 2 to 12. *Initial:* 0.5 mg/kg/day in divided doses, gradually increased, as needed and tolerated. *Maximum:* 3 mg/kg/day.

Route	Onset	Peak	Duration
P.O.	Up to several wk	6 wk to 6 mo	Unknown

Mechanism of Action

Depresses areas of the brain that control activity and aggression, including the cerebral cortex, hypothalamus, and limbic system by blocking postsynaptic dopamine$_2$ (D$_2$) receptors. Drug may relieve anxiety by indirectly reducing arousal and increasing filtration of internal stimuli to the brain stem reticular activating system.

Contraindications

Coma; concurrent use of drugs that inhibit the metabolism of thioridazine, such as fluoxetine, fluvoxamine, paroxetine, pindolol, and propranolol; concurrent use of drugs that prolong the QT interval; concurrent use of high doses of a CNS depressant; history of arrhythmias; hypersensitivity to thioridazine, other phenothiazines, or their components; prolonged QT interval; reduced cytochrome P450 2D6 activity; severe CNS depression; severe hypertensive or hypotensive cardiac disease

Interactions

DRUGS

amantadine, antihistamines, antimuscarinics, clozapine, cyclobenzaprine, diphenoxylate, disopyramide, maprotilene: Additive anticholinergic effects

amiodarone, bepridil, cisapride, disopyramide, erythromycin, flecainide, grepafloxacin, ibutilide, pimozide, probucol, procainamide, quinidine, sotalol, sparfloxacin, tocainide: Possibly prolonged QT interval

amphetamine, chlorpromazine, dextroamphetamine: Possibly decreased effects of these drugs and thioridazine

antacids, antidiarrheals (adsorbent), kaolin, rifabutin, rifampin, rifapentine: Reduced bioavailability of thioridazine

anxiolytics, benzodiazepines, clonidine, dronabinol, guanabenz, guanfacine, opioid analgesics, phenothiazines, sedative-hypnotics: Possibly increased CNS effects or hypotension

barbiturates, fosphenytoin, phenytoin, valproic acid: Increased CNS depression, lowered seizure threshold

bromocriptine: Possibly decreased effectiveness of bromocriptine

carbamazepine: Possibly decreased blood thioridazine level

charcoal: Reduced thioridazine absorption

dopamine, droperidol, haloperidol, metoclopramide, metyrosine: Possibly increased adverse CNS effects

ephedrine, epinephrine, norepinephrine, phenylephrine: Possibly severe hypotension, MI, or tachycardia

fluoxetine, fluvoxamine, other cytochrome P450 2D6 inhibitors, paroxetine, pindolol: Inhibited metabolism of thioridazine, leading to elevated blood thioridazine level

general anesthetics: Possibly potentiated CNS depression

guanadrel, guanethidine, methyldopa: Inhibited hypotensive effect of these drugs

levodopa, pergolide, pramipexole, ropinirole: Possibly inhibited antiparkinsonian response

lithium (high doses): Risk of encephalopathic syndrome (characterized by confusion, elevated liver function test results and fasting blood glucose level, extrapyramidal symptoms, fever, lethargy, leukocytosis, and weakness)

MAO inhibitors: Possibly exaggerated extrapyramidal reactions

methoxsalen, oral contraceptives, porfimer, sulfonamides, sulfonylureas, tetracyclines, thiazide diuretics, vitamin A analogues: Possibly increased photosensitivity

propranolol: Increased blood propranolol and thioridazine levels, increased CNS effects, hypotension

tramadol: Increased blood tramadol level, possibly increased risk of seizures

trazodone: Possibly additive hypotension

ACTIVITIES

alcohol use: Additive CNS effects

Adverse Reactions

CNS: Akathisia, altered temperature regulation, depression, dizziness, drowsiness, extrapyramidal reactions (dystonia, laryngospasm, motor restlessness, pseudoparkinsonism), headache, insomnia

CV: ECG changes, hypertension, hypotension, prolonged QT interval, torsades de pointes, ventricular tachycardia

EENT: Blurred vision, change in color perception, dry mouth, impaired night vision, mydriasis, photophobia

ENDO: Breast engorgement, galactorrhea

GI: Constipation, ileus, nausea

GU: Amenorrhea, decreased libido, ejaculation disorders, impotence, menstrual irregularities, priapism, urine retention

HEME: Agranulocytosis, anemia, aplastic anemia, eosinophilia, leukocytosis, leukopenia, pancytopenia, thrombocytopenia

SKIN: Hyperpigmentation, jaundice, photosensitivity

Other: Weight gain

Nursing Considerations

•**WARNING** Expect to give thioridazine only if patient has failed to respond to therapy with at least two other antipsychotic drugs because it may prolong the QT interval and has been associated with torsades de pointes and sudden death.

•Obtain baseline and serial ECG tracings and serum potassium levels, as ordered. Notify prescriber if QT interval is greater than 500 msec or if potassium level is abnormal, and expect to discontinue drug immediately.

•Frequently monitor blood pressure and assess for chest pain in patients with heart disease because thioridazine has caused hypotension and has precipitated angina on occasion. Also monitor urine output in patients with benign prostatic hyperplasia because drug can worsen urine retention.

•Be aware that high doses and large dosage changes in patient with a seizure disorder may lower seizure threshold. Institute seizure precautions, as appropriate, according to facility policy.

•Administer drug with food, milk, or a full glass of water to minimize GI distress.

•Measure oral suspension using calibrated measuring device. Dilute with 60 to 120 ml of fruit juice, distilled water, or acidified tap water immediately before administration.

•Don't administer thioridazine oral suspension with carbamazepine oral suspension; a rubbery orange precipitate may form in stool.

•To prevent contact dermatitis, don't let oral solution come in contact with skin.

•Administer antacid or adsorbent antidiarrheal at least 1 hour before or 2 hours after thioridazine.

•**WARNING** Be aware that thioridazine can cause neuroleptic malignant syndrome—most commonly in males. Signs and symptoms include altered level of consciousness, altered mental status, autonomic instability (diaphoresis, hypotension or hypertension, sinus tachycardia), hyperthermia, and severe extrapyramidal dysfunction. Acute renal failure, increased serum creatine phosphokinase level, and leukocytosis also have occurred. Notify prescriber immediately if such symptoms develop, and be prepared to discontinue therapy.

•Be aware that drug shouldn't be discontinued abruptly. Sudden withdrawal of thioridazine may produce transient dizziness, nausea, tremor, and vomiting.

•Assess for eye pain because drug's anticholinergic effects can worsen angle-closure glaucoma.

•Promptly investigate and report blurred vision, defective color perception, or impaired night vision because of the risk of pigmentary retinopathy.

•Expect prescriber to discontinue thioridazine and order CBC if patient experiences signs of infection. Also expect drug therapy to be stopped 48 hours before myelography and resumed 24 to 48 hours afterward.

•Monitor patient for signs and symptoms of tardive dyskinesia—such as uncontrollable movements of the arms, face, or legs—even after treatment stops. Notify prescriber if they develop.

PATIENT TEACHING

•Instruct patient to take thioridazine exactly as prescribed and not to stop taking drug without consulting prescriber because of the risk of withdrawal symptoms.

•Instruct patient to notify prescriber immediately if she develops unusual symptoms, such as dizziness, palpitations, and syncope, because they may indicate the presence of torsades de pointes.

•Advise patient not to take drug within 2 hours of an antacid.

•Caution patient to avoid alcohol use, which increases drug's sedative effects, and to avoid hazardous activities if drowsiness occurs.

•Urge patient to notify prescriber immediately if she experiences blurred vision, defective color perception, difficulty with nighttime vision, excessive drowsiness, nausea, sore throat, or other signs of infection. Treatment may be discontinued.

•Advise female patient to use effective contraception while taking drug because its fetal effects are unknown. Instruct her to inform prescriber immediately of known or suspected pregnancy.

•Because drug may alter temperature regulation, encourage patient to avoid exposure to extreme temperatures during therapy.

•Advise patient to wear protective dark glasses to minimize the effects of adverse vision reactions.

•If patient requires long-term therapy, explain the risk of tardive dyskinesia, and urge her to notify prescriber immediately if she develops uncontrollable movements of her arms, face, or legs.

•Instruct patient to tell other prescribers that she's taking thioridazine before she takes any new drug.

thiothixene

Navane

thiothixene hydrochloride

Navane, Thiothixene HCl Intensol

Class and Category

Chemical: Thioxanthene derivative
Therapeutic: Antipsychotic
Pregnancy category: Not rated

Indications and Dosages

➤ *To treat psychotic disorders, such as acute psychosis, psychotic depression, and schizophrenia*

CAPSULES (THIOTHIXENE), ORAL SOLUTION (THIOTHIXENE HYDROCHLORIDE)

Adults and children age 12 and older. *Initial:* 2 mg t.i.d. (for mild conditions) or 5 mg b.i.d.

(for more severe conditions), increased q wk, as needed. *Usual:* 10 to 40 mg/day in divided doses. *Maximum:* 60 mg/day (for severe conditions).

DOSAGE ADJUSTMENT For elderly patients, lowest effective dosage used for maintenance therapy; maximum dosage limited to 30 mg/day. For some patients, one daily dose possibly used for maintenance therapy.

I.M. INJECTION (THIOTHIXENE HYDROCHLORIDE)

Adults. *Initial:* 4 mg b.i.d. to q.i.d. *Optimal:* 4 mg q 6 to 12 hr. *Usual:* 16 to 20 mg/day in divided doses. *Maximum:* 30 mg/day.

Mechanism of Action
Increases dopamine turnover by blocking postsynaptic dopamine receptors in the mesolimbic system. Eventually, dopamine neurotransmission decreases, resulting in antipsychotic effects.

Contraindications
Blood dyscrasias, coma, hypersensitivity to thiothixene or its components, Parkinson's disease, severe CNS depression, shock, use of quinidine

Interactions
DRUGS
amphetamines: Decreased effectiveness of either drug
antacids, antidiarrheals (adsorbent): Possibly reduced bioavailability of thiothixene
antihistamines, tricyclic antidepressants: Additive anticholinergic effects, causing severe constipation, ileus, or increased intraocular pressure
bromocriptine: Possibly increased serum prolactin level and decreased effectiveness of bromocriptine
carbamazepine: Possibly decreased blood thiothixene level
dopamine: Decreased vasoconstrictive effect of dopamine (in high doses)
ephedrine, phenylephrine: Possibly reduced vasopressor response
epinephrine: Possibly epinephrine reversal, leading to severe hypotension, tachycardia, and possibly MI
erythromycin: Increased adverse effects of thiothixene
general anesthetics, opioid analgesics, tramadol: Additive CNS effects, increased risk of seizures

guanadrel, guanethidine: Possibly decreased antihypertensive effect of these drugs
levodopa: Possibly reduced effectiveness of levodopa
lithium: Possibly encephalopathic syndrome (with blood level exceeding 12 mEq/L)
MAO inhibitors: Possibly exaggerated extrapyramidal reactions
metaraminol, methoxamine, norepinephrine: Possibly reduced vasopressor response
pergolide: Possibly reduced effectiveness of pergolide
propranolol: Possibly seizures and increased hypotension
quinidine: Additive orthostatic hypotension, possibly prolonged QT interval

ACTIVITIES
alcohol use: Additive CNS effects, increased risk of seizures
smoking: Possibly decreased blood thiothixene level

Adverse Reactions
CNS: Agitation, akathisia, drowsiness, dystonia, fatigue, insomnia, light-headedness, neuroleptic malignant syndrome, paradoxical exacerbation of psychotic disorder, restlessness, seizures, syncope, tardive dyskinesia, weakness
CV: ECG changes, edema, hypotension, peripheral edema, tachycardia
EENT: Blurred vision, dry mouth, increased salivation, miosis, mydriasis, nasal congestion, retinopathy
ENDO: Breast engorgement, galactorrhea, hyperglycemia, hypoglycemia
GI: Anorexia, constipation, diarrhea, elevated liver function test results, ileus, increased appetite, nausea, vomiting
GU: Glycosuria, impotence, priapism
HEME: Agranulocytosis, anemia, eosinophilia, hemolytic anemia, leukocytosis, leukopenia, pancytopenia, thrombocytopenia
SKIN: Contact dermatitis, decreased sweating, photosensitivity, pruritus, rash
Other: Hyperuricemia, weight gain

Nursing Considerations
•Administer thiothixene capsules with food or milk if needed to minimize GI distress.
•Don't administer drug within 1 hr of an antacid.
•Dilute oral solution with 60 to 120 ml of fruit or tomato juice, milk, soup, water, or a carbonated beverage before administering.

Measure dose and administer using a cali-brated measuring device. Avoid spilling solu-tion on skin because drug may cause contact dermatitis.

• Avoid inadvertent I.V. administration of thiothixene injection solution. It's intended for I.M. use only.

• Be aware that I.M. administration usually is reserved for acute, severe agitation or for pa-tients who can't take oral preparations.

• Maintain patient in recumbent position for 30 minutes after I.M. injection to minimize orthostatic hypotension.

• Assess for early signs of potentially irre-versible tardive dyskinesia, a syndrome of involuntary rhythmic movements of the face, jaw, mouth, or tongue.

• **WARNING** Be aware that drug can precipi-tate neuroleptic malignant syndrome, a seri-ous condition characterized by altered men-tal status, arrhythmias, diaphoresis, hyper-pyrexia, muscle rigidity, and tachycardia, es-pecially in patients with hyperthyroidism or thyrotoxicosis. Symptoms may be severe enough to cause life-threatening respiratory depression.

• Monitor patient's serum calcium level be-cause hypocalcemia may lead to dystonic re-actions.

• Keep in mind that hypotension from thio-thixene may precipitate angina in patients with known cardiac disease.

• **WARNING** Be aware that drug-induced ad-verse CNS reactions may mimic or suppress neurologic signs and symptoms of CNS disor-ders, such as brain tumor, encephalitis, en-cephalopathy, meningitis, Reye's syndrome, and tetanus.

• Monitor for extrapyramidal symptoms—particularly dystonias—in children with acute illnesses, including CNS infections, de-hydration, gastroenteritis, measles, or vari-cella-zoster infections.

• Observe for signs of adverse hematologic reactions, such as sore throat and other symptoms of infection. If they occur, be pre-pared to obtain CBC, as ordered, and discon-tinue thiothixene, as prescribed.

• Implement seizure precautions in patients with a history of seizures or EEG abnormali-ties because thiothixene can lower the sei-zure threshold.

• Assess patient for eye pain because drug's anticholinergic effects may worsen angle-closure glaucoma. Assess patient with benign prostatic hyperplasia for urine retention.

PATIENT TEACHING

• Fully inform patient facing long-term thio-thixene therapy about risk of developing tar-dive dyskinesia.

• Advise patient to avoid exposure to sunlight or ultraviolet light, and to apply sunscreen when outdoors.

• Urge patient to avoid smoking or to begin a smoking cessation program while taking thio-thixene.

• Encourage patient to avoid extreme tem-perature changes during drug therapy to pre-vent hyperthermia or hypothermia caused by decreased sweating.

• Instruct patient to immediately report sore throat or other signs of infection to pre-scriber.

thyroid USP

Armour Thyroid, Thyrar, Thyroid Strong, Westhroid

Class and Category

Chemical: Porcine thyroid gland hormone
Therapeutic: Thyroid hormone replacement
Pregnancy category: A

Indications and Dosages

➤ *To treat hypothyroidism without myx-edema*

TABLETS

Adults and children. *Initial:* 60 mg/day, in-creased by 30 mg/day q mo p.r.n. *Mainte-nance:* 60 to 120 mg/day.

➤ *To treat hypothyroidism or myxedema in patients with cardiovascular disease*

TABLETS

Adults. *Initial:* 15 mg/day; daily dosage dou-bled q 2 wk, as indicated to achieve desired response, up to 180 mg/day. *Maintenance:* 60 to 180 mg/day.

➤ *To treat congenital hypothyroidism (cre-tinism) or severe hypothyroidism in chil-dren and infants*

TABLETS

Children and infants. *Initial:* 15 mg/day; daily dosage doubled q 2 wk, as indicated to achieve desired response, up to 180 mg/day. If desired response isn't achieved, dosage further increased by 30 to 60 mg/day. *Main-tenance:* Individualized.

Mechanism of Action

Stimulates growth and maturation of tissues, increases energy expenditure, and affects all enzyme actions through several mechanisms. Thyroid hormone:
- regulates cell differentiation and proliferation
- aids in myelination of nerves and development of axonal and dendritic processes in the nervous system
- enhances protein and carbohydrate metabolism by promoting metabolic processes that increase gluconeogenesis and protein synthesis and facilitate the mobilization of glycogen stores.

Contraindications

Acute MI not associated with hypothyroidism, hypersensitivity to thyroid USP or its components, obesity treatment, untreated thyrotoxicosis

Interactions
DRUGS

barbiturates, carbamazepine, phenytoin, rifampin: Possibly increased catabolism of thyroid hormone
cholestyramine, colestipol: Decreased effectiveness of thyroid hormone
corticosteroids: Decreased metabolism of corticosteroids
estrogens: Possibly increased circulating concentrations of thyroxine-binding globulin, decreased effectiveness of thyroid hormone
insulin, oral antidiabetic drugs: Possibly altered blood glucose control
ketamine: Risk of marked hypertension and tachycardia
oral anticoagulants: Altered anticoagulant effect
sympathomimetics: Increased adverse cardiovascular effects
tricyclic antidepressants: Increased therapeutic and toxic effects of both drugs

FOODS
all foods: Possibly altered absorption of thyroid hormone

Adverse Reactions

CNS: Headache, insomnia, nervousness, tremor
CV: Angina; arrhythmias, including atrial fibrillation and sinus tachycardia; palpitations
ENDO: Hyperthyroidism
GI: Diarrhea, vomiting
GU: Menstrual irregularities
SKIN: Alopecia, diaphoresis
Other: Heat intolerance, weight loss

Nursing Considerations
- Avoid administering oral thyroid hormone with food because it may alter drug absorption.
- Don't administer thyroid hormone within 5 hours of cholestyramine or colestipol. Simultaneous administration of these drugs can reduce hormone absorption.
- **WARNING** Be aware that thyroid hormone therapy can unmask or exacerbate symptoms of adrenal insufficiency, precipitate adrenal crisis in patients with uncontrolled adrenal insufficiency, and increase the risk of arrhythmias in patients with coronary artery disease.
- Frequently monitor blood glucose level because thyroid hormone therapy can unmask or exacerbate symptoms of other endocrine disorders and also may alter antidiabetic drug dosage requirements in patients with diabetes mellitus. Be aware that withdrawal of thyroid hormone can precipitate a hypoglycemic response in susceptible patients.

PATIENT TEACHING
- Instruct patient to take thyroid hormone on an empty stomach and at the same time each day.
- Advise her to inform prescriber immediately and seek medical attention if she experiences chest pain, nervousness, or sweating.
- Instruct patient who uses cholestyramine or colestipol not to take these drugs within 5 hours of thyroid dose.
- Inform patient that full effects may not be evident for 1 to 3 weeks.
- Instruct patient with diabetes mellitus to monitor blood glucose level frequently.

thyrotropin

(thyroid-stimulating hormone, TSH)

Thytropar

thyrotropin alfa

Thyrogen

Class and Category
Chemical: Recombinant glycoprotein of human TSH
Therapeutic: Diagnostic aid
Pregnancy category: C

Indications and Dosages

➤ *To provide diagnostic follow-up of patients with well-differentiated thyroid carcinoma*

I.M. INJECTION (THYROTROPIN ALFA)
Adults and adolescents age 16 and older.
0.9 mg q 24 hr for 2 doses or q 72 hr for 3 doses. Scanning or serum thyroglobulin testing performed 72 hr after last injection.

➤ *To provide differential diagnosis of subclinical hypothyroidism or low thyroid reserve*

I.M. OR S.C. INJECTION (THYROTROPIN)
Adults and adolescents age 16 and older.
10 IU q.d. for 1 to 3 days, followed by radioactive iodine study 24 hr after last injection. No response indicates thyroid failure; substantial response indicates pituitary failure.

➤ *To determine thyroid status in patients receiving thyroid hormone, to differentiate between primary and secondary hypothyroidism*

I.M. OR S.C. INJECTION (THYROTROPIN)
Adults and adolescents age 16 and older.
10 IU q.d. for 1 to 3 days.

➤ *To aid in diagnosing thyroid carcinoma remnant after surgery*

I.M. OR S.C. INJECTION (THYROTROPIN)
Adults and adolescents age 16 and older. 10 IU q.d. for 3 to 7 days.

Mechanism of Action

Stimulates production of thyroglobulin by active thyroid tissue and enhances the uptake of iodine, the synthesis of thyroid precursor hormones (monoiodotyrosine, diiodotyrosine, and levothyroxine), and the release of triiodothyronine (T_3) and thyroxine (T_4) from the thyroid gland into the systemic circulation. Thyrotropin also binds with thyroid cancer tissue and stimulates iodine uptake in radioactive iodine imaging to detect cancer cells in euthyroid patients after near-total or total thyroidectomy.

Contraindications

Coronary thrombosis, hypersensitivity to thyrotropin or its components, uncorrected adrenal insufficiency

Adverse Reactions

CNS: Asthenia, fever, headache, paresthesia
ENDO: Hyperthyroidism
GI: Nausea, vomiting
SKIN: Rash, urticaria
Other: Flulike symptoms

Nursing Considerations

•**WARNING** Be aware that thyrotropin therapy can unmask or exacerbate symptoms of adrenal insufficiency, precipitate adrenal crisis in patients with uncontrolled adrenal insufficiency, and increase the risk of arrhythmias in patients with coronary artery disease.
•Reconstitute thyrotropin solution with manufacturer-provided diluent, which contains no preservatives.
•**WARNING** Avoid inadvertent I.V. or intradermal injection of thyrotropin. I.V. administration may result in severe reactions, including diaphoresis, hypotension, nausea, tachycardia, and vomiting. Intradermal injection may damage tissue at injection site.
•Monitor for chest pain and increased heart rate, especially in patients with preexisting cardiac or coronary artery disease, including angina, hypertension, and recent acute MI, and in patients with residual thyroid tissue. Drug may significantly increase serum thyroid hormone level.

PATIENT TEACHING
•Advise patient to continue taking any thyroid hormone replacement while receiving injections of thyrotropin alfa unless otherwise directed by prescriber.
•For patient scheduled to undergo testing with radioactive iodine, instruct her to follow a low-iodine diet.
•Inform patient that testing may take 5 to 12 days to complete.

tiagabine hydrochloride

Gabitril

Class and Category

Chemical: Nipecotic acid derivative
Therapeutic: Anticonvulsant
Pregnancy category: C

Indications and Dosages

➤ *As adjunct to treat partial seizures*

TABLETS
Adults. *Initial:* 4 mg q.d.; increased by 4 mg/wk up to 16 mg/day, then dosage increased

by 4 to 8 mg q wk until desired response occurs. *Usual:* 32 to 56 mg/day. *Maximum:* 56 mg/day in 2 to 4 divided doses.
Children ages 12 to 18. *Initial:* 4 mg q.d. for 1 wk, then increased by 4 to 8 mg/wk until desired response occurs. *Maximum:* 32 mg/day in 2 to 4 divided doses.

DOSAGE ADJUSTMENT For patients with impaired hepatic function, dosage individualized and reduced, or dosing interval extended if needed, because of reduced drug clearance.

Mechanism of Action
May inhibit neuronal and glial uptake of gamma-aminobutyric acid (GABA), the major inhibitory neurotransmitter in the CNS. Tiagabine makes more GABA available in the CNS to open chloride channels in the postsynaptic membranes, thereby leading to membrane hyperpolarization and preventing transmission of nerve impulses.

Contraindications
Hypersensitivity to tiagabine or its components

Interactions
DRUGS
benzodiazepines, CNS depressants: Possibly additive CNS depression
carbamazepine, phenobarbital, phenytoin: Possibly decreased tiagabine effectiveness
ACTIVITIES
alcohol use: Possibly additive CNS depression

Adverse Reactions
CNS: Amnesia, anxiety, asthenia, ataxia, confusion, depression, dizziness, drowsiness, EEG abnormalities, hostility, impaired cognition, insomnia, light-headedness, paresthesia, seizures, tremor, weakness
EENT: Pharyngitis, stomatitis
GI: Abdominal pain, diarrhea, increased appetite, nausea, vomiting
GU: UTI
MS: Dysarthria
SKIN: Ecchymosis, rash

Nursing Considerations
•Administer tiagabine with food.
•WARNING Expect to taper dosage gradually as prescribed because abrupt discontinuation may increase seizure frequency. Be prepared to implement seizure precautions as needed.

PATIENT TEACHING
•Instruct patient to take tiagabine with food.
•Advise patient to avoid potentially hazardous activities until drug's CNS effects are known. Also urge her to avoid alcohol use during therapy.
•Caution patient who also takes CNS depressants that drug may increase depressant effect.
•Instruct patient not to stop taking tiagabine abruptly. Explain that prescriber usually tapers drug over 4 weeks to reduce the risk of withdrawal seizures.

ticarcillin disodium
Ticar

Class and Category
Chemical: Penicillin
Therapeutic: Antibiotic
Pregnancy category: B

Indications and Dosages
➤ *To treat moderate to severe infections, such as bacteremia, diabetic foot ulcers, empyema, intra-abdominal infections, lower respiratory tract infections (including pneumonia), lung abscess, peritonitis, pulmonary infections due to complications of cystic fibrosis (including bronchiectasis and pneumonia), septicemia, and skin and soft-tissue infections (including cellulitis) caused by susceptible organisms*

I.V. INFUSION
Adults and children. 200 to 300 mg/kg/day in divided doses q 4 to 6 hr. *Usual:* 3 g q 4 hr or 4 g q 6 hr.
➤ *To treat uncomplicated UTI*
I.V. INFUSION, I.M. INJECTION
Adults and children weighing 40 kg (88 lb) or more. 1 g q 6 hr.
Children over age 1 month and weighing less than 40 kg. 50 to 100 mg/kg/day in divided doses q 6 to 8 hr.
➤ *To treat complicated UTI*
I.V. INFUSION
Adults and children. 150 to 200 mg/kg in equally divided doses q 4 to 6 hr. *Usual:* 3 g q 6 hr.
DOSAGE ADJUSTMENT For patients with creatinine clearance of 30 to 60 ml/min/1.73 m^2,

T

2 g I.V. q 4 hr; with creatinine clearance of 10 to 30 ml/min/1.73 m^2, 2 g I.V. q 8 hr; with creatinine clearance of less than 10 ml/min/1.73 m^2, 2 g I.V. q 12 hr or 1 g I.M. q 6 hr.

Mechanism of Action

Inhibits bacterial cell wall synthesis by binding to specific penicillin-binding proteins located inside the bacterial cell wall. Ultimately, this leads to cell wall lysis and death.

Incompatibilities

Don't administer ticarcillin through same I.V. line as amikacin, gentamicin, or tobramycin. Don't administer within 1 hr of aminoglycosides.

Contraindications

Hypersensitivity to ticarcillin, penicillins, or their components

Interactions

DRUGS

aminoglycosides: Additive or synergistic activity against some bacteria, possibly mutual inactivation

anticoagulants: Possibly interference with platelet aggregation, prolonged PT

methotrexate: Prolonged blood methotrexate level, increased risk of methotrexate toxicity

probenecid: Prolonged blood ticarcillin level

Adverse Reactions

CV: Thrombophlebitis, vasculitis

GI: Elevated liver function test results, nausea, pseudomembranous colitis, vomiting

GU: Proteinuria

HEME: Anemia, eosinophilia, hemorrhage, leukopenia, neutropenia, prolonged bleeding time, thrombocytopenia

SKIN: Erythema nodosum, exfoliative dermatitis, pruritus, rash, toxic epidermal necrolysis, urticaria

Other: Anaphylaxis, hypernatremia, hypokalemia, injection site pain, superinfection

Nursing Considerations

• Obtain body fluid or tissue samples for culture and sensitivity testing, as ordered. Review test results, if possible, before giving first dose of ticarcillin.

• Don't inject more than 2 g of drug at any one I.M. injection site.

• Reconstitute each gram of ticarcillin with 4 ml of compatible diluent. Further dilute reconstituted I.V. solution to 10 to 100 mg/ml with compatible I.V. solution. To minimize vein irritation, don't exceed concentration of 100 mg/ml. Concentrations of 50 mg/ml or greater are preferred. Infuse appropriate I.V. dose over 30 to 120 minutes.

• Assess for local injection site reaction, including thrombophlebitis, during therapy.

• Be aware that ticarcillin may exacerbate symptoms in patients with a history of GI disease or colitis.

• For patients with renal impairment, implement seizure precautions, according to facility policy, because they're at increased risk for seizures.

• Assess patient for signs of pseudomembranous colitis, such as abdominal cramps and severe watery diarrhea. Also assess for other signs of superinfection, such as oral candidiasis and rash in breast-feeding infant.

• Monitor serum electrolyte levels for hypernatremia due to drug's high sodium content and for hypokalemia due to increased urinary potassium loss.

• **WARNING** Monitor patient's platelet count, PT, and APTT because ticarcillin may increase bleeding time and, in rare cases, may induce thrombocytopenia.

PATIENT TEACHING

• Instruct patient taking ticarcillin to report past allergies to penicillins and to notify prescriber immediately about adverse reactions, including fever.

• Advise patient to decrease sodium intake to reduce the risk of electrolyte imbalance.

ticarcillin disodium and clavulanate potassium

Timentin

Class and Category

Chemical: Penicillin

Therapeutic: Antibiotic combination

Pregnancy category: B

Indications and Dosages

➤ *To treat moderate to severe infections, such as appendicitis, bacteremia, bone and joint infections (including osteomyelitis), diabetic foot ulcers, diverticuli-*

tis, gynecologic infections (including endometritis), infectious arthritis, intra-abdominal infections, lower respiratory tract infections (including pneumonia), peritonitis, septicemia, skin and soft-tissue infections (including cellulitis), and UTIs caused by susceptible organisms; to manage febrile neutropenia

I.V. INFUSION

Adults and children age 12 and older weighing 60 kg (132 lb) or more. 3.1 g (3 g of ticarcillin and 100 mg of clavulanic acid) infused over 30 min q 4 to 6 hr.

Adults and children age 12 and older weighing less than 60 kg. 200 to 300 mg/kg/ day (based on ticarcillin content) in divided doses q 4 to 6 hr.

Children and infants over age 3 months. For mild to moderate infections, 200 mg/kg/day (based on ticarcillin content) in divided doses q 6 hr; for severe infections, 300 mg/kg/day (based on ticarcillin content) in divided doses q 4 to 6 hr.

➤ *To treat pulmonary infections caused by complications of cystic fibrosis, such as bronchiectasis or pneumonia*

I.V. INFUSION

Children. 350 to 450 mg/kg/day (based on ticarcillin content) in divided doses.

DOSAGE ADJUSTMENT For patients with renal impairment, loading dose of 3.1 g given, then dosage adjusted based on creatinine clearance.

Mechanism of Action

Inhibits bacterial cell wall synthesis by binding to specific penicillin-binding proteins located inside bacterial cell walls. In this way, ticarcillin ultimately leads to cell wall lysis and death. Clavulanic acid, which doesn't alter the action of ticarcillin, binds with bound and extracellular beta-lactamase, preventing beta-lactamase from inactivating ticarcillin.

Incompatibilities

Don't administer ticarcillin and clavulanate through same I.V. line as amikacin, gentamicin, or tobramycin. Don't administer within 1 hour of aminoglycosides.

Contraindications

Hypersensitivity to ticarcillin, clavulanic acid, or their components

Interactions

DRUGS

aminoglycosides: Additive or synergistic activity against some bacteria, possibly mutual inactivation

anticoagulants: Possibly interference with platelet aggregation

methotrexate: Prolonged blood methotrexate level, increased risk of methotrexate toxicity

probenecid: Prolonged blood ticarcillin level

Adverse Reactions

CV: Thrombophlebitis, vasculitis

GI: Elevated liver function test results, nausea, pseudomembranous colitis, vomiting

GU: Proteinuria

HEME: Anemia, eosinophilia, hemorrhage, leukopenia, neutropenia, prolonged bleeding time, thrombocytopenia

SKIN: Erythema nodosum, exfoliative dermatitis, pruritus, rash, toxic epidermal necrolysis, urticaria

Other: Anaphylaxis, hypernatremia, hypokalemia, infusion site pain

Nursing Considerations

• Keep in mind that 3.1 g of combination drug ticarcillin and clavulanate corresponds to 3 g of ticarcillin and 100 mg of clavulanic acid.

• Dilute reconstituted I.V. solution to concentration of 10 to 100 mg/ml with compatible I.V. solution. To minimize vein irritation, don't exceed concentration of 100 mg/ml. Concentrations of 50 mg/ml or greater are preferred. Infuse appropriate I.V. dose over 30 to 120 min.

• Know that ticarcillin and clavulanate may exacerbate symptoms in patients with a history of GI disease or colitis.

• For patients with renal impairment, implement seizure precautions, according to facility policy, because they're at increased risk for seizures.

• Assess patient for signs of pseudomembranous colitis, such as abdominal cramps and severe watery diarrhea. Also assess for other signs of superinfection, such as oral candidiasis and rash in breast-feeding infant.

• Monitor serum electrolyte levels for hypernatremia due to drug's high sodium content and for hypokalemia due to increased urinary potassium loss.

•WARNING Monitor patient's platelet count, PT, and APTT because drug may increase bleeding time and, in rare cases, may induce thrombocytopenia.

• Be aware that patient receiving high doses of ticarcillin may develop pseudoproteinuria.

PATIENT TEACHING

• Instruct patient taking ticarcillin and clavulanate to report past allergies to penicillins and to notify prescriber immediately about adverse reactions, including fever.

• Advise patient to decrease sodium intake to reduce the risk of electrolyte imbalance.

ticlopidine hydrochloride

Ticlid

Class and Category

Chemical: Thienopyridine derivative
Therapeutic: Antithrombotic, platelet aggregation inhibitor
Pregnancy category: B

Indications and Dosages

➤ *To reduce the risk of initial thrombotic CVA in patients who have experienced transient ischemic attack, to reduce the* risk of recurrent CVA in patients who have previously experienced thrombotic CVA

TABLETS

Adults. 250 mg b.i.d.

➤ *As adjunct to reduce the risk of subacute stent thrombosis after successful coronary stent implantation*

TABLETS

Adults. 250 mg b.i.d with antiplatelet doses of aspirin for up to 30 days after successful stent implantation.

Route	Onset	Peak	Duration
P.O.	2 to 4 days	8 to 11 days	1 to 2 wk

Contraindications

Coagulopathy, GI bleeding, hematologic disorders related to hematopoiesis (including history of thrombotic thrombocytopenic purpura, neutropenia, and thrombocytopenia), hemophilia, hypersensitivity to ticlopidine or its components, intracranial bleeding, retinal bleeding, severe hepatic disease

Mechanism of Action

Normally, platelets don't adhere to blood vessel walls. However, when a thrombotic CVA or other disorder damages blood vessel walls, platelets are activated and adhere within seconds. Once activated, platelets release adenosine diphosphate (ADP). This causes fibrinogen to bind to glycoprotein IIb/IIIa (GP IIb/IIIa) receptors on the surface of activated platelets and connect with other activated platelets. Then a thrombus forms.

Ticlopidine inhibits the release of ADP from activated platelets, which prevents fibrinogen from binding to GP IIb/IIIa receptors on the surface of activated platelets, as shown below. This action prevents platelets from aggregating to form a thrombus, which prevents thrombosis of an implanted stent or recurrence of CVA.

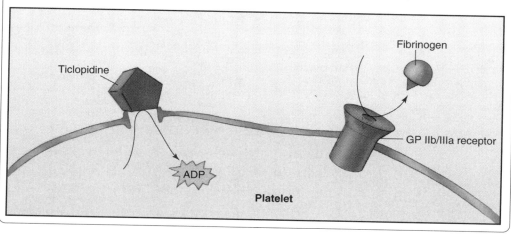

Interactions
DRUGS
aluminum- and magnesium-containing antacids: Possibly decreased peak blood ticlopidine level
antineoplastics, antithymocyte globulin, heparin, NSAIDs, oral anticoagulants, platelet aggregation inhibitors, salicylates, strontium-89 chloride, thrombolytics: Increased risk of bleeding
cimetidine: Reduced clearance of ticlopidine, increased risk of adverse reactions
cyclosporine, digoxin: Decreased blood level and possibly reduced effectiveness of these drugs
porfimer: Decreased effectiveness of porfimer photodynamic therapy
xanthines (aminophylline, oxytriphylline, theophylline): Decreased theophylline clearance, increased risk of toxicity

Adverse Reactions
CNS: Dizziness
CV: Hypercholesterolemia, vasculitis
EENT: Tinnitus
GI: Abdominal pain, anorexia, diarrhea, elevated liver function test results, flatulence, indigestion, nausea, vomiting
HEME: Agranulocytosis, aplastic anemia, hemolysis, hemolytic anemia, neutropenia, pancytopenia, thrombocytopenia, thrombotic thrombocytopenia, thrombotic thrombocytopenic purpura
SKIN: Pruritus, purpura, rash
Other: Hyponatremia, serum sickness-like reaction

Nursing Considerations
•Administer ticlopidine with food to maximize GI absorption and minimize any GI distress.
•Avoid I.M. injections of other drugs because excessive bleeding, bruising, or hematoma may occur.
•During first 3 months of therapy, monitor CBC every 2 weeks, as ordered (more frequently in patients with depressed neutrophil count).
•Be aware that ticlopidine therapy typically is used for patients with CVA or an increased risk of CVA who can't tolerate aspirin because of the risk of neutropenia or agranulocytosis.
•WARNING Be aware that ticlopidine therapy irreversibly affects platelet aggregation. Expect prescriber to discontinue drug 10 to 14 days before surgical procedures to prevent uncontrolled bleeding.

•Monitor serum cholesterol level during first month of ticlopidine therapy for expected increase. Hypercholesterolemia may persist for duration of treatment.
PATIENT TEACHING
•Advise patient to take ticlopidine with food.
•Inform patient that she may be at increased risk for infection because drug may decrease WBC or platelet count, especially in first 3 months of therapy.
•Advise patient to notify prescriber immediately if she experiences chills, fever, or sore throat.
•Encourage patient to keep scheduled appointments for blood tests to detect any abnormalities.
•Instruct patient to apply prolonged pressure to injured areas because bleeding may take longer than usual to stop. Urge her to immediately report to prescriber any unusual bleeding or bruising.

tiludronate disodium

(contains 200 mg of tiludronic acid per tablet)

Skelid

Class and Category
Chemical: Aminobiphosphonate
Therapeutic: Bone resorption inhibitor
Pregnancy category: C

Indications and Dosages
➤ *To treat Paget's disease in patients with serum alkaline phosphatase levels at least twice the upper limit of normal, who are symptomatic or at risk for future complications of the disease*
TABLETS
Adults. *Initial:* 400 mg of tiludronic acid q.d. 2 hr a.c. or p.c. for 3 mo. *Maximum:* 400 mg of tiludronic acid q.d.

Contraindications
Creatinine clearance less than 30 ml/min/ 1.73 m^2, esophageal abnormalities that delay esophageal emptying, hypersensitivity to tiludronate or its components

Interactions
DRUGS
aluminum- or magnesium-containing antacids, mineral supplements (such as calcium, iron),

salicylates, salicylate-containing compounds:
Decreased absorption of tiludronate
indomethacin: Possibly increased bioavailability of tiludronate
FOODS
all foods and beverages (except plain water):
Decreased absorption of tiludronate

> ## Mechanism of Action
> Reduces the activity of cells that cause bone loss and increases bone mass. Tiludronate may act by inhibiting osteoclast activity on newly formed bone resorption surfaces. This activity reduces the number of sites at which bone is remodeled. When bone formation exceeds bone resorption at these remodeling sites, bone mass increases. Tiludronate may also inhibit bone destruction by binding to hydroxyapatite crystals, which give bone its rigidity.

Adverse Reactions
CNS: Dizziness, headache
CV: Chest pain, edema
EENT: Cataracts, conjunctivitis, glaucoma, pharyngitis, rhinitis
GI: Diarrhea, esophageal irritation and ulceration, flatulence, indigestion, nausea, vomiting
MS: Arthralgia, back pain, myalgia
RESP: Cough, upper respiratory tract infection
SKIN: Rash
Other: Flulike symptoms

Nursing Considerations
•Be prepared to monitor serum calcium levels before, during, and after tiludronate therapy because drug may exacerbate such conditions as hyperparathyroidism, hypocalcemia, and vitamin D deficiency. Ensure adequate dietary intake of calcium and vitamin D during and after treatment. If hypocalcemia occurs, expect to administer a calcium supplement, as prescribed.
•**WARNING** Be aware that tiludronate may irritate upper GI mucosa, causing such adverse reactions as esophageal ulcer. To help minimize these reactions, have patient take drug with full glass of plain water and remain upright for at least 30 minutes afterward.

PATIENT TEACHING
•Instruct patient to take tiludronate with 6 to 8 oz of plain water and on an empty stomach (at least 2 hours before or after taking any beverages, food, other drugs, or mineral supplements, including mineral water) because food and beverages may severely reduce drug's therapeutic effect. Also, advise her to remain upright for at least 30 minutes after taking drug.
•Advise patient not to chew or suck on tablet to reduce the risk of esophageal irritation.
•Instruct patient to notify prescriber immediately if she develops signs or symptoms of esophageal irritation, such as difficulty swallowing or worsening heartburn, because these may indicate a serious esophageal disorder.
•Caution patient not to take salicylate-containing drugs, such as aspirin, during tiludronate therapy.

timolol maleate

Apo-Timol (CAN), Blocadren, Novo-Timol (CAN)

Class and Category
Chemical: Beta blocker
Therapeutic: Antihypertensive, MI prophylactic, vascular headache prophylactic
Pregnancy category: C

Indications and Dosages
➤ *To manage hypertension*
TABLETS
Adults. *Initial:* 10 mg b.i.d., increased q wk as prescribed. *Maintenance:* 20 to 40 mg/day in divided doses. *Maximum:* 60 mg/day.

➤ *To provide long-term prophylaxis after MI*
TABLETS
Adults. 10 mg b.i.d., beginning 1 to 4 wk after MI and continuing for at least 2 yr.

➤ *To prevent migraine headache*
TABLETS
Adults. *Initial:* 10 mg b.i.d. *Maintenance:* 20 mg/day in divided doses. *Maximum:* 30 mg/day; discontinued after 8 wk, as prescribed, if maximum dose is ineffective.

Route	Onset	Peak	Duration
P.O.	30 min	1 to 2 hr	4 to 8 hr

Mechanism of Action
Selectively blocks alpha$_1$ and beta$_2$ receptors in vascular smooth muscle and beta$_1$ receptors in the heart. This reduces peripheral vascular resistance and blood pressure and relieves migraine headaches. Timolol's potent beta blockade prevents the reflex tachycardia that typically occurs with most alpha blockers, and decreases cardiac excitability, cardiac output, and myocardial oxygen demand, thus preventing MI.

Contraindications
Acute bronchospasm; asthma; cardiogenic shock; children; COPD (severe); heart failure; hypersensitivity to timolol, other beta blockers, or their components; second- or third-degree AV block; severe sinus bradycardia

Interactions
DRUGS
allergen immunotherapy, allergenic extracts for skin testing: Increased risk of serious systemic adverse reactions or anaphylaxis
amiodarone: Additive depressant effect on cardiac conduction, negative inotropic effect
anesthetics (hydrocarbon inhalation): Increased risk of myocardial depression and hypotension
beta blockers: Additive beta blockade effects
calcium channel blockers, clonidine, diazoxide, guanabenz, reserpine, other hypotension-producing drugs: Additive hypotensive effect and, possibly, other beta blockade effects
cimetidine: Possibly interference with timolol clearance
estrogens: Decreased antihypertensive effect of timolol
fentanyl, fentanyl derivatives: Possibly increased risk of initial bradycardia after induction doses of fentanyl or derivative (with long-term timolol use)
glucagon: Possibly blunted hyperglycemic response
insulin, oral antidiabetic drugs: Possibly masking of tachycardia in response to hypoglycemia, impaired glucose control
lidocaine: Decreased lidocaine clearance, increased risk of lidocaine toxicity
MAO inhibitors: Increased risk of significant hypertension
neuromuscular blockers: Possibly potentiated and prolonged action of these drugs

NSAIDs: Possibly decreased hypotensive effect
phenothiazines: Increased blood levels of both drugs
phenytoin (parenteral): Additive cardiac depressant effect
sympathomimetics, xanthines: Possibly mutual inhibition of therapeutic effects

Adverse Reactions
CNS: Asthenia, CVA, decreased concentration, depression, dizziness, fatigue, hallucinations, headache, insomnia, nervousness, nightmares, paresthesia, syncope, vertigo
CV: Angina, arrhythmias, bradycardia, cardiac arrest, chest pain, edema, palpitations, Raynaud's phenomenon, vasodilation
EENT: Diplopia, dry eyes, eye irritation, ptosis, tinnitus, vision changes
ENDO: Hyperglycemia, hypoglycemia
GI: Abdominal pain, diarrhea, hepatomegaly, indigestion, nausea, vomiting
GU: Decreased libido, impotence
MS: Arthralgia, muscle weakness
RESP: Bronchospasm, cough, crackles, dyspnea
SKIN: Alopecia, diaphoresis, hyperpigmentation, pruritus, purpura, rash
Other: Weight loss

Nursing Considerations
•**WARNING** Be aware that timolol may mask signs and symptoms of acute hypoglycemia in diabetic patient. The drug also may mask certain signs of hyperthyroidism, such as tachycardia.
•Be aware that timolol may prolong hypoglycemia by interfering with glycogenolysis or may promote hyperglycemia by decreasing tissue sensitivity to insulin.
•Monitor blood pressure and cardiac output, as appropriate, for patient with a history of systolic heart failure or left ventricular dysfunction because timolol's negative inotropic effect can depress cardiac output.
•**WARNING** Be aware that timolol shouldn't be discontinued abruptly because this may produce MI, myocardial ischemia, severe hypertension, or ventricular arrhythmias, particularly in patient with known cardiovascular disease.
•Expect varied drug effectiveness in elderly patients; they may be less sensitive to drug's antihypertensive effect or more sensitive because of reduced drug clearance.
•Monitor for impaired circulation in elderly

patients with age-related peripheral vascular disease or patients with Raynaud's phenomenon. Such patients may experience exacerbated symptoms from increased alpha stimulation. Elderly patients also are at increased risk for beta blocker–induced hypothermia.
• If timolol exacerbates skin condition, such as psoriasis, notify prescriber.

PATIENT TEACHING
• Instruct patient taking timolol to inform prescriber of chest pain, fainting, light-headedness, or shortness of breath, which may indicate the need for dosage change.
• Caution patient not to stop taking drug abruptly. Timolol dosage must be tapered gradually under prescriber's supervison.
• Instruct patient with diabetes mellitus to monitor blood glucose level frequently during therapy.
• Warn patient with psoriasis about possible flare-ups of skin condition.

tinzaparin sodium

Innohep

Class and Category

Chemical: Low-molecular-weight heparin
Therapeutic: Anticoagulant, antithrombotic
Pregnancy category: B

Indications and Dosages

➤ *As adjunct to treat pulmonary thromboembolism and acute symptomatic deep vein thrombosis*

S.C. INJECTION
Adults. 175 anti-Xa IU/kg q.d. for at least 6 days. *Maximum:* 18,000 to 21,000 anti-Xa IU/day.

Route	Onset	Peak	Duration
S.C.	2 to 3 hr	4 to 6 hr	24 hr

Mechanism of Action

Potentiates the action of antithrombin III, a coagulation inhibitor. By binding with antithrombin III, tinzaparin rapidly binds with and inactivates clotting factors (primarily fibrin and factor Xa). Without thrombin, fibrinogen can't convert to fibrin and clots can't form.

Contraindications

Active major bleeding; heparin-induced thrombocytopenia (current or past); hypersensitivity to tinzaparin or its components, other low-molecular-weight heparins, sulfites, benzyl alcohol, or pork products

Interactions

DRUGS
alteplase, anistreplase, aspirin, dextran, dipyridamole, NSAIDs, oral anticoagulants, streptokinase, sulfinpyrazone, urokinase: Possibly increased risk of bleeding

Adverse Reactions

CNS: Confusion, dizziness, headache, insomnia, intracranial hemorrhage, paralysis
CV: Angina, hypertension, hypotension, tachycardia
EENT: Epistaxis, gingival bleeding, pharyngeal bleeding
GI: Constipation, elevated liver function test results, GI and retroperitoneal bleeding, hematemesis, nausea, vomiting
GU: Hematuria, genitourinary bleeding, prolonged or heavy menstrual bleeding, UTI
HEME: Anemia, thrombocytopenia, unusual bruising
MS: Back pain
RESP: Dyspnea, hemoptysis, pulmonary embolism
SKIN: Bleeding at puncture sites, surgical incision sites, or venous cutdown sites; rash
Other: Injection site hematoma, including itching, pain, redness, and swelling

Nursing Considerations

• Expect warfarin therapy to begin within 1 to 3 days of tinzaparin use.
• Monitor patient's INR. Expect tinzaparin therapy to be continued until INR reaches 2.0 for 2 consecutive days.
• **WARNING** Monitor for signs and symptoms of GI bleeding, including bloody or black, tarry stools; bloody or coffee-ground vomitus; and severe stomach pain. Notify prescriber immediately if patient develops any of these signs or symptoms.
• Assess tinzaparin injection site for signs and symptoms of hematoma, including deep, dark purple bruises under skin and itching, pain, redness, or swelling.
• Assess for signs and symptoms of intracranial bleeding (such as decreased level of consciousness), retroperitoneal bleeding (such as

abdominal pain or swelling and back pain), genitourinary bleeding (such as hematuria), or respiratory tract bleeding (such as hemoptysis). Notify prescriber immediately if patient develops any of these signs or symptoms.
•If serious bleeding (not controllable by local pressure) occurs, expect to discontinue any concomitant warfarin or antiplatelet drugs immediately.
•Expect to treat bleeding by administering 1 mg of protamine sulfate 1% solution I.V. per 100 anti-Xa IU of tinzaparin, as prescribed.
•If possible, avoid giving patient I.M. injections while she's receiving tinzaparin. If arterial puncture becomes necessary during tinzaparin therapy, expect to apply pressure after procedure and to monitor puncture site frequently for signs of bleeding.
•Monitor laboratory test results for elevated liver enzyme levels. If significant elevations persist or worsen, notify prescriber immediately.

PATIENT TEACHING
•Advise patient who is receiving tinzaparin to immediately report any bleeding, including from nose or gums.
•Instruct patient to limit physical activity during tinzaparin administration to reduce the risk of injury or bleeding.

tiopronin

Thiola

Class and Category
Chemical: Thiol compound
Therapeutic: Antiurolithic
Pregnancy category: C

Indications and Dosages
➤ *To prevent the formation of urinary cystine calculi*
TABLETS
Adults. 800 mg/day in 3 divided doses.
Children over age 9. 15 mg/kg in 3 divided doses.
DOSAGE ADJUSTMENT For patients with a history of hypersensitivity to penicillamine, therapy initiated at a reduced dosage; later dosage adjusted as prescribed, according to urine cystine level.

Route	Onset	Peak	Duration
P.O.	Rapid	Unknown	8 to 10 hr

Mechanism of Action
Inhibits the formation of urinary cystine calculi by undergoing thiol-disulfide exchange with cystine (cystine-cystine disulfide) to form a water-soluble compound, tiopronin-cystine disulfide.

Contraindications
History of agranulocytosis, aplastic anemia, or thrombocytopenia; hypersensitivity to tiopronin or its components

Interactions
DRUGS
bone marrow depressants: Increased risk of adverse hematologic effects
hepatotoxic drugs: Increased risk of adverse hepatotoxic effects
nephrotoxic drugs: Increased risk of adverse nephrotoxic effects

Adverse Reactions
CNS: Chills, fever
CV: Peripheral edema
EENT: Laryngeal edema, stomatitis
GU: Hematuria, proteinuria
HEME: Anemia, eosinophilia, leukopenia, thrombocytopenia
MS: Arthralgia
SKIN: Ecchymosis, jaundice, pruritus, rash, urticaria

Nursing Considerations
•Assess for signs of drug fever, which may occur during first month of tiopronin therapy.
•Be aware that drug may be stopped temporarily, then restarted at lower dose.
•Expect to monitor urine cystine level so dosage can be adjusted to keep cystine level below 250 g/ml.

PATIENT TEACHING
•Instruct patient to take tiopronin on an empty stomach, 1 hour before or 2 hours after meals, for faster drug absorption.
•Advise patient to drink at least 3 L of fluid daily to maintain a urine output of at least 2 L/day during therapy.
•Encourage patient to maintain a diet low in methionine, an essential amino acid found in eggs, cheese, fish, and milk.

tirofiban hydrochloride

Aggrastat

Class and Category
Chemical: Tyrosine derivative
Therapeutic: Platelet aggregation inhibitor
Pregnancy category: B

Indications and Dosages
➤ *To treat acute coronary syndrome*
I.V. INFUSION
Adults. 0.4 mcg/kg/min for 30 min, followed by 0.1 mcg/kg/min.
DOSAGE ADJUSTMENT For patients with creatinine clearance of less than 30 ml/min/1.73 m^2, infusion rate reduced by one-half.

Route	Onset	Peak	Duration
I.V.	Immediate	30 min	4 to 8 hr

Mechanism of Action
Binds to glycoprotein IIb/IIIa receptor sites on the surface of activated platelets. Circulating fibrinogen can bind to these receptor sites and link platelets together, forming a clot that eventually blocks a coronary artery. By binding to receptor sites, tirofiban prevents the normal binding of fibrinogen and other factors and inhibits platelet aggregation.

Incompatibilities
Don't infuse tirofiban in same I.V. line as any drug other than heparin.

Contraindications
Acute pericarditis; arteriovenous malformation; coagulopathy; CVA within previous 30 days, or history of hemorrhagic CVA; GI or GU bleeding; hemophilia; history of thrombocytopenia after tirofiban use; hypersensitivity to tirofiban or its components; intracranial aneurysm or mass, intracranial bleeding, retinal bleeding, aortic dissection, or any evidence of active abnormal bleeding within previous 30 days; major surgery or trauma within previous 6 weeks; severe uncontrolled hypertension (systolic blood pressure above 180 mm Hg, diastolic blood pressure above 110 mm Hg)

Interactions
DRUGS
antineoplastics, antithymocyte globulin, NSAIDs, oral anticoagulants, platelet aggregation inhibitors, strontium-89 chloride, thrombolytics: Increased risk of bleeding
levothyroxine, omeprazole: Increased rate of tirofiban clearance

porfimer: Decreased effectiveness of porfimer photodynamic therapy
salicylates: Increased risk of bleeding, possibly hypoprothrombinemia

Adverse Reactions
CNS: Chills, dizziness, fever, headache, intracranial hemorrhage
CV: Edema, hemopericardium, peripheral edema, sinus bradycardia
GI: Hematemesis, nausea, retroperitoneal bleeding, vomiting
GU: Hematuria, pelvic pain
HEME: Severe thrombocytopenia with chills, fever, and possibly fatal bleeding complications
RESP: Pulmonary hemorrhage
SKIN: Diaphoresis, rash, urticaria
Other: Allergic reaction, anaphylaxis, infusion site bleeding

Nursing Considerations
•**WARNING** Dilute 50-ml vial of tirofiban before use; don't dilute 500-ml container because it holds premixed solution ready for I.V. infusion. Don't use solution unless it's clear and the seal is intact.
•If prescribed, administer tirofiban with heparin for 48 to 108 hours. Expect to continue infusion throughout angiography and for 12 to 24 hours after angioplasty or atherectomy.
•**WARNING** If patient is also receiving a heparin infusion, expect to monitor APTT before treatment, 6 hours after heparin infusion starts, and regularly thereafter. Expect to adjust heparin dosage to maintain APTT at about two times the control. Notify prescriber immediately about an abnormally high APTT. Also, assess patient for signs and symptoms of abnormal bleeding and report them to prescriber immediately because potentially life-threatening bleeding may occur.
•After cardiac catheterization or percutaneous transluminal coronary angioplasty, maintain patient on bed rest and keep head of bed elevated. Ensure percutaneous site hemostasis at least 4 hours before discharge. Minimize invasive procedures, including epidural procedures, to reduce the risk of bleeding.
•Monitor platelet count, hemoglobin level, and hematocrit, as ordered. Expect to discontinue drug if platelet count is less than 90,000/mm^3, or to administer a platelet transfusion, as prescribed, if platelet count falls below 50,000/mm^3.

•Advise patient to immediately report any bleeding, bruising, headache, pain, or swelling during I.V. infusion of tirofiban.

tizanidine hydrochloride

Zanaflex

Class and Category
Chemical: Imidazoline
Therapeutic: Antispasmodic
Pregnancy category: C

Indications and Dosages
➤ *To manage acute and intermittent increases of muscle tone associated with spasticity*
TABLETS
Adults. 4 mg q 6 to 8 hr, p.r.n., increased gradually by 2 to 4 mg/dose, as needed and as prescribed. *Maximum:* 36 mg/day or 3 doses/day.

Route	Onset	Peak	Duration
P.O.	Unknown	1 to 2 hr	3 to 6 hr

Mechanism of Action
Reduces spasticity by decreasing the release of excitatory amino acids. This alpha$_2$-adrenergic agonist's action increases presynaptic inhibition of spinal motor neurons, with the greatest effects on polysynaptic pathways.

Contraindications
Hypersensitivity to tizanidine or its components

Interactions
DRUGS
acetaminophen: Delayed peak effects of acetaminophen
alpha$_2$-adrenergic agonists: Possibly significant hypotension
antihypertensives: Additive hypotensive effects
oral contraceptives: Decreased tizanidine clearance
ACTIVITIES
alcohol use: Increased adverse effects of tizanidine, additive CNS depression

Adverse Reactions
CNS: Anxiety, delusions, drowsiness, dyskinesia, fatigue, hallucinations, slurred speech
CV: Orthostatic hypotension
EENT: Dry mouth, pharyngitis, rhinitis
GI: Anorexia, constipation, diarrhea, elevated liver function test results, hepatic failure, hepatomegaly, nausea, vomiting
GU: Urinary frequency, UTI
MS: Muscle weakness
SKIN: Diaphoresis, jaundice, rash, ulceration

Nursing Considerations
•Monitor hepatic and renal function during first 6 months of tizanidine therapy and periodically thereafter.
•Expect prolonged drug use to inhibit salivary flow.
PATIENT TEACHING
•Suggest that patient use sugarless hard candy or gum and ice chips to relieve dry mouth.
•Advise patient to change position slowly to minimize effects of orthostatic hypotension.
•Instruct patient to avoid potentially hazardous activities until drug's CNS effects are known.
•Urge patient to avoid alcohol during drug therapy; caution her about its additive CNS effects.
•Advise patient to notify prescriber or dentist if dry mouth persists for longer than 2 weeks.

tobramycin sulfate

Nebcin, Tobi

Class and Category
Chemical: Aminoglycoside
Therapeutic: Antibiotic
Pregnancy category: D

Indications and Dosages
➤ *To treat bacteremia; bone and joint, gynecologic, intra-abdominal, lower respiratory tract, skin and soft-tissue, and urinary tract infections; endocarditis; meningitis; neonatal sepsis; pyelonephritis; and septicemia caused by susceptible strains of* Acinetobacter *sp.,* Aeromonas *sp.,* Citrobacter *sp.,* Enterobacter *sp.,* Escherichia coli, Haemophilus influenzae (beta lactamase–negative and –positive),* Klebsiella *sp.,* Morganella morganii, Proteus mirabilis, Proteus vulgaris, Providencia rettgeri, Pseudomonas aeruginosa, Salmonella *sp.,* Serratia *sp.,* Shigella *sp.,* Staphylococcus aureus, *and* Staphylococcus epidermidis; *to treat febrile neutropenia*

I.V. INFUSION, I.M. INJECTION

Adults. 3 to 6 mg/kg/day in divided doses q 8 to 12 hr.

Children over age 5. 2 to 2.5 mg/kg q 8 hr.

Children under age 5. 2.5 mg/kg q 8 to 16 hr.

Neonates over age 7 days weighing more than 2 kg (4.4 lb). 2.5 mg/kg q 8 hr.

Neonates over age 7 days weighing 1.2 to 2 kg (2.6 to 4.4 lb). 2.5 mg/kg q 8 to 12 hr.

Neonates age 7 days and under weighing 2 kg or more. 2.5 mg/kg q 12 hr.

Neonates age 7 days and under weighing 1.2 to 2 kg. 2.5 mg/kg q 12 to 18 hr.

Preterm neonates weighing 1 to 1.2 kg (2.2 to 2.6 lb). 2.5 mg/kg q 18 to 24 hr.

Preterm neonates weighing less than 1 kg. 3.5 mg/kg q 24 hr.

➤ *To treat pulmonary infection caused by* P. aeruginosa *in patients with cystic fibrosis*

I.V. INFUSION

Adults and children. 2.5 to 3.3 mg/kg q 8 hr; dosage adjusted to achieve peak blood drug level of 8 to 12 mcg/ml and trough blood drug level below 2 mcg/ml.

INHALATION

Adults and children over age 6. 1 ampule (300 mg) b.i.d. in alternating periods of 28 days on and 28 days off.

➤ *To treat meningitis caused by suscepti-ble organisms*

INTRATHECAL INJECTION

Adults. 4 to 8 mg q.d. in combination with parenteral therapy.

Children. 1 to 2 mg q.d. in combination with parenteral therapy.

➤ *To treat systemic infection*

INTRAPERITONEAL INFUSION

Adults and children. 1.5 to 2 mg/kg.

➤ *To treat dialysis-associated peritonitis in patients with end-stage renal disease*

INTRAPERITONEAL INFUSION

Adults and children. 4 to 8 mg/L in each dialysate exchange bag, increased, as pre-scribed, to 6 to 8 mg/L in documented *Pseu-domonas* infection or to 20 mg/L adminis-tered in one exchange bag q.d.

DOSAGE ADJUSTMENT For patients with renal impairment, dosage possibly reduced.

Incompatibilities

Don't mix tobramycin in same solution with parenteral aminoglycosides or beta-lactam antibiotics because mutual inactivation may result. Don't dilute or mix inhalation solu-tion in nebulizer with dornase alfa.

Mechanism of Action

Inhibits bacterial protein synthesis by binding irreversibly to one of two amino-glycoside-binding sites on the 30S riboso-mal subunit, resulting in bacteriostatic ef-fects. Bactericidal effects may stem from tobramycin's ability to accumulate within cells so that the intracellular drug level exceeds the extracellular level.

Contraindications

Concurrent cidofovir therapy; hypersensitiv-ity to tobramycin, aminoglycosides, sodium bisulfite, or their components

Interactions

DRUGS

acyclovir, aminoglycosides, amphotericin B, carboplatin, cisplatin, NSAIDs, vancomycin: Additive nephrotoxicity

carbenicillin, ticarcillin: Possibly inactivation of tobramycin

dimenhydrinate: Possibly masking of symp-toms of ototoxicity

ethacrynic acid, furosemide: Additive ototox-icity

general anesthetics, neuromuscular blockers: Possibly exaggerated neuromuscular blockade

Adverse Reactions

CNS: Confusion, dizziness, headache, leth-argy, neurotoxicity, vertigo

EENT: Hearing loss, tinnitus

GI: Diarrhea, elevated liver function test re-sults, nausea, vomiting

GU: Elevated BUN and serum creatinine lev-els, nephrotoxicity, oliguria, proteinuria, re-nal failure

HEME: Anemia, leukocytosis, leukopenia, neutropenia, thrombocytopenia

SKIN: Exfoliative dermatitis, pruritus, rash, urticaria

Other: Hypocalcemia, hypokalemia, hypomag-nesemia, hyponatremia, injection site pain

Nursing Considerations

•Obtain body fluid and tissue samples for culture and sensitivity testing before and during tobramycin treatment, as ordered. Re-view test results, if available, before therapy begins.

•After reconstituting drug with 30 ml of sterile or bacteriostatic water for injection, dilute further with NS or D_5W.
•Administer each I.V. dose over 20 to 60 minutes.
•**WARNING** Don't infuse tobramycin over less than 20 minutes because doing so may result in neuromuscular blockade and excessive peak blood drug level.
•Don't expose ampules for inhalation solution to intense light. Refrigerate them at 36° to 46° F (2° to 8° C).
•Because drug can cause bilateral and irreversible hearing loss, assess for early signs of cochlear and vestibular ototoxicity, including high-frequency hearing loss and vertigo.
•Monitor serum calcium, magnesium, potassium, and sodium levels to detect electrolyte imbalances.
•**WARNING** Be alert for allergic reactions, including anaphylaxis, because some forms of drug contain sodium bisulfite.
•Discontinue tobramycin therapy 7 days before starting cidofovir therapy, as prescribed.
•Assess for signs of nephrotoxicity, such as elevated BUN and serum creatinine levels.
•Expect dehydration to increase the risk of nephrotoxicity.
•**WARNING** Monitor patient with myasthenia gravis or parkinsonism for increased muscle weakness because of tobramycin's potential curare-like effect.

PATIENT TEACHING
•For tobramycin inhalation therapy, instruct patient to inhale over 10 to 15 minutes, using a handheld nebulizer with a compressor.
•Teach patient how to use nebulizer while sitting or standing upright and to breathe normally through its mouthpiece. Nose clips may help patient breathe through her mouth.
•Urge patient to immediately report high-frequency hearing loss and vertigo.
•Instruct female patient to notify prescriber immediately about known or suspected pregnancy because drug poses danger to fetus.

tocainide hydrochloride
Tonocard

Class and Category
Chemical: Lidocaine analogue
Therapeutic: Class IB antiarrhythmic
Pregnancy category: C

Indications and Dosages
➤ *To treat life-threatening, sustained ventricular tachycardia*
TABLETS
Adults. *Initial:* 400 mg q 8 hr. *Maintenance:* 1.2 to 1.8 g/day in divided doses q 8 hr.
DOSAGE ADJUSTMENT Dosage possibly reduced by 25% if creatinine clearance is 10 to 30 ml/min/1.73 m^2 and by 50% if creatinine clearance is less than 10 ml/min/1.73 m^2.

Route	Onset	Peak	Duration
P.O.	Unknown	0.5 to 2 hr	8 hr

Mechanism of Action
Combines with fast sodium channels in myocardial cell membranes, which inhibits sodium influx into cells and decreases ventricular depolarization, automaticity, and excitability during diastole.

Contraindications
Hypersensitivity to tocainide or its components, second- or third-degree AV block without ventricular pacemaker

Interactions
DRUGS
antiarrhythmics: Possibly additive cardiac effects, additive toxicity
beta blockers: Increased cardiac index, left ventricular pressures, and pulmonary artery wedge pressures
cimetidine: Possibly decreased blood tocainide level
rifampin: Accelerated hepatic metabolism of tocainide, reduced tocainide effectiveness

Adverse Reactions
CNS: Agitation, anxiety, ataxia, coma, confusion, depression, dizziness, fatigue, hallucinations, headache, mood changes, nervousness, paresthesia, psychosis, seizures, sleep disturbance, syncope, tremor, vertigo
CV: AV conduction disorders, bradycardia, chest pain, heart failure, hypertension, hypotension, palpitations, prolonged QT interval, PVCs, tachycardia, ventricular fibrillation
EENT: Blurred vision, vision changes
GI: Anorexia, diarrhea, nausea, vomiting
HEME: Agranulocytosis, anemia, aplastic anemia, bone marrow depression, hemolysis, leukopenia, neutropenia, thrombocytopenia

RESP: Pulmonary edema, fibrosis, and hypersensitivity (pneumonitis); respiratory arrest
SKIN: Diaphoresis, exfoliative dermatitis, pruritus, rash, skin lesions, urticaria

Nursing Considerations
•Monitor CBC with differential weekly during first 3 months of tocainide treatment and routinely thereafter to detect blood dyscrasias. Although rare, agranulocytosis, anemia, aplastic anemia, bone marrow depression, hemolysis, leukopenia, neutropenia, or thrombocytopenia may be fatal. Expect findings to normalize about 1 month after therapy stops.
•Maintain continuous cardiac monitoring or obtain periodic ECG tracings, as ordered, to assess drug effectiveness.
•Assess for tremor, a possible sign of maximum dosing.
•Assess for additive adverse cardiac effects, especially if tocainide is used with another antiarrhythmic.
•Be aware that tocainide is secreted in breast milk and has the potential to cause serious adverse reactions in breast-feeding infants.

PATIENT TEACHING
•Inform patient that electrophysiologic studies may be performed before tocainide therapy starts.
•Instruct patient to notify prescriber about tremor because dosage may need to be adjusted.
•Explain that chest X-rays may be needed if adverse pulmonary reactions occur.
•Inform patient that ambulatory monitoring may be needed to verify antiarrhythmic response.
•Stress the importance of keeping all scheduled appointments for follow-up laboratory blood tests.

tolazamide
Tolinase

Class and Category
Chemical: First-generation sulfonylurea
Therapeutic: Antidiabetic
Pregnancy category: C

Indications and Dosages
➤ *As adjunct to treat type 2 diabetes mellitus that's uncontrolled by diet and exercise*

TABLETS
Adults. *Initial:* 100 mg q.d. with breakfast if fasting blood glucose level is less than 200 mg/dl; 250 mg q.d. if fasting blood glucose level is more than 200 mg/dl. Dose adjusted q wk by 100 to 250 mg, if needed. Doses greater than 500 mg/day are divided and given q 12 hr. *Maximum:* 1,000 mg/day.
DOSAGE ADJUSTMENT If patient takes more than 40 U/day of insulin, initial dosage increased to 250 mg q.d. and insulin dosage decreased by 50%.

Route	Onset	Peak	Duration
P.O.	Unknown	3 to 4 hr	10 to 20 hr

Mechanism of Action
Stimulates insulin release from beta cells in the pancreas. Tolazamide also increases peripheral tissue sensitivity to insulin either by enhancing insulin binding to cellular receptors or by increasing the number of insulin receptors.

Contraindications
Diabetic coma; diabetic ketoacidosis; hypersensitivity to tolazamide, sulfonylureas, or their components; pregnancy; sole therapy for type 1 diabetes mellitus

Interactions
DRUGS
ACE inhibitors, anabolic steroids, androgens, azole antifungals, bromocriptine, chloramphenicol, clofibrate, disopyramide, guanethidine, H_2-receptor antagonists, insulin, magnesium salts, MAO inhibitors, methyldopa, octreotide, oxyphenbutazone, phenylbutazone, probenecid, quinidine, salicylates, sulfonamides, tetracycline, theophylline, tricyclic antidepressants, urinary acidifiers: Increased risk of hypoglycemia
asparaginase, calcium channel blockers, cholestyramine, clonidine, corticosteroids, danazol, diazoxide, estrogen, glucagon, hydantoins, isoniazid, lithium, morphine, nicotinic acid, oral contraceptives, phenothiazines, rifabutin, rifampin, sympathomimetics, thiazide diuretics, thyroid drugs, urinary alkalizers: Increased risk of hyperglycemia
beta blockers: Possibly hyperglycemia or masking of signs and symptoms of hypoglycemia

digoxin: Increased risk of digitalis toxicity
pentamidine: Initial hypoglycemia and then hyperglycemia if beta cell damage occurs
ACTIVITIES
alcohol use: Altered blood glucose control (usually hypoglycemia), possibly disulfiram-like reaction

Adverse Reactions
CNS: Dizziness, fatigue, headache, malaise, paresthesia, vertigo
ENDO: Hypoglycemia
GI: Anorexia, cholestasis, heartburn, nausea, vomiting
HEME: Agranulocytosis, aplastic anemia, hemolysis, hemolytic anemia, leukopenia, thrombocytopenia
MS: Muscle weakness
SKIN: Erythema, photosensitivity, pruritus, rash, urticaria

Nursing Considerations
• When switching an insulin-treated patient with type 2 diabetes, expect to start tolazamide at 100 mg q.d. if patient takes less than 20 U/day of insulin, or 250 mg q.d. if patient takes 20 to 40 U/day of insulin.
• Anticipate that patient receiving tolazamide may need temporary insulin treatment during periods of physiologic stress, such as fever, surgery, systemic infection, and trauma.
• For patient over age 65, expect to start tolazamide at 100 mg q.d.
• Assess elderly patients for signs of hypoglycemia because they're more susceptible to drug's hypoglycemic effect. Anticipate that hypoglycemia may be more difficult to detect.
• Assess patient with thyroid disease for altered blood glucose control because thyroid hormone increases GI absorption of glucose.
• Expect prescriber to stop tolazamide 2 weeks before pregnant patient delivers her neonate to minimize the risk of prolonged hypoglycemia in neonate.
PATIENT TEACHING
• Advise patient to avoid alcohol while taking tolazamide.
• Teach patient and family members how to monitor blood glucose level and how to recognize signs of hypoglycemia and hyperglycemia.
• Instruct patient to treat mild hypoglycemia with fruit juice or other simple sugars.

tolbutamide

Apo-Tolbutamide (CAN), Novo-Butamide (CAN), Orinase

Class and Category
Chemical: First-generation sulfonylurea
Therapeutic: Antidiabetic
Pregnancy category: C

Indications and Dosages
➤ *As adjunct to treat type 2 diabetes mellitus that's uncontrolled by diet and exercise*
TABLETS
Adults. *Initial:* 1 to 2 g/day in divided doses b.i.d. or t.i.d. *Maintenance:* 0.25 to 2 g/day. *Maximum:* 3 g/day.

Route	Onset	Peak	Duration
P.O.	Unknown	3 to 4 hr	6 to 12 hr

Mechanism of Action
Stimulates insulin release from beta cells in the pancreas. Tolbutamide also increases peripheral tissue sensitivity to insulin either by enhancing insulin binding to cellular receptors or by increasing the number of insulin receptors.

Contraindications
Diabetes complicated by pregnancy; diabetic coma; diabetic ketoacidosis; hypersensitivity to tolbutamide, sulfonylureas, or their components; sole therapy for type 1 diabetes mellitus

Interactions
DRUGS
ACE inhibitors, anabolic steroids, androgens, azole antifungals, bromocriptine, chloramphenicol, clofibrate, disopyramide, guanethidine, H_2-receptor antagonists, insulin, magnesium salts, MAO inhibitors, methyldopa, octreotide, oxyphenbutazone, phenylbutazone, probenecid, quinidine, salicylates, sulfonamides, tetracycline, theophylline, tricyclic antidepressants, urinary acidifiers: Increased risk of hypoglycemia
asparaginase, calcium channel blockers, cholestyramine, clonidine, corticosteroids, danazol, diazoxide, estrogen, glucagon, hydantoins, isoniazid, lithium, morphine, nicotinic acid, oral contraceptives, phenothiazines, ri-

T

fabutin, rifampin, sympathomimetics, thiazide diuretics, thyroid drugs, urinary alkalizers: Increased risk of hyperglycemia
beta blockers: Possibly hyperglycemia or masking of signs and symptoms of hypoglycemia
digoxin: Increased risk of digitalis toxicity
pentamidine: Initial hypoglycemia and then hyperglycemia if beta cell damage occurs
ACTIVITIES
alcohol use: Altered blood glucose control (usually hypoglycemia), possibly disulfiram-like reaction

Adverse Reactions
CNS: Dizziness, fatigue, headache, malaise, paresthesia, vertigo
ENDO: Hypoglycemia
GI: Anorexia, cholestasis, heartburn, nausea, vomiting
HEME: Agranulocytosis, aplastic anemia, hemolysis, hemolytic anemia, leukopenia, thrombocytopenia
MS: Muscle weakness
SKIN: Erythema, photosensitivity, pruritus, rash, urticaria

Nursing Considerations
•If patient takes 20 U or less of insulin/day, expect a possible transfer from insulin to tolbutamide therapy. If patient takes more than 20 U of insulin/day, expect to reduce insulin dosage as tolbutamide therapy starts.
•Anticipate that patient receiving tolbutamide may need temporary insulin treatment during periods of physiologic stress, such as fever, surgery, systemic infection, or trauma.
•Assess elderly patients for signs of hypoglycemia because they're more susceptible to drug's hypoglycemic effect. Anticipate that hypoglycemia may be more difficult to detect.
•Assess patient with thyroid disease for altered blood glucose control because thyroid hormone increases GI absorption of glucose.
•Expect prescriber to stop tolbutamide 2 weeks before pregnant patient delivers her neonate to minimize the risk of prolonged hypoglycemia in neonate.
PATIENT TEACHING
•Advise patient to avoid alcohol while taking tolbutamide.
•Teach patient and family members how to

monitor blood glucose level and how to recognize signs of hypoglycemia and hyperglycemia.
•Instruct patient to treat mild hypoglycemia with fruit juice or other simple sugars.

tolcapone
Tasmar

Class and Category
Chemical: Nitrobenzophenone
Therapeutic: Antidyskinetic
Pregnancy category: C

Indications and Dosages
➤ *As adjunct (with levodopa and carbidopa) to treat Parkinson's disease*
TABLETS
Adults. *Initial:* 100 mg t.i.d. *Maximum:* 200 mg t.i.d.

Mechanism of Action
Prolongs plasma half-life of levodopa by inhibiting catechol-*O*-methyltransferase (COMT), an enzyme responsible for metabolizing catecholamines—including dopa, dopamine, epinephrine, norepinephrine, and their hydroxylated metabolites. COMT inhibition reduces the amount of metabolizing enzyme for levodopa, which results in a more sustained plasma levodopa level. This action makes more levodopa available for diffusion into the CNS, where it is converted to dopamine.

Contraindications
Confusion, hyperpyrexia, or rhabdomyolysis with previous use of tolcapone; hepatic dysfunction; hypersensitivity to tolcapone or its components

Interactions
DRUGS
desipramine: Possibly increased frequency of adverse effects
levodopa: Increased levodopa bioavailability, with increased risk of orthostatic hypotension and syncope
MAO inhibitors: Possibly inhibited catecholamine metabolism

Adverse Reactions
CNS: Confusion, dizziness, drowsiness, dyskinesia, fatigue, fever, hallucinations, headache, lethargy, loss of balance

CV: Chest pain, orthostatic hypotension
EENT: Dry mouth
GI: Abdominal pain, anorexia, cholestasis, constipation, diarrhea, elevated liver function test results, vomiting
GU: Bright yellow urine, hematuria
MS: Muscle cramps, rhabdomyolysis
RESP: Dyspnea, upper respiratory tract infection
SKIN: Diaphoresis, jaundice

Nursing Considerations
•Monitor liver function test results, as ordered, during tolcapone therapy to detect hepatic impairment.
•Assess for hallucinations, especially in patient over age 75.
•Anticipate that drug may precipitate or exaggerate preexisting dyskinesia.
•Expect tolcapone to be discontinued if no improvement occurs after 3 weeks of therapy.
PATIENT TEACHING
•Inform patient that urine may turn bright yellow during tolcapone therapy.
•Advise patient to avoid potentially hazardous activities until drug's CNS effects are known.
•Urge patient to notify prescriber immediately about darkened urine, decreased appetite, fatigue, jaundice, lethargy, and right-sided abdominal pain.
•Caution patient not to stop taking drug abruptly. Explain that prescriber will supervise tapering of drug dosage.
•Urge patient to have regular follow-up appointments and laboratory tests.

tolmetin
Novo-Tolmetin (CAN), Tolectin DS, Tolectin 200, Tolectin 400 (CAN), Tolectin 600

Class and Category
Chemical: Pyrroleacetic acid derivative
Therapeutic: Anti-inflammatory
Pregnancy category: C (first trimester), Not rated (later trimesters)

Indications and Dosages
➤ *To relieve moderate pain from rheumatoid arthritis and osteoarthritis*
CAPSULES, TABLETS
Adults. *Initial:* 400 mg t.i.d. *Maintenance:* 600 to 1,800 mg/day in divided doses t.i.d. or

q.i.d. *Maximum:* 2,000 mg/day for rheumatoid arthritis, 1,600 mg/day for osteoarthritis.
➤ *To treat juvenile rheumatoid arthritis*
CAPSULES, TABLETS
Children over age 2. *Initial:* 20 mg/kg/day in divided doses t.i.d. or q.i.d. *Maintenance:* 15 to 30 mg/kg/day in divided doses. *Maximum:* 30 mg/kg/day.

Route	Onset	Peak	Duration
P.O.	Unknown	1 to 2 wk	Unknown

Mechanism of Action
Blocks the activity of cyclooxygenase, the enzyme needed to synthesize prostaglandins, which mediate the inflammatory response and cause local vasodilation, swelling, and pain. Prostaglandins also promote pain transmission from the periphery to the spinal cord. By blocking cyclooxygenase and inhibiting prostaglandins, tolmetin reduces inflammatory symptoms and relieves pain.

Contraindications
Angioedema, asthma, bronchospasm, nasal polyps, rhinitis, or urticaria caused by aspirin, iodides, or other NSAIDs

Interactions
DRUGS
ACE inhibitors, beta blockers: Decreased effectiveness of these drugs, possibly reduced renal function
alendronate, corticosteroids, other NSAIDs, salicylates: Increased risk of adverse GI effects
anticoagulants, platelet aggregation inhibitors, thrombolytics: Additive inhibition of platelet aggregation; prolonged bleeding time
antineoplastics, antithymocyte globulin, strontium-89 chloride: Increased risk of bleeding
cidofovir: Possibly nephrotoxicity
cyclosporine: Potentiated cyclosporine nephrotoxicity
digoxin: Increased blood digoxin level
lithium: Possibly lithium toxicity
methotrexate: Increased or prolonged blood methotrexate level
ACTIVITIES
alcohol use: Increased risk of adverse GI effects

Adverse Reactions

CNS: Depression, dizziness, drowsiness, fatigue, headache, weakness
CV: Chest pain, edema, hypertension, peripheral edema
EENT: Tinnitus
GI: Abdominal pain; constipation; diarrhea; elevated liver function test results; flatulence; gastritis; GI bleeding, perforation, or ulceration; hepatitis; indigestion; nausea; peptic ulcer disease; vomiting
GU: Dysuria, elevated BUN level, hematuria, interstitial nephritis, nephrotic syndrome, nephrotoxicity, proteinuria, UTI
HEME: Hemolytic anemia, prolonged bleeding time
SKIN: Jaundice, maculopapular rash, urticaria
Other: Weight gain or loss

Nursing Considerations

• Give tolmetin with food or milk to reduce adverse GI reactions.
• Assess for improvement within 7 days and progressive improvement over several successive weeks.
• Assess patients with heart failure, hypertension, or peripheral edema for fluid retention, which can worsen these conditions.
• Assess BUN and serum creatinine levels for abnormalities, as ordered, because long-term drug use may cause renal impairment.
• Assess invasive sites or wounds for bleeding and bruising caused by drug's effects on platelets.
• Be aware that tolmetin's anti-inflammatory effects may mask signs of infection.

PATIENT TEACHING

• Instruct patient to take drug with food or milk.
• Urge patient to limit sodium intake because drug may cause fluid retention.
• Caution patient to avoid alcohol during therapy.
• Advise patient to report unusual bleeding or bruising. Explain the risks of GI bleeding, perforation, and ulceration.
• Teach patient how to perform proper oral hygiene, and advise her to have needed dental work done before tolmetin therapy starts because of the increased risk of bleeding.

tolterodine tartrate

Detrol, Detrol LA

Class and Category

Chemical: Prodrug of 5-hydroxymethyl-tolterodine
Therapeutic: Antispasmodic
Pregnancy category: C

Indications and Dosages

➤ *To treat overactive bladder*
TABLETS
Adults. 2 mg b.i.d. Dosage reduced to 1 mg b.i.d. based on individual response and tolerance.
DOSAGE ADJUSTMENT Dosage reduced to 1 mg b.i.d. for patients with significant hepatic dysfunction and for patients who are also receiving cytochrome P450 3A4 inhibitors, such as clarithromycin, erythromycin, and the antifungals itraconazole, ketoconazole, and miconazole.
E.R. TABLETS
Adults. 4 mg q.d. Dosage reduced to 2 mg q.d. based on individual response and tolerance.

Mechanism of Action

Exerts antimuscarinic (atropine-like) and potent direct antispasmodic (papaverine-like) actions on smooth muscle in the bladder, which decreases detrusor muscle contractions. This helps reduce urinary frequency and urgency as well as urge-related incontinence.

Contraindications

Gastric retention, hypersensitivity to tolterodine tartrate or its components, uncontrolled angle-closure glaucoma, urine retention

Interactions

DRUGS

clarithromycin, erythromycin, itraconazole, ketoconazole, miconazole: Possibly increased blood tolterodine level
fluoxetine: Possibly decreased tolterodine metabolism

Adverse Reactions

CNS: Dizziness, fatigue, headache, somnolence
CV: Chest pain, hypertension
EENT: Abnormal vision, dry eyes, dry mouth
GI: Abdominal pain, constipation, diarrhea, flatulence, indigestion, nausea
GU: Dysuria, urine retention, UTI
Other: Flulike symptoms

Nursing Considerations

•**WARNING** Monitor patients with a history of bladder outflow obstruction for decreased urine output or bladder distention because tolterodine poses a risk of urine retention.
•Monitor patients with a history of GI obstructive disorders, such as pyloric stenosis, for abdominal distention or bloating because of increased risk of gastric retention.
•Be aware that drug's antimuscarinic effects may produce blurred vision, dizziness, and drowsiness. If these occur, institute fall precautions according to institution policy.

PATIENT TEACHING

•Instruct patient taking tolterodine to immediately report to prescriber difficulty urinating or infrequent urination.
•Advise patient not to drive or perform activities that require high level of alertness until drug's CNS and vision effects are known. Instruct her to notify prescriber if dizziness or blurred vision persists.
•Encourage patient to use sugarless candy, gum, or ice to relieve dry mouth. Advise her to notify prescriber or dentist if dry mouth persists or worsens over 2 weeks.

topiramate

Topamax

Class and Category

Chemical: Sulfamate-substituted monosaccharide
Therapeutic: Anticonvulsant
Pregnancy category: C

Indications and Dosages

➤ *As adjunct to treat partial seizures and primary generalized tonic-clonic seizures*

CAPSULES, TABLETS

Adults and adolescents age 17 and older. *Initial:* 25 to 50 mg/day in divided doses b.i.d. for 1 wk. Increased by 25 to 50 mg/day q wk. *Maintenance:* 200 to 400 mg/day in divided doses b.i.d. *Maximum:* 1,600 mg/day.
Children ages 2 to 16. *Initial:* 25 mg or less q h.s. for 1 wk. Increased q 1 to 2 wk by 1 to 3 mg/kg/day in divided doses q 12 hr, as prescribed. *Usual:* 5 to 9 mg/kg/day in divided doses q 12 hr.

➤ *As adjunct to treat seizures associated with Lennox-Gastaut syndrome*

CAPSULES, TABLETS

Children ages 2 to 16. 25 mg h.s. for 1 wk. Increased q 1 to 2 wk by 1 to 3 mg/kg/day in divided doses q 12 hr, as prescribed. *Usual:* 5 to 9 mg/kg/day in divided doses q 12 hr.

DOSAGE ADJUSTMENT For patients with moderate to severe renal impairment, dosage possibly reduced by 50%.

Mechanism of Action

May block the spread of seizures through its ability to reduce the length and frequency of excitatory transmission. Topiramate increases the availability of the inhibitory neurotransmitter gamma-aminobutyric acid by blocking voltage-sensitive sodium channels. This action promotes the movement of chloride ions into neurons.

Contraindications

Hypersensitivity to topiramate or its components

Interactions

DRUGS

antihistamines, barbiturates, benzodiazepines, CNS depressants, opioid analgesics, skeletal muscle relaxants, tricyclic antidepressants: Additive CNS depression
carbamazepine: Decreased blood topiramate level
carbonic anhydrase inhibitors: Increased risk of renal calculus formation
digoxin: Possibly decreased blood digoxin level
ethinyl estradiol: Increased risk of breakthrough bleeding
oral contraceptives: Increased risk of breakthrough bleeding, decreased contraceptive efficacy
phenobarbital: Altered blood phenobarbital level
phenytoin: Decreased blood topiramate level
probenecid: Possibly blocked renal tubular reabsorption of topiramate and decreased blood topiramate level
valproic acid: Decreased blood levels of both drugs

ACTIVITIES

alcohol use: Additive CNS depression

Adverse Reactions

CNS: Agitation, anxiety, ataxia, confusion, decreased concentration, depression, dizziness, fatigue, headache, irritability, memory loss, mood changes, nervousness, paresthesia, psychomotor slowing, slurred speech, somnolence, syncope

CV: Cardiac arrest, hot flashes, hypotension, palpitations, vasodilation
EENT: Diplopia, gingivitis, hearing loss, nystagmus, pharyngitis, rhinitis, secondary angle-closure glaucoma with acute myopia, taste perversion, vision changes
ENDO: Breast pain
GI: Abdominal pain, anorexia, constipation, diarrhea, flatulence, gastroenteritis, indigestion, nausea, vomiting
GU: Dysmenorrhea, dysuria, menstrual irregularities, renal calculi, UTI, vaginitis
HEME: Leukopenia
MS: Arthralgia, back pain, muscle weakness
RESP: Bronchitis, cough, upper respiratory tract infection
SKIN: Acne, alopecia
Other: Weight gain or loss

Nursing Considerations
• Give capsule with water and have patient swallow it whole. If needed, open capsules and empty contents onto a spoonful of soft food. Discard unused portion.
• Never store food sprinkled with drug for use at a later time.
• **WARNING** Anticipate an increase in seizure activity if therapy stops abruptly. Implement seizure precautions, as appropriate, according to facility policy.
• If patient reports ocular pain or decreased visual acuity, notify prescriber immediately because topiramate may cause increased intraocular pressure and secondary angle-closure glaucoma. Expect to discontinue drug immediately to avoid permanent vision loss.
• If patient has a history of renal calculi, assess for signs of recurrence.

PATIENT TEACHING
• Instruct patient to swallow topiramate tablets whole.
• Urge patient to avoid potentially hazardous activities until drug's CNS effects are known.
• Advise female patient of possible breakthrough bleeding. If she takes an oral contraceptive, encourage her to use another form of contraception during therapy.

torsemide
Demadex

Class and Category
Chemical: Anilinopyridine sulfonylurea derivative

Therapeutic: Antihypertensive, diuretic
Pregnancy category: B

Indications and Dosages
➤ *To treat edema in heart failure*
TABLETS, I.V. INJECTION
Adults. *Initial:* 10 to 20 mg q.d., adjusted by doubling, as prescribed, to achieve desired effect. *Maximum:* 200 mg q.d.
➤ *To treat edema in chronic renal failure*
TABLETS, I.V. INJECTION
Adults. *Initial:* 20 mg q.d., adjusted by doubling, as prescribed, to achieve desired effect. *Maximum:* 200 mg q.d.
➤ *To treat ascites, alone or with amiloride or spironolactone*
TABLETS, I.V. INJECTION
Adults. *Initial:* 5 to 10 mg q.d. *Maximum:* 40 mg q.d.
➤ *To manage hypertension*
TABLETS
Adults. *Initial:* 5 mg q.d., increased to 10 mg q.d. after 4 to 6 wk, as prescribed, if response is inadequate. *Maximum:* 10 mg q.d.

Route	Onset	Peak	Duration
P.O.	1 hr	1 to 2 hr	6 to 8 hr
I.V.	10 min	1 hr	6 to 8 hr

Mechanism of Action
Blocks active sodium and chloride reabsorption in the ascending loop of Henle by promoting rapid excretion of water, sodium, and chloride. Torsemide also increases the production of renal prostaglandins, increasing the plasma renin level and renal vasodilation. As a result, systolic and diastolic blood pressures fall, reducing preload and afterload.

Contraindications
Hypersensitivity to torsemide, sulfonamides, or their components

Interactions
DRUGS
ACE inhibitors, antihypertensives: Additive hypotension
amiloride, spironolactone, triamterene: Possibly counteracted torsemide-induced hypokalemia
amphotericin B: Increased risk of nephrotoxicity and severe, prolonged hypokalemia or hypomagnesemia

cisplatin: Increased risk of significant hypokalemia or hypomagnesemia, possibly permanent ototoxicity
cortisone, fluorocortisone, hydrocortisone: Increased risk of sodium retention and hypokalemia
digoxin: Increased risk of arrhythmias and digitalis toxicity due to hypokalemia or hypomagnesemia
indomethacin: Possibly decreased diuretic and antihypertensive effects of torsemide and increased risk of renal failure
lithium: Possibly lithium toxicity
metolazone, thiazide diuretics: Increased risk of severe fluid and electrolyte loss
neuromuscular blockers: Possibly increased neuromuscular blockade due to hypokalemia
probenecid: Possibly decreased diuretic effect of torsemide
quinidine and other ototoxic drugs: Increased risk of ototoxicity
salicylates: Increased risk of salicylate toxicity
ACTIVITIES
alcohol use: Additive diuresis and, possibly, dehydration

Adverse Reactions

CNS: Dizziness, drowsiness, fatigue, headache, insomnia, lethargy, nervousness, restlessness, weakness
CV: Chest pain, ECG abnormalities, edema, hypotension, tachycardia
EENT: Dry mouth, hearing loss, ototoxicity, pharyngitis, rhinitis, tinnitus
GI: Constipation, diarrhea, indigestion, nausea, thirst, vomiting
GU: Azotemia (prerenal), oliguria, urinary frequency
MS: Muscle spasms, myalgia
RESP: Cough
Other: Hypochloremia, hypokalemia, hypomagnesemia, hyponatremia, hypovolemia

Nursing Considerations

•Inject I.V. torsemide slowly over 2 minutes. Flush I.V. line with NS before and after administration.
•Don't exceed 200 mg in a single I.V. dose.
•Monitor serum electrolyte levels, as ordered, and fluid intake and output to detect hypovolemia.
•WARNING Expect torsemide-induced electrolyte imbalances, such as hypokalemia and hypomagnesemia, to increase the risk of toxicity and fatal arrhythmias in a patient

who takes a digitalis glycoside. Hypokalemia also potentiates neuromuscular blockade effects of nondepolarizing neuromuscular blockers.
PATIENT TEACHING
•Advise patient to change position slowly to minimize effects of orthostatic hypotension.
•Instruct patient to notify prescriber at once about drowsiness, dry mouth, hearing changes, lethargy, muscle pain, nausea, restlessness, thirst, vomiting, or weakness.
•Advise diabetic patient to monitor her blood glucose level frequently because torsemide may increase it.

tramadol hydrochloride

Ultram

Class and Category
Chemical: Cyclohexanol
Therapeutic: Analgesic
Pregnancy category: C

Indications and Dosages
➤ *To relieve moderate to moderately severe pain*
TABLETS
Adults and adolescents over age 16. 50 to 100 mg q 4 to 6 hr, p.r.n. *Maximum:* 400 mg/day.
DOSAGE ADJUSTMENT For patients with hepatic impairment, dosage reduced to 50 mg q 12 hr. For patients age 75 or older, maximum dosage reduced to 300 mg/day. For patients with a creatinine clearance of 30 ml/min/1.73 m^2 or less, dosage interval increased to q 12 hr and maximum dosage limited to 200 mg/day.

Route	Onset	Peak	Duration
P.O.	1 hr	2 to 3 hr	7 to 14 hr

Mechanism of Action
Binds with mu receptors and inhibits the reuptake of norepinephrine and serotonin, which may account for tramadol's analgesic effect.

Contraindications
Alcohol intoxication; excessive use of central-acting analgesics, hypnotics, opioids, or other psychotropic drugs; hypersensitivity to tramadol or its components; use within 14 days of MAO inhibitor therapy

Interactions
DRUGS
amiodarone, cimetidine, clomipramine, desipramine, fluphenazine, haloperidol, propafenone, quinidine, ritonavir, thioridazine: Decreased analgesia, increased adverse effects of tramadol
amphetamines, antipsychotics, bupropion, cyclobenzaprine, dextroamphetamine, MAO inhibitors, naloxone, tricyclic antidepressants: Increased risk of seizures
barbiturates, benzodiazepines, opioid analgesics, sedative-hypnotics, tranquilizers: Additive CNS depression
carbamazepine: Increased tramadol metabolism
general anesthetics: Increased CNS and respiratory depression
phenothiazines, rifampin: Additive CNS depression, increased risk of seizures
selective serotonin-reuptake inhibitors: Increased risk of serotonin syndrome and seizures
warfarin: Possibly increased INR
ACTIVITIES
alcohol use: Additive CNS depression

Adverse Reactions
CNS: Agitation, dizziness, emotional lability, euphoria, fatigue, hallucinations, headache, hypertonia, nervousness, somnolence, tremor, vertigo, weakness
CV: Vasodilation
EENT: Dry mouth, vision changes
GI: Anorexia, constipation, diarrhea, indigestion, nausea, vomiting
GU: Urinary frequency, urine retention
SKIN: Diaphoresis, pruritus, rash
Other: Physical and psychological dependence

Nursing Considerations
•Be aware that tramadol is a synthetic analogue of codeine and therefore poses a risk of drug abuse.
•To help prevent adverse GI reactions, expect to titrate tramadol to lowest effective analgesic dosage, as prescribed.
•Anticipate that drug may hinder assessment of acute abdominal conditions and obscure evidence of increasing intracranial pressure.
PATIENT TEACHING
•Instruct patient to observe prescribed dose limits and dosing intervals to prevent respiratory depression and seizures.
•Instruct patient to avoid potentially hazardous activities until drug's CNS effects are known.
•Advise patient to avoid alcohol while taking tramadol.

tramadol hydrochloride and acetaminophen
Ultracet

Class and Category
Chemical: Cyclohexanol (tramadol), aminophenol derivative (acetaminophen)
Therapeutic: Opioid analgesic (tramadol), nonnarcotic analgesic (acetaminophen)
Pregnancy category: C

Indications and Dosages
➤ *To provide short-term management of acute pain*
TABLETS
Adults. *Initial:* 75 mg tramadol and 650 mg acetaminophen q 4 to 6 hr, p.r.n. *Maximum:* 300 mg tramadol and 2,600 mg acetaminophen/day for up to 5 days.
DOSAGE ADJUSTMENT Dosing interval increased to 12 hr and maximum dose reduced to 75 mg tramadol and 650 mg acetaminophen/dose in patients with creatinine clearance of less than 30 ml/min/1.73 m^2.

Route	Onset	Peak	Duration
P.O.	In 1 hr	Unknown	Unknown

Mechanism of Action
Binds with mu receptors and inhibits the reuptake of norepinephrine and serotonin, which may account for tramadol's analgesic effect. Acetaminophen blocks the activity of cyclooxygenase, an enzyme necessary for prostaglandin synthesis. Prostaglandins, important mediators in the inflammatory response, cause local vasodilation, swelling, and pain.

Contraindications
Acute intoxication with alcohol, centrally acting analgesics, hypnotics, narcotics, opioids, or psychotropic drugs; hypersensitivity to tramadol, other opioids, acetaminophen, or components of these drugs

Interactions
DRUGS
acetaminophen-containing products: Increased risk of hepatotoxicity
carbamazepine: Increased tramadol metabolism and risk of seizures; possibly significantly reduced analgesic effect of tramadol
CNS depressants: Increased risk of CNS and respiratory depression

cytochrome P450 2D6 inhibitors, such as amitriptyline, fluoxetine, and paroxetine: Possibly inhibited tramadol metabolism
digoxin: Possibly digitalis toxicity, although rare
MAO inhibitors, selective serotonin reuptake inhibitors: Increased risk of seizures and serotonin syndrome
neuroleptics, opioids, tricyclic antidepressants: Increased risk of seizures
quinidine: Increased blood tramadol level
warfarin: Possibly elevated PT and altered effects of warfarin
FOODS
any food: Possibly delayed peak plasma time
ACTIVITIES
alcohol use: Increased risk of CNS and respiratory depression

Adverse Reactions
CNS: Dizziness, insomnia, seizures, somnolence
EENT: Dry mouth
GI: Anorexia, constipation, diarrhea, hepatotoxicity, nausea
GU: Prostate disorder
RESP: Respiratory depression
SKIN: Increased sweating, pruritus
Other: Hypersensitivity, physical and psychological dependence

Nursing Considerations
•Be aware that tramadol and acetaminophen shouldn't be given to patients with a history of anaphylactoid reactions to codeine or other opioid analgesics.
•After patient receives first dose, assess her for allergic reactions, including angioedema, bronchospasm, pruritus, Stevens-Johnson syndrome, toxic epidermal necrolysis, and urticaria. Also assess patient for signs and symptoms of anaphylaxis, such as dyspnea and hypotension.
•If patient has respiratory depression, frequently assess her respiratory status for signs of further respiratory depression. Be aware that tramadol and acetaminophen shouldn't be given to patient with respiratory depression; instead, she should receive an alternative nonopioid analgesic.
•If patient develops respiratory depression, expect to treat it as an overdose by administering naloxone. Assess patient for seizures because naloxone may increase this risk. Institute seizure precautions according to facility protocol.
•Frequently assess respiratory status of pa-

tients with increased intracranial pressure or head trauma because they may experience exaggerated carbon dioxide retention and secondary elevation of CSF pressure, both of which may cause respiratory depression. Also, because tramadol and acetaminophen can cause pupillary constriction, be aware that this effect may obscure the existence or extent of underlying intracranial complications in these patients.
•**WARNING** Assess patients with epilepsy, a history of seizures, or a risk of seizures, such as those with head trauma, metabolic disorders, alcohol or drug withdrawal, and CNS infections, for seizure activity because they have an increased risk of seizures while taking tramadol and acetaminophen.
•Be aware that tramadol and acetaminophen shouldn't be stopped abruptly because this may cause acute withdrawal symptoms, including anxiety, diarrhea, increased sweating, insomnia, nausea, pain, piloerection, rigors, tremors, and upper respiratory symptoms. Instead, when prescriber determines that drug is no longer needed, expect drug to be tapered.
•Because tramadol and acetaminophen may lead to physical and psychological dependence and abuse, assess patient for evidence of dependence or abuse, such as drug-seeking behavior. Be aware that drug shouldn't be used in patients with a history of dependence on other opioids because dependence may recur.
•Avoid giving tramadol and acetaminophen to patients with acute abdominal conditions because drug may mask important signs and symptoms and interfere with assessment of the abdomen.
•Monitor liver function test results, as appropriate, and notify prescriber of abnormal results. Be aware that this drug combination isn't recommended for patients with hepatic impairment.
PATIENT TEACHING
•Tell patient to avoid potentially hazardous activities until drug's adverse effects are known.
•Warn patient to avoid alcohol while taking tramadol and acetaminophen.
•Warn patient to avoid other drugs that contain tramadol or acetaminophen, including OTC preparations.
•Urge patient to notify prescriber if she becomes pregnant, thinks she might be pregnant, or is trying to become pregnant.

•Caution patient that taking more of this drug than prescribed or taking it more often than prescribed can lead to serious adverse reactions, including respiratory depression, seizures, hepatotoxicity, and death.

trandolapril

Mavik

Class and Category

Chemical: ACE inhibitor (non-sulfhydryl-containing)
Therapeutic: Antihypertensive, vasodilator
Pregnancy category: C (first trimester), D (later trimesters)

Indications and Dosages

➤ *To manage hypertension*

TABLETS

Adults. *Initial:* 1 mg q.d., increased q wk based on clinical response. Dosage may be given in two daily doses if antihypertensive effect diminishes before 24 hr. *Usual:* 2 to 4 mg/day. *Maximum:* 8 mg/day.

DOSAGE ADJUSTMENT Initial dosage increased to 2 mg q.d. for blacks with hypertension. Initial dosage reduced to 0.5 mg for patients also receiving a diuretic, those with a creatinine clearance of less than or equal to 30 ml/min/1.73 m², and those with cirrhosis.

➤ *To treat heart failure after MI*

TABLETS

Adults. *Initial:* 1 mg q.d. *Usual:* 4 mg or more q.d. *Maximum:* 8 mg/day.

Route	Onset	Peak	Duration
P.O.	2 hr	8 hr	24 hr

Contraindications

History of angioedema related to previous treatment with ACE inhibitor, hypersensitivity to trandolapril or its components

Interactions

DRUGS

allopurinol, bone marrow depressants (such as methotrexate), corticosteroids (systemic), cytostatic drugs, procainamide: Increased risk of potentially fatal neutropenia or agranulocytosis
antacids: Decreased blood trandolapril level
cyclosporine, potassium-containing drugs, potassium-sparing diuretics, potassium supplements: Increased risk of hyperkalemia

diuretics, other antihypertensives: Increased hypotensive effects
lithium: Increased blood lithium level and risk of lithium toxicity
NSAIDs, sympathomimetics: Possibly reduced antihypertensive effects

FOODS

high-potassium diet, low-sodium milk, potassium-containing salt substitutes: Increased risk of hyperkalemia

ACTIVITIES

alcohol use: Possibly increased hypotensive effect

Adverse Reactions

CNS: Dizziness, fatigue, fever, headache
CV: Hypotension, orthostatic hypotension
EENT: Loss of taste
GI: Diarrhea, nausea
GU: Decreased libido, impotence
MS: Myalgia
RESP: Cough, dyspnea, upper respiratory tract infection
SKIN: Pruritus, rash
Other: Angioedema

Nursing Considerations

•WARNING Closely monitor blood pressure during first 2 weeks of trandolapril therapy and whenever dosage is adjusted, especially in patients with heart failure, hyponatremia, or severe volume or sodium loss. If excessive hypotension occurs, notify prescriber immediately, place patient in supine position, and prepare to infuse I.V. normal saline solution, as prescribed.

•WARNING Be alert for signs and symptoms of angioedema. If swelling of tongue, glottis, or larynx causes airway obstruction, notify prescriber and be prepared to discontinue drug and administer emergency measures, including S.C. epinephrine 1:1,000 (0.3 to 0.5 ml).

•Continue to monitor patient's blood pressure to assess drug's long-term effectiveness.

PATIENT TEACHING

•Instruct patient to notify prescriber immediately and stop taking trandolapril if she experiences swelling of face, eyes, lips, or tongue or has difficulty breathing.

•Explain that drug may cause dizziness and light-headedness, especially during first few days of therapy. Advise patient to avoid driving and other potentially hazardous activities until drug's CNS effects are known and to notify prescriber immediately if she faints.

• Inform female patient of childbearing age about risks of taking trandolapril during pregnancy, especially during second and third trimesters. Urge her to use effective contraceptive method and to notify prescriber immediately if she becomes or thinks she might be pregnant.

• Advise patient planning to undergo surgery or anesthesia to inform specialist that she's taking trandolapril.

• Instruct patient to consult prescriber before using potassium supplements or salt substitutes containing potassium.

• Inform patient about possible loss of taste, which may result in weight loss. Reassure her that loss of taste is usually reversed after 2 to 3 months.

trandolapril and verapamil hydrochloride

Tarka

Class and Category
Chemical: ACE inhibitor (non–sulfhydryl-containing) (trandolapril), phenylalkylamine derivative (verapamil)
Therapeutic: Antihypertensive
Pregnancy category: C (first trimester), D (later trimesters)

Indications and Dosages
➤ *To manage hypertension*
E.R. TABLETS
Adults. *Initial:* 1 mg trandolapril and 240 mg verapamil, 2 mg trandolapril and 180 mg verapamil, 2 mg trandolapril and 240 mg verapamil, or 4 mg trandolapril and 240 mg verapamil q.d. *Maximum:* 4 mg trandolapril and 240 mg verapamil.
DOSAGE ADJUSTMENT Patients with hepatic impairment given 30% of normal dosage. Dosage may also be reduced in patients with cirrhosis and those with creatinine clearance less than 30 ml/min/1.73 m².

Route	Onset	Peak	Duration
P.O.	1 to 2 hr	Unknown	24 hr

Contraindications
Cardiogenic shock; history of angioedema related to previous treatment with ACE inhibitor; hypersensitivity to trandolapril, other ACE inhibitors, verapamil, or their components; hypotension; severe heart failure; severe left ventricular dysfunction; sick sinus syndrome or second- or third-degree AV block (unless artificial pacemaker is in place)

Mechanism of Action
Trandolapril is the prodrug for trandolaprilat, which reduces blood pressure by inhibiting the conversion of angiotensin I to angiotensin II. Angiotensin II is a potent vasoconstrictor that stimulates the renal cortex to secrete aldosterone. Decreased release of aldosterone reduces sodium and water retention and increases their excretion, thereby reducing blood pressure. Trandolapril may also inhibit renal and vascular production of angiotensin II.

Verapamil inhibits calcium entry into coronary and vascular smooth-muscle cells by blocking slow calcium channels in cell membranes. The resulting decrease in the intracellular calcium level inhibits smooth-muscle cell contractions and decreases myocardial oxygen demand by relaxing coronary and vascular smooth muscle, reducing peripheral vascular resistance, and decreasing systolic and diastolic blood pressures.

Interactions
DRUGS
anesthetics (inhaled): Enhanced cardiodepressive effects of verapamil
beta blockers: Increased risk of heart failure, hypotension, and severe bradycardia
carbamazepine, cyclosporine, theophylline: Possibly increased blood levels of these drugs and increased risk of toxicity
cimetidine: Decreased metabolism and increased blood level of verapamil
digoxin: Increased blood level of digoxin and risk of digitalis toxicity
disopyramide, flecainide: Possibly additive negative inotropic effects
diuretics: Increased risk of hypotension
lithium: Increased risk of lithium-induced neurotoxicity
neuromuscular blockers: Prolonged recovery from neuromuscular blockade
phenobarbital: Increased verapamil clearance

tranylcypromine sulfate

potassium-sparing diuretics, potassium sup-plements: Increased risk of hyperkalemia
quinidine: Increased risk of quinidine tox-icity, increased QT interval, additive negative inotropic effects
rifampin: Decreased bioavailability of oral verapamil
Foods
all foods: Decreased verapamil bioavailability
high-potassium diet, potassium-containing salt substitutes: Increased risk of hyper-kalemia

Adverse Reactions
CNS: Dizziness, fatigue
CV: AV block, bradycardia, junctional rhythm, orthostatic hypotension
EENT: Dry mouth
GI: Constipation
RESP: Cough
Other: Angioedema

Nursing Considerations
•Be aware that disopyramide and flecainide should not be given within 48 hours before or 24 hours after trandolapril and verapamil because additive negative inotropic effects can result.
•WARNING Closely monitor blood pressure during first 2 weeks of drug therapy and whenever drug dosage or accompanying di-uretic dosage is adjusted, especially in pa-tients with heart failure, hyponatremia, or severe volume or sodium loss. If excessive hypotension occurs, notify prescriber imme-diately, place patient in supine position, and prepare to infuse I.V. normal saline solution, as prescribed.
•WARNING Be alert for signs and symptoms of angioedema. If swelling of tongue, glottis, or larynx causes airway obstruction, notify prescriber and be prepared to discontinue drug and administer emergency measures, including S.C. epinephrine 1:1,000 (0.3 to 0.5 ml).
•Assess for bradycardia and hypotension, which may indicate AV block, and notify prescriber if heart rate or blood pressure declines significantly.
•Continue to monitor blood pressure to as-sess drug's long-term effectiveness.
PATIENT TEACHING
•Instruct patient not to crush or chew E.R. trandolapril and verapamil tablet, but in-form her that she may break tablet in half to aid in swallowing.

•Advise patient to take drug with food.
•Direct patient to monitor pulse rate before taking drug and to notify prescriber if pulse rate falls below 50 beats/min or as instructed by prescriber.
•Instruct patient to notify prescriber imme-diately and stop taking drug if she experi-ences swelling of face, eyes, lips, or tongue or has difficulty breathing.
•Explain that drug may cause dizziness and light-headedness, especially during first few days of therapy. Urge patient to avoid potentially hazardous activities until drug's adverse CNS effects are known and to notify prescriber immediately if she faints.
•Inform female patient of childbearing age about risks of taking trandolapril and ver-apamil during pregnancy, especially during second and third trimesters. Urge her to use effective contraception and to notify pre-scriber immediately if she becomes or thinks she might be pregnant.
•Advise patient planning to undergo surgery or anesthesia to inform specialist that she's taking trandolapril and verapamil.
•Instruct patient to consult prescriber before using potassium supplements or salt substi-tutes containing potassium.
•Encourage patient to increase dietary fiber intake to prevent constipation. Advise her to notify prescriber if constipation persists.

tranylcypromine sulfate
Parnate

Class and Category
Chemical: Nonhydrazine derivative
Therapeutic: Antidepressant
Pregnancy category: Not rated

Indications and Dosages
➤ *To treat major depressive episodes with-out melancholia*
TABLETS
Adults and adolescents over age 16. 30 mg/day in divided doses. After first 2 wk, in-creased by 10 mg q 1 to 2 wk, as prescribed. *Maintenance:* 10 to 40 mg/day. *Maximum:* 60 mg/day.
DOSAGE ADJUSTMENT For elderly patients, initial dosage possibly reduced to 2.5 to 5 mg/day and increased by 2.5 to 5 mg q 3 to 4 days, as prescribed; maximum dosage limited

to 45 mg/day. Alternative therapies should be carefully considered for patients over age 60.

Route	Onset	Peak	Duration
P.O.	7 to 10 days	4 to 8 wk	10 days

Mechanism of Action
Reversibly binds to MAO, reducing its activity and resulting in increased levels of neurotransmitters, including dopamine, epinephrine, and norepinephrine. This regulation of CNS neurotransmitters helps ease depression.

Contraindications
Cardiovascular disease; cerebrovascular disease; heart failure; hepatic disease; history of headaches; hypersensitivity to tranylcypromine or its components; hypertension; pheochromocytoma; severe renal impairment; use of anesthetics, antihypertensives, bupropion, buspirone, carbamazepine, CNS depressants, cyclobenzaprine, dextromethorphan, meperidine, other MAO inhibitors, selective serotonin-reuptake inhibitors, sympathomimetics, or tricyclic antidepressants

Interactions
DRUGS
amoxapine, bupropion, maprotiline, selective serotonin-reuptake inhibitors, trazodone, tricyclic antidepressants: Increased risk of severe hypertensive crisis, increased anticholinergic effects
anticonvulsants: Additive CNS depression
antihistamines: Possibly prolonged anticholinergic and CNS depressant effects
antipsychotics: Additive anticholinergic, hypotensive, and sedative effects
beta blockers: Possibly worsened bradycardia
bromocriptine: Increased blood prolactin level and interference with bromocriptine effects
buspirone: Increased blood pressure
dextroamphetamine, isometheptene, local anesthetics, naphazoline, oxymetazoline, psychostimulants, sympathomimetics, tetrahydrozoline, xylometazoline: Increased risk of severe hypertensive reaction
dextromethorphan, tryptophan: Increased risk of serotonin syndrome
diuretics: Additive hypotensive effects
doxapram: Increased vasopressor effects
furazolidone, procarbazine, selegiline: Increased risk of severe hyperpyretic or hypertensive crisis, seizures, or death

guanadrel, guanethidine: Increased risk of moderate to severe hypertension
insulin, oral antidiabetic drugs: Possibly prolonged hypoglycemic response
levodopa: Increased vasopressor effects, hypertension, adverse cardiovascular effects
meperidine: Increased risk of coma, diaphoresis, excitation, hypertension, rigidity, severe respiratory depression, shock, and, possibly death
methyldopa: Increased risk of hallucinations
metrizamide, tramadol: Increased risk of seizures
succinylcholine: Possibly prolonged succinylcholine effects
FOODS
aged cheese; avocadoes; bananas; fava or broad beans; cured sausage (bologna, pepperoni, salami, and summer sausage) or other meat; overripe fruit; pickled fish, meats, or poultry; protein extract; smoked fish, meats, or poultry; soy sauce; yeast extract; and other foods high in pressor amines, such as tyramine: Increased risk of sudden, severe hypertension
caffeine-containing beverages and foods: Increased risk of severe hypertensive crisis and dangerous arrhythmias
ACTIVITIES
alcohol-containing products that also may contain tyramine, such as beer (including reduced-alcohol and alcohol-free beer), wine (red and white), sherry, hard liquor, liqueurs: Increased risk of hypertensive crisis

Adverse Reactions
CNS: Anxiety, chills, dizziness, drowsiness, fever, headache, insomnia, intracranial hemorrhage, paresthesia, restlessness, tremor, weakness
CV: Bradycardia, chest pain, edema, hypertensive crisis, orthostatic hypotension, palpitations, tachycardia
EENT: Blurred vision, dry mouth, mydriasis, photophobia, tinnitus
GI: Abdominal pain, anorexia, constipation, diarrhea, nausea, vomiting
GU: Ejaculation disorders, impotence, urine retention
HEME: Agranulocytosis, anemia, leukopenia, thrombocytopenia
MS: Muscle spasms, myoclonus, neck stiffness
SKIN: Clammy skin, diaphoresis

Nursing Considerations
• Monitor patient's blood pressure during tranylcypromine therapy to detect hyperten-

sive crisis and to decrease the risk of orthostatic hypotension.

•WARNING Notify prescriber immediately if patient experiences signs of hypertensive crisis (drug's most serious adverse effect), such as chest pain, headache, neck stiffness, and palpitations. Expect to stop drug immediately if such signs occur.

•Anticipate that therapeutic response may not occur for up to 4 weeks.

•Expect drug to aggravate symptoms of Parkinson's disease, including muscle spasms, myoclonic movement, and tremor.

•Keep dietary restrictions in place for at least 2 weeks after stopping tranylcypromine because of the slow recovery from drug's enzyme-inhibiting effects.

•Ideally, expect to stop drug 10 days before elective surgery, as prescribed, to avoid hypotension.

•Be aware that abrupt cessation of drug can precipitate original symptoms.

•Frequently assess diabetic patient's blood glucose level to detect possible loss of blood glucose control.

•Anticipate that coadministration with a selective serotonin-reuptake inhibitor may cause confusion, seizures, severe hypertension, and other, less severe symptoms.

•Monitor severely depressed patient for suicidal tendencies. Take safety measures and notify prescriber immediately.

•Assess patient for sudden insomnia. If it develops, notify prescriber and be prepared to administer drug early in the day.

PATIENT TEACHING

•Instruct patient to avoid foods that contain cheese and that are high in tyramine, such as anchovies, avocadoes, bananas, beer, canned figs, caviar, Chianti wine, chocolate, dried fruit, fava beans, liqueurs, meat tenderizers, overripe fruit, pickled herring, raspberries, sauerkraut, sherry, sour cream, soy sauce, yeast extract, and yogurt while taking tranylcypromine.

•Urge patient to continue dietary restrictions for at least 2 weeks after therapy stops.

•Advise patient to notify prescriber immediately about chest pain, dizziness, headache, nausea, neck stiffness, palpitations, rapid heart rate, sweating, and vomiting.

•Urge patient to avoid alcohol and excessive caffeine intake during therapy.

•Suggest that patient change position slowly to minimize effects of orthostatic hypotension.

•Advise patient to avoid potentially hazardous activities until drug's CNS effects are known.

•Advise patient not to take other prescription or OTC drugs without consulting prescriber.

•Caution patient not to stop taking drug abruptly to avoid recurrence of original symptoms.

•Instruct female patient to use effective contraception during tranylcypromine therapy to prevent fetal abnormalities. Urge her to notify prescriber immediately about known or suspected pregnancy.

trazodone hydrochloride

Desyrel, Trazon, Trialodine

Class and Category

Chemical: Triazolopyridine derivative
Therapeutic: Antidepressant, anxiolytic
Pregnancy category: C

Indications and Dosages

➤ *To treat major depression, with or without generalized anxiety*

TABLETS

Adults. *Initial:* 150 mg/day in divided doses, increased by 50 mg/day q 3 to 4 days, p.r.n., as prescribed. *Maximum:* 400 mg/day for outpatients, 600 mg/day for inpatients.

Children ages 6 to 18. *Initial:* 1.5 to 2 mg/kg/day in divided doses, increased q 3 to 4 days, p.r.n., as prescribed. *Maximum:* 6 mg/kg/day in divided doses.

Route	Onset	Peak	Duration
P.O.	1 to 2 wk	Unknown	Unknown

Mechanism of Action

Blocks serotonin reuptake along the presynaptic neuronal membrane, causing an antidepressant effect. Trazodone exerts an alpha-adrenergic blocking action and produces modest histamine blockade, causing a sedative effect. It also inhibits the vasopressor response to norepinephrine, which reduces blood pressure.

Contraindications

Hypersensitivity to trazodone or its components, recovery from acute MI

Interactions
DRUGS
anticonvulsants: Decreased seizure threshold
antihypertensives: Increased risk of excessive hypotension
anxiolytics, brompheniramine, carbinoxamine, chlorpheniramine, clemastine, dimenhydrinate, diphenhydramine, doxylamine, general anesthetics, methdilazine, opioid analgesics, phenothiazines, sedative-hypnotics, skeletal muscle relaxants: Increased CNS depression, increased risk of respiratory depression and hypotension
barbiturates: Decreased seizure threshold and barbiturate effectiveness, increased drowsiness
buspirone, selective serotonin-reuptake inhibitors, tricyclic antidepressants: Possibly excessive serotonergic stimulation
clonidine: Interference with clonidine's antihypertensive effect
digoxin: Possibly increased blood digoxin level and risk of digitalis toxicity
MAO inhibitors: Increased serotonin-related effects
warfarin: Decreased anticoagulation response
ACTIVITIES
alcohol use: Increased CNS depression, increased risk of respiratory depression and hypotension

Adverse Reactions
CNS: Dizziness, drowsiness, fatigue, headache, light-headedness, nervousness, syncope, tremor
CV: Arrhythmias, hypotension, orthostatic hypotension, palpitations
EENT: Blurred vision, dry mouth
GI: Constipation, indigestion, nausea, vomiting
GU: Anorgasmy, ejaculation disorders, increased libido, priapism
SKIN: Pruritus, rash

Nursing Considerations
• Administer trazodone shortly after a meal or light snack to reduce nausea.
• Give larger portion of daily dose at bedtime if drowsiness occurs.
• Because trazadone's mechanism of action is similar to that of selective serotonin-reuptake inhibitors, expect high doses (6 to 8 mg/kg) to increase blood serotonin level and low doses (0.05 to 1 mg/kg) to decrease blood serotonin level.
• Expect most patients who respond to trazodone to do so by the end of the second week.

• Closely monitor depressed patient for suicidal thoughts. Notify prescriber if they occur and take suicide precautions, according to facility policy.
• Be aware that adverse CNS reactions usually improve after a few weeks of therapy.
• **WARNING** Be aware that trazodone therapy may increase the risk of priapism.
PATIENT TEACHING
• Urge patient to avoid taking trazodone on an empty stomach because doing so may increase dizziness or light-headedness.
• Caution patient to avoid potentially hazardous activities during therapy.
• Advise patient not to fast during therapy because of the increased risk of adverse CNS reactions.
• Instruct male patient to notify prescriber immediately about priapism.

treprostinil sodium
Remodulin

Class and Category
Chemical: Prostaglandin, tricyclic benzidene analog
Therapeutic: Vasodilator
Pregnancy category: B

Indications and Dosages
➤ *To treat pulmonary artery hypertension in patients with New York Heart Association Class II to IV symptoms in order to diminish exercise-induced symptoms*
S.C. INFUSION
Adults. *Initial:* 1.25 ng/kg/min. *Maintenance:* Infusion rate increased in increments of no more than 1.25 ng/kg/min each wk for first 4 wk, and in increments of no more than 2.5 ng/kg/min each wk thereafter, as needed. *Maximum:* 40 ng/kg/min.
DOSAGE ADJUSTMENT If initial dosage isn't tolerated or if patient has mild to moderate hepatic insufficiency, decrease initial dose to 0.625 ng/kg/min (ideal body weight).

Contraindications
Hypersensitivity to treprostinil, its components, or structurally related compounds

Interactions
DRUGS
anticoagulants: Increased risk of bleeding
antihypertensives, diuretics, other vasodilators: Increased risk of hypotension

Mechanism of Action

Acts directly on pulmonary and systemic arterial vascular beds to produce vasodilation. The vasodilatory effects reduce right and left ventricular afterload and increase cardiac output and stroke volume. These effects improve symptoms of pulmonary hypertension, such as dyspnea, and enable patients with pulmonary hypertension to walk greater distances with less discomfort.

Adverse Reactions

CNS: Anxiety, dizziness, headache, restlessness
CV: Edema, hypotension, vasodilatation
EENT: Jaw pain
GI: Diarrhea, nausea, vomiting
SKIN: Pruritus, rash
Other: Infusion site pain or reaction (erythema, induration, rash)

Nursing Considerations

•Assess patient's ability to care for a subcutaneous catheter and use an infusion pump. Discuss findings with prescriber before starting treprostinil therapy.
•Be aware that drug shouldn't be diluted before administering it.
•Calculate infusion rate using the following formula:
   Infusion Rate (ml/hr) = Dose (ng/kg/min) × Weight (kg) × [0.00006/treprostinil dosage strength concentration (mg/ml)]
or refer to charts in package insert to find infusion delivery rate for dosage prescribed.
•**WARNING** Don't abruptly stop treprostinil infusion or make sudden large reductions in dose because symptoms of pulmonary hypertension may worsen.
•Assess patient frequently for drug effectiveness and for adverse reactions. Know that the goal of chronic dosage adjustments is to find a dose that will improve symptoms of pulmonary hypertension, such as dyspnea and fatigue, while minimizing the drug's adverse effects, such as headache, nausea, vomiting, restlessness, anxiety, and infusion site pain or reaction.
•Monitor patients with mild to moderate hepatic insufficiency closely for adverse reactions, especially after dosage increases, because treprostinil is metabolized primarily by the liver.
•Be aware that patient must be discharged with a backup infusion pump, it should be

one that's adjustable to about 0.002 ml/hr and has occlusion/no delivery, low battery, programming error, and motor malfunction alarms. Also, the pump should have a delivery accuracy of ±6% or better, be positive-pressure driven, and have a reservoir made of polyvinyl chloride, polypropylene, or glass. Make sure patient has additional S.C. infusion sets to prevent potential interruptions in drug delivery.

PATIENT TEACHING
•Explain to patient that treprostinil is infused continuously through an S.C. catheter via an infusion pump.
•Teach patient to operate and maintain the S.C. infusion pump and to recognize the drug's adverse effects.
•Tell patient that a single vial of the drug shouldn't be used beyond 14 days after opening and that once the drug is placed in the pump's reservoir, it shouldn't be used after 72 hours.
•Instruct patient to store treprostinil vials at room temperature (about 25° C [77° F]).
•Inform patient that drug will be needed for prolonged periods, possibly years. Stress the importance of not discontinuing drug abruptly or making sudden large reductions in dosage without consulting prescriber because symptoms could worsen.
•Ensure patient understands that treprostinil use doesn't preclude the subsequent use of an I.V. therapy.
•Ensure that patient has emergency contact information for potential problems or questions about administering treprostinil at home.

triamcinolone

Aristocort, Aristopak, Atolone, Kenacort, Nasacort AQ

triamcinolone acetonide

Azmacort, Cenocort A-40, Cinonide-40, Kenaject-40, Kenalog-10, Kenalog-40, Ken-Jec-40, Nasacort, Robalog, Tac-3, Triam-A, Triamonide, Tri-Kort, Trilog

triamcinolone diacetate

Acetocot, Amcort, Aristocort, Aristocort Forte, Articulose-LA, Cenocort Forte, Cinalone 40, Clinacort, Kenacort Diacetate, Tilone, Tramacort-D, Triam-Forte, Triamolone 40, Tristoject

triamcinolone hexatonide

Aristospan

Class and Category

Chemical: Synthetic glucocorticoid
Therapeutic: Anti-inflammatory, immunosuppressant
Pregnancy category: C (nasal and oral inhalation), Not rated (oral and parenteral)

Indications and Dosages

➤ *To prevent bronchospasm or provide long-term corticosteroid treatment to control asthma*

ORAL INHALATION (TRIAMCINOLONE ACETONIDE)
Adults and children age 12 and older. *Initial:* 2 metered sprays (200 mcg) t.i.d. or q.i.d. *Maintenance:* Individualized dosage given b.i.d. *Maximum:* 16 metered sprays/day in divided doses.
Children ages 6 to 11. 2 to 4 metered sprays (200 to 400 mcg) b.i.d. to q.i.d. *Maximum:* 12 metered sprays/day.

➤ *To treat acute rheumatic carditis, berylliosis, and Hodgkin's disease; as adjunct to treat fulminating or disseminated pulmonary tuberculosis (with appropriate antituberculosis therapy)*

SYRUP (TRIAMCINOLONE DIACETATE), TABLETS (TRIAMCINOLONE)
Adults and children age 12 and older. *Initial:* 4 to 48 mg/day as a single dose or in divided doses. Some patients may require an initial dose of 60 mg.
Children under age 12. 0.42 to 1.7 mg/kg/day as a single dose or in divided doses.

I.M. INJECTION (TRIAMCINOLONE ACETONIDE)
Adults and children age 12 and older. 40 to 80 mg q 4 wk, as needed.
Children ages 6 to 11. 40 mg q 4 wk, as needed, or 30 to 200 mcg/kg q 1 to 7 days.

I.M. INJECTION (TRIAMCINOLONE DIACETATE)
Adults and children age 12 and older. 40 mg q wk, or 4 to 7 times the daily P.O. dose as a single injection q 4 days to q 4 wk.
Children ages 6 to 11. 40 mg/wk.

➤ *To relieve inflammation caused by acute gouty arthritis, acute nonspecific tenosynovitis, acute or subacute bursitis, epicondylitis, osteoarthritis, posttraumatic osteoarthritis, rheumatoid arthritis, and synovitis*

SYRUP (TRIAMCINOLONE DIACETATE)
Adults and children age 12 and older. 4 to 48 mg/day as a single dose or in divided doses, adjusted, as prescribed, to lowest effective dose based on clinical response.

TABLETS (TRIAMCINOLONE)
Adults and children age 12 and older. 8 to 16 mg/day in divided doses t.i.d. or q.i.d., adjusted, as prescribed, to lowest effective dose based on clinical response.

SYRUP (TRIAMCINOLONE DIACETATE), TABLETS (TRIAMCINOLONE)
Children ages 6 to 11. 0.42 to 1.7 mg/kg/day as a single dose or in divided doses, adjusted, as prescribed, based on clinical response.

I.M. INJECTION (TRIAMCINOLONE ACETONIDE)
Adults and children age 12 and older. 40 to 80 mg q 4 wk.
Children ages 6 to 11. 40 mg q 4 wk.

I.M. INJECTION (TRIAMCINOLONE DIACETATE)
Adults and children age 6 and older. 40 mg q wk as a single injection, repeated q 4 wk, if needed.

INTRA-ARTICULAR OR INTRABURSAL INJECTION (TRIAMCINOLONE ACETONIDE)
Adults and children age 6 and older. 2.5 to 15 mg, as needed.

INTRA-ARTICULAR OR INTRASYNOVIAL INJECTION (TRIAMCINOLONE DIACETATE)
Adults. 5 to 40 mg, repeated as prescribed q 1 to 8 wk, as needed.

INTRA-ARTICULAR INJECTION (TRIAMCINOLONE HEXATONIDE)
Adults. 2 to 20 mg, repeated as prescribed q 3 to 4 wk, as needed.

➤ *To treat primary (Addison's disease) or secondary adrenocortical insufficiency*

SYRUP (TRIAMCINOLONE DIACETATE)
Adults and children age 12 and older. 4 to 12 mg/day as a single dose or in divided doses.

SYRUP (TRIAMCINOLONE DIACETATE), TABLETS (TRIAMCINOLONE)
Children ages 6 to 11. 0.12 mg (base)/kg/day as a single dose or in divided doses.

➤ *To treat inflammatory dermatoses*

TABLETS (TRIAMCINOLONE)
Adults and children age 12 and older. 8 to 16 mg/day. *Usual:* 1 to 2 mg/day.

➤ *To treat disseminated lupus erythematosus*

TABLETS (TRIAMCINOLONE)
Adults and children age 12 and older. 20 to 30 mg/day. *Usual:* 3 to 30 mg/day.

T

> *To treat nephrotic syndrome*

TABLETS (TRIAMCINOLONE)
Adults and children age 12 and older. 16 to 20 mg/day.

> *To relieve symptoms of perennial and seasonal allergic rhinitis*

TABLETS (TRIAMCINOLONE)
Adults and children age 12 and older. 8 to 12 mg/day. *Usual:* 2 to 6 mg/day.
Children ages 6 to 11. 0.42 to 1.7 mg/kg/day as a single dose or in divided doses.

NASAL INHALATION (NASACORT)
Adults and children age 12 and older. *Initial:* 220 mcg/day in 2 sprays (55 mcg each)/nostril. *Maintenance:* 110 mcg/day in 1 spray (55 mcg each)/nostril. *Maximum:* 440 mcg or 8 sprays/day.

NASAL INHALATION (NASACORT AQ)
Adults and children age 12 and older. *Initial:* 110 mcg/day in 2 sprays (55 mcg each)/nostril. *Maintenance:* 55 mcg/day in 1 spray/nostril. *Maximum:* 220 mcg or 4 sprays/day.
Children ages 6 to 11. 110 mcg/day in 1 spray (55 mcg each)/nostril. *Maximum:* 220 mcg or 4 sprays/day.

> *To treat chronic idiopathic thrombocytopenic purpura*

TABLETS (TRIAMCINOLONE)
Adults and children age 12 and older. 0.8 mg/kg/day.

Route	Onset	Peak	Duration
P.O. (tablets)	Unknown	1 to 2 hr	2.25 days
I.M. (acetonide)	24 to 48 hr	Unknown	1 to 6 wk
I.M. (diacetate)	Slow	Unknown	4 days to 4 wk
Inhalation	12 hr	3 to 4 hr	Unknown
Intra-articular, intrabursal (acetonide)	Unknown	Unknown	Several wk
Intra-articular, intrasynovial (diacetate)	Unknown	Unknown	1 to 8 wk

Incompatibilities
Don't mix triamcinolone hexacetonide with parenteral local anesthetics because precipitation can occur.

Mechanism of Action
Inhibits the release of prostaglandins and leukotrienes, thus reducing immediate and late-phase allergic responses in chronic asthma. Triamcinolone also:
• decreases peribronchial edema and mucus secretion by inhibiting the binding of allergens to immunoglobulin E antibodies on the surface of mast cells, thereby inactivating the release of chemotactic substances
• decreases inflammation by interfering with leukocyte adhesion to capillary walls
• inhibits the release of leukocytic acid hydrolases, preventing macrophage accumulation at the infection site
• inhibits histamine and kinin release, preventing the formation of scar tissue.

Contraindications
Acute status asthmaticus (inhalation form), hypersensitivity to triamcinolone or its components, live-virus vaccine therapy, systemic fungal infection

Interactions
DRUGS
amphotericin B, ethacrynic acid, furosemide, thiazide diuretics: Increased potassium-wasting effect, severe hypokalemia
aspirin: Increased blood salicylate level, increased risk of salicylate toxicity
barbiturates, carbamazepine, phenytoin, rifampin: Increased triamcinolone metabolism
cholinesterase inhibitors: Increased risk of severe muscle weakness in patients with myasthenia gravis
digitalis glycosides: Increased risk of arrhythmias and digitalis toxicity
estrogens: Increased triamcinolone effects
insulin, oral antidiabetic drugs: Increased blood glucose level
isoproterenol: Increased risk of cardiotoxicity
live-virus vaccines: Decreased antibody response, increased risk of neurologic complications
neuromuscular blockers: Increased risk of hypokalemia and enhanced neuromuscular blockade
NSAIDs: Increased risk of adverse GI effects
toxoids: Decreased resistance to toxoids

Adverse Reactions

CNS: Emotional lability, exacerbated psychosis, headache, insomnia, restlessness, seizure, vertigo
CV: Edema, heart failure, hypertension
EENT: Dry mouth, glaucoma, hoarseness, nasal irritation (inhalation form), oropharyngeal candidiasis, pharyngitis, posterior subcapsular cataracts, secondary ocular infection, sinusitis, sneezing
ENDO: Cushing's syndrome, diabetes mellitus
GI: Abdominal pain, constipation, diarrhea, esophageal ulceration, gastritis, vomiting
GU: Cystitis, renal disease, UTI, vaginitis
MS: Bursitis, muscle wasting or weakness, myalgia, osteoporosis, tenosynovitis
RESP: Bronchospasm (inhalation form), chest congestion
SKIN: Ecchymosis, petechiae (parenteral form), photosensitivity, rash, striae, urticaria
Other: Angioedema; facial edema; herpes infection; impaired wound healing; injection site atrophy, induration, pain, soreness, and sterile abscess; weight gain

Nursing Considerations

•Give oral form of triamcinolone with meals to minimize GI distress.
•Use calibrated device to measure liquid doses.
•If necessary, crush tablets and mix with food or fluids.
•Shake I.M. suspension thoroughly before drawing it into syringe.
•Be aware that specialized training may be required to administer parenteral forms of triamcinolone.
•Don't administer parenteral forms of triamcinolone I.V.
•Be aware that triamcinolone may reactivate tuberculosis in patients with a history of the disease.
•**WARNING** Assess patient for signs and symptoms of adrenal insufficiency (fatigue, hypotension, lassitude, nausea, vomiting, and weakness) during times of stress, such as infection, surgery, or trauma. Notify prescriber immediately if you detect these signs and symptoms because adrenal insufficiency may be life-threatening.

PATIENT TEACHING
•Caution patient not to adjust triamcinolone dosage without consulting prescriber.
•Instruct patient to dispose of aerosol canister after 240 uses because dosage may not be correct after that time.
•Inform patient that maximum benefit may not occur for up to 2 weeks.
•Advise patient to notify prescriber immediately if asthma fails to respond to inhaled drug because additional systemic therapy may be needed.
•Caution patient to avoid exposure to people with chickenpox or measles throughout therapy and for 12 months afterward.
•Advise patient to have periodic eye examinations during long-term therapy, which can cause glaucoma or ocular nerve damage.

triamterene

Dyrenium

Class and Category

Chemical: Pterdine derivative
Therapeutic: Diuretic
Pregnancy category: B

Indications and Dosages

➤ *To treat edema in cirrhosis, heart failure, and nephrotic syndrome*

CAPSULES
Adults. *Initial:* 25 to 100 mg/day. *Maximum:* 300 mg/day.

Route	Onset	Peak	Duration
P.O.	2 to 4 hr	1 to several days	7 to 9 hr

Mechanism of Action
Inhibits sodium reabsorption in distal convoluted tubules and cortical collecting ducts, causing sodium and water loss and enhancing potassium retention.

Contraindications

Anuria, diabetic nephropathy or renal disease linked to renal insufficiency, hyperkalemia (potassium level of 5.5 mEq/L or more), hypersensitivity to triamterene or its components, severe hepatic dysfunction

Interactions
DRUGS
ACE inhibitors, amiloride, angiotensin-II receptor antagonists, cyclosporine, heparin, potassium-containing drugs, potassium salts, potassium supplements, spironolactone: Increased risk of hyperkalemia
amantadine: Decreased amantadine clearance, possibly amantadine toxicity

antihypertensives: Increased antihypertensive effect
diuretics: Increased diuretic effect
folic acid: Possibly antagonized action of folic acid
indomethacin: Increased risk of renal impairment
lithium: Increased risk of lithium toxicity
NSAIDs: Decreased diuretic effect of triamterene, increased risk of hyperkalemia
oral antidiabetic drugs: Altered blood glucose control

Adverse Reactions

CNS: Dizziness, fatigue, headache, weakness
EENT: Dry mouth
ENDO: Hyperglycemia, hypoglycemia
GI: Diarrhea, nausea, vomiting
GU: Azotemia, elevated BUN and serum creatinine levels, renal calculi
SKIN: Jaundice, photosensitivity, rash

Nursing Considerations

•Be aware that triamterene shouldn't be given to patient with creatinine clearance below 10 ml/min/1.73 m^2 because this condition increases the risk of drug-induced hyperkalemia.
•Monitor serum potassium level during therapy, especially in patient with renal impairment or diabetes mellitus. Also monitor BUN and serum creatinine levels to assess renal function and prevent hyperkalemia.
•Monitor for irregular heartbeat, usually the first sign of hyperkalemia.
•If you suspect hyperkalemia, obtain an ECG tracing, as ordered. A widened QRS complex or an arrhythmia requires prompt additional therapy.
•Monitor laboratory test results and assess for signs of metabolic or respiratory acidosis, which may occur suddenly in patient with cardiac disease or uncontrolled diabetes mellitus.
•Monitor patient's serum uric acid and sodium levels, as ordered, because drug may reduce uric acid clearance and increase the risk of gout and hyperuricemia. It also may worsen preexisting hyponatremia.
•Monitor CBC with differential because drug may increase the risk of megaloblastic anemia in patient with folic acid deficiency.

PATIENT TEACHING
•Advise patient to take triamterene with food or milk.

•Instruct patient to avoid exposure to excessive heat or sunlight to prevent dehydration and, possibly, photosensitivity.
•Explain to patient with a history of gout that drug may increase the risk of an attack.
•Advise patient to notify prescriber about ineffective diuresis and unexplained weight gain during therapy.

triazolam

Alti-Triazolam (CAN), Apo-Triazo (CAN), Gen Triazolam (CAN), Halcion, Novo-Triolam (CAN)

Class, Category, and Schedule

Chemical: Benzodiazepine
Therapeutic: Sedative-hypnotic
Pregnancy category: X
Controlled substance: Schedule IV

Indications and Dosages

➤ *To provide short-term management of insomnia*

TABLETS
Adults. 0.125 to 0.25 mg h.s. *Maximum:* 0.5 mg/day (for patients with inadequate response to usual dose).
DOSAGE ADJUSTMENT For elderly or debilitated patients, initial dosage reduced to 0.125 mg h.s. and maximum dosage limited to 0.25 mg/day.

Route	Onset	Peak	Duration
P.O.	15 to 30 min	Unknown	Unknown

Mechanism of Action

Potentiates the effects of the inhibitory neurotransmitter gamma-aminobutyric acid, which increases the inhibition of the ascending reticular activating system and produces varying levels of CNS depression, including sedation, hypnosis, skeletal muscle relaxation, anticonvulsant activity, and coma.

Contraindications

Hypersensitivity to triazolam or its components, ketoconazole or itraconazole therapy, pregnancy

Interactions

DRUGS
anxiolytics, barbiturates, brompheniramine, carbinoxamine, cetirizine, chlorpheniramine,

clemastine, cyproheptadine, dimenhydrinate, diphenhydramine, doxylamine, general anesthetics, methdilazine, opioid analgesics, sedative-hypnotics, phenothiazines, promethazine, tramadol, tricyclic antidepressants, trimeprazine: Increased sedation, respiratory depression
cimetidine, diltiazem, disulfiram, erythromycin, probenecid, verapamil: Increased sedation
fluconazole: Increased blood triazolam level and effects
flumazenil: Increased risk of withdrawal symptoms
itraconazole, ketoconazole: Delayed triazolam elimination
oral contraceptives: Increased blood triazolam level

FOODS
grapefruit juice: Increased blood triazolam level and sedation

ACTIVITIES
alcohol use: Increased sedation, respiratory depression

Adverse Reactions
CNS: Anxiety, ataxia, confusion, depression, dizziness, drowsiness, fatigue, headache, insomnia, nightmares, syncope, talkativeness, tremor, vertigo
Other: Physical and psychological dependence

Nursing Considerations
•Be aware that triazolam shouldn't be discontinued abruptly, even after only 1 to 2 weeks of therapy. Doing so can cause withdrawal symptoms, including abdominal cramps, confusion, depression, diaphoresis, hyperacusis, insomnia, irritability, nausea, nervousness, paresthesia, perceptual disturbances, photophobia, tachycardia, tremor, and vomiting.
•**WARNING** Assess patient for signs of physical and psychological dependence, and notify prescriber if they occur.
•Monitor respiratory rate and depth and ABG results, as appropriate, because drug may worsen ventilatory failure in patient with pulmonary disease, such as severe COPD, respiratory depression, or sleep apnea. Use drug cautiously in patients with acute intermittent porphyria, myasthenia gravis, and severe renal impairment because it may aggravate these conditions.
•Take safety precautions for elderly patients because drug may impair cognitive and motor function and increase the risk for falls.

•Use triazolam cautiously in patients with advanced Parkinson's disease because drug may worsen cognition, coordination, and psychosis.

PATIENT TEACHING
•Instruct patient to take triazolam exactly as prescribed and not to stop taking it abruptly because of the risk of withdrawal symptoms.
•Caution patient about possible drowsiness.
•Urge patient to avoid alcohol because it increases drug's sedative effects.
•Advise patient to notify prescriber about excessive drowsiness, known or suspected pregnancy, or nausea.

trifluoperazine hydrochloride

Apo-Trifluoperazine (CAN), PMS-Trifluoperazine (CAN), Stelazine, Stelazine Concentrate

Class and Category
Chemical: Piperazine phenothiazine
Therapeutic: Antianxiety, antipsychotic
Pregnancy category: Not rated

Indications and Dosages
➤ *To treat psychotic disorders*
SYRUP, TABLETS
Adults and adolescents. *Initial:* 2 to 5 mg b.i.d., increased gradually, as needed. *Maintenance:* 15 to 20 mg/day. *Maximum:* 40 mg/day.
Children age 6 and older. *Initial:* 1 mg q.d. or in divided doses b.i.d., increased gradually, as needed.
I.M. INJECTION
Adults and adolescents. 1 to 2 mg q 4 to 6 hr, as needed. *Maximum:* 10 mg/day.
Children age 6 and older. 1 mg q.d. or in divided doses b.i.d., as needed.
➤ *To relieve anxiety*
SYRUP, TABLETS, I.M. INJECTION
Adults and adolescents. *Initial:* 1 to 2 mg/day, increased gradually, as needed. *Maximum:* 6 mg/day for 12 wk.

Contraindications
Blood dyscrasias; bone marrow depression; cerebral arteriosclerosis; coma; coronary artery disease; hepatic dysfunction; hypersensitivity to trifluoperazine, other phenothiazines, or their components; myeloproliferative disorders; severe hypertension or hypotension; significant CNS depression; subcortical brain damage; use of high doses of CNS depressants

T

Mechanism of Action

Blocks postsynaptic dopamine receptors, increasing dopamine turnover and decreasing dopamine neurotransmission. This action may depress the areas of the brain that control activity and aggression, including the cerebral cortex, hypothalamus, and limbic system. Trifluoperazine may relieve anxiety by indirectly reducing arousal and increasing the filtering of internal stimuli to the reticular activating system.

Interactions

DRUGS

adsorbent antidiarrheals, aluminum- and magnesium-containing antacids: Possibly inhibited absorption of oral trifluoperazine
amantadine, anticholinergics, antidyskinetics, antihistamines: Possibly intensified adverse anticholinergic effects, increased risk of trifluoperazine-induced hyperpyrexia
amphetamines: Decreased stimulant effect of amphetamines, decreased antipsychotic effect of trifluoperazine
anticonvulsants: Lowered seizure threshold
antithyroid drugs: Increased risk of agranulocytosis
apomorphine: Possibly decreased emetic response to apomorphine, additive CNS depression
appetite suppressants: Decreased effects of appetite suppressants
astemizole, cisapride, disopyramide, erythromycin, pimozide, probucol, procainamide, quinidine: Prolonged QT interval, increased risk of ventricular tachycardia
beta blockers: Increased blood levels of both drugs, possibly leading to additive hypotensive effect, arrhythmias, irreversible retinopathy, and tardive dyskinesia
bromocriptine: Impaired therapeutic effects of bromocriptine
CNS depressants: Additive CNS depression
ephedrine, metaraminol: Decreased vasopressor response to ephedrine
epinephrine: Blocked alpha-adrenergic effects of epinephrine
extrapyramidal reaction–causing drugs (droperidol, haloperidol, metoclopramide, metyrosine, risperidone): Increased severity and frequency of extrapyramidal reactions
hepatotoxic drugs: Increased risk of hepatotoxicity

hypotension-producing drugs: Possibly severe hypotension with syncope
levodopa: Decreased antidyskinetic effect of levodopa
lithium: Reduced absorption of oral trifluoperazine, possibly encephalopathy and additive extrapyramidal effects
MAO inhibitors, maprotiline, tricyclic antidepressants: Possibly prolonged and intensified sedative and anticholinergic effects, increased blood level of antidepressants, impaired trifluoperazine metabolism, increased risk of neuroleptic malignant syndrome
mephentermine: Decreased antipsychotic effect of trifluoperazine and vasopressor effect of mephentermine
methoxamine, phenylephrine: Decreased vasopressor effect and shortened duration of action of these drugs
metrizamide: Increased risk of seizures
opioid analgesics: Increased risk of CNS and respiratory depression, orthostatic hypotension, severe constipation, and urine retention
ototoxic drugs: Possibly masking of some symptoms of ototoxicity, such as dizziness, tinnitus, and vertigo
phenytoin: Lowered seizure threshold; inhibited phenytoin metabolism, possibly leading to phenytoin toxicity
photosensitizing drugs: Possibly additive photosensitivity and intraocular photochemical damage to choroid, lens, or retina
thiazide diuretics: Possibly hyponatremia and water intoxication

ACTIVITIES

alcohol use: Increased CNS and respiratory depression, increased hypotensive effect

Adverse Reactions

CNS: Akathisia, altered temperature regulation, dizziness, drowsiness, extrapyramidal reactions (dystonia, pseudoparkinsonism, tardive dyskinesia)
CV: Hypotension, orthostatic hypotension, tachycardia
EENT: Blurred vision, dry mouth, nasal congestion, ocular changes (deposits of fine particles in cornea and lens), pigmentary retinopathy
ENDO: Galactorrhea, gynecomastia
GI: Constipation, epigastric pain, nausea, vomiting
GU: Ejaculation disorders, menstrual irregularities, urine retention

SKIN: Contact dermatitis, decreased sweating, photosensitivity, pruritus, rash
Other: Injection site irritation and sterile abscess, weight gain

Nursing Considerations
•Use trifluoperazine cautiously in patients with glaucoma because of drug's anticholinergic effect.
•Before administration, observe parenteral solution, which may turn slightly yellow without altering its potency. Don't use solution if discoloration is pronounced or precipitate is present.
•For I.M. administration, inject drug slowly and deep into upper outer quadrant of the buttocks. Keep patient in a supine position for 30 minutes after injection to minimize hypotensive effect.
•Rotate I.M. injection sites to avoid irritation and sterile abscesses.
•**WARNING** Monitor closely for tardive dyskinesia, which may continue after treatment stops. Signs include uncontrolled movements of arms, body, cheeks, jaw, legs, mouth, or tongue. Notify prescriber if such signs occur.
•Closely monitor elderly patients and severely ill or dehydrated children. They're at increased risk for certain adverse CNS reactions.
•To prevent contact dermatitis, avoid skin contact with oral or injection solution.

PATIENT TEACHING
•Instruct patient to take trifluoperazine exactly as prescribed and not to stop taking drug abruptly or without consulting prescriber.
•Advise patient to take drug with food or a full glass of milk or water to minimize adverse GI reactions.
•Urge patient to consult prescriber before using other drugs because of possible interactions.
•Instruct patient to notify prescriber immediately if she experiences difficulty swallowing or speaking and tongue protrusion.
•Caution patient to avoid alcohol during therapy.
•Advise patient to avoid potentially hazardous activities until drug's CNS effects are known.
•Instruct patient to change position slowly to minimize effects of orthostatic hypotension.
•Urge patient to avoid exposure to the sun and extreme heat because drug may cause photosensitivity and interfere with thermoregulation. Encourage her to wear sunscreen when outdoors.

triflupromazine
Vesprin

Class and Category
Chemical: Phenothiazine
Therapeutic: Antiemetic, antipsychotic
Pregnancy category: Not rated

Indications and Dosages
➤ *To treat psychotic disorders*
I.M. INJECTION
Adults and adolescents. 60 mg, as needed. *Maximum:* 150 mg/day.
Children age 30 months and older. 0.2 to 0.25 mg/kg, as needed. *Maximum:* 10 mg/day.
➤ *To treat nausea and vomiting*
I.V. INJECTION
Adults. 1 mg, p.r.n. *Maximum:* 3 mg/day.
I.M. INJECTION
Adults and adolescents. 5 to 15 mg q 4 hr. *Maximum:* 60 mg/day.
Children age 30 months and older. 0.2 to 0.25 mg/kg, p.r.n. *Maximum:* 10 mg/day.

Mechanism of Action
Blocks postsynaptic dopamine receptors, increasing dopamine turnover and decreasing dopamine neurotransmission. This action may depress the areas of the brain that control activity and aggression, including the cerebral cortex, hypothalamus, and limbic system. Triflupromazine also prevents nausea and vomiting by inhibiting or blocking dopamine receptors in the medullary chemoreceptor trigger zone and, peripherally, by blocking the vagus nerve in the GI tract.

Contraindications
Blood dyscrasias, bone marrow depression, cerebral arteriosclerosis, coma or severe CNS depression, concurrent use of large amount of CNS depressants, coronary artery disease, hepatic dysfunction, hypersensitivity to phenothiazines, severe hypertension or hypotension, subcortical brain damage

Interactions

DRUGS

amantadine, anticholinergics, antidyskinetics, antihistamines: Possibly intensified adverse anticholinergic effects, increased risk of triflupromazine-induced hyperpyrexia

amphetamines: Decreased stimulant effect of amphetamines, decreased antipsychotic effect of triflupromazine

anticonvulsants: Lowered seizure threshold

antithyroid drugs: Increased risk of agranulocytosis

apomorphine: Possibly decreased emetic response to apomorphine, additive CNS depression

appetite suppressants: Decreased anorectic effect of appetite suppressants

astemizole, cisapride, disopyramide, erythromycin, pimozide, probucol, procainamide, quinidine: Prolonged QT interval, increased risk of ventricular tachycardia

beta blockers: Increased blood levels of both drugs, possibly leading to additive hypotensive effect, arrhythmias, irreversible retinopathy, and tardive dyskinesia

bromocriptine: Impaired therapeutic effects of bromocriptine

CNS depressants: Additive CNS depression

ephedrine: Decreased vasopressor response to ephedrine

epinephrine: Blocked alpha-adrenergic effects of epinephrine

extrapyramidal reaction–causing drugs (droperidol, haloperidol, metoclopramide, metyrosine, risperidone): Increased severity and frequency of extrapyramidal reactions

hepatotoxic drugs: Increased risk of hepatotoxicity

hypotension-producing drugs: Possibly severe hypotension with syncope

levodopa: Decreased antidyskinetic effect of levodopa

lithium: Possibly encephalopathy and additive extrapyramidal effects

MAO inhibitors, maprotiline, tricyclic antidepressants: Increased CNS depression, impaired triflupromazine metabolism, increased risk of neuroleptic malignant syndrome

mephentermine: Possibly antagonized antipsychotic effect of triflupromazine and vasopressor effect of mephentermine

metaraminol: Decreased vasopressor effect of metaraminol

methoxamine, phenylephrine: Decreased vasopressor effect and shortened duration of action of these drugs

metrizamide: Increased risk of seizures

opioid analgesics: Increased risk of CNS and respiratory depression, orthostatic hypotension, severe constipation, and urine retention

ototoxic drugs: Possibly masking of symptoms of ototoxicity, such as dizziness, tinnitus, and vertigo

phenytoin: Lowered seizure threshold; inhibited phenytoin metabolism, possibly leading to phenytoin toxicity

photosensitizing drugs: Possibly additive photosensitivity and intraocular photochemical damage to choroid, lens, or retina

thiazide diuretics: Possibly hyponatremia and water intoxication

ACTIVITIES

alcohol use: Increased CNS and respiratory depression, increased hypotensive effect

Adverse Reactions

CNS: Akathisia, altered temperature regulation, dizziness, drowsiness, extrapyramidal reactions (dystonia, pseudoparkinsonism, tardive dyskinesia)

CV: Hypotension, orthostatic hypotension, tachycardia

EENT: Blurred vision, dry mouth, nasal congestion, ocular changes (deposits of fine particles in cornea and lens), pigmentary retinopathy

ENDO: Galactorrhea, gynecomastia

GI: Constipation, epigastric pain, nausea, vomiting

GU: Ejaculation disorders, menstrual irregularities, urine retention

SKIN: Decreased sweating, photosensitivity, pruritus, rash

Other: Injection site irritation and sterile abscess, weight gain

Nursing Considerations

• Use triflupromazine cautiously in patients with glaucoma because of drug's anticholinergic effects.

• Before administration, observe parenteral solution, which may turn slightly yellow without altering potency. Don't use solution if discoloration is pronounced or precipitate is present.

• Don't let solution come in contact with your skin because contact dermatitis may occur.

• For I.M. administration, slowly inject drug deep into upper outer quadrant of buttocks. Keep patient supine for 30 minutes afterward to minimize hypotensive effect.
• Rotate I.M. injection sites to avoid irritation and sterile abscesses.
• **WARNING** Monitor closely for tardive dyskinesia, which may continue after treatment stops. Signs include uncontrolled movements of arms, body, cheeks, jaw, legs, mouth, or tongue. Notify prescriber if all signs occur.
• Closely monitor elderly patients and severely ill or dehydrated children. They're at increased risk for certain adverse CNS reactions.

PATIENT TEACHING
• Instruct patient to change position slowly to minimize effects of orthostatic hypotension.
• Urge patient to avoid potentially hazardous activities until drug's CNS effects are known.
• Instruct patient to notify prescriber immediately if she experiences difficulty swallowing or speaking and tongue protrusion.
• Caution patient to avoid alcohol during therapy.
• Urge patient to avoid exposure to the sun and extreme heat because drug may cause photosensitivity and interfere with thermoregulation. Encourage her to wear sunscreen when outdoors.

trihexyphenidyl hydrochloride

Apo-Trihex (CAN), Artane, PMS Trihexyphenidyl (CAN), Trihexane, Trihexy

Class and Category
Chemical: Tertiary amine
Therapeutic: Antidyskinetic
Pregnancy category: C

Indications and Dosages
➤ *To treat parkinsonism*
ELIXIR, TABLETS
Adults. *Initial:* 1 to 2 mg on day 1, divided into 3 equal doses and given with meals. Total daily dose increased by 2 mg q 3 to 5 days until desired response or maximum dose is reached. *Maximum:* 15 mg/day.
E.R. CAPSULES
Adults. 5 mg after breakfast; additional 5 mg 12 hr later, if needed. *Maximum:* 15 mg/day.

➤ *To treat drug-induced extrapyramidal symptoms*
TABLETS
Adults. 1 mg/day, increased to 5 to 15 mg/day, as prescribed, to control symptoms.

Route	Onset	Peak	Duration
P.O.	1 hr	Unknown	6 to 12 hr

Mechanism of Action
Blocks acetylcholine's action at cholinergic receptor sites. This restores the brain's normal dopamine and acetylcholine balance, which relaxes muscle movement and decreases drooling, rigidity, and tremor. Trihexyphenidyl also may inhibit dopamine reuptake and storage, which prolongs dopamine's action.

Contraindications
Achalasia, bladder neck or prostatic obstruction, glaucoma, hypersensitivity to trihexyphenidyl or its components, megacolon, myasthenia gravis, pyloric or duodenal obstruction, stenosing peptic ulcer

Interactions
DRUGS
amantadine, anticholinergics, MAO inhibitors: Increased anticholinergic effects
antidiarrheals (adsorbent): Possibly decreased therapeutic effects of trihexyphenidyl
chlorpromazine: Decreased blood chlorpromazine level
CNS depressants: Increased sedative effect
levodopa: Increased efficacy of levodopa
ACTIVITIES
alcohol use: Increased sedation

Adverse Reactions
CNS: Confusion, drowsiness
EENT: Blurred vision; dry eyes, mouth, nose, or throat; mydriasis
GI: Constipation, nausea, vomiting
GU: Dysuria, urine retention
SKIN: Decreased sweating

Nursing Considerations
• Use trihexyphenidyl cautiously in patients with cardiovascular, hepatic, or renal disorders. Patients with cardiovascular disorders, such as atherosclerosis, hypertension, and ischemic heart disease, are at risk for tachycardia and coronary ischemia from drug's

positive chronotropic effects. Hepatic and renal dysfunction increase the risk of adverse reactions.

•Before therapy begins, assess patient's muscle rigidity and tremor to establish a baseline. During therapy, reassess patient to detect improvement in these signs and evaluate drug effectiveness.

PATIENT TEACHING

•Instruct patient to take trihexyphenidyl after meals.

•Teach patient not to break or chew E.R. capsules.

•Instruct patient to use calibrated device to measure elixir.

•Advise patient to avoid potentially hazardous activities until drug's CNS effects are known.

•Advise patient with dry eyes or increased contact lens awareness to use lubricating drops or stop wearing contact lenses during drug therapy.

trimethobenzamide hydrochloride

Benzacot, Tebamide, Tigan, Tribenzagan, Trimazide

Class and Category

Chemical: Ethanolamine derivative
Therapeutic: Antiemetic
Pregnancy category: Not rated

Indications and Dosages

➤ *To treat nausea and vomiting*

CAPSULES

Adults and adolescents. 250 mg q 6 to 8 hr, p.r.n.
Children weighing 15 to 45 kg (33 to 99 lb). 100 to 200 mg q 6 to 8 hr, p.r.n.

I.M. INJECTION

Adults and adolescents. 200 mg q 6 to 8 hr, p.r.n.

RECTAL SUPPOSITORIES

Adults and adolescents. 200 mg q 6 to 8 hr, p.r.n.
Children weighing 15 to 45 kg. 100 to 200 mg q 6 to 8 hr, p.r.n.
Children weighing less than 15 kg. 100 mg q 6 to 8 hr, p.r.n.

Contraindications

Children (I.M. injection); hypersensitivity to trimethobenzamide, benzocaine, or their components; infants and neonates (suppositories)

Mechanism of Action

Prevents or stops nausea and vomiting by blocking dopamine receptors and emetic impulses at the chemoreceptor trigger zone, the area in the brain that controls vomiting.

Interactions

DRUGS

apomorphine: Decreased emetic response to apomorphine, increased CNS effects
barbiturates, belladonna alkaloids, phenothiazines: Increased risk of coma, extrapyramidal reactions, opisthotonos, and seizures
CNS depressants: Possibly enhanced effects of both drugs
ototoxic drugs: Masked signs of ototoxicity

Adverse Reactions

CNS: Dizziness, drowsiness, headache
EENT: Blurred vision
GI: Diarrhea
MS: Muscle cramps
Other: Injection site burning, irritation, pain, redness, or swelling

Nursing Considerations

•Use trimethobenzamide cautiously in patients who are dehydrated and those with an electrolyte imbalance, encephalitis, encephalopathy, gastroenteritis, or high fever.

•Be aware that drug shouldn't be used in children who have viral illnesses because they're at increased risk for Reye's syndrome, characterized by abrupt onset of irrational behavior; lethargy; persistent, severe vomiting; progressive encephalopathy leading to coma; seizures; and, possibly, death.

•To minimize injection site irritation, inject trimethobenzamide deep into a large muscle mass, using the Z-track technique to block solution from escaping along the injection route.

•Moisten rectal suppository with water or water-soluble lubricant before insertion. If suppository is too soft, refrigerate it for 30 minutes or run cold water over it before removing the wrapper.

PATIENT TEACHING

•Teach patient how to insert a trimethobenzamide suppository, if necessary.

•Inform patient that drug may cause blurred vision, dizziness, and drowsiness. Advise her to avoid potentially hazardous activities until drug's CNS effects are known.

•Inform patient's parents that drug may cause Reye's syndrome, and urge them to notify prescriber immediately if they notice decreased level of consciousness, irrational behavior, lethargy, or severe vomiting.

trimethoprim

Proloprim, Trimpex

Class and Category

Chemical: Dihydrofolic acid analogue
Therapeutic: Antibiotic
Pregnancy category: C

Indications and Dosages

➤ *To treat UTIs caused by* Enterobacter *sp.,* Escherichia coli, Klebsiella pneumoniae, Proteus mirabilis, *and coagulase-negative staphylococci, including* Staphylococcus saprophyticus

TABLETS

Adults and children age 12 and older. 100 mg q 12 hr or 200 mg q.d. for 10 days.

DOSAGE ADJUSTMENT For patients with creatinine clearance of 15 to 30 ml/min/1.73 m², dosage usually reduced by 50%.

Mechanism of Action

Inhibits the formation of tetrahydrofolic acid, the metabolically active form of folic acid, in susceptible bacteria. This depletes the level of folate, an essential component of bacterial development, thereby interfering with production of bacterial nucleic acid and protein.

Contraindications

Hypersensitivity to trimethoprim or its components, megaloblastic anemia caused by folate deficiency, severe renal impairment (creatinine clearance of less than 15 ml/min/1.73 m²)

Interactions

DRUGS

bone marrow depressants: Increased risk of leukopenia, thrombocytopenia
cyclosporine: Increased risk of nephrotoxicity
dapsone: Increased blood levels and risk of adverse effects (especially methemoglobinemia) of both drugs
folate antagonists: Increased risk of megaloblastic anemia

phenytoin: Decreased phenytoin metabolism, increased risk of phenytoin toxicity
procainamide: Increased blood levels of procainamide and its metabolite, *N*-acetylprocainamide
rifampin: Increased elimination and decreased effectiveness of trimethoprim
warfarin: Increased anticoagulant activity of warfarin

Adverse Reactions

CNS: Fever, headache
EENT: Glossitis
GI: Abdominal pain, anorexia, diarrhea, elevated liver function test results, epigastric pain, nausea, vomiting
GU: Elevated BUN and serum creatinine levels
HEME: Leukopenia, megaloblastic anemia, methemoglobinemia, neutropenia, thrombocytopenia
SKIN: Exfoliative dermatitis, pruritus, rash

Nursing Considerations

•Obtain urine specimen, as ordered, before trimethoprim therapy starts.
•Give drug on an empty stomach to enhance absorption.
•Evaluate laboratory test values for folic acid deficiency and signs of bone marrow depression.

PATIENT TEACHING

•Instruct patient to complete entire course of trimethoprim therapy, as prescribed, even if she feels better beforehand.
•Advise patient to take drug with food or milk if GI distress occurs.
•Instruct patient to notify prescriber if she experiences rash, severe fatigue, sore throat, or unusual bleeding or bruising.

trimipramine maleate

Apo-Trimip (CAN), Novo-Tripramine (CAN), Rhotrimine (CAN), Surmontil

Class and Category

Chemical: Dibenzazepine derivative
Therapeutic: Antidepressant
Pregnancy category: C

Indications and Dosages

➤ *To treat depression*

CAPSULES

Adults in inpatient settings. *Initial:* 100 mg/day in divided doses, increased gradually in

a few days to 200 mg/day. *Maximum:* 300 mg/day in 2 to 3 wk.
Adolescents in inpatient settings. *Initial:* 50 mg/day in divided doses, increased as needed. *Maximum:* 100 mg/day.
Adults in outpatient settings. *Initial:* 75 mg/day in divided doses, increased gradually up to 150 mg/day, as needed. *Maintenance:* 50 to 150 mg/day. *Maximum:* 200 mg/day.
Adolescents in outpatient settings. *Initial:* 50 mg/day in divided doses, increased as needed. *Maximum:* 100 mg/day.
DOSAGE ADJUSTMENT For elderly patients, initial dosage reduced to 50 mg/day in divided doses, and maximum dosage limited to 100 mg/day.

Route	Onset	Peak	Duration
P.O.	2 to 3 wk	Unknown	Unknown

Mechanism of Action
Inhibits the reuptake of norepinephrine at presynaptic neurons, thus increasing its concentration in synapses. This action may elevate mood and relieve depression.

Contraindications
Hypersensitivity to trimipramine, other dibenzazepine tricyclic antidepressants, or their components; recovery period after an MI; use within 14 days of therapy with an MAO inhibitor or other tricyclic antidepressant

Interactions
DRUGS
amantadine, anticholinergics, antidyskinetics, antihistamines: Increased anticholinergic effects, especially confusion, hallucinations, and nightmares
anticonvulsants: Increased CNS depression, lowered seizure threshold (with high doses of trimipramine), decreased anticonvulsant effect
antithyroid drugs: Increased risk of agranulocytosis
barbiturates, carbamazepine: Decreased blood level and therapeutic effects of trimipramine
bupropion, clozapine, cyclobenzaprine, haloperidol, loxapine, maprotiline, molindone, phenothiazines, thioxanthenes: Intensified and prolonged sedative and anticholinergic effects of both drugs, increased risk of seizures

cimetidine: Decreased trimipramine metabolism, possibly leading to trimipramine toxicity
clonidine: Decreased hypotensive effect and increased CNS depressant effect of clonidine
CNS depressants: Increased hypotension and CNS and respiratory depression
disulfiram, etchlorvynol: Transient delirium, increased risk of CNS depression (with ethchlorvynol)
fluoxetine: Increased blood trimipramine level
guanadrel, guanethidine: Decreased hypotensive effect
MAO inhibitors: Increased risk of death, hyperpyrexia, hypertensive crisis, and severe seizures
methylphenidate: Decreased methylphenidate effects, increased blood trimipramine level
metrizamide: Increased risk of seizures
naphazoline (ophthalmic), oxymetazoline (nasal or ophthalmic), phenylephrine (nasal or ophthalmic), xylometazoline (nasal): Increased vasopressor effect of these drugs
oral anticoagulants: Increased anticoagulant activity
phenothiazines: Increased blood trimipramine level, decreased phenothiazine metabolism
pimozide, probucol: Increased risk of arrhythmias, possibly prolonged QT interval
sympathomimetics: Increased risk of arrhythmias, hyperpyrexia, and severe hypertension
thyroid hormones: Increased therapeutic and toxic effects of both drugs
ACTIVITIES
alcohol use: Increased hypotension and CNS and respiratory depression

Adverse Reactions
CNS: Anxiety, ataxia, confusion, CVA, delirium, dizziness, drowsiness, excitement, extrapyramidal reactions, hallucinations, headache, insomnia, nervousness, nightmares, parkinsonism, seizures, tremor
CV: Arrhythmias, orthostatic hypotension
EENT: Blurred vision, dry mouth, increased intraocular pressure, taste perversion, tinnitus, tongue swelling
ENDO: Gynecomastia, syndrome of inappropriate ADH secretion
GI: Constipation, diarrhea, heartburn, ileus, increased appetite, nausea, vomiting
GU: Sexual dysfunction, testicular swelling, urine retention

HEME: Agranulocytosis, bone marrow depression
RESP: Wheezing
SKIN: Alopecia, diaphoresis, jaundice, photosensitivity, pruritus, rash, urticaria
Other: Facial edema, weight gain

Nursing Considerations
•Expect to gradually reduce dosage, as prescribed, before electroconvulsive therapy.
PATIENT TEACHING
•Instruct patient to take the last dose of trimipramine early in the evening to avoid insomnia.
•Advise patient to avoid potentially hazardous activities until drug's CNS effects are known.
•Encourage patient to change position slowly to minimize effects of orthostatic hypotension.
•Urge patient to avoid alcohol during therapy.
•Advise patient to avoid excessive exposure to sunlight and to wear sunscreen when she's outdoors.
•Instruct patient to notify prescriber about unusual bruising and signs of infection.
•Suggest that patient use sugarless gum or hard candy to relieve dry mouth.

tromethamine

Tham

Class and Category
Chemical: Organic amine
Therapeutic: Alkalinizer
Pregnancy category: C

Indications and Dosages
➤ *To treat metabolic acidosis associated with cardiac arrest*
I.V. INFUSION
Adults and children. 3.6 to 10.8 g (111 to 333 ml) of 0.3 M solution.
I.V INJECTION
Adults and children. If chest is opened, 2 to 6 g injected directly into open ventricular cavity.
➤ *To treat metabolic acidosis during cardiac bypass surgery*
I.V. INFUSION
Adults and children. 9 ml (2.7 mEq or 0.32 g) of 0.3 M solution/kg as a single dose. *Usual:* 500 ml (150 mEq or 18 g) infused over 1 hr. *Maximum:* 500 mg/kg over 1 hr.

Mechanism of Action
Combines with hydrogen ions and their associated acid anions, including lactic, pyruvic, and carbonic acid, to form salts that are excreted in urine. Tromethamine exerts additional alkalinizing effects by acting as an osmotic diuretic, promoting the excretion of alkaline urine that contains increased amounts of carbon dioxide and electrolytes.

Contraindications
Anuria, chronic respiratory acidosis, hypersensitivity to tromethamine or its components, uremia

Interactions
DRUGS
amphetamines, quinidine, other pH-dependent drugs: Altered excretion of these drugs

Adverse Reactions
CNS: Fever
CV: Vasospasm
ENDO: Hypoglycemia
GI: Hepatic necrosis (hemorrhagic)
RESP: Respiratory depression
Other: Hypervolemia; infusion site infection, phlebitis, or venous thrombosis; metabolic alkalosis

Nursing Considerations
•Evaluate blood pH, blood glucose, and serum bicarbonate and electrolyte levels, and partial pressure of arterial carbon dioxide before, during, and after tromethamine therapy, as ordered.
•Be aware that, except in life-threatening situations, tromethamine therapy is limited to 1 day because of the risk of alkalosis.
•**WARNING** Be aware that exceeding the recommended dosage can cause alkalosis, respiratory depression, and reduced carbon dioxide level.
•Expect I.V. administration to increase the risk of hypervolemia and subsequent pulmonary edema.
•Assess infusion site frequently for signs of infiltration, which may cause inflammation, necrosis, thrombosis, tissue sloughing, and vasospasm.
•Be aware that patients with renal failure have an increased risk of developing hyperkalemia. For such patients, be prepared to monitor ECG continuously and assess serum potassium level frequently.

• Monitor blood glucose level frequently during and after therapy because rapid administration can cause hypoglycemia for several hours.

PATIENT TEACHING

• Inform family members that patient's vital signs and laboratory test results will be measured frequently to monitor her progress.

tubocurarine chloride

Class and Category

Chemical: Isoquinoline derivative
Therapeutic: Anticonvulsant
Pregnancy category: C

Indications and Dosages

➤ *To manage muscle contractions of seizures associated with electroshock therapy*

I.V. INJECTION

Adults. 157 mcg/kg (0.157 mg/kg) over 30 to 90 sec, given just before electroshock therapy. Expect initial dose to be 3 mg less than calculated total dose.

➤ *To produce skeletal muscle paralysis during anesthesia*

I.V. OR I.M. INJECTION

Adults. *Initial:* 6 to 9 mg. *Maintenance:* 3 to 4.5 mg in 3 to 5 min. if needed. For prolonged procedures, 3-mg supplemental doses given.

Infants and children. 500 mcg/kg I.V.

Neonates. *Initial:* 250 to 500 mcg/kg I.V. *Maintenance:* One-fifth to one-sixth of initial dose if needed.

➤ *To facilitate endotracheal intubation and aid controlled respiration during mechanical ventilation*

I.V. INJECTION

Adults. *Initial:* 16.5 mcg/kg. *Maintenance:* Dosage individualized based on patient response.

Mechanism of Action

Tubocurarine reduces the intensity of skeletal muscle contractions caused by electrically induced seizures. Normally, when a nerve impulse arrives at a somatic motor nerve terminal, it triggers acetylcholine (ACh) stored in synaptic vesicles to be released into the neuromuscular junction. The released ACh binds with nicotinic receptors embedded in the skeletal muscle motor endplate, as shown below left, triggering muscle cell depolarization and contraction.

Tubocurarine is a nondepolarizing neuromuscular blocker that acts as a competitive antagonist of ACh. By binding to the nicotinic receptors, as shown below right, it prevents transmission of the action potential at the neuromuscular junction, thereby sustaining skeletal muscle relaxation and eliminating the peripheral muscular manifestations of seizures. The drug has no effect on the CNS processes involved with seizures because it doesn't cross the blood-brain barrier.

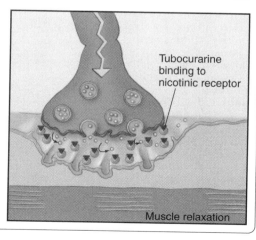

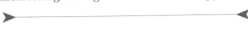

➤ *To aid in the diagnosis of myasthenia gravis*

I.V. INJECTION

Adults. 4 to 33 mcg/kg. After 2 to 3 min, 1.5 mg of neostigmine is given I.V. to terminate the test.

Route	Onset	Peak	Duration
I.V.	1 min	2 to 5 min	20 to 40 min

Incompatibilities

Don't mix tubocurarine with barbiturates, such as methohexital or thiopental, because a precipitate may form.

Contraindications

Hypersensitivity to tubocurarine or its components, patients in whom histamine release may be dangerous

Interactions

DRUGS

alfentanil, fentanyl, sufentanil: Prevented or reversed muscle rigidity caused by these drugs

aminoglycosides, anesthetics, capreomycin, citrate-anticoagulated blood, clindamycin, lidocaine (I.V.), lincomycin, polymyxins, procaine (I.V.), trimethaphan: Additive neuromuscular blocking effects

beta blockers, calcium salts: Prolonged and enhanced effects of tubocurarine

magnesium salts, procainamide, quinidine: Enhanced blockade effects

opioid analgesics: Additive histamine release effects, additive respiratory depressant effects, worsened bradycardia and hypotension

Adverse Reactions

CV: Arrhythmias, bradycardia, edema, hypotension, shock, tachycardia

RESP: Bronchospasm

SKIN: Erythema, flushing, itching, rash

Other: Anaphylaxis

Nursing Considerations

•If patient has a history of CV disease or is hypotensive, monitor her for further decrease in blood pressure.

•Monitor patient for bronchospasm and hypotension because tubocurarine may cause increased histamine release.

•Keep emergency equipment and drugs nearby in case respiratory depression occurs.

PATIENT TEACHING

•Explain the need for frequent hemodynamic monitoring during tubocurarine therapy.

➤ ◀

T

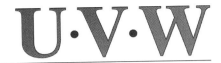

urea
(carbamide)

Ureaphil

Class and Category
Chemical: Carbonic acid diamide salt
Therapeutic: Antiglaucoma, diuretic
Pregnancy category: C

Indications and Dosages
➤ *To reduce cerebral edema and intracranial pressure*
I.V. INFUSION
Adults and children age 2 and older. 500 mg to 1.5 g/kg as 30% solution in D_5W, $D_{10}W$, or 10% invert sugar solution infused over 30 min to 2 hr at 4 or 6 ml/min, according to manufacturer's instructions. *Maximum:* 2 g/kg/day.
Children under age 2. 100 mg to 1.5 g/kg as 30% solution in D_5W, $D_{10}W$, or 10% invert sugar solution infused over 30 min to 2 hr at 4 or 6 ml/min, according to manufacturer's instructions.

➤ *To treat malignant or secondary glaucoma*
I.V. INFUSION
Adults. 500 mg to 1.5 g/kg as 30% solution in D_5W, $D_{10}W$, or 10% invert sugar solution infused over 30 min to 2 hr at 4 or 6 ml/min, according to manufacturer's instructions. *Maximum:* 2 g/kg/day.
DOSAGE ADJUSTMENT Dosage reduced or drug withheld for patients with renal impairment if BUN level rises to 75 mg/dl or more or if diuresis fails to occur within 2 hr after administration.

Route	Onset	Peak	Duration
I.V.	10 min	1 to 2 hr	3 to 10 hr*

Contraindications
Active intracranial bleeding, hepatic failure, hypersensitivity to urea or its components, renal impairment, severe dehydration

_____

* For diuresis; 5 to 6 hr for reduced intraocular pressure.

Mechanism of Action
Elevates blood plasma osmolality, creating an osmotic effect that increases the movement of water from the brain, CSF, and anterior portion of the eyes into interstitial fluid and plasma. This action reduces cerebral edema, intracranial pressure, CSF volume, and intraocular pressure. Large doses inhibit the reabsorption of water and solutes in the renal tubules and induce diuresis by affecting the osmotic pressure gradient of the glomerular filtrate.

Interactions
DRUGS
carbonic anhydrase inhibitors, other diuretics: Additive diuretic and intraocular pressure–reducing effects
lithium: Increased renal excretion of lithium

Adverse Reactions
CNS: Agitation, confusion, fever, headache, hyperthermia, nervousness, subarachnoid hemorrhage, subdural hematoma, syncope
CV: Tachycardia
EENT: Dry mouth, intraocular hemorrhage
GI: Nausea, thirst, vomiting
GU: Elevated BUN level
HEME: Hemolysis
SKIN: Blemishes, extravasation with tissue necrosis and sloughing
Other: Dehydration, hypokalemia, hyponatremia, infusion site phlebitis or thrombosis

Nursing Considerations
•To obtain maximum reduction of intracranial or intraocular pressure, expect to give urea 60 minutes before ocular or intracranial surgery.
•Don't mix urea with invert sugar solution if patient has fructose intolerance from aldolase deficiency.
•Avoid infusing drug into leg veins to reduce risk of phlebitis and thrombosis.
•Discard unused portion of drug after 24 hours.
•Be aware that rapid administration may cause hemolysis, increased capillary bleeding, and, in patients with glaucoma, intraocular hemorrhage.
•Maintain adequate hydration to minimize adverse reactions. Assess for signs of dehydration, including dry mucous membranes or tenting.

•Monitor BUN and serum electrolyte levels as well as fluid intake and output during urea therapy because prolonged use can cause diuresis.

PATIENT TEACHING

•Instruct patient to notify prescriber immediately about difficulty breathing or shortness of breath because drug can cause transient increases in circulatory volume, leading to circulatory overload, exacerbations of heart failure, or pulmonary edema.

•Advise patient to expect increased urine output.

•Encourage patient to remain on bed rest during therapy.

urokinase

Abbokinase, Abbokinase Open-Cath

Class and Category

Chemical: Renal enzymatic protein
Therapeutic: Thrombolytic
Pregnancy category: B

Indications and Dosages

➤ *To treat acute coronary artery thrombosis*

INTRACORONARY INFUSION

Adults. 6,000 IU/min until artery is maximally opened (up to 2 hr may be required). *Usual:* 500,000 IU.

➤ *To treat acute pulmonary thromboembolism*

I.V. INFUSION

Adults. *Initial:* 4,400 IU/kg over 10 min, followed by 4,400 IU/kg/hr for about 12 hr.

➤ *To clear I.V. catheter occlusion*

INSTILLATION

Adults and children. 5,000 IU/ml instilled into occluded line.

Route	Onset	Peak	Duration
I.V.	Unknown	20 min to 2 hr	4 hr
Intracoronary	Unknown	Unknown	4 hr

Incompatibilities

Don't administer I.V. urokinase through the same I.V. line as other drugs or add other drugs to urokinase solution.

Mechanism of Action

Indirectly promotes conversion of plasminogen to plasmin, an enzyme that breaks down fibrin clots, fibrinogen, and other plasma proteins, including procoagulant factors V and VIII.

Contraindications

Arteriovenous malformation, bleeding disorder, CVA during previous 2 months, hypersensitivity to urokinase or its components, internal bleeding, intracranial aneurysm, intracranial or intraspinal surgery during previous 2 months, intracranial tumor, recent cardiopulmonary resuscitation, recent trauma, severe uncontrolled hypertension (systolic blood pressure of 200 mm Hg or higher, or diastolic blood pressure of 110 mm Hg or higher)

Interactions

DRUGS

antifibrinolytics (aminocaproic acid, aprotinin): Mutual antagonism
antihypertensives: Increased risk of severe hypotension
cefamandole, cefoperazone, cefotetan, plicamycin, valproic acid: Increased risk of hypoprothrombinemia and severe hemorrhage
corticosteroids, ethacrynic acid, salicylates (nonacetylated): Increased risk of GI ulceration and bleeding
enoxaparin, heparin, NSAIDs, oral anticoagulants, platelet-aggregation inhibitors: Increased risk of hemorrhage
thiotepa: Increased therapeutic effects of thiotepa

Adverse Reactions

CNS: Chills, CVA, fever, headache
CV: Arrhythmias, including tachycardia; chest pain; hypertension; hypotension
GI: Nausea, vomiting
HEME: Unusual bleeding
MS: Back pain, myalgia
RESP: Dyspnea, hypoxemia, wheezing
SKIN: Cyanosis, ecchymosis, flushing, pruritus, rash, urticaria
Other: Anaphylaxis, metabolic acidosis

Nursing Considerations

•To prevent foaming, don't shake urokinase when reconstituting. Consult with pharmacist about giving drug through 0.45-micron or smaller cellulose membrane filter.

• Assess baseline hematocrit, platelet count, thrombin time, APTT, PT, and INR as ordered.
• Monitor heart rate and rhythm by continuous ECG during therapy, especially during rapid lysis of coronary thrombi, because arrhythmias can occur with reperfusion.
• Monitor blood pressure for hypotension. If hypotension occurs, notify prescriber and expect to reduce infusion rate.
• Check for bleeding at puncture sites and in urine and stool. Check for intracranial bleeding by performing frequent neurologic assessments.
• After arterial puncture is performed, apply pressure for at least 30 minutes and then apply pressure dressing. Check frequently for bleeding during therapy.
• To prevent bleeding and associated complications, avoid venipunctures; use an external blood pressure cuff to measure blood pressure; give acetaminophen (not aspirin), as prescribed, for fever; and handle patient as little as possible.
• **WARNING** If serious bleeding begins and can't be controlled with local pressure, stop the infusion immediately and notify prescriber.

PATIENT TEACHING
• Instruct patient to remain on bed rest during urokinase therapy.
• Inform patient that minor bleeding may occur at wounds or puncture sites.

ursodiol

(ursodeoxycholic acid)

Actigall, Ursofalk (CAN)

Class and Category
Chemical: Naturally occurring bile acid
Therapeutic: Cholelitholytic
Pregnancy category: B

Indications and Dosages
➤ *To prevent gallstone formation in obese patients during rapid weight loss*
CAPSULES
Adults and adolescents. 300 mg b.i.d. Alternatively, 8 to 10 mg/kg/day in divided doses b.i.d or t.i.d.
➤ *To dissolve gallstones*
CAPSULES
Adults and adolescents. 8 to 10 mg/kg/day in divided doses b.i.d. or t.i.d.

Mechanism of Action
Suppresses hepatic synthesis, biliary secretion, and intestinal reabsorption of cholesterol. Prolonged use promotes dissolution of gallstones.

Contraindications
Acute cholangiitis; gallstone complications (such as biliary GI fistula; biliary obstruction; calcified, radiopaque, or radiotranslucent bile-pigment gallstones; cholecystitis; pancreatitis); hypersensitivity to ursodiol, other bile acids, or their components

Interactions
DRUGS
aluminum-containing antacids, cholestyramine, colestipol: Decreased absorption and therapeutic effects of ursodiol
clofibrate, estrogens, neomycin, oral contraceptives, progestins: Interference with ursodiol's therapeutic effects
FOODS
any foods: Increased dissolution of drug

Adverse Reactions
CNS: Anxiety, depression, fatigue, headache, sleep disturbance
EENT: Metallic taste, rhinitis, stomatitis
GI: Abdominal pain, cholecystitis, constipation, diarrhea, flatulence, indigestion, nausea, vomiting
MS: Arthralgia, back pain, myalgia
RESP: Cough
SKIN: Alopecia, diaphoresis, dry skin, pruritus, rash, urticaria

Nursing Considerations
• Administer ursodiol with food to increase drug dissolution.
• Administer aluminum-containing antacids, cholestyramine, and colestipol at least 1 hour before or 4 hours after ursodiol because they may decrease drug's effects.
• Expect drug to be discontinued if gallstones haven't partially dissolved after 12 months of therapy.
PATIENT TEACHING
• Instruct patient to take ursodiol with meals.
• Advise patient to take aluminum-containing antacids at least 1 hour before or 4 hours after ursodiol to avoid impaired absorption.
• Urge patient to notify prescriber immediately if signs of acute cholecystitis develop, such as acute right-upper-quadrant abdominal pain.

•Inform patient that he may need to take ursodiol for a prolonged period before gallstones dissolve.

valdecoxib

Bextra

Class and Category
Chemical: Benzenesulfonamide
Therapeutic: Antidysmenorrheal, antirheumatic
Pregnancy category: C

Indications and Dosages
➤ *To relieve signs and symptoms of osteoarthritis and adult rheumatoid arthritis*
TABLETS
Adults. 10 mg q.d.
➤ *To treat pain and other symptoms of primary dysmenorrhea*
TABLETS
Adults. 20 mg b.i.d. as needed.

Mechanism of Action
Inhibits the enzymatic activity of cyclooxygenase-2 (COX-2), the enzyme needed to convert arachidonic acid to prostaglandins. Prostaglandins are responsible for mediating the inflammatory response and causing local vasodilation, swelling, and pain. They also play a role in peripheral pain transmission to the spinal cord. By inhibiting COX-2 activity and prostaglandin production, this NSAID reduces inflammatory symptoms and relieves pain.

Contraindications
Allergic reaction (such as anaphylaxis or angioedema) to aspirin or other NSAIDs, hypersensitivity to valdecoxib or its components

Interactions
DRUGS
ACE inhibitors: Possibly decreased antihypertensive effect of these drugs
aspirin: Increased risk of GI ulceration and other GI complications
dextromethorphan, lithium: Possibly elevated blood levels of these drugs
fluconazole, ketoconazole: Increased blood valdecoxib level

furosemide, thiazide diuretics: Decreased diuretic effect of these drugs
warfarin: Possibly increased INR and risk of bleeding
ACTIVITIES
alcohol and tobacco use: Increased risk of GI bleeding

Adverse Reactions
CNS: Dizziness, headache, neuralgia, paresthesia, tremor, vertigo
CV: Angina, arrhythmias, heart failure, hypertension, peripheral edema
EENT: Sinusitis, taste perversion
GI: Abdominal distention or pain, constipation, diarrhea, dry mouth, duodenal or gastric ulcer, elevated liver function test results, flatulence, gastritis, GI bleeding, hematemesis, hematochezia, indigestion, melena, nausea
GU: Amenorrhea, dysmenorrhea, increased BUN and serum, creatinine levels, menorrhagia, menstrual bloating, vaginal hemorrhage
HEME: Anemia, thrombocytopenia
MS: Back pain, fractures, myalgia
RESP: Upper respiratory tract infection
SKIN: Ecchymosis, rash
Other: Flulike symptoms

Nursing Considerations
•Expect to rehydrate dehydrated patients before administering valdecoxib to decrease the risk of adverse renal reactions.
•**WARNING** Be aware that serious GI tract ulceration and bleeding can occur without warning or symptoms. Assess patient frequently, especially if she has a history of GI bleeding or ulcers. Administer valdecoxib with food to minimize the risk of these complications.
•Monitor liver function test results because in rare cases elevations may progress to severe hepatic reactions, including fatal hepatitis, hepatic necrosis, and hepatic failure.
•Monitor intake and output, especially in patients with edema, heart failure, or hypertension, because drug may cause fluid retention.
•Monitor BUN and serum creatinine levels in patients with heart failure or a history of impaired renal function because drug may cause renal failure.
•Monitor hemoglobin level and hematocrit, especially in patients on long-term valdecoxib therapy who exhibit signs or symptoms of anemia, such as pale skin or tiredness.

•Be aware that drug may mask fever and inflammation from other medical conditions.

PATIENT TEACHING
•Advise patient to notify prescriber if pain continues or is poorly controlled with valdecoxib.
•Urge patient to avoid smoking and alcohol use during valdecoxib therapy because these activities may increase the risk of adverse GI reactions.
•Instruct patient to notify prescriber immediately if she experiences a rash, shortness of breath, difficulty breathing, or black and tarry stools or if she vomits coffee-ground material.
•Advise patient to report weight gain or swelling of extremities, which may indicate fluid retention, or signs of hepatotoxicity, such as tiredness, nausea, yellow skin, or flu-like symptoms.

valproic acid

Alti-Valproic (CAN), Depakene, Deproic (CAN), Dom-Proic (CAN), Med-Valproic (CAN), Novo-Valproic (CAN), Nu-Valproic (CAN), PMS-Valproic Acid (CAN)

valproate sodium

Depacon

divalproex sodium

Depakote, Depakote Sprinkle, Epival (CAN)

Class and Category

Chemical: Carboxylic acid derivative
Therapeutic: Anticonvulsant
Pregnancy category: D

Indications and Dosages

➤ *To treat simple or complex absence seizures, complex partial seizures, myoclonic seizures, and generalized tonic-clonic seizures as monotherapy*

CAPSULES, DELAYED-RELEASE SPRINKLE CAPSULES, DELAYED-RELEASE TABLETS, SYRUP, I.V. INFUSION (VALPROIC ACID, VALPROATE SODIUM, DIVALPROEX SODIUM)

Adults and adolescents. *Initial:* 10 to 15 mg/kg/day in divided doses b.i.d. or t.i.d., increased by 5 to 10 mg/kg/day q wk, as needed and as prescribed. *Maximum:* 60 mg/kg/day.
Children. *Initial:* 15 to 45 mg/kg/day in divided doses b.i.d. or t.i.d., increased by 5 to

10 mg/kg/day q wk, as needed and as prescribed.

➤ *As adjunct to treat simple or complex absence seizures, complex partial seizures, myoclonic seizures, and generalized tonic-clonic seizures*

CAPSULES, DELAYED-RELEASE SPRINKLE CAPSULES, DELAYED-RELEASE TABLETS, SYRUP, I.V. INFUSION (VALPROIC ACID, VALPROATE SODIUM, DIVALPROEX SODIUM)

Adults and adolescents. 10 to 30 mg/kg/day in divided doses, increased by 5 to 10 mg/kg/day q wk, as needed and as prescribed.
Children. 30 to 100 mg/kg/day in divided doses, as prescribed.

➤ *To treat acute manic phase of bipolar disorder*

DELAYED-RELEASE TABLETS (DIVALPROEX SODIUM)

Adults. *Initial:* 750 mg/day in divided doses. *Maximum:* 60 mg/kg/day.

➤ *To prevent migraine headache*

DELAYED–RELEASE TABLETS, TABLETS (DIVALPROEX SODIUM)

Adults. 250 mg q 12 hr, increased p.r.n. *Maximum:* 1 g/day.

Mechanism of Action

May decrease seizure activity by blocking the reuptake of gamma-aminobutyric acid (GABA), the most common inhibitory neurotransmitter in the brain. GABA is known to suppress the rapid firing of neurons by inhibiting voltage-sensitive sodium channels.

Contraindications

Hepatic dysfunction; hypersensitivity to valproic acid, valproate sodium, divalproex sodium, or their components; urea cycle disorders

Interactions

DRUGS
aspirin, heparin, NSAIDs, oral anticoagulants, thrombolytics: Increased inhibition of platelet aggregation and risk of bleeding
barbiturates, primidone: Increased blood levels of both drugs, additive CNS effects
carbamazepine: Possibly decreased valproic acid effectiveness
cholestyramine: Decreased bioavailability of valproic acid
clonazepam: Increased risk of absence seizures
CNS depressants: Increased CNS depression

diazepam: Inhibited diazepam metabolism
ethosuximide: Unpredictable blood ethosuximide level
felbamate: Impaired valproic acid metabolism and increased blood drug level
haloperidol, loxapine, MAO inhibitors, maprotiline, phenothiazines, thioxanthenes, tricyclic antidepressants: Increased CNS depression, lowered seizure threshold
lamotrigine: Decreased lamotrigine clearance
mefloquine: Decreased blood levels of valproic acid, divalproex, and valproate sodium; increased risk of seizures
phenytoin: Increased risk of phenytoin toxicity, loss of seizure control

ACTIVITIES
alcohol use: Additive CNS depression

Adverse Reactions
CNS: Agitation, ataxia, confusion, depression, dizziness, drowsiness, euphoria, hallucinations, headache, hyperesthesia, lack of coordination, lethargy, loss of seizure control, paresthesia, psychosis, sedation, tremor, vertigo, weakness
EENT: Diplopia, nystagmus, pharyngitis, spots before eyes
ENDO: Galactorrhea, hyperglycemia
GI: Abdominal pain, anorexia, constipation, diarrhea, elevated liver function test results, hepatotoxicity, increased appetite, indigestion, nausea, pancreatitis, vomiting
GU: Menstrual irregularities
HEME: Eosinophilia, hematoma, leukopenia, prolonged bleeding time, thrombocytopenia
MS: Dysarthria
SKIN: Alopecia, diaphoresis, erythema multiforme, jaundice, petechiae, photosensitivity, pruritus, rash, Stevens-Johnson syndrome
Other: Facial edema, hyperammonemia, injection site pain, weight gain or loss

Nursing Considerations
•Give oral valproic acid or divalproex with food to minimize GI irritation, if necessary.
•Administer drug at least 2 hours before or 6 hours after cholestyramine.
•Don't mix syrup with carbonated beverages; doing so may produce an unpleasant-tasting mixture and irritate the mouth and throat.
•Don't break or allow patient to chew delayed-release tablets.
•As needed, sprinkle contents of delayed-release sprinkle capsules on small amount of semisolid food just before administration. Instruct patient not to chew contents of delayed-release sprinkle capsules.
•For I.V. administration, dilute prescribed dose with at least 50 ml of compatible diluent and infuse over 60 minutes.
•Be aware that patient should be switched from I.V. to P.O. form of valproic acid as soon as possible.
•Be aware that patient with hypoalbuminemia or another protein-binding deficiency is at increased risk for valproic acid toxicity.
•Assess for signs and symptoms of decreased hepatic function, including anorexia, facial edema, jaundice, lethargy, loss of seizure control, malaise, vomiting, and weakness.
•Monitor liver function test results, as ordered. Assess for signs and symptoms of hepatotoxicity during first 6 months of treatment, especially in children under age 2. Notify prescriber immediately if you suspect hepatotoxicity.
•Monitor platelet count, as ordered, for signs of thrombocytopenia, and notify prescriber if they appear.
•Be aware that hyperammonemia may occur even if patient's liver function test results are normal. Monitor ammonia levels, as ordered. If patient develops unexplained lethargy, vomiting, or changes in mental status with an increase in ammonia level or if asymptomatic ammonia elevations are detected and persist, expect valproic acid to be discontinued.

PATIENT TEACHING
•Instruct patient to swallow capsules whole to prevent irritation to mouth and throat. However, delayed-release sprinkle capsules may be opened and contents mixed with food for easier swallowing. Instruct patient not to chew contents of delayed-release sprinkle capsules.
•Advise patient to avoid potentially hazardous activities during therapy because drug may affect mental and motor performance.
•Caution patient to avoid alcohol during therapy.
•Urge female patient to notify prescriber immediately about suspected or known pregnancy.
•Advise patient to notify prescriber if tremor develops during therapy; occurence of tremor may be dose-related.

valsartan

Diovan

Class and Category

Chemical: Nonpeptide tetrazole derivative
Therapeutic: Antihypertensive
Pregnancy category: C (first trimester), D (later trimesters)

Indications and Dosages

➤ *To manage hypertension, alone or with other antihypertensives*

CAPSULES

Adults. *Initial:* 80 or 160 mg q.d., increased as needed and prescribed. *Maximum:* 320 mg/day.

➤ *To treat class II to IV heart failure in patients who are intolerant of ACE inhibitors*

CAPSULES

Adults. *Initial:* 40 mg b.i.d., increased to 80 mg b.i.d. and then 160 mg b.i.d., as needed and prescribed. *Maximum:* 320 mg/day.

Route	Onset	Peak	Duration
P.O.	2 hr	6 hr	24 hr

Mechanism of Action

Blocks the hormone angiotensin II from binding to the receptor sites in vascular smooth muscle, adrenal glands, and other tissues. This action inhibits angiotensin II's vasoconstrictive and aldosterone-secreting effects, thereby reducing blood pressure.

Contraindications

Hypersensitivity to valsartan or its components

Interactions

DRUGS

antihypertensives, diuretics: Additive hypotensive effect
potassium salts, potassium-sparing diuretics: Possibly hyperkalemia

FOODS

potassium-containing salt substitutes: Possibly hyperkalemia

Adverse Reactions

CNS: Dizziness, fatigue, headache, insomnia
CV: Edema
EENT: Pharyngitis, rhinitis, sinusitis
GI: Abdominal pain, diarrhea, indigestion, nausea, vomiting
MS: Arthralgia
RESP: Cough, upper respiratory tract infection
Other: Hyperkalemia, viral infection

Nursing Considerations

•Be aware that valsartan shouldn't be given to patients who have hypovolemia or are taking a diuretic because of the increased risk of severe hypotension from volume depletion.
•Use valsartan cautiously during second and third trimesters of pregnancy because of the risk of serious adverse effects on fetus.
•Monitor blood pressure frequently during therapy.
•Be aware that maximal blood pressure reduction typically occurs after 4 weeks.
•Monitor serum potassium level because drug may elevate potassium level by blocking aldosterone secretion.

PATIENT TEACHING

•Instruct patient to take valsartan exactly as prescribed at the same time each day to maintain therapeutic effect.
•Advise patient to avoid potentially hazardous activities until drug's CNS effects are known.
•Advise patient to avoid using potassium-containing salt substitutes without consulting prescriber.
•Instruct female patient of childbearing age to use reliable birth control during therapy and to notify prescriber immediately about known or suspected pregnancy.
•Urge patient to keep follow-up appointments with prescriber to monitor progress.

vancomycin hydrochloride

Vancocin

Class and Category

Chemical: Tricyclic glycopeptide derivative
Therapeutic: Antibiotic
Pregnancy category: B (oral), C (parenteral)

Indications and Dosages

➤ *To treat pseudomembranous colitis caused by* Clostridium difficile *and enterocolitis caused by staphylococci*

CAPSULES, ORAL SOLUTION

Adults and adolescents. 125 to 500 mg q 6 hr for 7 to 10 days. *Maximum:* 2 g/day.

Children. 10 mg/kg (up to 125 mg) q 6 hr for 7 to 10 days. *Maximum:* 2 g/day.
➤ *To treat bacterial endocarditis caused by methicillin-resistant* Staphylococcus aureus
I.V. INFUSION
Adults. 30 mg/kg/day in equally divided doses b.i.d. for 4 to 6 wk. *Maximum:* 2 g/day.
➤ *As adjunct to treat bacterial endocarditis caused by methicillin-resistant* S. aureus *in patients with prosthetic heart valve*
I.V. INFUSION
Adults. 30 mg/kg/day in equally divided doses b.i.d. to q.i.d. for 6 wk or longer in conjunction with rifampin and gentamicin. *Maximum:* 2 g/day.
➤ *To treat bacterial endocarditis caused by* Streptococcus bovis *or* Streptococcus viridans
I.V. INFUSION
Adults. 30 mg/kg/day in equally divided doses b.i.d. for 4 wk. *Maximum:* 2 g/day.
➤ *As adjunct to treat bacterial endocarditis caused by enterococci*
I.V. INFUSION
Adults. 30 mg/kg/day in equally divided doses b.i.d. for 4 to 6 wk in conjunction with gentamicin. *Maximum:* 2 g/day.
➤ *To treat bacterial septicemia, bone and joint infections, pneumonia, and skin and soft-tissue infections caused by* Staphylococcus, *including methicillin-resistant strains, and life-threatening infections*
I.V. INFUSION
Adults and children age 12 and older. 500 mg q 6 hr or 1 g q 12 hr infused over at least 60 min. *Maximum:* 4 g/day.
Children ages 1 month to 12 years. 10 mg/kg q 6 hr or 20 mg/kg q 12 hr infused over at least 60 min.
Neonates ages 1 week to 1 month. *Initial:* 15 mg/kg followed by 10 mg/kg q 8 hr infused over at least 60 min.
Neonates under age 1 week. *Initial:* 15 mg/kg followed by 10 mg/kg q 12 hr infused over at least 60 min.

Mechanism of Action
Inhibits bacterial RNA and cell wall synthesis; alters permeability of bacterial membranes, causing cell wall lysis and cell death.

Incompatibilities
Don't administer I.V. vancomycin through the same I.V. line as other drugs. Don't add vancomycin to albumin-containing solutions, alkaline solutions, aminophylline, amobarbital sodium, aztreonam, cefepime, ceftazidime, chloramphenicol sodium succinate, chlorothiazide sodium, dexamethasone sodium phosphate, foscarnet sodium, heparin sodium, methicillin sodium, penicillin G, pentobarbital sodium, phenobarbital sodium, piperacillin sodium and tazobactam sodium, secobarbital sodium, and sodium bicarbonate. Drug may form precipitate with heavy metals.

Contraindications
Hypersensitivity to vancomycin or its components

Interactions
DRUGS
aminoglycosides (amikacin, gentamicin, tobramycin), amphotericin B, bacitracin (parenteral), bumetanide, capreomycin, carmustine, cidofovir, cisplatin, cyclosporine, ethacrynic acid, furosemide, paromomycin, pentamidine (parenteral), polymyxins, salicylates (parenteral), streptozocin: Additive nephrotoxicity or ototoxicity
antihistamines, buclizine, cyclizine, meclizine, phenothiazines, thioxanthenes, trimethobenzamide: Masked symptoms of ototoxicity
cholestyramine, colestipol: Decreased antibacterial activity of oral vancomycin
dexamethasone: Decreased penetration of vancomycin into CSF
nephrotoxic drugs: Increased risk of nephrotoxicity

Adverse Reactions
CNS: Chills, dizziness, vertigo
CV: Hypotension
EENT: Ototoxicity
GI: Nausea
GU: Nephrotoxicity
HEME: Eosinophilia, neutropenia
RESP: Dyspnea, wheezing
SKIN: Exfoliative dermatitis; extravasation with pain, tenderness, thrombophlebitis, and tissue necrosis; pruritus; rash; toxic epidermal necrolysis; urticaria
Other: Anaphylaxis, drug-induced fever, injection site inflammation, superinfection

Nursing Considerations

•To reconstitute 500-mg vial of vancomycin for I.V. use, add 10 ml of sterile water for injection; further dilute with at least 100 ml of compatible I.V. solution. For 1-g vial of dry, sterile powder, add 20 ml of sterile water for injection; further dilute with at least 200 ml of compatible I.V. solution.

•**WARNING** Infuse over at least 1 hour. Rapid administration may cause hypotension or transient "red man syndrome," characterized by chills; fainting; fever; flushing of face, neck, upper arms, and torso; hypotension; nausea; tachycardia; and vomiting.

•Monitor blood vancomycin levels, as ordered; be aware that therapeutic levels are 10 to 15 mcg/ml trough and 30 to 40 mcg/ml peak.

•Monitor CBC results and serum creatinine and BUN levels during therapy.

•Monitor I.V. infusion site for signs and symptoms of extravasation, including necrosis, pain, tenderness, and thrombophlebitis. If extravasation occurs, discontinue infusion immediately and notify prescriber.

•Monitor hearing during therapy. Transient or permanent ototoxicity may occur if patient receives an excessive amount of drug, has an underlying hearing loss, or receives concurrent aminoglycosides.

•Monitor patient receiving prolonged therapy for signs of superinfection, such as severe diarrhea and white patches on tongue.

PATIENT TEACHING

•Instruct patient to use calibrated device to measure doses of oral solution.

•Advise patient to notify prescriber if no improvement occurs after a few days.

•Instruct patient to complete full course of vancomycin, as prescribed.

•Caution patient to consult prescriber before taking any drug to control diarrhea because that condition may signal superinfection.

•Instruct patient to keep follow-up appointments to monitor progress during and after treatment.

vasopressin

(antidiuretic hormone [ADH])

Pitressin, Pressyn (CAN)

Class and Category

Chemical: Polypeptide hormone
Therapeutic: Antidiuretic
Pregnancy category: C

Indications and Dosages

➤ *To prevent or control symptoms of central diabetes insipidus caused by insufficient ADH*

I.M. OR S.C. INJECTION

Adults. 5 to 10 U b.i.d. or t.i.d., as needed.
Children. 2.5 to 10 U t.i.d. or q.i.d., as needed.

➤ *To prevent or treat abdominal distention*

I.M. INJECTION

Adults. 5 U, increased to 10 U q 3 to 4 hr, as needed.

Route	Onset	Peak	Duration
I.M., S.C.	Unknown	Unknown	2 to 8 hr

Contraindications

Chronic nephritis with nitrogen retention, hypersensitivity to vasopressin or its components

Interactions

DRUGS

carbamazepine, chlorpropamide, clofibrate, fludrocortisone, tricyclic antidepressants: Increased antidiuretic effect
demeclocycline, lithium, norepinephrine: Decreased antidiuretic effect

Adverse Reactions

CNS: Dizziness, headache, light-headedness, tremor
CV: Angina, MI
EENT: Circumoral pallor
ENDO: Water intoxication
GI: Abdominal cramps, diarrhea, eructation, flatulence, intestinal hypermotility, nausea, vomiting
SKIN: Diaphoresis, pallor
Other: Allergic reaction

Nursing Considerations

•Use vasopressin with extreme caution in patients with coronary artery disease because drug may cause angina or MI; in those with hypertension because drug may increase blood pressure; and in those with asthma, epilepsy, heart failure, or migraine headache because rapid increases in extracellular fluid may pose risks.

Mechanism of Action

Vasopressin, a synthetic form of antidiuretic hormone, treats diabetes insipidus by decreasing urine output and raising urine osmolality. When vasopressin attaches to vasopressin$_2$ (V_2) receptors on cell membranes in the nephron's collecting duct, it activates the enzyme adenyl cyclase to convert adenosine triphosphate (ATP) to cyclic adenosine monophosphate (cAMP). This action increases the collecting duct's permeability and enhances water reabsorption into the blood.

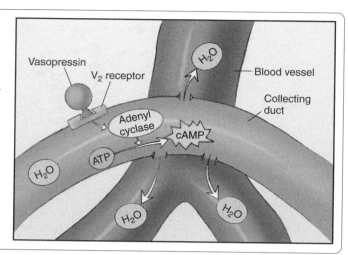

•Monitor fluid and electrolyte balance during vasopressin therapy. Monitor intake and output at least every 8 hours, and assess for signs and symptoms of water intoxication and hyponatremia, including anuria, confusion, drowsiness, headache, listlessness, and weight gain.

PATIENT TEACHING

•Teach patient how to administer vasopressin; emphasize the need to rotate injection sites.
•Urge patient to notify prescriber immediately if he experiences signs of possible water intoxication, including anuria, confusion, drowsiness, headache, listlessness, and unexplained weight gain.
•Inform patient that abdominal cramps, nausea, and skin blanching will subside after a few minutes and can be minimized by drinking one or two glasses of water.

venlafaxine hydrochloride

Effexor, Effexor XR

Class and Category

Chemical: Phenylethylamine derivative
Therapeutic: Antidepressant
Pregnancy category: C

Indications and Dosages

➤ *To treat and prevent relapse of major depression*

E.R. CAPSULES

Adults. 75 mg q.d. (for some patients, 37.5 mg q.d. for 4 to 7 days before increasing to 75 mg/day), then increased by 75 mg/day q 4 days, as prescribed. *Maximum:* 225 mg/day.

TABLETS

Adults. 75 mg/day in divided doses b.i.d. or t.i.d., increased by 75 mg/day q 4 days, as prescribed. *Maximum:* 375 mg/day (225 mg/day for outpatients).

➤ *To treat generalized anxiety disorder*

E.R. CAPSULES

Adults. 75 mg q.d. (for some patients, 37.5 mg q.d. for 4 to 7 days before increasing to 75 mg/day), and then increased by 75 mg/day q 4 days, as prescribed. *Maximum:* 225 mg/day.

DOSAGE ADJUSTMENT Initial daily dose decreased by 25% to 50% for patients with mild to moderate renal impairment and by 50% for patients with hepatic impairment.

Route	Onset	Peak	Duration
P.O.	2 wk	Unknown	Unknown

Contraindications

Hypersensitivity to venlafaxine or its components, use within 14 days of MAO inhibitor therapy

Inhibits neuronal reuptake of serotonin and norepinephrine, along with its active metabolite, *O*-desmethylvenlafaxine. These actions raise serotonin and norepinephrine levels at nerve synapses, elevating mood and reducing depression.

Interactions
DRUGS
amitriptyline, clomipramine, desipramine, doxepin, haloperidol, imipramine, nortriptyline, protriptyline, trazodone: Possibly serotonin syndrome
cimetidine: Decreased clearance and increased blood level of venlafaxine
MAO inhibitors: Increased risk of hypertension; hyperthermia; mental status changes, including coma and delirium; muscle rigidity; and severe myoclonus

Adverse Reactions
CNS: Agitation, anxiety, asthenia, chills, confusion, delusions, dizziness, dream disturbances, drowsiness, headache, insomnia, mood changes, paresthesia, tremor
CV: Chest pain, hypertension, palpitations, sinus tachycardia
EENT: Blurred vision, dry mouth, rhinitis, tinnitus
GI: Abdominal pain, anorexia, constipation, diarrhea, flatulence, indigestion, nausea, vomiting
GU: Decreased libido, ejaculation disorders, impotence
SKIN: Diaphoresis
Other: Weight loss

Nursing Considerations
•Monitor blood pressure frequently during venlafaxine therapy because drug may cause dose-related increase in supine diastolic pressure. Expect to reduce or stop drug, as prescribed, if increase develops.
•Assess for suicidal ideation; implement suicide precautions, according to facility policy, as appropriate.
•WARNING Be aware that drug shouldn't be discontinued abruptly because doing so may cause asthenia, dizziness, headache, insomnia, and nervousness.
PATIENT TEACHING
•Instruct patient not to crush or chew E.R. capsules.
•Caution patient to avoid potentially hazardous activities until drug's CNS effects are known.
•Advise patient to avoid alcohol during venlafaxine therapy.
•Advise patient to weigh herself daily and to notify prescriber about significant weight loss.
•Advise patient not to stop taking drug abruptly.

verapamil

Apo-Verap (CAN), Calan, Isoptin, Novo-Veramil (CAN), Nu-Verap (CAN)

verapamil hydrochloride

Calan SR, Isoptin SR, Verelan

Class and Category
Chemical: Phenylalkylamine derivative
Therapeutic: Antianginal, antiarrhythmic, antihypertensive
Pregnancy category: C

Indications and Dosages
➤ *To treat chronic angina pectoris*
TABLETS (VERAPAMIL)
Adults and adolescents age 15 and older. *Initial:* 80 to 120 mg t.i.d., increased q day or wk, as needed and prescribed. *Maximum:* 480 mg/day in divided doses.
Infants and children up to age 15. 4 to 8 mg/kg/day in divided doses.
➤ *To manage hypertension*
E.R. CAPSULES (VERAPAMIL HYDROCHLORIDE)
Adults and adolescents. *Initial:* 240 mg/day, increased q day or wk, as needed and prescribed. *Maximum:* 480 mg/day.
E.R. TABLETS (VERAPAMIL HYDROCHLORIDE)
Adults and adolescents. *Initial:* 180 mg q.d., increased q day or wk, as needed and prescribed, according to following schedule: 240 mg q.d. in the morning; 180 mg q 12 hr or 240 mg in the morning and 120 mg in the evening; then 240 mg q 12 hr. *Maximum:* 480 mg/day in divided doses.
TABLETS (VERAPAMIL)
Adults and adolescents age 15 and older. *Initial:* 80 to 120 mg t.i.d., increased q day or wk, as needed and prescribed. *Maximum:* 480 mg/day in divided doses.
Infants and children up to age 15. 4 to 8 mg/kg/day in divided doses.

➤ *To prevent or treat supraventricular tachycardia*

TABLETS (VERAPAMIL)

Adults and adolescents age 15 and older. *Initial:* 80 to 120 mg t.i.d., increased q day or wk, as needed and prescribed. *Maximum:* 480 mg/day in divided doses.

DOSAGE ADJUSTMENT Initial P.O. dosage possibly reduced to 40 mg t.i.d. (120 mg/day for E.R. tablets or capsules) for elderly patients and those with impaired hepatic or left ventricular function.

I.V. INJECTION (VERAPAMIL HYDROCHLORIDE)

Adults and adolescents age 15 and older. *Initial:* 5 to 10 mg slowly over 2 min; then 10 mg, as prescribed, if response isn't adequate after 30 min.

Children ages 1 to 15. *Initial:* 100 to 300 mcg/kg slowly over 2 min, up to maximum of 5 mg; then 10 mg, as prescribed, if response isn't adequate after 30 min.

Infants up to age 1. *Initial:* 100 to 200 mcg/kg slowly over 2 min.

DOSAGE ADJUSTMENT I.V. drug administered over 3 minutes in elderly patients.

Route	Onset	Peak	Duration
P.O.	1 to 2 hr	30 to 90 min	6 to 8 hr
P.O. (E.R.)	1 to 2 hr	30 to 90 min	Unknown
I.V.	1 to 5 min	3 to 5 min	10 min to 6 hr

Mechanism of Action

Inhibits calcium movement into coronary and vascular smooth-muscle cells by blocking slow calcium channels in cell membranes. The resulting decrease in the intracellular calcium level has the following effects:
• inhibits smooth-muscle cell contractions
• decreases myocardial oxygen demand by relaxing coronary and vascular smooth muscle, reducing peripheral vascular resistance, and decreasing systolic and diastolic pressures
• slows AV conduction time and prolongs AV nodal refractoriness
• interrupts reentry circuit in AV nodal reentrant tachycardias.

Incompatibilities

Don't mix I.V. verapamil with albumin, amphotericin B injection, hydralazine hydrochloride injection, nafcillin, or sulfamethoxazole and trimethoprim injection. Solutions with pH above 6.0 cause precipitation.

Contraindications

Cardiogenic shock, concomitant use of beta blockers (with I.V. verapamil), hypersensitivity to verapamil or its components, hypotension, severe heart failure unless secondary to supraventricular tachycardia that responds to verapamil, severe left ventricular dysfunction, sick sinus syndrome or second- or third-degree heart block unless artificial pacemaker is in place, ventricular tachycardia (with I.V. verapamil)

Interactions
DRUGS

alpha blockers, antihypertensives, general anesthetics (hydrocarbon), prazosin: Hypotensive effects
beta blockers: Increased risk of heart failure, hypotension, and severe bradycardia
calcium supplements: Decreased response to verapamil
carbamazepine, cyclosporine, theophylline, valproate: Increased risk of toxicity from these drugs
cimetidine: Decreased metabolism and increased blood level of verapamil
dantrolene: Increased risk of hyperkalemia and myocardial depression
digoxin: Increased blood digoxin level and risk of digitalis toxicity
disopyramide, flecainide: Additive negative inotropic effects
lithium: Increased risk of neurotoxicity
neuromuscular blockers: Prolonged recovery from neuromuscular blockade
NSAIDs, sympathomimetics: Decreased antihypertensive effect of verapamil
phenobarbital: Increased verapamil clearance
procainamide: Increased Q-T interval, additive negative inotropic effects
protein-bound drugs (hydantoins, salicylates, sulfonamides, sulfonylureas, and warfarin and other oral anticoagulants): Altered blood levels of these drugs
quinidine: Increased risk of quinidine toxicity, increased Q-T interval, additive negative inotropic effects

rifampin: Decreased bioavailability of oral verapamil

ACTIVITIES
alcohol use: Increased blood alcohol level and prolonged CNS effects

Adverse Reactions
CNS: Dizziness, fatigue, headache
CV: Angina, AV conduction disorders, brady-cardia, claudication, heart failure, hypoten-sion, peripheral edema, tachycardia
GI: Constipation, nausea
GU: Galactorrhea, menstrual irregularities
RESP: Dyspnea, pulmonary edema, wheezing
SKIN: Flushing, rash

Nursing Considerations
•Administer I.V. verapamil with compatible so-lutions, including Ringer's injection, D_5W, or NS.
•Maintain continuous ECG monitoring and keep emergency resuscitative equipment and drugs readily available during I.V. therapy.
•Assess patient with hypertrophic cardiomy-opathy for early development of hypotension and pulmonary edema because second-degree AV block and sinus arrest can result.
•Assess for bradycardia and hypotension, and notify prescriber if heart rate or blood pressure declines significantly.
•Be aware that disopyramide or flecainide shouldn't be given within 48 hours before or 24 hours after verapamil because additive negative inotropic effects can result.
•Institute measures to prevent constipation, including a high-fiber diet and a stool soft-ener, as prescribed.

PATIENT TEACHING
•Instruct patient not to crush or chew ver-apamil E.R. tablets or capsules. Inform her that she may break E.R. tablets in half if necessary to aid swallowing.
•Direct patient to check her pulse rate be-fore taking verapamil and to notify prescrib-er if it's below 50 beats/minute or as instruc-ted by prescriber.
•Caution patient about possible dizziness and the need to avoid potentially hazardous activities until drug's CNS effects are known.
•Inform patient that adverse skin reactions may subside with continued use. Advise her to notify prescriber if rash persists.
•Encourage patient to increase dietary fiber intake to help prevent constipation. Advise her to notify prescriber if problem becomes persistent or severe.

voriconazole
Vfend

Class and Category
Chemical: Triazole
Therapeutic: Antifungal
Pregnancy category: D

Indications and Dosages
➤ *To treat invasive aspergillosis; to treat serious fungal infections caused by* Scedosporium apiospermum *and* Fusar-ium sp., *including* Fusarium solani, *in patients intolerant of or refractory to other therapy*

I.V. INFUSION
Adults and children age 12 and older. *Initial:* 6 mg/kg over 1 to 2 hr at a rate not to ex-ceed 3 mg/kg/hr q 12 hr for 2 doses. *Mainte-nance:* 4 mg/kg over 1 to 2 hr at a rate not to exceed 3 mg/kg/hr q 12 hr.

TABLETS
Adults and children age 12 and older weigh-ing 40 kg (88 lb) or more. *Maintenance:* 200 mg q 12 hr, increased to 300 mg q 12 hr, as needed, and taken at least 1 hr before or after a meal.
Adults and children age 12 and older weigh-ing less than 40 kg. *Maintenance:* 100 mg q 12 hr, increased to 150 mg q 12 hr, as needed, and taken at least 1 hr before or after a meal.
DOSAGE ADJUSTMENT If patient can't tolerate treatment, I.V. maintenance dose may be re-duced to 3 mg/kg q 12 hr and oral mainte-nance dose reduced by 50 mg steps to a mini-mum of 200 mg q 12 hr (or to 100 mg q 12 hr for patients weighing less than 40 kg). For coadministration with phenytoin, mainte-nance dose may be increased to 5 mg/kg I.V. q 12 hr or from 200 mg to 400 mg P.O. q 12 hr (100 mg to 200 mg q 12 hr for patients weighing less than 40 kg). For patients with mild to moderate hepatic cirrhosis, standard loading dose should be used, but mainte-nance dose should be halved for I.V. or P.O. administration. For patients with moderate to severe renal insufficiency (creatinine clear-ance greater than 50 ml/min), only the oral form should be administered, if possible.

Incompatibilities
Don't infuse into the same line or cannula with other drugs, including parenteral nutri-tion, to prevent an increase in subvisible

particulate matter. Avoid infusion with blood products and any electrolyte supplements. Don't dilute with 4.2% sodium bicarbonate infusion because the mildly alkaline nature of the diluent causes slight degradation of voriconazole after 24 hours of storage at room temperature.

> ## Mechanism of Action
> Prevents fungal ergosterol biosynthesis by inhibiting fungal cytochrome P450–mediated 14 alpha-lanosterol demethylation. The loss of ergosterol in the fungal cell wall renders the fungal cell inactive.

Contraindications
Coadministration with long-acting barbiturates, carbamazepine, CYP3A4 substrates (astemizole, cisapride, pimozide, quinidine, or terfenadine), ergot alkaloids, rifabutin, rifampin, or sirolimus; hypersensitivity to voriconazole or its components; galactose intolerance, glucose-galactose malabsorption, or Lapp lactase deficiency (oral form only contains lactose)

Interactions
DRUGS
benzodiazepines: Possibly prolonged sedative effect of benzodiazepines
calcium channel blockers; HMG-CoA reductase inhibitors, such as lovastatin; omeprazole; sirolimus: Possibly increased plasma concentrations of these drugs, leading to increased risk of adverse reactions and toxicity
carbamazepine, long-acting barbiturates, phenytoin, rifampin: Decreased plasma voriconazole concentration
coumarin, warfarin: Possibly increased PTT
cyclosporine, sirolimus, tacrolimus: Increased serum concentrations of these drugs and risk of toxicity, especially nephrotoxicity
CYP3A4 substrates (astemizole, cisapride, pimozide, quinidine, terfenadine): Increased plasma concentrations of these drugs, which may lead to prolonged QT-interval and rare occurrences of torsades de pointes
ergot alkaloids (ergotamine, dihydroergotamine): May increase plasma concentration of ergot alkaloids leading to ergotism
HIV protease inhibitors (amprenavir, nelfenavir, saquinavir), non-nucleoside reverse transcriptase inhibitors (delavirdine, efavirenz):

Possibly inhibited metabolism of these drugs and voriconazole
rifabutin: Increased rifabutin plasma concentration; decreased voriconazole plasma concentrations
sulfonylureas: Possibly increased plasma concentrations of sulfonylureas and increased risk of hypoglycemia
vinca alkaloids: Possibly increased risk of neurotoxicity

Adverse Reactions
CNS: Chills, dizziness, fever, hallucinations, headache
CV: Chest pain, hypertension, hypotension, peripheral edema, tachycardia, vasodilation
EENT: Abnormal or blurred vision, altered or enhanced visual perception, change in color perception, chromatopsia, dry mouth, eye hemorrhage, photophobia, visual disturbances
GI: Abdominal pain, cholestatic jaundice, diarrhea, elevated hepatic enzyme levels and liver function test results, increased bilirubin and SGOT or SGPT, jaundice, nausea, vomiting
GU: Abnormal kidney function, acute renal failure, elevated serum creatinine level
HEME: Anemia, leukopenia, pancytopenia, thrombocytopenia
RESP: Respiratory disorders
SKIN: Erythema multiforme, maculopapular rash, photosensitivity, pruritus, rash, Stevens-Johnson syndrome, toxic epidermal necrolysis
Other: Anaphlaxis *(I.V. form),* elevated alkaline phosphatase, hypokalemia, hypomagnesemia, sepsis

Nursing Considerations
• Use voriconazole cautiously in patients with known hypersensitivity to other azoles.
• Determine if patient has any problems with galactose intolerance, Lapp lactase deficiency, or glucose-galactose malabsorption before starting therapy because voriconazole tablets contain lactose and shouldn't be given to patients with these conditions.
• Obtain specimens for fungal culture and other relevant laboratory studies (including histopathology), as ordered, before giving first dose. Expect to begin drug before test results are known.
• Assess patient's liver function, including bilirubin, as ordered, at the start of

voriconazole therapy and periodically thereafter. Be aware that drug may be discontinued if liver abnormalities occur.

•For I.V. infusion, reconstitute powder with 19 ml of water for injection to obtain 20 ml of concentrate that contains 10 mg/ml of voriconazole. Use a standard 10-ml nonautomated syringe to ensure that exact amount of water is injected into vial. Shake the vial until all powder is dissolved. Further dilute so that final concentration is not less than 0.5 mg/ml nor more than 5 mg/ml. This requires withdrawing and discarding at least an equal volume of diluent from the infusion bag or bottle before instillation of concentrate.

•Discard partially used vials after mixing. If infusion isn't administered immediately, store at 2° to 8° C (37° to 46° F) for no longer than 24 hours.

•Administer I.V. infusion over 1 to 2 hours at a rate that doesn't exceed 3 mg/kg/hr.

•Monitor renal function, especially serum creatinine level, when administering I.V. form of voriconazole because drug may accumulate in body when creatinine clearance is less than 50 ml/min, increasing the risk of adverse reactions.

•WARNING Observe patient receiving I.V. voriconazole closely for anaphylactoid-type reactions—such as flushing, fever, sweating, tachycardia, chest tightness, dyspnea, faintness, nausea, pruritus and rash—which may occur immediately after starting the infusion. Stop the infusion if these reactions occur, and notify prescriber immediately.

•Monitor patient closely throughout therapy for skin rash, which may indicate a serious cutaneous reaction, such as Stevens-Johnson syndrome. If a rash occurs, notify prescriber, and expect that drug may be discontinued.

•Monitor cyclosporine, tacrolimus, and warfarin closely for elevated levels when voriconazole is coadministered with any of these drugs.

•Monitor diabetic patients also taking sulfonylureas closely for hypoglycemia, and check blood glucose levels regularly.

•Be aware that voriconazole dosage will need to be adjusted when co-administered with phenytoin. Expect to monitor plasma phenytoin levels and observe patient closely for phenytoin-related adverse reactions.

•Assess patient's visual function, including visual acuity, visual field, and color perception, if voriconazole therapy continues longer than 28 days.

PATIENT TEACHING

•Instruct patient taking oral voriconazole to take the tablets at least 1 hour before or 1 hour after a meal.

•Inform female patient of possible fetal risk, and stress the importance of avoiding pregnancy. Tell her to use an effective form of contraception throughout therapy and to notify the prescriber immediately if pregnancy is suspected.

•Caution patient not to drive at night and to avoid potentially hazardous activities because drug may cause visual disturbances, including blurring or photophobia.

•Advise patient to avoid exposure to direct sunlight or UV light and to wear sunscreen when outdoors.

warfarin sodium

Coumadin

Class and Category

Chemical: Coumarin derivative
Therapeutic: Anticoagulant
Pregnancy category: X

Indications and Dosages

➤ *To prevent or treat pulmonary embolism; recurrent MI; thromboembolic complications from atrial fibrillation, heart valve replacement, or MI; and venous thrombosis (and its extension)*

TABLETS

Adults. *Initial:* 2 to 5 mg/day for 2 to 4 days. *Usual:* 2 to 10 mg/day based on target PT and INR results. *Maximum:* Determined by target PT and INR results, as prescribed.

I.V. INJECTION

Adults. *Initial:* 2 to 5 mg/day infused over 1 to 2 min. *Usual:* 2 to 10 mg/day infused over 1 to 2 min. *Maximum:* Determined by target PT and INR results, as prescribed.

DOSAGE ADJUSTMENT For patients with hepatic dysfunction, dosage reduced to 0.1 mg/kg, as prescribed. For elderly patients, dosage possibly reduced based on PT and INR results.

Route	Onset	Peak	Duration
P.O.	24 hr	3 to 4 days	2 to 5 days
I.V.	Unknown	3 to 4 days	2 to 5 days

U
V
W

Mechanism of Action

Interferes with the liver's ability to synthesize vitamin K-dependent clotting factors, depleting clotting factors II (prothrombin), VII, IX, and X. This action, in turn, interferes with the clotting cascade. By depleting vitamin K-dependent clotting factors and interfering with the clotting cascade, warfarin prevents coagulation.

Incompatibilities

Don't mix warfarin in solution with amikacin sulfate, epinephrine hydrochloride, metaraminol tartrate, oxytocin, promazine hydrochloride, tetracycline hydrochloride, or vancomycin hydrochloride.

Contraindications

Bleeding or bleeding tendencies; blood dyscrasias; cerebral or dissecting aneurysm; cerebrovascular hemorrhage; diverticulitis; eclampsia or preeclampsia; history of warfarin-induced necrosis; hypersensitivity to warfarin or its components; malignant or severe uncontrolled hypertension; malnutrition and emaciation; mental state or condition that leads to lack of patient cooperation; pericardial effusion; pericarditis; polyarthritis; pregnancy; prostatectomy; recent or planned neurosurgery, ophthalmic surgery, or spinal puncture; severe hepatic or renal disease

Interactions

DRUGS

acetaminophen, aminoglycosides, amiodarone, androgens, beta blockers, capecitabine, cephalosporins, chloral hydrate, chloramphenicol, chlorpropamide, cimetidine, clofibrate, corticosteroids, cyclophosphamide, dextrothyroxine, diflunisal, disulfiram, erythromycin, fluconazole, gemfibrozil, glucagon, hydantoins, ifosfamide, influenza virus vaccine, isoniazid, ketoconazole, loop diuretics, lovastatin, metronidazole, miconazole, mineral oil, moricizine, nalidixic acid, NSAIDs, omeprazole, penicillins, phenylbutazones, propafenone, propoxyphene, quinidine, quinine, quinolones, salicylates, streptokinase, sulfamethoxazole-trimethoprim, sulfinpyrazone, sulfonamides, tamoxifen, tetracyclines, thyroid hormones, urokinase, vitamin E: Increased anticoagulant effect of warfarin, increased risk of bleeding

aminoglutethimide, barbiturates, carbamazepine, cholestyramine, dicloxacillin, estrogens, ethchlorvynol, etretinate, glutethimide, griseofulvin, nafcillin, oral contraceptives, rifampin, spironolactone, sucralfate, thiazide diuretics, trazodone, vitamin C, vitamin K: Decreased anticoagulant effect of warfarin

atorvastatin, pravastatin: Increased or decreased anticoagulant effect of warfarin

herbal remedies (including bromelains, danshen, dong quai, garlic, ginkgo biloba, and ginseng): Increased anticoagulant effect of warfarin, increased risk of bleeding

I.V. lipid emulsion, other medical products that contain soybean oil: Possibly decreased vitamin K absorption and increased anticoagulant effect of warfarin

nicotine patch: Altered response to warfarin

FOODS

certain multivitamins, enteral feedings, vitamin–K-rich foods: Decreased effects of warfarin

ACTIVITIES

alcohol use: Increased risk of hypoprothrombinemia

smoking, smoking cessation: Altered response to warfarin

Adverse Reactions

CNS: Intracranial hemorrhage, weakness
EENT: Epistaxis, intraocular hemorrhage
GI: Abdominal cramps and pain, diarrhea, hepatitis, nausea, vomiting
GU: Hematuria, vaginal bleeding (abnormal)
HEME: Potentially fatal hemorrhage (from any tissue or organ)
SKIN: Alopecia, ecchymosis, jaundice, petechiae, pruritus, purple-toe syndrome, tissue necrosis

Nursing Considerations

• Reconstitute parenteral warfarin just before administration with 2.7 ml of sterile water for injection to yield 2 mg/ml. Then administer slowly over 1 to 2 minutes through peripheral I.V.

• Expect to administer another parenteral anticoagulant, such as heparin or enoxaparin, with oral warfarin for at least 3 days, or until desired response occurs, before giving warfarin only.

• Avoid I.M. injections during warfarin therapy, if possible, because they can result in bleeding, bruising, and hematoma.

• Monitor INR (daily in acute care setting) and assess for therapeutic effects, as prescribed. Therapeutic INR levels are 2.0 to 3.0 for bioprosthetic heart valve, nonvalvular atrial fibrillation, and venous thromboembolism, and 2.5 to 3.5 after MI and for mechanical heart valve.

• Expect treatment to last up to 12 weeks for bioprosthetic heart valve, 1 to 3 months for nonvalvular atrial fibrillation or venous thromboembolism, and for rest of life after MI and for mechanical heart valve replacement.

• **WARNING** Be aware of the increased risk for intracranial hemorrhage if patient has cerebral ischemia (such as recent transient ischemic attack or minor ischemic CVA) and INR of 3 to 4.5. As prescribed, withhold next warfarin dose and give vitamin K if INR exceeds 4 because of the risk of bleeding.

• Assess for occult bleeding if patient receives I.V. lipid emulsion or other medical product that contains soybean oil. Such products can decrease vitamin K absorption and increase warfarin's anticoagulant effect.

PATIENT TEACHING

• Explain that warfarin therapy aims to prevent thrombosis by decreasing clotting ability while avoiding the risk of spontaneous bleeding.

• Instruct patient to take drug exactly as prescribed at the same time each evening.

• Urge patient to keep weekly follow-up appointments for blood tests after discharge until PT and INR levels are stabilized.

• Advise patient to avoid alcohol during warfarin therapy.

• Urge patient to take precautions against bleeding, such as using an electric shaver and a soft-bristled toothbrush. Advise him to continue these precautions for 2 to 5 days after therapy stops, as directed, because anticoagulant effect may persist during this time.

• Caution patient to avoid activities that could cause traumatic injury and bleeding.

• Advise patient to eat consistent amounts of vitamin K–rich foods, such as dark green, leafy vegetables.

• Urge patient to notify prescriber immediately about unusual bleeding and any unexplained symptoms, such as abnormal vaginal bleeding; dizziness; easy bruising; gum bleeding; headache; nosebleeds; prolonged bleeding from cuts; red, black, or tarry stool; red or dark brown urine; swelling; and weakness.

• Advise patient to consult prescriber before taking other drugs—including OTC drugs and herbal remedies—during therapy.

• Instruct female patient of childbearing age to stop taking warfarin and notify prescriber immediately about known or suspected pregnancy.

• Explain that drug may cause reversible purple-toe syndrome and that this syndrome isn't harmful.

• Urge patient to carry medical identification that reveals he's taking warfarin therapy.

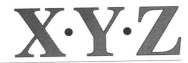

zafirlukast

Accolate

Class and Category

Chemical: Peptide leukotriene receptor antagonist
Therapeutic: Antiasthmatic
Pregnancy category: B

Indications and Dosages

➤ *To treat chronic asthma*

TABLETS

Adults and children over age 11. 20 mg b.i.d.
Children ages 5 to 11. 10 mg b.i.d.

Route	Onset	Peak	Duration
P.O.	1 wk	Unknown	Unknown

Mechanism of Action

Inhibits the selective binding of cysteinyl leukotrienes (arachidonic acid derivatives that usually mediate inflammation in asthma and other inflammatory disorders) by competitively blocking receptor sites. This action causes bronchial relaxation and decreases vascular leakage and edema, mucus secretion, eosinophil movement, and bronchial hyperresponsiveness.

Contraindications

Hypersensitivity to zafirlukast or its components

Interactions

DRUGS

alprazolam, amitriptyline, calcium channel blockers, carbamazepine, citalopram, corticosteroids, cyclosporine, diazepam, diclofenac, ibuprofen, imipramine, irbesartan, lidocaine, lovastatin, midazolam, phenytoin, quinidine, simvastatin, tolbutamide, tolterodine, triazolam: Inhibited metabolism and, possibly, additive adverse effects of these drugs
aspirin: Increased blood zafirlukast level
erythromycin, terfenadine: Decreased response to zafirlukast
sildenafil: Increased adverse effects of sildenafil
theophylline: Decreased blood zafirlukast level
warfarin: Prolonged PT

FOODS

any food: Possibly decreased bioavailability of zafirlukast

Adverse Reactions

CNS: Asthenia, dizziness, fever, headache
GI: Abdominal pain, diarrhea, elevated liver function test results, indigestion, nausea, vomiting
MS: Back pain, myalgia
Other: Generalized pain

Nursing Considerations

•Be aware that zafirlukast shouldn't be used to treat bronchospasm during an acute asthma attack or status asthmaticus; it can't relieve symptoms quickly enough.
•Assess respiratory rate, depth, and quality as well as breath sounds before and during treatment to evaluate response to therapy.
•If patient is being weaned from corticosteroids while taking zafirlukast, monitor her for Churg-Strauss syndrome, a rare allergic reaction characterized by eosinophilia, fever, myalgia, and weight loss as well as cardiac complications, neuropathy, and worsening pulmonary symptoms.

PATIENT TEACHING

•Instruct patient to take drug exactly as prescribed, in evenly spaced doses, every day. Stress the need to take drug even during symptom-free periods and acute exacerbations.
•Instruct patient to take drug on an empty stomach at least 1 hour before or 2 hours after meals.
•Advise patient to continue using rescue inhalants, as prescribed, for acute attacks.
•Teach patient how to use peak-flow meter to monitor pulmonary function.

zaleplon

Sonata

Class, Category, and Schedule

Chemical: Imidazopyridine derivative
Therapeutic: Sedative-hypnotic
Pregnancy category: C
Controlled substance: Schedule IV

Indications and Dosages

➤ *To provide short-term treatment of insomnia*

CAPSULES

Adults up to age 65. 10 mg/day h.s., as prescribed, for up to 35 days. *Usual:* 10 mg/day h.s. for 7 to 10 days. *Maximum:* 20 mg/day.

X
Y
Z

DOSAGE ADJUSTMENT For elderly patients and those who have hepatic impairment or take cimetidine, dosage possibly reduced to 5 mg/day.

Route	Onset	Peak	Duration
P.O.	30 min	Unknown	4 hr

Mechanism of Action
Selectively binds with type 1 benzodiazepine (BZ1 or omega$_1$) receptors on the gamma-aminobutyric acid-A receptor complex. This binding produces muscle relaxation and sedation as well as anti-anxiety and anticonvulsant effects.

Contraindications
Hypersensitivity to zaleplon or its components

Interactions
DRUGS

amitriptyline; amoxapine; azatadine; benzodiazepines; brompheniramine; chlorpheniramine; clemastine; clomipramine; clozapine; cyproheptadine; dexchlorpheniramine; diphenhydramine; doxepin; entacapone; haloperidol; hydroxyzine; imipramine; maprotiline; mirtazapine; molindone; nefazodone; nortriptyline; olanzapine; opioid analgesics; other anxiolytics, sedatives, and hypnotics; phenindamine; phenothiazines; pimozide; pramipexole; promethazine; quetiapine; risperidone; ropinirole; thioridazine; trazodone; trimipramine; tripelennamine: Possibly additive CNS depression
carbamazepine, phenobarbital, phenytoin, rifampin: Reduced zaleplon effects
cimetidine: Increased blood zaleplon level
flumazenil: Reversal of zaleplon's sedative effect

FOODS
high-fat foods: Prolonged absorption time and reduced effectiveness of zaleplon

ACTIVITIES
alcohol use: Increased CNS depression

Adverse Reactions
CNS: Amnesia, anxiety, depression, dizziness, drowsiness, fever, hallucinations, hypertonia, insomnia, paresthesia, seizures, tremor, vertigo
EENT: Dry mouth, gingivitis, glossitis, mouth ulcers, stomatitis
GI: Anorexia, colitis, constipation, eructation, esophagitis, flatulence, gastritis, gastroenteritis, increased appetite, indigestion, melena, nausea, rectal bleeding, vomiting

MS: Back pain
SKIN: Photosensitivity, pruritus, rash
Other: Physical and psychological dependence

Nursing Considerations
• Administer zaleplon just before bedtime because its onset of action is rapid.
• Avoid giving drug with or after a heavy, high-fat meal because decreased absorption may reduce drug's effects.
• **WARNING** Anticipate an increased risk of suicidal ideation in patient with major depression who takes zaleplon. Implement suicide precautions, as appropriate, according to facility policy.
• Monitor patient for signs of drug abuse because zaleplon has an abuse potential similar to that of benzodiazepines and benzodiazepine-like hypnotics.
PATIENT TEACHING
• Inform patient that zaleplon is for short-term use only. Advise her not to use drug for anything other than insomnia.
• Caution patient not to exceed prescribed dosage.
• Instruct patient to take zaleplon immediately before bedtime or right after experiencing difficulty falling asleep because of rapid onset of action.
• Teach patient alternative measures for relaxation and sleep induction.
• Advise patient to consult prescriber before taking other CNS depressants.
• Urge patient to avoid alcohol during zaleplon therapy.
• Warn patient that zaleplon contains FD & C Yellow No. 5 (tartrazine), which can cause an allergic reaction, especially in those with an aspirin sensitivity. Instruct patient to report any allergic reactions, such as rash or difficulty breathing, to prescriber.
• Instruct patient to notify prescriber if inability to sleep continues. Dosage may need to be adjusted.

zileuton
Zyflo

Class and Category
Chemical: Leukotriene inhibitor
Therapeutic: Antiasthmatic
Pregnancy category: C

Indications and Dosages
➤ *To treat chronic asthma*

TABLETS
Adults and adolescents. 600 mg q.i.d. *Maximum:* 2,400 mg/day.

Route	Onset	Peak	Duration
P.O.	2 hr	Unknown	Unknown

> **Mechanism of Action**
> Inhibits the formation of leukotrienes found mainly in neutrophils, eosinophils, monocytes, macrophages, and mast cells. Normally, leukotrienes augment neutrophil and eosinophil migration, neutrophil and monocyte aggregation, leukocyte adhesion, capillary permeability, and smooth-muscle contraction. By inhibiting leukotriene formation, zileuton causes bronchial relaxation and decreases vascular leakage and edema, mucus secretion, eosinophil movement, and bronchial hyperresponsiveness.

Contraindications
Hepatic impairment, hypersensitivity to zileuton or its components

Interactions
DRUGS
propranolol, terfenadine: Increased effects of these drugs
theophylline: Doubled blood theophylline level
warfarin: Prolonged PT and INR

Adverse Reactions
CNS: Asthenia, dizziness, fever, headache, hypertonia, insomnia, malaise, nervousness, somnolence
CV: Chest pain
EENT: Conjunctivitis
GI: Abdominal pain, constipation, flatulence, indigestion, nausea, vomiting
GU: UTI, vaginitis
MS: Arthralgia, myalgia, neck pain or rigidity
SKIN: Pruritus
Other: Lymphadenopathy

Nursing Considerations
•Be aware that zileuton shouldn't be used to treat bronchospasm during an acute asthma attack or status asthmaticus; it can't relieve symptoms quickly enough.
•Monitor serum ALT level, as ordered, usually before treatment starts, once a month for 3 months, every 2 to 3 months for remainder of first year, and periodically thereafter during therapy.

•Monitor results of liver and pulmonary function tests and CBC periodically during therapy.
PATIENT TEACHING
•Advise patient to take drug exactly as prescribed, in evenly spaced doses, every day. Stress the importance of taking drug even during symptom-free periods and acute exacerbations.
•Instruct patient to continue using rescue inhalants, as prescribed, for acute attacks.
•Teach patient how to use peak-flow meter to determine and monitor pulmonary function.

zinc acetate

(contains 25 or 50 mg of elemental zinc per capsule)
Galzin

zinc chloride

(contains 1 mg of elemental zinc per ml for I.V. infusion)

zinc gluconate

(contains 1.4 mg of elemental zinc per lozenge; 1.4, 2, 4, 7, 8, 10, 11, 13, 31, 50, or 52 mg of elemental zinc per tablet)
Orazinc

zinc sulfate

(contains 25 or 50 mg of elemental zinc per capsule; 15, 25, 45, or 50 mg of elemental zinc per tablet; 50 mg of elemental zinc per E.R. tablet; and 1 or 5 mg of elemental zinc per ml for I.V. infusion)
Orazinc, Verazinc, Zinc 15, Zinc-220, Zinca-Pak, Zincate

Class and Category
Chemical: Trace element, mineral
Therapeutic: Copper absorption inhibitor, nutritional supplement
Pregnancy category: A (oral), C (I.V.)

Indications and Dosages
➤ *To prevent zinc deficiency based on U.S. and Canadian recommended daily allowances*
CAPSULES, E.R. TABLETS, LOZENGES, TABLETS
Male adults and children age 11 and older. 15 mg (9 to 12 mg Canadian) of elemental zinc daily.
Female adults and children age 11 and older. 12 mg (9 mg Canadian) of elemental zinc daily.

Pregnant females. 15 mg (15 mg Canadian) of elemental zinc daily.
Breast-feeding females. 16 to 19 mg (15 mg Canadian) of elemental zinc daily.
Children ages 7 to 10. 10 mg (7 to 9 mg Canadian) of elemental zinc daily.
Children ages 4 to 6. 10 mg (5 mg Canadian) of elemental zinc daily.
Children from birth to age 3. 5 to 10 mg (2 to 4 mg Canadian) of elemental zinc daily.
I.V. INFUSION
Adults and children. 2.5 to 4 mg q.d. added to total parenteral nutrition (TPN) solution. *Maximum:* 12 mg/day.
Children from birth to age 5. 100 mcg/kg/day added to TPN solution.
Premature infants weighing up to 3 kg. 300 mcg/kg/day added to TPN solution.

➤ *To treat zinc deficiency*
CAPSULES, E.R. TABLETS, LOZENGES, TABLETS
Adults and children. Dosage individualized based on severity of deficiency.
I.V. INFUSION
Adults and adolescents. 2.5 to 4 mg q.d. added to TPN solution. *Maximum:* 12 mg/day.
Children from birth to age 5. 100 mcg/kg/day added to TPN solution.
Premature infants weighing up to 3 kg. 300 mcg/kg/day added to TPN solution.

➤ *As adjunct maintenance therapy for patients previously treated for Wilson's disease*
CAPSULES
Adults. 50 mg t.i.d.
Pregnant females. 25 mg t.i.d., increased to 50 mg t.i.d. if drug effectiveness decreases.
Children age 10 and older. 25 mg t.i.d., increased to 50 mg t.i.d. if drug effectiveness decreases.

Contraindications
Hypersensitivity to zinc or its components

Interactions
DRUGS
copper supplements: Impaired copper absorption (with large doses of zinc)
oral iron supplements, oral phosphate salts, penicillamine, phosphorus-containing drugs: Decreased zinc absorption
quinolones, tetracyclines: Decreased absorption and possibly decreased effectiveness of these antibiotics

thiazide diuretics: Increased urinary excretion of zinc
zinc-containing preparations: Increased blood zinc level
FOODS
fiber- or phylate-containing foods (such as bran, whole-grain breads, cereal), phosphorus-containing foods (including milk, poultry): Decreased zinc absorption

Mechanism of Action
Necessary for proper functioning of more than 200 metalloenzymes (enzymes containing tightly bound zinc atoms as an integral part of their structure), including carbonic anhydrase, carboxypeptidase A, alcohol dehydrogenase, alkaline phosphatase, and RNA polymerase. Zinc also helps maintain nucleic acid, protein, and cell membrane structure and is essential for certain physiologic functions, including cell growth and division, sexual maturation and reproduction, dark adaptation and night vision, wound healing, host immunity, and taste acuity. This mineral also provides cellular antioxidant protection by scavenging free radicals.

In addition, zinc acetate interferes with intestinal absorption of copper and produces a protein that binds with copper, preventing its transfer to the blood. Bound copper is then excreted in stools, thus decreasing copper toxicity in Wilson's disease.

Adverse Reactions
None with usual dosages

Nursing Considerations
•**WARNING** Don't administer I.V. zinc preparations that contain benzyl alcohol to neonates or premature infants because this preservative may cause a fatal toxic syndrome characterized by metabolic acidosis and CNS, respiratory, circulatory, and renal function impairment.
•Administer oral zinc supplements 1 hour before or 2 to 3 hours after meals; at least 2 hours after administering oral iron supplements (to prevent decreased zinc absorption) or copper supplements (to prevent decreased copper absorption); and at least 6 hours before or 2 hours after administering quinolone or tetracycline antibiotics (to prevent decreased absorption of these drugs).

•Monitor patient receiving long-term zinc therapy for sideroblastic anemia, which may result from zinc-induced copper deficiency and is characterized by anemia, leukopenia, neutropenia, granulocytopenia, and bone marrow problems. Be aware that these effects are reversible after zinc is discontinued.
•Monitor patient with preexisting copper deficiency for exacerbation of this condition because zinc therapy can further decrease serum copper level.
•Assess for signs and symptoms of zinc deficiency, such as growth retardation, hypogonadism, delayed sexual maturation, alopecia, impaired wound healing, skin lesions, immune deficiencies, behavioral disturbances, night blindness, and impaired sense of taste.
•Monitor blood alkaline phosphatase (ALP) level monthly, as ordered, because ALP level may increase during zinc therapy.

PATIENT TEACHING
•Explain to patient why she needs a zinc supplement.
•Instruct patient to take zinc on an empty stomach, at least 1 hour before or 2 hours after meals. Caution her not to take zinc within 2 hours of iron or copper supplements or phosphorus-containing drugs.
•Instruct patient to allow zinc lozenge to dissolve in mouth slowly and completely, not to swallow it whole or chew it. Advise her not to take zinc lozenges more often than directed.
•Caution patient to keep lozenges out of children's reach to prevent choking.

ziprasidone hydrochloride

Geodon

ziprasidone mesylate

Geodon for Injection

Class and Category
Chemical: Benzisoxazole derivative
Therapeutic: Antipsychotic
Pregnancy category: C

Indications and Dosages
➤ *To treat schizophrenia*
CAPSULES
Adults. *Initial:* 20 mg b.i.d. Dosage increased as indicated q 2 or more days. *Usual:* 20 to 80 mg b.i.d. *Maximum:* 100 mg b.i.d.

I.M. INJECTION
Adults. *Initial:* 10 to 20 mg. 10 mg dose may be administered q 2 hr up to maximum dose; 20 mg dose may be administered q 4 hr up to maximum dose. *Maximum:* 40 mg/day.

Mechanism of Action
Selectively blocks serotonin and dopamine receptors in the mesocortical tract of the CNS, thereby suppressing psychotic symptoms.

Incompatibilities
Don't mix injection form with drugs or solvents other than sterile water for injection.

Contraindications
Concomitant use of other drugs that prolong QT interval, history of arrhythmia, hypersensitivity to ziprasidone or its components, known history of QT-interval prolongation, recent acute MI, uncompensated heart failure

Interactions
DRUGS
antihypertensives: Additive antihypertensive effects
carbamazepine: Possibly decreased blood ziprasidone level
CNS depressants: Increased CNS depressant effects
dopamine agonists, levodopa: Decreased therapeutic effects of these drugs
drugs that prolong QT interval (including quinidine, dofetilide, pimozide, sotalol, thioridazine, and sparfloxacin): Increased risk of prolonged QT or QTc interval, torsades de pointes, and sudden death
ketoconazole: Possibly increased blood ziprasidone level
FOODS
all foods: Increased ziprasidone absorption

Adverse Reactions
CNS: Agitation, akathisia, amnesia, anxiety, asthenia, dizziness, dystonia, extrapyramidal reactions, headache, hypertonia, insomnia, neuroleptic malignant syndrome, paresthesia, personality or speech disorder, somnolence, tremor
CV: Bradycardia, hypertension, orthostatic hypotension, prolonged QT or QTc interval, vasodilation
EENT: Abnormal vision, dry mouth, increased salivation, rhinitis
ENDO: Dysmenorrhea

X
Y
Z

GI: Abdominal pain, anorexia, constipation, diarrhea, dyspepsia, dysphagia, indigestion, nausea, rectal bleeding, vomiting
MS: Arthralgia, back pain, dysarthria
RESP: Cough, upper respiratory tract infection
SKIN: Furunculosis, rash, sweating
Other: Accidental injury, flulike syndrome, injection site pain, weight gain

Nursing Considerations

•Protect ziprasidone injection vials from light. Reconstitute injection form by adding 1.2 ml of sterile water for injection to vial and shaking vigorously until all of drug is dissolved. Each ml of reconstituted solution contains 20 mg ziprasidone. Discard any unused portion. Administer only by I.M. route.
•Store reconstituted drug for 24 hours protected from light; if refrigerated, drug may be stored for up to 7 days protected from light.
•Administer I.M. form cautiously to patients with impaired renal function.
•**WARNING** Assess for abnormal cardiac rhythm in patients with hypokalemia or hypomagnesemia. Be aware that such symptoms as dizziness, palpitations, and syncope may indicate life-threatening torsades de pointes in these patients. Be prepared to discontinue ziprasidone in patients whose QTc interval is greater than 500 msec.
•Monitor patient, especially elderly females, for involuntary dyskinetic movements, which may progress to irreversible tardive dyskinesia. If symptoms develop, notify prescriber immediately and be prepared to discontinue drug.
•Monitor patient for signs and symptoms of neuroleptic malignant syndrome, a rare but potentially fatal adverse reaction. Signs and symptoms include hyperpyrexia, muscle rigidity, altered mental status, irregular pulse, blood pressure changes, tachycardia, diaphoresis, arrhythmia, myoglobinuria (rhabdomyolysis), and acute renal failure. Notify prescriber immediately if patient develops any of these signs or symptoms.

PATIENT TEACHING
•Instruct patient to take ziprasidone with food to increase drug's absorption.
•Advise patient to avoid potentially hazardous activities until drug's CNS effects are known.
•Instruct patient to rise slowly from seated or lying position to minimize effects of orthostatic hypotension.

zoledronic acid

Zometa

Class and Category

Chemical: Bisphosphonate
Therapeutic: Antihypercalcemic, bone resorption inhibitor
Pregnancy category: D

Indications and Dosages

➤ *To treat hypercalcemia caused by cancer*
I.V. INFUSION
Adults. 4 mg infused over at least 15 min. After 7 days, retreatment with 4 mg if serum calcium level doesn't remain at or return to normal. *Maximum:* 4 mg/dose.

➤ *As adjunct treatment for patients with multiple myeloma or bony metastasis who are receiving standard antineoplastic therapy*
I.V. INFUSION
Adults. 4 mg infused over at least 15 min q 3 to 4 wk.

Mechanism of Action

Inhibits osteoclastic bone resorption and induces osteoclast cellular breakdown. By binding to bone, zoledronic acid also blocks the osteoclastic resorption of mineralized bone and cartilage. Hypercalcemia from cancer is caused by osteoclastic hyperactivity that leads to excessive bone resorption. As bone is resorbed, excessive amounts of calcium are released into the blood, which results in polyuria, GI disturbances, progressive dehydration, and a decreasing glomerular filtration rate. This, in turn, results in increased renal resorption of calcium, setting up a cycle of worsening hypercalcemia. Zoledronic acid interrupts this process.

Incompatibilities

Don't mix zoledronic acid with calcium-containing I.V. solutions, such as lactated Ringer's solution.

Contraindications

Hypersensitivity to zoledronic acid, other bisphosphonates, or their components

Interactions

DRUGS
aminoglycosides: Possibly additive serum calcium–lowering effect
loop diuretics, such as furosemide: Possibly increased risk of hypocalcemia

Adverse Reactions

CNS: Chills, fever

EENT: Conjunctivitis
GI: Nausea, vomiting
GU: Elevated serum creatinine level
MS: Arthralgia, myalgia
Other: Hypocalcemia, hypomagnesemia, hypophosphatemia, infusion site redness and swelling

Nursing Considerations
• Be aware that zoledronic acid isn't indicated to treat hypercalcemia from hyperparathyroidism or other non-tumor-related conditions.
• Expect to aggressively hydrate hypercalcemic patient with I.V. NS before and throughout zoledronic acid therapy, as prescribed, to achieve and maintain a urine output of about 2 L/day.
• **WARNING** During hydration, frequently monitor fluid intake and output and assess patient, especially one with heart failure, for life-threatening signs and symptoms of overhydration.
• Reconstitute zoledronic acid by adding 5 ml of sterile water for injection to drug vial to yield a solution that contains 4 mg of zoledronic acid. Be sure that drug is completely dissolved before withdrawing it. Further dilute drug in 100 ml of NS and infuse over no less than 15 minutes.
• Before giving drug, inspect the reconstituted and diluted solution and discard if particles or discoloration are present.
• Refrigerate reconstituted drug at 2° to 8° C (36° to 46° F) and discard it after 24 hours.
• Administer drug as a single I.V. solution in a separate I.V. line.
• **WARNING** Be aware that a single dose of zoledronic acid shouldn't exceed 4 mg and shouldn't be infused over less than 15 minutes because this may lead to significant renal function deterioration, which may progress to renal failure.
• **WARNING** Assess patient's renal status, including renal function test results, as ordered, before and during zoledronic acid therapy to detect deterioration in renal function. For patient with a normal serum creatinine level who develops an increase of 0.5 mg/dl within 2 weeks of receiving drug, expect to withhold next dose until serum creatinine level is within 10% of patient's baseline value. For patient with an abnormal serum creatinine level who develops an increase of 1.0 mg/dl within 2 weeks of receiving drug, expect to

withhold next dose until serum creatinine level is within 10% of patient's baseline value.
• Monitor serum calcium, magnesium, and phosphate levels, as ordered, throughout zoledronic acid therapy. If hypocalcemia, hypomagnesemia, or hypophosphatemia occurs, expect to administer appropriate short-term supplemental therapy, as prescribed.
• Assess aspirin-sensitive asthma patients for worsening of respiratory symptoms during zoledronic acid therapy because other bisphosphonates have caused bronchoconstriction in these patients.
• Store drug at 25° C (77° F).
PATIENT TEACHING
• Teach patient the importance of consuming a nutritious diet, including adequate amounts of calcium and vitamin D.
• Advise patient to alert prescriber about muscle or bone pain.

zolmitriptan
Zomig, Zomig ZMT

Class and Category
Chemical: Selective 5-hydroxytryptamine agonist
Therapeutic: Antimigraine
Pregnancy category: C

Indications and Dosages
➤ *To treat acute migraine headache with or without aura*
DISINTEGRATING TABLETS
Adults. 2.5 mg, repeated q 2 hr p.r.n. *Maximum:* 10 mg in 24 hr or 3 headaches/mo.
TABLETS
Adults. 2.5 mg or less, repeated q 2 hr p.r.n. *Maximum:* 10 mg in 24 hr or 3 headaches/mo.
DOSAGE ADJUSTMENT Dosage reduced for patients with hepatic impairment.

Mechanism of Action
Binds to receptors on intracranial blood vessels and sensory nerves in the trigeminal-vascular system to stimulate negative feedback, which halts the release of serotonin. In this way, zolmitriptan selectively constricts inflamed and dilated cranial blood vessels in the carotid circulation and inhibits the production of proinflammatory neuropeptides.

X
Y
Z

[]

Contraindications

Basilar or hemiplegic migraine, cardiovascular disease, concurrent use of ergotamine-containing drugs, hypersensitivity to zolmitriptan or its components, ischemic heart disease, Prinzmetal's angina, symptomatic Wolff-Parkinson-White syndrome or other accessory pathway conduction disorder, use of another 5-hydroxytryptamine agonist within past 24 hours, use within 14 days of MAO inhibitor therapy

Interactions
DRUGS

acetaminophen: Delayed peak effect of acetaminophen (by 1 hour)
cimetidine: Prolonged zolmitriptan half-life
ergot alkaloids: Prolonged vasoconstriction
fluoxetine, fluvoxamine, paroxetine, sertraline: Hyperreflexia, lack of coordination, and weakness
MAO inhibitors: Increased zolmitriptan effects
naratriptan, rizatriptan, sumatriptan: Prolonged zolmitriptan effects
oral contraceptives, propranolol: Increased blood zolmitriptan level

Adverse Reactions

CNS: Asthenia, dizziness, hyperesthesia, paresthesia, somnolence, vertigo
CV: Angina, hypertension, palpitations
EENT: Dry mouth
GI: Dysphagia, indigestion, nausea, vomiting
MS: Myalgia; myasthenia; pain, pressure, or tightness in jaw, neck, or throat
SKIN: Diaphoresis, flushing

Nursing Considerations

•WARNING Expect an increased risk of vasoconstriction, which may lead to vascular and colonic ischemia with abdominal pain and bloody diarrhea, especially if patient has peripheral vascular disease (including Raynaud's phenomenon) or ischemic bowel disease.
•Monitor elderly patients and those with hepatic impairment for hypertension. If blood pressure rises significantly, notify prescriber immediately.
PATIENT TEACHING
•Instruct patient to consult prescriber before using zolmitriptan to treat more than three headaches in 30 days.
•Advise patient not to remove disintegrating tablet from blister pack until just before use. Instruct her to peel open pack, place disintegrating tablet on her tongue to dissolve it, and then swallow it with saliva.

zolpidem

Ambien

Class, Category, and Schedule

Chemical: Imidazopyrine derivative
Therapeutic: Antianxiety, sedative-hypnotic
Pregnancy category: B
Controlled substance: Schedule IV

Indications and Dosages

➤ *To provide short-term treatment of insomnia*
TABLETS
Adults. 10 mg h.s. for 7 to 10 days. *Maximum:* 20 mg/day.
DOSAGE ADJUSTMENT For elderly or debilitated patients and those with hepatic impairment, dosage possibly reduced to 5 mg h.s., with a maximum of 5 mg/day for nursing facility residents.

> ### Mechanism of Action
> May potentiate the effects of GABA and other inhibitory neurotransmitters. Zolpidem binds to specific benzodiazepine receptor sites in the limbic and cortical areas of the CNS. By binding to these receptor sites, zolpidem increases GABA's inhibitory effects and blocks cortical and limbic arousal and preserves deep sleep (stages 3 and 4).

Contraindications

Hypersensitivity to zolpidem or its components, ritonavir therapy

Interactions
DRUGS

azole antifungals: Increased CNS activity and additive adverse effects of zolpidem
barbiturates, chlorpromazine, general anesthetics, opioid agonists, other CNS depressants, phenothiazines, tramadol, tricyclic antidepressants: Possibly increased CNS depression and reduced psychomotor function
bupropion: Increased blood zolpidem level, possibly visual hallucinations and loss of alertness
desipramine, imipramine: Increased risk of visual hallucinations and reduced alertness
flumazenil: Antagonized sedative effect of zolpidem

haloperidol: Increased CNS depression
nevirapine: Decreased blood zolpidem level
rifabutin, rifampin: Increased zolpidem clearance
selective serotonin-reuptake inhibitors: Increased risk of delusions, disorientation, and hallucinations

FOODS
all foods: Increased time to peak blood zolpidem level, decreased effects of zolpidem

ACTIVITIES
alcohol use: Increased CNS depression

Adverse Reactions
CNS: Amnesia, dizziness, drowsiness, headache, lethargy, paradoxical CNS stimulation (including agitation, euphoria, hallucinations, hyperactivity, and nightmares)
GI: Constipation, diarrhea, indigestion, nausea, vomiting
Other: Withdrawal symptoms

Nursing Considerations
•Administer zolpidem just before bedtime because drug has a rapid onset of action.
•Expect patient to receive no more than a 1-month supply of drug for outpatient therapy.
•**WARNING** If zolpidem is withdrawn abruptly (especially after prolonged therapy), monitor for withdrawal symptoms, such as abdominal cramps or discomfort, fatigue, flushing, inconsolable crying, light-headedness, nausea, nervousness, panic attack, rebound insomnia, and vomiting.
•Expect drug to produce anticonvulsant and muscle relaxant effects at high doses.
•If patient receives other CNS depressants, expect to administer reduced zolpidem dosage, as prescribed.

PATIENT TEACHING
•Caution patient to take drug exactly as prescribed and not to increase dosage unless directed by prescriber.
•Instruct patient to take zolpidem immediately before bedtime on an empty stomach.
•Advise patient to notify prescriber immediately about abdominal cramps or discomfort, fatigue, flushing, inconsolable crying, light-headedness, nausea, nervousness, panic attack, and vomiting.

zonisamide
Zonegran

Class and Category
Chemical: Benzisoxazole derivative, sulfonamide
Therapeutic: Anticonvulsant
Pregnancy category: C

Indications and Dosages
➤ *As adjunct to treat partial seizures*
CAPSULES
Adults. *Initial:* 100 mg q.d. Dosage increased by 100 mg/day q 2 wk, as needed. *Usual:* 200 to 400 mg/day. *Maximum:* 600 mg/day.

Mechanism of Action
May stop the spread of seizures and suppress their foci by blocking sodium channels and reducing voltage-dependent, inward currents from calcium channels. This action stabilizes neuronal membranes and suppresses synchronized neuronal hyperactivity.

Contraindications
Hypersensitivity to sulfonamides, zonisamide, or their components

Interactions
DRUGS
carbamazepine, phenobarbital, phenytoin, valproate: Possibly decreased blood zonisamide level
CNS depressants: Additive CNS depressant effects
FOODS
grapefruit juice: Possibly decreased metabolism of zonisamide

Adverse Reactions
CNS: Agitation, ataxia, dizziness, irritability, somnolence
GI: Anorexia

Nursing Considerations
•**WARNING** Monitor results of CBC and other laboratory tests for signs of blood dyscrasias because zonisamide is a sulfonamide and can be absorbed systemically. Systemic absorption may result in life-threatening reactions, including toxic epidermal necrolysis, Stevens-Johnson syndrome, fulminant hepatic necrosis, agranulocytosis, aplastic anemia, and other blood dyscrasias.
•Be aware that patients receiving doses of 300 mg/day or more are at increased risk for

X
Y
Z

adverse CNS reactions, including decreased concentration, fatigue, drowsiness, and impaired speech.

• Monitor serum creatinine and BUN levels for signs of abnormally decreased glomerular filtration rate (GFR). Expect some decrease in GFR during first 4 weeks of treatment and a return to baseline within 2 to 3 weeks after drug is discontinued.

• Monitor patient for signs and symptoms of renal calculi.

• Be aware that zonisamide should not be discontinued abruptly because doing so may increase the frequency of seizures.

PATIENT TEACHING

• Inform patient that zonisamide is usually prescribed with other anticonvulsants and that she should continue to take all drugs as prescribed.

• Instruct patient to swallow capsules whole, and not to chew them or break them open.

• Inform patient that prescriber may have to adjust dosage over several weeks or months before a stable dose is achieved.

• Advise patient to use caution when driving or performing other activities that require mental alertness because zonisamide commonly causes somnolence, dizziness, and decreased concentration, particularly during first month of therapy.

• Advise patient to wear a medical identification bracelet or necklace with information about her seizure disorder.

• Unless contraindicated, encourage patient to drink 6 to 8 glasses of water each day to prevent kidney stones.

• Advise patient to rise slowly from a lying or seated position to reduce the risk of dizziness.

Appendices

Oral Antidiabetic Combinations

Oral antidiabetic drugs are prescribed, along with life-style changes such as diet and exercise, to manage type 2 diabetes mellitus. A combination of two different types of oral antidiabetic drugs may be prescribed to simplify a patient's drug regimen, enhance drug actions, and, ultimately, provide a patient with better control of his blood glucose level.

The following chart lists the generic and trade names of oral antidiabetic combination drugs, the usual adult dosages for use as monotherapy, and the usual adult dosages for use with patients whose blood glucose levels aren't adequately controlled with one oral antidiabetic drug taken by itself.

Further information about the mechanisms of action, interactions, adverse reactions, and nursing considerations can be found for the specific oral antidiabetic drugs in the alphabetical drug monographs.

GENERIC AND TRADE NAMES AND CHEMICAL CLASSES	USUAL ADULT DOSAGE AS INITIAL THERAPY	USUAL ADULT DOSAGE WHEN PREVIOUS THERAPY HAS FAILED
glipizide and metformin hydrochloride METAGLIP *Chemical:* Sulfonylurea (glipizide), dimethylbiguanide (metformin)	*Initial:* For blood glucose levels less than 280 mg/dL, 2.5 mg/250 mg tab q.d. with a meal; for blood glucose levels of 280 to 320 mg/dL, 2.5 mg/500 mg tab b.i.d. with meals. Dosage increased by one tab/day q 2 wk, as needed and prescribed. *Maximum:* 10 mg/1000mg or 10 mg/2000 mg daily in divided doses.	*Initial:* 2.5 mg/500 mg or 5 mg/500 mg b.i.d. with morning and evening meals (starting dosage shouldn't exceed daily doses of glipizide or metformin already being taken). Dosage increased in increments of no more than 5 mg/500 mg. *Maximum:* 20 mg/2,000 mg daily.
glyburide and metformin hydrochloride Glucovance *Chemical:* Sulfonylurea (glyburide), dimethylbiguanide (metformin)	*Initial:* 1.25 mg/250 mg tab q.d. or b.i.d. Dosage increased by 1.25 mg/250 mg/day q 2 wk, as needed.	*Initial:* 2.5 mg/500 mg tab or 5 mg/500 mg tab b.i.d. Dosage increased, as prescribed, by 5 mg/500 mg/day. *Maximum:* 20 mg/2,000 mg daily.
rosiglitazone maleate and metformin hydrochloride Avandamet *Chemical:* Thiazolidinedione (rosiglitazone), dimethylbiguanide (metformin)	Safety and efficacy as initial therapy hasn't been established.	•If previous metformin dose was 1,000 mg/day, give 1 tab of 2 mg/500 mg b.i.d., as prescribed. •If previous metformin dose was 1,000 to 2,000 mg, dosage must be individualized. •If previous metformin dose was 2,000 mg/day, give 2 tabs of 1 mg/500 mg b.i.d., as prescribed. •If previous rosiglitazone dose was 4 mg/day, give 1 tab of 2 mg/500 mg b.i.d., as prescribed. •If previous rosiglitazone was 8 mg/day, give 1 tab of 4 mg/500 mg b.i.d. •Dosage adjustment required when switching from existing combination therapy.*

* When switching from combination of rosiglitazone and metformin as separate tablets, usual starting dose is the dose of rosiglitazone and metformin already being taken. For additional blood glucose control, daily dose may be increased in increments of 4 mg rosiglitazone and/or 500 mg metformin, up to maximum daily dose of 8 mg/2,000 mg.

Insulin Preparations

For each category of insulin, the following chart lists the species; common trade names; onset, peak, and duration; and key nursing considerations.

CATEGORY, SPECIES, AND TRADE NAMES	KEY NURSING CONSIDERATIONS

Rapid-acting insulin

Onset: 15 min **Peak:** 30 to 90 min **Duration:** In 6 hr

Human •Humalog •NovoLog (insulin aspart)	•Mix rapid-acting insulin with other insulin types, if needed. Administer immediately after mixing. •When mixing rapid-acting insulin with a longer-acting insulin, always draw the rapid-acting insulin into the syringe first to avoid dosage errors. •Administer only by the S.C. route, up to 15 minutes (for Humalog) or 5 to 10 minutes (for NovoLog) before a meal. •Be aware that 1 U of rapid-acting insulin has the same glucose-lowering ability as 1 U of short-acting insulin. •Be aware that rapid-acting insulin is available as a cartridge for use with the B-D Pen, NovoPen, NovoPen 1.5, or NovolinPen. •Be aware that the absorption rate of rapid-acting insulin may slow when this type of insulin is mixed in a syringe with human isophane insulin (NPH). Monitor the blood glucose level frequently.

Short-acting insulin

Onset: 30 min **Peak:** 2 to 5 hr **Duration:** 6 to 8 hr

Human •Humulin R •Humulin-R (CAN) •Humulin R (concentrated), U-500 •Novolin ge Toronto (CAN) •Novolin ge Toronto Penfill (CAN) •Novolin R •Novolin R PenFill •Novolin R Prefilled •Velosulin BR •Velosulin Human (CAN) Pork •Regular Iletin II •Regular (concentrated), Iletin II, U-500 •Regular Insulin (pork) •Regular Insulin (purified pork)	•Don't use short-acting insulin if it's cloudy, discolored, or unusually viscous. •Use the U-500 strength to treat insulin resistance, as prescribed. •Mix short-acting insulin with other insulin types, if needed. However, don't mix phosphate-buffered insulin with a zinc-containing insulin because the short-acting insulin's effectiveness may be reduced. •Administer by the S.C., I.M., or I.V. route, as prescribed. Use a continuous S.C. infusion pump, if ordered. For an insulin pump, phosphate-buffered insulin is preferred over nonphosphate-buffered insulin. The catheter tubing and reservoir insulin should be changed every 48 hours or as specified by the pump manufacturer. •When administering S.C. or I.M. injections, give the short-acting insulin 15 to 30 minutes before a meal or bedtime snack.

(continued on page 918)

Insulin Preparations (continued)

CATEGORY, SPECIES, AND TRADE NAMES	KEY NURSING CONSIDERATIONS

Intermediate-acting insulin

Onset: 1 to 3 hr **Peak:** 4 to 15 hr **Duration:** 18 to 24 hr

Human
•Humulin L
•Humulin-L (CAN)
•Humulin N
•Humulin-N (CAN)
•Novolin ge Lente (CAN)
•Novolin ge NPH (CAN)
•Novolin ge NPH Penfill (CAN)
•Novolin L
•Novolin N
•Novolin N PenFill
•Novolin N Prefilled
Pork
•Lente (purified pork)
•Lente Iletin II (purified pork)
•Lente Iletin II (pork) (CAN)
•NPH Iletin II
Beef and pork
•Lente Iletin (CAN)
•NPH Iletin (CAN)

•Don't use intermediate-acting insulin if it contains precipitate that is clumped or granular or that clings to the sides of the vial.
•Roll the vial gently between your palms to mix; don't shake it. Also gently turn the prefilled syringe up and down several times before using to achieve a uniform mixture.
•Administer by S.C. injection only, 30 minutes before a meal or bedtime snack.
•Be aware that intermediate-acting insulin rarely produces a blood glucose level that's as close to normal as possible. So expect to mix it with a short-acting insulin, as prescribed, for optimum blood glucose control.

Long-acting insulin

Onset: 4 to 6 hr **Peak:** 8 to 20 hr **Duration:** 24 to 28 hr

Human
•Humulin U Ultralente
•Humulin-U (CAN)
•Lantus (insulin glargine)
•Novolin ge Ultralente (CAN)

•Don't use long-acting insulin if it contains precipitate that is clumped or granular or that clings to the sides of the vial.
•As prescribed, mix long-acting insulin with other insulin types—usually a short-acting insulin—if needed. Be aware that Lantus must not be diluted or mixed with another insulin or solution and that the drug is slowly released over 24 hours (maintaining a relatively constant blood level). It has a slower onset of action and no pronounced peak.
•Roll the vial gently between your palms to obtain a uniform mixture; don't shake it.
•Administer by the S.C. route only, 30 to 60 minutes before a meal or bedtime snack.

Combination insulins

Onset: 30 min **Peak:** 2 to 12 hr **Duration:** 18 to 24 hr

Human
•Humalog Mix 75/25 Pen
•Humulin 10/90 (CAN)
•Humulin 20/80 (CAN)
•Humulin 30/70 (CAN)
•Humulin 40/60 (CAN)

•Don't use combination insulin if it contains precipitate that is clumped or granular.
•Roll the vial gently between your palms to mix; don't shake it. Also gently turn the prefilled syringe up and down several times before using to achieve a uniform mixture.

Insulin Preparations (continued)

CATEGORY, SPECIES, AND TRADE NAMES	KEY NURSING CONSIDERATIONS

Combination insulins (continued)

Onset: 30 min **Peak:** 2 to 12 hr **Duration:** 18 to 24 hr *(continued)*

Human *(continued)*
•Humulin 50/50
•Humulin 70/30
•Novolin 70/30
•Novolin 70/30 PenFill
•Novolin 70/30 Prefilled
•Novolin ge 10/90 Penfill (CAN)
•Novolin ge 20/80 Penfill (CAN)
•Novolin ge 30/70 (CAN)
•Novolin ge 30/70 Penfill (CAN)
•Novolin ge 40/60 Penfill (CAN)
•Novolin ge 50/50 Penfill (CAN)

•Administer combination insulin by the S.C. route only, 30 minutes before a meal.
•Be aware that Canadian and American products contain the same insulin ratio but express it differently. For example, the Canadian Humulin 30/70 and the American Humulin 70/30 both contain 30 units of a short-acting insulin and 70 units of an intermediate-acting insulin. Canadian products list the short-acting insulin first; American products list it second.

Nasal, Ophthalmic, and Otic Drugs

Although less commonly prescribed than oral drugs, drugs instilled into the nostrils, eyes, or ears are frequently brought into the clinical setting by patients with chronic conditions. In most cases, the patient or a family member has administered these preparations at home. Your patient teaching should include a review of proper administration and storage of these drugs. Have the patient or a family member demonstrate proper use of the drug to make sure it will be administered correctly at home. Use this time to reassess the patient's ability to continue self-medication. Also, instruct him to report any changes in the condition being treated, either negative or positive. A properly educated patient not only ensures safe drug administration, but also is more likely to detect adverse reactions that require a dosage reduction or drug discontinuation, thus preventing the development of more serious health problems.

The following chart lists the generic and trade names, FDA-approved indications, and usual adult dosages for those nasal, ophthalmic, and otic preparations you're most likely to see in your practice setting. The drugs are divided according to administration route, and the ophthalmic drugs are further subdivided according to therapeutic use.

GENERIC AND TRADE NAMES	INDICATIONS	USUAL ADULT DOSAGES
Nasal drugs		
beclomethasone dipropionate Beconase, Vancenase, Vancenase Pockethaler **beclomethasone dipropionate mono-hydrate nasal suspension** Beconase AQ, Vancenase AQ	To treat nasal inflammation	0.042 to 0.05 mg (1 metered spray) in each nostril b.i.d. to q.i.d. (solution), or 0.042 to 0.1 mg (1 or 2 metered sprays) in each nostril q.d. to b.i.d. (suspension)
budesonide nasal aerosol Rhinocort	To treat nasal inflammation	0.064 mg (2 metered sprays) in each nostril b.i.d., or 0.128 mg (4 metered sprays) in each nostril q.d.
budesonide nasal spray Rhinocort Aqua	To treat nasal inflammation	0.032 mg (1 metered spray) in each nostril q.d.
dexamethasone sodium phosphate nasal aerosol Dexacort Turbinaire	To treat nasal inflammation	0.2 mg (2 metered sprays) in each nostril b.i.d. to t.i.d.
ephedrine sulfate Pretz-D, Vicks Vatronol	To treat nasal congestion	2 or 3 gtt of solution in each nostril q 4 hr p.r.n.
flunisolide nasal solution Nasalide, Nasarel, Rhinalar (CAN)	To treat nasal inflammation	0.05 mg (2 metered sprays) in each nostril b.i.d. to t.i.d.
fluticasone propionate nasal suspension Flonase	To treat nasal inflammation	0.1 mg (2 metered sprays) in each nostril q.d., or 0.05 mg (1 metered spray) in each nostril b.i.d.

Nasal, Ophthalmic, and Otic Drugs (continued)

GENERIC AND TRADE NAMES	INDICATIONS	USUAL ADULT DOSAGES
Nasal drugs (continued)		
mometasone furoate nasal suspension Nasonex	To treat nasal inflammation	0.1 mg (2 metered sprays) in each nostril q.d., tapered to 0.05 mg (1 metered spray) q.d.
naphazoline hydrochloride Privine	To treat nasal inflammation	1 or 2 gtt or sprays in each nostril at least 6 hr apart
oxymetazoline hydrochloride Afrin, Allerest 12 Hour Nasal Spray, Chlorphed-LA, Dristan Long Lasting, Duramist Plus, Duration, 4-Way Long Lasting Spray, Genasal Spray, NeoSynephrine 12 Hour Nasal Spray, Nostrilla, NTZ Long Acting Decongestant Nasal Spray, Sinarest 12 Hour Nasal	To treat nasal inflammation	2 or 3 gtt or sprays in each nostril b.i.d.
phenylephrine hydrochloride Alconefrin Nasal Drops 12, Alconefrin Nasal Drops 25, Alconefrin Nasal Drops 50, Doktors, Duration, Neo-Synephrine, Nostril, Rhinall, Sinex	To treat nasal inflammation	2 or 3 gtt or 1 or 2 sprays in each nostril q 4 hr p.r.n. up to 5 days
triamcinolone acetonide Nasacort	To treat nasal inflammation	0.11 mg (2 metered sprays) in each nostril q.d., tapered to 0.055 mg (1 metered spray) in each nostril q.d.
triamcinolone acetonide nasal spray Tri-Nasal Spray	To treat nasal inflammation	0.1 mg (2 metered sprays) in each nostril q.d.
triamcinolone nasal suspension Nasacort AQ	To treat nasal inflammation	0.11 mg (2 metered sprays) in each nostril q.d., tapered to 0.055 mg (1 metered spray) in each nostril q.d.

(continued on page 922)

Nasal, Ophthalmic, and Otic Drugs (continued)

GENERIC AND TRADE NAMES	INDICATIONS	USUAL ADULT DOSAGES
Nasal drugs *(continued)*		
xylometazoline hydrochloride Decongest Nasal Spray (CAN), Inspire Nasal Spray, Inspire Nasal Spray M-D Pump, Otrivin Nasal Spray	To treat nasal congestion	2 or 3 gtt or sprays in each nostril q 8 to 10 hr p.r.n.
Ophthalmic antibiotics		
bacitracin AK-Tracin	To treat surface bacterial infections affecting the conjunctiva and cornea	Small amount of ointment applied to conjunctival sac p.r.n.
chloramphenicol AK-Chlor, Chloromycetin, Chloroptic, Chloroptic S.O.P., Diochloram, Dioptic (CAN), Pentamycetin (CAN), Sopamycetin (CAN)	To treat surface bacterial infections affecting the conjunctiva and cornea	1 or 2 gtt in eye q 3 to 6 hr and p.r.n.; or small amount of ointment applied to lower conjunctival sac q 3 to 6 hr and p.r.n. for at least 48 hr after eye resumes normal appearance
ciprofloxacin hydrochloride Ciloxan	To treat corneal ulcers due to *Pseudomonas aeruginosa, Staphylococcus aureus, Staphylococcus epidermidis, Streptococcus pneumoniae,* and possibly *Serratia marcescens* and *Streptococcus viridans*	2 gtt in affected eye q 15 min for first 6 hr, then 2 gtt q 30 min for remainder of first day; on day 2, 2 gtt in affected eye q 1 hr; on days 3 to 14, 2 gtt in affected eye q 4 hr
	To treat bacterial conjunctivitis due to *Haemophilus influenzae, S. aureus, S. epidermidis,* and possibly *S. pneumoniae*	1 or 2 gtt in conjunctival sac of affected eye q 2 hr while awake for first 2 days, then 1 or 2 gtt q 4 hr while awake for next 5 days; or ½-inch strip of ointment applied in affected eye t.i.d. for 2 days, then b.i.d. for next 5 days
erythromycin Ilotycin	To treat acute or chronic conjunctivitis and other eye infections	1 cm of ointment applied in infected eye up to 6 times/day, depending on severity of infection
	To treat chlamydial ophthalmic infections (trachoma)	Small amount applied in each eye b.i.d. for 2 mo; or b.i.d. on first 5 days of each month for 6 mo

Nasal, Ophthalmic, and Otic Drugs *(continued)*

GENERIC AND TRADE NAMES	INDICATIONS	USUAL ADULT DOSAGES
Ophthalmic antibiotics *(continued)*		
gentamicin sulfate Garamycin, Genoptic, Gentacidin, Gentak	To treat blepharitis, blepharoconjunctivitis, conjunctivitis, corneal ulcers, dacryocystitis, keratoconjunctivitis, or meibomianitis due to susceptible organisms	1 or 2 gtt in eye q 4 hr or, for severe infection, up to 2 gtt/hr; alternatively, ointment applied to lower conjunctival sac b.i.d. or t.i.d.
levofloxacin 0.5% Quixin	To treat bacterial conjunctivitis	On days 1 and 2: 1 or 2 gtt in affected eye q 2 hr while awake, up to 8 times/day; on days 3 to 7: 1 or 2 gtt in affected eye q 4 hr while awake, up to 4 times/day
norfloxacin Chibroxin	To treat superficial ocular infections involving the conjunctiva or cornea due to susceptible microorganisms	1 gtt 4 times/day for up to 7 days
ofloxacin 0.3% Ocuflox	To treat conjunctivitis due to *Staphylococcus aureus, Staphylococcus epidermidis, Streptococcus pneumoniae, Enterobacter cloacae, Haemophilus influenzae, Proteus mirabilis, Pseudomonas aeruginosa,* and *Propionibacterium acnes*	1 or 2 gtt in conjunctival sac q 2 to 4 hr while awake for first 2 days, then 1 gtt q.i.d. for up to 5 more days
	To treat bacterial corneal ulcers due to *S. aureus, S. epidermidis, S. pneumoniae, E. cloacae, H. influenzae, P. mirabilis, P. aeruginosa, Serratia marcescens,* and *P. acnes*	1 or 2 gtt q 30 min while awake and 1 or 2 gtt 4 to 6 hr after retiring for 2 days; then 1 or 2 gtt/hr while awake for up to 7 more days; then 1 gtt q.i.d. from 7th, 8th, or 9th day until end of treatment
polymyxin B sulfate	To treat superficial eye infections involving the conjunctiva or cornea caused by *Pseudomonas* or other gram-negative organisms	1 to 3 gtt of 0.1% to 0.25% (10,000 to 25,000 U/ml) q 1 hr; or up to 10,000 U in lower conjunctival sac q.d.

(continued on page 924)

Nasal, Ophthalmic, and Otic Drugs (continued)

GENERIC AND TRADE NAMES	INDICATIONS	USUAL ADULT DOSAGES
Ophthalmic antibiotics *(continued)*		
sulfacetamide sodium 10% AK-Sulf, Bleph-10, Ocusulf-10, Sodium Sulamyd 10%, Sulf-10 **sulfacetamide sodium 15%** Isopto Cetamide **sulfacetamide sodium 30%** Sodium Sulamyd 30%	To treat inclusion conjunctivitis, corneal ulcers, and chlamydial infections	1 or 2 gtt solution (10%) in lower conjunctival sac q 2 to 3 hr during day, less often at night; or 1 or 2 gtt (15%) in lower conjunctival sac q 1 to 2 hr; or 1 gtt (30%) in lower conjunctival sac q 2 hr; or 1.25 to 2.5 cm ointment (10%) into conjunctival sac q.i.d. and h.s.
	To treat trachoma	2 gtt (30%) in lower conjunctival sac q 2 hr in combination with systemic sulfonamide or tetracycline
tobramycin AKTob, Tobrex	To treat superficial ocular infections involving the conjunctiva or cornea	1 gtt q 1 to 4 hr, depending on severity of infection; or thin strip of ointment applied to lower conjunctival sac q 8 to 12 hr for mild to moderate infections or q 3 to 4 hr for severe infections
Ophthalmic anti-inflammatory drugs		
dexamethasone Maxidex **dexamethasone sodium phosphate** AK-Dex, Boldex, Dexair, R.O. Dexasone (CAN)	To treat allergic conjunctivitis; corneal injury from chemical or thermal burns or from penetration of foreign bodies; inflammatory conditions of the anterior segment of globe, conjunctiva, cornea, or eyelids; iridocyclitis; suppression of graft rejection after keratoplasty; and uveitis	1 or 2 gtt of suspension or solution or 1.25 to 2.5 cm of ointment in conjunctival sac from q 1 hr (in severe disease) to 6 times/day; or ointment may be applied t.i.d. or q.i.d., then tapered to b.i.d., and then q.d.
diclofenac sodium 0.1% Voltaren, Voltaren Ophtha (CAN)	To treat postoperative inflammation after removal of cataract	1 gtt in conjunctival sac q.i.d., beginning 24 hr after surgery and continuing through first 2 wk of postoperative period
	To treat photophobia in incisional refractive surgery	1 or 2 gtt in operative eye 1 hr before surgery; then 1 or 2 gtt 15 min after surgery, followed by 1 gtt q.i.d., beginning 4 to 6 hr after surgery, for up to 3 days p.r.n.

Nasal, Ophthalmic, and Otic Drugs (continued)

GENERIC AND TRADE NAMES	INDICATIONS	USUAL ADULT DOSAGES
Ophthalmic anti-inflammatory drugs *(continued)*		
fluorometholone Fluor-Op, FML Forte, FML Liquifilm, FML S.O.P. **fluorometholone acetate** Eflone, Flarex	To treat inflammatory and allergic conditions of the anterior uvea, conjunctiva, cornea, or sclera	1 or 2 gtt suspension in conjunctival sac b.i.d. to q.i.d. or, in severe conditions, up to q 2 hr during first 1 to 2 days p.r.n.; or thin strip of ointment applied to conjunctival sac q.d. to t.i.d.
flurbiprofen sodium Ocufen	To inhibit intraoperative miosis	1 gtt in affected eye q 30 min, beginning 2 hr before surgery, up to total of 4 gtt
ketorolac tromethamine Acular	To relieve ocular itching due to seasonal allergic conjunctivitis	1 gtt in conjunctival sac of each eye q.i.d.
	To treat postoperative inflammation in patients who have undergone cataract extraction	1 gtt in operative eye q.i.d., beginning 24 hr after cataract surgery and continuing through first 2 wk of postoperative period
loteprednol etabonate Alrex, Lotemax	To provide temporary relief of seasonal allergic conjunctivitis and to treat steroid-responsive inflammatory conditions of the palpebral and bulbar conjunctiva, cornea, and anterior segment of the globe	1 gtt of 0.2% suspension in affected eyes q.i.d.; or 1 or 2 gtt of 0.5% suspension in conjunctival sac of affected eye q.i.d. up to 1 gtt/hr
	To treat postoperative inflammation following ocular surgery	1 or 2 gtt in conjunctival sac of operated eye q.i.d., beginning 24 hr after surgery and continuing through first 2 wk of postoperative period
medrysone HMS Liquifilm	To treat allergic conjunctivitis, episcleritis, ephinephrine sensitivity, and vernal conjunctivitis	1 gtt into conjunctival sac up to q 4 hr
prednisolone acetate suspension Econopred, Econopred Plus, Pred Forte, Pred Mild **prednisolone sodium phosphate solution** AK-Pred, Inflamase Forte, Inflamase Mild	To treat inflammation of the anterior segment of globe, cornea, and palpebral and bulbar conjunctiva	1 or 2 gtt in conjunctival sac b.i.d. to q.i.d. (suspension) or up to 6 times/day (solution)

(continued on page 926)

Nasal, Ophthalmic, and Otic Drugs (continued)

GENERIC AND TRADE NAMES	INDICATIONS	USUAL ADULT DOSAGES
Ophthalmic anti-inflammatory drugs (continued)		
rimexolone Vexol	To treat anterior uveitis	1 or 2 gtt in conjunctival sac of affected eye q 1 hr while awake in first week; 1 gtt q 2 hr while awake in second week; then tapered until uveitis is resolved
	To treat postoperative inflammation after ocular surgery	1 or 2 gtt in conjunctival sac of affected eye q.i.d., beginning 24 hr after surgery and continuing through first 2 wk of postoperative period
Ophthalmic cycloplegic mydriatics		
atropine sulfate Atropisol, Isopto Atropine, Minims Atropine (CAN)	To treat acute iritis or uveitis	1 gtt up to q.i.d.; or small strip of ointment applied to conjunctival sac up to b.i.d.
	To produce dilation for cycloplegic refraction	1 or 2 gtt of 1% solution 1 hr before refraction
cyclopentolate hydrochloride AK-Pentolate, Cyclogyl, Minims Cyclopentolate (CAN), Pentolair	To produce mydriasis and cycloplegia required in specific diagnostic procedures	1 gtt of 0.5%, 1%, or 2% solution in each eye; then 1 or 2 gtt in 5 to 10 min p.r.n.
homatropine hydrobromide Isopto Homatropine, Minims Homatropine (CAN)	To dilate pupils for cycloplegic refraction	1 or 2 gtt in each eye, repeated in 5 to 10 min for 2 or 3 doses p.r.n.
	To treat uveitis	1 or 2 gtt in each eye q 3 to 4 hr
scopolamine hydrobromide Isopto Hyoscine	To dilate pupils for cycloplegic refraction	1 or 2 gtt of 0.25% solution 1 hr before refraction
	To treat iritis or uveitis	1 or 2 gtt of 0.25% solution q.d. to q.i.d.
tropicamide Mydriacyl, Opticyl, Tropicacyl	To dilate pupils for cycloplegic refraction	1 gtt of 1% solution, repeated in 5 min; additional 1 gtt in 20 to 30 min p.r.n.
Ophthalmic miotics		
acetylcholine chloride Miochol-E	To produce papillary miosis in anterior segment surgery	0.5 to 2 ml gently into anterior chamber before or after sutures secured

Nasal, Ophthalmic, and Otic Drugs (continued)

GENERIC AND TRADE NAMES	INDICATIONS	USUAL ADULT DOSAGES
Ophthalmic miotics (continued)		
carbachol 0.01% Carbastat, Miostat **carbachol 0.75%, 1.5%, 2.25%, 3%** Carboptic, Isopto Carbachol	To produce papillary miosis in ocular surgery To treat open-angle glaucoma	0.5 ml (solution) into anterior chamber before or after sutures secured 1 or 2 gtt up to t.i.d.
pilocarpine Ocusert Pilo	To treat primary open-angle glaucoma	1 or 2 gtt up to q.i.d.; or 1-cm ribbon of 4% gel applied h.s.; or 1 Ocusert Pilo system (20 or 40 mcg/hr) q 7 days
pilocarpine hydrochloride Adsorbocarpine, Akarpine, Isopto Carpine, Miocarpine (CAN), Pilocar, Pilopine HS, Pilostat	To treat acute angle-closure glaucoma as emergency therapy	1 gtt of 2% solution q 5 to 10 min for 3 to 6 doses; then 1 gtt q 1 to 3 hr until pressure is controlled
pilocarpine nitrate Pilagan, P.V. Carpine Liquifilm (CAN)	To treat mydriasis due to mydriatic or cycloplegic drug therapy	1 gtt of 1% solution
Ophthalmic vasoconstrictors		
naphazoline hydrochloride Ak-Con, Albalon Liquifilm, Allerest, Clear Eyes, Comfort Eye Drops, Degest 2, Nafazair, Naphcon, Naphcon Forte, Vasocon Regular	To treat ocular congestion, irritation, or itching	1 gtt of 0.1% solution q 3 to 4 hr; or 1 gtt of 0.012% to 0.03% solution up to q.i.d.
oxymetazoline hydrochloride OcuClear, Visine L.R.	To provide relief from eye redness due to minor eye irritations	1 or 2 gtt in conjunctival sac b.i.d. to q.i.d. (at least 6 hr apart)
phenylephrine hydrochloride Ak-Dilate, Ak-Nefrin, Isopto Frin, Mydfrin, Phenoptic, Prefrin Liquifilm, Relief Eye Drops for Red Eyes	To produce mydriasis without cycloplegia To produce mydriasis and vasoconstriction To treat chronic mydriasis To treat posterior adhesion of iris	1 gtt of 2.5% or 10% solution before eye exam, then repeated in 1 hr p.r.n. 1 gtt of 2.5% or 10% solution as single dose 1 gtt of 2.5% or 10% solution b.i.d. or t.i.d. 1 gtt of 2.5% or 10% solution as single dose

(continued on page 928)

Nasal, Ophthalmic, and Otic Drugs (continued)

GENERIC AND TRADE NAMES	INDICATIONS	USUAL ADULT DOSAGES
Ophthalmic vasoconstrictors *(continued)*		
proparacaine hydrochloride Alcaine, Ophthaine, Ophthetic	To provide deep anesthesia during cataract extraction	1 gtt q 5 to 10 min for 5 to 7 doses
	To provide anesthesia during removal of eye sutures	1 or 2 gtt 2 to 3 min before procedure
	To provide anesthesia during removal of foreign bodies	1 or 2 gtt in affected eye before surgery
	To provide anesthesia during tonometry	1 or 2 gtt immediately before measurement
tetracaine Pontocaine	To provide eye anesthesia (short term)	1 or 2 gtt p.r.n.
tetrahydrozoline hydrochloride Collyrium Fresh Eye Drops, Eyesine, Murine Plus, Optigene 3, Tetrasine, Visine Moisturizing, Visine Extra	To treat conjunctival congestion, irritation, and allergic conditions	1 or 2 gtt of 0.05% solution up to q.i.d. or as directed
Miscellaneous ophthalmic drugs		
apraclonidine hydrochloride Iopidine	To prevent or control elevated intraocular pressure (IOP) before and after ocular laser surgery	1 gtt of 1% solution 1 hr before laser surgery on anterior segment; then 1 drop immediately after surgery
azelastine hydrochloride 0.05% Optivar	To treat itching of the eye associated with allergic conjunctivitis	1 gtt in affected eye b.i.d.
betaxolol hydrochloride Betoptic, Betoptic S	To treat chronic open-angle glaucoma or ocular hypertension	1 or 2 gtt of 0.5% solution or 0.25% suspension b.i.d.
bimatoprost 0.03% Lumigan	To reduce elevated IOP in patients with open-angle glaucoma or ocular hypertension who can't tolerate or have insufficiently responded to other IOP-lowering medications	1 gtt in affected eye q.d. in evening

Nasal, Ophthalmic, and Otic Drugs (continued)

GENERIC AND TRADE NAMES	INDICATIONS	USUAL ADULT DOSAGES
Miscellaneous ophthalmic drugs (continued)		
brimonidine tartrate Alphagan, Alphagan P	To reduce IOP in open-angle glaucoma or ocular hypertension	1 gtt in affected eye t.i.d., about 8 hr apart
carteolol hydrochloride Ocupress	To treat chronic open-angle glaucoma or intraocular hypertension	1 gtt in conjunctival sac of affected eye b.i.d.
dipivefrin hydrochloride Ophto-Dipivefrin (CAN), Propine	To reduce IOP in chronic open-angle glaucoma	1 drop of 0.1% solution q 12 hr
dorzolamide hydrochloride Trusopt	To treat increased IOP in ocular hypertension or open-angle glaucoma	1 gtt in conjunctival sac of affected eye t.i.d.
emedastine difumarate Emadine	To treat allergic conjunctivitis	1 gtt in affected eye up to q.i.d.
fluorescein sodium AK-Fluor, Fluorescite, Fluor-I-Strip, Fluor-I-Strip-A.T., Ful-Glo, Funduscein-10, Funduscein-25, Ophthifluor	To diagnose corneal abrasions and foreign bodies, fit hard contact lenses, determine lacrimal patency, and assist in fundus photography and applanation tonometry	1 or 2 gtt of 2% solution followed by irrigation; or moisten strip with sterile water, then touch conjunctiva or fornix with moistened tip, and flush with irrigating solution; have patient blink several times after application
ketotifen fumarate Zaditor	To treat allergic conjunctivitis	1 gtt in affected eye b.i.d. q 8 to 12 hr
latanoprost Xalatan	To reduce IOP in ocular hypertension or open-angle glaucoma	1 gtt in conjunctival sac of affected eye q.d. in evening
levobetaxolol hydrochloride 0.5% Betaxon	To lower IOP in chronic open-angle glaucoma or ocular hypertension	1 gtt in affected eye b.i.d.
levobunolol hydrochloride AKBeta, Betagan, Novo-Levobunolol (CAN)	To treat chronic open-angle glaucoma or ocular hypertension	1 or 2 gtt of 0.5% solution q.d. or 0.25% solution b.i.d.
metipranolol hydrochloride OptiPranolol	To reduce IOP in ocular hypertension or chronic open-angle glaucoma	1 gtt in affected eye b.i.d.

(continued on page 930)

Nasal, Ophthalmic, and Otic Drugs (continued)

GENERIC AND TRADE NAMES	INDICATIONS	USUAL ADULT DOSAGES
Miscellaneous ophthalmic drugs (continued)		
sodium chloride, hypertonic Adsorbonac, AK-NaCl, Muro-128, Muroptic-5	To provide temporary relief from corneal edema	1 or 2 gtt q 3 to 4 hr; or 6 mm of ointment applied q 3 to 4 hr
timolol hemihydrate Betimol **timolol maleate** Apo-Timop (CAN), Timoptic **timolol maleate extended-release solution** Timoptic-XE	To reduce IOP in ocular hypertension or open-angle glaucoma	1 gtt of 0.25% or 0.5% solution in affected eye b.i.d., then 1 gtt q.d.; or 1 gtt extended-release solution in affected eye q.d.
travoprost 0.004% Travatan	To reduce elevated IOP in patients with open-angle glaucoma or ocular hypertension who can't tolerate or have insufficiently responded to other IOP-lowering medications	1 gtt in affected eye q.d. in evening
unoprostone isopropyl 0.15% Rescula	To reduce elevated IOP in patients with open-angle glaucoma or ocular hypertension who can't tolerate or have insufficiently responded to other IOP-lowering medications	1 gtt in affected eye b.i.d.
Otic drugs		
antipyrine and benzocaine A/B Otic, Allergen, Analgesic Otic, Antiben, Auralgan, Aurodex, Auroto, Dolotic, Ear Drops, Earache Drops (CAN), Otocalm	To relieve pain and provide anesthesia of the ear To assist in cerumen removal	Fill ear canal and occlude q 1 to 2 hr until relief is obtained. Fill ear canal and occlude b.i.d to t.i.d for 2 to 3 days; then irrigate ear canal.
carbamide peroxide Auro Ear Drops, Debrox, Murine Ear	To assist in removal of impacted cerumen	5 to 10 gtt in affected ear and occlude for 15 min; then remove with warm water b.i.d. for up to 4 days.
chloramphenicol Chloromycetin	To treat external ear canal infections	2 or 3 gtt in affected ear b.i.d. to t.i.d.

Nasal, Ophthalmic, and Otic Drugs *(continued)*

GENERIC AND TRADE NAMES	INDICATIONS	USUAL ADULT DOSAGES
Otic drugs *(continued)*		
triethanolamine polypeptide oleate-condensate Cerumenex	To soften impacted cerumen	Fill affected ear canal with solution, plug with cotton for 15 to 30 min, and then flush with warm water.

Selected Antihypertensive Combinations

Antihypertensive drugs are used along with lifestyle changes to manage hypertension. Antihypertensive combinations, which commonly include one or two antihypertensives and a diuretic, are used to simplify patients' drug regimens and, in some cases, to enhance drug actions.

The chart below lists the generic and trade names; functional classes; usual adult dosages;

ANTIHYPERTENSIVE COMBINATION TRADE NAMES	ANTIHYPERTENSIVE GENERIC NAMES	DIURETIC GENERIC NAMES
Aldoril-15	methyldopa 250 mg	hydrochlorothiazide (HCTZ) 15 mg
Aldoril-25	methyldopa 250 mg	HCTZ 25 mg
Aldoril D30	methyldopa 500 mg	HCTZ 30 mg
Aldoril D50	methyldopa 500 mg	HCTZ 50 mg
Apresazide 25/25	hydralazine hydrochloride (HCl) 25 mg	HCTZ 25 mg
Apresazide 50/50	hydralazine HCl 50 mg	HCTZ 50 mg
Apresazide 100/50	hydralazine HCl 100 mg	HCTZ 50 mg
Atacand HCT 16/12.5	candesartan cilexetil 16 mg	HCTZ 12.5 mg
Atacand HCT 32/12.5	candesartan cilexetil 32 mg	HCTZ 12.5 mg
Avalide-150	irbesartan 150 mg	HCTZ 12.5 mg
Avalide-300	irbesartan 300 mg	HCTZ 12.5 mg
Capozide 25/15	captopril 25 mg	HCTZ 15 mg
Capozide 25/25	captopril 25 mg	HCTZ 25 mg
Capozide 50/15	captopril 50 mg	HCTZ 15 mg
Capozide 50/25	captopril 50 mg	HCTZ 25 mg
Diovan HCT 80/12.5	valsartan 80 mg	HCTZ 12.5 mg
Diovan HCT 160/12.5	valsartan 160 mg	HCTZ 12.5 mg
Diovan HCT 160/25	valsartan 160 mg	HCTZ 25 mg
Dyazide	triamterene 37.5 mg	HCTZ 25 mg
Hyzaar 50/12.5	losartan potassium 50 mg	HCTZ 12.5 mg
Hyzaar 100/25	losartan potassium 100 mg	HCTZ 25 mg
Inderide 80/25	propranolol HCl 80 mg	HCTZ 25 mg
Inderide LA 80/50	propranolol HCl 80 mg	HCTZ 50 mg
Inderide LA 120/50	propranolol HCl 120 mg	HCTZ 50 mg
Inderide LA 160/50	propranolol HCl 160 mg	HCTZ 50 mg

to antihypertensive combinations, review the individual drug monographs for the specific antihypertensives and diuretics that they contain.

ADULT DOSAGES	ONSET, PEAK, AND DURATION
b.i.d or t.i.d b b.i.d. ab q.d. tab q.d.	**Onset:** Unknown **Peak:** 4 to 6 hr **Duration:** 12 to 24 hr
cap q.d. or b.i.d. 1 cap q.d. or b.i.d. 1 cap q.d. or b.i.d.	**Onset:** 20 to 30 min **Peak:** 1 to 2 hr **Duration:** 2 to 4 hr
1 tab q.d. or b.i.d. 1 tab q.d.	**Onset:** 1 to 2 wk **Peak:** Within 4 wk **Duration:** Unknown
1 tab q.d. 1 tab q.d.	**Onset:** Unknown **Peak:** Unknown **Duration:** Unknown
ACE inhibitor and thiazide diuretic — 1 tab q.d. to t.i.d. 1 tab q.d. or b.i.d. 1 tab q.d. to t.i.d. 1 tab q.d. or b.i.d.	**Onset:** 15 to 60 min **Peak:** 60 to 90 min **Duration:** 6 to 12 hr
ACE inhibitor and thiazide diuretic — 1 or 2 tabs q.d. 1 tab q.d. 1 tab q.d.	**Onset:** 2 hr **Peak:** 6 hr **Duration:** 24 hr
Potassium-sparing diuretic and thiazide diuretic — 1 or 2 caps or tabs q.d.	**Onset:** 2 to 4 hr **Peak:** 1 day **Duration:** 7 to 9 hr
ACE inhibitor and thiazide diuretic — 1 or 2 tabs q.d. 1 tab q.d.	**Onset:** Unknown **Peak:** 6 hr **Duration:** 24 hr or more
Beta blocker and thiazide diuretic — 1 or 2 tabs b.i.d. 1 cap q.d. 1 cap q.d. 1 cap q.d.	**Onset:** Unknown **Peak:** 1 to 1.5 hr **Duration:** Unknown

(continued on page 934)

Selected Antihypertensive Combinations (continued)

ANTIHYPERTENSIVE COMBINATION TRADE NAMES	ANTIHYPERTENSIVE GENERIC NAMES	DIURETIC GENERIC NAMES
Lopressor HCT 50/25	metoprolol tartrate 50 mg	HCTZ 25 mg
Lopressor HCT 100/25	metoprolol tartrate 100 mg	HCTZ 25 mg
Lopressor HCT 100/50	metoprolol tartrate 100 mg	HCTZ 50 mg
Lotensin HCT 5/6.25	benazepril HCl 5 mg	HCTZ 6.25 mg
Lotensin HCT 10/12.5	benazepril HCl 10 mg	HCTZ 12.5 mg
Lotensin HCT 20/12.5	benazepril HCl 20 mg	HCTZ 12.5 mg
Lotensin HCT 20/25	benazepril HCl 20 mg	HCTZ 25 mg
Lotrel 2.5/10	amlodipine 2.5 mg, benazepril HCl 10 mg	none
Lotrel 5/10	amlodipine 5 mg, benazepril HCl 10 mg	none
Lotrel 5/20	amlodipine 5 mg, benazepril HCl 20 mg	none
Lotrel 10/20	amlodipine 10 mg, benazepril HCl 20 mg	none
Maxzide 37.5/25	triamterene 37.5 mg	HCTZ 25 mg
Maxzide 75/50	triamterene 75 mg	HCTZ 50 mg
Micardis HCT 40/12.5	telmisartan 40 mg	HCTZ 12.5 mg
Micardis HCT 80/12.5	telmisartan 80 mg	HCTZ 12.5 mg
Moduretic	amiloride 5 mg	HCTZ 50 mg
Prinzide 10/12.5	lisinopril 10 mg	HCTZ 12.5 mg
Prinzide 20/12.5	lisinopril 20 mg	HCTZ 12.5 mg
Prinzide 20/25	lisinopril 20 mg	HCTZ 25 mg
Timolide 10/25	timolol maleate 10 mg	HCTZ 25 mg
Uniretic 15/25	moexipril HCl 15 mg	HCTZ 25 mg
Vaseretic 5/12.5	enalapril maleate 5 mg	HCTZ 12.5 mg
Vaseretic 10/25	enalapril maleate 10 mg	HCTZ 25 mg

FUNCTIONAL CLASSES	USUAL ADULT DOSAGES	ONSET, PEAK, AND DURATION
Beta blocker and thiazide diuretic	1 or 2 tabs q.d. or 1 tab b.i.d. 1 or 2 tabs q.d. or 1 tab b.i.d. 1 or 2 tabs q.d. or 1 tab b.i.d.	**Onset:** 1 hr **Peak:** 1 to 2 hr **Duration:** Unknown
ACE inhibitor and thiazide diuretic	1 tab q.d. 1 tab q.d. 1 tab q.d. 1 tab q.d.	**Onset:** 1 hr **Peak:** 2 to 4 hr **Duration:** 24 hr
ACE inhibitor and calcium channel blocker	1 or 2 caps q.d. 1 cap q.d. 1 cap q.d. 1 cap q.d.	**Onset:** Unknown **Peak:** Unknown **Duration:** 24 hr
Potassium-sparing diuretic and thiazide diuretic	1 tab q.d. 1 tab q.d.	**Onset:** 2 to 4 hr **Peak:** 1 day **Duration:** 7 to 9 hr
Angiotensin II receptor antagonist and thiazide diuretic	1 tab q.d. or b.i.d. 1 tab q.d. or b.i.d.	**Onset:** Within 3 hr **Peak:** In 4 wk **Duration:** Several days to 1 wk
Potassium-sparing diuretic and thiazide diuretic	1 or 2 tabs q.d.	**Onset:** 2 hr **Peak:** 6 to 10 hr **Duration:** 24 hr
ACE inhibitor and thiazide diuretic	1 or 2 tabs q.d. 1 or 2 tabs q.d. 1 or 2 tabs q.d.	**Onset:** 1 hr **Peak:** 6 hr **Duration:** 24 hr
Beta blocker and thiazide diuretic	1 tab b.i.d. or 2 tabs q.d.	**Onset:** Unknown **Peak:** 1 to 2 hr **Duration:** Unknown
Potassium-sparing diuretic and thiazide diuretic	1 or 2 tabs q.d.	**Onset:** 1 hr **Peak:** 3 to 6 hr **Duration:** 24 hr
ACE inhibitor and thiazide diuretic	1 tab q.d. or b.i.d. 1 tab q.d. or b.i.d.	**Onset:** 1 hr **Peak:** 4 to 6 hr **Duration:** 24 hr

(continued on page 936)

Selected Antihypertensive Combinations (continued)

ANTIHYPERTENSIVE COMBINATION TRADE NAMES	ANTIHYPERTENSIVE GENERIC NAMES	DIURETIC GENERIC NAMES
Zestoretic 10/12.5	lisinopril 10 mg	HCTZ 12.5 mg
Zestoretic 20/12.5	lisinopril 20 mg	HCTZ 12.5 mg
Zestoretic 20/25	lisinopril 20 mg	HCTZ 25 mg
Ziac 2.5/6.25	bisoprolol fumarate 2.5 mg	HCTZ 6.25 mg
Ziac 5/6.25	bisoprolol fumarate 5 mg	HCTZ 6.25 mg
Ziac 10/6.25	bisoprolol fumarate 10 mg	HCTZ 6.25 mg

FUNCTIONAL CLASSES	USUAL ADULT DOSAGES	ONSET, PEAK, AND DURATION
ACE inhibitor and thiazide diuretic	1 or 2 tabs q.d. 1 or 2 tabs q.d. 1 or 2 tabs q.d.	**Onset:** 1 hr **Peak:** 6 hr **Duration:** 24 hr
Beta blocker and thiazide diuretic	1 or 2 tabs q.d. 1 or 2 tabs q.d. 1 or 2 tabs q.d.	**Onset:** Unknown **Peak:** Unknown **Duration:** Unknown

Antihistamines

Antihistamines are generally used to relieve immediate hypersensitivity reactions. They're also used as sedatives, antiemetics (especially in motion sickness), antitussives, antidyskinetics, and adjuncts to preoperative or postoperative analgesia.

Antihistamines are contraindicated in patients who are receiving drugs that prolong the QT interval (including some macrolide antibiotics, quinidine, itraconazole, ketoconazole, mibefradil, and zileuton). They're also contraindicated in patients who are hypersensitive to antihistamines or their components.

The chart below includes the trade names; usual dosages; and onset, peak, and duration for the antihistamines your patient is most likely to use daily or intermittently to control the symptoms of allergic rhinitis. When caring for a patient who takes an antihistamine, individualize your plan of care but be sure to include these general interventions:

•Use antihistamines cautiously in patients with a history of glaucoma, peptic ulcer, or urine retention because the drugs' anticholinergic effects may exaggerate these conditions.

•Before antihistamine therapy, assess the patient for hypokalemia and correct the imbalance, as prescribed, to reduce the risk of arrhythmias.

•Before antihistamine therapy, obtain a detailed medication history to help prevent drug interactions.

•Administer antihistamines with food if they cause GI distress.

•Instruct the patient to avoid alcohol and other CNS depressants during antihistamine use because the combination can cause additive CNS depression.

•Monitor blood pressure because the drugs' anticholinergic effects may cause hypertension.

GENERIC AND TRADE NAMES	USUAL ADULT DOSAGE	ONSET, PEAK, AND DURATION
acrivastine Semprex-D (also includes pseudoephedrine)	8 mg P.O. q 4 to 6 hr	**Onset:** 30 min **Peak:** Unknown **Duration:** 6 to 8 hr
azatadine Optimine Trinalin Repetabs (also includes pseudoephedrine)	1 to 2 mg P.O. q 8 to 12 hr 1 tablet P.O. q 12 hr	**Onset:** 15 to 60 min **Peak:** 4 hr **Duration:** 12 hr
azelastine Astelin	2 sprays (137 mcg/spray) in each nostril b.i.d.	**Onset:** In 3 hr **Peak:** Unknown **Duration:** 12 hr
cetirizine Zyrtec	5 to 10 mg P.O. q.d.	**Onset:** 30 to 60 min **Peak:** 1 hr **Duration:** Up to 24 hr
desloratadine Clarinex Clarinex Reditabs	5 mg P.O. q.d. 5 mg P.O. q.d.	**Onset:** Unknown **Peak:** Unknown (Clarinex); 3 hr (Clarinex Reditabs) **Duration:** Unknown
fexofenadine Allegra	60 mg P.O. b.i.d. or 180 mg P.O. q.d.	**Onset:** 1 hr **Peak:** 2 to 3 hr **Duration:** 12 hr
loratadine Claritin	10 mg P.O. q.d.	**Onset:** 1 to 3 hr **Peak:** 8 to 12 hr **Duration:** At least 24 hr

Topical Drugs

Topical preparations consist of an active drug prepared in a specified medium that promotes absorption through the skin. Media are commonly chosen based on drug solubility; rate of drug release; ability to hydrate the outer skin layer; ability to enhance penetration; drug stability; and interactions between the chosen medium, skin, and active ingredient. Topical media include aerosols, creams, gels, lotions, powders, tinctures, and wet dressings. Aerosols, gels, lotions, and tinctures are convenient for applications to the scalp and hairy areas. Acutely inflamed areas are best treated with drying preparations, such as lotions, tinctures, and wet dressings. Chronic inflammations do well with applications of lubricating preparations, including creams and ointments.

Because of its physical properties, the skin can act as a holding area for many drugs, allowing for slow penetration and prolonged duration of action. However, when administering topical or transdermal drugs that aren't prescribed for a specific location, keep in mind that penetration properties may vary in different areas of the skin. For example, the scrotum, face, axillae, and scalp are more permeable than the extremities, and ventral surfaces are generally more permeable than dorsal surfaces.

Topical agents are classified as antibacterials, antifungals (the largest group), antivirals, corticosteroids, retinoids, and other miscellaneous preparations.

•*Antibacterials* may be useful in the early treatment of minor skin infections and wounds. Minor skin infections may respond well to topical drugs applied at the infection site. Minor wounds should be treated at the site and in the immediately surrounding area to prevent other pathogens from colonizing the area.

•*Antifungals* are usually used to treat mucocutaneous infections, such as tineas, primarily ringworm and athlete's foot. Systemic use of antifungals is limited by their potentially toxic adverse effects, most commonly renal damage. Most fungi are completely resistant to conventional antibacterial drugs.

•*Antivirals* are used to inhibit viral replication. They work by targeting any one of the steps involved in viral replication: penetration into susceptible host cells; uncoating of the virus nucleic acid; synthesis of regulatory proteins, RNA and DNA, and structural proteins; assembly of viral particles; and release of the virus from the cell. Topical antivirals such as pencyclovir can shorten the duration of lesions, lessen lesion pain, and minimize viral shedding.

•*Corticosteroids* reduce the signs and symptoms of inflammation. Topical corticosteroids cause vasoconstriction, probably by suppressing cell degranulation. They also cause decreased cell permeability by reducing histamine release from basal and mast cells.

•*Retinoids,* typically derivatives of vitamin A, are very effective in treating acne vulgaris. When applied to the skin, retinoids remain primarily in the dermis; less than 10% of the drug is absorbed into the circulation. Prolonged use of retinoids promotes new dermal growth, new blood vessel formation, and thickening of the epidermis.

•*Miscellaneous topical drugs* are used to treat a variety of topical skin conditions, including dry skin, ichthyosis, parasitic infestations, psoriasis, and unwanted hair growth.

Before you apply a topical preparation, clean the site and let it dry. Use gloves or a finger cot during application to prevent the drug from being absorbed through your own skin. Inform your patient of any expected discomfort, such as temporary stinging or burning. After application, cover the site only if required; some topical drugs shouldn't be covered with an occlusive dressing. Be sure to teach the patient and a family member correct administration technique. Also, review possible adverse reactions, highlighting those that should be reported to the prescriber. Stress the importance of compliance with the drug regimen because some topical drugs require weeks or months of therapy to eradicate the underlying condition.

The following chart includes the generic and trade names of many commonly prescribed topical drugs as well as their FDA-approved indications and usual adult dosage.

(continued on page 940)

Topical Drugs (continued)

GENERIC AND TRADE NAMES	INDICATIONS	USUAL ADULT DOSAGES
Antibacterials		
azelaic acid cream Azelex, Finevin	To treat mild to moderate inflammatory acne vulgaris	Gently massage thin film into affected area b.i.d., morning and evening.
bacitracin Baciguent	To treat topical infections, abrasions, cuts, and minor burns or wounds	Apply thin film to affected area q.d. to t.i.d. up to 3 wk.
benzoyl peroxide Benoxyl 10 Lotion, Benzac AC Wash, BenzaShave 5 Cream, Clearasil Maximum Strength, Desquam-E 2.5 Gel, Fostex 10 BPO Gel, PanOxyl 10 Bar, Triaz	To treat mild to moderate inflammatory acne vulgaris	Apply to affected area q.d., gradually increasing to b.i.d. or t.i.d.
clindamycin phosphate Cleocin, Cleocin T Gel, Cleocin T Lotion, Clinda-Derm, Dalacin, Dalacin T Topical Solution (CAN)	To treat inflammatory acne vulgaris To treat bacterial vaginosis	Apply to affected area b.i.d., morning and evening. Insert 1 applicatorful (100 mg) intravaginally q h.s. for 7 days.
erythromycin Akne-Mycin, A/T/S, Erycette, EryDerm, Erygel, Erymax, Ery-Sol (CAN), ETS (CAN), Sans-Acne (CAN), Staticin, T-Stat (CAN)	To treat inflammatory acne vulgaris	Apply to affected areas b.i.d., morning and evening.
erythromycin 3% and benzoyl peroxide 5% Benzamycin	To treat moderate inflammatory acne	Apply to affected areas b.i.d., morning and evening.
gentamicin sulfate Garamycin, G-myticin	To prevent or treat superficial skin infections due to susceptible bacteria; to treat superficial burns	Rub small amount gently into skin t.i.d. or q.i.d.
metronidazole MetroCream, MetroGel, MetroGel-Vaginal	To treat inflammatory papules and pustules of acne rosacea To treat bacterial vaginosis	Apply thin film to affected area b.i.d., morning and evening. Insert 1 applicatorful (37.5 mg) intravaginally q h.s. or b.i.d. for 5 days.

and onset, peak, and duration for commonly used antihypertensive combinations. For information about the mechanisms of action, interactions, adverse reactions, and nursing considerations related to antihypertensive combinations, review the individual drug monographs for the specific antihypertensives and diuretics that they contain.

FUNCTIONAL CLASSES	USUAL ADULT DOSAGES	ONSET, PEAK, AND DURATION
Centrally acting antiadrenergic and thiazide diuretic	1 tab b.i.d or t.i.d 1 tab b.i.d. 1 tab q.d. 1 tab q.d.	**Onset:** Unknown **Peak:** 4 to 6 hr **Duration:** 12 to 24 hr
Peripherally acting arterial dilator and thiazide diuretic	1 cap q.d. or b.i.d. 1 cap q.d. or b.i.d. 1 cap q.d. or b.i.d.	**Onset:** 20 to 30 min **Peak:** 1 to 2 hr **Duration:** 2 to 4 hr
Angiotensin II receptor antagonist and thiazide diuretic	1 tab q.d. or b.i.d. 1 tab q.d.	**Onset:** 1 to 2 wk **Peak:** Within 4 wk **Duration:** Unknown
ACE inhibitor and thiazide diuretic	1 tab q.d. 1 tab q.d.	**Onset:** Unknown **Peak:** Unknown **Duration:** Unknown
ACE inhibitor and thiazide diuretic	1 tab q.d. to t.i.d. 1 tab q.d. or b.i.d. 1 tab q.d. to t.i.d. 1 tab q.d. or b.i.d.	**Onset:** 15 to 60 min **Peak:** 60 to 90 min **Duration:** 6 to 12 hr
ACE inhibitor and thiazide diuretic	1 or 2 tabs q.d. 1 tab q.d. 1 tab q.d.	**Onset:** 2 hr **Peak:** 6 hr **Duration:** 24 hr
Potassium-sparing diuretic and thiazide diuretic	1 or 2 caps or tabs q.d.	**Onset:** 2 to 4 hr **Peak:** 1 day **Duration:** 7 to 9 hr
ACE inhibitor and thiazide diuretic	1 or 2 tabs q.d. 1 tab q.d.	**Onset:** Unknown **Peak:** 6 hr **Duration:** 24 hr or more
Beta blocker and thiazide diuretic	1 or 2 tabs b.i.d. 1 cap q.d. 1 cap q.d. 1 cap q.d.	**Onset:** Unknown **Peak:** 1 to 1.5 hr **Duration:** Unknown

(continued on page 934)

Selected Antihypertensive Combinations (continued)

ANTIHYPERTENSIVE COMBINATION TRADE NAMES	ANTIHYPERTENSIVE GENERIC NAMES	DIURETIC GENERIC NAMES
Lopressor HCT 50/25	metoprolol tartrate 50 mg	HCTZ 25 mg
Lopressor HCT 100/25	metoprolol tartrate 100 mg	HCTZ 25 mg
Lopressor HCT 100/50	metoprolol tartrate 100 mg	HCTZ 50 mg
Lotensin HCT 5/6.25	benazepril HCl 5 mg	HCTZ 6.25 mg
Lotensin HCT 10/12.5	benazepril HCl 10 mg	HCTZ 12.5 mg
Lotensin HCT 20/12.5	benazepril HCl 20 mg	HCTZ 12.5 mg
Lotensin HCT 20/25	benazepril HCl 20 mg	HCTZ 25 mg
Lotrel 2.5/10	amlodipine 2.5 mg, benazepril HCl 10 mg	none
Lotrel 5/10	amlodipine 5 mg, benazepril HCl 10 mg	none
Lotrel 5/20	amlodipine 5 mg, benazepril HCl 20 mg	none
Lotrel 10/20	amlodipine 10 mg, benazepril HCl 20 mg	none
Maxzide 37.5/25	triamterene 37.5 mg	HCTZ 25 mg
Maxzide 75/50	triamterene 75 mg	HCTZ 50 mg
Micardis HCT 40/12.5	telmisartan 40 mg	HCTZ 12.5 mg
Micardis HCT 80/12.5	telmisartan 80 mg	HCTZ 12.5 mg
Moduretic	amiloride 5 mg	HCTZ 50 mg
Prinzide 10/12.5	lisinopril 10 mg	HCTZ 12.5 mg
Prinzide 20/12.5	lisinopril 20 mg	HCTZ 12.5 mg
Prinzide 20/25	lisinopril 20 mg	HCTZ 25 mg
Timolide 10/25	timolol maleate 10 mg	HCTZ 25 mg
Uniretic 15/25	moexipril HCl 15 mg	HCTZ 25 mg
Vaseretic 5/12.5	enalapril maleate 5 mg	HCTZ 12.5 mg
Vaseretic 10/25	enalapril maleate 10 mg	HCTZ 25 mg

Topical Drugs (continued)

GENERIC AND TRADE NAMES	INDICATIONS	USUAL ADULT DOSAGES
Antibacterials *(continued)*		
mupirocin Bactroban, Bactroban Cream, Bactroban Nasal	To treat impetigo	Apply to affected areas t.i.d. for 1 to 2 wk.
	To treat secondary infections of traumatic skin lesions due to *Staphylococcus aureus* and *Streptococcus pyogenes*	Apply thin film and cover with an occlusive dressing t.i.d. for 10 days.
	To eradicate nasal colonization of methicillin-resistant S. aureus	Apply half of the contents of a unit-dose tube to each nostril b.i.d. for 5 days.
neomycin sulfate Myciguent	To prevent or treat superficial bacterial infections	Rub fingertip-size dose into affected area q.d. to t.i.d.
nitrofurazone Furacin	As adjunct to treat third-degree burns and to treat infection in skin grafts	Apply directly to lesions or on gauze; repeat p.r.n.
povidone-iodine Betadine, Betadine Cream, Betadine Spray	To disinfect wounds and burns	Apply or spray to affected area p.r.n.
silver sulfadiazine Flamazine (CAN), Silvadene, Thermazine	To prevent and treat bacterial and fungal infection in second- and third-degree burns	Apply 1/16-inch layer aseptically q.d. to b.i.d to clean, debrided burns; reapply promptly if removed.
sulfacetamide sodium 10% Klaron	To treat acne vulgaris	Apply thin film b.i.d.
sulfacetamide sodium 10% and sulfur 5% Sulfacet-R	To treat acne rosacea, acne vulgaris, and seborrheic dermatitis	Apply thin film, and massage into affected area q.d. to t.i.d.
tetracycline hydrochloride Achromycin, Topicycline	To treat acne vulgaris	Rub solution into affected area b.i.d.
	To prevent or treat superficial skin infections due to susceptible bacteria	Apply to affected area b.i.d. (morning and evening) or t.i.d.

(continued on page 942)

Topical Drugs (continued)

GENERIC AND TRADE NAMES	INDICATIONS	USUAL ADULT DOSAGES
Antifungals		
amphotericin B Fungizone	To treat cutaneous or mucocutaneous candidal infections	Apply liberally and rub in gently b.i.d. to q.i.d. for 1 to 3 wk (interdigital lesions and paronychias), for 2 to 4 wk (perianal candidiasis or glabrous lesions), or for several months (onychomycoses).
butenafine hydrochloride 1% Mentax	To treat tinea corporis, tinea cruris, or tinea versicolor	Apply to affected and immediately surrounding area q.d. for 2 wk.
	To treat interdigital tinea pedis due to *Epidermophyton floccosum, Trychophyton mentagrophytes,* or *T. rubrum*	Apply to affected and immediately surrounding area q.d. for 4 wk or b.i.d. for 1 wk.
butoconazole nitrate Femstat	To treat vulvovaginal mycotic infections caused by *Candida* species	Insert 1 applicatorful (100 mg) intravaginally q h.s. for 3 days; may repeat course for total of 6 days.
Gynazole-1	To treat vulvovaginal infections caused by *Candida albicans*	Insert 1 applicatorful (100 mg) intravaginally once anytime day or night.
ciclopirox olamine 1% Loprox	To treat candidiasis due to *Candida albicans;* tinea corporis, tinea cruris, and tinea pedis due to *E. floccosum, T. mentagrophytes, T. rubrum,* or *Microsporum canis;* tinea versicolor due to *Malassezia furfur;* onychomycosis due to *T. rubrum;* and seborrheic dermatitis	Massage gently into affected and surrounding area b.i.d., morning and evening.
ciclopirox olamine 8% Penlac	To treat onychomycosis of the fingernails and toenails	Apply evenly to entire nail surface and surrounding 5 mm of skin q h.s. for up to 48 wk.
clotrimazole Canesten (CAN), Gyne-Lotrimin, Lotrimin, Mycelex, Mycelex-7, Mycelex-G, Mycelex OTC, Trivagizole 3	To treat superficial fungal infections (tinea corporis, tinea cruris, tinea pedis, tinea versicolor, candidiasis)	Apply thin film and massage into affected and surrounding area b.i.d., morning and evening, for 2 to 4 wk.
	To treat vulvovaginal candidiasis	Insert 100-mg vaginal tablet q h.s. for 7 days; or 500-mg vaginal tablet q h.s. for 1 day; or 1 applicatorful intravaginally q h.s. for 7 days (or 3 days if using Trivagizole 3).

Topical Drugs (continued)

GENERIC AND TRADE NAMES	INDICATIONS	USUAL ADULT DOSAGES
Antifungals *(continued)*		
clotrimazole *(continued)*	To treat oropharyngeal candidiasis	Dissolve oral troche over 15 to 30 min 5 times/day for 14 days.
	To prevent oropharyngeal candidiasis	Dissolve oral troche over 15 to 30 min t.i.d. for duration of chemotherapy or until corticosteroid dosage is reduced to maintenance levels.
econazole nitrate Ecostatin (CAN), Spectazole	To treat tinea corporis, tinea cruris, tinea pedis, tinea versicolor, cutaneous candidiasis	Rub into affected area q.d. or b.i.d for at least 2 wk.
	To treat cutaneous candidiasis	Rub into affected area b.i.d. for 2 wk.
gentian violet Genapax	To treat candidiasis	Insert 1 intravaginal tampon t.i.d. to q.i.d. for 12 days; or apply 1% or 2% solution to affected area q.d. to b.i.d. for 3 days.
haloprogin Halotex	To treat tinea corporis, tinea cruris, tinea manuum, and tinea pedis due to *E. floccosum, M. canis, T. mentagrophytes, T. rubrum,* or *T. tonsurans;* to treat tinea versicolor due to *M. furfur*	Apply liberally to affected area b.i.d. for 2 to 3 wk or, for intertriginous lesions, up to 4 wk.
ketoconazole Nizoral	To treat tinea corporis, tinea cruris, and tinea versicolor due to susceptible organisms; to treat cutaneous candidiasis	Apply thin film to affected and immediately surrounding area and cover with an occlusive dressing q.d. for at least 2 wk.
	To treat tinea pedis	Apply to affected and immediately surrounding area q.d. for 6 wk; or apply shampoo to wet hair, lather, massage for 1 min, leave drug on scalp for 3 min, then rinse and repeat 2 times/wk for 4 weeks (with at least 3 days between shampoos), then intermittently p.r.n.
	To treat seborrheic dermatitis	Apply to affected and immediately surrounding area b.i.d. for 4 wk.

(continued on page 944)

Topical Drugs (continued)

GENERIC AND TRADE NAMES	INDICATIONS	USUAL ADULT DOSAGES
Antifungals (continued)		
miconazole nitrate Femizol-M, Fungoid, Micatin, Monistat-Derm, Monistat 3, Monistat 7, Ony-Clear Nail	To treat tinea corporis, tinea cruris, tinea pedis; cutaneous candidiasis; and common dermatophyte infections	Apply cream sparingly (or powder or spray liberally) over affected area. b.i.d. for 2 to 4 wk.
	To treat tinea versicolor	Apply sparingly to affected area q.d. for 2 wk.
	To treat vulvovaginal candidiasis	Insert 1 applicatorful (100 mg) or vaginal suppository (100 mg) h.s. for 7 days, and repeat p.r.n.; or insert vaginal suppository (200 mg) h.s. for 3 days.
	To treat onychomycosis	Brush tincture on affected areas of nail surface, beds, and edges and under nail surface b.i.d. for up to several mo; or spray on clean, dry, affected nails, holding actuator down for 1 or 2 sec.
naftifine hydrochloride Naftin	To treat tinea corporis, tinea cruris, and tinea pedis	Apply cream to affected area q.d.; or apply gel to affected area b.i.d., morning and evening.
nystatin Mycostatin, Nadostine (CAN), Nilstat	To treat cutaneous and mucocutaneous infections due to *C. albicans*	Apply cream to affected area b.i.d. or as indicated; or apply powder b.i.d. or t.i.d.; or insert 1 or 2 lozenges (200,000 to 400,000 units) 4 to 5 times/day for up to 48 hr after symptoms have subsided or 14 days; or insert 4 to 6 ml (400,000 to 600,000 units) of oral suspension in mouth q.i.d. (one-half of dose in each side of mouth) and retain as long as possible before swallowing.
	To treat vulvovaginal candidiasis	Insert 1 intravaginal tablet (100,000 units) or 1 applicatorful (100,000 to 500,000 units) q.d. or b.i.d. for 14 days.
oxiconazole nitrate Oxistat, Oxizold (CAN)	To treat tinea corporis, tinea cruris, and tinea pedis caused by *E. floccosum, T. mentagrophytes,* or *T. rubrum*	Apply to affected and surrounding area q.d. or b.i.d. for 2 wk (tinea corporis and tinea cruris) or for 4 wk (tinea pedis).
	To treat tinea versicolor caused by *M. furfur*	Apply cream to affected and surrounding area q.d. for 2 wk.

Topical Drugs *(continued)*

GENERIC AND TRADE NAMES	INDICATIONS	USUAL ADULT DOSAGES
Antifungals *(continued)*		
selenium sulfide Selsun	To treat tinea versicolor	Apply to scalp, lather with small amount of water, wait 10 min, then rinse, q 7 days.
	To treat dandruff and seborrheic scalp dermatitis	Massage into wet scalp, wait 2 to 3 min, rinse, and repeat 2 times/wk for 2 wk, then p.r.n.
sulconazole nitrate Exelderm	To treat tinea corporis, tinea cruris, and tinea pedis (cream only) caused by *E. floccosum, M. canis, T. mentagrophytes,* or *T. rubrum;* to treat tinea versicolor	Massage small amount gently into affected and surrounding areas q.d. or b.i.d. (tinea pedis) for up to 6 wk.
terbinafine hydrochloride Lamisil Solution	To treat tinea versicolor	Apply to affected area b.i.d. for 1 wk.
Lamisil AT Cream	To treat tinea corporis, tinea cruris, and tinea pedis	Apply thin film to affected area b.i.d. for 1 wk or 2 wk (plantar tinea pedis).
Lamisil AT Solution	To treat interdigital tinea pedis, tinea corporis, and tinea cruris	Apply between the toes b.i.d. for 1 wk (interdigital tinea pedis) or to affected area q.d. for 1 wk (tinea corporis and tinea cruris).
terconazole Terazol 3, Terazol 7	To treat vulvovaginal candidiasis	Insert 1 applicatorful (20 mg) intravaginally h.s. for 3 days (0.4%) or 1 applicatorful (40 mg) for 7 days (0.8%); or insert 80-mg vaginal suppository h.s. for 3 consecutive days.
tioconazole GyneCure Ovules (CAN), Vagistat-1	To treat vulvovaginal candidiasis	Insert 1 applicatorful (300 mg) or 1 suppository (300 mg) intravaginally h.s. as a single dose.

(continued on page 946)

Topical Drugs (continued)

GENERIC AND TRADE NAMES	INDICATIONS	USUAL ADULT DOSAGES
Antifungals *(continued)*		
tolnaftate Absorbine Footcare, Aftate for Athlete's Foot, Aftate for Jock Itch, Dr. Scholl's Athlete's Foot, Genaspore, NP-27, Pitrex, Quinsana Plus, Tinactin, Ting, Zeasorb-AF	To treat tinea capitis, corporis, cruris, manuum, pedis, and versicolor	Apply 1% aerosol, cream, gel, powder, or solution to affected and surrounding areas b.i.d.; continue for 2 wk after symptoms subside or up to 6 wk.
Antivirals		
acyclovir Zovirax	To treat mucocutaneous herpes simplex in immunocompromised patients	Apply cream to affected area using finger cot or rubber glove 4 to 6 times a day for 10 days. Apply ointment to affected area using finger cot or rubber glove q 3 hr (6 times/day) for 7 days.
docosanol Abreva	To treat recurrent oral-facial herpes simplex	Apply cream gently and completely to affected area 5 times daily, starting with first visible sign of lesion and continuing until lesion is healed.
penciclovir Denavir	To treat recurrent herpes labialis of lips and face	Apply q 2 hr while awake for 4 days.
Corticosteroids		
alclometasone dipropionate Aclovate	To treat corticosteroid-responsive dermatoses	Apply thin film to affected area and massage b.i.d. to t.i.d.
amcinonide Cyclocort	To treat corticosteroid-responsive dermatoses	Apply thin film to affected area and massage b.i.d. (ointment, lotion) or b.i.d. to t.i.d. (cream).
betamethasone benzoate Beben (CAN), Uticort	To treat corticosteroid-responsive dermatoses	Apply thin film or a few drops to affected area q.d. to b.i.d. up to 45 g/wk (ointment, cream), 50 g/wk (gel), or 50 ml (lotion).
betamethasone dipropionate Diprolene, Diprosone, Topilene (CAN)	To treat corticosteroid-responsive dermatoses	Apply thin film or a few drops to affected area q.d. to b.i.d. up to 45 g/wk (ointment, cream), 50 g/wk (gel), or 50 ml (lotion).

Topical Drugs (continued)

GENERIC AND TRADE NAMES	INDICATIONS	USUAL ADULT DOSAGES
Corticosteroids (continued)		
betamethasome valerate Luxiq	To treat corticosteroid-responsive dermatoses	Apply foam to scalp, and massage until foam disappears, b.i.d.
clobetasol propionate Dermovate (CAN), Temovate	To treat corticosteroid-responsive dermatoses	Apply thin film to affected area and rub in gently b.i.d. to t.i.d., up to 50 g/wk, for 2 wk.
Olux	To treat corticosteroid-responsive dermatoses of scalp	Apply to affected area of scalp b.i.d., once in morning and once at night, for 2 wk.
desonide Desowen, Tridesilon	To treat corticosteroid-responsive dermatoses	Apply thin film to affected area b.i.d. to q.i.d.
diflorasone diacetate Florone, Maxiflor, Psorcon	To treat corticosteroid-responsive dermatoses	Apply thin film to affected area q.d. to q.i.d.
fluocinolone acetonide Bio-Syn, Fluocet, Fluoderm (CAN), Fluolar (CAN), Fluonid (CAN), Fluonide (CAN), Flurosyn, Synalar, Synalar-HP, Synamol (CAN), Synemol	To treat corticosteroid-responsive dermatoses	Apply thin film to affected area b.i.d. to q.i.d.
fluocinonide Lidemol (CAN), Lidex	To treat corticosteroid-responsive dermatoses	Apply thin film to affected area b.i.d. to q.i.d.
flurandrenolide Cordran, Cordran Tape, Drenison (CAN)	To treat corticosteroid-responsive dermatoses	Apply thin film to affected area and massage b.i.d. to t.i.d.; or apply tape q 12 to 24 hr.
fluticasone propionate Cutivate	To treat atopic dermatitis and corticosteroid-responsive dermatoses	Apply thin film q.d. (atopic dermatitis) or b.i.d. (dermatoses).
halcinonide Halog	To treat corticosteroid-responsive dermatoses	Apply sparingly and massage q.d. to t.i.d.
halobetasol propionate Ultravate	To treat corticosteroid-responsive dermatoses	Apply thin film to affected area and rub in gently q.d. to b.i.d., up to 50 g/wk, for 2 wk.

(continued on page 948)

Topical Drugs (continued)

GENERIC AND TRADE NAMES	INDICATIONS	USUAL ADULT DOSAGES
Corticosteroids *(continued)*		
hydrocortisone 0.25% Cetacort, Cort-Dome **hydrocortisone 0.5%** Bactine, Cetacort, Cortate (CAN), Cort-Dome, Cortifair, Delacort, DermiCort, Dermtex HC, Emo-Cort (CAN), Hydro-Tex, Hytone, MyCort, Sential (CAN), S-T Cort **hydrocortisone 1%** Ala-Cort, Allercort, Alphaderm, Acticort 100, Barriere-HC (CAN), Beta-HC, Cetacort, Cort-Dome, Cortifair, Cortril, Dermacort, Emo-Cort (CAN), Gly-Cort, Hi-Cor 1.0, Hydro-Tex, Hytone, LactiCare-HC, Lemoderm, Nutracort, Penecort, Prevex-HC (CAN), Rederm, Sarna HC (CAN), Synacort, Unicort (CAN) **hydrocortisone 2%** Ala-Scalp HP **hydrocortisone 2.5%** Allercort, Anusol-HC, Emo-Cort (CAN), Hi-Cor 2.5, Hytone, LactiCare-HC, Lemoderm, Nutracort, Penecort, Synacort **hydrocortisone acetate 0.1%** Corticreme (CAN) **hydrocortisone acetate 0.5%** 9-1-1, Corticaine, Cortacet (CAN), Cortaid, Cortoderm (CAN), FoilleCort, Gynecort, Hyderm (CAN), Lanacort, Novohydrocort (CAN), Pharma-Cort	To treat corticosteroid-responsive dermatoses	Apply thin film (aerosol foam, cream, lotion, ointment, solution) to affected area q.d. to q.i.d.

Topical Drugs (continued)

GENERIC AND TRADE NAMES	INDICATIONS	USUAL ADULT DOSAGES
Corticosteroids *(continued)*		
hydrocortisone acetate 1% Cortaid, Cortef Feminine Itch, Corticreme (CAN), Cortoderm (CAN), Hyderm (CAN), Maximum Strength Cortaid, Novohydrocort (CAN) **hydrocortisone acetate topical aerosol foam** Epifoam	To treat corticosteroid-responsive dermatoses	Apply thin film (aerosol foam, cream, lotion, ointment, solution) to affected area q.d. to q.i.d.
hydrocortisone acetate dental paste Orabase-HCA	To treat inflamed oral mucosa	Apply to oral mucosa b.i.d. to t.i.d. after meals and h.s.
hydrocortisone butyrate Locoid **hydrocortisone valerate** Westcort	To treat corticosteroid-responsive dermatoses	Apply to affected area b.i.d. to t.i.d.
hydrocortisone acetate, polymyxin B sulfate, and neomycin sulfate Cortisporin	To treat corticosteroid-responsive dermatoses (short term)	Apply sparingly and massage b.i.d. to q.i.d.
hydrocortisone and iodoquinol Vytone	To treat corticosteroid-responsive dermatoses with mild bacterial or fungal infection (short term)	Apply to affected area q.d. to t.i.d.
mometasone furoate Elocom (CAN), Elocon	To treat corticosteroid-responsive dermatoses	Apply thin film or a few drops to affected area q.d.
prednicarbate Dermatop	To treat corticosteroid-responsive dermatoses	Apply thin film to affected area b.i.d.
triamcinolone acetonide 0.025% Aristocort, Aristocort A, Aristocort D (CAN), Flutex, Kenac, Kenalog, Kenonel, Triacet, Triaderm (CAN), Trianide Mild (CAN)	To treat corticosteroid-responsive dermatoses	Apply thin film (cream) to affected area b.i.d. to q.i.d.; 0.025% lotion or ointment q.d. or b.i.d; 0.1% lotion or ointment q.d.; or 0.5% ointment q.d.

(continued on page 950)

Topical Drugs (continued)

GENERIC AND TRADE NAMES	INDICATIONS	USUAL ADULT DOSAGES
Corticosteroids *(continued)*		
triamcinolone acetonide 0.1% Aristocort, Aristocort A, Aristocort R (CAN), Delta-Tritex, Flutex, Kenac, Kenalog, Kenalog-H, Kenonel, Triacet, Triaderm (CAN), Trianide Regular (CAN) **triamcinolone acetonide 0.5%** Aristocort, Aristocort A, Aristocort C (CAN), Flutex, Kenalog, Kenonel, Triacet	To treat corticosteroid-responsive dermatoses	Apply thin film (cream) to affected area b.i.d. to q.i.d.; 0.025% lotion or ointment q.d. or b.i.d; 0.1% lotion or ointment q.d.; or 0.5% ointment q.d.
triamcinolone acetonide dental paste Kenalog in Orabase, Oracort, Oralone	To treat inflammatory or ulcerative oral lesions	Apply to oral mucosa b.i.d. to t.i.d. after meals and h.s.
triamcinolone acetonide topical aerosol Kenalog	To treat corticosteroid-responsive dermatoses	Spray affected area t.i.d. to q.i.d.
Retinoids		
adapalene Differin	To treat acne vulgaris	Apply to affected area q h.s.
tazarotene 0.05%, 0.1% Tazorac	To treat plaque psoriasis	Apply thin film to affected area q h.s.
tazarotene 0.1% Tazorac	To treat facial acne vulgaris or plaque psoriasis	Apply thin film to affected area q h.s.
tretinoin Avita, Retin-A, Retin-A Micro, Stieva-A (CAN)	To treat acne vulgaris	Apply sparingly to clean, dry affected area q h.s.

Topical Drugs (continued)

GENERIC AND TRADE NAMES	INDICATIONS	USUAL ADULT DOSAGES
Miscellaneous topical drugs		
ammonium lactate Lac-Hydrin	To treat dry skin and ichthyosis	Apply to affected area, and rub in b.i.d.
anthralin Anthranol 1 (CAN), Drithocreme, Dritho-Scalp	To treat chronic psoriasis	Apply sparingly and massage into affected lesions q.d.
	To treat chronic scalp psoriasis	Apply only to lesions q.d. for 1 wk.
chlorhexidine Hibiclens	To clean skin wounds	Rinse area, apply minimal amount to cover, then wash and rinse thoroughly.
chloroxine Capitrol	To treat dandruff and seborrheic dermatitis	Massage into wet scalp, wait 3 min, rinse, and repeat 2 times/wk.
clotrimazole and betamethasone dipropionate 0.05%, 1% Lotrisone	To treat symptomatic inflammatory tinea corporis, tinea cruris, and tinea pedis	Massage cream gently into affected and surrounding skin areas b.i.d. for 2 wk (tinea corporis, tinea cruris) or for 4 wk (tinea pedis).
coal tar Zetar, Zetar Shampoo	To treat psoriasis	Add 15 to 20 ml to lukewarm bath, immerse affected area for 15 to 20 min, and rinse thoroughly 3 to 7 times/wk.
	To treat dandruff or scalp seborrhea	Massage into wet scalp, rinse, repeat application and wait 5 min, then rinse again.
crotamiton Eurax	To treat scabies	Massage into cleansed body from chin to soles of feet, and reapply after 24 hr; change bed linens next day, and bathe 48 hr after second dose; repeat in 7 to 10 days if new lesions appear.
diclofenac sodium 3% Solaraze	To treat actinic keratoses	Massage gel gently onto affected lesion areas b.i.d. for 60 to 90 days.
doxepin hydrochloride Zonalon	To treat pruritus associated with dermatitis and chronic lichen simplex	Apply thin film to affected area q.i.d. (q 3 to 4 hr) for up to 8 days.

(continued on page 952)

Topical Drugs (continued)

GENERIC AND TRADE NAMES	INDICATIONS	USUAL ADULT DOSAGES
Miscellaneous topical drugs *(continued)*		
eflornithine Vaniqa	To retard unwanted hair growth	Apply thin film to affected area of face and chin b.i.d. (at least 8 hr apart); don't wash treated area for at least 4 hr.
hexachlorophene pHisoHex	To treat skin preoperatively	Rinse area, apply minimal amount to cover, then wash and rinse thoroughly.
imiquimod Aldara	To treat external genital and perianal warts	Apply thin layer to affected area and rub in 3 times/wk h.s. for up to 16 wk; remove with soap and water after 6 to 10 hr.
lidocaine and prilocaine EMLA	For local anesthesia	Apply 1 disk or thick layer of 2.5-g cream occlusively for at least 1 hr.
permethrin 1% Nix	To prevent or treat head lice	Wash and dry hair, saturate scalp with 1% cream, leave on hair for 10 min, then rinse; remove nits with provided comb; repeat in 7 days if living mites are still present.
permethrin 5% Acticin, Elimite	To treat scabies	Massage 5% cream into skin from head to soles of feet, and remove after 8 to 10 hr; repeat in 14 days if living mites are still present.
pyrethrum extract and piperonyl butoxide 4% Rid Mousse	To treat head, pubic, and body lice	Apply to dry hair or affected body area. Massage through all hairy areas until hair is wet. Leave on hair for 10 min; then wash with warm water and soap or shampoo. Repeat in 7 to 10 days.
tacrolimus Protopic	To treat moderate to severe atopic dermatitis in patients unresponsive to other therapies	Apply thin layer to affected areas b.i.d., rubbing in gently and completely. Continue for 1 wk after signs and symptoms have disappeared.

Equianalgesic Doses for Opioid Agonists

An equianalgesic dose of a synthetic opioid agonist is the dose that produces the same level of
analgesia as 10 mg of I.M. or S.C. morphine, the
prinicipal opioid obtained from opium poppies. If
your patient is switched from one opioid to another, expect to use the equianalgesic dose to decrease the risk of adverse reactions while increasing the likelihood of adequate pain relief. The
chart below compares equianalgesic doses (oral
and parenteral) for adults and children who weigh
50 kg (110 lb) or more.

OPIOID	ORAL DOSE	PARENTERAL DOSE
codeine	200 mg (Not recom- mended dose)	120 to 130 mg
hydrocodone	30 mg	Not applicable
hydromorphone	7.5 mg	1.5 mg
levorphanol	4 mg	2 mg
meperidine	300 mg	75 to 100 mg
morphine (around-the-clock dosing)	30 mg	10 mg
morphine (single or intermittent dosing)	60 mg	10 mg
oxycodone	30 mg	Not applicable

Interferons

Interferons are classified as biological response modifiers or antineoplastics. They fall into three major categories—alpha, beta, and gamma—which are described below.

The chart on the following pages lists the trade names, indications, usual adult dosages, adverse reactions, and nursing considerations for these interferons.

Interferon alpha

Highly purified proteins produced by a recombinant DNA process, drugs in this category exhibit antiviral and antitumor activity. Antiviral activity depends on their inhibition of viral protein synthesis. Antitumor activity results from their ability to exert a cytostatic effect, reducing the rate of cell proliferation by delaying RNA and protein production.

This delay induces cells to enter a resting stage. These drugs also increase the activity of human natural killer (NK) cells, which have the ability to lyse certain tumor cells and normal targets. They also selectively increase the number of cytotoxic T-cells, thereby affecting tumor growth. Phagocytic activity of macrophages also is increased.

INTERFERON ALFACON
This specific form of interferon is produced by fermentation of genetically engineered *Escherichia coli*. It's structurally and functionally related to interferon beta and has greater biological activity than other interferon alfas.

Interferon beta

Produced by fibroblasts and epithelial cells, drugs in this category neutralize the activity of endoge-

GENERIC AND TRADE NAMES	INDICATIONS AND USUAL ADULT DOSAGES
Interferon alpha drugs	
peginterferon alfa-2b PEG-Intron	*As monotherapy to treat patients with chronic hepatitis C who have compensated liver disease and have never received an interferon alpha:* 1 mcg/kg/wk S.C. for 1 year.
	As adjunct to treat patients with chronic hepatitis C who have compensated liver disease and have never received an interferon alpha: 1.5 mcg/kg/wk S.C. with ribavirin 800 mg/day P.O. in two divided doses.
recombinant interferon alfa-2a Roferon-A	*To treat hairy cell leukemia:* 3 million U/day I.M. or S.C. for 16 to 24 wk, followed by 3 million U 3 times/wk for maintenance.
	To treat AIDS-associated Kaposi's sarcoma: 36 million U/day I.M. or S.C. for 10 to 12 wk; alternatively, 3 million U/day I.M. or S.C. on days 1 to 3, 9 million U/day on days 4 to 6, 18 million U/day on days 7 to 9, and 36 million U/day for remainder of 10- to 12-wk induction period, followed by 36 million U 3 times/wk for maintenance.
recombinant interferon alfa-2b Intron A	*To treat hairy cell leukemia:* 2 million U/m² I.M. or S.C. 3 times/wk.
	To treat condyloma acuminatum: 1 million U (using only the 10-million U/ml strength) intralesionally at base of wart (up to 5 warts/course) 3 times/wk on alternate days for 3 wk. If response is inadequate 12 to 16 wk after initial treatment, repeat course, as prescribed.
	To treat AIDS-associated Kaposi's sarcoma: 30 million U/m² (using 50 million-U/ml strength) I.M. or S.C. 3 times/wk.
	To treat chronic, active hepatitis B and C: 3 million U I.M. or S.C. 3 times/wk.

nous interferon gamma (IFNG), the substance that may be responsible for triggering the autoimmune process that leads to multiple sclerosis. In multiple sclerosis, an initial viral infection may stimulate IFNG production by T-lymphocytes. Then IFNG induces macrophages to produce proteinases that degrade the myelin sheath around the spinal cord. Cytotoxic T-cells then move to the site of inflammation, recognizing antigens as receptor sites, where they attack the tissue affected by IFNG, resulting in progressive neurologic dysfunction. Interferon beta drugs interfere with IFNG production by lymphocytes and the mRNA transcription caused by IFNG. As a result, cytotoxic T-cells can't locate receptor sites and cause further damage in the CNS.

Interferon gamma

Produced from genetically engineered *Escherichia coli,* this type of interferon is chemically and therapeutically distinct from interferon alpha. Drugs in this category have potent phagocyte-activating properties. By enhancing oxidative metabolism, they produce toxic oxygen metabolites in phagocytes, which permits more efficient killing of certain fungi, bacteria, and protozoal microbes. Enhanced antibody-dependent cellular cytotoxicity and NK-cell activity reduce the risk of developing a serious infection in patients with chronic disease. These drugs also stimulate production of cytokines, such as interleukin-1-beta, and regulate the immune system by suppressing the IgE level and inhibiting collagen production.

ADVERSE REACTIONS	NURSING CONSIDERATIONS
CNS: Dizziness, fatigue, headache **CV:** Hypotension **EENT:** Dry mouth **GI:** Anorexia, diarrhea, hepatotoxicity, nausea, vomiting **HEME:** Anemia, leukopenia, thrombocytopenia **SKIN:** Alopecia, rash **Other:** Flulike symptoms	•Use interferon alpha drugs cautiously in patients with renal impairment and in elderly patients. •Be aware that cross-sensitivity may occur among alfa interferons. •Be aware that interferon alfa-2a, -2b, and -n3 aren't interchangeable. •Be aware that patients who are sensitive to mouse immunoglobulin also may be sensitive to recombinant interferon alfa-2a. •Unless contraindicated, ensure that patient is well hydrated at the start of and throughout therapy to reduce the risk of hypotension. •Reconstitute by adding 3 ml of diluent provided by manufacturer and swirling gently to dissolve. •Don't shake vial. •Be aware that reconstitution of interferon alfa-n3 is not necessary and that cross-sensitivity to mouse immunoglobulin, egg protein, or neomycin may occur. •Implement bleeding and infection-control measures, according to facility policy. •Administer acetaminophen, as prescribed, to prevent or treat fever and headache.

(continued on page 956)

Interferons *(continued)*

GENERIC AND TRADE NAMES	INDICATIONS AND USUAL ADULT DOSAGES
Interferon alpha drugs *(continued)*	
recombinant interferon alfa-2b Intron A *(continued)*	*To treat chronic hepatitis B:* 5 million U/day or 10 million U 3 times/wk I.M. or S.C. for 16 wk. *To treat malignant melanoma:* 20 million U/m^2 as I.V. infusion for 5 consecutive days/wk for 4 wk, followed by 10 million U/m^2 S.C. 3 times/wk for 48 wk.
interferon alfa-n3 Alferon N	*To treat condyloma acuminatum:* 250,000 U intralesionally at base of wart 2 times/wk for up to 8 wk.
Interferon alfacon drugs	
interferon alfacon-1 Infergen	*To treat chronic, active hepatitis C:* 9 mcg S.C. 3 times/wk, at intervals of at least 48 hours, for 24 wk. If inadequate response or relapse occurs, 15 mcg 3 times/wk for 6 mo.
Interferon beta drugs	
interferon beta-1a Avonex	*To treat relapsing forms of multiple sclerosis:* 30 mcg I.M. once/wk.
interferon beta-1b Betaseron	*To treat relapsing forms of multiple sclerosis:* 0.25 mg S.C. q.o.d.
Interferon gamma drugs	
interferon gamma-1b Actimmune	*To treat chronic granulomatous disease or to delay progression of severe, malignant osteopetrosis in patients with body surface area greater than 0.5 m^2:* 50 mcg/m^2 (1.5 million IU/m^2) S.C. three times/wk. *To treat chronic granulomatous disease or to delay progression of severe, malignant osteopetrosis in patients with body surface area of 0.5 m^2 or less:* 1.5 mcg/kg/dose S.C. three times/wk.

ADVERSE REACTIONS	NURSING CONSIDERATIONS
(See page 955.)	*(See page 955.)*
CNS: Anxiety, confusion, decreased concentration, depression, insomnia, nervousness **EENT:** Abnormal vision **HEME:** Leukopenia, thrombocytopenia	•Be aware that use of interferon alfacon-1 isn't recommended for patients with autoimmune hepatitis or psychiatric disorders. •Be aware that cross-sensitivity may occur with other interferon alfa drugs or *Escherichia coli*–derived products. •Don't shake vial. •Implement bleeding and infection-control measures, according to facility policy. •Monitor patient for signs and symptoms of vision abnormalities.
CNS: Fatigue, headache, weakness **GI:** Diarrhea, nausea **HEME:** Anemia, unusual bleeding or bruising **Other:** Flulike symptoms, infection	•Use beta interferons with extreme caution in patients with depression or seizure disorder. •Be aware that cross-sensitivity may occur with natural or recombinant interferon beta or human albumin. •Reconstitute following manufacturer's directions and refrigerate. Use interferon beta-1a within 6 hours of reconstitution. Use interferon beta-1b within 3 hours of reconstitution. •Implement bleeding and infection-control measures, according to facility policy.
CNS: Fatigue, headache **GI:** Diarrhea, nausea, vomiting **HEME:** Leukopenia **SKIN:** Rash **Other:** Flulike symptoms	•Use gamma interferon cautiously in patients previously exposed to cytotoxic drugs or radiation therapy. •Be aware that cross-sensitivity may occur with *Escherichia coli*–derived products. •Discard vial if left at room temperature for more than 12 hours. •Implement bleeding and infection-control measures, according to facility policy. •Administer acetaminophen, as prescribed, to prevent or treat headache and fever.

Selected Antivirals

Antivirals are used to treat and manage viral infections, including influenza, human immunodeficiency virus (HIV), herpes simplex virus (HSV) I and II, herpes zoster, and cytomegalovirus (CMV) infections.

The following chart lists the generic and trade names, indications, and usual adult dosages for some commonly used antivirals. Although you must individualize your care for a patient who receives an antiviral, be sure to include these general interventions in your plan of care:
•Administer antivirals to your patient on an empty stomach, if prescribed, to enhance absorption.
•Avoid administering HIV drugs all at once.
•If a patient takes an antacid, administer it 1 hour before or 2 hours after an antiviral because antacids may reduce antiviral absorption.
•Monitor hepatic enzyme levels to detect elevations and help prevent hepatotoxicity.
•Monitor BUN and serum creatinine levels to detect signs of impaired renal function.
•Monitor I.V. injection site for pain or phlebitis, which may result from the high pH of reconstituted solutions.
•Assess an immunosuppressed patient for signs and symptoms of opportunistic infections during antiviral therapy.
•Inform a female patient that oral contraceptives may be ineffective when administered with HIV drugs. Suggest alternate contraceptive methods.

GENERIC AND TRADE NAMES	INDICATIONS	USUAL ADULT DOSAGES
Antivirals used for HIV infection		
abacavir sulfate Ziagen	To treat HIV infection	300 mg P.O. b.i.d.
abacavir sulfate, lamivudine, and zidovudine Trizivir	To treat HIV-1 infection	1 tablet P.O. b.i.d.
amprenavir Agenerase	To treat HIV infection	1,200 mg P.O. b.i.d.
delavirdine Rescriptor	To treat HIV infection	400 mg P.O. t.i.d.
didanosine Videx, Videx EC	To treat HIV infection in patients who haven't had success with zidovudine and who weigh 60 kg (132 lb) or more	200 mg P.O. q 12 hr or 250 mg buffered powder P.O. q 12 hr (Videx); or 400 mg P.O. q.d. (Videx EC).
	To treat HIV infection in patients who haven't had success with zidovudine and who weigh less than 60 kg	125 mg P.O. q 12 hr or 167 mg buffered powder P.O. q 12 hr (Videx); or 250 mg P.O. q.d. (Videx EC).
efavirenz Sustiva	To treat HIV infection	600 mg P.O. q.d.
indinavir Crixivan	To treat HIV infection	800 mg P.O. q 8 hr.

Selected Antivirals (continued)

GENERIC AND TRADE NAMES	INDICATIONS	USUAL ADULT DOSAGES
Antivirals used for HIV infection (continued)		
lamivudine (3TC, lamivudine triphosphate) Epivir	To treat HIV infection in patients who weigh 50 kg (110 lb) or more	150 mg P.O. b.i.d.
	To treat HIV infection in patients who weigh less than 50 kg	2 mg/kg P.O. b.i.d.
lamivudine and zidovudine (3TC/AZT, 3TC/ZDV) Combivir	To treat HIV infection in patients who weigh 50 kg or more	150 mg of lamivudine and 300 mg of zidovudine P.O. b.i.d.
lopinavir and ritonavir Kaletra	To treat HIV infection in patients who weigh more than 40 kg (88 lb) and don't take nevirapine or efavirenz	400 mg lopinavir and 100 mg ritonavir (3 capsules or 5 ml) b.i.d.
	As adjunct to treat HIV infection in patients who weigh more than 50 kg and take nevirapine or efavirenz	533 mg lopinavir and 133 mg ritonavir (4 capsules or 6.5 ml) b.i.d.
nelfinavir Viracept	To treat HIV infection	750 mg P.O. t.i.d.
nevirapine Viramune	To treat HIV infection	200 mg P.O. q.d. for 14 days.
ritonavir Norvir	To treat HIV infection	600 mg P.O. b.i.d.
saquinavir Fortovase, Invirase	To treat HIV infection	600 mg P.O. t.i.d. (Invirase) or 1,200 mg P.O. t.i.d. (Fortovase).
stavudine Zerit	To treat HIV infection in patients who weigh 60 kg or more	40 mg P.O. q 12 hr.
	To treat HIV infection in patients who weigh less than 60 kg	30 mg P.O. q 12 hr.
tenofovir Viread	To treat HIV infection	300 mg P.O. q.d.
zalcitabine HIVID	To treat HIV infection	0.75 mg P.O. q 8 hr.
zidovudine (AZT, ZDV) Apo-Zidovudine (CAN), Novo-AZT (CAN), Retrovir	To treat HIV infection	100 mg P.O. q 4 hr while awake, up to 600 mg/day; or 1 to 2 mg/kg I.V. over 1 hr q 4 hr, up to 6 times/day or 6 mg/kg/day.

(continued on page 960)

Selected Antivirals (continued)

GENERIC AND TRADE NAMES	INDICATIONS	USUAL ADULT DOSAGES
Antivirals used for herpes virus infection		
acyclovir Zovirax	To treat HSV encephalitis	10 mg/kg I.V. over 1 hr q 8 hr for 10 days.
	To treat HSV genitalis	200 mg P.O. q 4 hr while awake, up to 5 times/day, for 10 days.
	To treat herpes zoster infection	800 mg P.O. q 4 hr while awake, up to 5 times/day, for 7 to 10 days; or 10 mg/kg I.V. over 1 hr q 8 hr for 7 days.
famciclovir Famvir	To treat HSV genitalis	125 mg P.O. b.i.d. for 5 days.
	To treat herpes zoster infection	500 mg P.O. q 8 hr for 7 days.
foscarnet Foscavir	To treat acyclovir-resistant HSV I and II infections	90 mg/kg I.V. q 12 hr, or 60 mg/kg q 8 hr for 2 to 3 wk.
idoxuridine Herplex Liquifilm, Stoxil	To treat HSV keratitis	1 cm applied to conjunctiva q 4 hr while awake, up to 5 times/day; or 1 gtt of 0.1% solution q hr during daytime and q 2 hr during nighttime for 7 to 10 days.
penciclovir Denavir	To treat HSV labialis	1% cream applied to lips q 2 hr while awake for 4 days.
valacyclovir Valtrex	To treat HSV genitalis	1 g P.O. b.i.d. for 10 days for initial episode; 500 mg P.O. b.i.d. for 3 days for recurrent episodes.
	To suppress recurrent HSV genitalis	1 g P.O. q.d.; alternatively, 500 mg P.O. q.d. for patients with a history of nine or fewer recurrences/year.
	To treat herpes zoster infection	1 g P.O. t.i.d. for 7 days.
vidarabine Vira-A	To treat acute viral conjunctivitis and recurrent epithelial keratitis caused by HSV infection	1.25 cm applied to conjunctiva q 3 hr until re-epithelialized, then 1.25 cm b.i.d. for 7 days.
Antivirals used for CMV infections		
cidofovir Vistide	To treat CMV retinitis	5 mg/kg I.V. over 1 hr q wk for 2 wk.

Selected Antivirals (continued)

GENERIC AND TRADE NAMES	INDICATIONS	USUAL ADULT DOSAGES
Antivirals used for CMV infections (continued)		
foscarnet Foscavir	To treat CMV infection	90 mg/kg I.V. q 12 hr, or 60 mg/kg q 8 hr for 2 to 3 wk.
ganciclovir Cytovene	To treat CMV infection	5 mg/kg I.V. over 1 hr q 12 hr for 14 to 21 days. *Maintenance:* 1,000 mg P.O. t.i.d.
valganciclovir hydrochloride Valcyte	To treat CMV retinitis	900 mg P.O. b.i.d. for 21 days. *Maintenance:* 900 mg P.O. q.d.
Antivirals used for influenza infection		
oseltamivir phosphate Tamiflu	To treat uncomplicated, acute infections caused by influenza virus A or B in adults who have had symptoms for no more than 2 days	75 mg P.O. b.i.d. for 5 days, starting within 2 days after symptoms begin. *Maximum:* 75 mg b.i.d. for 5 days.
	To prevent influenza following close contact with infected individual	75 mg P.O. q.d. for 7 days, starting within 2 days of exposure
	To prevent influenza during a community outbreak	75 mg P.O. q.d. during period of potential exposure
rimantadine Flumadine	To prevent respiratory infections caused by influenza virus A	100 mg P.O. b.i.d.
	To treat respiratory infections caused by influenza virus A	100 mg P.O. b.i.d. for 5 to 7 days from onset of symptoms.
zanamivir Relenza	To treat infections caused by influenza virus A or B	2 inhalations (10 mg) q 12 hr for 5 days.

Vitamins

As you know, an adequate daily intake of vitamins is essential to vital bodily functions, such as embryonic development (vitamin A), regulation of serum calcium and phosphate (vitamin D), and blood clotting (vitamin K).

Vitamins are classified as one of two types: fat soluble (vitamins A, D, E, and K) and water soluble (vitamin C and all forms of vitamin B). Fat-soluble vitamins can accumulate in body tissue over time; when excessive amounts are ingested through diet or sup-

GENERIC AND TRADE NAMES	RECOMMENDED DAILY INTAKE
vitamin A **(retinol)** Aquasol A	**Adult men and boys over age 10.** 1,000 mcg/day. **Adult women and girls over age 10.** 800 mcg/day. **Pregnant women.** 800 mcg/day. (900 mcg/day [CAN].) **Breast-feeding women.** 1,200 to 1,300 mcg/day. (1,200 mcg/day [CAN].) **Children ages 7 to 10.** 700 mcg/day. (700 to 800 mcg/day [CAN].) **Children ages 4 to 7.** 500 mcg/day. **Neonates and children to age 4.** 375 to 400 mcg/day. (400 mcg/day [CAN].)
vitamin B$_1$ **(thiamine hydrochloride)** Betaxin (CAN), Bewon (CAN), Biamine	**Adult men and boys over age 10.** 1.2 to 1.5 mg/day. (0.8 to 1.3 mg/day [CAN].) **Adult women and girls over age 10.** 1 to 1.1 mg/day. (0.8 to 0.9 mg/day [CAN].) **Pregnant women.** 1.5 mg/day. (0.9 to 1 mg/day. [CAN].) **Breast-feeding women.** 1.6 mg/day. (1 to 1.2 mg/day [CAN].)

plementation, severe and life-threatening toxicity can develop. Water-soluble vitamins don't accumulate in the body; they are excreted daily so that toxicity is not usually a concern with excessive intake.

The following chart lists the generic and trade names of fat-soluble and water-soluble vitamins, the recommended daily intake to prevent vitamin deficiency, dosages when deficiency occurs, other indications and dosages for vitamin therapy, and guidelines for parenteral administration of vitamins.

OTHER INDICATIONS AND DOSAGES	PARENTERAL ADMINISTRATION GUIDELINES
To treat vitamin A deficiency **CAPSULES, ORAL SOLUTION, TABLETS** **Adults and adolescents.** Dosage individualized based on severity of deficiency, as prescribed. **I.M. INJECTION** **Adults and children age 8 and older.** 15,000 to 30,000 retinol equivalent (RE)/day (50,000 to 100,000 IU/day) for 3 days, followed by 15,000 RE/day (50,000 IU/day) for 2 wk. **Children ages 1 to 8.** 1,500 to 4,500 RE/day (5,000 to 15,000 IU/day) for 10 days; for severe deficiency, 5,250 to 10,500 RE/day (17,500 to 35,000 IU/day) for 10 days. **Infants to age 1 year.** 1,500 to 3,000 RE/day (5,000 to 10,000 IU/day) for 10 days; for severe deficiency, 2,250 to 4,500 RE/day (7,500 to 15,000 IU/day) for 10 days. **I.V. INFUSION** **Adults and children.** Dosage individualized as part of total parenteral nutrition solution, as prescribed. *To treat xerophthalmia* **CAPSULES, ORAL SOLUTION, TABLETS** **Children age 1 and older.** 60,000 RE (200,000 IU) as a single dose. Dose repeated on day 2 and again in 4 wk. **Children ages 6 months to 1 year.** 30,000 RE (100,000 IU) as a single dose. Dose repeated on day 2 and again in 4 wk. *As an adjunct to treat measles* **CAPSULES, ORAL SOLUTION, TABLETS** **Children age 1 and older.** 60,000 RE (200,000 IU) as a single dose when measles are diagnosed. **Children ages 6 months to 1 year.** 30,000 RE (100,000 IU) as a single dose when measles are diagnosed.	•Be aware that anaphylaxis and death have occurred after I.V. administration of vitamin A; I.V. administration is restricted to special solutions, such as in total parenteral solution. Typically, parenteral administration of vitamin A is by I.M. injection. •Take precautions to protect vitamin A solution from exposure to light because it's light sensitive.
To treat vitamin B$_1$ deficiency (beriberi) **ELIXIR, TABLETS** **Adults.** 5 to 10 mg t.i.d. **Children and infants.** 10 mg/day. **I.V. OR I.M. INJECTION** **Adults.** *Initial:* 5 to 100 mg q 8 hr, switched to P.O. vitamin B$_1$ therapy as soon as possible and continued for total of 1 mo.	•Be aware that I.V. administration of vitamin B$_1$ has caused severe and life-threatening reactions, especially with repeat administration. Monitor patient closely for angioedema, GI bleeding, respiratory distress, throat tightness, urticaria, vascular collapse, and weakness during and after administration.

(continued on page 964)

Vitamins (continued)

GENERIC AND TRADE NAMES	RECOMMENDED DAILY INTAKE
vitamin B$_1$ *(continued)*	**Children ages 7 to 10.** 1 mg/day. (0.8 to 1 mg/day [CAN].) **Children ages 4 to 7.** 0.9 mg/day. (0.7 mg/day [CAN].) **Children ages 1 to 4.** 0.3 to 0.7 mg/day. (0.3 to 0.6 mg/day [CAN].)
vitamin B$_3$ **(niacin)** Endur-Acin, Nia-Bid, Niac, Niacels, Niacor, Nico-400, Nicobid Tempules, Nicolar, Nicotinex Elixir, Novo-Niacin (CAN), Slo-Niacin	**Adult men and boys age 11 and older.** 15 to 20 mg/day. (14 to 23 mg/day [CAN].) **Adult women and girls age 11 and older.** 13 to 15 mg/day. (14 to 16 mg/day [CAN].) **Pregnant women.** 17 mg/day. (14 to 16 mg/day [CAN].) **Breast-feeding women.** 20 mg/day. (14 to 16 mg/day [CAN].) **Children ages 7 to 11.** 13 mg/day. (14 to 18 mg/day [CAN].) **Children ages 4 to 7.** 12 mg/day. (13 mg/day [CAN].) **Neonates and children to age 4.** 5 to 9 mg/day. (4 to 9 mg/day [CAN].)
vitamin B$_6$ **(pyridoxine hydrochloride)** Beesix, Doxine, Nestrex, Pyri, Rodex, Vita-bee 6	**Adult men and boys age 11 and older.** 1.7 to 2 mg/day. **Adult women and girls age 11 and older.** 1.4 to 1.6 mg/day. **Pregnant women.** 2.2 mg/day. **Breast-feeding women.** 2.1 mg/day. **Children ages 7 to 10.** 1.4 mg/day. **Children ages 4 to 6.** 1.1 mg/day. **Neonates and children to age 3.** 0.3 to 1 mg/day.

OTHER INDICATIONS AND DOSAGES

PARENTERAL ADMINISTRATION GUIDELINES

To treat Wernicke's encephalopathy
I.V. OR I.M. INJECTION
Adults. *Initial:* 100 mg I.V. *Maintenance:* 50 to 100 mg I.V. or I.M. q.d. until normal recommended daily intake is achieved.

•Rotate sites for I.M. administration of vitamin B₁ to help prevent tenderness and induration that may occur following administration.
•I.M. administration may be painful; use the Z-track method of administration
•Because of incompatibilities, don't add parenteral vitamin B₁ to alkaline or neutral solutions; also, don't mix it with oxidizing and reducing agents, including barbiturates, carbonates, citrates, and copper
•Take precautions to protect vitamin B₁ solution from exposure to light because it's light sensitive.

To treat vitamin B₃ deficiency
E.R. CAPSULES, E.R. TABLETS, ORAL SOLUTION, TABLETS
Adults and children age 11 and older. Dosage individualized based on severity of deficiency, as prescribed. *Maximum:* 6 g/day.
I.V. INJECTION
Adults and children age 11 and older. 25 to 100 mg at least b.i.d.
Children to age 11. Up to 300 mg q.d.
I.M. INJECTION
Adults and children age 11 and older. 50 to 100 mg at least 5 times/day.
Children to age 11. Dosage individualized based on severity of deficiency.

To treat hyperlipidemia (niacin only)
E.R. CAPSULES, E.R. TABLETS, ORAL SOLUTION, TABLETS
Adults. *Initial:* 1,000 mg t.i.d. Dosage increased by 500 mg/day q 2 to 4 wk, as needed. *Maintenance:* 1 to 2 g t.i.d. *Maximum:* 6 g/day.
DOSAGE ADJUSTMENT To reduce or prevent facial flushing, initial dosage reduced to 100 mg/day (tab) or 500 mg/day (E.R. tab), and then gradually increased to 3 to 4 g/day.

•Be aware that I.V. administration of vitamin B₃ may cause CNS or CV adverse reactions, such as arrhythmias, dizziness, headache, peripheral vasodilation, and syncope. Rate of I.V. administration shouldn't exceed 2 mg/min, regardless of method of I.V. administration.
•Vitamin B₃ must be diluted for I.V. administration. For direct injection, dilute to a concentration of 2 mg/ml; for intermittent or continuous infusion, dilute dose in 500 ml of NS or other compatible solution
•Give I.M. injection following routine I.M. administration guidelines. Vitamin B₃ doesn't need to be diluted for I.M. injection.
•Be aware that parenteral administration shouldn't be used to treat hyperlipidemia.

To treat vitamin B₆ deficiency
E.R. CAPSULES, TABLETS
Adults and children. Dosage individualized based on severity of deficiency, as prescribed.
E.R. TABLETS
Adults. Dosage individualized based on severity of deficiency, as prescribed.
I.V. INFUSION
Adults and children. Dosage individualized as part of total parenteral nutrition.

•Be aware that S.C. or I.M. administration of vitamin B₆ may cause injection site burning or stinging. Before giving injection, alert patient that this adverse effect may occur.
•Know that I.V. administration is given as part of a multivitamin solution; follow the guidelines for administering an I.V. multivitamin solution as recommended for the product being used.

(continued on page 966)

Vitamins (continued)

GENERIC AND TRADE NAMES	RECOMMENDED DAILY INTAKE
vitamin B$_6$ *(continued)*	*(See page 964.)*
vitamin B$_9$ **(folic acid)** Apo-Folic (CAN), Folvite, Novo-Folacid (CAN)	**Adult men and boys age 11 and older.** 150 to 400 mcg/day. (150 to 220 mcg/day [CAN].) **Adult women and girls age 11 and older.** 150 to 400 mcg/day. (145 to 190 mcg/day [CAN].) **Pregnant women.** 400 to 800 mcg/day. (445 to 475 mcg/day [CAN].) **Breast-feeding women.** 260 to 800 mcg/day. (245 to 275 mcg/day [CAN].) **Children ages 7 to 11.** 100 to 400 mcg/day. (125 to 180 mcg/day [CAN].) **Children ages 4 to 7.** 75 to 400 mcg/day. (90 mcg/day [CAN].) **Neonates and children to age 4.** 25 mcg/day. (50 to 80 mcg/day [CAN].)
vitamin B$_{12}$ **(cyanocobalamin, hydroxycobalamin)**	**Adults age 19 and older.** 2.4 mcg/day. **Pregnant women.** 2.6 mcg/day. **Breast-feeding women.** 2.8 mcg/day. **Adolescents ages 14 to 19.** 2.4 mcg/day. **Children ages 9 to 14.** 1.8 mcg/day. **Children ages 4 to 9.** 1.2 mcg/day. **Children ages 1 to 4.** 0.9 mcg/day. **Infants ages 6 to 12 months.** 0.4 mcg/day. **Neonates and infants to 6 months.** 0.5 mcg/day.

OTHER INDICATIONS AND DOSAGES

To treat pyridoxine dependency syndrome
I.V. OR I.M. INJECTION
Adults and children age 11 and older. 30 to 600 mg q.d.
Infants with seizures. *Initial:* 10 to 100 mg, then individualized based on severity of deficiency, as prescribed.

To treat drug-induced pyridoxine deficiency
I.V. OR I.M. INJECTION
Adults and children age 11 and older. 50 to 200 mg/day for 3 wk, then 25 to 100 mg/day, as needed.

To treat vitamin B$_9$ deficiency
TABLETS
Adults and children. Dosage individualized based on severity of deficiency, as prescribed.
I.V. INFUSION, I.M. OR S.C. INJECTION
Adults and children. 0.25 to 1 mg q.d. until hematologic response occurs.

To treat vitamin B$_{12}$ deficiency caused by nutritional intake imbalance (not for use to treat pernicious anemia)
LOZENGES, TABLETS
Adults and children. Dosage individualized based on severity of deficiency, as prescribed.

To treat vitamin B$_{12}$ deficiency caused by pernicious anemia; malabsorption disorders (tropical or nontropical sprue, partial or total gastrectomy, regional enteritis, gastroenterostomy, ileal resection); or malignancies, granulomas, strictures, or anastomoses involving the ileum.
S.C. INJECTION (CYANOCOBALAMIN)
Adults. *Initial:* 30 mcg q.d. for 5 to 10 days, then switched to I.M. administration for maintenance therapy.

PARENTERAL ADMINISTRATION GUIDELINES

•Vitamin B$_6$ may increase AST (SGOT) levels. Be aware that at least one manufacturer warns against I.V. administration of vitamin B$_6$ to patients with heart disease.
•Take precautions to protect vitamin B$_6$ solution from exposure to light because it's light sensitive.

•Be aware that some vitamin B$_9$ solutions contain benzyl alcohol. Don't administer these solutions to neonates or immature infants because of a risk of fatal toxic syndrome, which may include CNS, respiratory, circulatory, and renal impairment and metabolic acidosis.
•Unless ordered otherwise, dilute 5 mg/ml of vitamin B$_9$ with with 49 ml of sterile water for injection to provide a solution containing 0.1 mg of vitamin/ml.
•Know that parenteral administration may cause anaphylaxis. Parenteral administration should be used only in patients with severe vitamin deficiency or in those with severely impaired GI absorption.
•Be aware that S.C. administration should be injected deeply.
•Take precautions to protect vitamin B$_9$ solution from exposure to light because it's light sensitive.

•Be aware that parenteral vitamin B$_{12}$ solution is incompatible with many drugs, including ascorbic acid, chlorpromazine hydrochloride, dextrose, heavy metals, phytonadione, prochlorperazine edisylate, warfarin sodium, oxidizing or reducing agents, and alkaline or strongly acidic solutions. Do not administer vitamin with other drugs.
•Know that both cyanocobalamin and hydroxycobalamin may be administered by I.M. injection, but only cyanocobalamin may be administered as an S.C. injection. Be alert to which form is being administered to ensure correct route of administration.

(continued on page 968)

Vitamins (continued)

GENERIC AND TRADE NAMES	RECOMMENDED DAILY INTAKE
vitamin B$_{12}$ *(continued)*	*(See page 966.)*
vitamin C **(ascorbic acid)** Ascorbic Acid, Cecon Drops, Cenolate, Cevi-Bid, Vicks Vitamin C Drops	**Adult men.** 90 mg/day. **Adult women.** 75 mg/day. **Pregnant women age 19 and older.** 85 mg/day. **Breast-feeding women age 19 and older.** 120 mg/day. **Adolescent boys ages 14 to 19.** 75 mg/day. **Adolescent girls ages 14 to 19.** 65 mg/day. **Pregnant girls ages 14 to 19.** 80 mg/day. **Breast-feeding girls ages 14 to 19.** 115 mg/day. **Children ages 9 to 14.** 45 mg/day. **Children ages 4 to 9.** 25 mg/day. **Children ages 1 to 4.** 15 mg/day. **Infants ages 7 to 12 months.** 50 mg/day. **Neonates and infants to age 7 months.** 40 mg/day. DOSAGE ADJUSTMENT Recommended daily intake for people who smoke is 100 mg/day because of an increased utilization of vitamin C. Recommended daily intake should be increased to promote wound healing and for those with a chronic illness, fever, hemovascular disorder, or infection; the amount of vitamin C increase depends on the severity of the underlying condition.

OTHER INDICATIONS AND DOSAGES

PARENTERAL ADMINISTRATION GUIDELINES

Children. *Initial:* 1,000 to 5,000 mcg given in single daily doses of 100 mcg over 2 or more wk. *Maintenance:* 60 or more mcg/mo.

I.M. INJECTION (CYANOCOBALAMIN OR HYDROXYCOBAL-AMIN)
Adults. *Initial:* 30 mcg q.d. for 5 to 10 days. *Maintenance:* 100 to 200 mcg q mo.
Children. *Initial:* 1,000 to 5,000 mcg, given in single daily doses of 100 mcg over 2 or more wk. *Maintenance:* 60 or more mcg/mo.
DOSAGE ADJUSTMENT Dosage adjusted, as needed, to maintain normal hematologic morphology and an erythrocyte count greater than 4.5 million/mm^3.

To treat familial selective B$_{12}$ malabsorption
I.M. INJECTION (CYANOCOBALAMIN)
Adults. *Initial.* 1 mg/wk for 3 wk. *Maintenance:* 250 mcg/mo.

To treat hereditary deficiency of transcobalamin II
I.M. INJECTION (CYANOCOBALAMIN)
Adults. 1 to 2 mg/wk.

- Be aware that S.C. administration of cyanocobalamin should be injected deeply.
- Know that vitamin B$_{12}$ is excreted more rapidly after I.V. injection; I.V. administration isn't recommended.
- Take precautions to protect vitamin B$_{12}$ solution from exposure to light because it's light sensitive.

To treat vitamin C deficiency (scurvy)
E.R. CAPSULES; LOZENGES; ORAL SOLUTION;
E.R. TABLETS; TABLETS; S.C., I.M., OR I.V. INJECTION
Adults. 100 to 250 mg q.d. or b.i.d. until skeletal changes and signs and symptoms of hemorrhagic disorder are reversed (usually within 2 to 21 days).
ORAL SOLUTION; TABLETS; S.C., I.M., OR I.V. INJECTION
Infants and children. 100 to 300 mg/day in divided doses until skeletal changes and signs and symptoms of hemorrhagic disorder are reversed (usually within days).

- Be aware that I.M. injection is the preferred parenteral route for administering vitamin C, although it may be administered I.V. or S.C. when necessary.
- Rotate sites for I.M. and S.C. administration to help prevent transient mild soreness that may occur following administration. Inform patient that this adverse effect may occur.
- If giving I.V. vitamin C, avoid rapid administration to prevent faintness or dizziness.
- Administer vitamin C solution by itself because it's incompatible with many drugs.
- Be aware that vitamin C solution rapidly oxidizes in air and in alkaline solutions. Take precautions to protect vitamin solution from exposure to air and light.
- Open vitamin C ampules carefully because increased pressure may develop after prolonged storage.

(continued on page 970)

Vitamins (continued)

GENERIC AND TRADE NAMES	RECOMMENDED DAILY INTAKE
vitamin D$_2$ (ergocalciferol) Calciferol, Calciferol Drops, Drisdol, Drisdol Drops, Ostoforte (CAN), Radiostol Forte (CAN)	**Adults and children ages 11 and older.** 200 to 400 IU/day. (100 to 200 IU/day [CAN].) **Pregnant and breast-feeding women.** 400 IU/day. (200 to 300 IU/day [CAN].) **Children ages 7 to 11.** 400 IU/day. (100 to 200 IU/day [CAN].) **Children ages 4 to 7.** 400 IU/day. (200 IU/day [CAN].) **Neonates and children to age 4.** 300 to 400 IU/day. (200 to 400 IU/day [CAN].)
vitamin E (alpha tocopherol) Amino-Opti-E, Aquasol E, E-Complex 600, E-Vitamin succinate, Liqui-E, Pheryl E, Vita-Plus E, Webber Vitamin E (CAN)	**Adult men and adolescent boys.** 16.7 IU/day. (10 to 16.7 IU/day [CAN].) **Adult women and adolescent girls.** 13 IU/day. (8.3 to 11.7 IU/day [CAN].) **Pregnant women.** 16.7 IU/day. (13 to 15 IU/day [CAN].) **Breast-feeding women.** 18 to 20 IU/day. (15 to 16.7 IU/day [CAN].) **Children ages 7 to 10.** 11.7 IU/day. (10 to 13 IU/day [CAN].) **Children ages 4 to 7.** 11.7 IU/day. (8.3 IU/day [CAN].) **Infants and children to age 4.** 5 to 10 IU/day. (5 to 6.7 IU/day [CAN].)

OTHER INDICATIONS AND DOSAGES

To treat vitamin D$_2$ deficiency
CAPSULES, ORAL SOLUTION, TABLETS
Adults and children. Dosage individualized based on severity of deficiency, as prescribed.

To treat vitamin D-resistant rickets
CAPSULES, ORAL SOLUTION, TABLETS
Adults. 12,000 to 150,000 IU q.d.

To treat vitamin D-dependent rickets
CAPSULES, ORAL SOLUTION, TABLETS
Adults. 10,000 to 60,000 IU q.d. *Maximum:* 150,000 IU q.d.
Children. 3,000 to 10,000 IU q.d. *Maximum:* 50,000 IU q.d.

To treat osteomalacia caused by long-term anticonvulsant use
CAPSULES, ORAL SOLUTION, TABLETS
Adults. 1,000 to 4,000 IU q.d.
Children. 1,000 IU q.d.

To treat familial hypophosphatemia
CAPSULES
Adults. 50,000 to 100,000 IU q.d.

To treat hypoparathyroidism
CAPSULES
Adults. 50,000 to 150,000 IU q.d.
Children. 50,000 to 200,000 IU q.d.

To treat intestinal malabsorption
I.M. INJECTION
Adults and children. 10,000 IU q.d.

To treat vitamin E deficiency
CAPSULES (ADULTS ONLY), ORAL SOLUTION, TABLETS
Adults and children. Dosage individualized based on severity of deficiency, as prescribed.

PARENTERAL ADMINISTRATION GUIDELINES

•Be aware that vitamin D$_2$ is usually given orally. However, I.M. injection may be required for patients with GI, liver, or biliary disease associated with malabsorption of vitamin D analogs.
Take precautions to protect parenteral vitamin D$_2$ solution from exposure to light because light causes it to decompose.

Vitamin E isn't administered parenterally.

(continued on page 972)

Vitamins (continued)

GENERIC AND TRADE NAMES	RECOMMENDED DAILY INTAKE
vitamin K$_1$ **(phytonadione)** AquaMEPHYTON, Mephyton	*Recommended daily intake hasn't been established for vitamin K$_1$. However, adequate intake is suggested as follows:* **Adult men age 19 and older.** 120 mcg/day. **Adult women age 19 and older, pregnant and breast-feeding women.** 90 mcg/day. **Adolescents ages 14 to 19.** 75 mcg/day. **Children ages 9 to 14.** 60 mcg/day. **Children ages 4 to 9.** 55 mcg/day. **Children ages 1 to 4.** 30 mcg/day. **Infants ages 7 to 12 months.** 2.5 mcg/day. **Neonates and infants to age 7 months.** 2 mcg/day.

OTHER INDICATIONS AND DOSAGES

To prevent hypoprothrombinemia during pro-longed use of total parenteral nutrition
I.M. INJECTION
Adults. 5 to 10 mg/wk.
Children. 2 to 5 mg/wk.

To prevent hypoprothrombinemia in infants with diets deficient in vitamin K (less than 100 mcg/L)
I.M. INJECTION
Infants. 1 mg/mo.

To treat anticoagulant-induced hypoprothrombinemia
TABLETS, I.M. OR S.C. INJECTION
Adults. 2.5 to 25 mg, repeated 12 to 48 hr after P.O. dose or 6 to 8 hr after S.C. or I.M. dose, as prescribed. *Maximum:* 50 mg/dose.
Children. 2.5 to 10 mg S.C. or I.M., repeated in 6 to 8 hr, as prescribed.
Infants. 1 to 2 mg S.C. or I.M., repeated in 4 to 8 hr, as prescribed.

To treat hypoprothrombinemia from other causes
TABLETS, I.M. OR S.C. INJECTION
Adults. 2 to 25 mg. *Usual:* 25 mg. *Maximum:* 50 mg/dose.
Children. 5 to 10 mg S.C. or I.M.
Infants. 2 mg S.C. or I.M.

To prevent hemorrhagic disease in neonates
I.M. OR S.C. INJECTION
Neonates. 0.5 to 1 mg within 1 hr after birth, repeated in 6 to 8 hr, as prescribed.

To treat hemorrhagic disease in neonates
I.M. OR S.C. INJECTION
Neonates. 1 mg (or higher dose if mother took an oral anticoagulant or anticonvulsant during pregnancy).

PARENTERAL ADMINISTRATION GUIDELINES

• Be aware that severe adverse reactions, including anaphylaxis, cardiac and respiratory arrest, hypersensitivity, and shock, may occur during or immediately after I.M. or I.V. administration of vitamin K_1, even if it's diluted to avoid rapid infusion. Administer vitamin by S.C. route whenever possible.
• If vitamin K_1 must be administered I.V., do not exceed rate of 1 mg/min, as prescribed.
• Be aware that some vitamin K_1 solutions contain benzyl alcohol. Don't administer these solutions to neonates or immature infants because of a risk of fatal toxic syndrome, which may include CNS, respiratory, circulatory, and renal impairment and metabolic acidosis.
• Take precautions to protect vitamin K_1 solution from exposure to light because it's light sensitive.

Antineoplastic Drugs

Antineoplastic drugs have become the standard of treatment for most types of cancer today. Most of these drugs work by inhibiting cell proliferation, thereby leading to cell death. They're most effective at killing cells that are actively dividing. Cell-specific antineoplastics exert their actions during one or more phases of the cell cycle. S-phase antineoplastics interfere with deoxyribonucleic acid (DNA) synthesis; M-phase drugs interfere with the formation of microtubules and disrupt mitosis. Most antineoplastics impair DNA in one of the following four ways:

•preventing separation of DNA strands
•inhibiting DNA repair
•mimicking DNA bases
•disrupting the triplicate codons or producing oxygen free radicals that damage the DNA.

Antineoplastic drugs are cytotoxic, which means that they affect both neoplastic cells and normal cells. As a result, they may cause serious and sometimes life-threatening adverse reactions. Antineoplastics are most harmful to normal cells that exhibit rapid activity and growth, such as bone marrow tissue, the epithelium of the GI mucosa, and hair follicles. When they suppress bone marrow activity, the patient may develop leukopenia, thrombocytopenia, or anemia. When the drugs affect the GI mucosa, the patient may experience nausea, vomiting, anorexia, bowel dysfunction, and mucosal ulcerations. When they affect the hair follicles, the result is hair loss (alopecia), one of the most common adverse reactions; although not life-threatening, hair loss can be emotionally traumatic for patients, especially women.

Drug Classification

Antineoplastics are classified according to their mechanism of action.

•*Alkylating drugs,* the first drugs developed to fight cancer, are most effective against slow-growing tumors. These agents can damage tissue at the injection site and produce systemic toxicity. They can damage cells during all stages of growth, causing mitotic arrest. Because their actions are not limited to neoplastic cells, they also cause myelosuppression, a predictable adverse reaction. They can also result in secondary tumor development, even years after the initial therapy.

•*Antibiotic antineoplastics* originated from a genus of fungus-like bacteria called *Streptomyces*. Their classification is based on their origin, not on mechanism of action, toxicity, pharmacokinetics, or varying clinical indications. Many of these drugs bind to specific bases and block DNA synthesis to interfere with cell replication.

•*Antimetabolites* are cell-cycle-specific drugs that act by preventing synthesis of nucleotides or inhibiting enzymes by mimicking nucleotides. These drugs are often more effective when used in combination.

•*Antimitotic antineoplastics* disrupt the formation of microtubule structures within the cell during mitosis. This breakdown of microtubule production stops the formation of the mitotic spindle, inhibiting cellular reproduction.

•*Biological response modifiers* alter tumor-host metabolic and immunologic relationships.

•*Antineoplastic enzymes* interfere with the breakdown of extracellular asparagine, an endogenous enzyme that leukemic cells depend on for their survival. The rapid depletion of asparagine eventually kills leukemic cells by fragmenting them into membrane-bound particles that are eliminated by phagocytosis.

•*Hormonal antineoplastics* act as agonists to inhibit tumor cell growth or as antagonists to compete with endogenous growth-promoting hormones. Steroid hormones form specific receptor complexes that bind to certain nuclear proteins necessary for DNA transcription.

•*Miscellaneous antineoplastics* act in a variety of ways, such as by destroying microtubules that are essential for tumor cell structure before mitosis and by inhibiting topoisomerase, the enzyme that affects the degree of supercoiling in DNA by cutting one or both strands. This inhibition causes DNA strands to break and synthesizes toxic compounds that inhibit DNA strand repair.

The following chart lists the generic and common trade names of common antineoplastic drugs, which are grouped according to mechanism of action. It also includes FDA-approved indications and the usual adult dosage for each drug.

Antineoplastic Drugs (continued)

GENERIC AND TRADE NAMES	INDICATIONS	USUAL ADULT DOSAGES
Alkylating drugs		
busulfan Busulfex, Myleran	To provide palliative treatment of chronic myelocytic leukemia	*Initial:* 0.06 mg/kg P.O. q.d. until WBC count falls below 15,000/mm^3. *Usual:* 4 to 8 mg P.O. q.d. (but may range from 1 to 12 mg P.O. q.d.) *Maintenance:* 1 to 3 mg q.d. During remission, treatment resumed when WBC count reaches 50,000/mm^3; or 0.8 mg/kg I.V. over 2 hr q 6 hr for 4 days for a total of 16 doses as an adjunct with cyclophosphamide
carmustine (BCNU) BiCNU, Gliadel Wafer	To treat primary brain tumors and glioblastoma multiforme	Up to 8 implants per surgical procedure
	To treat primary brain tumors, Hodgkin's disease, non-Hodgkin's lymphoma, and multiple myeloma	150 to 200 mg/m^2 by slow I.V. infusion as a single dose q 6 to 8 wk; or 75 to 100 mg/m^2 by slow I.V. infusion q.d. for 2 days q 6 wk; or 40 mg/m^2 by slow I.V. infusion q.d. for 5 days q 6 wk
chlorambucil Leukeran	To provide palliative treatment of chronic lymphocytic leukemia, Hodgkin's disease, malignant lymphomas (including lymphosarcoma and giant follicular lymphoma), and non-Hodgkin's lymphoma	0.1 to 0.2 mg/kg/day as a single dose or in divided doses for 3 to 6 wk. *Usual:* 4 to 10 mg/day as a single dose or in divided doses for 3 to 6 wk
cyclophosphamide Cytoxan, Neosar, Procytox (CAN)	To treat acute lymphocytic leukemia, acute nonlymphocytic leukemia, chronic lymphocytic leukemia, chronic myelocytic leukemia, breast cancer, epithelial ovarian cancer, Hodgkin's disease, multiple myeloma, neuroblastoma, non-Hodgkin's lymphoma, and retinoblastoma	1 to 5 mg/kg P.O. q.d.; or 40 to 50 mg/kg I.V. in divided doses over 2 to 5 days; or 10 to 15 mg/kg I.V. q 7 to 10 days; or 3 to 5 mg/kg I.V. 2 times/wk; or 1.5 to 3 mg/kg I.V. q.d.
ifosfamide IFEX	To treat germ cell testicular tumors	1.2 g/m^2/day by I.V. infusion for 5 days q 3 wk
lomustine (CCNU) CeeNU	To treat primary brain tumors and Hodgkin's disease	100 to 130 mg/m^2 P.O. as a single dose q 6 wk

(continued on page 976)

Antineoplastic Drugs (continued)

GENERIC AND TRADE NAMES	INDICATIONS	USUAL ADULT DOSAGES
Alkylating drugs *(continued)*		
mechlorethamine hydrochloride (nitrogen mustard) Mustargen	To treat Hodgkin's disease, non-Hodgkin's lymphoma, and mycosis fungoides	0.4 mg/kg I.V. as a single dose or in divided doses over 2 to 4 days
	To treat malignant pericardial, peritoneal, or pleural effusions	0.4 mg/kg (peritoneal or pleural effusion); 0.2 mg/kg into affected cavity (pericardial effusion)
melphalan (L-phenylalanine mustard) Alkeran **melphalan hydrochloride** Alkeran	To treat multiple myeloma	0.15 mg/kg P.O. q.d. for 7 days, followed by 0.05 mg/kg q.d. after 3-wk period of no drug; or 0.1 to 0.15 mg/kg q.d. for 2 to 3 wk or 0.25 mg/kg for 4 days, followed by 2 to 4 mg q.d. after 2- to 4-wk period of no drug
	To treat epithelial ovarian cancer	0.2 mg/kg P.O. q.d. for 5 days, repeated q 4 to 5 wk
streptozocin Zanosar	To treat islet cell or pancreatic carcinoma	500 mg/m^2 I.V. for 5 days q 6 wk, or 1,000 mg/m^2 I.V. q wk for 2 wk
temozolomide Temodar	To treat astrocytoma	150 mg/m^2 P.O. q.d. for first 5 days of 28-day cycle, followed by 100 to 200 mg/m^2 P.O. q.d. for first 5 days of subsequent 28-day cycles
thiotepa (TESPA, triethylenethio-phosphoramide, TSPA) Thioplex	To treat breast cancer, epithelial ovarian cancer, and malignant pericardial or pleural effusions	0.6 to 0.8 mg/kg into affected cavity q 1 to 4 wk
	To treat breast cancer, epithelial ovarian cancer, and Hodgkin's disease	0.3 to 0.4 mg/kg I.V. q 1 to 4 wk, or 0.2 mg/kg for 4 to 5 days q 2 to 3 wk
	To treat bladder tumors	30 to 60 mg mixed in 30 to 60 ml of distilled water and instilled into bladder q wk for 4 wk
Antibiotic antineoplastics		
bleomycin sulfate Blenoxane	To treat non-Hodgkin's lymphoma, squamous cell carcinoma, and testicular cancer	0.25 to 0.5 unit/kg or 10 to 20 units/m^2 1 to 2 times/wk I.V., I.M., or S.C.; or 0.25 unit/kg or 15 units/m^2 q.d. by I.V. infusion over 24 hr
	To treat Hodgkin's disease	0.25 to 0.5 unit/kg I.V., I.M., or S.C., or 10 to 20 units/m^2 1 to 2 times/wk

Antineoplastic Drugs (continued)

GENERIC AND TRADE NAMES	INDICATIONS	USUAL ADULT DOSAGES
Antibiotic antineoplastics *(continued)*		
bleomycin sulfate *(continued)*	To treat squamous cell carcinoma of the cervix, head and neck, penis, or vulva	30 to 60 units by arterial infusion over 1 to 24 hr
cisplatin Platinol, Platinol-AQ	To treat bladder cancer	50 to 70 mg/m^2 by I.V. infusion as a single dose q 3 to 4 wk in combination with other agents
	To treat advanced ovarian cancer	75 to 100 mg/m^2 by I.V. infusion as a single dose q 21 days in combination with paclitaxel
	To treat testicular cancer	20 mg/m^2 by I.V. infusion q.d. for 5 days in combination with bleomycin and etoposide; repeated q 3 wk for two or more cycles
dactinomycin (actinomycin-D) Cosmegen	To treat Ewing's sarcoma, gestational trophoblastic or Wilms' tumors, rhabdomyosarcoma, sarcoma botryoides, and testicular cancer or tumors	0.5 mg I.V. q.d. for 5 days; may repeat after 3 wk
	To treat Ewing's sarcoma and sarcoma botryoides	0.05 mg/kg for lower extremity or pelvis; 0.035 mg/kg for upper extremity as an isolation-perfusion
daunorubicin hydrochloride Cerubidine	To treat acute lymphocytic leukemia	45 mg/m^2 q.d. for first 3 days of a 32-day course of vincristine, prednisone, and asparaginase combination therapy
	To treat acute nonlymphocytic leukemia	45 mg/m^2 q.d. for first 3 days of first course of cytarabine combination therapy and first 2 days of second course of cytarabine combination therapy
daunorubicin, liposomal DaunoXome	To treat AIDS-related Kaposi's sarcoma	40 mg/m^2 I.V. over 60 min q 2 wk

(continued on page 978)

Antineoplastic Drugs (continued)

GENERIC AND TRADE NAMES	INDICATIONS	USUAL ADULT DOSAGES
Antibiotic antineoplastics *(continued)*		
doxorubicin hydrochloride Adriamycin PFS, Adriamycin RDF, Rubex	To treat acute lymphocytic leukemia, acute nonlymphocytic leukemia; bladder, breast, gastric, epithelial ovarian, or thyroid cancer; Hodgkin's disease; neuroblastoma or Wilms' tumor; non-Hodgkin's lymphoma; small-cell lung carcinoma; and soft-tissue sarcoma or osteosarcoma	60 to 75 mg/m^2 I.V. as single dose q 21 days; or 25 to 30 mg/m^2 I.V. q.d. for 2 to 3 days q 3 to 4 wk; or 20 mg/m^2 q wk; or 40 to 60 mg/m^2 q 21 to 28 days in combination with other chemotherapeutic drugs
doxorubicin, liposomal Caelyx (CAN), Doxil	To treat AIDS-related Kaposi's sarcoma	20 mg/m^2 I.V. over 30 min q 3 wk as tolerated
epirubicin hydrochloride Ellence	To treat breast cancer	100 to 120 mg/m^2 by I.V. infusion over 3 to 5 min via a free-flowing I.V. solution as a single dose on day 1 or in divided doses on days 1 and 8, repeated q 3 to 4 wk for 6 cycles in combination with other chemotherapy agents
idarubicin hydrochloride Idamycin	To treat acute nonlymphocytic leukemia	12 mg/m^2/day I.V. over 10 to 15 min for 3 days in combination with cytarabine therapy
mitomycin (mitomycin-C) Mutamycin	To treat gastric or pancreatic cancer	20 mg/m^2 as a single dose q 6 to 8 wk
pentostatin (2′-deoxycoformycin) Nipent	To treat hairy cell leukemia	4 mg/m^2 by rapid I.V. injection or diluted for infusion over 20 to 30 min as a single dose q other wk
plicamycin (mithramycin) Mithracin	To treat testicular cancer	0.025 to 0.03 mg/kg I.V. q.d. over 4 to 6 hr for 8 to 10 days
	To treat hypercalcemia and hypercalciuria	0.015 to 0.025 mg/kg I.V. q.d. over 4 to 6 hr for 3 to 4 days; may repeat dose q wk as needed
valrubicin Valstar	To treat bladder cancer	800 mg q wk for 6 wk into affected cavity

Antineoplastic Drugs (continued)

GENERIC AND TRADE NAMES	INDICATIONS	USUAL ADULT DOSAGES
Antimetabolites		
capecitabine Xeloda	To treat locally advanced or metastatic breast cancer or metastatic colorectal cancer	1,250 mg/m^2 P.O. after a meal b.i.d. (morning and evening) for 2 wk, followed by 1-wk rest period; dose repeated in 3-wk cycles
cladribine (2-CdA, 2-chlorodeoxy-adenosine) Leustatin	To treat hairy cell leukemia	0.1 mg/kg/day by continuous I.V. infusion for 7 days
cytarabine (ARA-C, cytosine arabinoside) Cytosar, Cytosar-U	To treat acute nonlymphocytic leukemia	Initially, 100 mg/m^2/day by continuous I.V. infusion for 7 days, alone or in combination with other agents; or 100 mg/m^2 I.V. q 12 hr on days 1 to 7, then consult manufacturer's literature for specific dosing; or high-dose therapy of 2 to 3 g/m^2 I.V over 1 to 3 hr for 2 to 6 days, then consult manufacturer's literature for specific dosing
	To treat meningeal leukemia	30 mg/m^2 intrathecally as a single dose q.d. for 4 days
	To prevent or treat acute lymphocytic leukemia and chronic myelocytic leukemia	Consult manufacturer's literature for specific dosage.
cytarabine, liposomal DepoCyt, Depro Tech	To treat lymphomatous meningitis	Initially, 50 mg intrathecally (intraventricular or lumbar puncture) over 1 to 5 min q 14 days for two doses (wk 1 and 3); then 50 mg intrathecally q 14 days for three doses (wk 5, 7, and 9), followed by 1 50-mg dose at wk 13; then 50 mg intrathecally q 28 days for four doses (wk 17, 21, 25, and 29) in combination with dexamethasone 4 mg P.O. or I.V. b.i.d. for 5 days

(continued on page 980)

Antineoplastic Drugs (continued)

GENERIC AND TRADE NAMES	INDICATIONS	USUAL ADULT DOSAGES
Antimetabolites *(continued)*		
floxuridine (fluorodeoxyuridine) FUDR	To treat colorectal or hepatic cancer	0.1 to 0.6 mg/kg/day by continuous intra-arterial infusion for 14 to 21 days, followed by 2 wk of no drug; dose repeated in 5-wk cycles
fludarabine phosphate Fludara	To treat chronic lymphocytic leukemia	25 mg/m^2 I.V. infused over 30 min for 5 days; cycle repeated q 28 days
fluorouracil (5-fluorouracil, 5-FU) Adrucil, Carac, Efudex, Fluoroplex	To treat colorectal, breast, gastric, or pancreatic cancer	7 to 12 mg/kg/day I.V. for 4 days, followed by no drug for 3 days, then 7 to 10 mg/kg q 3 to 4 days for total of 2 wk; or 12 mg/kg/day for 4 days, followed by 1 day of no drug, then 6 mg/kg q.o.d. for 4 or 5 days, for total of 12 days; thereafter, 7 to 12 mg/kg/day I.V. q 7 to 10 days
	To treat multiple actinic (solar) keratoses	0.5% cream (face, anterior scalp), 1% cream (head, neck, chest), or 2% to 5% cream (hands) applied to skin q.d. to b.i.d. to cover lesions
	To treat superficial basal cell carcinoma	5% cream applied to skin b.i.d. for up to 12 wk to cover lesions
hydroxyurea Droxia, Hydrea	To treat epithelial ovarian cancer	60 to 80 mg/kg P.O. as a single dose q 3 days alone or with radiation therapy; or 20 to 30 mg/kg P.O. q.d.
	To treat resistant chronic myelocytic leukemia	20 to 30 mg/kg P.O. q.d. or in divided doses b.i.d.
mercaptopurine (6-mercaptopurine, 6-MP) Purinethol	To treat acute lymphocytic leukemia or acute nonlymphocytic leukemia	2.5 mg/kg/day or 80 to 100 mg/m^2/day (rounded off to nearest 25 mg) P.O. as a single dose or in divided doses, followed by 1.5 to 2.5 mg/kg/day P.O. or 50 to 100 mg/m^2/day

Antineoplastic Drugs *(continued)*

GENERIC AND TRADE NAMES	INDICATIONS	USUAL ADULT DOSAGES
Antimetabolites *(continued)*		
methotrexate (amethopterin) methotrexate sodium	To treat chorioadenoma destruens, choriocarcinoma, or hydatidiform mole	15 to 30 mg/day P.O. or I.M. for 5 days; repeat three to five times with 2 to 3 wk between courses
	To treat acute lymphocytic leukemia or meningeal leukemia	Initially, 3.3 mg/m²/day P.O., I.M., or I.V. in combination with prednisone or other drug; as maintenance dose, 30 mg/m²/wk P.O. or I.M. in two divided doses or 2.5 mg/kg I.V. q 14 days
	To treat Burkitt's lymphoma (stage I or II)	10 to 25 mg/day P.O. for 4 to 8 days, followed by no drug for 7 to 10 days; course repeated as needed
	To treat Burkitt's lymphoma (stage III)	Same as for stage I or II in combination with other drug
	To treat lymphosarcoma (stage III)	0.625 to 2.5 mg/kg/day P.O.
	To treat mycosis fungoides	2.5 to 10 mg/day P.O. for weeks or months; or 50 mg I.M. q wk or 25 mg I.M. 2 times/wk
	To treat osteosarcoma	12 g/m² by I.V. infusion over 12 hr, followed by leucovorin rescue on weeks 4, 5, 6, 7, 11, 12, 15, 16, 29, 30, 44, and 45 after surgery in combination with bleomycin, cisplatin, cyclophosphamide, dactinomycin, and doxorubicin
	To treat breast or head and neck cancer and non-small-cell or small-cell lung carcinoma	Consult manufacturer's literature for specific dosing.
thioguanine (6-TG, 6-thioguanine) Lanvis (CAN), Tabloid	To treat acute nonlymphocytic leukemia or chronic myelogenous leukemia	2 to 3 mg/kg P.O. as a single dose a.c., followed by 2 mg/kg/day P.O. for 5 to 7 days or until remission
Antimitotic antineoplastics		
docetaxel Taxotere	To treat breast cancer	60 to 100 mg/m² by I.V. infusion over 1 hr q 3 wk
	To treat non-small-cell lung carcinoma	75 mg/m² by I.V. infusion over 1 hr q 3 wk

(continued on page 982)

Antineoplastic Drugs (continued)

GENERIC AND TRADE NAMES	INDICATIONS	USUAL ADULT DOSAGES
Antimitotic antineoplastics *(continued)*		
paclitaxel Taxol	To treat ovarian cancer	135 or 175 mg/m^2 by I.V. infusion over 3 or 24 hr q 21 days
	To treat breast cancer	175 mg/m^2 by I.V. infusion over 3 or 24 hr q 21 days
	To treat AIDS-related Kaposi's sarcoma	135 mg/m^2 by I.V. infusion over 3 or 24 hr q 21 days; or 100 mg/m^2 by I.V. infusion over 3 or 24 hr q 14 days
	To treat non-small-cell lung carcinoma	135 mg/m^2 by I.V. infusion over 3 or 24 hr, followed by cisplatin 75 mg/m^2 I.V. q 21 days
vinblastine sulfate (VLB) Velban, Velbe (CAN)	To treat breast cancer, Hodgkin's disease, lymphomas, Kaposi's sarcoma, Letterer-Siwe disease, mycosis fungoides, non-Hodgkin's lymphoma, testicular cancer, and trophoblastic gestational tumors	0.15 to 0.2 mg/kg I.V. q wk
vincristine sulfate (VCR) Oncovin, Vincasar PFS	To treat acute lymphocytic leukemia, Hodgkin's disease, lymphomas, neuroblastoma, non-Hodgkin's lymphoma, rhabdomyosarcoma, and Wilms' tumor	0.01 to 0.03 mg/kg I.V.; or 0.4 to 1.4 mg/m^2 I.V. q wk as a single dose
vinorelbine tartrate Navelbine	To treat non-small-cell lung carcinoma	30 mg/m^2 I.V. over 6 to 10 min q wk alone, or 25 mg/m^2 I.V. over 6 to 10 min q wk in combination with cisplatin 100 mg/m^2 q 4 wk
Biological response modifiers		
aldesleukin (IL-2, interleukin-2) Proleukin	To treat renal cancer and metastatic melanoma	600,000 IU/kg by I.V. infusion over 15 min q 8 hr for 14 doses, followed by 9 days of no drug; then repeat course of 14 doses for total of 28 doses
alemtuzumab Campath	To treat B-cell chronic lymphocytic leukemia	*Initial:* 3 mg I.V. over 2 hr daily, then increased to 10 mg I.V. over 2 hr daily. *Maintenance:* 30 mg I.V. over 2 hr 3 times/wk on alternate days for up to 12 wk

Antineoplastic Drugs (continued)

GENERIC AND TRADE NAMES	INDICATIONS	USUAL ADULT DOSAGES
Biological response modifiers *(continued)*		
bacillus Calmette-Guérin (BCG) live, Connaught strain ImmuCyst (CAN), TheraCys	To treat bladder cancer	81 mg (reconstitute and dilute with 50 ml preservative-free NSS to 53 ml or less) instilled into bladder for 1 to 2 hr q wk for 6 wk, then as a single-dose treatment at 3, 6, 12, 18, and 24 mo
bacillus Calmette-Guérin, Tice strain TICE BCG		50 mg (reconstitute and dilute with 50 ml preservative-free NSS to 50 ml or less) for 1 to 2 hr q 6 wk; may repeat once, followed by single-dose treatment q mo for 6 to 12 mo
denileukin diftitox Ontak	To treat cutaneous or T-cell lymphomas, including mycosis fungoides	9 or 18 mcg/kg/day by I.V. infusion over at least 15 min for 5 days; repeated q 21 days
interferon alfa-2a, recombinant Roferon-A	To treat hairy cell leukemia	3 million U/day I.M. or S.C. for 16 to 24 wk, followed by 3 million U 3 times/wk
	To treat AIDS-related Kaposi's sarcoma	36 million U/day I.M. or S.C. for 10 to 12 wk; or 3 million U/day I.M. or S.C. on days 1 to 3, 9 million U/day on days 4 to 6, 18 million U/day on days 7 to 9, and 36 million U/day from day 10 until completion of 10- to 12-wk course; maintenance dose, 36 million U 3 times/wk
interferon alfa-2b, recombinant Intron A	To treat hairy cell leukemia	2 million U/m^2 I.M. or S.C. 3 times/wk
	To treat AIDS-related Kaposi's sarcoma	30 million U/m^2 I.M. or S.C. 3 times/wk
	To treat malignant melanoma	20 million U/m^2 by I.V. infusion on days 1 to 5 q wk for 4 wk, followed by 10 million U/m^2 I.V. 3 times/wk for 48 wk

(continued on page 984)

Antineoplastic Drugs (continued)

GENERIC AND TRADE NAMES	INDICATIONS	USUAL ADULT DOSAGES
Biological response modifiers (*continued*)		
levamisole hydrochloride Ergamisol	To treat colorectal cancer	Beginning 7 to 30 days after surgery, 50 mg P.O. q 8 hr for 3 days, repeated q 2 wk for 1 yr, in combination with fluorouracil 450 mg/m² by rapid I.V. infusion q.d. for 5 days, starting with first or second course of levamisole
Antineoplastic enzymes		
asparaginase Colaspase, Elspar, Kidrolase (CAN)	To treat acute lymphocytic leukemia	200 IU/kg I.V. q.d. for 28 days
pegaspargase (PEG-L-asparaginase) Oncaspar	To treat acute lymphoblastic leukemia in adults up to age 21	2,500 IU/m² I.M. or I.V. q 14 days
Hormonal antineoplastics		
anastrozole Arimidex	To treat breast cancer	1 mg P.O. q.d.
bicalutamide Casodex	To treat prostate cancer	50 mg P.O. q.d. in combination with luteinizing hormone-releasing hormone (LHRH) analog or after surgical castration
estramustine phosphate sodium Emcyt	To treat prostate cancer	600 mg/m²/day P.O. in three divided doses 1 hr a.c. or 2 hr p.c.; or 14 mg/m²/day in three or four divided doses 1 hr a.c. or 2 hr p.c.
exemestane Aromasin	To treat postmenopausal breast cancer	25 mg P.O. q.d. p.c.
flutamide Euflex (CAN), Eulexin	To treat prostate cancer	250 mg P.O. q 8 hr
goserelin acetate Zoladex, Zoladex LA, Zoladex 3-Month	To treat breast cancer	3.6 mg S.C. into upper abdominal wall q 28 days
	To treat prostate cancer	3.6 mg S.C. into upper abdominal wall q 28 days; or 10.8 mg S.C. q 12 wk

Antineoplastic Drugs (continued)

GENERIC AND TRADE NAMES	INDICATIONS	USUAL ADULT DOSAGES
Hormonal antineoplastics *(continued)*		
letrozole Femara	To treat breast cancer	2.5 mg P.O. q.d.
leuprolide acetate Lupron, Lupron Depot, Lupron Depot-3 Month, Lupron Depot-4 Month, Viadur	To treat prostate cancer	*Regular:* 1 mg S.C. q.d.; *depot:* 7.5 mg q mo; or 22.5 mg q 3 mo; or 30 mg q 4 mo; *implant:* 1 q 12 mo
medroxyprogesterone acetate Depo-Provera	To treat endometrial or renal cancer	400 to 1,000 mg q wk until stable, then 400 mg or more q mo
megestrol acetate Megace	To treat breast cancer	160 mg/day P.O. q.d. or in divided doses
	To treat endometrial cancer	40 to 320 mg P.O. q.d. or in divided doses
nilutamide Anandron (CAN), Nilandron	To treat prostate cancer	300 mg P.O. q.d. up to 30 days, then 150 mg P.O. q.d.
tamoxifen citrate Apo-Tamox (CAN), Gen-Tamoxifen (CAN), Nolvadex, Nolvadex-D (CAN), Novo-Tamoxifen (CAN), Tamofen (CAN), Tamone (CAN)	To prevent breast cancer or reduce the risk of invasive breast cancer in women with ductal carcinoma in situ	20 mg P.O. q.d. for 5 yr
	To treat breast cancer (node-negative or node-positive)	10 mg P.O. b.i.d. or, in metastatic disease, 10 to 20 mg P.O. b.i.d.
testolactone Teslac	To treat breast cancer	250 mg P.O. q.i.d.
toremifene citrate Fareston	To treat breast cancer	60 mg P.O. q.d.
triptorelin pamoate Trelstar LA	To provide palliative treatment of advanced prostate cancer	11.25 mg I.M. q 84 days

(continued on page 986)

Antineoplastic Drugs (continued)

GENERIC AND TRADE NAMES	INDICATIONS	USUAL ADULT DOSAGES
Miscellaneous antineoplastics		
arsenic trioxide Trisenox	To treat acute promyelocytic leukemia	*Induction:* 0.15 mg/kg I.V. daily until bone marrow remission occurs. *Maximum:* 60 doses. *Consolidation:* Begun 3 to 6 wk after completion of induction, 0.15 mg/kg I.V. daily for 25 doses over up to 5 wk
bexarotene Targretin	To treat cutaneous manifestations of cutaneous T-cell lymphoma	300 mg/m^2 P.O. q.d. with food; after 8 wk, may increase to 400 mg/m^2 P.O. q.d. with food, as needed and tolerated.
Targretin Gel	To treat cutaneous lesions of cutaneous T-cell lymphoma (stages IA and IB)	Apply generously to cover only lesions q.o.d. on 1st wk; then increased as tolerated to q.d. on 2nd wk, b.i.d. on 3rd wk, t.i.d on 4th wk and, finally, q.i.d. on 5th wk
dacarbazine DTIC (CAN), DTIC-Dome	To treat Hodgkin's disease	150 mg/m^2 I.V. q.d. for 5 days in combination with other drugs; may repeat q 28 days; or 375 mg/m^2 q 15 days in combination with other drugs
	To treat malignant melanoma	2 to 4.5 mg/kg I.V. q.d. for 10 days and q 28 days thereafter; or 250 mg/m^2 I.V. q.d. for 5 days and q 21 days thereafter
etoposide (VP-16) Toposar, VePesid	To treat germ-cell testicular tumors	50 to 100 mg/m^2/day I.V. on days 1 through 5 up to 100 mg/m^2 I.V. on days 1, 3, and 5; course repeated q 3 to 4 wk
	To treat small-cell lung carcinoma	35 mg/m^2/day I.V. for 4 days up to 50 mg/m^2/day I.V. for 5 days, repeated q 3 to 4 wk; or 70 mg/m^2/day P.O. for 4 days to 100 mg/m^2/day P.O. for 5 days, repeated q 3 to 4 wk

Antineoplastic Drugs (continued)

GENERIC AND TRADE NAMES	INDICATIONS	USUAL ADULT DOSAGES
Miscellaneous antineoplastics *(continued)*		
etoposide phosphate Etopophos	To treat germ-cell testicular tumors	50 to 100 mg/m^2/day by I.V. infusion on days 1 through 5 to 100 mg/m^2/day by I.V. infusion on days 1, 3, and 5; course repeated q 3 to 4 wk
	To treat small-cell lung carcinoma	35 mg/m^2/day by I.V. infusion for 4 days to 50 mg/m^2/day by I.V. infusion for 5 days, repeated q 3 to 4 wk
gemcitabine hydrochloride Gemzar	To treat non-small-cell lung carcinoma	1,000 mg/m^2 by I.V. infusion over 30 min q.d. on days 1, 8, and 15 q 28 days in combination with cisplatin 100 mg/m^2 on day 28; or 1,250 mg/m^2 I.V. q.d. on days 1 and 8 q 21 days in combination with cisplatin 100 mg/m^2 I.V. on day 21
	To treat pancreatic cancer	1,000 mg/m^2 by I.V. infusion over 30 min q wk for 7 wk, followed by 1 wk of no drug; then q wk for 3 wk, followed by 1 wk of no drug; then repeat 4-wk cycle
gemtuzumab ozogamicin Mylotarg	To treat first relapse in patients with CD33-positive acute myeloid leukemia who are age 60 or older and who are not candidates for cytotoxic therapy	9 mg/m^2 by I.V. infusion over 2 hr; repeated in 14 days
imatinib mesylate Gleevec	To treat chronic myeloid leukemia in accelerated phase or blast crisis, or in chronic phase after failure of interferon-alpha therapy	400 mg P.O. q.d. with food (chronic phase) or 600 mg P.O. q.d. with food (accelerated phase or blast crisis); after 3 mo, dosage may be increased to 600 mg P.O. q.d. (chronic phase) or 800 mg P.O. given in 2 divided doses of 400 mg (accelerated phase or blast crisis), as needed.

(continued on page 988)

Antineoplastic Drugs (continued)

GENERIC AND TRADE NAMES	INDICATIONS	USUAL ADULT DOSAGES
Miscellaneous antineoplastics *(continued)*		
irinotecan hydrochloride Camptosar	To treat colorectal cancer	125 mg/m^2 I.V. over 90 min q wk for 4 wk, followed by 2 wk of no drug, then repeat 6-wk cycle; or 240 to 350 mg/m^2 I.V. over 90 min q 3 wk
mitotane (o,p'-DDD) Lysodren	To treat adrenocortical carcinoma	2 to 6 g P.O. q.d. in divided doses t.i.d. or q.i.d.
mitoxantrone hydrochloride Novantrone	To treat hormone-refractory prostate cancer	12 to 14 mg/m^2 I.V. q 21 days
	To treat acute nonlymphocytic leukemia	12 mg/m^2 by I.V. infusion through free-flowing NSS or D$_5$W solution over 3 min q.d. on days 1 and 3, in combination with cytarabine 100 mg/m^2/day by continuous I.V. infusion on days 1 to 7; if response is inadequate, second course at same dosage may be given
porfimer sodium Photofrin	To treat esophageal cancer and non-small-cell lung carcinoma	2 mg/kg I.V. over 3 to 5 min, followed by laser light illumination and debridement of tumor; may repeat course q 30 days three times
procarbazine hydrochloride Matulane, Natulan (CAN)	To treat Hodgkin's disease	2 to 4 mg/kg/day (rounded to nearest 50 mg) P.O. as a single dose or in divided doses for 1 wk, followed by 4 to 6 mg/kg/day until leukopenia, thrombocytopenia, or maximal response occurs
rituximab Rituxan	To treat non-Hodgkin's lymphomas	375 mg/m^2/day by I.V. infusion q wk for 4 or 8 doses
topotecan hydrochloride Hycamtin	To treat ovarian cancer and small-cell lung carcinoma	1.5 mg/m^2 I.V. over 30 min q.d. for 5 days, repeated q 21 days
trastuzumab Herceptin	To treat breast cancer	4 mg/kg I.V. over 90 min, followed by 2 mg/kg I.V. over 30 min q 7 days

Drug Formulas and Calculations

When administering drugs, you must be familiar with drug formulas and calculation methods to ensure that your patient receives the prescribed drug in the correct dosage, strength, or flow rate. This appendix will provide you with a quick review of how to calculate the strength of a solution, drug dosages, and I.V. flow rates.

Calculating the Strength of a Solution

Most solutions come prepared in the required strength by the pharmacy or medical supply source. But sometimes only the concentrated form is available, and you'll need to dilute the solution or solid to administer the prescribed strength.

When a solid form of a drug is used to prepare a solution, the drug must be completely dissolved. Solid drug forms, such as tablets, crystals, and powders, are considered 100% strength. (An exception to this is boric acid, which is only 5% at full strength.) The final diluted solution is stated in terms of liquid measurement. To prepare a solution, you'll need to add the prescribed solid or liquid form of the drug (the solute) to the prescribed amount of diluent (the solvent). Two of the most common diluents used in the clinical setting are normal saline solution and sterile water.

You can use two formulas to calculate the strength of a solution, as shown in the examples below.

Method 1: Calculating percentage and volume
Use the following formula:

$$\frac{\text{Weaker solution}}{\text{Stronger solution}} = \frac{\text{Solute}}{\text{Solvent}}$$

Example: You need to dilute a stock solution of 100% strength to a 5% solution. How much solute will you need to add to obtain 500 ml of the 5% solution?

Calculate as follows:

$$\frac{5\ (\%)\ \text{(weaker solution)}}{100\ (\%)\ \text{(stronger solution)}} = \frac{\text{X (g) (solute)}}{500\ \text{ml (solvent)}}$$

$$100\ \text{X} = (500)(5)\ \text{or}\ 2,500$$

$$\text{X} = 25\ \text{g}$$

Answer: You'll need to add 25 g of solute to each 500 ml of solvent to prepare a 5% solution.

Method 2: Calculating percentage and volume
Use the following formula:

$$\frac{\text{(Desired strength)}}{\text{(Available strength)}} \times \frac{\text{Total amount of}}{\text{desired solution}} = \text{X} \frac{\text{(amount of undiluted drug}}{\text{needed to make solution)}}$$

Example: You need to make 100 ml of a 20% solution, using an 80% solution. How much of the 80% solution must you add to the sterile water to yield a final volume of 100 ml of a 20% solution?

Calculate as follows:

$$\frac{20\ (\%)\ \text{(Desired strength)}}{80\ (\%)\ \text{(Available strength)}} \times \frac{100\ \text{ml (Total amount}}{\text{of desired solution)}} = \text{X}$$

$$\frac{0.20}{0.80} = 0.25$$

$$0.25 \times 100\ \text{(ml)} = \text{X}$$

$$\text{X} = 25\ \text{ml of 80\% solution}$$

Answer: You'll need to add 25 ml of the 80% solution to the water to make a final volume of 100 ml of a 20% solution.

(continued on page 990)

Drug Formulas and Calculations (continued)

Calculating Drug Dosages

You may be required to calculate drug dosages when you need to administer a drug that's available only in one measure, but prescribed in another. You should also be prepared to convert various units of measure, such as milligrams (mg) to grains (gr), and dry measurements to liquid. You can use three common methods of ratio and proportion to calculate drug dosages, as shown in the examples below.

CALCULATING ORAL DRUG DOSAGES

Example: You need to give a patient 0.25 mg of digoxin, which comes only in 0.125-mg tablets. How many tablets will you need to give him to attain the proper dosage?

Method 1: Using labeled amount of drug

In this method, true proportions between the drug label and the prescribed dose are used to determine ratio and proportion. The drug label, which states the amount of drug in one unit of measurement—in this case, 0.125-mg in each tablet of digoxin—is the first ratio, expressed as follows:

$$\text{milligrams : tablets} = \text{milligrams : tablets}$$
$$0.125 \text{ mg (amount of drug) : 1 tablet (unit of measure)}$$

The prescribed dose—in this case, 0.25-mg—is the second ratio; it must be stated in the same order and units of measure as the first, as follows:

$$0.125 \text{ mg : 1 tablet} = 0.25 \text{ mg : X (tablets)}$$

Calculate as follows:

$$0.125 \text{ X} = 0.25$$
$$\text{X} = \frac{0.25}{0.125}$$
$$\text{X} = 2$$

Answer: You'll need to give the patient 2 tablets of digoxin 0.125 mg.

Be sure to use critical thinking to assess whether your answer is correct. Because the amount of drug prescribed is greater than the amount of drug in one tablet, it's reasonable to expect the required number of tablets to be greater than one.

Method 2: Using an established formula

To determine the correct number of digoxin tablets to give using this method, use the following formula:

$$\frac{\text{Prescribed dose}}{\text{Dose available}} \times \text{Quantity (unit of measure)} = \text{X (unknown quantity to be given)}$$

Calculate as follows:

$$\frac{0.25 \text{ mg}}{0.125 \text{ mg}} \times 1 \text{ tablet} = \text{X (number of 0.125-mg tablets)}$$
$$\frac{0.25}{0.125} = 2\text{X}$$
$$2 = \text{X}$$

Answer: You'll need to give the patient 2 tablets of digoxin 0.125 mg.

Drug Formulas and Calculations (continued)

Method 3: Calculating according to proportion size

This method uses the same components as method #1, but the ratio is based on proportions according to size. To determine the correct number of digoxin tablets to give using this method, use the following formula:

$$\frac{\text{smaller}}{\text{larger}} = \frac{\text{smaller}}{\text{larger}}$$

Substitute 0.125 into the smaller part and 0.25 into the greater part of the first ratio. Critical thinking leads us to believe that you'll need more than 1 tablet of the weaker 0.125-mg strength to equal the stronger 0.25 mg. Set up the proportion as follows:

$$\frac{0.125 \text{ mg}}{0.25 \text{ mg}} = \frac{1 \text{ (tablet)}}{X \text{ (tablets)}}$$

Calculate as follows:

$$0.125 \text{ X} = 0.25$$
$$X = \frac{0.25}{0.125}$$
$$X = 2 \text{ tablets}$$

Answer: You'll need to give the patient 2 tablets of digoxin 0.125 mg.

CALCULATING PARENTERAL DRUG DOSAGES

The same methods used for calculating oral drugs and solutions can be used for preparing parenteral injections.

Example: You need to administer a prescribed dose of 1 mg morphine sulfate from a unit-dose cartridge containing 4 mg per 2 ml. How many milliliters will you need to give to equal the prescribed dose of 1 mg?

Method 1: Using labeled amount of drug

Using the same ratio as for oral drugs, the drug label—in this case, 4 mg—is the first ratio, and the prescribed dose—in this case, 1 mg—is the second ratio, expressed as follows:

$$4 \text{ mg (the amount of drug)} : 2 \text{ ml (the unit of measure)}$$

Calculate as follows:

$$4 \text{ mg} : 2 \text{ ml} = 1 \text{ mg} : X \text{ ml}$$
$$4X = 2$$
$$X = \frac{2}{4}$$
$$X = 0.5 \text{ ml}$$

Answer: You'll need to give 0.5 ml of morphine sulfate to equal the prescribed dose of 1 mg.

Method 2: Using an established formula

Use this formula:

$$\frac{\text{Prescribed dose}}{\text{Dose available}} \times \text{Quantity (unit of measure)} = X \text{ (unknown quantity to be given)}$$

(continued on page 992)

Drug Formulas and Calculations (continued)

Calculate as follows:

$$\frac{1 \text{ mg}}{4 \text{ mg}} \times 2 \text{ ml} = X \text{ (number of ml)}$$

$$\frac{4}{2} = 0.5$$

Answer: You'll need to give 0.5 ml of morphine sulfate to equal the prescribed dose of 1 mg.

Method 3: Calculating according to proportion size
To determine the correct amount of morphine sulfate to give using this method, use the following formula:

smaller : greater = smaller : greater

milligrams : milligrams = milliliters : milliliters

Critical thinking leads us to believe that 1 mg is less than 4 mg and that you'll need less than 2 ml to give 1 mg of the drug; therefore, 1 mg goes into the smaller part of the first ratio, and X goes into the smaller part of the second ratio. Set up the proportion as follows:

$$1 \text{ mg} : 4 \text{ mg} = X \text{ (ml)} : 2 \text{ ml}$$

$$4X = 2$$

$$X = \frac{2}{4}$$

$$X = 0.5$$

Answer: You'll need to give 0.5 ml of morphine sulfate to equal the prescribed dose of 1 mg.

Calculating I.V. Flow Rates

When an I.V. solution is delivered by gravity, you must calculate the number of drops needed per minute for proper infusion. To calculate I.V. flow rates, you need to know three things:
•the drip factor—or the number of drops contained in 1 ml for the type of I.V. set you'll be using. This information is provided on the individual package label.

•the amount and type of fluid that you'll infuse as prescribed on the physician's order sheet
•the infusion duration time in minutes.
    Once you've gathered this information, you can calculate the I.V. flow rate using the following equation:

$$\frac{\text{Total number of ml}}{\text{Total number of minutes}} \times \text{drip factor (gtt/ml)} = \text{flow rate (gtt/min)}$$

Example 1: If the physician prescribes 1,000 ml of D₅W to infuse over 10 hours, and the drip rate for your administration set delivers 15 drops (gtt) per ml, calculate as follows:

$$\frac{1,000 \text{ ml}}{10 \text{ hours} \times 60 \text{ minutes}} \times 15 \text{ gtt/ml} = X \text{ gtt/minute}$$

$$\frac{1,000 \text{ ml}}{600 \text{ minutes}} \times 15 \text{ gtt/ml} = X \text{ gtt/minute}$$

Drug Formulas and Calculations (continued)

$$1.67 \text{ ml/minute} \times 15 \text{ gtt/ml} = X \text{ gtt/minute}$$
$$25.05 \text{ gtt/minute} = X$$

Answer: To infuse, round off 25.05 to 25 gtt/minute or according to your institution's policy.

Example 2: If the physician prescribes 500 ml of 0.45% NS to infuse over 2 hours, and the drip rate for your administration set delivers 10 gtt/ml, calculate as follows:

$$\frac{500 \text{ ml}}{2 \text{ hours} \times 60 \text{ minutes}} \times 10 \text{ gtt/ml} = X \text{ gtt/minute}$$

$$\frac{500 \text{ ml}}{120 \text{ minutes}} \times 10 \text{ gtt/ml} = X \text{ gtt/minute}$$

$$4.17 \text{ ml/minute} \times 10 \text{ gtt/ml} = X \text{ gtt/minute}$$
$$41.7 \text{ gtt/minute} = X$$

Answer: To infuse, round off 41.7 to 42 gtt/minute or according to your institution's policy.

Note: When preparing for I.V. administration using a controlled infusion device, the electronic flow-regulator will either count drops using an electronic eye or use a controlled pumping action to deliver the fluid in milliliters. Your final calculation will be based on the unit of measure used by the device: drops per minute, or ml per hour.

Weights and Equivalents

The following three tables show approximate equivalents among the various systems of measurement.

Table 1: Liquid Equivalents Among Household, Apothecaries', and Metric Systems

HOUSEHOLD	APOTHECARIES'	METRIC
1 teaspoon (tsp)	1 fluid dram (fʒ)	5 milliliters (ml)
1 tablespoon (tbs)	0.5 fluid ounce (fʒ)	15 ml
2 tbs (1 ounce [1 oz])	1 fluid ounce	30 ml
1 cupful	8 fluid ounces	240 ml
1 pint (pt)	16 fluid ounces	473 ml
1 quart (qt)	32 fluid ounces	946 ml (1 liter)

Table 2: Solid Equivalents Among Apothecaries' and Metric Systems

APOTHECARIES'	METRIC
15 grains (gr)	1 gram (g) (1,000 milligrams [mg])
10 gr	0.6 g (600 mg)
7.5 gr	0.5 g (500 mg)
5 gr	0.3 g (300 mg)
3 gr	0.2 g (200 mg)
1.5 gr	0.1 g (100 mg)
1 gr	0.06 g (60 mg) or 0.065 g (65 mg)
0.75 gr	0.05 g (50 mg)
0.5 gr	0.03 g (30 mg)
0.25 gr	0.015 g (15 mg)
1/60 gr	0.001 g (1 mg)
1/100 gr	0.6 mg
1/120 gr	0.5 mg
1/150 gr	0.4 mg

Weights and Equivalents (continued)

**Table 3: Solid Equivalents Among Avoirdupois, Apothecaries',
and Metric Systems**

AVOIRDUPOIS	APOTHECARIES'	METRIC
1 gr	1 gr	0.065 g
15.4 gr	15 gr	1 g
1 ounce (1 oz)	480 gr	28.35 g
437.5 gr	1 oz	31 g
1 pound (lb)	1.33 lb	454 g
0.75 lb	1 lb	373 g
2.2 lb	2.7 lb	1 kilogram (kg)

Compatible Drugs in a Syringe

The chart below lets you know at a glance whether particular drugs are compatible for at least 15 minutes when mixed together in a syringe for immediate administration. However, keep in mind that drugs listed as compatible when mixed in a syringe may not be compatible when prepared for other routes of administration. Drug combinations prepared for immediate administration usually require a more concentrated solution than those prepared for infusion.

(**Key:** C = Compatible; I = Incompatible; n/a = Compatibility information not available; no recommendations can be given.)

	atropine	chlorpromazine	dexamethasone	diazepam	diphenhydramine	droperidol	furosemide	glycopyrrolate	haloperidol	heparin	hydromorphone
atropine		C	n/a	n/a	C	C	n/a	C	I	n/a	C
chlorpromazine	C		n/a	n/a	C	C	n/a	C	n/a	I	C
dexamethasone	n/a	n/a		n/a	I	n/a	n/a	n/a	n/a	n/a	C
diazepam	n/a	n/a	n/a		n/a	n/a	n/a	I	n/a	I	n/a
diphenhydramine	C	C	I	n/a		C	n/a	C	I	n/a	C
droperidol	C	C	n/a	n/a	C		I	C	n/a	I	n/a
furosemide	n/a	n/a	n/a	n/a	n/a	I		n/a	n/a	C	n/a
glycopyrrolate	C	C	I	C	C	C	n/a		C	n/a	C
haloperidol	n/a	n/a	n/a	n/a	C	n/a	n/a	n/a		I	C
heparin	C	I	n/a	I	n/a	I	C	n/a	I		n/a
hydromorphone	C	C	n/a	n/a	C	n/a	n/a	C	C	n/a	
hydroxyzine	C	C	n/a	n/a	C	C	n/a	C	I	n/a	C
ketorolac	n/a	n/a	n/a	I	n/a	n/a	n/a	n/a	I	n/a	I
lidocaine	n/a	n/a	n/a	n/a	n/a	n/a	n/a	C	n/a	C	n/a
lorazepam	n/a	n/a	n/a	n/a	n/a	n/a	n/a	n/a	n/a	n/a	C
meperidine	C	C	n/a	C	C	C	n/a	C	n/a	I	n/a
metoclopramide	C	C	n/a	n/a	C	C	I	n/a	n/a	C	C
midazolam	C	C	n/a	n/a	C	n/a	n/a	C	C	n/a	C
morphine	C	C	n/a	n/a	C	C	n/a	C	I	C*	n/a
pentobarbital	C	I	n/a	n/a	I	I	n/a	I	n/a	n/a	C
prochlorperazine	C	n/a	n/a	n/a	C	C	n/a	C	n/a	n/a	I
ranitidine	C	I	C	n/a	C	n/a	n/a	C	n/a	n/a	C
scopolamine	C	C	n/a	n/a	C	C	n/a	C	n/a	n/a	C

* Compatible only with morphine doses of 1 mg, 2 mg, and 5 mg.

hydroxyzine	ketorolac	lidocaine	lorazepam	meperidine	metoclopramide	midazolam	morphine	pentobarbital	prochlorperazine	ranitidine	scopolamine
C	n/a	n/a	n/a	C	C	C	C	C	C	C	C
C	n/a	n/a	n/a	C	C	C	I	I	C	C	C
n/a	n/a	n/a	n/a	n/a	C	n/a	n/a	n/a	n/a	C	n/a
n/a	I	n/a	n/a	n/a	n/a	n/a	n/a	n/a	n/a	I	n/a
C	n/a	n/a	n/a	C	C	C	C	I	C	C	C
C	n/a	n/a	n/a	C	C	C	C	I	C	n/a	C
n/a	n/a	n/a	n/a	n/a	I	n/a	n/a	n/a	n/a	n	n/a
C	n/a	C	n/a	C	n/a	C	C	I	C	C	C
I	I	n/a	n/a	n/a	n/a	n/a	I	n/a	n/a	n/a	n/a
n/a	n/a	C	n/a	I	C	n/a	C	n/a	n/a	n	n/a
C	I	n/a	C	n/a	n/a	C	n/a	C	I	C	C
	I	C	n/a	C	C	C	C	I	C	C	C
I		n/a	n/a	n/a	n/a	n/a	n/a	n/a	I	n/a	n/a
C	n/a		n/a	n/a	C	n/a	n/a	n/a	n/a	n/a	n/a
n/a	n/a	n/a		n/a	n/a	n/a	n/a	n/a	n/a	I	n/a
C	n/a	n/a	n/a		C	C	I	I	C	C	C
n/a	n/a	C	n/a	C		C	C	n/a	C	C	C
C	n/a	n/a	n/a	C	C		C	I	I	I	C
C	n/a	n/a	n/a	n/a	C	C		I	C	C	C
I	n/a	n/a	n/a	I	I	I	I		I	I	C
C	I	n/a	n/a	C	C	I	C	I		C	C
I	n/a	n/a	I	C	C	I	C	I	C		C
C	n/a	n/a	n/a	C	C	C	C	C	C	C	

Abbreviations

The following abbreviations, which are common to nursing practice, are used throughout the book.

ABG	arterial blood gas		EEG	electroencephalogram
a.c.	before meals		EENT	eyes, ears, nose, and throat
ACE	angiotensin-converting enzyme		ENDO	endocrine
ADH	antidiuretic hormone		E.R.	extended-release
AIDS	acquired immunodeficiency syndrome		$°F$	degrees Fahrenheit
ALT	alanine aminotransferase		FDA	Food and Drug Administration
ANA	antinuclear antibodies		g	gram
APTT	activated partial thromboplastin time		GFR	glomerular filtration rate
AST	aspartate aminotransferase		GI	gastrointestinal
ATP	adenosine triphosphate		gtt	drop
AV	atrioventricular		GU	genitourinary
b.i.d.	twice a day		H_1	histamine$_1$
BUN	blood urea nitrogen		H_2	histamine$_2$
$°C$	degrees Celsius		HDL	high-density lipoprotein
cAMP	cyclic adenosine monophosphate		HEME	hematologic
(CAN)	Canadian drug trade name		HIV	human immunodeficiency virus
cap	capsule		HPV	human papilloma virus
CBC	complete blood count		hr	hour
cGMP	cyclic guanosine monophosphate		h.s.	at bedtime
CK	creatine kinase		HSV	herpes simplex virus
Cl	chloride		HZV	herpes zoster virus
cm	centimeter		I.D.	intradermal
CMV	cytomegalovirus		IgA	immunoglobulin A
CNS	central nervous system		IgE	immunoglobulin E
COPD	chronic obstructive pulmonary disease		I.M.	intramuscular
C.R.	controlled-release		INR	international normalized ratio
CSF	cerebrospinal fluid		IU	international unit
CV	cardiovascular		I.V.	intravenous
CVA	cerebrovascular accident		IVPB	intravenous piggyback
D_5LR	dextrose 5% in lactated Ringer's solution		kg	kilogram
D_5NS	dextrose 5% in normal saline solution		KIU	kallikrein inactivator units
$D_5/0.2NS$	dextrose 5% in quarter-normal saline solution		L	liter
$D_5/0.45NS$	dextrose 5% in half-normal saline solution		LA	long-acting
D_5W	dextrose 5% in water		LD	lactate dehydrogenase
$D_{10}W$	dextrose 10% in water		LDL	low-density lipoprotein
$D_{50}W$	dextrose 50% in water		LR	lactated Ringer's solution
dl	deciliter		M	molar
DNA	deoxyribonucleic acid		m^2	square meter
DS	double-strength		MAO	monoamine oxidase
EC	enteric-coated		mcg	microgram
ECG	electrocardiogram		mEq	milliequivalent
			mg	milligram
			MI	myocardial infarction
			min	minute
			ml	milliliter
			mm	millimeter
			mm^3	cubic millimeter

Abbreviations (continued)

mmol	millimole		q.d.	every day
mo	month		q.i.d.	four times a day
MS	musculoskeletal		q.o.d.	every other day
Na	sodium		RBC	red blood cell
NaCl	sodium chloride		REM	rapid eye movement
NG	nasogastric		RESP	respiratory
NPH	human isophane insulin		RNA	ribonucleic acid
NPO	nothing by mouth		RSV	respiratory syncytial virus
NS	normal saline solution		SA	sinoatrial
0.225NS	quarter-normal saline (0.225%) solution		S.C.	subcutaneous
0.45NS	half-normal saline (0.45%) solution		sec	second
NSAID	nonsteroidal anti-inflammatory drug		S.L.	sublingual
OTC	over the counter		S.R.	sustained-release
p.c.	after meals		stat	immediately
PCA	patient-controlled analgesia		supp	suppository
P.O.	by mouth		tab	tablet
P.R.	by rectum		T_3	triiodothyronine
p.r.n.	as needed		T_4	thyroxine
PSVT	paroxysmal supraventricular tachycardia		t.i.d.	three times a day
PT	prothrombin time		U	units
PTCA	percutaneous transluminal coronary angioplasty		USP	United States Pharmacopeia
PVC	premature ventricular contraction		UTI	urinary tract infection
q	every		VLDL	very low-density lipoprotein
			WBC	white blood cell
			wk	week

Index

- **Generic and alternate names:** lowercase initial letter
- **Trade names:** uppercase initial letter
- **Illustrations:** *i* after page number
- **Tables:** *t* after page number

A

abacavir sulfate, 956*t*
abacavir sulfate, lamivudine, and zidovudine, 956*t*
Abbokinase, 886
Abbokinase Open-Cath, 886
abciximab, 17–18
Abelcet, 65
Abenol, 20
Abitrate, 214
A/B Otic, 928*t*
Abreva, 944*t*
Absorbine Footcare, 944*t*
Absorption 2–4
acarbose, 18–19
Accolate, 903
AccuNeb, 29
Accupril, 745
Accutane, 460
acebutolol hydrochloride, 19–20
Aceon, 677
Acephen, 20
Aceta Elixir, 20
acetaminophen, 20–21
Acetaminophen Uniserts, 20
Aceta Tablets, 20
Acetazolam, 22
acetazolamide, 22–23
Acetocot, 868
acetohexamide, 23–24
acetohydroxamic acid, 25
acetylcholine chloride, 924*t*
acetylcysteine, 25–27
acetylsalicylic acid, 81–83
Achromycin, 823, 939*t*
Achromycin V, 823
Acilac, 472
AcipHex, 750
Aclovate, 944*t*
Acova, 79
acrivastine, 936*t*
Act, 350
Acticin, 950*t*

Acticort 100, 946*t*
Actigall, 887
Actimmune, 954*t*
actinomycin-D, 975*t*
Actiprofen Caplets, 430
Actiq, 358
Activase, 40
Activase rt-PA, 40
Activella, 335
Actonel, 763
Actos, 694
Actron, 468
Acular, 923*t*
acyclovir, 944t, 958*t*
Adalat, 616
Adalat CC, 616
Adalat PA, 616
Adalat XL, 616
adamantanamine hydro-chloride, 42–44
adapalene, 948*t*
Adderall, 62
Adderall XR, 62
Adenocard, 27
adenosine, 27–28
ADH, 893–894
Adrenalin, 313
Adrenalin Chloride Solution, 313
adrenaline, 313–316
Adriamycin PFS, 976*t*
Adriamycin RDF, 976*t*
Adrucil, 978*t*
Adsorbocarpine, 925*t*
Adsorbonac, 928*t*
Adverse reaction, 5–6
Advil, 430
AeroBid, 370
AeroBid-M, 370
Aerolate, 826
Aerolate III, 826
Aerolate Jr., 826
Aerolate Sr., 826
Aerosporin, 701
Afko-Lube, 287

Afko-Lube Lax, 287
Afrin, 919*t*
Aftate for Athlete's Foot, 944*t*
Aftate for Jock Itch, 944*t*
Agenerase, 956*t*
Aggrastat, 847
Aggrenox, 83
Agonists, 5
Agrylin, 72
A-hydroCort, 424
Airet, 29
Akarpine, 925*t*
AKBeta, 927*t*
AK-Chlor, 920*t*
Ak-Con, 925*t*
AK-Dex, 922*t*
Ak-Dilate, 925*t*
AK-Fluor, 927*t*
Akineton, 115
Akineton Lactate, 115
AK-NaCl, 928*t*
Ak-Nefrin, 925*t*
Akne-Mycin, 938*t*
AK-Pentolate, 924*t*
AK-Pred, 923*t*
AK-Sulf, 922*t*
AKTob, 922*t*
AK-Tracin, 920*t*
Ak-Zol, 22
Ala-Cort, 946*t*
Ala-Scalp HP, 946*t*
alatrofloxacin mesylate, 28–29
Albalon Liquifilm, 925*t*
Albert Docusate, 287
Albert Glyburide, 403
albuterol, 29–30, 30*i*
albuterol sulfate, 29–30
Alcaine, 926*t*
alclometasone dipropionate, 944*t*
Alconefrin Nasal Drops 12, 687, 919*t*
Alconefrin Nasal Drops 25, 687, 919*t*

O

NOTES

Body Mass Index Calculation

Body mass index (BMI) is a formula used to determine obesity; it's calculated by dividing a person's weight in kilograms by height in meters squared (kg/m^2), A BMI of 25 or higher increases your patient's risk of developing hypertension, cardiovascular disease, type 2 diabetes mellitus, and stroke. It also increases the risk that he won't respond effectively to the usual drug dosages. If your patient has an abnormal BMI, be prepared to make dosage adjustments that are individualized based on body weight, as prescribed.

The table below will help you find your patient's BMI easily. The table converts pounds to kilograms and inches to meters, and then it shows the BMI. To use it, simply find the patient's height on either side of the table, then move across the row to the weight that matches your patient's *most closely*. At the bottom of the column containing the weight, you'll find the BMI for that patient. For example, the BMI for a patient who is 70″ tall and weighs 208 lb is 30.

WEIGHT (POUNDS)

HEIGHT (INCHES)																		
58	91	96	100	105	110	115	119	124	129	134	138	143	148	153	158	162	167	172
59	94	99	104	109	114	119	124	128	133	138	143	148	153	158	163	168	173	178
60	97	102	107	112	118	123	128	133	138	143	148	153	158	163	168	174	179	184
61	100	106	111	116	122	127	132	137	143	148	153	158	164	169	174	180	185	190
62	104	109	115	120	126	131	136	142	147	153	158	164	169	175	180	186	191	196
63	107	113	118	124	130	135	141	146	152	158	163	169	175	180	186	191	197	203
64	110	116	122	128	134	140	145	151	157	163	169	174	180	186	192	197	204	209
65	114	120	126	132	138	144	150	156	162	168	174	180	186	192	198	204	210	216
66	118	124	130	136	142	148	155	161	167	173	179	186	192	198	204	210	216	223
67	121	127	134	140	146	153	159	166	172	178	185	191	198	204	211	217	223	230
68	125	131	138	144	151	158	164	171	177	184	190	197	203	210	216	223	230	236
69	128	135	142	149	155	162	169	176	182	189	196	203	209	216	223	230	236	243
70	132	139	146	153	160	167	174	181	188	195	202	209	216	222	229	236	243	250
71	136	143	150	157	165	172	179	186	193	200	208	215	222	229	236	243	250	257
72	140	147	154	162	169	177	184	191	199	206	213	221	228	235	242	250	258	265
73	144	151	159	166	174	182	189	197	204	212	219	227	235	242	250	257	265	272
74	148	155	163	171	179	186	194	202	210	218	225	233	241	249	256	264	272	280
75	152	160	168	176	184	192	200	208	216	224	232	240	248	256	264	272	279	287
76	156	164	172	180	189	197	205	213	221	230	238	246	254	263	271	279	287	295
	19	20	21	22	23	24	25	26	27	28	29	30	31	32	33	34	35	36

BODY MASS INDEX